Medicinal Chemistry

Second Edition

Medicinal Chemistry

Second Edition

Balkishen Razdan PhD

former Dean
Postgraduate Studies and Research
Birla Institute of Technology
Mesra, Ranchi, Jharkhand
and
former Director
S Bhagwan Singh Postgraduate Institute
of Biomedical Sciences and Research
Balawal, Dehradun, Uttarakhand

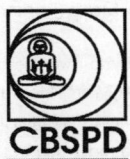

CBSPD

CBS Publishers & Distributors Pvt Ltd

New Delhi • Bengaluru • Chennai • Kochi • Kolkata • Lucknow • Mumbai
Hyderabad • Jharkhand • Nagpur • Patna • Pune • Uttarakhand

Medicinal Chemistry

Second Edition

ISBN: 978-93-87964-05-1

Copyright © Author and Publisher

Second Edition: 2019

Reprint: 2022, **2025**

First Edition: 2010

Published by Satish Kumar Jain and produced by Varun Jain for
CBS Publishers & Distributors Pvt Ltd
4819/XI Prahlad Street, 24 Ansari Road, Daryaganj, New Delhi 110 002, India.
Ph: 011-23289259, 23266838   Website: www.cbspd.com
                                   e-mail: delhi@cbspd.com
Corporate Office: 204 FIE, Industrial Area, Patparganj, Delhi 110 092
Ph: 011-4934 4934   Fax: 011-4934 4935   e-mail: publishing@cbspd.com; publicity@cbspd.com

Branches

- **Bengaluru:** Seema House 2975, 17th Cross, K.R. Road, Banasankari 2nd Stage, Bengaluru 560 070, Karnataka, India
  Ph: +91-80-26771678/79   Fax: +91-80-26771680   e-mail: bangalore@cbspd.com
- **Chennai:** Subbaraya Street, Shenoy Nagar, Chennai 600 030, Tamil Nadu, India
  Ph: +91-44-26680620/26681266   e-mail: chennai@cbspd.com
- **Kochi:** 42/1325, 1326, Power House Road, Opp KSEB, Ernakulam 682 018, Kochi, Kerala, India
  Ph: +91-484-4059061-65, 67   Fax: +91-484-4059065   e-mail: kochi@cbspd.com
- **Kolkata:** 147, Hind Ceramics Compound, 1st Floor, Nilgunj road, Belghoria, Kolkata 700056, West Bengal, India
  Ph: 033-25633055/56   e-mail: kolkata@cbspd.com
- **Lucknow:** Basement, Khushnuma Complex, 7-Meerabai Marg (Behind Jawahar Bhawan), Lucknow-226 001, Uttar Pradesh, India.
  Ph: +0552-4000032   e-mail:tiwari.lucknowi@cbspd.com
- **Mumbai:** PWD shed, Gala No. 25/26, Ramchandra Bhatt Marg, Next to JJ Hospital Gate No. 2, OPP. Union Bank of India, Noorbaug, Mumbai-400009, Maharashtra, India
  Ph: 022-66661880/89   e-mail: mumbai@cbspd.com

Representatives

• **Hyderabad**	0-9885175004	• **Jharkhand**	0-9811541605	• **Nagpur**	0-8692091830
• **Patna**	0-9334159340	• **Pune**	0-9664372571	• **Uttarakhand**	0-9716462459

Printed at: SRK Graphic, Delhi, India

Preface to the Second Edition

THE GENERAL plan of the second edition of this book is the same as the first edition. However, in this edition, opportunity has been taken to incorporate the latest developments in various areas and three new chapters, namely:

1. Antiemetic Agents,
2. Drugs Used for Constipation, Diarrhea, and Inflammatory Bowel Diseases, and
3. Vitamins.

The other features included in this edition are:

1. Glossary of medical terms
2. Compound index.

As indicated earlier, this book is meant for undergraduate students of pharmacy and students of other streams who offer medicinal chemistry as one of the electives.

Once again, I take the opportunity of thanking my beloved brother, my wife, and childen for supporting and encouraging me while working on the manuscript. I am also thankful to all my students working as teachers in various institutions and readers of this book for their suggestions. I also take this opportunity of thanking Mr Naveen Sharma, Dr Monica Sachdeva, and Dr Dilip K Gupta, for the material which they have provided to incorporate in this edition.

I am also thankful to CBS Publishers & Distributors. I would like to put on record the sincere efforts of Mr YN Arjuna (Senior Vice President Publishing, Editorial and Publicity) and his team comprising Ms Ritu Chawla (AGM Production), Mr Parmod Kumar, Ms Sanjubala Tripathy and Mr Manish Raj, for bringing out the book in the present form.

Balkishen Razdan

Preface to the First Edition

THIS BOOK is an outcome of teaching medicinal chemistry to the students of postgraduate and undergraduate students of pharmacy for the last four decades. The project was conceived about five years back and could be completed only now.

With the advances in molecular biology, developments in medicinal chemistry are taking place at a rapid pace. I have tried to incorporate the latest developments in the book. This book is meant for undergraduate students of pharmacy and students from other streams who offer medicinal chemistry as one of the course.

Sufficient care has been taken so that there are no errors/mistakes in the text as well as in chemical structures. However, in case if there are some, I would be grateful to the readers to inform me/publisher about any such mistakes/errors which they may notice in the book.

I am grateful to my beloved brother, my wife and my children for their moral and material support throughout the preparation of the manuscript of this book. Without their inspiration, constant encouragement and support it would not have been possible to complete this task.

Last but not the least, I would like to thank CBS Publishers & Distributors for bringing out this edition.

Balkishen Razdan

Contents

Preface to the Second Edition   *v*
Preface to the First Edition   *vii*

Section I DRUGS AFFECTING SYNAPTIC AND NEUROEFFECTOR JUNCTIONAL SITES

1. Adrenergic Drugs   **3–49**

Biosynthesis, Storage, and Release of Norepinephrine   4
Adrenergic Receptors   6
Drugs Affecting Norepinephrine Biosynthesis   9
Drugs Affecting Norepinephrine Storage   10
Drugs Affecting Norepinephrine Release   10
Drugs Acting on Adrenergic Receptors—Agonists   12
Drugs Acting on Adrenergic Receptors—Antagonists (Blockers)   15
Individual Compounds   20

2. Cholinergic Drugs   **50–101**

Acetylcholine Synthesis and Release   51
Acetylcholine Receptors   51
Muscarinic Agonists   55
Nicotinic Agonists   56
Acetylcholinesterase Inhibitors   56
Cholinergic Blockers   59
Individual Compounds   70

Section II DRUGS AFFECTING CENTRAL NERVOUS SYSTEM

3. General Anesthetics   **105–116**

Characteristics of an Ideal Anesthetic   106
Inhalation Anesthetics   106
Intravenous Anesthetics   110
Adjuvants to Anesthetics   114
Theories and Mechanism of Action of General Anesthetics   114

4. Local Anesthetics   **117–137**
Ester Type Local Anesthetics   117
Amide Type Local Anesthetics   121
Miscellaneous Compounds   122
Mechanism of Action   123
Adminstration of Local Anesthetics   124
Individual Compounds   125

5. Sedatives and Hypnotics   **138–160**
Barbiturates   138
Piperidinediones   141
Benzodiazepines   141
Nonbezodiazepine $GABA_A$ Receptor Agonists   142
Miscellaneous Compounds   143
Individual Compounds   144

6. Neuroleptics and Anxiolytic Agents   **161–198**
Neuroleptics   161
Anxiolytic Agents   166
Individual Compounds   170

7. Antiepileptic Drugs   **199–215**
Characteristics of an Ideal Antiepileptic Drug   199
Antiepileptic Drugs   200
Individual Compounds   204

8. Opioid Analgesics   **216–244**
Opium and Morphine Analogs   216
Synthetic Opioids   219
Narcotic Antagonists as Analgesics   224
Endogenous Opioid Peptides   224
Opioid Receptors   225
Individual Compounds   226

9. Antiparkinsonian Drugs   **245–254**
Parkinsonism and Dopamine   245
Individual Compounds   249

10. Central Nervous System Stimulants   **255–286**
Analeptics   255
Psychomotor Stimulants   256
Antidepressant Drugs   258
Psychotomimetics and Hallucinogens   262
Individual Compounds   263

Section III DRUG THERAPY OF INFLAMMATION

11. Antihistaminics and Antiulcer Agents   **289–334**
  Biosynthesis, Storage, and Release of Histamine   290
  Pharmacological Effects   290
  Histamine Release Inhibitors   291
  H_1-Receptor Antagonists   291
  Histamine Release Inhibitors with H_1-Receptor Antagonistic Activity   297
  Antiulcer Agents   298
  Individual Compounds   301

12. Analgesics, Antipyretics, and Nonsteroidal Anti-Inflammatory Drugs   **335–375**
  Analgesic, Antipyretic, and Nonsteroidal Anti-Inflammatory Drugs (NSAIDs) 338
  Cyclooxygenase-2 (Cox-2) Inhibitors   345
  Disease Modifying Antirheumatoid Drugs (DMARDs)   346
  Drugs Used in Gout   347
  Individual Compounds   349

Section IV RENAL AND CARDIOVASCULAR DRUGS

13. Diuretics   **379–407**
  Water and Osmotic Agents   381
  Acidifing Salts   381
  Organomercurials   382
  Phenoxyacetic Acids   383
  Purines and Related Heterocyclics   384
  Sulphonamides   385
  Aldosterone Antagonists and Inhibitors   389
  High Ceiling Diuretics   391
  Potassium Sparing Diuretics   391
  Individual Compounds   392

14. Antihypertensive Drugs   **408–437**
  Antihypertensive Drugs   409
  Individual Compounds   420

15. Antianginal, Antiarrhythmic, and Cardiotonic Drugs   **438–471**
  Antianginal Drugs   438
  Antiarrhythmic Drugs   443
  Cardiotonic Drugs   445
  Individual Compounds   452

Section V DRUGS ACTING ON BLOOD

16. Anticoagulants, Antiplatelet, and Thrombolytics Drugs   **475–496**

Blood Coagulation   475
Anticoagulants   478
Antiplatelet Drugs   482
Thrombolytic Drugs   485
Individual Compounds   485

Section VI HORMONES AND ANTIHORMONAL DRUGS

17. Steroids and Steroidal Drugs   **499–588**

Cholesterol   500
Phytosterols and Mycosterols   501
Bile Acids   501
Sex Hormones   503
Adrenal Cortex Hormones   517
Individual Compounds   521

18. Hypoglycemic Agents   **589–606**

Insulin and Related Analogs   589
Oral Hypoglycemic Agents   593
Individual Compounds   596

19. Thyroid and Antithyroid Drugs   **607–611**

Biosynthesis of Thyroid Hormones   607
Mechanism of Action of Thyroid Hormones   608
Hypothyroidism   609
Hyperthyroidism   609
Individual Compounds   610

Section VII DRUGS AFFECTING GASTROINTESTINAL FUNCTIONS

20. Antiemetic Agents   **615–624**

Antiemetic Agents   615
Individual Compounds   619

21. Drugs Used for Constipation, Diarrhea, and in Inflammatory Bowel Diseases   **625–641**

Drugs Used for Constipation   625
Drugs Used for Diarrhea   629
Drugs Used in Inflammatory Bowel Diseases   631
Individual Compounds   633

Section VIII CHEMOTHERAPY—DRUGS USED IN PARASITIC INFECTIONS

22. Antiprotozoal Drugs I: Chemotherapy of Malaria   645–667
Antimalarial Drugs   647
Individual Compounds   660

23. Antiprotozoal Drugs II   668–682
Chemotherapy of Amoebiasis   668
Chemotherapy of Trypanosomiasis   672
Chemotherapy of Leishmaniasis   675
Chemotherapy of Trichomoniasis   675
Chemotherapy of Giardiasis   675
Individual Compounds   675

24. Drugs Used in Helminthiasis   683–692
Anthelmintic Drugs   684
Individual Compounds   688

Section IX CHEMOTHERAPY—DRUGS USED IN MICROBIAL INFECTIONS

25. Sulphonamides and Quinolones   695–719
Sulphonamides   695
Dihydrofolate Reductase Inhibitors   700
Quinolones   702
Individual Compounds   704

26. Antibiotics   720–726
Chemical Classification   720

27. β-Lactam Antibiotics   727–788
Penicillins   727
Carbapenems   735
Cephalosporins   737
Carbacephems and Oxacephems   742
Monobactams   743
Indivdiual Compounds   743

28. Peptide Antibiotics   789–791
Individual Compounds   789

29. Macrolide Antibiotics   792–794
Individual Compounds   793

30. Aminoglycoside Antibiotics   795–799
Individual Compounds   796

31. Tetracycline Antibiotics   800–806
Individual Compounds   802

32. Miscellaneous Antibiotics   807–810
    Chloramphenicol   807
    Individual Compounds   809

33. Chemotherapy of Acid-Fast Infections   811–824
    Tuberculosis   811
    Leprosy   818
    Individual Compounds   818

34. Antifungal Agents   825–846
    Antifungal Agents   825
    Individual Compounds   831

35. Antiviral Agents   847–881
    Virus Life History   847
    Approaches for Prevention of Viral Infections   849
    Antiviral Agents   850
    Individual Compounds   858

Section X CHEMOTHERAPY—DRUGS USED IN CANCER

36. Anticancer Agents   885–919
    Alkylating Agents   886
    DNA Cross Linking Agents – Organoplatinum Complexes   892
    Antimetabolites   892
    Antibiotics   896
    Plant Products   898
    Hormones and Antihormones   900
    Inhibitors of Protein Kinases   901
    Miscellaneous Compounds   903
    Individual Compounds   903

Section XI DIAGNOSTIC AGENTS

37. Diagnostic Agents   923–934
    Radiopaque Substances   923
    Individual Compounds   924

Section XII VITAMINS

38. Vitamins   937–995
    Fat Soluble Vitamins   937
    Water Soluble Vitamins   959

    Glossary   997–1012
    Subject Index   1013–1020
    Compound Index   1021–1041

Section I
Drugs Affecting Synaptic
and
Neuroeffector Junctional Sites

ADRENERGIC DRUGS

AUTONOMIC NERVOUS SYSTEM is broadly classified into two divisions, the sympathetic and parasympathetic. Norepinephrine [noradrenaline, (1)] is the neurotransmitter between the nerve endings and the effector organ in case of sympathetic or adrenergic nervous system, while acetylcholine (2) is the neurotransmitter in case of parasympathetic or cholinergic nervous system.

(1)   (2)

Adrenergic drugs are the substances which modify the activity of sympathetic nervous system. Substances which increase the activity are known as sympathomimetic or adrenergic stimulants. Substances which decrease the sympathetic activity are known as adrenergic blockers or sympatholytics. Both types of substances have clinical applications and are used in asthama, cardiac arrhythmias, ischemic heart diseases, control of blood pressure, glaucoma, nasal decongestants, etc.

After its release from sympathetic nerve endings, norepinephrine (1) interacts with specific presynaptic and postsynaptic adrenergic receptors.

Epinephrine [adrenaline, (3)] is another endogenous sympathomimetic agent which after its synthesis is stored in adrenal medulla. Unlike norepinephrine (1), epinephrine (3) is not released from sympathetic nerve endings and is a neurohormone. It is secreted along with norepinephrine (1) by the adrenal medulla.

(3)

3

BIOSYNTHESIS, STORAGE, AND RELEASE OF NOREPINEPHRINE

Biosynthesis of norepinephrine (1) takes place in adrenergic neurons (Fig. 1.1). The biosynthesis takes place from L-tyrosine which is taken up by the adrenergic neurons by an active transport system. In the adrenergic neurons, tyrosine hydroxylase converts this into dihydroxyphenylalanine (dopa). In the next step, dopa is converted to dopamine by dopa decarboxylase. The dopamine

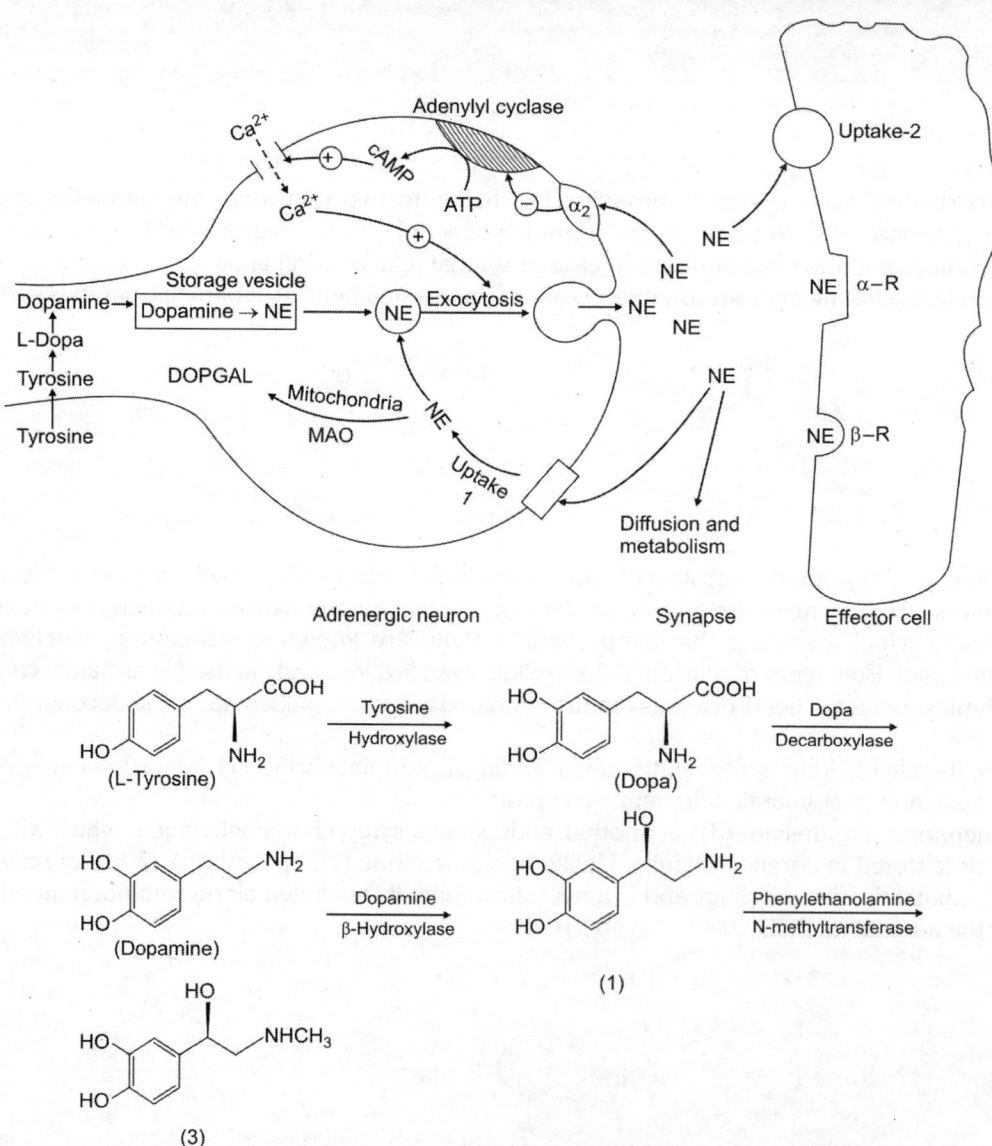

Fig. 1.1: Biosynthesis, storage, and release of norepinephrine (1).

formed is then taken up by the active transport into the storage vesicles where it is converted to norepinephrine (1) by the action of dopamine β-hydroxylase which introduces hydroxyl group at β-position in R configuration. The norepinephrine (1) is stored along with ATP in storage vesicles in the ratio of 4:1 complex, respectively. In this synthesis, the first step, i.e. conversion of tyrosine to dopa, is the rate limiting step.

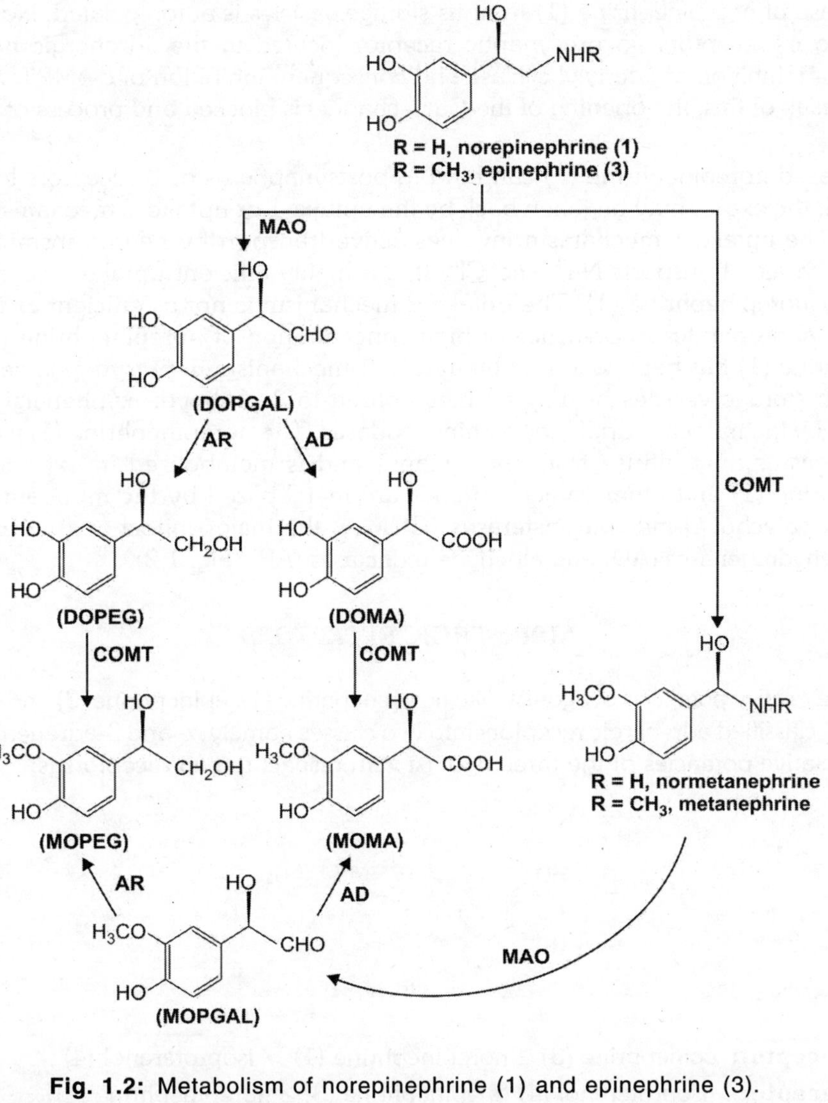

Fig. 1.2: Metabolism of norepinephrine (1) and epinephrine (3).

(MAO, monoamine oxidase; COMT, catechol-O-methyltransferase; AR, aldehyde reductase; AD, aldehyde dehydrogenase; DOPGAL, 3, 4-dihydroxyphenylglycoaldehyde; DOPEG, 3, 4-dihydroxyphenylethyleneglycol; DOMA, 3, 4-dihydroxymandelic acid; MOPEG, 3-methoxy-4-hydroxyphenylethyleneglycol; MOMA, 3-methoxy-4-hydroxymandelic acid; MOPGAL, 3-methoxy-4-hydroxyphenylglycoaldehyde.)

The norepinephrine (1) formed is converted to epinephrine (3) by the action of phenylethanolamine-N-methyltransferase which is located in adrenal medulla.

The release of norepinephrine [NE, (1)] into the synapse takes place by a process of exocytosis. Depolarization promotes opening of voltage dependent Ca^{2+} channel and consequent influx of Ca^{2+}. The Ca^{2+} promote the fusion of the storage vesicles to the neuronal cell membrane and by the process of exocytosis the neurotransmitter along with ATP is spilled into the synapse.

The release of norepinephrine (1) from its storage vesicles is autoregulated. Norepinephrine (1) binds to α_2-receptors—a presynaptic receptor located in the adrenergic neurons. This results in the inhibition of adenylyl cyclase and consequent inhibition of c-AMP formation from ATP. As a result of this, the opening of the Ca^{2+} channel is blocked and process of exocytosis is prevented.

The released norepinephrine (1) can bind to postsynaptic α- or β-receptors located in the effector cell, the excess may be taken back by the uptake-1 or uptake-2 mechanism or may be degraded. The uptake-1 mechanism involves active transport by neurotransmitter transport protein which also transports Na^+ and Cl^-. It is a highly efficient uptake mechanism and is selective for norepinephrine (1). The uptake-2 mechanism is not as efficient as the uptake-1 mechanism and operates in presence of high concentration of norepinephrine (1). After the norepinephrine (1) has been taken up by uptake-1 mechanism in presynaptic neuron, it may be stored in storage vesicles or may be metabolized to 3, 4-dihydroxyphenylglycoaldehyde (DOPGAL) by the mitochondrial monoamine oxidases. The norepinephrine (1) which escapes uptake processes may diffuse from the synapse and is metabolized in extraneuronal site. Norepinephrine (1) and other catecholamines are metabolized by the monoamine oxidases (MAO) and catechol-O-methyltransferases (COMT), the major mitochondrial enzymes, and aldehyde dehydrogenases (AD) and aldehyde reductases (AR) (Fig. 1.2)

ADRENERGIC RECEPTORS

Based on the relative potencies of agonists like norepinephrine (1), epinephrine (3) and isoproterenol (4), Ahlquist classified adrenergic receptors into two classes namely α- and β-adrenergic receptors. Thus, the relative potencies of the three agonist with respect to two receptors is:

(4)

α-receptor: epinephrine (3) $\geq$ norepinephrine (1) > isoproterenol (4)

β-receptor: isoproterenol (4) > epinephrine (3) $\geq$ norepinephrine (1)

With the use of other agonist and antagonists, it has been possible to classify the two receptors further and these include α_1- and α_2-receptors and β_1-, β_2-, and β_3-receptors. At present, six types of α-receptors are known and these are designated as α_{1A}, α_{1B}, α_{1C}, α_{2A}, α_{2B} and α_{2C}.

Both α_1- and α_2-adrenergic receptors are guanine-nucleotide-regulatory protein (G-protein) linked receptors. However, they differ in second messenger system. In case of α_1-adrenergic receptor, the Gs-protein is coupled to phospholipase C. Activation of the α_1-receptor results in activation of phospholipase C which hydrolyses phosphatidylinositol-4, 5-diphosphate [PIP$_2$, (5)] into diacylglycerol [DAG, (6)] and inositol triphosphate [IP$_3$, (7)]. Both of these function as second messengers. Production of DAG (6) results in activation of membrane-bound protein kinase C,which causes phosphorylation of protein. IP$_3$ (7) on the other hand, causes release of Ca^{2+} from intracellular stores, the endoplasmic reticulum. The endoplasmic reticulum is coupled to calcium channel, which open after IP$_3$ (7) binds to receptor in endoplasmic reticulum. Increased free intracellular Ca^{2+} results in smooth muscle contraction, increased force of contraction of cardiac muscle and transmitter release.

R = arachidonic acid
R' = Fatty acid

(5)   (6)   (7)

α_2-Adrenoreceptors are G$_i$-linked. Activation of these receptors results in inhibition of adenylyl cyclase. This leads to lowering of c-AMP levels.

In summary, the stimulation of α_1-receptors results in vasoconstriction, relaxation of gastrointestinal smooth muscles, salivary secretion and hepatic glycogenolysis, while stimulation of α_2-receptors results in inhibition of transmitter release, both norepinephrine (1) and acetylcholine (2), platelet aggregation, contraction of vascular smooth muscles and inhibition of insulin release.

All the three types of β-receptors are linked to guanine nucleotide protein Gs and the second messenger in all the three subtypes of β-receptors is adenylyl cyclase, which catalyzes the formation of c-AMP from ATP. The increased levels of c-AMP result in activation of protein kinase which phosphorylates myosin-light-chain kinase, thereby inhibiting the contraction. Activation of β-receptors also reduces the intracellular Ca^{2+} through its efflux.

The effect of stimulation of β_1-receptors results in increased cardiac rate and force, β_2-receptor stimulation leads to bronchial dilation, vasodilation, relaxation of visceral smooth muscles and hepatic glycogenolysis. The stimulation of β_3-receptors results in lipolysis.

The distribution of various classes of adrenergic receptors and the effect of their stimulation on some organs is summarized in Table 1.1.

Table 1.1: Distribution of adrenergic receptors in various organs and response obtained after stimulation

SN.	Organ	Major Receptor Type	Response after stimulation
1.	Heart	β_1	Increase rate and force
2.	Blood vesels	α_1, α_2	Constriction
3.	Lungs	β_2	Relaxation
4.	G.I. tract	α_1, β_2	Decreased motility
5.	Uterus		
	pregnant	α_1	Constriction
	nonpregnant	β_2	Relaxation
6.	Liver	α_1, β_2	Incneased Glycogenolysis and Gluconeogenesis
7.	Eye radial muscle	α_1	Contraction
8.	Skeletal muscle	β_2	Tremors, Glucogenolysis and increase speed of constriction

From the studies on structure-activity relationships on norepinephrine (1) and its analogs, certain generalisations can be made with regard to requirements of structure for the adrenergic activity and these are:

1. A phenylethylamine moiety, with an amino group separated from phenyl group by two carbons, is necessary for the activity.

(1)

2. For agonist activity, the amino group should be 1° or 2°.
3. Compounds containing an alkyl group on amino nitrogen have lower α-agonist activity and higher β-agonist activity.
4. Increase in the bulk of alkyl group at amino nitrogen also reduces the α-agonist activity and increases the β-agonist activity.
5. For direct-acting compounds, hydroxyl group at position 3 and 4 in the phenyl ring and a hydroxyl group at β-position is necessary. The hydroxyl group at β-position should have a proper orientation. Compounds having hydroxyl group at β-position with R-configuration have maximum activity.
6. Removal of β-hydroxyl group reduces the affinity for the receptors. Similar removal of phenolic hydroxyl groups also results in compounds which are devoid of affinity or have very weak affinity for adrenergic receptors.
7. Modification of phenolic hydroxyl groups results in compounds resistant to COMT.

8. Introduction of an alkyl group (methyl, ethyl) at α-position reduces receptor agonist activity at both α- and β-receptors. There is also increase in duration of action because such compounds are resistant to MAO and they also have greater CNS activity. α-Alkylation also affects selectivity towards receptor. Thus, α-substitution in case of β-agonist gives selective β_2-agonist, similarly in case of α-agonist such a substitution results in α_2-agonists.
9. Modification of side chain as well as phenolic hydroxyl groups results in compound which are β-adrenoreceptor antagonist.

As will be evident, these generalizations account for various drugs acting directly or indirectly. The various types of adrenergic drugs can be classified as:

1. Drugs affecting norepinephrine biosynthesis,
2. drugs affecting norepinephrine storage,
3. drugs affecting norepinephrine release, and
4. drugs affecting adrenergic receptors, agonists and antagonists.

DRUGS AFFECTING NOREPINEPHRINE BIOSYNTHESIS

Reduction in the norepinephrine (1) concentration would lead to reduction in adrenergic stimulation. Inhibitors for all the steps involved in the biosynthesis of norepinephrine (Fig. 1.1) are known but only few have gained the clinical acceptance.

α-Methyltyrosine, commonly called metyrosine (8) is a competitive inhibitor of tyrosine hydroxylase, which is involved in the hydroxylation of tyrosine (Fig. 1.1), the rate limiting step of

(8)

biosynthesis of norepinephrine (1). Although the (–) isomer possesses the inhibitory activity, but racemic mixture is used in clinical practice. Metyrosine (8) is used in preoperative management of pheochromocytoma, a disease characterized by a tumor in adrenal medulla. Although these tumors are benign, but a large amount of norepinephrine is produced and patients suffer hypertensive episode. Metyrosine (8) reduces the frequency and the severity of these episodes.

Methyldopa (9), which competes with dopa (Fig. 1.1) for dopa decarboxylase, is taken up by adrenergic neurons and decarboxylated and hydroxylated as dopa (Fig. 1.1) and converted to α-methylnorepinephrine (10). In contrast to norepinephrine (1), α-methylnorepinephrine (10) is not metabolized by MAO in adrenergic neurons and acts as a false neurotransmitter. It is released in the same way as norepinephrine (1) from the neuron and binds to α-receptor. It is less active at α_1-receptors but is more active at presynaptic α_2-receptors, binding to which results in inhibition of transmitter release. The side effects include sedation and may cause immune hemolytic reaction. It is mainly used for hypertension in late pregnancy.

(9)

(10)

DRUGS AFFECTING NOREPINEPHRINE STORAGE

Reserpine (11) is an alkaloid obtained form various species of *Rauwolfia* belonging to family *Apocynaceae*. Reserpine (11) binds to the ATP-driven monoamine transporter which transports norepinephrine (1) into the storage vesicles. The norepinephrine (1) is thus not transported and it gets destroyed by the MAO in the cytoplasm. Further, there is a gradual loss of already stored norepinephrine (1) by the sympathetic activity. This results in net loss of norepinephrine (1) from sympathetic neuron. Reserpine (11) also causes depletion of serotonin and dopamine from the neurons in brain.

(11)

The onset of reserpine (11) action is slow and a sustained effect. Earlier it was used for hypertension, but now it is not used because of the side effects, mainly depression, which is caused by impairment of noradrenergic transmission and serotonin in brain.

DRUGS AFFECTING NOREPINEPHRINE RELEASE

Norepinephrine (1) release from its stores can either be blocked or enhanced. Drugs which block the norepinephrine (1) release from its storage vesicles are known as noradrenergic neuron blocking agents. While as drugs which enhance the release of norepinephrine (1) from its storage sites are known as indirect acting sympathomimetics.

Noradrenergic Neuron Blocking Agents

Noradrenergic neuron blocking agents include bretylium tosylate (12), guanadrel (13), and guanethidine (14). These agents enter the adrenergic neuron by uptake-1 mechanism and inhibit the release of norepinephrine (1).

(12)

(13) (14)

Bretylium tosylate (12) is used as an antiarrhythmic agent. Its mechanism of action is not known Guanadrel (13) and guanethidine (14) are used in hypertension. They do not have central effects.

Indirect Acting Sympathomimetics

The indirect acting sympathomimetics are a class of phenylpropylamines that enhance the release of endogeneous norepinephrine (1) from its storage vesicles and do not have any direct action on adrenergic receptors. They enter adrenergic neuron by uptake-1 mechanism, after which they are transported to norepinephrine (1) storage vesicles by vesicular monoamine transporter in exchange of norepinephrine (1). No exocytosis is involved. After escaping into cytosol, part of norepinephrine (1) is metabolized by MAO and rest of it escapes, in exchange for indirectly acting amine by uptake-1 mechanism, to interact with postsynaptic adrenergic receptors. They also reduce reuptake of norepinephrine (1). Although they stimulate adrenergic nervous system, the response, however, differs from drugs which act directly by binding to the adrenergic receptors. Some of these differences are:

1. Indirectly acting sympathomimetics are less effective when the norepinephrine (1) storage sites are depleted by reserpine (11),
2. they are also central nervous system stimulants,
3. many of these compounds are effective anorexics, and
4. they are effective as nasal decongestants.

Some of these compounds are amphetamine (15), benzphetamine (16), hydroxyamphetamine (17), methamphetamine (18), phentermine (19), chlorphentermine (20), mephentermine (21), methoxyphentermine (22), and pholedrine (23).

(15), R = R' = R" = Y = H

(17), R = R' = R" = H, Y = OH

(19), R = CH_3, R' = R" = Y = H

(21), R = R' = CH_3, R" = Y = H

(23), R = R" = H, R' = CH_3, Y = OH

(16), R = Y = H, R' = $CH_2C_6H_5$, R" = CH_3

(18), R = R" = Y = H, R' = CH_3

(20), R = CH_3, R' = R" = H, Y = Cl

(22), R = CH_3, R' = R" = H, Y = OCH_3

None of the indirectly acting sympathomimetics contains a catechol moiety or a hydroxyl group at β-carbon atom. This enables them to pass the blood-brain barrier, as a result of which they possess significant CNS stimulant activity. Further, all of these compounds possess a methyl group at α-carbon atom. Phenylethylamines with a methyl group at α-carbon are poor substrates for MAO. Moreover this confers increased oral activity on the compounds.

Indirectly acting sympathomimetics are mainly used as nasal decongestants.

Sympathomimetics with Mixed Action

Some the phenylalkylamines have shown to increase the levels of norepinephrine (1) by interacting directly with the adrenergic receptors as well as indirectly by increasing the release of norepinephrine (1) from its storage sites. Some of these are ephedrine (24), metaraminol (25), phenylethanolamine (26), phenylpropanolamine (27), and tyramine (28).

(24), R = OH, R' = R" = CH$_3$, Y = H;   (25), R = Y = OH, R' = CH$_3$, R" = H

(26), R = OH, R' = R" = Y = H   (27), R = OH, R' = CH$_3$, R" = Y = H

(28)

All of these drugs have very weak action on adrenergic receptors and their main adrenergic action is through action on storage sites of norepinephrine (1) as in case of indirectly acting sympathomimetics, discussed earlier. As is evident from the structures of indirectly acting amines and amines with mixed activity, there does not seem to be stringent structural requirements for the action.

Ephedrine (24) has two asymmetric centres and can exist in 4 stereoisomers, DL-erythro (29) and DL-threo (30). Ephedrine (24) is the naturally occurring D(–)-erythro-isomer. It is 36 times more active than D(–)-threo form, which is commonly called D(–)-pseudoephedrine. The relative pressor activities of D-(–) ephedrine, L-(+)-ephedrine, L-(+)-pseudoephedrine, and D-(–)-pseudoephedrine are 36, 11, 7, and 1, respectively.

(29)   (30)

DRUGS ACTING ON ADRENERGIC RECEPTORS—AGONISTS

The endogenous catecholamines, norepinephrine (1) and epinephrine (3) are potent stimulants of α- and β-adrenergic receptors. Both drugs are equipotent at β$_1$-receptor. Norepinephrine (1) is a potent agonist of α-adrenergic receptor and has little action on β$_2$-receptors, however, it is less potent than epinephrine (3) on the α-receptors of most of the organs.

α$_1$-Adrenergic Receptor Agonists

Mephentermine (21) and metaraminol (25) have mixed actions, acting directly by binding to

α_1-receptor and indirectly by increasing the release of norepinephrine (1) from its storage sites. Other phenylethanolamines which have α_1-adrenergic agonist activity include methoxamine (31) and phenylephrine (32). Among the imidazoline analogs, naphazoline (33), oxymetazoline (34), tetrahydrozoline (35), and xylometazoline (36) are some of the compounds having α_1-agonist activity.

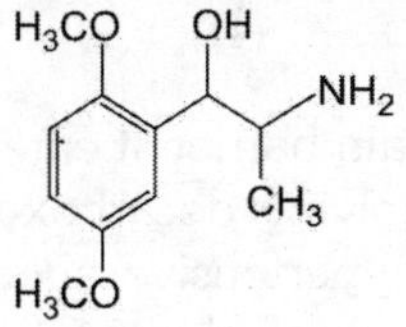

(31)

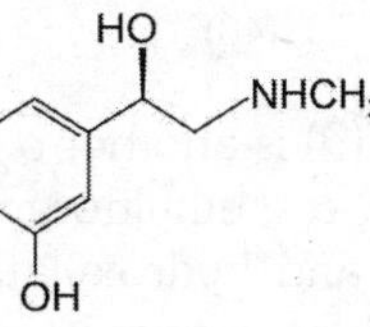

(32)

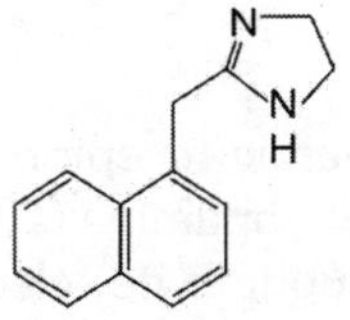

(33)

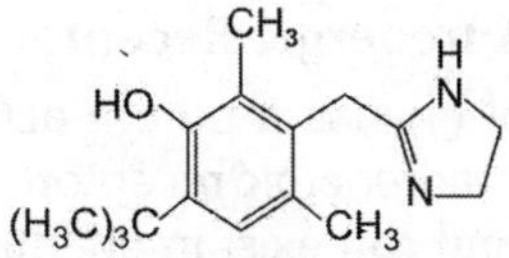

(34)

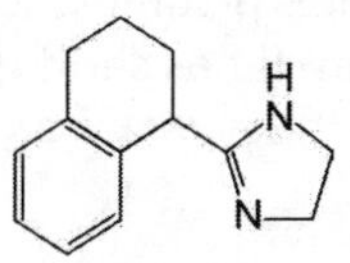

(35)

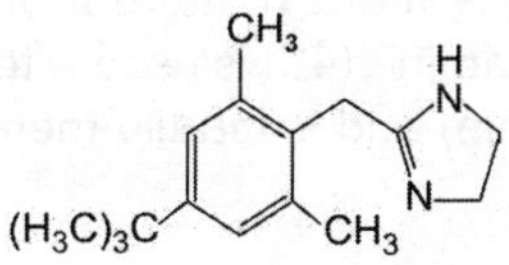

(36)

Activation of α_1-adrenergic receptors results in vasoconstriction and consequent increase in blood pressure. All these drugs are used in hypotension and as nasal decongestants.

α_2-Adrenergic Receptor Agonists

α_2-Adrenergic agonists include clonidine (37), apraclonidine (38), and brimonidine (39). Structure-activity relation studies on clonidine (37) has shown that imidazoline ring is not necessary for antihypertensive effect. These studies have resulted in two useful compounds guanabenz (40) and guanfacine (41). These compounds act by stimulating the α_2-adrenergic receptor and imidazoline-I_1 receptors in CNS. All this results in inhibition of sympathetic output and consequent decrease in peripheral resistance.

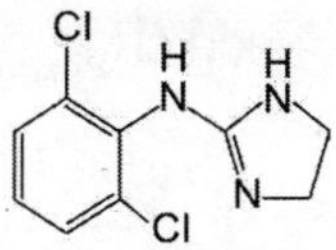

(37)

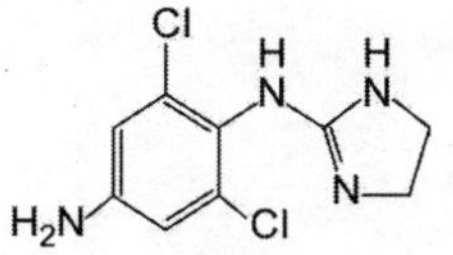

(38)

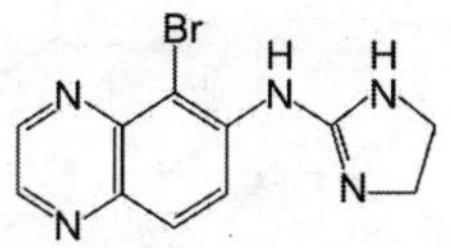

(39)

(40)

(41)

Methyldopa (9) is another α_2-agonist. After crossing blood-brain barrier, it enters CNS where it is converted to α-methylnorepinephrine (10) in two steps involving decarboxylation by dopa decarboxylase and hydroxylation by β-hydroxylase (see antihypertensive agents). Binding of α-methylnorepinephrine to α_2-receptors results in decrease in peripheral resistance.

All the α_2-agonists are used as antihypertensives clinically.

β_1- and β_2 Adrenergic Receptor Agonists

Isoproterenol (4) has a potent action on both β_1- and β_2-adrenergic receptors with a very low affinity for α_1-adrenergic receptors. Dobutamine (42), an analog of dopamine (43), has a centre of asymmetry and can exist in enantiomeric form. It was earlier thought to be selective β_1-agonists. Recent studies have shown that (–) isomer is an agonist at α_1- and β-receptors, while (+) – isomer is an antagonist at α_1-receptor and an agonist at β-receptors. The β-agonistic activity of (+) – isomer is about 10 times more than (–) isomer. The net result is β-stimulation by the racemic form. Dobutamine (42) is used after surgery for cardiac stimulation. It has short duration of action (half-life 2 min) and is readily metabolised by COMT.

(42)

(43)

Dopamine (43) is a catecholamine which acts on dopamine receptors as well as on β_1-adrenergic receptor. It is usually used in shock, myocardial infarction, and congestive heart failure.

β_2-Adrenergic Receptor Agonists

The β_2-adrenergic agonists include, clenbuterol (44) metaproterenol (45), terbutaline (46), salbutamol (47), salmeterol (48), pirbuterol (49), and bitolterol (50).

(44)

(45)

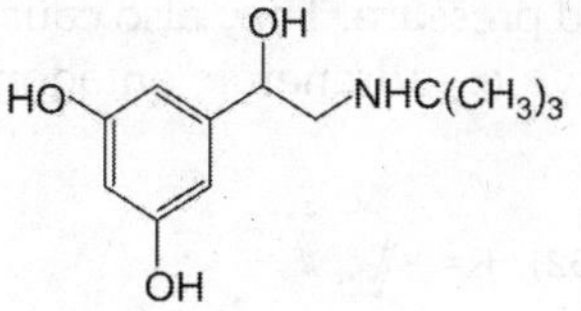

OH
HO NHC(CH₃)₃

OH

(46)

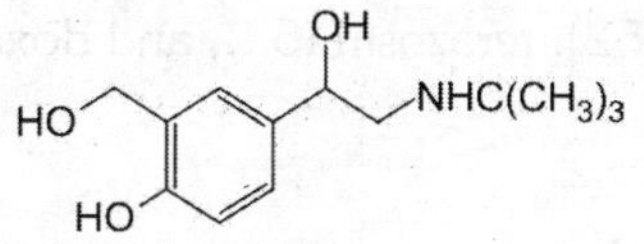

OH
HO NHC(CH₃)₃

HO

(47)

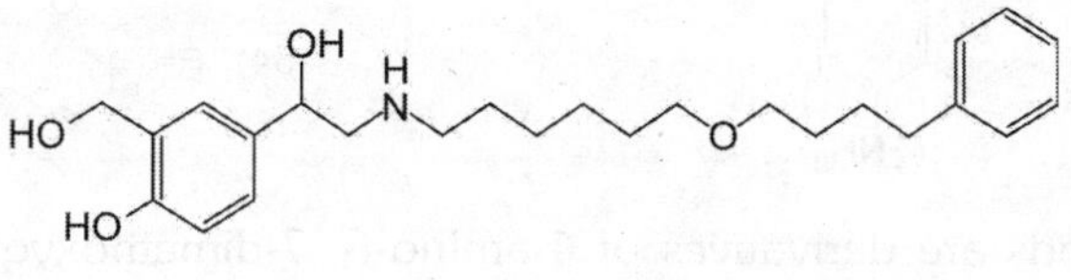

OH H
HO N O

HO

(48)

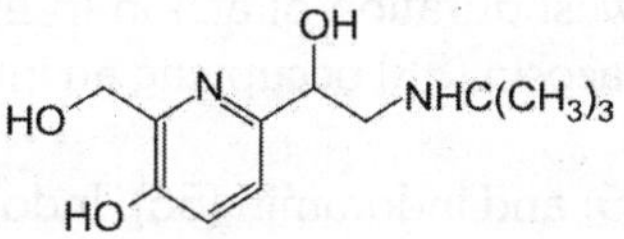

OH
HO N NHC(CH₃)₃

HO

(49)

OH
NHC(CH₃)₃
O
O
CH₃
H₃C
O
O

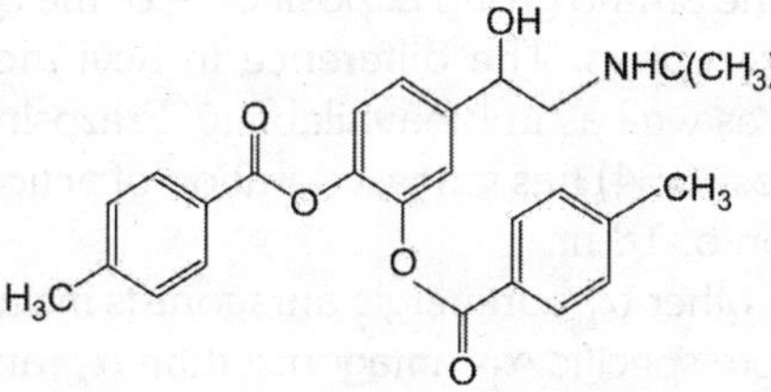

(50)

Increasing of bulk of the alkyl group at amino nitrogen leads to enhanced β-activity as compared to α-activity. All the β₂-agonists have been used for asthama. Since one of the major side effects of antiasthamatics is stimulation of heart caused by β₁-agonist activity, efforts have been made to have selective β₂-agonist. This selectivity has been achieved by having non-catechol moiety attached to ethanolamine residue excepting bitolterol (50). This has also resulted in oral activity as well as longer duration of action because they are not the substrates for enzymes which metabolize catecholamines.

Bitolterol (50) which is catecholamine diester of 4-methylbenzoic acid is actually a prodrug, esterases hydrolyse (50) to colterol (51) which is the active form of bitolterol (50).

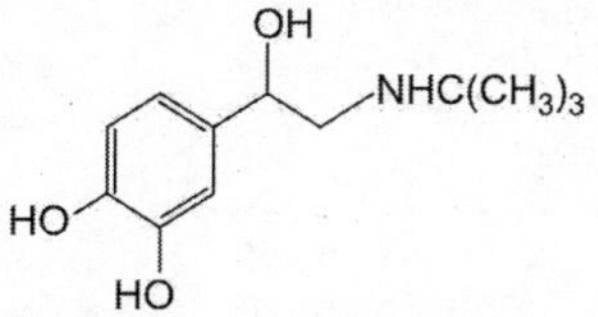

OH
NHC(CH₃)₃

HO

HO

(51)

All the β₂-adrenergic agonists are used in asthma for dilation of bronchi.

DRUGS ACTING ON ADRENERGIC RECEPTORS—ANTAGONISTS (BLOCKERS)

α₁-Adrenergic Receptor Antagonists (Blockers)

Blockade of α₁-adrenergic receptors results in vasodilation (inhibition of vasoconstriction by norepinephrine and epinephrine) with consequent fall in blood pressure. They also cause relaxation of smooth muscles of bladder and neck. Some of the selective α_1-adrenergic antagonists include prazosin (52), terazosin (53), and doxazosin (54).

(52), R=

(53), R=

(54), R=

All of these compounds are derivatives of 4-amino-6, 7-dimethoxyquinazoline containing a piperazine moiety at position 2. The structural difference is in the acyl moiety on N- 4 of piperazine ring. The amino group at position 4 of the quinazoline nucleus seems to be essential for the affinity of α_1-receptors. The difference in acyl moiety results in differences in half-life and duration of action as well as in bioavailability. Prazosin (52) has the lowest duration of action (3 hr) while as doxazosin (54) has longest duration of action (36 hr) with terazosin (53) occupying an intermediate position of 18 hr.

The other α_1-adrenergic antagonists include tamsulosin (55) and indoramin (56). Indoramin (56) is a more specific α_1- antagonist than α_2- antagonist. It also blocks H_1- and serotonin receptors.

(55)

(56)

Corynanthine (57) is a stereoisomer of *allo*-yohimbine (58). It is a selective α_1-adrenergic antagonist.

(57)

(58)

Nonspecific α_2-Adrenergic Receptor Antagonists (Blockers)

allo-Yohimbine (58) an indole alkaloid has been obtained from the bark of *Pausinystlia johimbe* and roots of *Rauwolfia* species. *allo*-Yohimbine (58) through blockade of α_2-receptors in CNS increases the heart rate and blood pressure.

Other nonspecific α_2-adrenergic antagonist include phenoxybenzamine (59), phentolamine (60), and tolazoline (61). Phenoxybenzamine (59) contains a β-haloalkylamine moiety which is found in many alkylating agents. Because of this, it alkylates α-receptors and reversibly inactivates both α_1- as well as α_2-receptors. It causes decrease in peripheral resistance which is due to α_1-blockade. However, α_2-blockade results in enhanced release of norepinephrine (1) and inhibition of uptake of norepinephrine (1) into the adrenergic nerve terminals and extraneuronal tissues. It is used in pheochromocytoma and for patients whose tumors cannot be operated upon.

(59)　　　　　　　　　(60)　　　　　　　　　(61)

Phentolamine (60) and tolazoline (61) are the imidazoline analogs. Both block α_1- and α_2-adrenergic receptors. Both have vasodilatory effect due to blockade of α_1-receptor. α_2-Blockade leads to norepinephrine (1) release. Phentolamine (60) is used for control of hypertension in pheochromocytoma.

Tolazoline (61) has a weak antagonistic activity. It also stimulates gastric acid secretion and has histamine like effects. It is used in newborn babies who have pulmonary hypertension.

Ergot alkaloids are obtained from dried sclerotium of the fungus *Claviceps purpurea* that grows on rye plants. All the alkaloids are derivatives of (+)-lysergic acid (62). Two groups of alkaloids are present in ergot and these are water insoluble alkaloids ergotamine (63), ergosine (64), ergocristine (65), α-ergocryptine (66), and ergocornine (67). The other group is the water soluble alkaloid ergonovine (68). The members of water insoluble group, i.e. ergotamine (63), ergosine (64), ergocristine (65), α-ergocryptine (66), and ergocornine (67) are α-adrenergic blocking agent. They also cause a rise in blood pressure by constriction of peripheral blood vessels. One of the important pharmacological actions of these alkaloids for which they are used therapeutically is stimulation of smooth muscles of uterus.

(62)

	R	R'
(63),	CH_3	H_2C-phenyl
(64),	CH_3	$CH_2CH(CH_3)_2$
(65),	$CH(CH_3)_2$	H_2C-phenyl
(66),	$CH(CH_3)_2$	$CH_2CH(CH_3)_2$
(67),	$CH(CH_3)_2$	$CH(CH_3)_2$

(68)

Selective β₁-Adrenergic Receptor Antagonists (Blockers)

The selective β_1-adrenergic blocking agents include acebutolol (69), atenolol (70), betaxolol (71), bisoprolol (72), esmolol (73), metoprolol (74), and practolol (75). β_1-Blockers are used for hypertension, cardiac arrhythmia, angina and myocardial infarction. Since β_1-antagonists do not block β_2-receptors, they can be safely used in case of asthma patients. Moreover, there is no reflex sympathetic activity because of blockade of vascular β_2-receptors, which is observed in non-specific β-blockers. However, the cardioselectivity is observed only in low doses.

	R	R'
(69),	$COCH_3$	$NHCO(CH_2)_2CH_3$
(70),	H	CH_2CONH_2
(71),	H	$CH_2CH_2OCH_2-\triangleleft$
(72),	H	$CH_2O(CH_2)_2OCH(CH_3)_2$
(73),	H	$CH_2CH_2COOCH_3$
(74)	H	$CH_2CH_2OCH_3$
(75),	H	$NHCOCH_3$

Non-selective β-Adrenergic Receptor Antagonists (Blockers)

Dichloroisoproterenol (76) was the first compound which had β-blocking activity. It is an analog of isoproterenol (4) in which the two phenolic groups have been replaced by chlorine. Dichloroisoproterenol (76) in addition to β-blocking activity also possesses β-agonist activity. Pronethalol (77) in which the dichlorophenyl ring is replaced by naphthalene ring was the next β-blocker. However, because it caused thymic tumor, it was withdrawn from clinical testing. Continued search for β-blockers, resulted in the syntheses of aryloxypropylamine class of compounds, first of which was propranolol (78). Some other compounds in this series include carteolol (79), levobunolol (80), metipranolol (81), nadolol (82), penbutolol (83), pindolol (84), and timolol (85).

All of these compounds show high stereoselectivity. The configuration of the carbon carrying hydroxyl group should be S in order to show the β-blocking activity. However, most of these compounds are used as racemic mixtures. β-Adrenergic blockers are used in hypertension, angina, and in supraventricular and ventricular arrhythmias. Since most of these compounds block both β_1- and β_2-receptors, they are contraindicated in patients with asthama and bronchitis. Carteolol (79), metipranolol (81) and timolol (85) are used in glaucoma to reduce the intraocular pressure with no effect on pupil size.

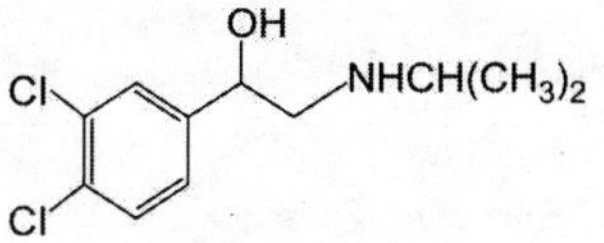

(76)

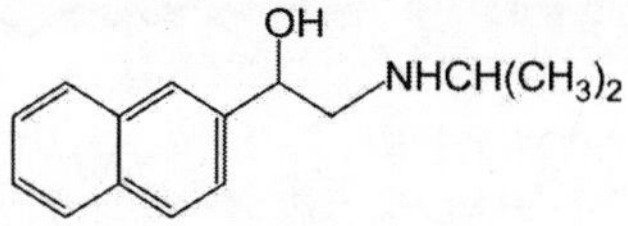

(77)

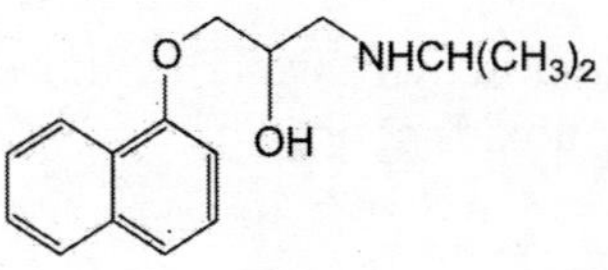

(78)

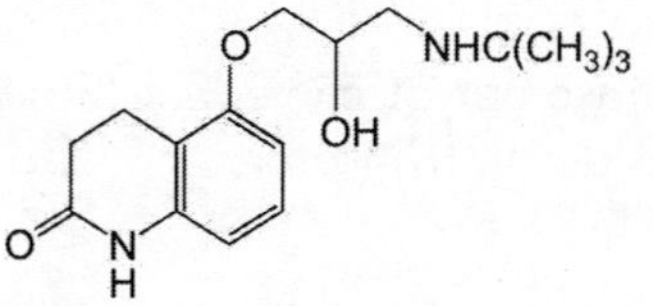

(79)

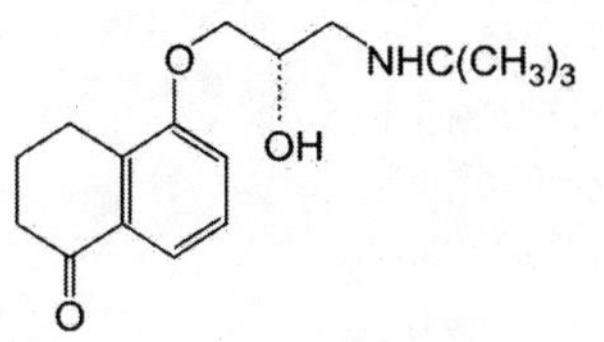

(80)

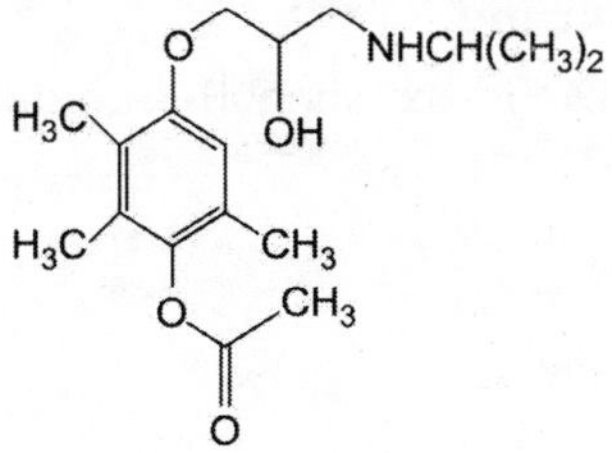

(81)

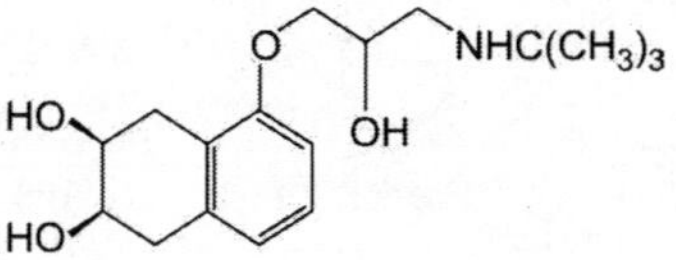

(82)

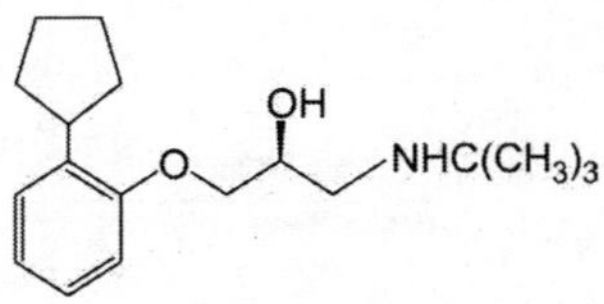

(83)

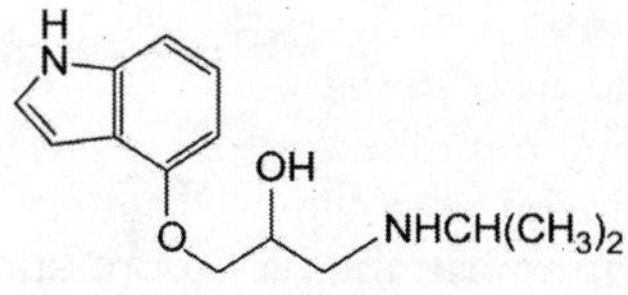

(84)

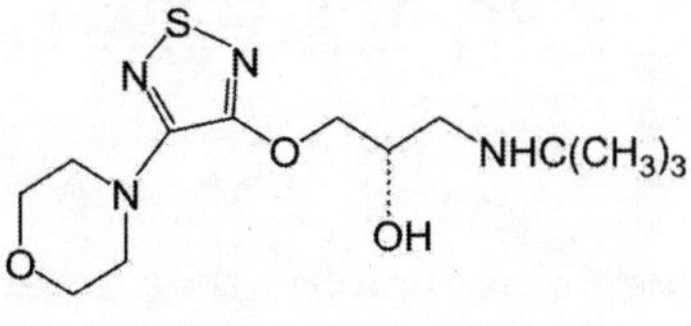

(85)

Mixed α- and β-Adrenergic Receptor Antagonists (Blockers)

Compounds possessing α_1- and β-adrenergic receptor blocking activity have been developed. As antihypertensive, they have advantage over non-specific β-blockers. Thus, α_1-blockade produces vasodilation while as non-specific β-blockade would prevent reflex vasoconstriction which usually follows vasodilation. Compounds of this type include carvedilol (86) and labetalol (87). Carvedilol (86) possesses aryloxypropanolamine moiety while labetalol (87) is an analog of arylethanolamine.

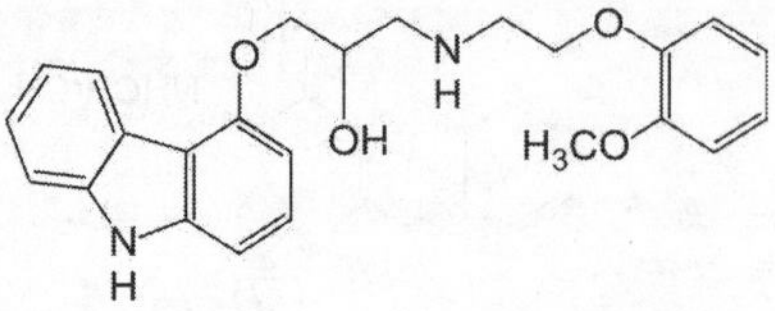

(86)

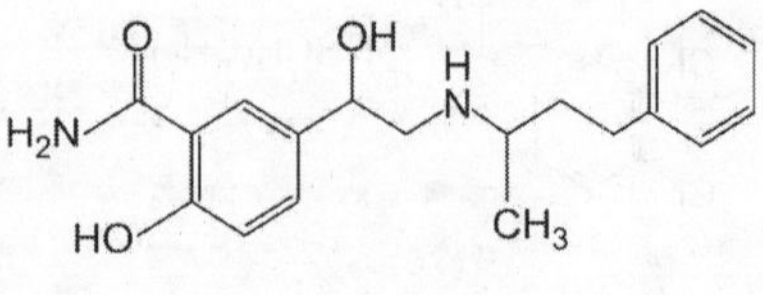

(87)

The (S)-isomer of carvedilol (86) possesses the β-blocking activity while as the α_1-blocking activity resides in (R)-isomer. It is also reported to possess antioxidant activity.

INDIVIDUAL COMPOUNDS

ENDOGENOUS CATECHOLAMINES

Norepinephrine

(R)-1-(3,4-Dihydroxyphenyl)-2-aminoethanol

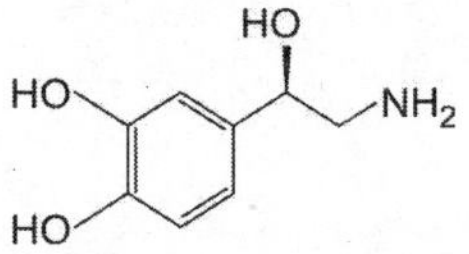

Synthesis

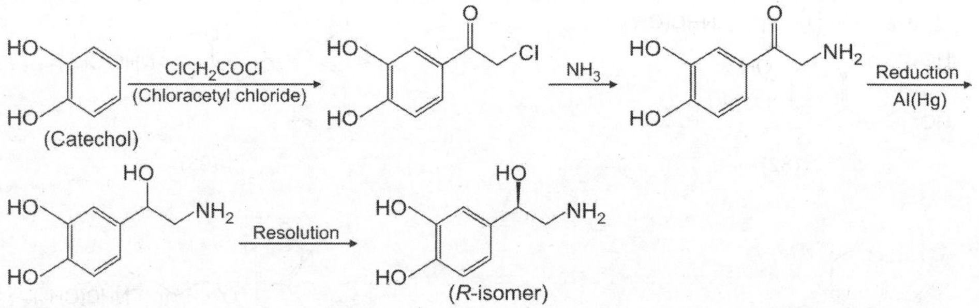

Norepinephrine is more active at α-receptor. It is used to maintain the blood pressure in acute hypotensive states such as shock, hemorrhage. It is administered by intravenous route, sodium bisulphite is used as an antioxidant in the formulation.

Epinephrine

(R)-1-(3,4-Dihydroxyphenyl)-2-methylaminoethanol

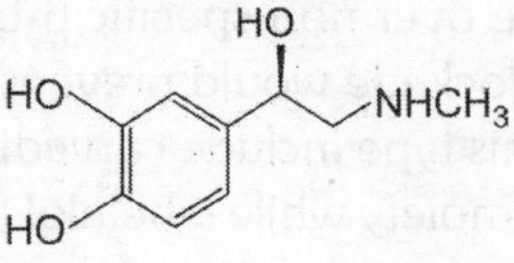

Synthesis

(Catechol) → (via ClCH$_2$COCl, Chloracetyl chloride) → (via CH$_3$NH$_2$, Methyl amine) → (Reduction Al(Hg))

(via Resolution) → (R-isomer)

It stimulates both α- and β-adrenergic receptors. It is used in hemorrhage and as a nasal decongestant. Its vasoconstrictor property is used for prolonging the local anesthetic activity (α-receptors stimulation). It is also used to relax bronchial muscles in asthma (β$_2$-agonist activity). It has also found use in open-angle glaucoma. Use of epinephrine in eye results in irritation which is because of phenolic groups. Drugs in which phenolic groups are masked have been developed and include epinephryl borate (88) and dipivefrin (89). Dipivefrin (89) is a pivalic acid diester of epinephrine (3). It is a prodrug of epinephrine and is hydrolyzed in cornea and innerchamber by the esterases. It has a short duration of action.

(88)

(89)

Dopamine

4-(2-Aminoethyl)pyrocatechol

Synthesis

(Catechol) → (via ClCH$_2$CH$_2$Cl/AlCl$_3$, Ethylene chloride/Aluminium chloride) → (via NH$_3$)

Dopamine is used intravenously in treatment of shock. It increases blood flow to kidney which results in increase in filtration rate, sodium ion excretion, and consequent increase in urine output. This action of dopamine on renal blood vessels is due to interaction with dopamine D$_1$-receptors. Dopamine in higher doses stimulates β$_1$-receptors. It is not given orally because it is metabolized fast by MAO and COMT.

DRUGS AFFECTING NOREPINEPHRINE STORAGE

Reserpine

See **ANTIHYPERTENSIVE DRUGS**

DRUGS AFFECTING NOREPINEPHRINE RELEASE : NORADRENERGIC NEURON BLOCKING AGENTS

Bretylium Tosylate

See **ANTIANGINAL, ANTIARRHYTHMIC, AND CARDIOTONIC DRUGS**

Guanadrel and Guanethidine

See **ANTIHYPERTENSIVE DRUGS**

DRUGS AFFECTING NOREPINEPHRINE RELEASE : INDIRECT ACTING SYMPATHOMIMETICS

Amphetamine

(±)-1-Phenyl-2-aminopropane

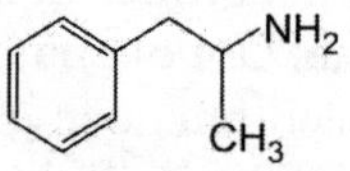

Synthesis

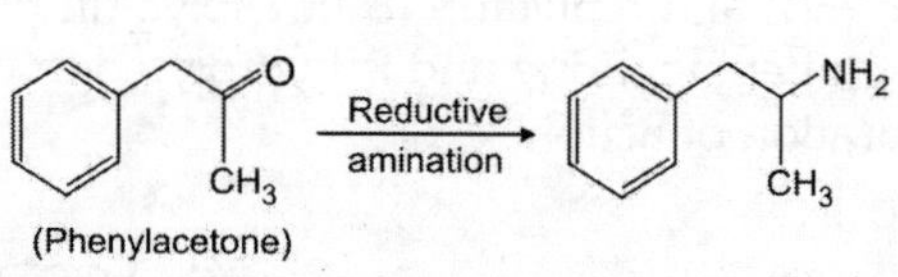

(Phenylacetone)

It is an indirect acting sympathomimetic with CNS stimulating effect. Dexamphetamine, the dextro-isomer, is more powerful CNS stimulant. It is used in obesity, narcolepsy.

Benzphetamine

(*S*)-(+)-*N*-Benzyl-*N*,α-dimethylphenylethlamine

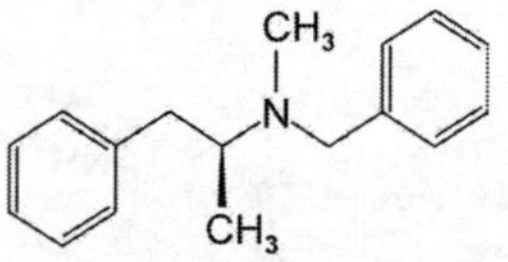

Synthesis

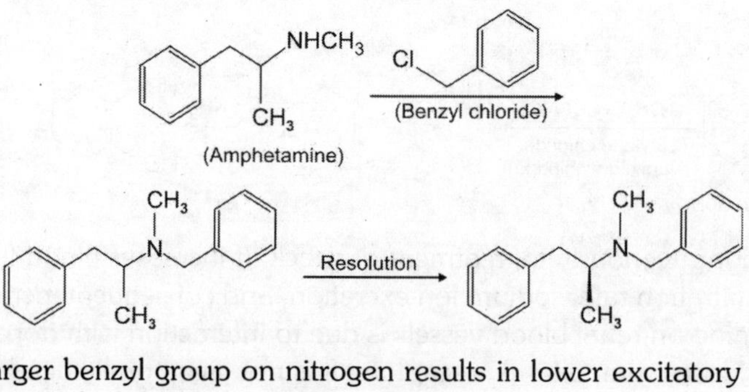

(Amphetamine)   (Benzyl chloride)

Introduction of larger benzyl group on nitrogen results in lower excitatory effects. It is used as appetite reducing agent which has lower CNS excitatory effects.

Hydroxyamphetamine

(±)-4-(2-Aminopropyl)phenol

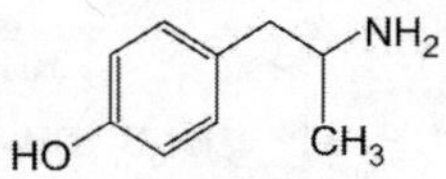
NH2
HO
CH3

Synthesis

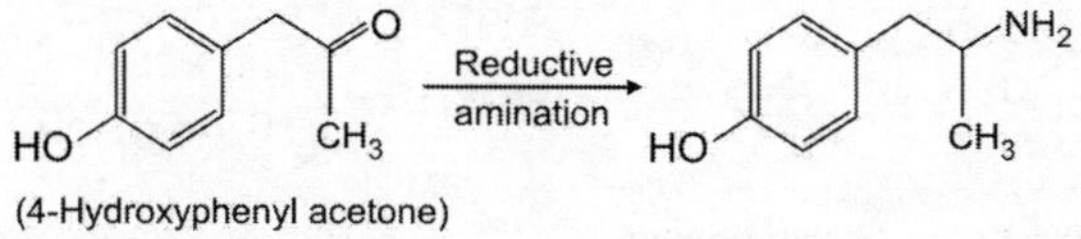
O
HO
CH3
(4-Hydroxyphenyl acetone)
Reductive
amination
NH2
HO
CH3

It has little or no CNS stimulating action. It is used in ophthalmology along with cholinergic blocking agents to produce mydriatic effect.

Methamphetamine

(*S*)-(+)-*N*,α-Dimethylphenethylamine

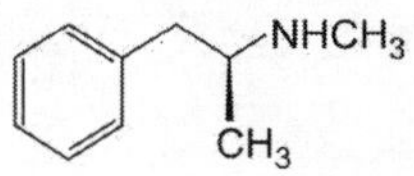
NHCH3
CH3

Synthesis

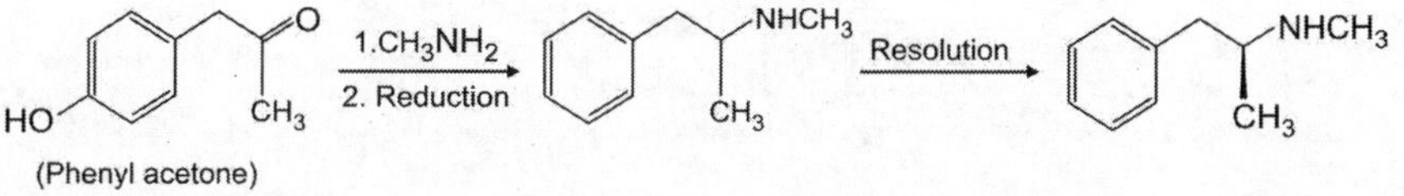
O
HO
CH3
(Phenyl acetone)
1.CH3NH2
2. Reduction
NHCH3
CH3
Resolution
NHCH3
CH3

It has similar action as amphetamine (15), but with more pronounced CNS stimulating action than peripheral action.

Phentermine

α,α-Dimethylphenylethylamine

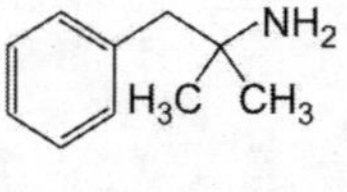
NH2
H3C
CH3

Synthesis

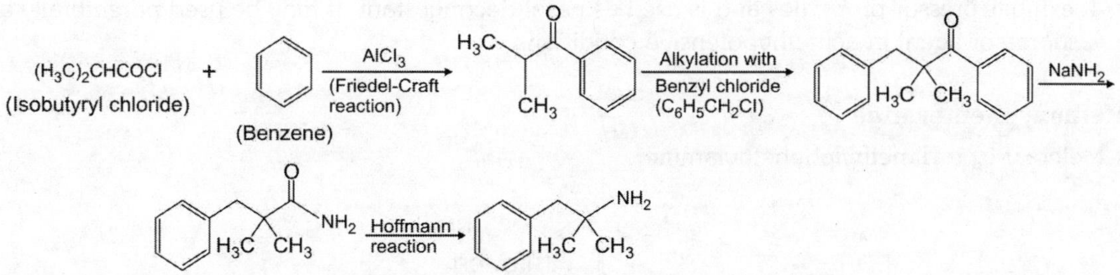
(H3C)2CHCOCl
(Isobutyryl chloride)
+
(Benzene)
AlCl3
(Friedel-Craft
reaction)
H3C
O
CH3
Alkylation with
Benzyl chloride
(C6H5CH2Cl)
O
H3C
CH3
NaNH2
O
NH2
H3C
CH3
Hoffmann
reaction
NH2
H3C
CH3

Phentermine is used as appetite suppressant.

Chlorphentermine

4-Chloro-α,α-dimethylphenethylamine

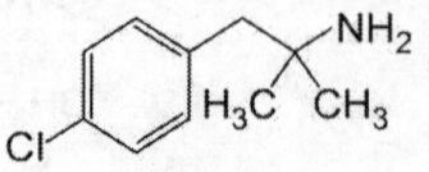

Synthesis

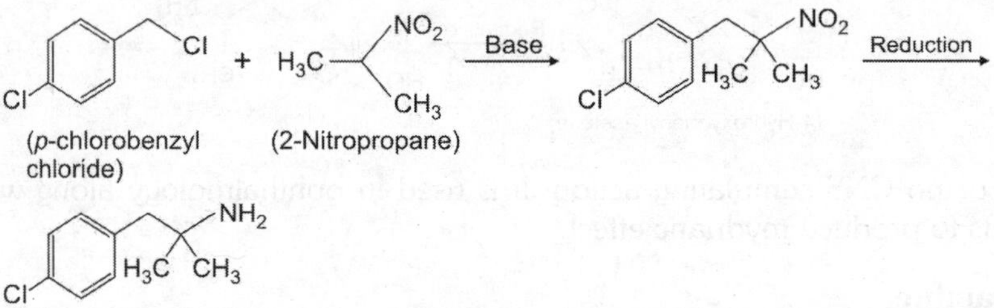

Similar action as phentermine (19).

Mephentermine

N,α,α-Trimethylphenethylamine

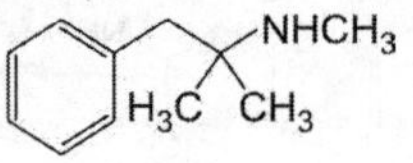

Synthesis

(Phentermine)

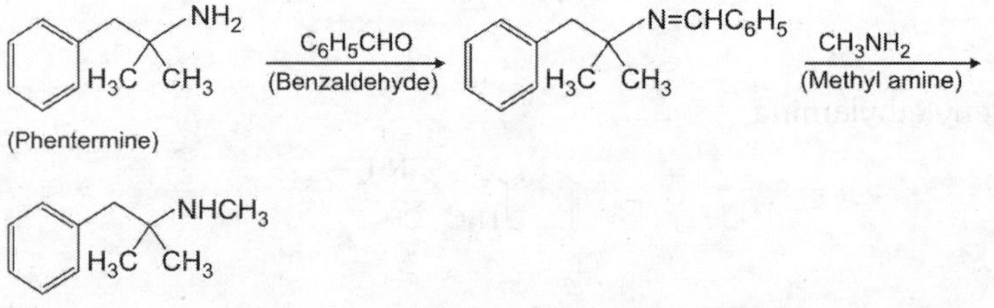

It exhibits pressor properties and is used as nasal decongestant. It may be used parenterally as a vasopressor agent in acute hypotensive conditions.

Methoxyphentermine

4-Methoxy-α, α-dimethylphenethylamine

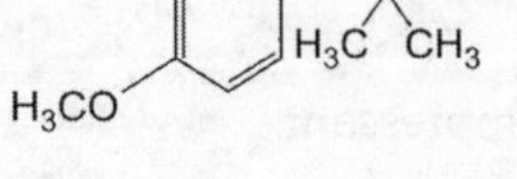

Synthesis

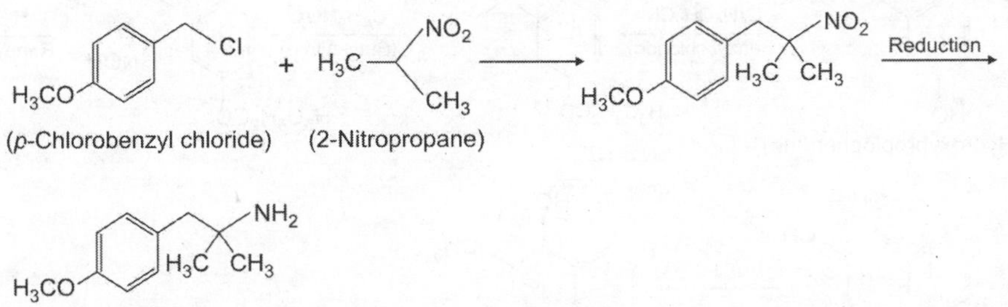
(p-Chlorobenzyl chloride)
(2-Nitropropane)
Reduction

Similar action as phentermine (19).

DRUGS AFFECTING NOREPINEPHRINE RELEASE: SYMPATHOMIMETICS WITH MIXED ACTIONS

Ephedrine

(1*R*,2*S*)-2-Methylamino-1-phenylpropan-1-ol

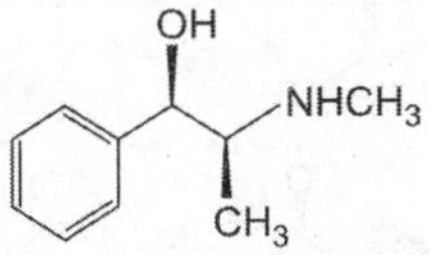

Synthesis

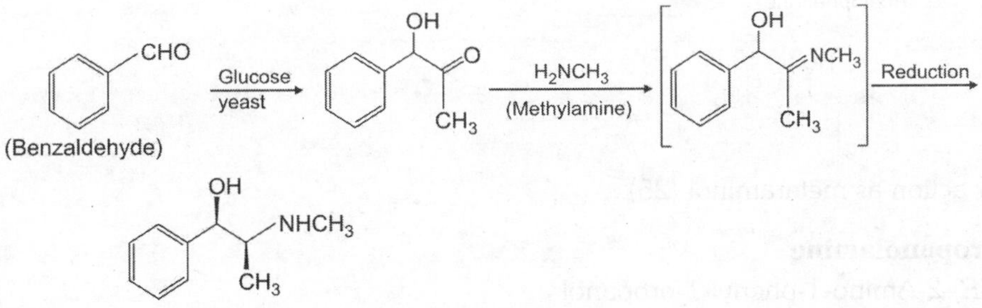
(Benzaldehyde)
Glucose
yeast
H_2NCH_3
(Methylamine)
Reduction

Metaraminol

(1*R*,2*S*)-2-Amino-1-(*m*-hydroxyphenyl)-1-propanol

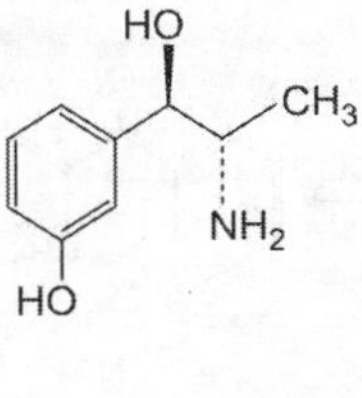

Synthesis

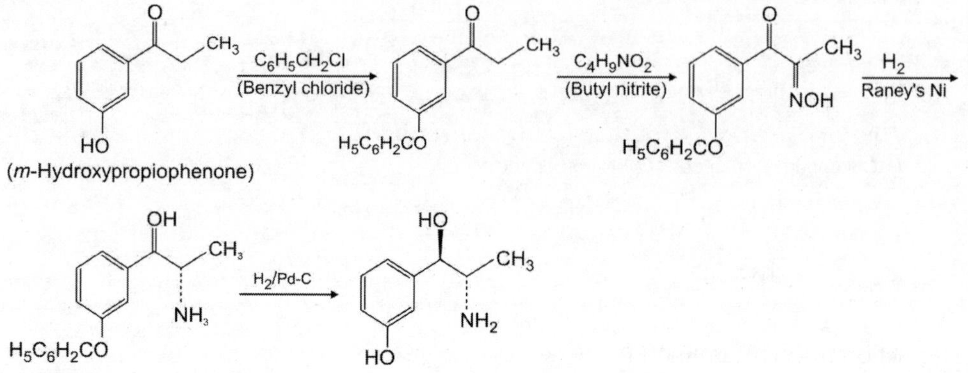

(m-Hydroxypropiophenone)

It is used as nasal decongestant and appetite suppressant.

Phenylethanolamine

β-Hydroxyphenylethylamine

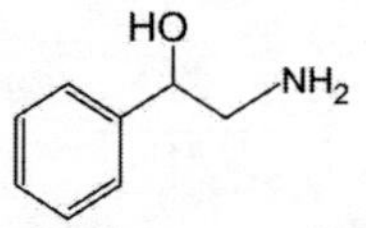

Synthesis

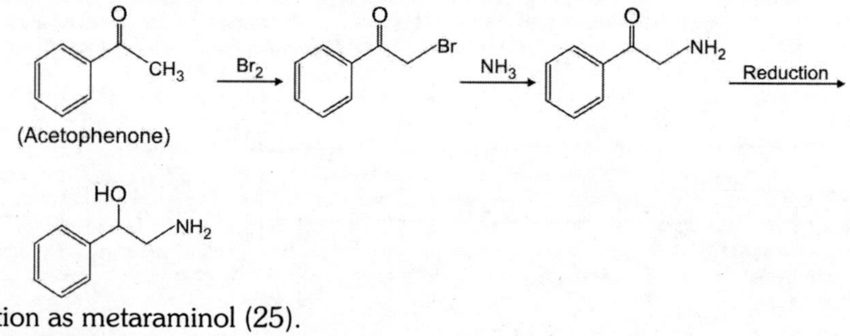

(Acetophenone)

Similar action as metaraminol (25).

Phenylpropanolamine

(1RS, 2SR)-2-Amino-1-phenyl-1-propanol

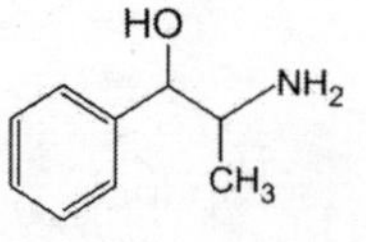

Synthesis

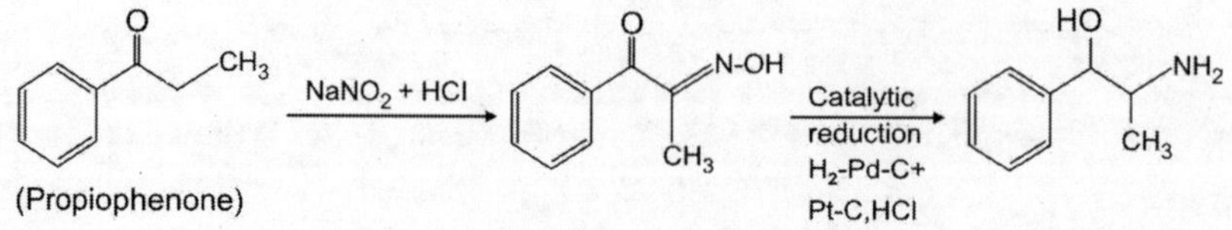

(Propiophenone)

It has a slightly higher vasopressor action and lower toxicity than ephedrine (24). It is used as nasal decongestant and appetite suppressant.

Tyramine

4-Hydroxyphenylethylamine

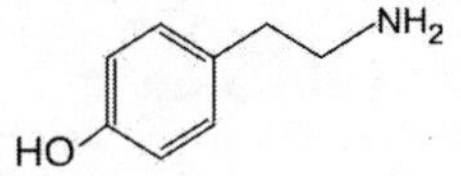

Synthesis

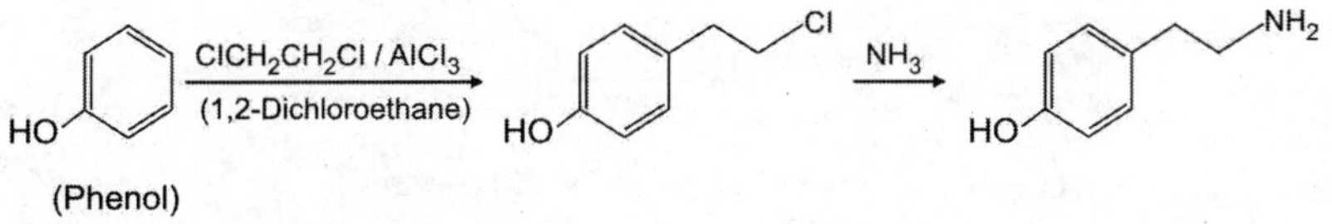

It has similar action as amphetamine (15).

DRUGS ACTING ON ADRENERGIC RECEPTORS : α_1-AGONISTS

Methoxamine

2-Amino-1-(2,5-dimethoxyphenyl)propan-1-ol

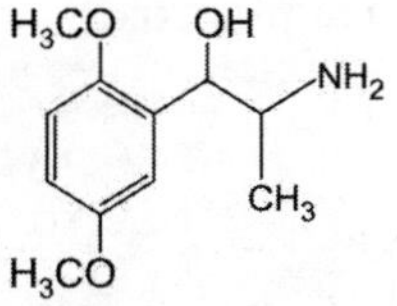

Synthesis

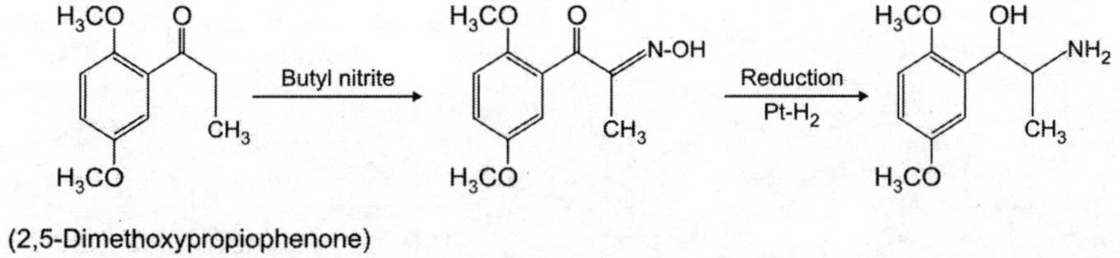

(2,5-Dimethoxypropiophenone)

It is a potent vasoconstrictor without stimulant action on heart. It is used for maintaining blood pressure during surgery in myocardial shock and other hypotensive conditions associated with hemorrhage, trauma and surgery, it is also used topically for nasal congestion.

Phenylephrine

(*R*)-1-(3-Hydroxyphenyl)-2-methylaminoethanol

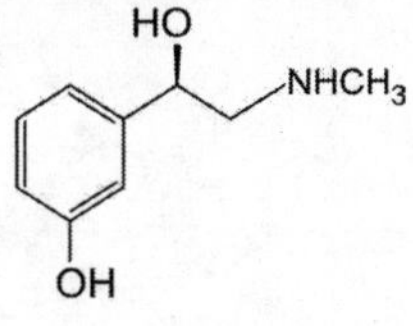

Synthesis

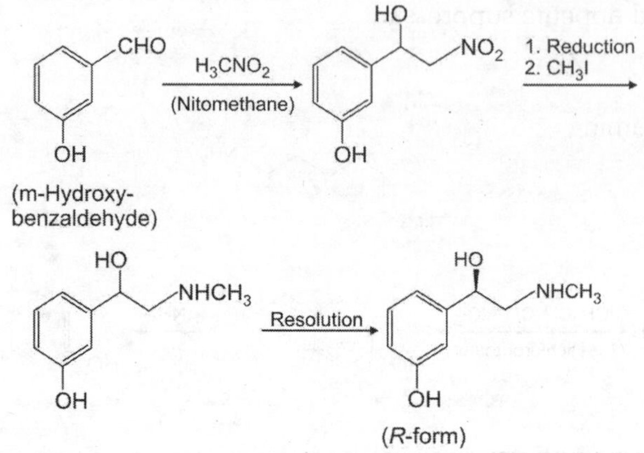

(m-Hydroxy-benzaldehyde)

(R-form)

It is an α_1-agonist and is active when given orally. When applied to mucous membrane it reduces congestion and swelling and is therefore mainly used as nasal decongestant. It is nontoxic and is also used as mydriatic.

Naphazoline

4, 5-Dihydro-2-(1-naphthenylmethyl)-1 *H*-imidazole

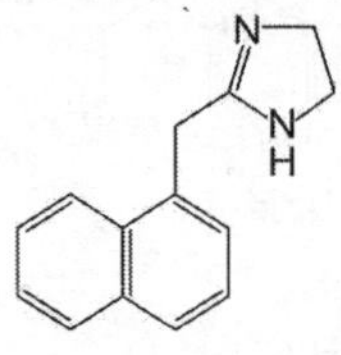

Synthesis

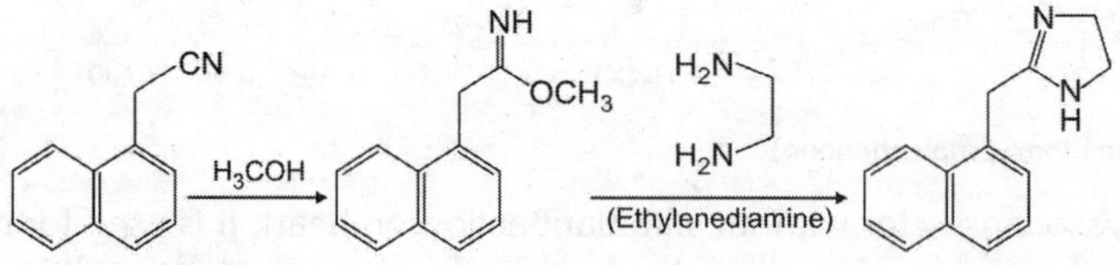

(1-Naphthyl acetonitrile)

It is used as nasal decongestant.

Oxymetazoline

6-*tert*-Butyl-3-(2-imidazolin-2ylmethyl)-2, 4-dimethylphenol

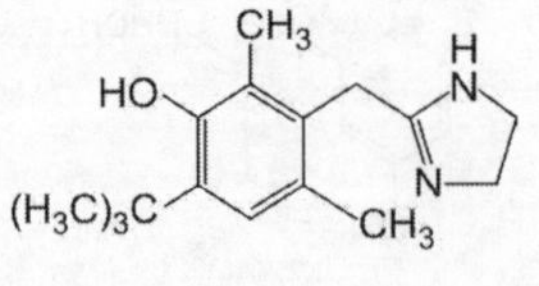

Synthesis

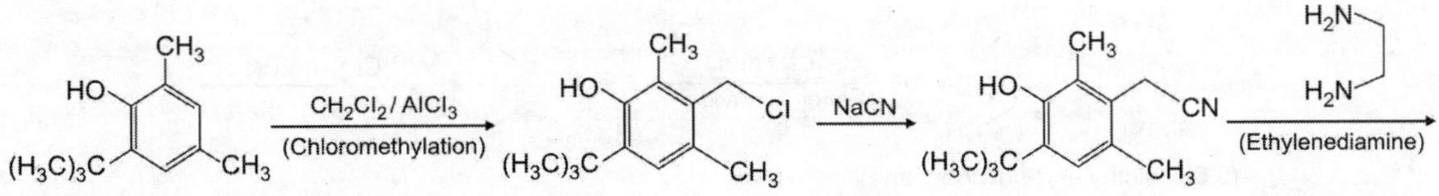

(2-Hydroxy-3-*tert*-butyl
5-methyltoluene)

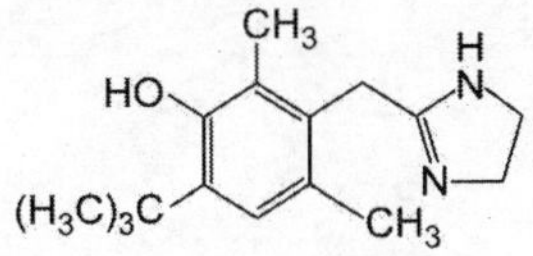

It is used as nasal decongestant.

Tetrahydrozoline
2-(1, 2, 3, 4-Tetrahydro-1-naphthylenyl)-2 imidazoline

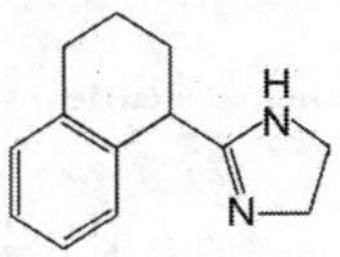

Synthesis

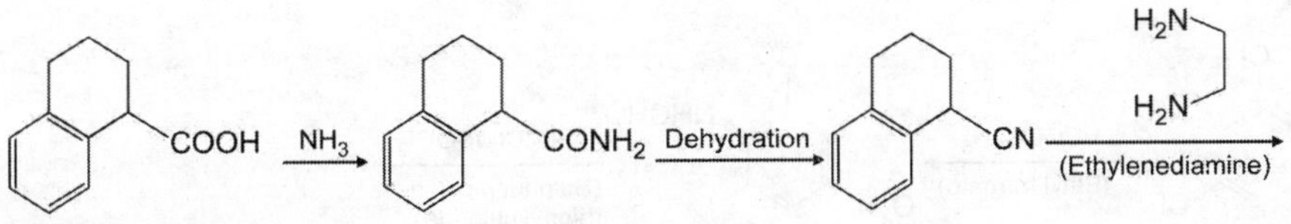

(Tetraline-1-carboxylic acid)

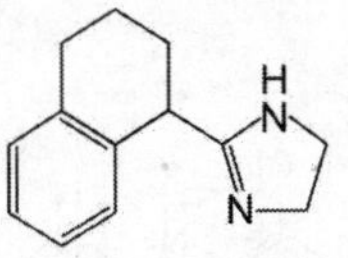

It is used as nasal decongestant.

Xylometazoline
2-(4-*tert*-Butyl-2, 6-dimethylbenzyl)-2-imidazoline

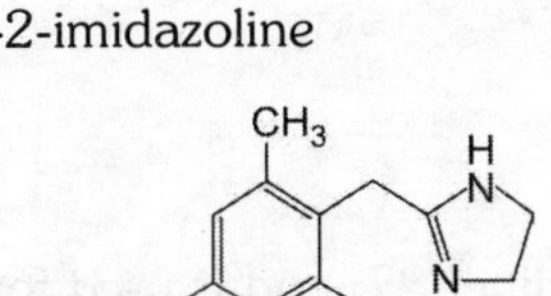

Synthesis

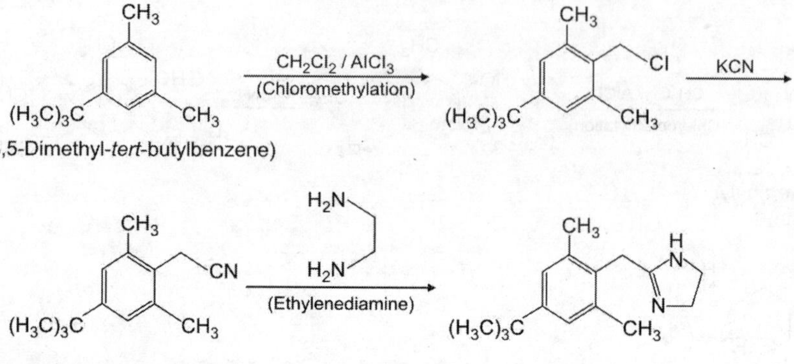

(3,5-Dimethyl-*tert*-butylbenzene)

It is used as nasal decongestant.

DRUGS ACTING ON ADRENERGIC RECEPTORS : α_2-AGONISTS

Clonidine

See **ANTHYPERTENSIVE DRUGS**

Apraclonidine

2-[(4-Amino-2,6-dichlorophenyl)imino]imidazolidine

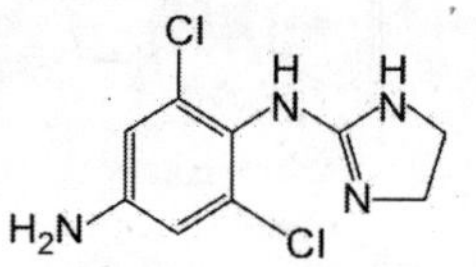

Synthesis

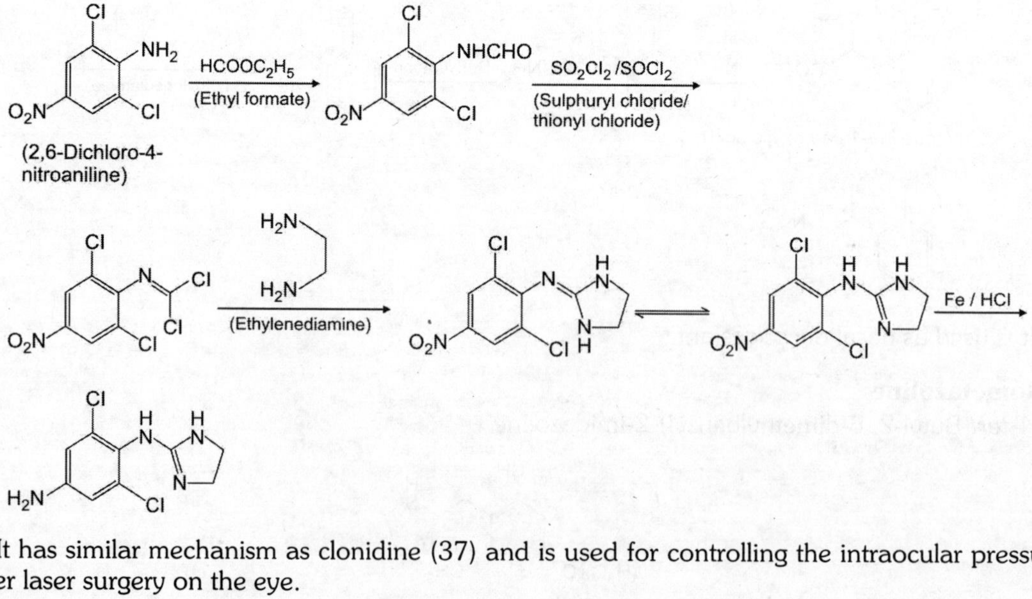

(2,6-Dichloro-4-
nitroaniline)

It has similar mechanism as clonidine (37) and is used for controlling the intraocular pressure after laser surgery on the *eye*.

Brimonidine

5-Bromo-N-(4,5-dihydro-1H-imidazol-2-yl)-6-quinoxalinamine

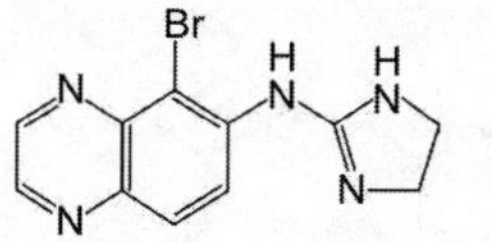

Synthesis

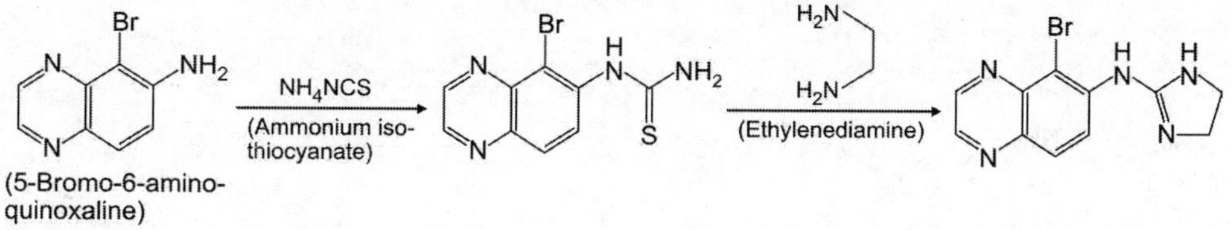

Similar action as apraclonidine (38).

Guanabenz, Guanfacine, and Methyldopa as Methyldopate Hydrochloride
See **ANTIHYPERTENSIVE DRUGS**

DRUGS ACTING ON ADRENERGIC RECEPTORS : β_1- AND β_2-AGONISTS
Isoproterenol

1-(3, 4-Dihydroxyphenyl)-2-isopropylaminoethanol

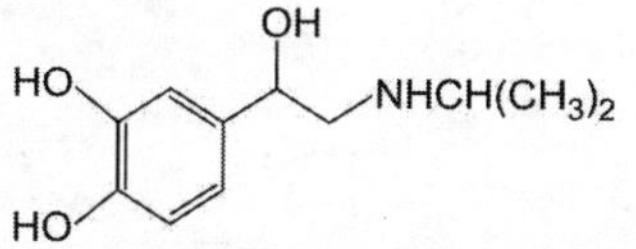

Synthesis

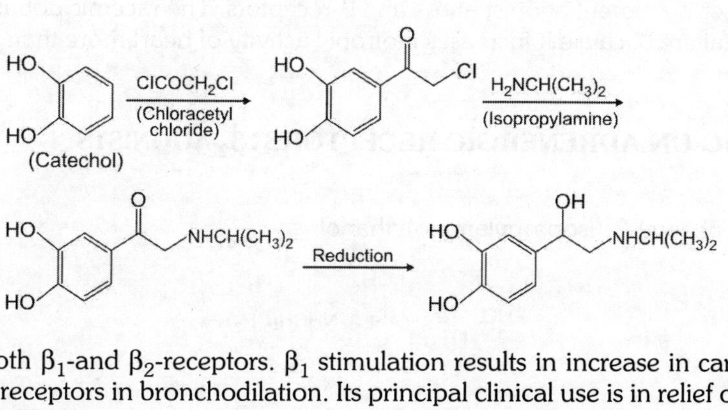

It stimulates both β_1-and β_2-receptors. β_1 stimulation results in increase in cardiac output and stimulation of β_2-receptors in bronchodilation. Its principal clinical use is in relief of bronchospasm associated with asthma.

Dobutamine

3,4-Dihydroxy-N-[3-(4-hydroxyphenyl)-1-methylpropyl]-β-phenylethylamine

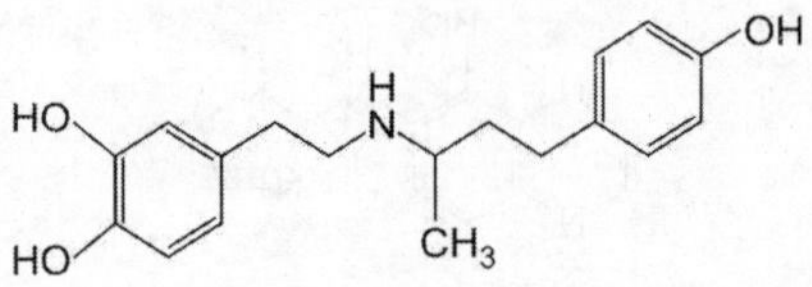

Synthesis

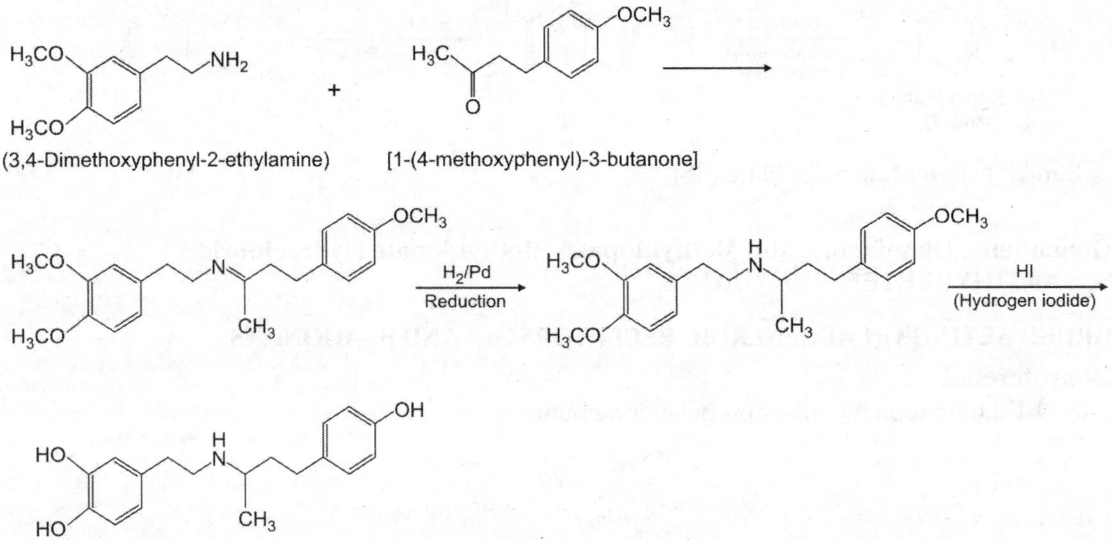

(3,4-Dimethoxyphenyl-2-ethylamine)   [1-(4-methoxyphenyl)-3-butanone]

It is structurally a derivative of dopamine (43) and has one asymmetric carbon atom. The dextro-isomer is a potent agonist of β_1- and β_2-receptors and antagonist at α_1-receptor. The levorotatory isomer is a potent agonist at α_1- and β-receptors. The racemic dobutamine is used in congestive heart failure because it increases inotropic activity of heart more than the chronotropic activity.

DRUGS ACTING ON ADRENERGIC RECEPTORS : β_2-AGONISTS

Metaproterenol

1-(3,5-Dihydroxyphenyl)-2-(isopropylamino)ethanol

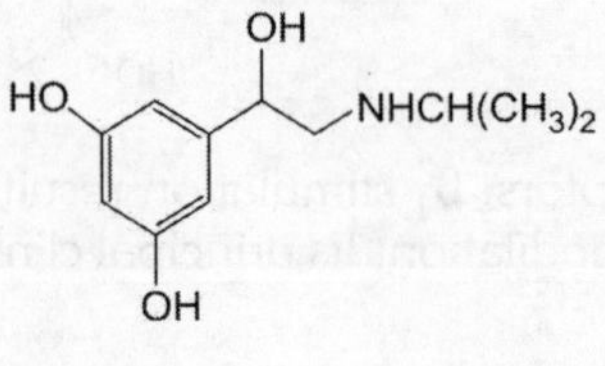

Synthesis

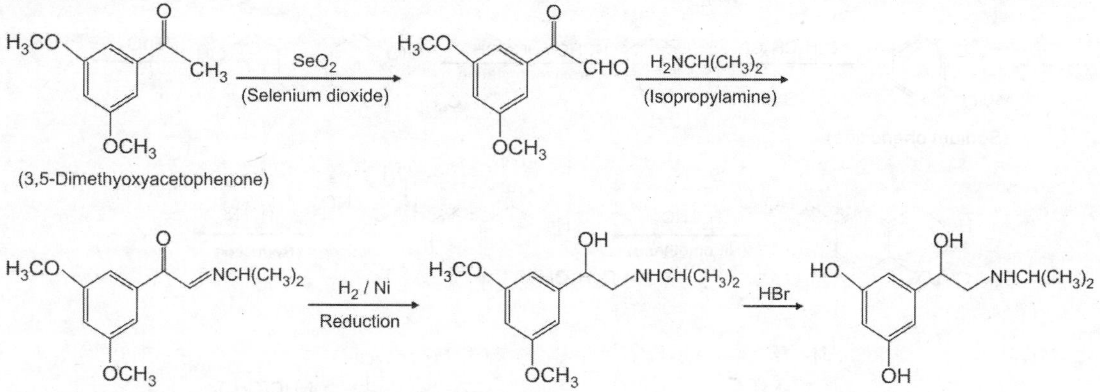

(3,5-Dimethyoxyacetophenone)

It is β_2-agonist and is used as bronchodilator.

Terbutaline

1-(3,5-Dihydroxyphenyl)-2-(*tert*-butylamino)ethanol

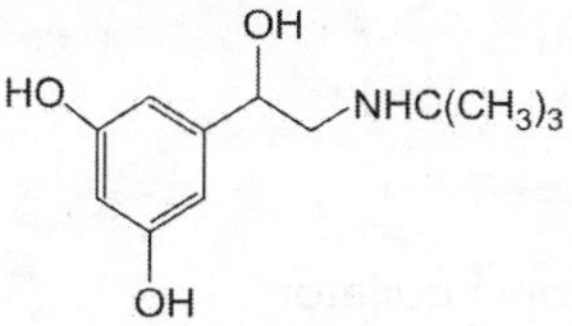

Synthesis

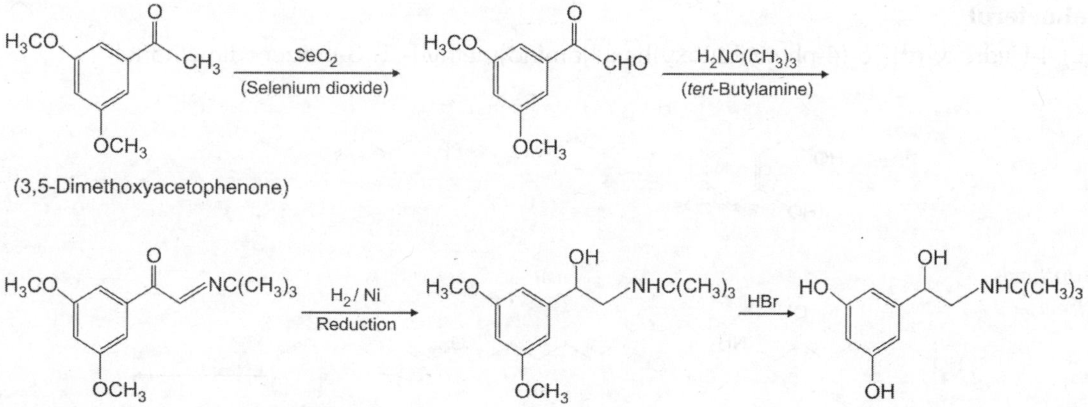

(3,5-Dimethoxyacetophenone)

It is used as a bronchodilator

Salbutamol

1-(4-Hydroxy-3-hydroxymethylphenyl)-2-(*tert*-butylamino)ethanol.

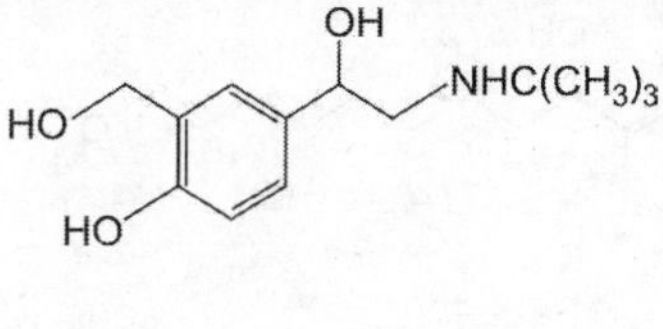

Synthesis

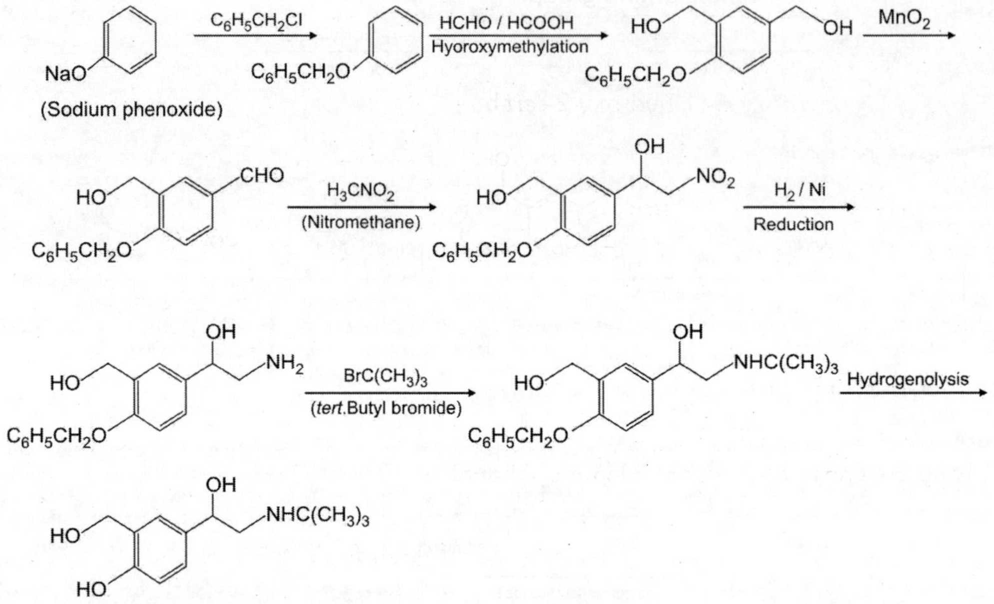

It is a β_2-agonist and is used as bronchodilator.

Salmeterol

($\pm$)-4-Hydroxy-α^1[[[6-(4-phenylbutoxy)hexyl]amino]methyl]- 1, 3-benzenedimethanol

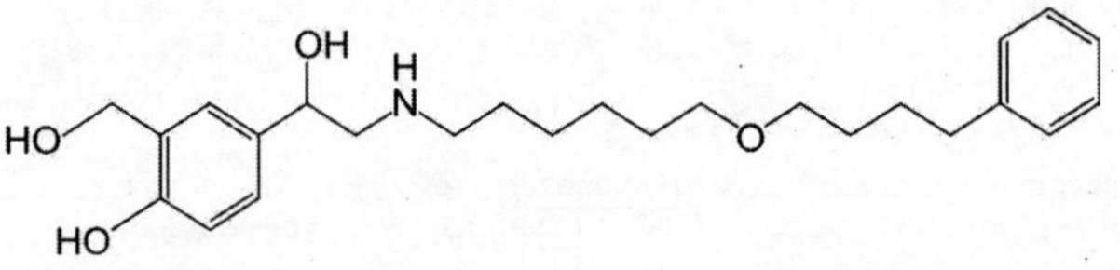

Synthesis

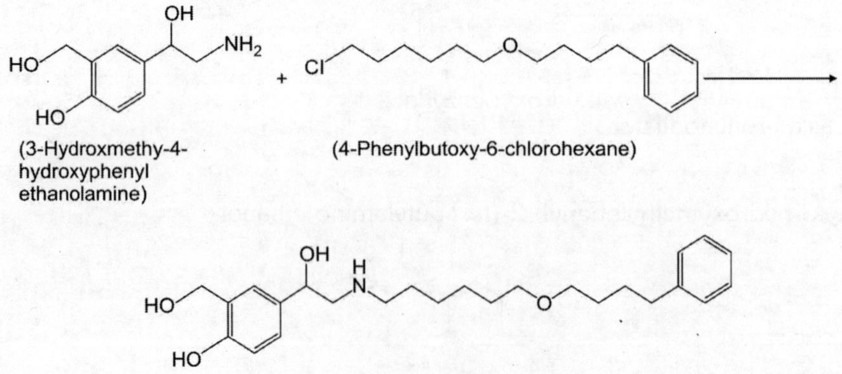

(3-Hydroxmethy-4-
hydroxyphenyl
ethanolamine)

(4-Phenylbutoxy-6-chlorohexane)

It is used as a bronchodilator. It has a longer duration of action, about 12 hr, which is because of phenylalkyloxyalkyl group on the amino group.

Pirbuterol

2-Hydroxymethyl-3-hydroxy-6-(1-hydroxy-2-$tert$-butylaminoethyl)pyridine

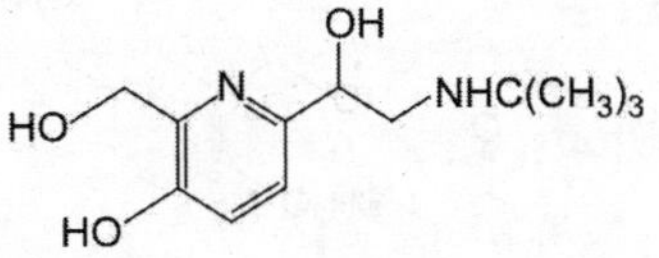

Synthesis

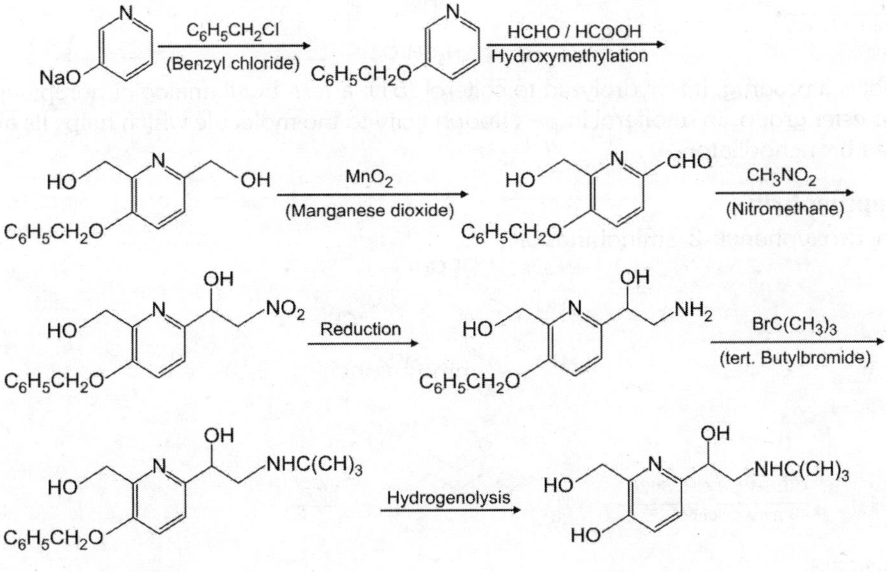

Used as bronchodilator.

Bitolterol

α-[($tert$-Butylamino)methyl]-3,4-dihydroxybenzyl alcohol 3,4-di-p-toluate

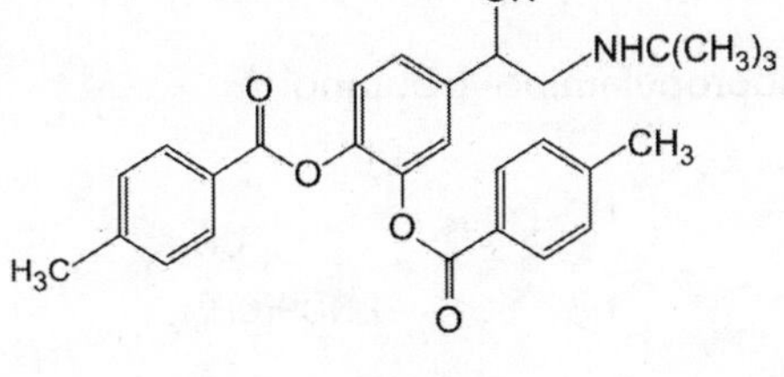

Synthesis

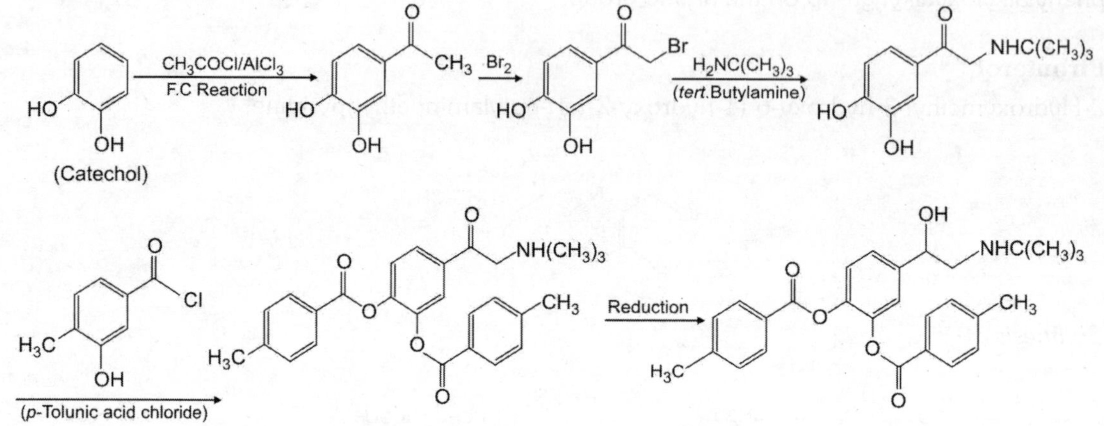

Bitolterol is a prodrug. It is hydrolyzed to colterol (51), a *tert*- butyl analog of norepinephrine (1). The two ester groups in bitolterol impart lipophilicity to the molecule which helps its absorption. It is used as bronchodilator.

Ethylnorepinephrine

1-(3,4-Dihydroxyphenyl)-2-aminobutanol-1

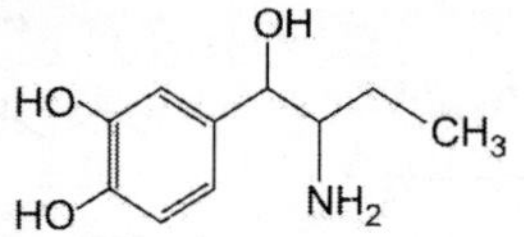

Synthesis

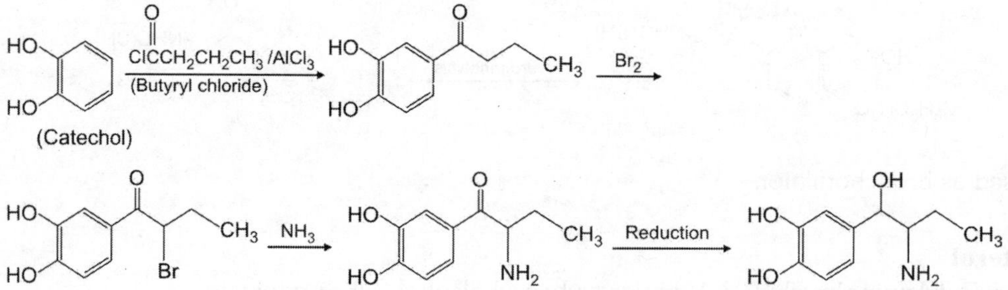

It is used as a bronchodilator.

Isoetharine

1-(3,4-Dihydroxyphenyl)-2-isopropylamino-1-butanol

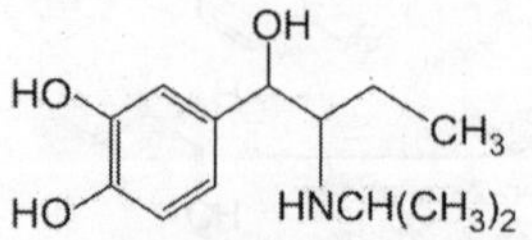

Synthesis

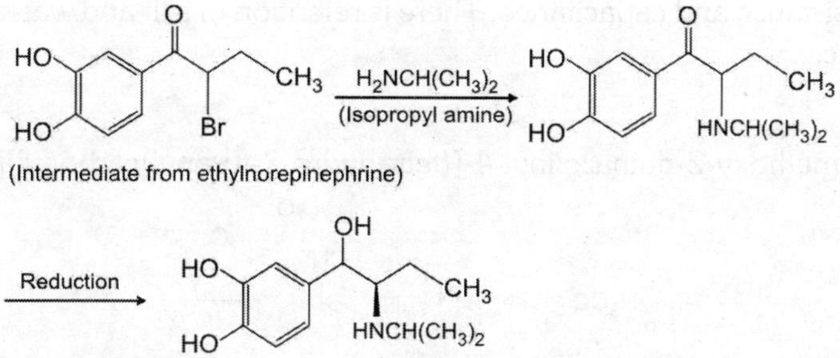

It is used as a bronchodilator.

DRUGS ACTING ON ADRENERGIC RECEPTORS : α_1-ANTAGONISTS (BLOCKERS)

Prazosin

2-[4-(2-Furoyl)-piperazin-1-yl]-4-amino-6,7-dimethoxyquinazoline

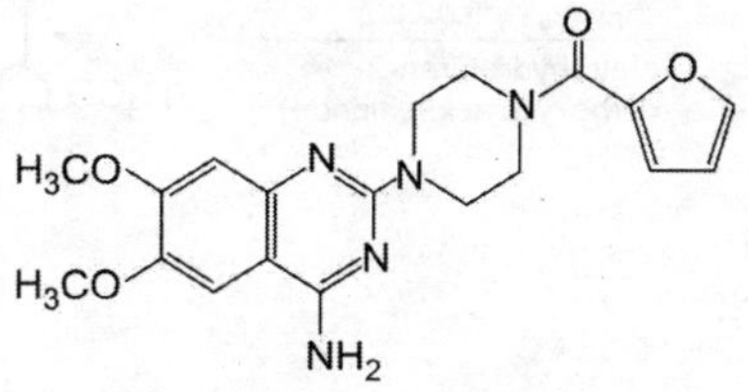

Synthesis

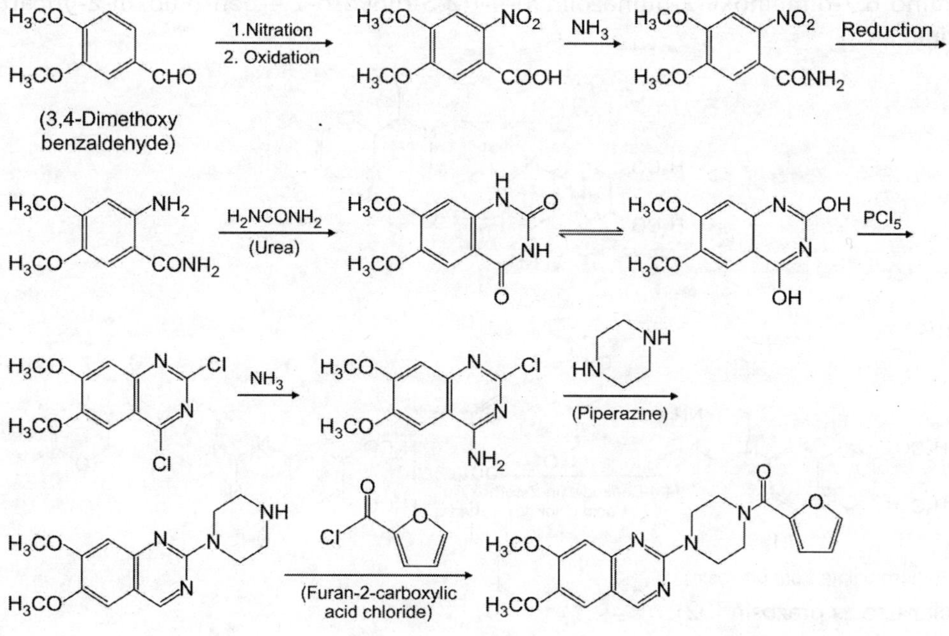

It causes α_1-blockade selectively without blocking the α_2-receptor. It reduces arterial blood pressure by dilating both resistance and capacitance. There is retention of salt and water. It is effective when used with a diuretic.

Terazosin

1-(4-Amino-6,7-dimethoxy-2-quinazolinyl-4-[(tetrahydro-2-furanyl)carbonyl]piperazine

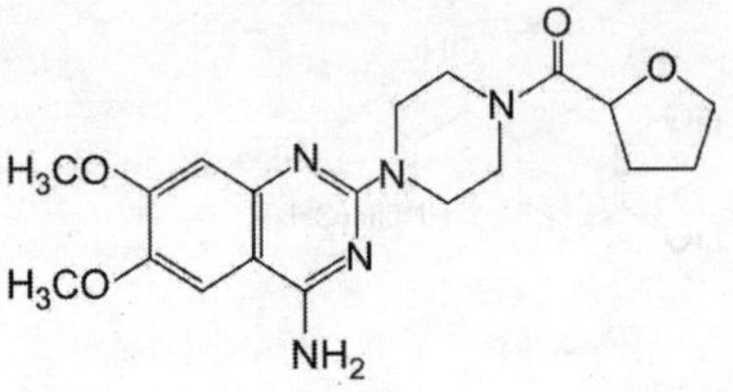

Synthesis

(Tetrahydrofuran-2-carboxylic acid chloride)

(Intermediate from prazosin)

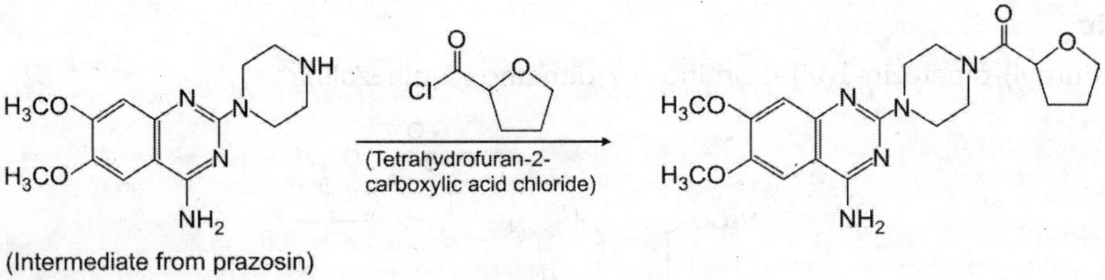

Action similar to prazosin (52).

Doxazosin

1-(4-Amino-6,7-dimethoxy-2-quinazolinyl)-4-[(2,3-dihydro-1,4-benzodioxin-2-yl)carbonyl]-piperazine.

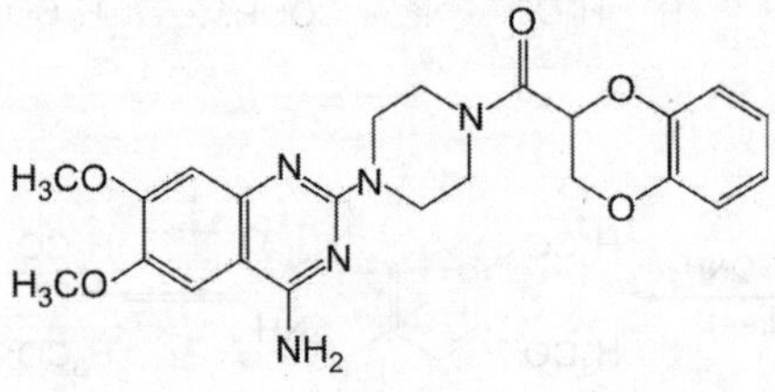

Synthesis

(1,4-Benzodioxin-2-carboxylic acid chloride)

(Intermediate from prazosin)

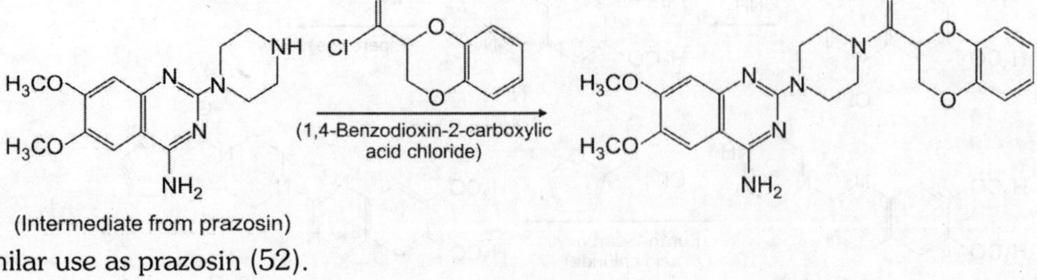

Similar use as prazosin (52).

Indoramin

3-[2-(4-Benzamidopiperidino)ethyl]indole

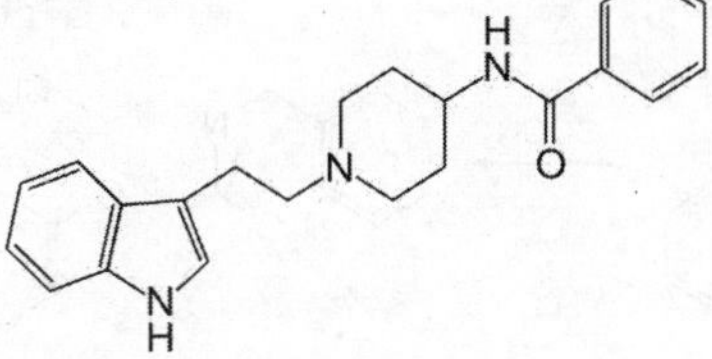

Synthesis

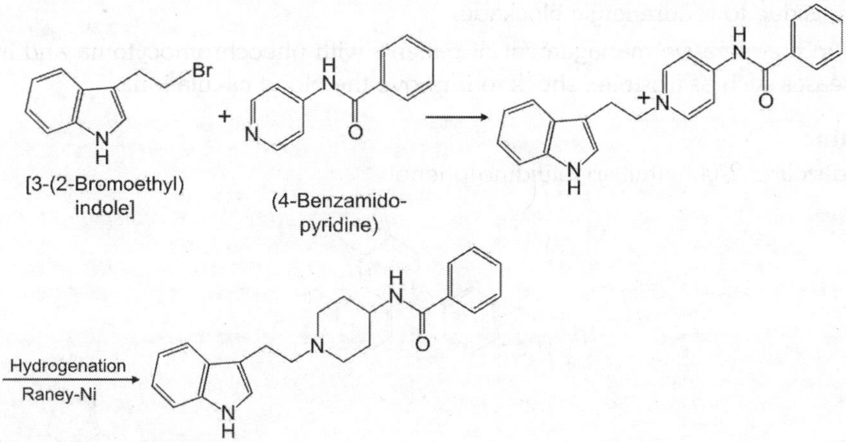

[3-(2-Bromoethyl)
indole]

(4-Benzamido-
pyridine)

Hydrogenation
Raney-Ni

Used as antihypertensive agent.

DRUGS ACTING ON ADRENERGIC RECEPTORS : NONSPECIFIC α_2-ANTAGONISTS (BLOCKERS)

Phenoxybenzamine

N-Phenoxyisopropyl-*N*-benzyl-β-chloroethylamine

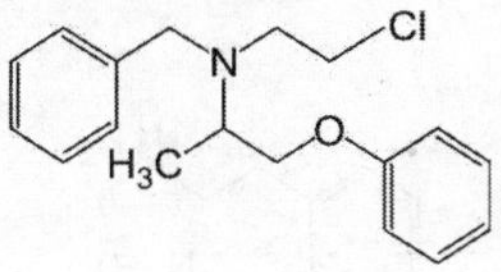

Synthesis

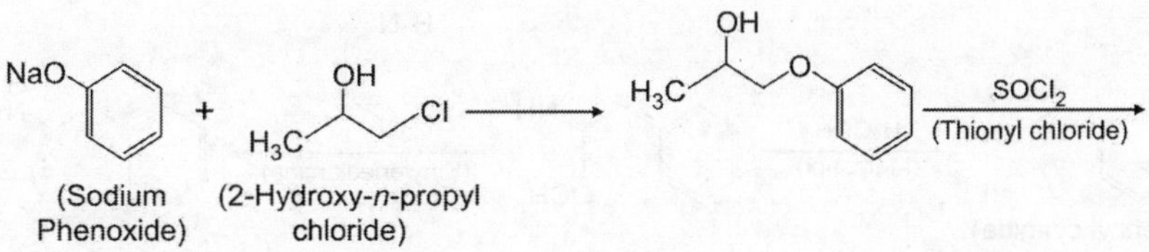

(Sodium
Phenoxide)

(2-Hydroxy-*n*-propyl
chloride)

SOCl₂
(Thionyl chloride)

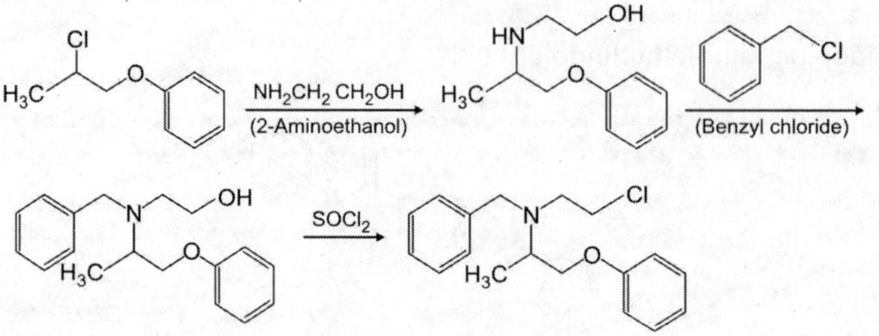

Phenoxybenzamine blocks selectively the excitatory responses of smooth muscle and heart muscle. It also blocks acetylcholine, histamine and serotonin receptors. Its primary effect, that is vasodilation, is due to α-adrenergic blockade.

It is used in preoperative management of patients with pheochromocytoma and in peripheral vascular diseases such as frostbite, shock to improve the blood circulation.

Phentolamine

3-[N-(2-imidazoline-2-ylmethyl)-p-toluidino]phenol

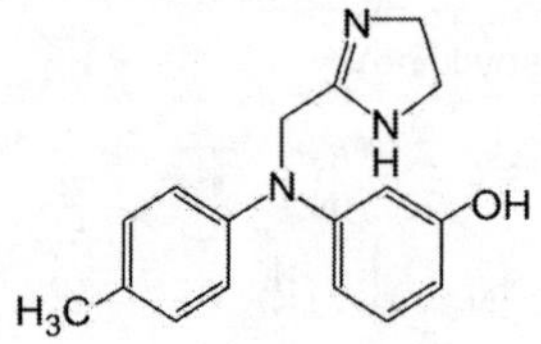

Synthesis

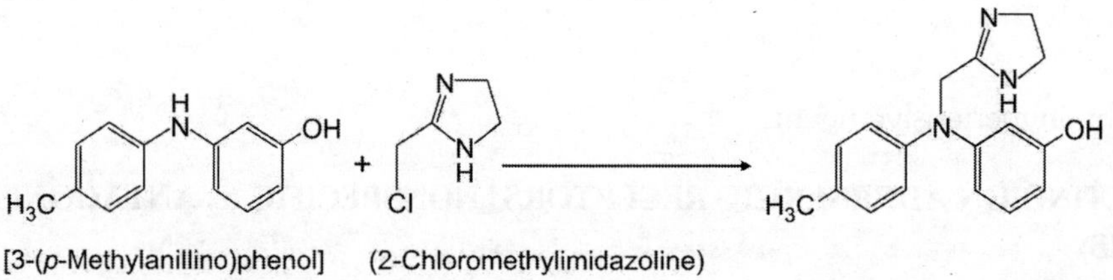

[3-(p-Methylanillino)phenol]   (2-Chloromethylimidazoline)

It is used as hydrochloride and mesylate salt to regulate the blood pressure in pheochromocytoma.

Tolazoline
2-Benzyl-2-imidazoline

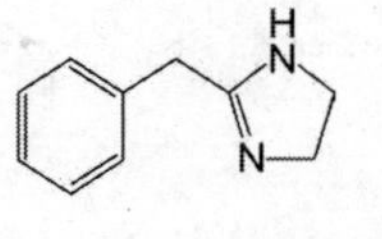

Synthesis

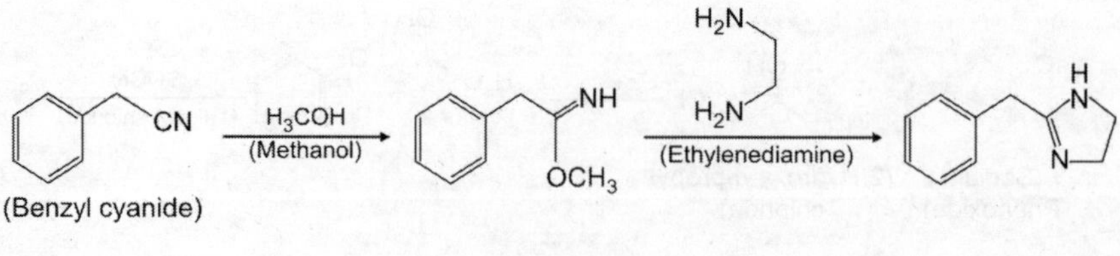

(Benzyl cyanide)

Tolazoline has direct vasodilatory effect on vascular smooth muscle. It has agonistic activity on histamine and acetylcholine receptors which might be contributing to its vasodilatory action.

DRUGS ACTING ON ADRENERGIC RECEPTORS : SELECTIVE β_1-ANTAGONISTS (BLOCKERS)

Acebutolol

1-(2-Acetyl-4-n-butyramidophenoxy)-2-hydroxy-3-isopropylaminopropane

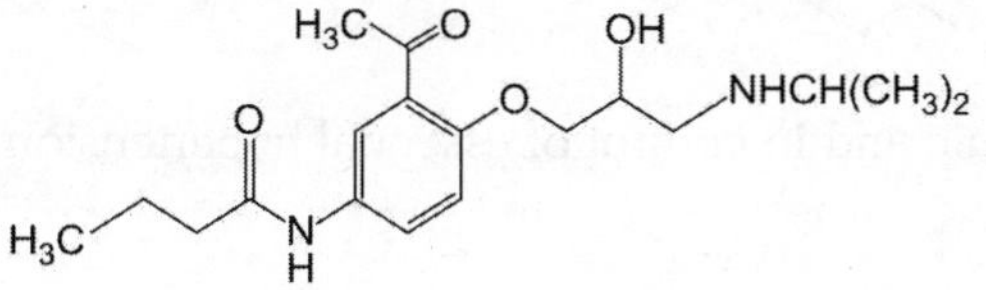

Synthesis

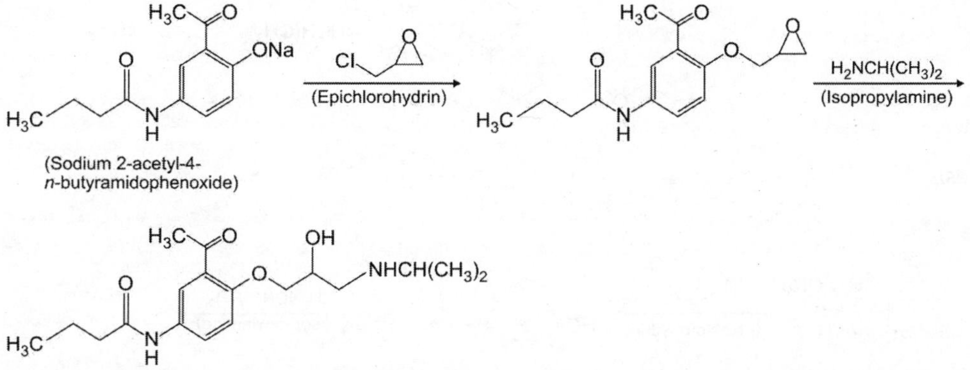

(Sodium 2-acetyl-4-n-butyramidophenoxide)

It is a β_1-adrenoreceptors blocker and is used in cardiac arrhythmias, angina pectoris, and in essential & neurovascular hypertension.

Atenolol

4-(2-Hydroxy-3-isopropylaminopropoxy)phenylacetamide

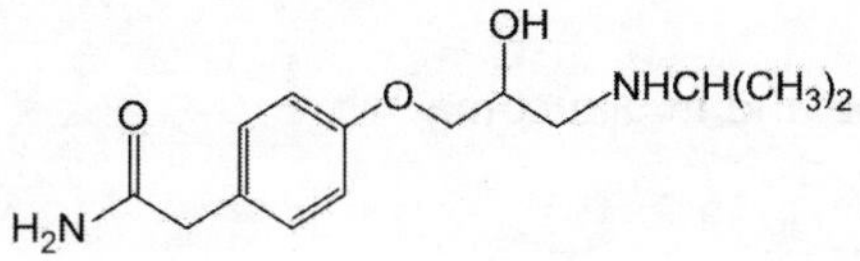

Synthesis

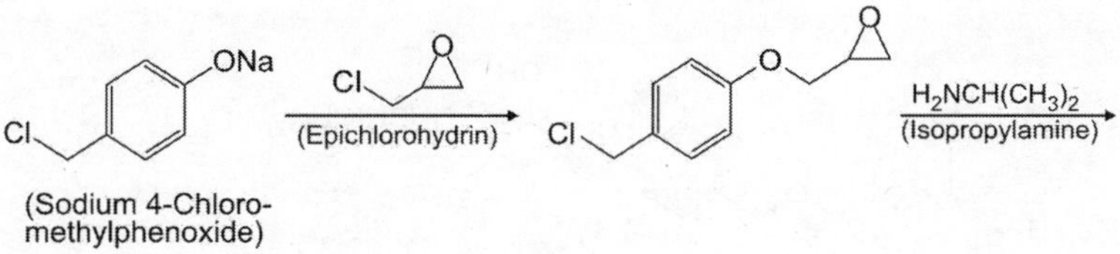

(Sodium 4-Chloro-methylphenoxide)

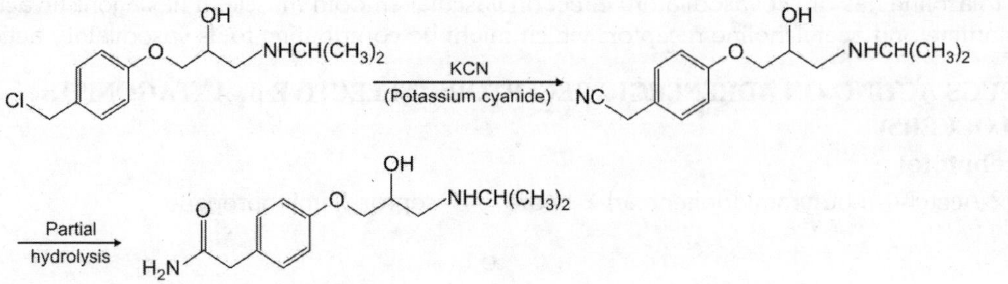

It is used as antiarrhythmic and in control of essential hypertension.

Betaxolol

($\pm$)-1-(Isopropylamino)-3-[*p*-(cyclopropylmethoxyethyl) phenoxy]-2-propanol

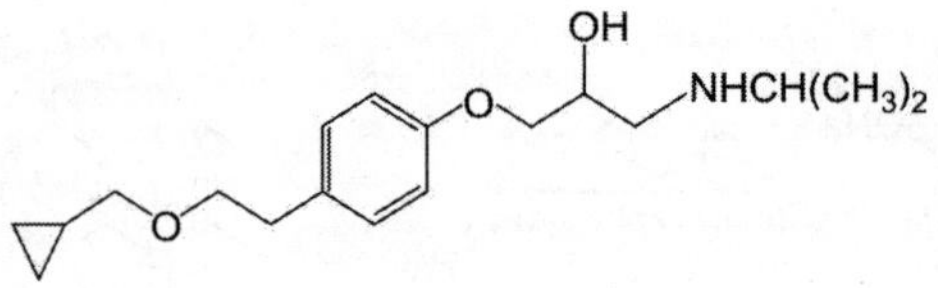

Synthesis

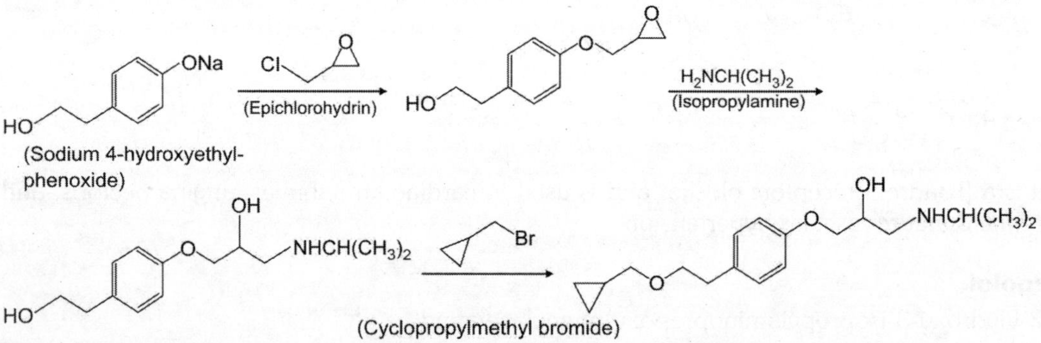

It is used as antihypertensive and in glaucoma.

Bisoprolol

($\pm$)-1-[[α-(2-Isopropoxyethoxy)-*p*-tolyl]oxy]-3-(isopropylamino)-2-propanol

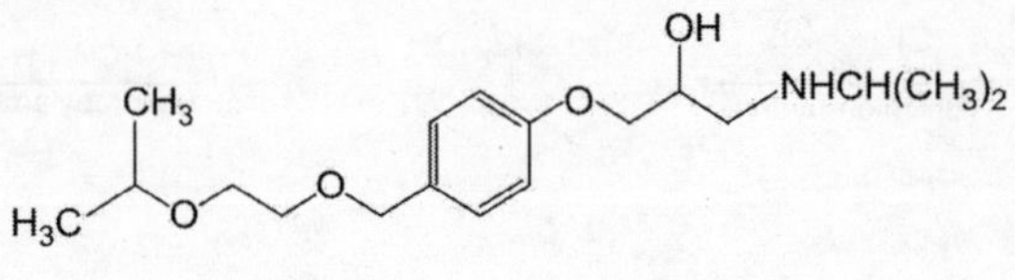

Synthesis

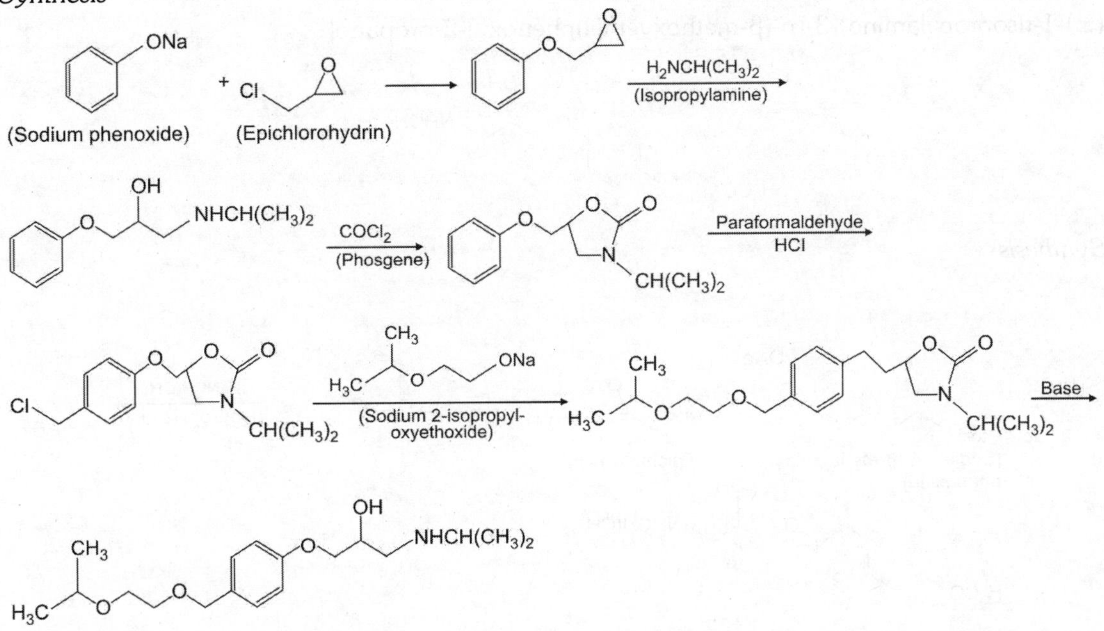

It is a β_1-adrenoreceptor blocker and is used in cardiac arrhythmias, angina pectoris, and in essential and neurovascular hypertension.

Esmolol

($\pm$)-Methyl 3-[4-[2-hydroxy-3-(isopropylamino)propoxy]phenyl]propionate

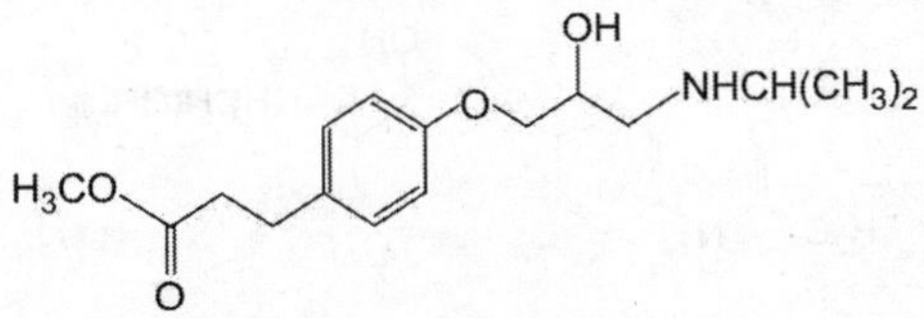

Synthesis

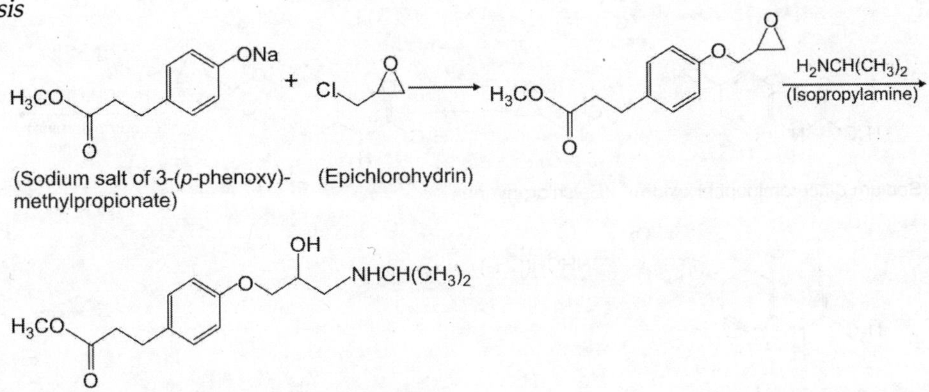

Similar action and used as acebutolol (69).

Metoprolol

(±)-1-(Isopropylamino)-3-[p-(β-methoxyethyl)phenoxy]-2-propanol

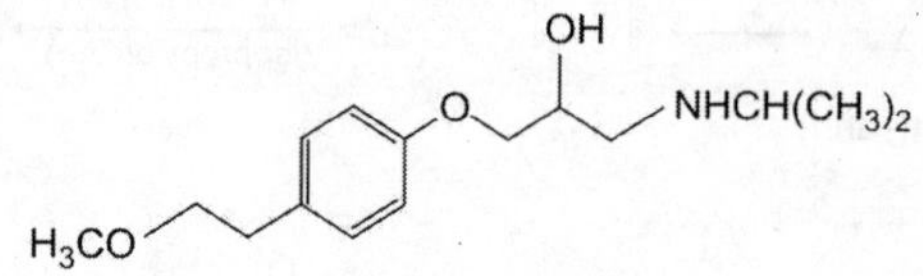

Synthesis

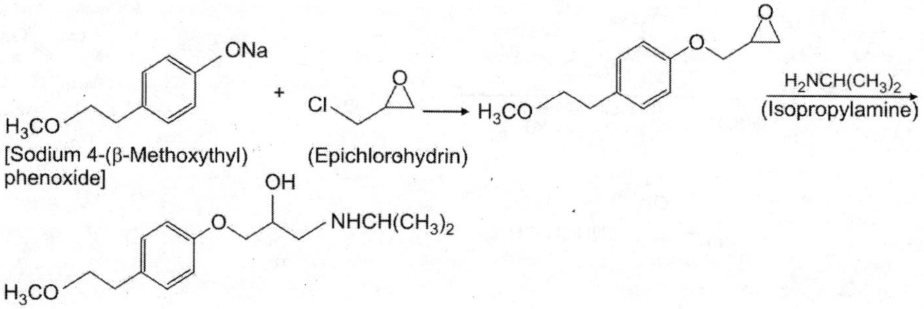

[Sodium 4-(β-Methoxythyl) phenoxide]   (Epichlorohydrin)

Similar action and use as acebutolol (69).

Practolol

1-(4-Acetamidophenoxy)-3-isopropylamino-2-propanol

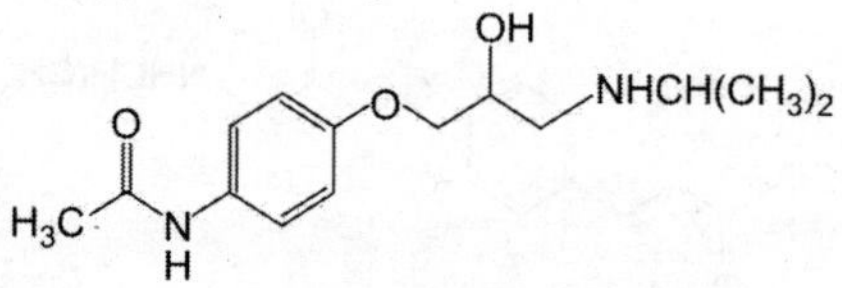

Synthesis

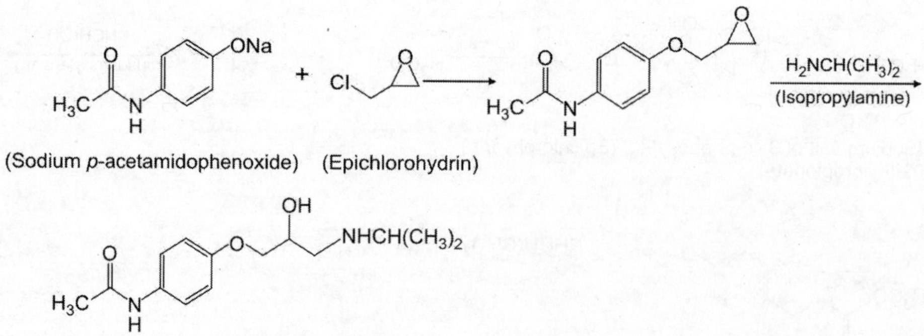

(Sodium *p*-acetamidophenoxide)   (Epichlorohydrin)

Similar action and use as acebutolol (69).

DRUGS ACTING ON ADRENERGIC RECEPTORS : NONSELECTIVE β-ANTAGONISTS (BLOCKERS)

Pronethalol

1-(2´-Naphthyl)-2-isopropylaminoethanol

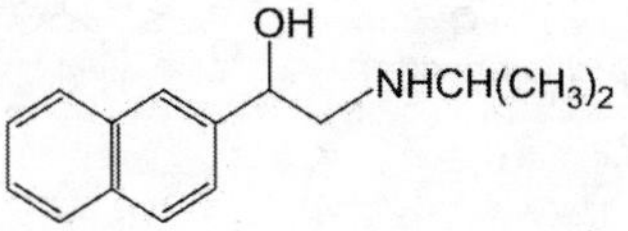

Synthesis

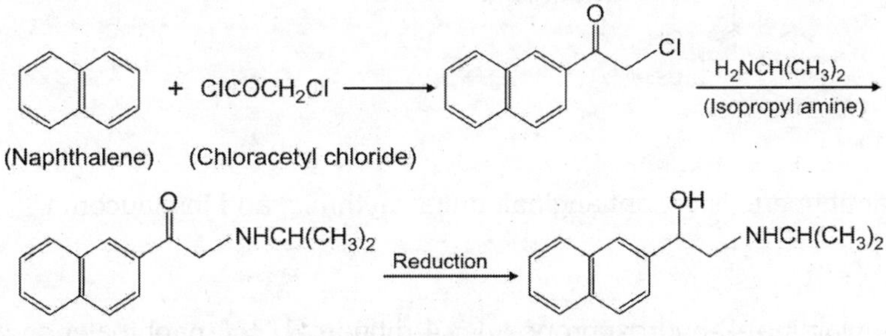

It is used as antianginal, antiarrhythmic, and anihypertensive agents.

Propranolol

1-Isopropylamino-3-(1-naphthyloxy)-propan-2-ol

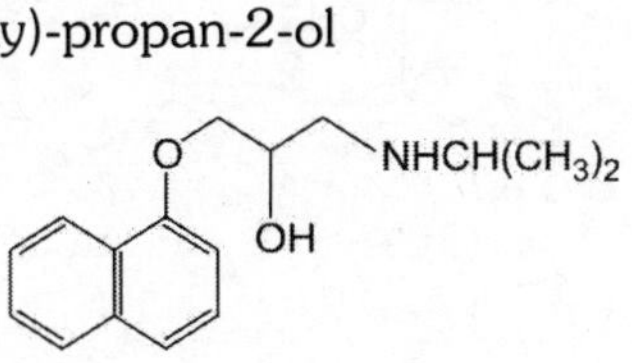

Synthesis

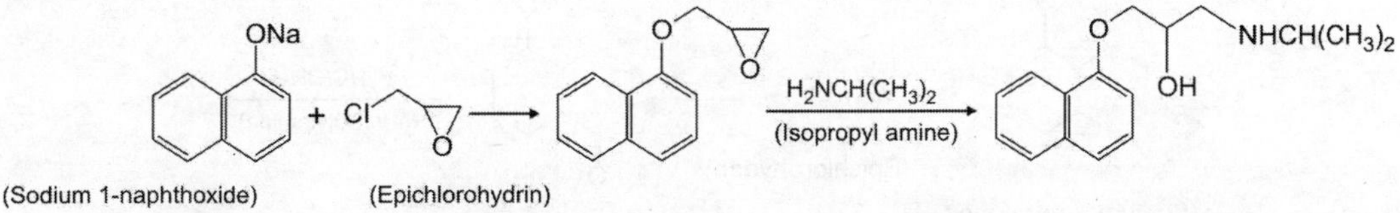

It blocks β-receptors of heart resulting in slowing of heart. Its antihypertensive action is partly due to reduced cardiac output as well as suppression of renin release from kidney.

Carteolol

5-[3-(*tert*-Butylamino)-2-hydroxypropoxy]-3,4-dihydrocarbostyril

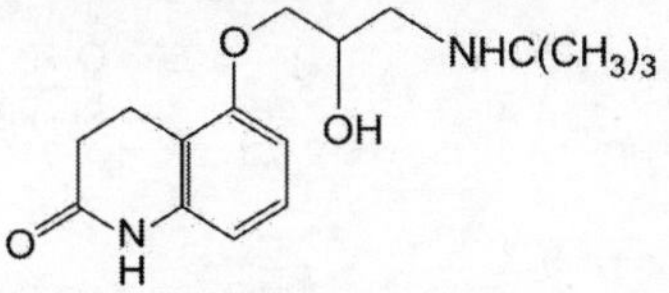

Synthesis

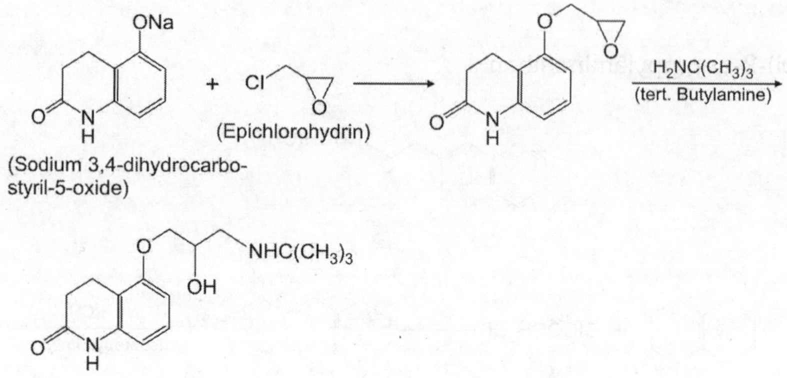
ONa
Cl
(Epichlorohydrin)
(Sodium 3,4-dihydrocarbo-
styril-5-oxide)
$H_2NC(CH_3)_3$
(tert. Butylamine)
$NHC(CH_3)_3$
OH

It is used as antihypertensive, antianginal, antiarrhythmic, and in glaucoma.

Levobunolol

(–)-5-[3-(*tert*-Butylamino)-2-hydroxypropoxy]-3,4-dihydro-1(2*H*)-naphthalenone

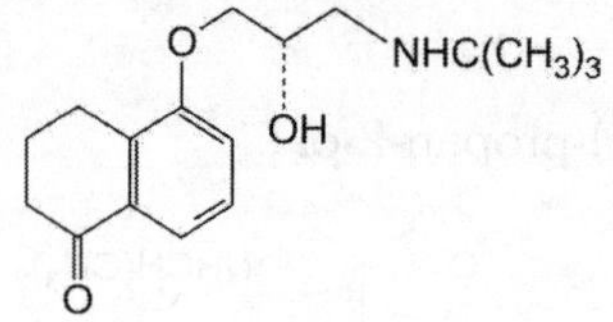
$NHC(CH_3)_3$
OH

Synthesis

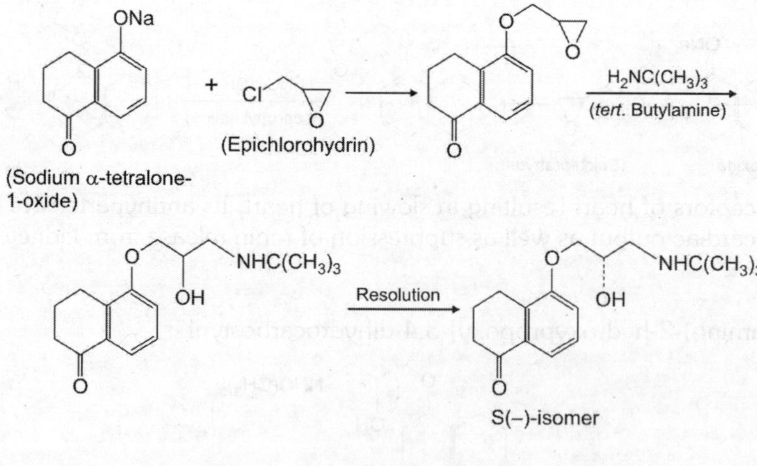
ONa
Cl
(Epichlorohydrin)
$H_2NC(CH_3)_3$
(*tert*. Butylamine)
(Sodium α-tetralone-
1-oxide)
$NHC(CH_3)_3$
OH
Resolution
S(–)-isomer

It is used in glaucoma.

Metipranolol

1-(4-Hydroxy-2,3,5-trimethylphenoxy)-3-(isopropylamino)-2-propanol 4-acetate

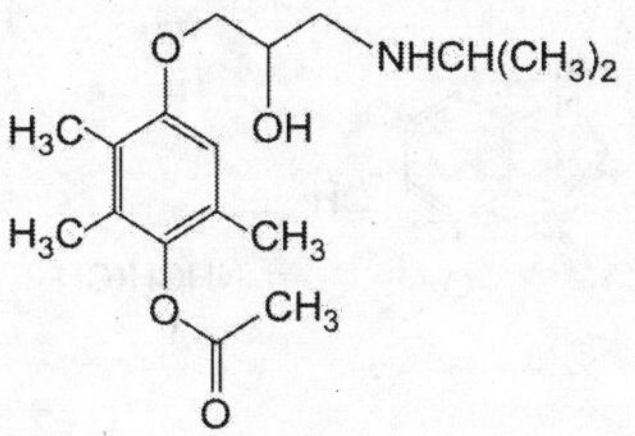

Synthesis

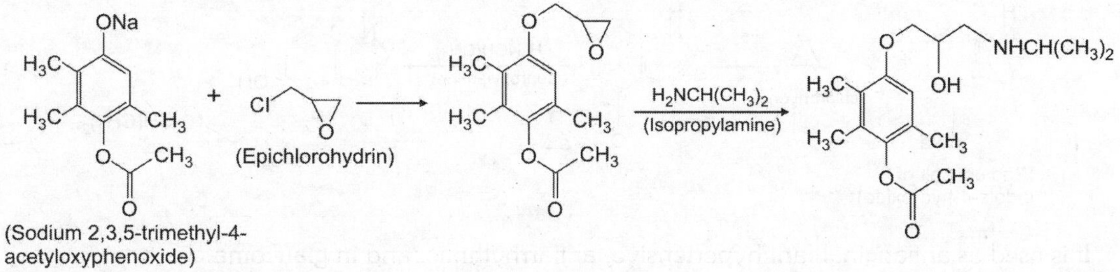

(Sodium 2,3,5-trimethyl-4-acetyloxyphenoxide)

It is used as antihypertensive, and in glaucoma.

Nadolol

1-(*tert*-Butylamino)-3-[(5,6,7,8-tetrahydro-*cis*-6,7-dihydroxy-1-naphthyl)oxy]-2-propanol

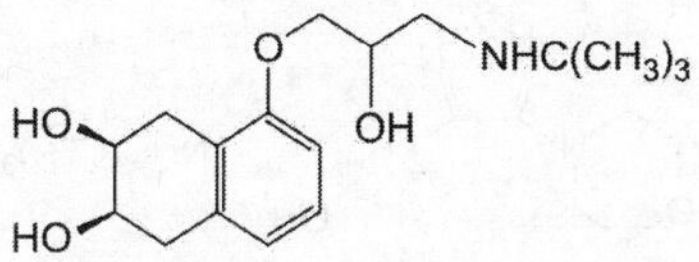

Synthesis

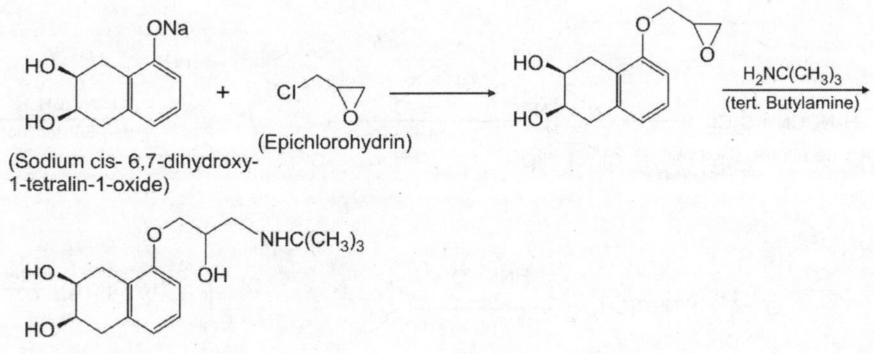

(Sodium cis- 6,7-dihydroxy-1-tetralin-1-oxide)

It is used as antianginal and antihypertensive.

Pindolol

4-[2-Hydroxy-3-(isopropylamino)propoxy]indole

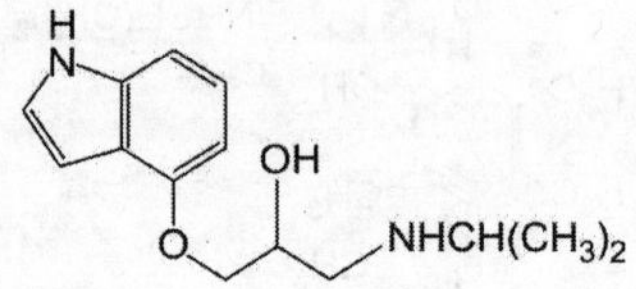

Synthesis

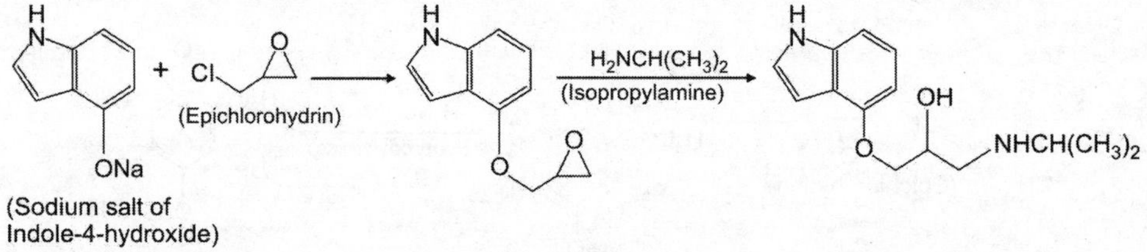

(Sodium salt of
Indole-4-hydroxide)

It is used as antianginal, antihypertensive, antiarrhythmic, and in glaucoma.

Timolol

(−)-3-Morpholino-4-(3-*tert*-butylamino-2-hydroxypropoxy)-1,2,5-thiadiazole

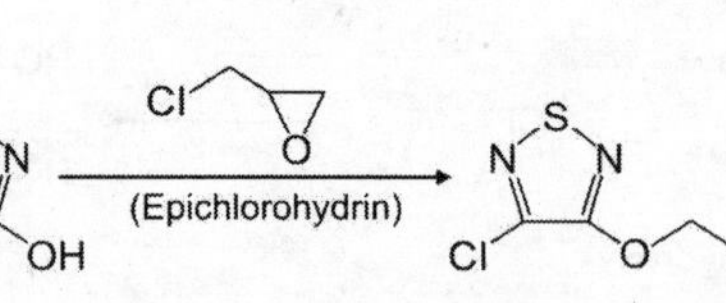

Synthesis

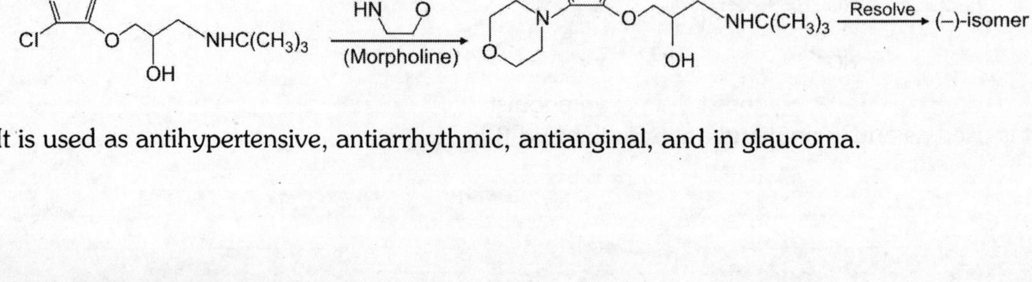

It is used as antihypertensive, antiarrhythmic, antianginal, and in glaucoma.

DRUGS ACTING ON ADRENERGIC RECEPTORS : MIXED α- AND β-ANTAGONISTS (BLOCKERS)

Carvedilol

1-(9H-Carbazol-4-yloxy)-3-[[2-(2-methoxyphenoxy)ethyl]amino]-2-propanol

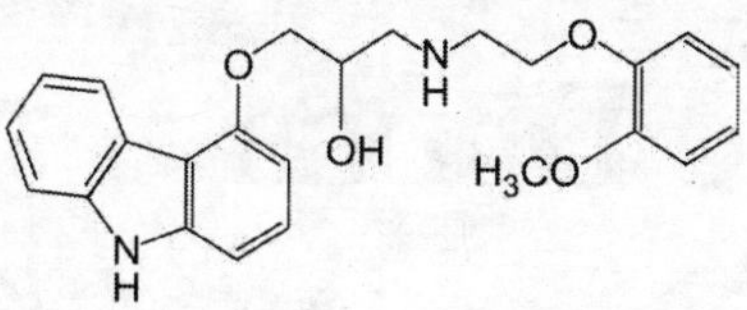

Synthesis

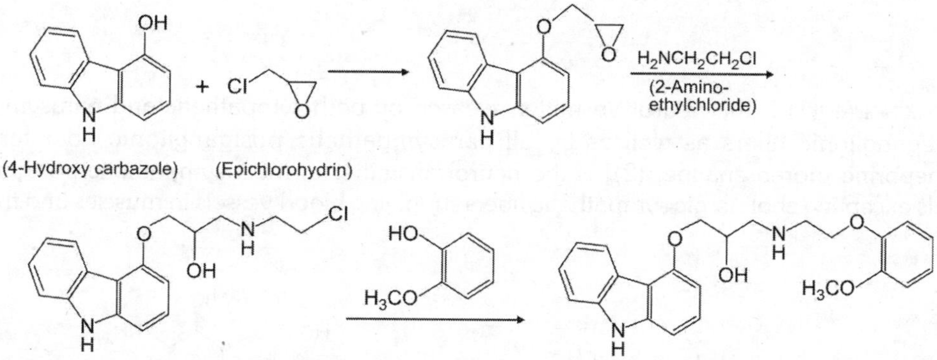

(4-Hydroxy carbazole)   (Epichlorohydrin)

It is used as antihypertensive agent.

Labetalol

(±)-2-Hydroxy-5-[1-hydroxy-2-[(1-methyl-3-phenylpropyl)amino]ethyl]benzamide

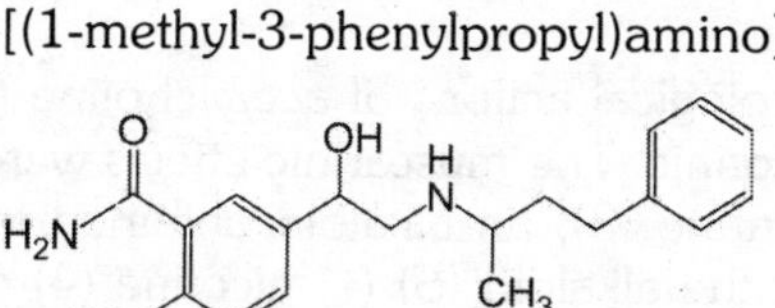

Synthesis

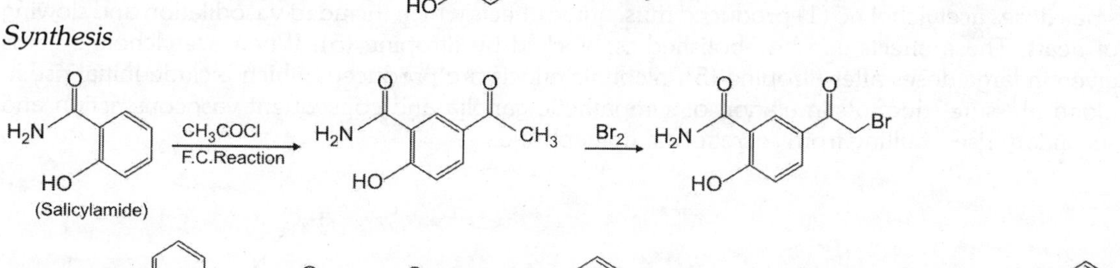

(Salicylamide)

(4-Phenylbutyl-2-amine)

It is more potent β-antagonist than α-antagonist. It is used clinically as antihypertensive agent. α-Receptor blockade produces-vasodilation and β-blockade produces tachycardia.

CHOLINERGIC DRUGS

A CETYLCHOLINE (1) is the neurotransmitter released by both sympathetic and parasympathetic preganglionic fibers as well as by all parasympathetic postganglionic fiber terminals. Norepinephrine [noradrenaline, (2)] is the neurotransmitter at most sympathetic postganglionic terminals excepting cholinergic sympathetic fibers supplying blood vessels in muscles and the sweat glands.

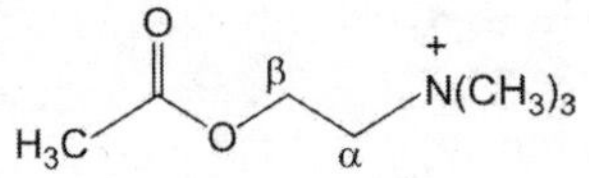

(1)

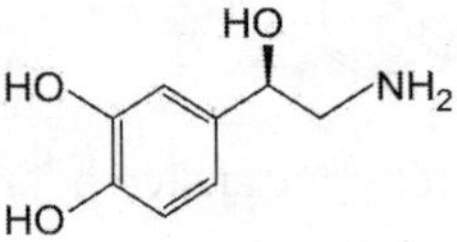

(2)

While studying the pharmacological actions of acetylcholine (1), Dale identified two types of actions, the muscarinic and nicotinic. The muscarinic effects were similar to the effects produced by the (2S, 3R, 5S) (+)-muscarine (3), an alkaloid obtained from *Amanita muscaria* while as nicotinic effects were similar to the alkaloid (S) (–)-nicotine (4) obtained from tobacco. Thus, in small doses acetylcholine (1) produced muscarinic effects which included vasodilation and slowing of heart. These effects can be abolished or blocked by atropine (5). When acetylcholine (1) is given in large doses after atropine (5), nicotinic effects are produced, which include initial rise in blood pressure due to stimulation of sympathetic ganglia and consequent vasoconstriction and secondary rise resulting from secretion of epinephrine.

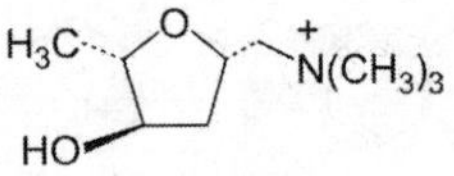

(3)

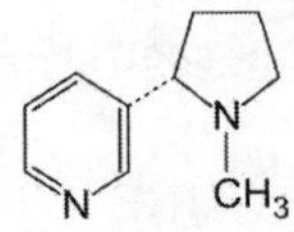

(4)

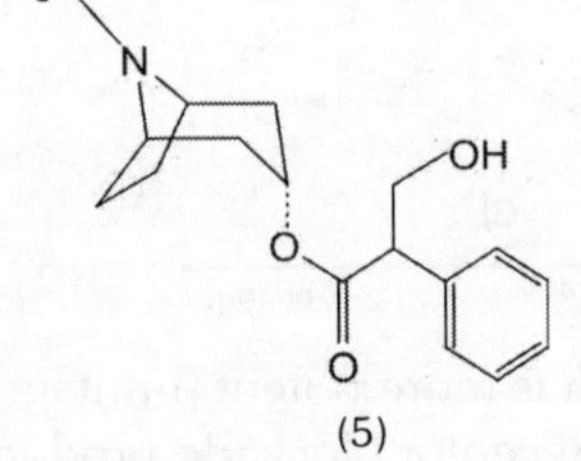

(5)

The muscarinic actions are similar to the action produced by acetylcholine (1) on postganglionic parasympathetic nerve endings with the exception of action on blood vessels and sweat glands.

Although blood vessels do not have parasympathetic innervation yet acetylcholine (1) causes vasodilation which is because it causes release of smooth muscle relaxant, nitric oxide, from endothelial cell. The stimulation of sweat glands by acetylcholine (1) is because these glands are innervated by cholinergic fibers of sympathetic systems.

The nicotinic effects are due to stimulation of sympathetic and parasympathetic ganglia, motor end plate of voluntary muscle and secretory cells of adrenal medulla.

ACETYLCHOLINE SYNTHESIS AND RELEASE

Acetylcholine (1) is synthesised in the nerve terminal from choline. The choline is transported into nerve terminal by active transport system. It is next acylated by choline acetyltransferase which transfers acyl group of acetyl CoA to choline. The acetylcholine (1) so formed is next stored in storage vesicles. The stored acetylcholine (1) is released in synapse by exocytosis which is triggered by the calcium entry into the nerve terminal (Fig. 2.1). The released acetylcholine (1) combines with the receptors. Some of it is hydrolysed by acetylcholinesterase which is present in basement membrane of nerve terminal. The choline so formed is transported back to nerve terminal for the synthesis of acetylcholine (1).

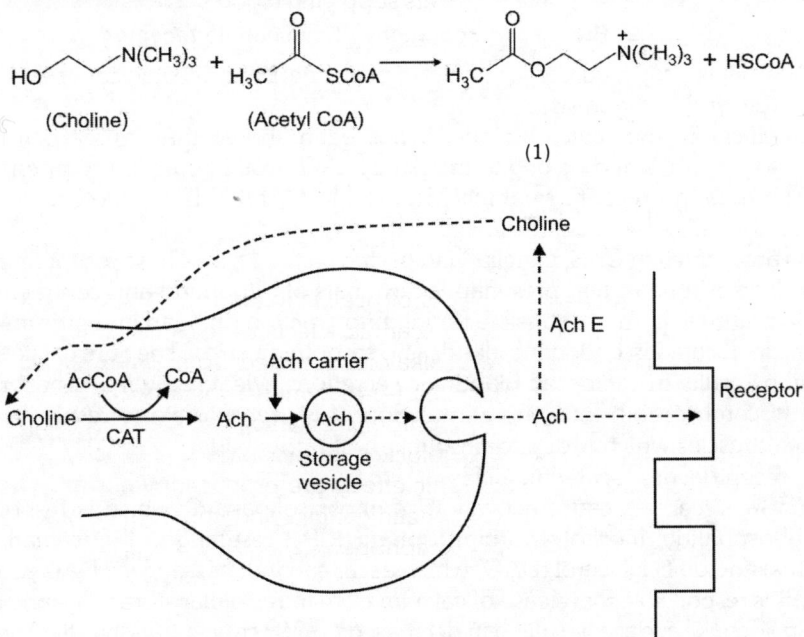

Fig. 2.1: Biosynthesis of acetylcholine (1).

(CAT–Choline acetyltransferase; Ach–acetylcholine; AchE–acetylcholinesterase.)

ACETYLCHOLINE RECEPTORS

The two major classes of acetylcholine receptors include muscarinic and nicotinic receptors.

Muscarinic Receptors

The earlier concept of muscarinic receptors was based on the studies on acetylcholine (1), muscarine (3), muscarone (6), and 1, 3-dioxolane (7). Based on this, it was proposed that the muscarinic receptor contained two sites, one anionic site and another esteratic site (Fig. 2.2). At the anionic site, the quaternary nitrogen was held and at the esteratic site the ester oxygen formed a hydrogen bonding. The two sites were about two carbons away from each other. Some workers proposed that muscarinic receptors must be similar to active site on acetylcholinesterase, the enzyme responsible for the hydrolysis of acetylcholine (1). This proposal was, however, rejected because interaction of cholinergic ligands with muscarinic receptors did not lead to chemical change of the ligands.

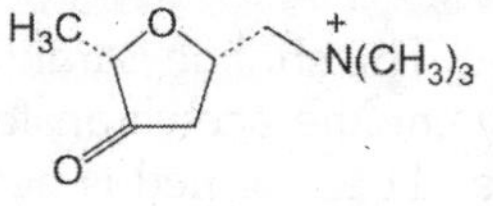

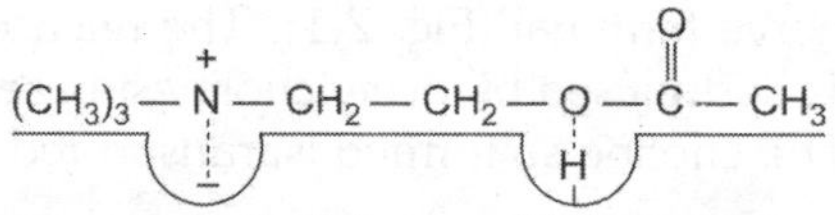

Fig. 2.2: Proposed topography of muscarinic receptor.

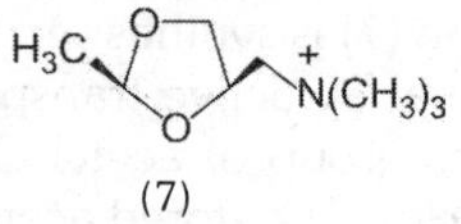

None of the models proposed earlier could explain the pharmacological effects produced by muscarinic agonists and antagonists.

With the advances in molecular biology, it has been shown that muscarinic receptors are membrane bound receptors and belong to the family of G-protein-coupled receptors. At least five distinct types of muscarinic receptors namely M_1, M_2, M_3, M_4 and M_5 are known. Out of these, M_1, M_2 and M_3 receptors have been characterized.

M_1-receptors are located in CNS, ganglia, and gastric parietal cells. These receptors are excitatory.

M_2-receptors occur in heart and presynaptic terminals of peripheral and central neurons. They are inhibitory in nature and are responsible for inhibitory action on heart and presynaptic neurons.

M_3-receptors are located in endocrine glands and smooth muscles. They are excitatory in nature. Their stimulation results in increased glandular secretion (sweat, salivary, and bronchial) and contraction of visceral smooth muscles. Stimulation of M_3-receptors also results in relaxation of vascular smooth muscles which is due to production of nitric oxide.

M_4- and M_5-receptors are located in CNS.

M_1-, M_3- and M_5-receptors cause activation of phospholipase C, which is responsible for the hydrolysis of phosphatidyl inositol-4, 5-biphosphate (PIP_2) resulting in the formation of inositol triphosphate (IP_3) and diacylglycerol (DAG) which act as second messengers. DAG activates protein kinase C and IP_3 is responsible for release of calcium from intracellular stores. M_2- and M_4- receptors act by inhibiting adenylyl cyclase, resulting in decreased c-AMP concentrations affecting the enzymes involved in energy metabolism, cell division, ion channels, etc.

Nicotinic Receptors

Two types of nicotinic receptors have been identified. These are muscle and neuronal type. Muscle type known as N_M are located at neuromuscular junction. The neuronal type known as N_N are located at autonomic ganglia and CNS. Both type of receptors are ligand-gated ion channels. The channels in case of N_M receptors are made up of five subunits (α_2, β, ε, & δ). Each subunit is composed of four hydrophobic trans-membrane spanning α-helical regions (M_1, M_2, M_3 & M_4). In case of N_N receptors, the channels are entirely composed of α-, β-subunits. Seven different α-subunit types ($\alpha_2 - \alpha_8$) and three β-subunit types ($\beta_2 - \beta_4$) have been detected in neuronal tissues. The acetylcholine (1) binding site in both type of receptors is located at α-subunits.

The distribution of various classes of cholinergic receptors and the effects observed after their stimulation are summarized in Table 2.1.

Table 2.1: Cholinergic receptors, their location, and effects observed after stimulation.

Receptors	Location	Response after excitation	Mechanism
Muscarinic M_1	CNS, exocrine glands (gastric, salivary)	CNS excitation, gastric and salivary secretion	Stimulation of phospholipase C. Increased IP_3, DAG and K^+ conductance.
Muscarinic M_2	heart, atria, smooth muscles, GI. tract, CNS	cardiac inhibition, tremors, hypothermia	Inhibition of adenylyl cyclase. K^+ channel opening
Muscarinic M_3	exocrine glands (salivary and gastric) smooth muscles (G.I tract and eye) blood vessels (endothelium)	Increased salivary and gastric secretion. Contraction of smooth muscles, ocular accommodation Vasodilation	As in M_1
Muscarinic M_4	CNS	As in M_2	As in M_2
Muscarinic M_5	CNS	As in M_3	As in M_1
Nicotinic N_M	Skeletal muscle at neuromuscular junction	End-plate depolarization, skeletal muscle contraction	Opening of Na^+/K^+ channels
Nicotinic N_N	Autonomic ganglia Adrenal medulla	Depolarization Secretion of catecholamines	Opening of Na^+/K^+ channels

ACETYLCHOLINE—STEREOCHEMISTRY AND STRUCTURE-ACTIVITY RELATIONSHIP

Acetylcholine (1) can assume number of conformations. According to NMR studies, the preferred conformation in aqueous solution is gauche (1a). The electrostatic attraction between the quarternary nitrogen and the carbonyl oxygen stabilises this conformation. However, studies on *cis*- and *trans*-2-acetoxycyclopropyl-1-trimethylammonium iodides, (8) and (9), respectively, have shown that acetylcholine (1) interacts with muscarinic receptors in its less favoured conformation—anticlinal (eclipsed) (1b) conformation.

(1a)

$$(CH_3)_3\overset{+}{N}\diagdown\diagup OCOCH_3 \qquad (CH_3)_3\overset{+}{N}\diagdown\diagup H$$
$$H \qquad\qquad H \qquad\qquad\qquad H \qquad\qquad OCOCH_3$$

(8)　　　　　　　　　　　　　　　(9)

$$\overset{+}{N}(CH_3)_3$$

(b)

(1b)

Acetylcholine (1) is a poor therapeutic agent. It is rapidly hydrolyzed in gastrointestinal tract after oral administration. When given parenterally it is rapidly hydrolyzed by tissue cholinesterases. Structural modifications of acetylcholine (1) have been carried out to find out the structural requirements for cholinergic activities and these include:

1. Alteration of quarternary ammonium head,
2. substitution of acetyl group with other acyl groups,
3. alteration of alkylene chain connecting the quarternary head with ester group, and
4. substitution or elimination of ester groups.

Alteration of Quarternary Ammonium Head

For maximum activity, the nitrogen has to be quarternary. Primary, secondary, and tertiary analogs have much less muscarinic activity. Successive replacement of methyl groups on the quarternary nitrogen by ethyl group results in decrease in activity and the triethyl analog is antagonistic.

Replacement of nitrogen by other atoms such as phosphorus, arsenic, antimony results in compounds which have much less activity.

These studies have shown that for optimum activity trimethylammonium head is necessary.

Substitution of Acetyl Group with other Acyl Groups

The cholinergic activity of choline is enhanced by its esterification with acetic acid. Replacement of acetyl group with other acyl groups has resulted in compounds which either possess lower activity or have altogether different pharmacological activity. The carbamate ester of choline, carbachol (10), possesses greater nicotinic activity than acetylcholine (1). It is, however, more toxic and is used only when other drugs do not respond. It has been found useful in glaucoma.

$$H_2N \diagdown \overset{O}{\underset{O}{\|}} \diagdown O \diagdown \overset{+}{N}(CH_3)_3 \quad Cl^-$$

(10)

Alteration of Alkylene Chain Connecting Quarternary Head with Ester Group

For optimum activity, the size of alkylene bridge has to be 2 carbons, i.e. an ethylene bridge. Substitution at the α- and β-positions has resulted in some useful compounds.

(11)   (12)

Substitution by methyl group on α-carbon atom results in decrease in muscarinic activity, while as substitution by methyl groups at β-carbon, resulting in acetyl β-methylcholine chloride or methacholine chloride (11), shows higher activity than acetylcholine (1). However, substitution by higher alkyl groups at the same position results in compounds with lower activity. Introduction of methyl group at β-position also results in asymmetry in the molecule. Out of the two isomers, S(+)-acetyl β-methylcholine has been found to be more active than R(–)-isomer. Futher, S(+)-isomer is hydrolysed faster and R(–)-isomer has been found to be inhibitor of acetylcholinesterase. In the racemic mixture, the hydrolysis of more active S(+)-isomer is inhibited by R(–)-isomer. The acetate ester, methacholine chloride (11) and its carbamate analog, bethanechol chloride (12), have found use in clinical practice. They have longer duration of action and are resistant to hydrolysis in the gastrointestinal tract, thus permitting the use of these agents by oral route.

Other modifications such as introduction of double bond or triple bond results in compounds which have either low activity or are inactive.

Substitution or Elimination of Ester Group

Most of the cholinergic agents used in clinical practice are esters. Replacement of ester with ether and ketonic groups, usually results in lower muscarinic as well as nicotinic activity. Thus, choline ethyl ether (13) and its β-methyl analog (14) possesses lower muscarinic activity. The reversed ester of acetylcholine (1), methyl β-trimethylammonium propionate (15) possesses a strong muscarinic activity and moderate nicotinic activity. It is poor substrate of acetylcholinesterases and does not inhibit the enzyme.

(13)   (14)   (15)

MUSCARINIC AGONISTS

The muscarinic agonists include acetylcholine (1), muscarine (3), carbachol (10), methacholine chloride (11), bethanechol chloride (12) and pilocarpine (16). The effects observed on administration of a muscarinic agonist include slowing of heart, reduced cardiac output, and dilation of blood vessels leading to fall in arterial blood pressure. The action on smooth muscles results in contraction. The peristaltic activity of gastrointestinal tract is increased. Stimulation of exocrine glands results in increased sweating, lacrimation, salivation and bronchial secretions. Muscarinic agonists activate the constrictor pupillae muscle and thus lower the intraocular pressure in glaucoma.

(16)

The clinical use of muscarinic agonists is in the treatment of glaucoma. Pilocarpine (16) is the most effective muscarinic agonist in glaucoma. Bethanechol chloride (12) is used in bladder emptying and to stimulate gastrointestinal motility.

NICOTINIC AGONISTS

Nicotinic receptor agonists affect ganglion and motor endplate receptors. Some of these agonists are nicotine (4), lobeline (17) suxamethonium chloride [succinylcholine chloride, (18)], and decamethonium (19).

(17)   (18)   (19)

Nicotine stimulates and then blocks the autonomic ganglia and central nervous system. Lobeline (17) stimulates autonomic ganglia and sensory nerve terminals, suxamethonium (18) and decamethonium (19) cause depolarisation block of neuromuscular junction. Suxamethonium (18) is the only compound used clinically as muscle relaxant.

ACETYLCHOLINESTERASE INHIBITORS

Acetylcholinesterase (AchE) is an enzyme which hydrolyses acetylcholine (1) to acetic acid and choline. Inhibition of acetylcholinesterase, thus, results in preservation of endogenous acetylcholine (1), resulting in parasympathetic stimulation.

The inhibition of acetylcholinesterase could be achieved by competitive and noncompetitive inhibition. In the competitive inhibition, acetylcholine (1) and inhibitor compete for the enzyme acetylcholinesterase. This type of inhibition is reversible, while as non-competitive inhibition is irreversible.

The active site of the acetylcholinesterase is composed of an anionic and an esteratic site. The anionic site is believed to be the ω–carboxylic group of aminodicarboxylic acid. Both aspartic and glutamic acids have been isolated form the site. At the esteratic site, the oxygen of the acyloxy group is believed to bind with hydroxyl of serine through hydrogen bonding. For hydrolysis, nucleophilic attack on carbonyl carbon is necessary. It is assumed that hydroxyl of serine is involved in this. Since hydroxyl group of serine as such is not capable of hydrolysing the ester, it gets activated by imidazole. The imidazole accepts proton from the hydroxyl group of serine, the alkoxy group then acts as a nucleophile.

The nucleophilic attack is followed by splitting of ester and liberation of choline (Fig. 2.3).

(1) AchE — Ser — OH + $H_3CCOCH_2CH_2\overset{+}{N}(CH_3)_3$ ⟶ AchE — Ser — O — C — $OCH_2CH_2\overset{+}{N}(CH_3)_3$ ⟶

AchE — Ser — $OCCH_3$ + $HOCH_2CH_2\overset{+}{N}(CH_3)_3$

(Choline)

$$(2) \quad \text{AchE} - \text{Ser} - \overset{\overset{\displaystyle O}{\|}}{\text{O}}\text{CCH}_3 \xrightarrow{\text{H}_2\text{O}} \text{H}_3\text{CCOOH} + \text{AchE} - \text{Ser} - \text{OH}$$

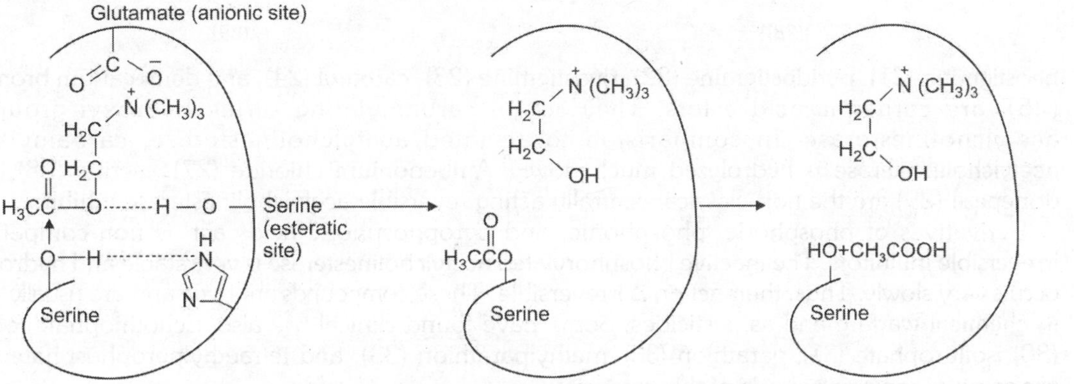

Fig. 2.3: Mechanism of hydrolysis of acetylcholine (1) by acetylcholinesterase.

The various reversible inhibitors of acetylcholinesterase include, physostigmine (20), neostigmine (21), pyridostigmine (22), rivastigmine (23), carbaryl (24), demecarium bromide (25), edrophonium chloride (26), ambenonium chloride (27) tacrine (28), and donepezil (29). Physostigmine (20),

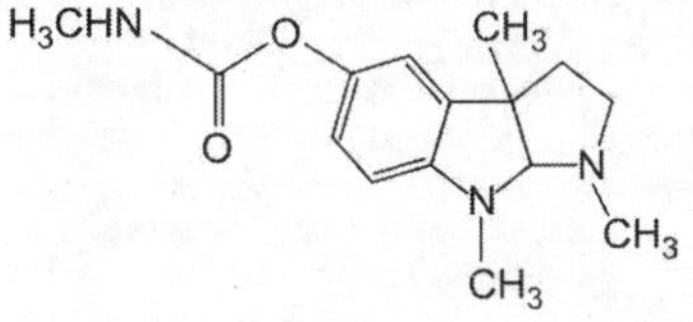

(20)

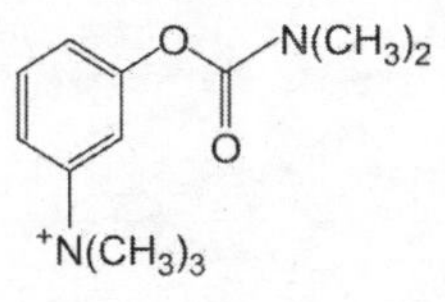

(21)

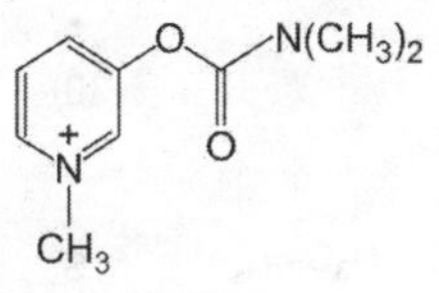

(22)

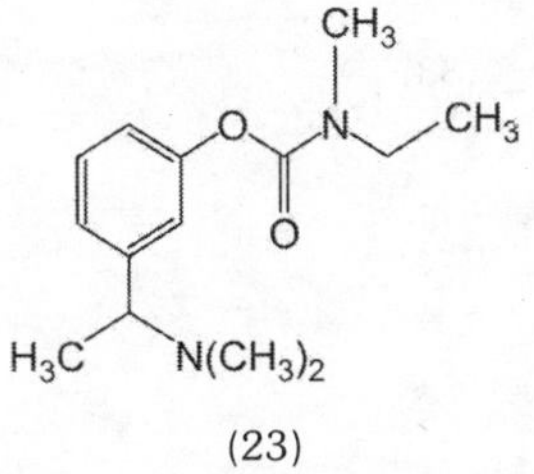

(23)

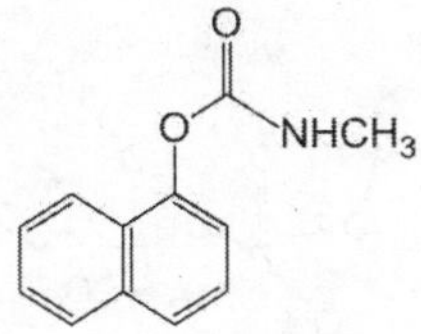

(24)

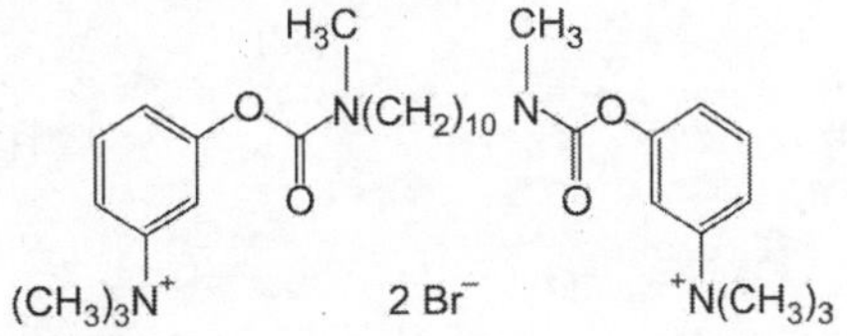

(25)

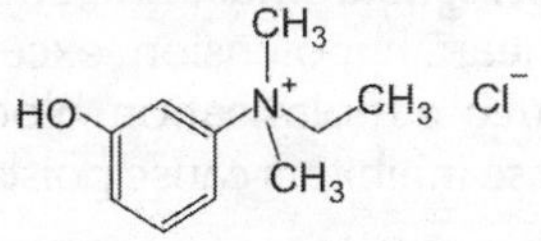

(26)

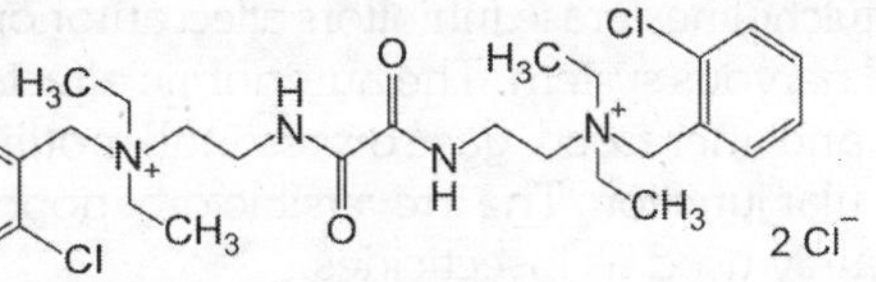

(27)

(28)   (29)

neostigmine (21), pyridostigmine (22), rivastigmine (23), carbaryl (24), and demecarium bromide (25), are carbamic acid esters. They act by carbamylating serine hydroxyl group of acetylcholinesterase. In comparision to acylated acetylcholinesterase, carbamylated acetylcholinesterase is hydrolyzed much slowly. Ambenonium chloride (27), tacrine (28), and donepezil (29) are the non-classical centrally acting reversible acetylcholinesterase inhibitors.

Derivatives of phosphoric, phosphonic, and pyrophosphoric acids act as non-competitive irreversible inhibitors. The inactive phosphorylated acetylcholinesterase is very stable and hydrolysis occurs very slowly. Thus, their action is irreversible. These compounds are toxic and are usually used in chemical warfare and as pesticides. Some have found clinical use also. Echothiophate iodide (30) isoflurophate (31), parathion (32), methylparathion (33), and tetraethylpyrophosphate (34) are some of the compounds of this category.

(30)   (31)

(32)   (33)

(34)

The acetylcholinesterase inhibitors affect autonomic cholinergic synapses, neuromuscular junction, and central nervous system. The autonomic effects include slowing of heart, hypotension, excessive secretion, and increased gastrointestinal motility. They also produce depolarisation block at neuromuscular junction. The irreversible organophosphate cholinesterase inhibitors cause poisoning and are mainly used as insecticides.

The anticholinesterases are used in myasthenia gravis and glaucoma.

CHOLINERGIC BLOCKERS

The three types of peripheral cholinergic receptors which are stimulated by acetylcholine (1) are located at:

1. Parasympathetic postganglionic nerve endings in smooth muscle,
2. the sympathetic and parasympathetic ganglia, and
3. the neuromuscular junctions in skeletal muscle.

The drugs used to block each of these include:

1. Parasympatholytics, anticholinergics or cholinolytics. They block parasymapathetic postganglionic terminals.
2. Ganglionic blocking agents, they block the autonomic ganglion, both sympathetic and parasympthetic.
3. Neuromuscular blocking agents or curare-form drugs, they block the neuromuscular junction.

PARASYMPATHOLYTICS

Parasympatholytics, also known as parasympathetic postganglionic blocking agents, block the action of muscarine (3) and therefore they are also known as antimuscarinic agents.

Clinically, parasympatholytics are used as antispasmodics and as mydriatics and cycloplegic. Spasm of gastrointestinal tract may be caused by not only acetylcholine (1), but also by histamine, serotonin, and barium chloride. Antispasmodics are the drugs which block the spasm caused by acetylcholine (1). In addition to antispasmodic effect, the parasympatholytics have action on other organs which include heart, secretory glands like sweat and salivary glands, ititic, and ciliary muscles.

Mydriatics are the drugs that dilate the pupil while as cycloplegics partially or completely paralyze the accommodation. The size of the pupil is controlled by the dilator muscle, which are sympathetically innervated, and the constrictor muscle which are parasympathetically innervated. Administration of parasympatholytics results in paralysis of constrictor muscle, thus allowing the pupil to widen. The widened pupil can then be examined by the ophthalmologists.

Mydriatics and cyloplegics are administered locally in concentrations which do not show side effects as in case of antispasmodics.

In addition to reduction of salivation and perspiration, parasympatholytics also reduce gastric secretion, a property which has led to their use in peptic ulcers. They are usually used in combination with CNS depressants or with a neuroleptic drugs.

Anticholinergics have also been used in Parkinsonism, a disease characterised by degeneration of dopaminergic neurons.

The various classes of drugs used as parasympatholytics include:

1. Solanaceous alkaloids.
2. Semisynthetic analogs of solanaceous alkaloids.
3. Synthetic parasympatholytics.

Solanaceous Alkaloids

The alkaloids (–)- hyoscyamine (35), atropine (5) (which is (±) –hyoscyamine) and scopolamine (36) are the best known naturally occurring antimuscarinic agents. These alkaloids have been isolated from *Hyoscyamus niger*, *Atropa belladonna*, and *Datura stramonium* belonging to *Solanacea* family.

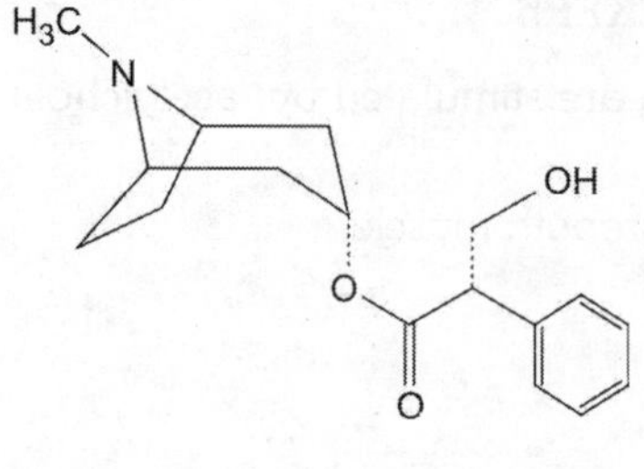

(35) 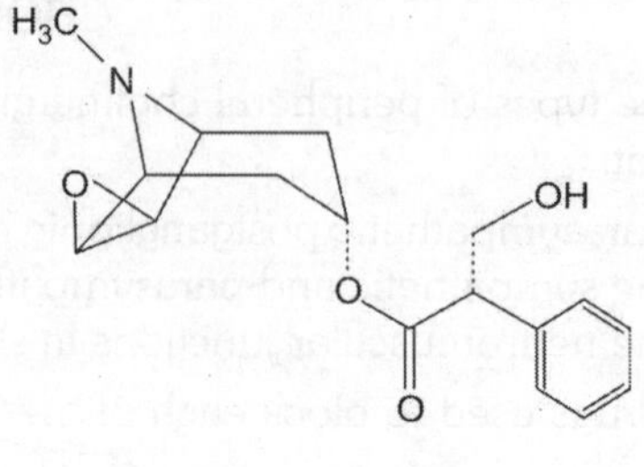　　　　　　　　　　　　　　　　　　　(36)

The alkaloids are tropic acid esters of bicyclic amino alcohols, tropine [3α-hydroxy tropane, (37)] and scopine [6,7-β-epoxy – 3α–hydroxy tropane, (38)].

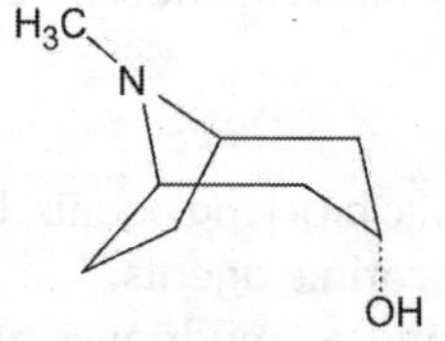

(37) 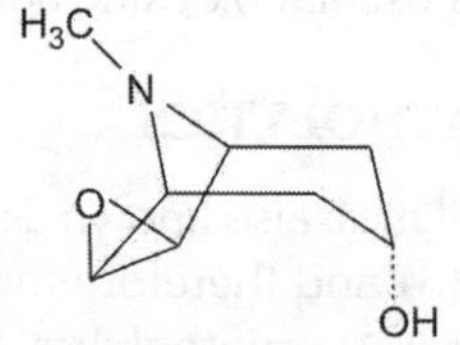　　　　　　　　　　　　　　　　　　　(38)

Atropine (5) and related compounds are competitive antagonists of acetylcholine (1) at muscarinic receptor. They differ in their action on CNS. In the doses used in clinical practice, atropine (5) causes mild vagal excitation as a result of stimulation of medulla. With higher doses of atropine (5), there is increased CNS stimulation. Scopolamine (36) in therapeutic doses causes CNS depression resulting in drowsiness, amnesia and dreamless sleep.

Semisynthetic Analogs of Solanaceous Alkaloids

These include esters of tropine (37) and scopine (38) with acids other that tropic acid and quarternary analogs of atropine (5). Among the esters synthesized, the homatropine [mandelyl ester, (39)] has survived as a therapeutic agent.

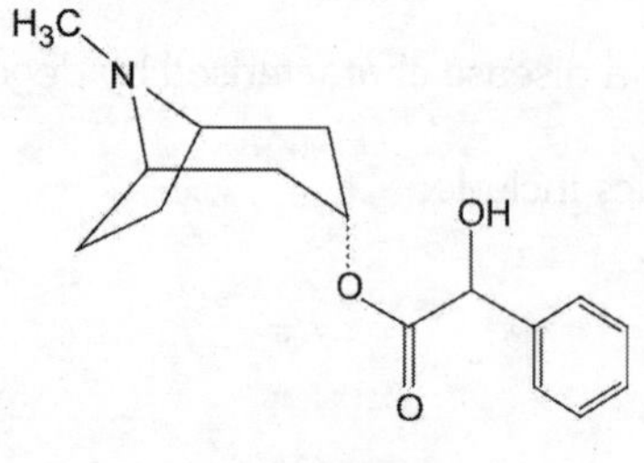

(39) 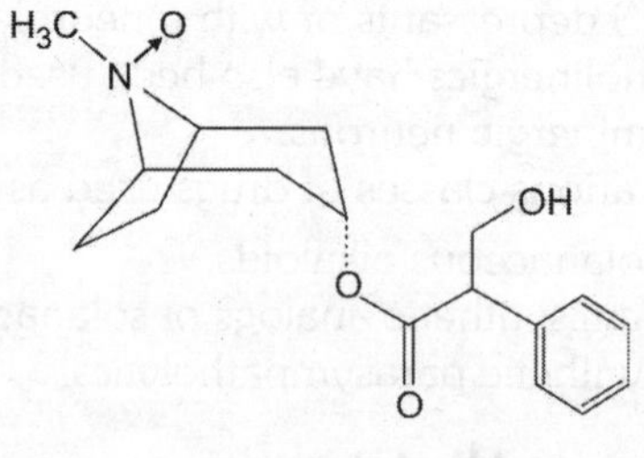　　　　　　　　　　　　　　　　　　　(40)

The quarternary analogs include atropine N-oxide (40), atropine methylnitrate (or methylbromide) (41), ipratropium bromide (42), scopolamine N-oxide (43), scopolamine methobromide (44), and homatropine methobromide (45).

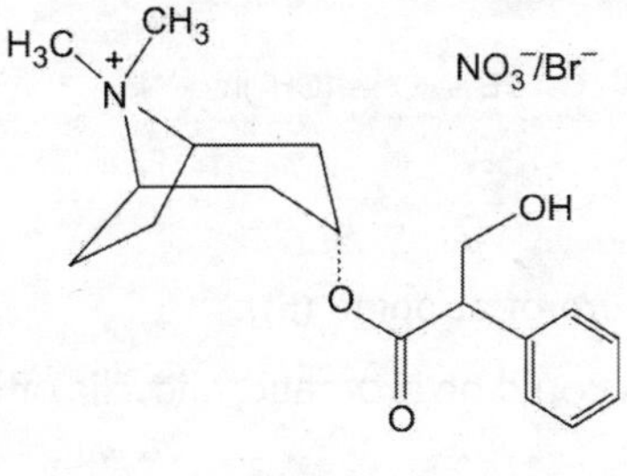

(41)

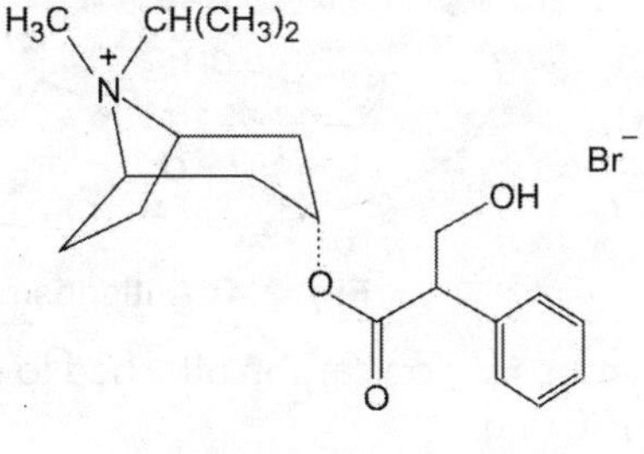

(42)

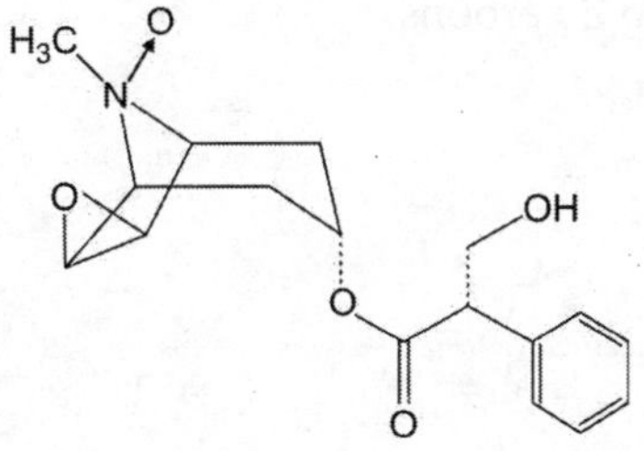

(43)

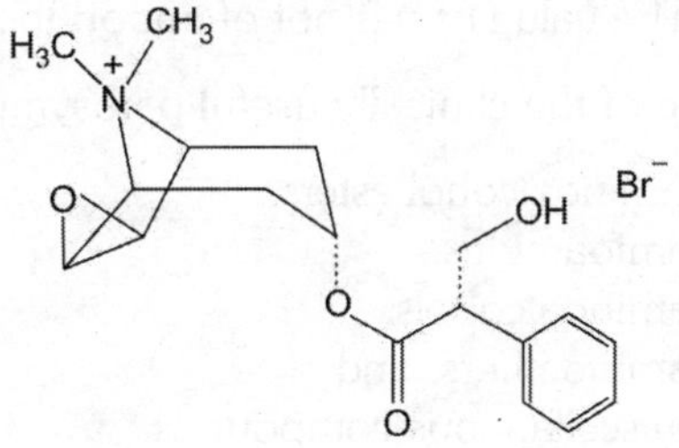

(44)

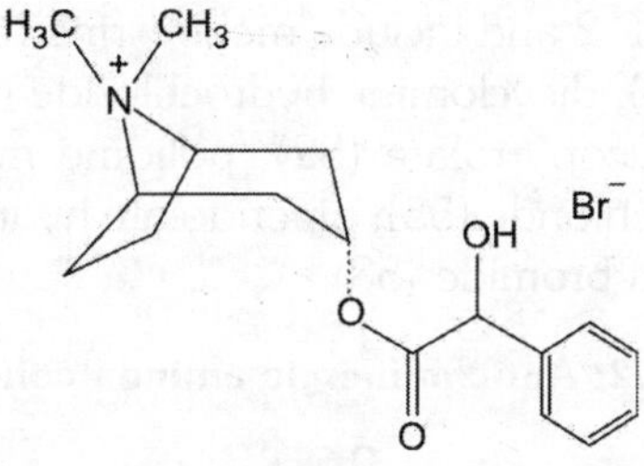

(45)

Quarternary ammonium salts of these alkaloids have advantage over the free base. They do not have central action as they cannot penetrate the blood-brain barrier. Further they have a prolonged action on gastrointestinal tract because the salts are not readily absorbed.

N-oxides have longer duration of action because they are hydrolysed slowly to tertiary bases. They are also claimed to be less toxic.

The choice between the base and salt depends on its use. Thus, for ophthalmic use, bases are better because they are absorbed faster than the quarternary salts. For antispasmodic action, salts are better because they are less readily absorbed from gastrointestinal tract and remain there for prolonged period.

Synthetic Parasympatholytics

The moiety responsible for activity in atropine (5) is as shown in Fig. 2.4 (encircled portion). Structure activity relationship has shown that:

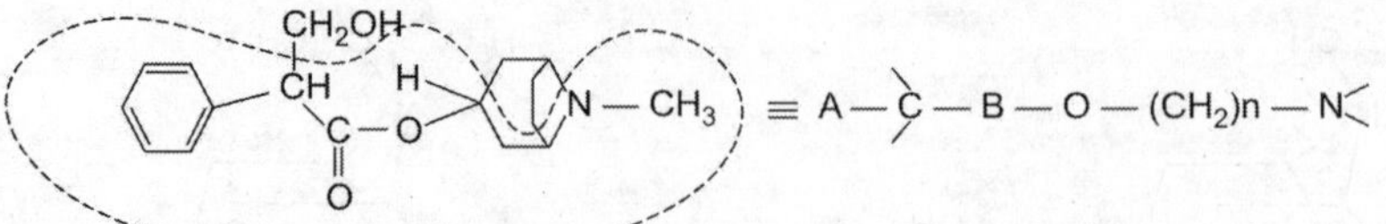

Fig. 2.4: Antispasmodic pharmacophore of atropine (5).

(a) Groups (A) on carbon attached to carbonyl ester (B) could be aromatic, alicyclic or heterocyclic ring.

(b) The ester group (B) could be replaced by either oxygen or could be absent.

(c) The nitrogen could be part of a ring or aliphatic tertiary amino group.

(d) The value of n is not of importance, it could be 2 to 3 carbons.

Some of the clinically useful parasympatholytics include:

(a) Aminoalcohol esters,

(b) amioamides,

(c) aminoalcohols,

(d) aminoethers, and

(e) miscellaneous compounds.

Aminoalcohol Esters

Some of these are given in Table 2.2 and include mebeverine (46), oxyphenonium bromide (47), cyclopentolate hydrochloride (48), dicyclomine hydrochloride (49), methantheline bromide (50), propantheline bromide (51), glycopyrrolate (52), polidine methylsulphate (53), mepenzolate bromide (54), eucatropine hydrochloride (55), piperidolate hydrochloride (56), oxyphencyclimine hydrochloride (57), and clidinium bromide (58).

Table 2.2: Anticholinergic aminoalcohol esters

$$R - \overset{\overset{\textstyle O}{\|}}{C} - O - R'$$

	R	R'	Use
(46)	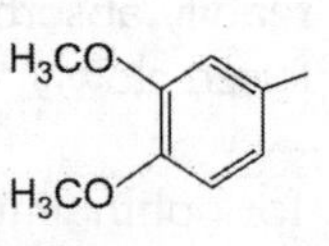 H₃CO—, H₃CO— (dimethoxyphenyl)	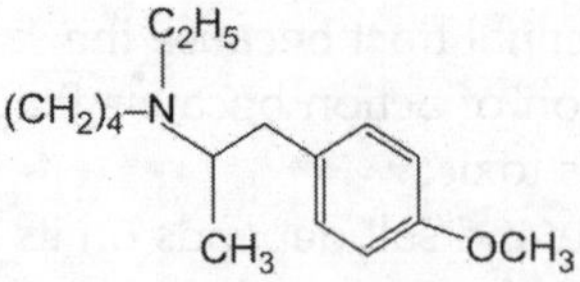 $(CH_2)_4$–N with C_2H_5 and CH_3, phenyl–OCH₃	Antispasmodic
(47)	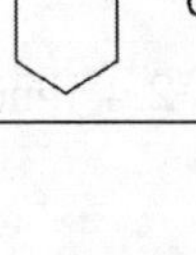 (phenyl cyclohexyl) OH	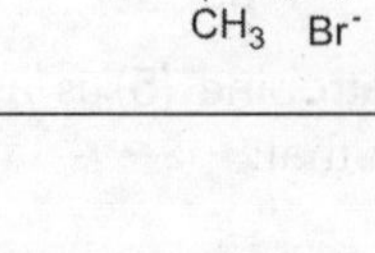 H_2C–N⁺ with C_2H_5, C_2H_5, CH_3 Br⁻	Antispasmodic

Contd.

Table 2.2: Anticholinergic aminoalcohol esters (Contd.)

$$R - \overset{\overset{\displaystyle O}{\|}}{C} - O - R'$$

R	R'	Use
(48)		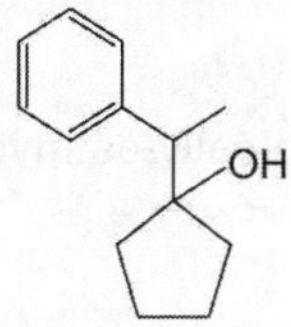 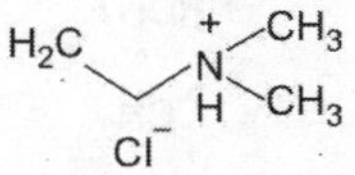 Cycloplegic and mydrlatic
(49)		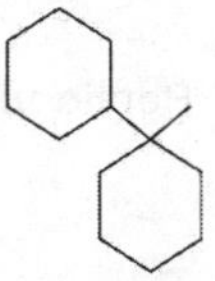 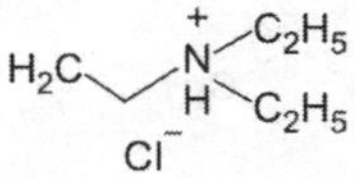 Antispasmodic
(50)		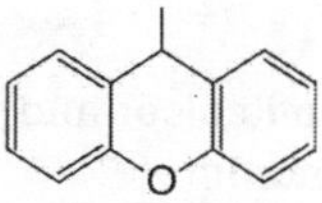 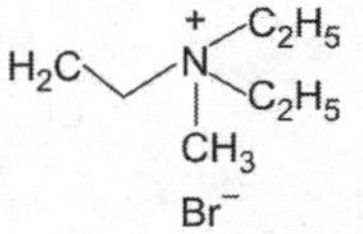 Antispasmodic
(51)		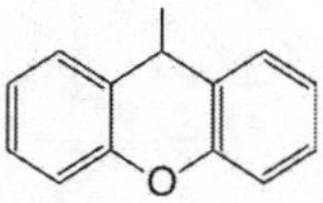 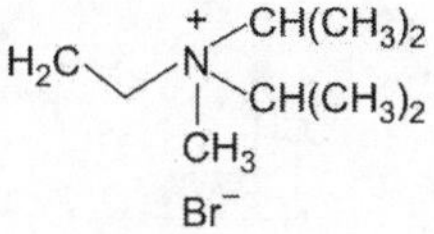 Antispasmodic
(52)		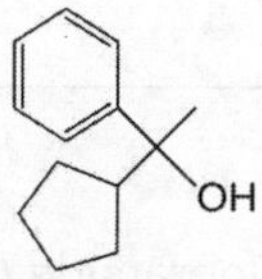 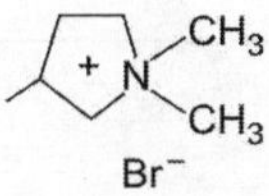 Peptic ulcer and in hyperacidity
(53)		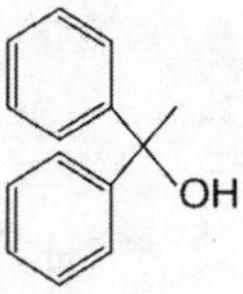 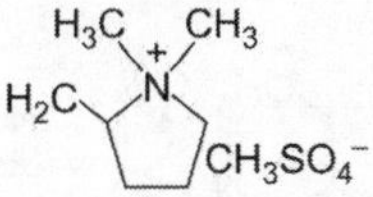 Peptic ulcer and in hyperacidity
(54)		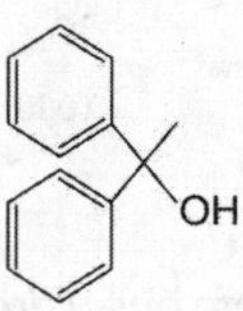 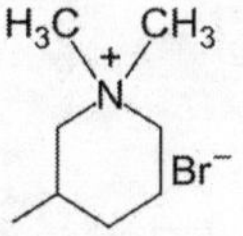 Antispasmodic

Contd.

Table 2.2: Anticholinergic aminoalcohol esters (Contd.)

$$R - \overset{\overset{\displaystyle O}{\|}}{C} - O - R'$$

R	R'	Use
(55)		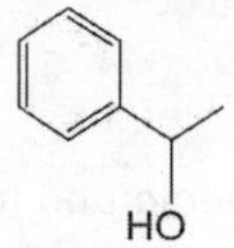 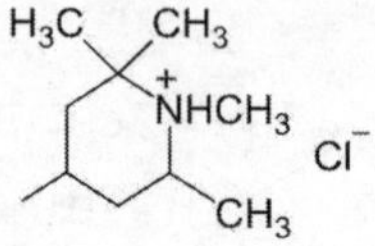 Topically as mydriatic
(56)		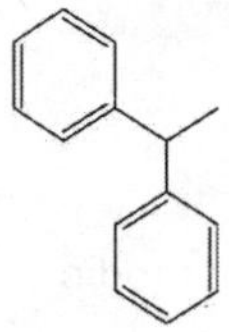 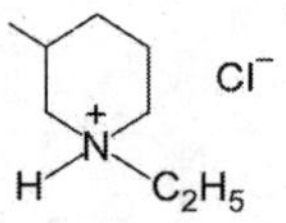 Peptic ulcer
(57)		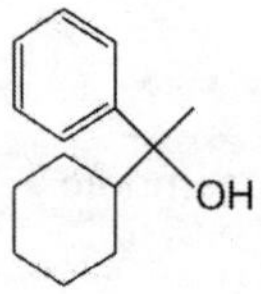 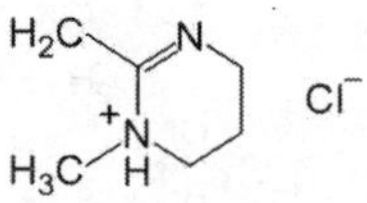 Peptic ulcer and functional bowel syndrome
(58)		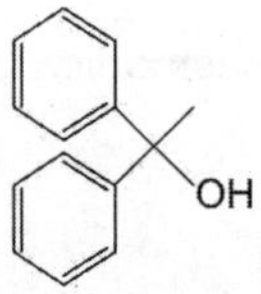 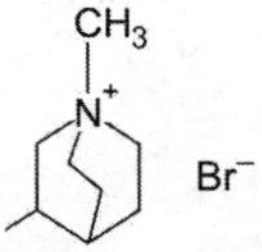 Peptic ulcer and hyperchlorhydlria

Aminoamides

These include isopropamide iodide (59), tropicamide (60), and metoclopramide (61). They have also bulky groups as in other anticholinergics.

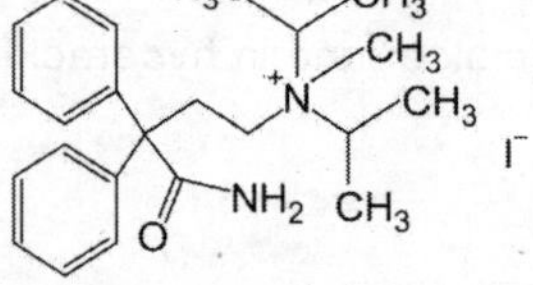

(59) 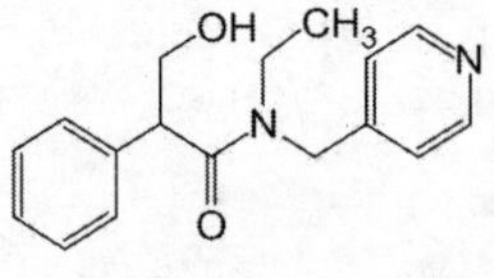   (60) 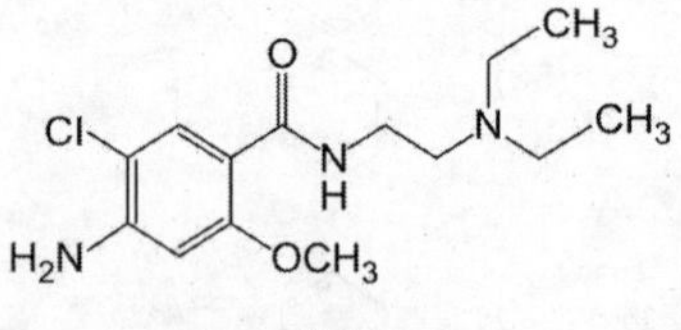   (61)

Aminoalcohols

These parasympatholytics have an aminoalcohol moiety. Further, there are bulky groups around the alcoholic group. Some of these compounds include tridihexethyl chloride (62), procyclidine hydrochloride

(63) trihexyphenidyl hydrochloride (64), and biperiden (65). As bases they are mainly used as antiparkinsonian drugs. Quaternization destroys antiparkinsonian activity because the salt cannot pass the blood-brain barrier. As salts, they are used mainly as anticholinergics.

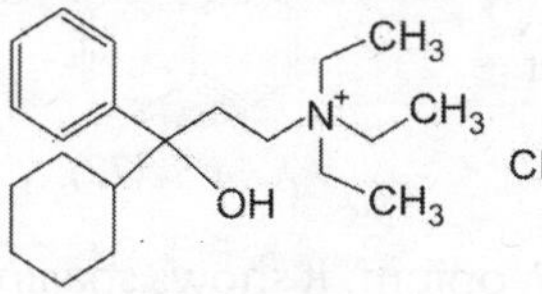

(62)

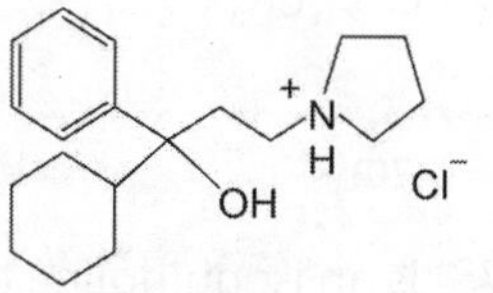

(63)

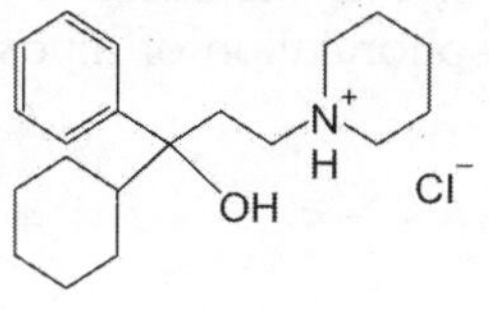

(64)

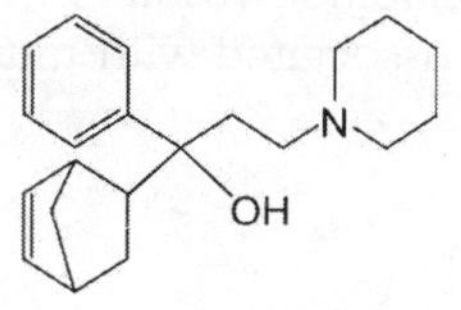

(65)

Aminoethers

The amino ethers include benztropine mesylate (66), chlorphenoxamine (67), and orphenadrine (68). They are closely related to antihistaminic, such as diphenhydramine (69) and possess antihistaminic activity also. They have been mainly used as antiparkinsonian drugs rather than conventional anticholinergics, i.e. mydriatics and spasmolytics.

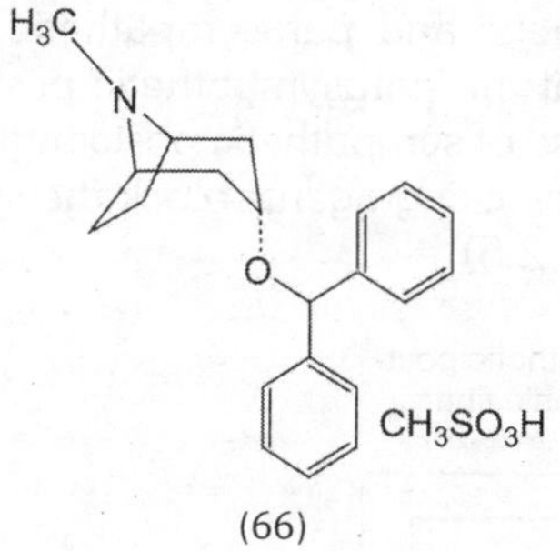

(66)

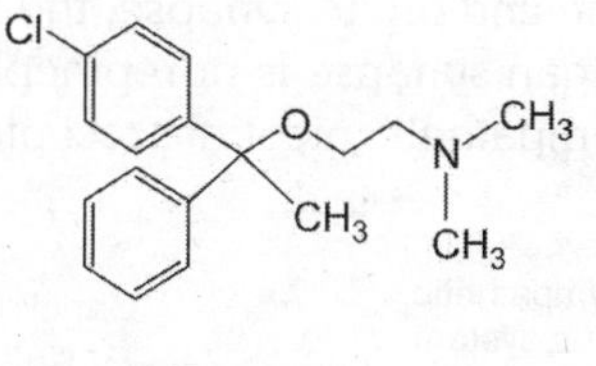

(67)

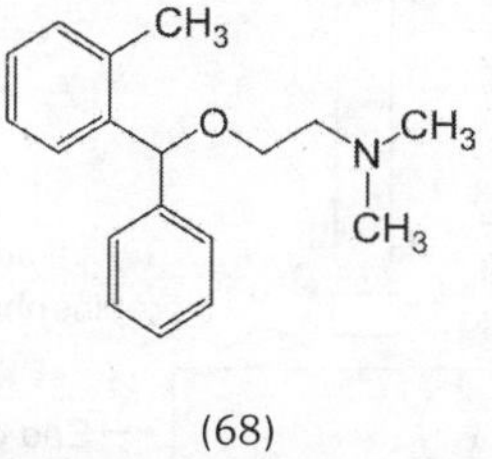

(68)

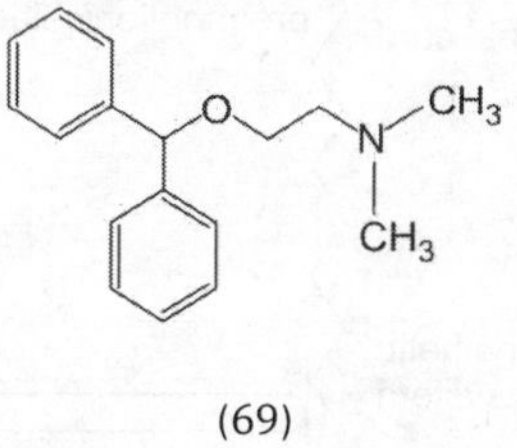

(69)

Miscellaneous Compounds

Some of these include diphemanil methylsulphate (70), a phenothiazine derivative, ethopropazine hydrochloride (71), and thioxanthene analog, methixene (72). All of them contain bulky groups.

(70)   (71)   (72)

Papaverine (73) is an isoquinoline type of alkaloid isolated from opium. It shows spasmolytic effect by inhibiting the enzyme phosphodiesterase which is responsible for destruction of c-AMP and c-GMP. This inhibition results in higher concentration of these. The increased levels of c-AMP and c-GMP is associated with muscle relaxation through phosphorylation of myosin light chain kinase.

(73)

GANGLIONIC BLOCKING AGENTS

Acetylcholine (1) is the neurotransmitter at both sympathetic and parasympathetic ganglionic synapses. While acetylcholine (1) is the neurotransmitter at the parasympathetic postganglionic fiber and the end organ synapse, the neurotransmitter in case of sympathetic postganglionic fibers and end organ synapse is norepinephrine (2). Ganglionic blocking agents block the sympathetic and parasympathetic nicotinic receptors in the ganglia (Fig. 2.5).

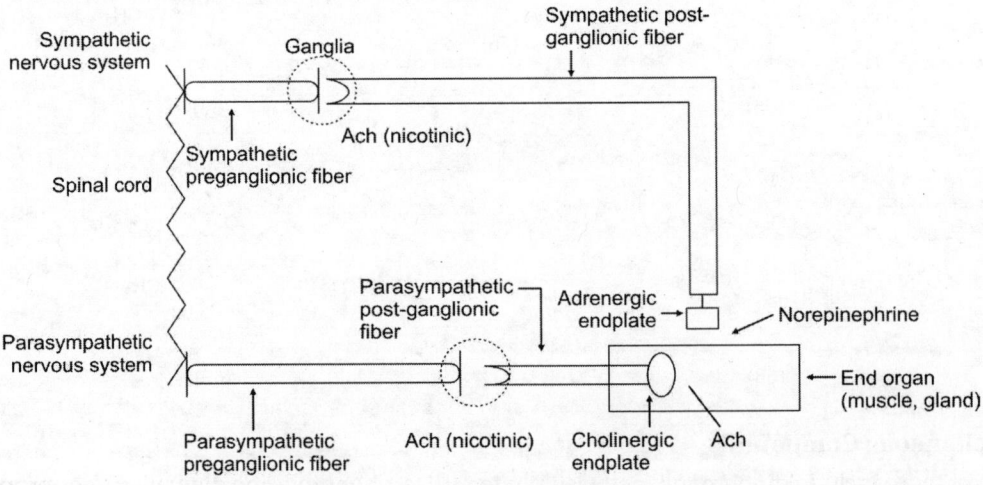

Fig. 2.5: Ganglionic transmission.

Nicotine (4) after initial stimulation blocks the autonomic ganglia. Lobeline (17) and 1,1-Dimethyl-4-phenylpiperazinium iodide [DMPP, (74)] stimulate the autonomic ganglia. None of these are clinically used. The block of autonomic ganglia by using nicotinic receptor antagonist results in hypotension, loss of cardiovascular reflexes, inhibition of secretions, gastrointestinal paralysis, and impaired micturition.

(74)

Ganglionic blocking agents have been classified into:
- (a) Depolarizing ganglionic blocking agents.
- (b) Non-depolarizing competitive ganglionic blocking agents.
- (c) Non-depolarizing non-competitive ganglionic blocking agents.

Nicotine (4) in smaller doses causes stimulation of autonomic ganglion, but in larger doses brings about a ganglionic blockade. This blockade is characterized initially by depolarization followed by competitive antagonism.

Non-depolarizing competitive ganglionic blocking agents compete with acetylcholine (1). They have the affinity for nicotinic receptor but not the intrinsic activity to stimulate it and thus block the receptor. Mecamylamine (75), tetraethylammonium (76), hexamethonium (77), and trimethaphan camsylate (78) are some of the competitive non-depolarizing ganglionic blockers. Mecamylamine (75) is both competitive as well as non-competitive non-depolarizing ganglionic blocker.

(75)

$(C_2H_5)_4\overset{+}{N}$

(76)

$(CH_3)_3\overset{+}{N}(CH_2)_6\overset{+}{N}(CH_3)_3$

(77)

(78)

Quarternary compounds also possess curare-like activity. However, structure-activity relationship has shown that when the value of n in (79) is 5 to 6, the compound is predominantly a ganglionic blocking agents while as when the value of n in (79) is 9 to 12, it possesses curare-like activity.

$$(CH_3)_3\overset{+}{N}(CH_2)_n\ \overset{+}{N}(CH_3)_3$$

(79)

Ganglionic blocking agents have no clinical use. They were earlier used as antihypertensives. However, since they also block parasympathetic ganglion, it results in serious side effect. Further, they also cause postural hypotension.

NEUROMUSCULAR BLOCKING AGENTS

The arrival of an impulse at the motor nerve terminal results in influx of calcium and release of acetylcholine(1). The acetylcholine (1) then diffuses through the synaptic cleft and binds to the nicotinic receptors located on the motor-end-plate. This interaction of acetylcholine (1) with nicotinic receptors leads to increased permeability of membrane in the end-plate to sodium. With the increase of intracellular sodium, membrane depolarizes. This is known as end-plate potential. When end-plate potential reaches threshold level, an action potential is generated in the adjacent membrane region which is conducted all along the muscle. This depolarization results in contraction of muscle fiber and is known as excitation-contraction coupling. The released acetylcholine (1) is destroyed by the acetylcholinesterase.

The neuromuscular transmission can be blocked either presynaptically by blocking the synthesis or relase of acetylcholine (1) or postsynaptically. The drugs which are used clinically act postsynaptically.

Neuromuscular blocking agents are mainly used as adjunct in surgical procedures for relaxation of muscles.

Drugs used as neuromuscular blocking agents acting postsynaptically are of two types:

(a) Non-depolarizing blocking agents, and
(b) depolarizing blocking agents.

Non-depolarizing Blocking Agents

These drugs compete with acetylcholine (1) for the nicotinic receptors. With most of receptors blocked by the drugs and decrease in effective acetycholine-receptor combinations small end-plate potential is generated which is not sufficient to initiate the propagated action potential. This results in paralysis of neuromuscular transmission and cosequently excitation-contraction coupling and the muscle is relaxed.

Examples of non-depolarizing neuromuscular blocking agents are tubocurarine chloride (80), metocurine iodide (81), gallamine triethiodide (82), pancuronium bromide (83), pipecurium bromide (84), vecuronium bromide (85), atracurium besylate (86), doxacurium chloride (87), and mivacurium chloride (88).

(80)   (81)   (82)

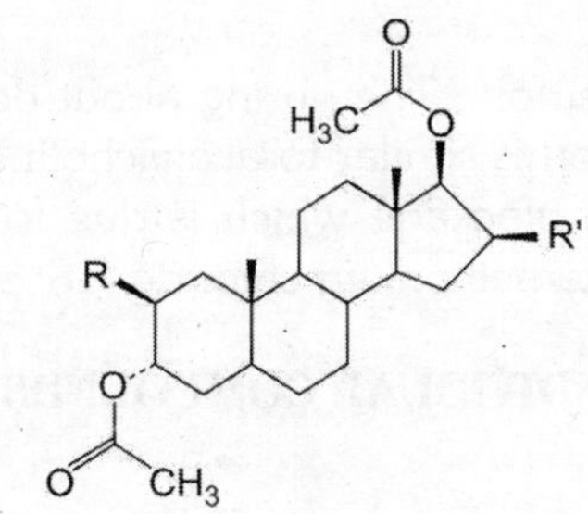

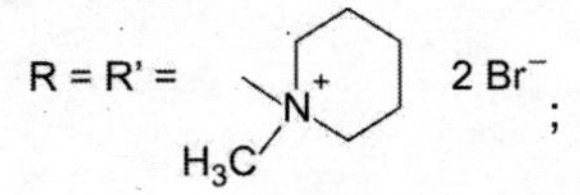

R = R' = (83)   2 Br⁻ ;   R = R' = (84)   2 Br⁻ ;   R = (85)   R' =   Br⁻

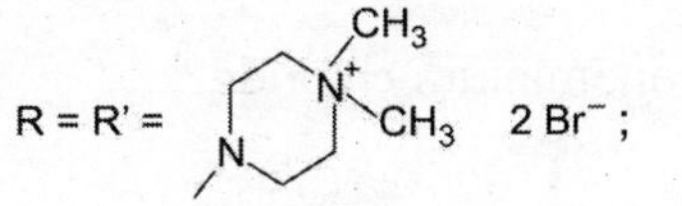

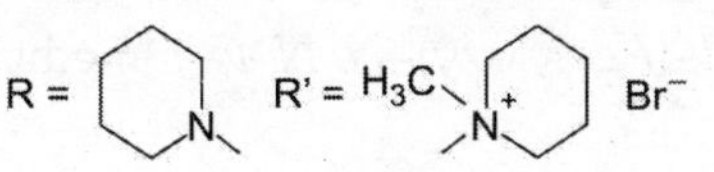

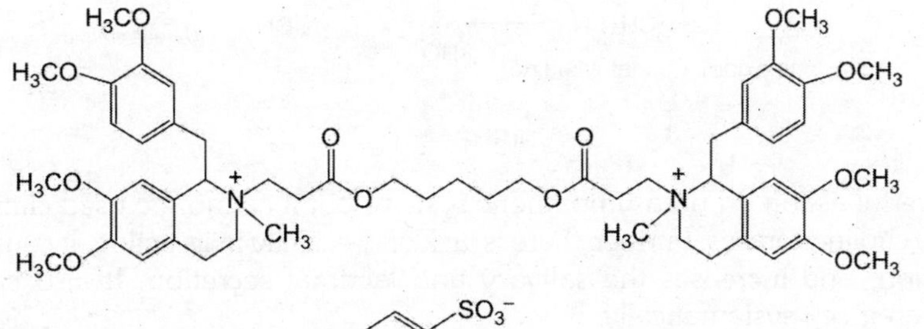

(86)

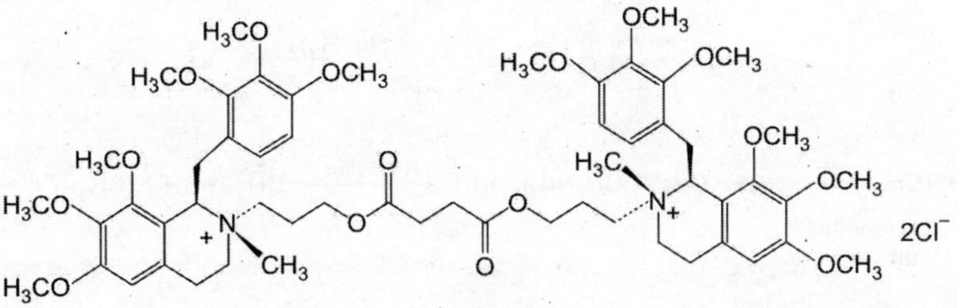

(87)

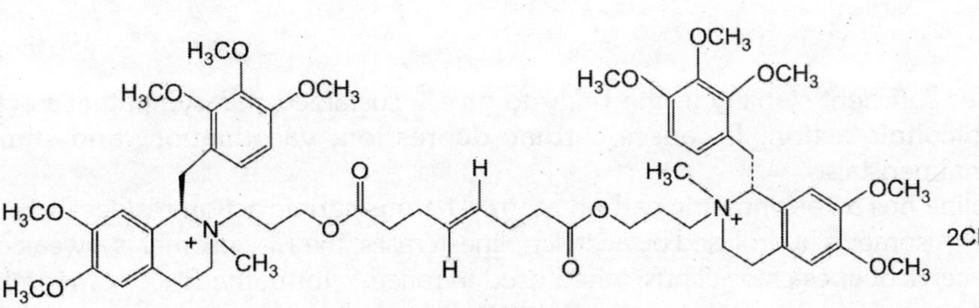

(88)

Depolarizing Blocking Agents

These are agonists at nicotinic receptors. They bring about depolarization of membrane of the muscle end-plate. This depolarization is similar to acetylcholine (1). If the drug is used in higher concentration there is eventually a blockade which is due to tachyphylaxis or desensitization. Examples in this category include suxamethonium chloride (18) and decamethonium (19).

INDIVIDUAL COMPOUNDS

MUSCARINIC AGONISTS

Acetylcholine Chloride

2–(Acetyloxy)–N, N, N–trimethylethanaminium chloride

Synthesis

It exerts powerful action on parasympathetic system, but it cannot be used clinically because it is hydrolysed by cholinesterases. Further, there is lack of specificity in its action. It causes vasodilation, cadiac depression, and increases the salivary and lacrimal secretion. It also causes bronchial constriction when given systematically.

Methacholine Chloride

(2-Acetoxypropyl) trimethylammonium chloride

Synthesis

It possesses sufficient stability in the body to give a sustained parasympathetic action. It has almost no nicotinic action. It causes cardiac depression, vasodilation, and stimulation of gastrointestinal peristalsis.

Methacholine has an asymmetric carbon atom. The muscarinic action resides in $S(+)$- isomer. While the $S(+)$-isomer is hydrolysed by acetylcholinesterases, the $R(-)$–isomer is a weak competitive inhibitor of acetylcholinesterase. Thus, when used in racemic form, the $R(-)$–isomer reinforces the muscarinic action of $S(+)$–isomer by preventing its hydrolysis.

Carbachol

Carbamylcholine chloride

$$H_2N-\overset{O}{\overset{\|}{C}}-O-CH_2CH_2-\overset{+}{N}(CH_3)_3Cl^-$$

Synthesis

$$COCl_2 + HOCH_2CH_2\overset{+}{N}(CH_3)_3Cl^- \longrightarrow ClCOCH_2CH_2\overset{+}{N}(CH_3)_3Cl^- \overset{NH_3}{\longrightarrow} H_2N-\overset{O}{\overset{\|}{C}}-O-CH_2CH_2-\overset{+}{N}(CH_3)_3Cl^-$$

(Phosgene)   (Choline chloride)

Carbachol is non-specific in its action on various muscarinic receptors. It also possesses nicotinic action. It is hydrolysed by cholinesterases very slowly. It also has a stimulant action on autonomic ganglia. Carbachol is used for reducing the intraocular pressure in glaucoma.

Bethanechol Chloride

β-Methylcholine carbamate chloride

$$H_2N-\overset{O}{\overset{\|}{C}}-O-\overset{CH_3}{\underset{}{CH}}-CH_2-\overset{+}{N}(CH_3)_3Cl^-$$

Synthesis

$$COCl_2 + HO\overset{CH_3}{\underset{}{CH}}CH_2\overset{+}{N}(CH_3)_3Cl^- \longrightarrow ClCO\overset{CH_3}{\underset{}{CH}}CH_2\overset{+}{N}(CH_3)_3Cl^- \overset{NH_3}{\longrightarrow} H_2N-\overset{O}{\overset{\|}{C}}-O-\overset{CH_3}{\underset{}{CH}}-CH_2-\overset{+}{N}(CH_3)_3Cl^-$$

(Phosgene)   (β–Methylcholine chloride)

It is similar in action as methacholine chloride (11). However, being a carbamate ester it is hydrolysed showly than the corresponding acetate ester. It is used in the relief of urinary retention and abdominal distention after surgery. It is never administered intramuscularly or intravenously as there is danger of overstimulation of cholinergic system.

Pilocarpine

(3S-cis)-3-Ethyldihydro-4-[(1-methyl-1H-imidazol-5yl)methyl]-2(3H)-furanone

Pilocarpine is an alkaloid obtained from *Pilocarpus jamborandi* and *Pilocarpus microphyllus*. It is used as nitrate or hydrochloride salt. Pilocarpine mimics the actions of muscarine (3). Its molecular architecture and interatomic distances of its functional groups in certain conformations are smiliar to those found in muscarine (3). It causes profound sweating, salivation, and gastric secretion. It is used in treatment of glaucoma to reduce the intraocular pressure.

ACETYLCHOLINESTERASE INHIBITORS : REVERSIBLE

Physostigmine

(3αS-cis)-1,2,3,3a,8,8a,-Hexahydro-1,3a,8-timehylpyrrolo[2,3-b]indol-5-ol methylcarbamate

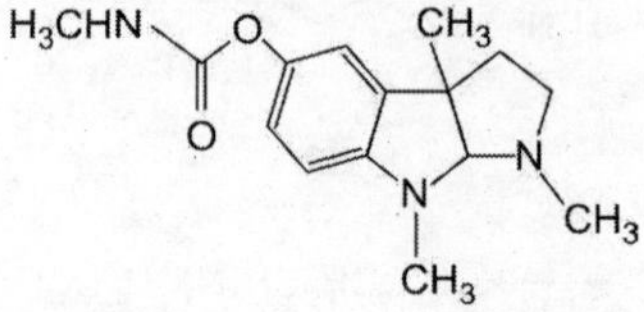

Physostigmine is an alkaloid obtained from *Physostigma venenosum* and is used as salicylate or sulphate salt. It is a reversible antagonist of cholinesterase used in glaucoma to decrease the intraocular pressure. It also causes stimulation of intestinal musculature and is used in condition of depressed intestinal motility.

Neostigmine Bromide

(3-Dimethylcarbamoxyphenyl)trimethylammonium bromide

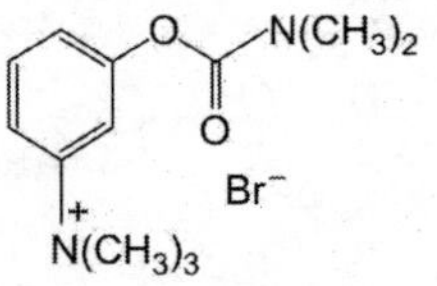

Synthesis

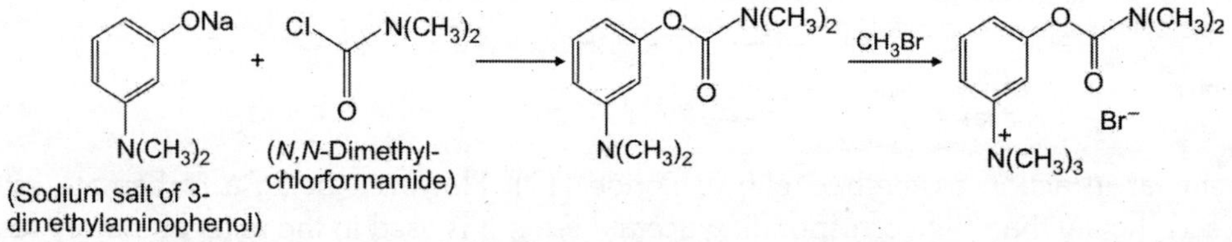

It is also used as methylsulphate salts. It has a greater miotic action, fewer, and less unpleasant effects than physostigmine (20). It is used to prevent atony of intestinal, skeletal, and bladder musculature. It is also used in myasthenia gravis.

Pyridostigmine Bromide

3-Hydroxy-1-methylpyridinium bromide dimethylcarbamate

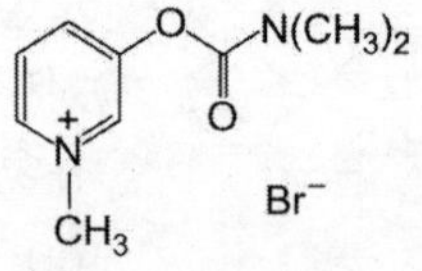

Synthesis

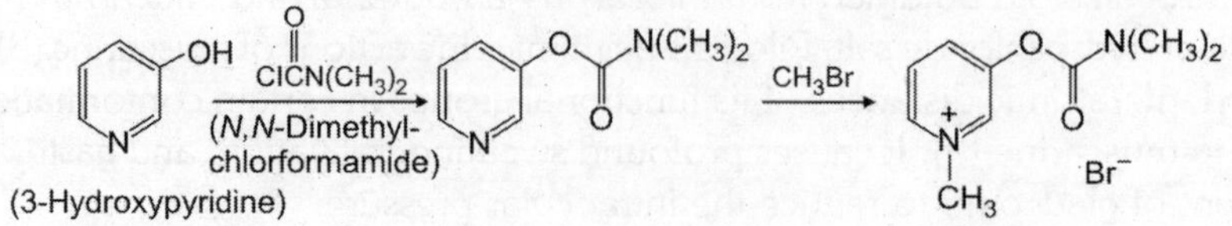

It is 1/5th as active as neostigmine (21). It is used in myasthenia gravis and has a longer duration of action. It has less muscarinic effects on gastrointestinal tract.

Rivastigmine

(3-Methylethylcarbamoyloxy)-α-dimethylaminoethyl benzene

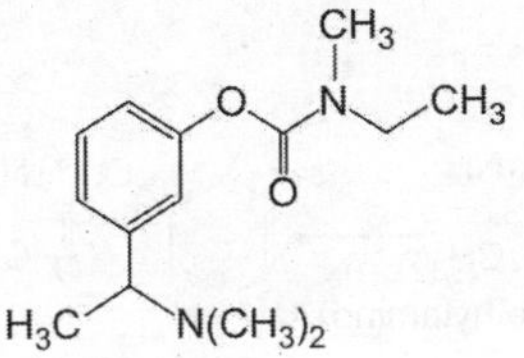

Synthesis

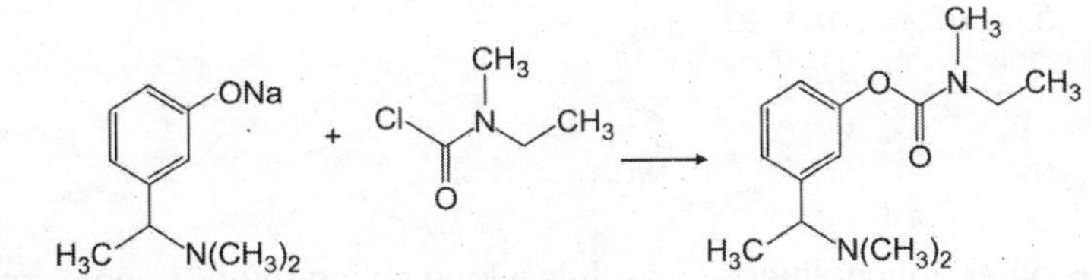

[Sodium3-(α-dimethyl-
aminoethyl)phenoxide]

(*N*-Ethyl-*N*-mehyl-
chlorformamide)

It is a centrally acting acetylcholinesterase inhibitor used for Alzheimer's disease. It has a lower liver toxicity.

Carbaryl

Methyl carbamic acid 1-naphthyl ester

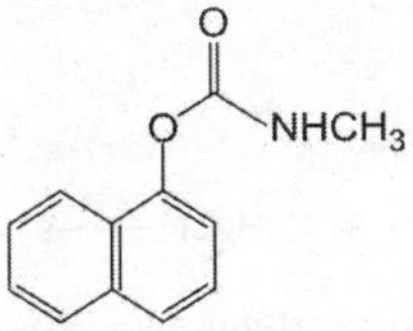

Synthesis

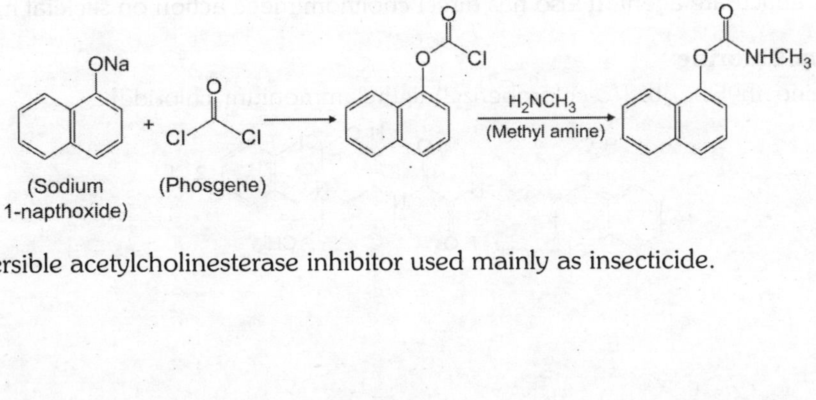

(Sodium
1-napthoxide)

(Phosgene)

H₂NCH₃
(Methyl amine)

It is a reversible acetylcholinesterase inhibitor used mainly as insecticide.

Demecarium Bromide

(*m*-Hydroxyphenyl)trimethylammonium bromide decamethylenebis(methylcarbamate)

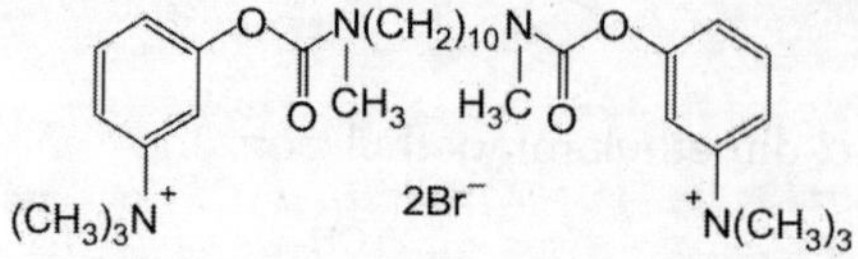

Synthesis

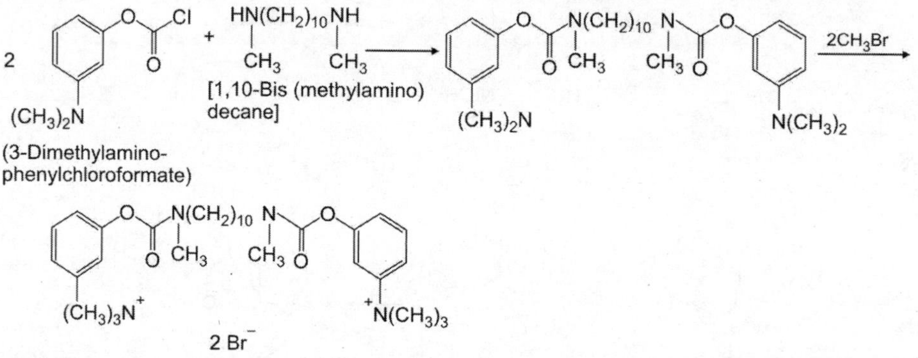

It is as active as other anticholinesterases. It is a long acting miotic agent used for treatment of glaucoma.

Edrophonium Chloride

Ethyl (*m*-hydroxyphenyl)dimethylammonium chloride

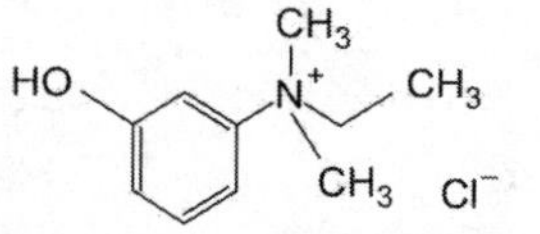

Synthesis

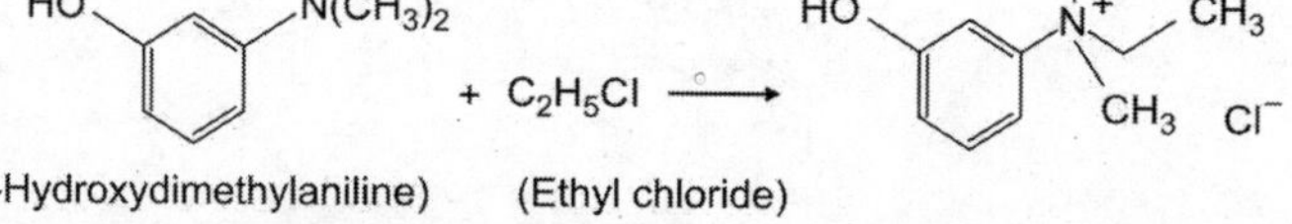

(*m*-Hydroxydimethylaniline)   (Ethyl chloride)

It is a reversible cholinesterase inhibitor with rapid onset of action which is of shorter duration. It is a specific anticurare agent. It also has direct cholinomimetic action on skeletal muscles.

Ambenonium Chloride

[Oxalylbis(iminoethylene)]bis[(*o*-chlorobenzyl)diethylammonium chloride]

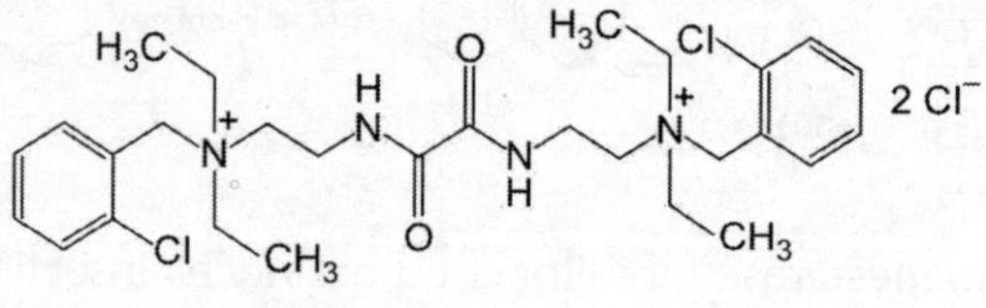

Synthesis

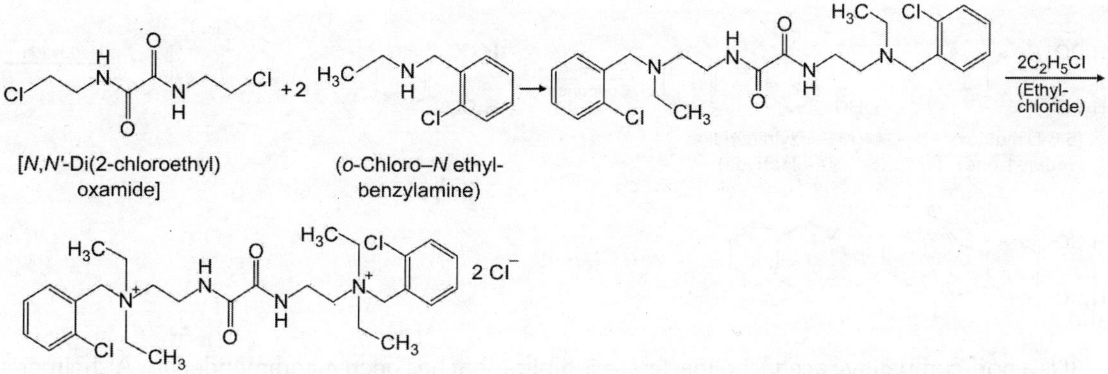

[*N,N'*-Di(2-chloroethyl) oxamide]

(*o*-Chloro–*N* ethyl- benzylamine)

2C$_2$H$_5$Cl (Ethyl- chloride)

2 Cl$^-$

Ambenonium chloride is used for myasthenia gravis in patients who do not respond to neostigmine (21) and pyridostigmine (22). It suppresses the activity of acetylcholinesterases and possesses long duration of action.

Tacrine

9-Amino-1,2,3,4,-tetrahydroacridine

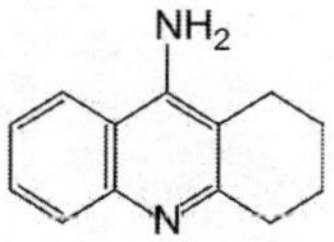

Synthesis

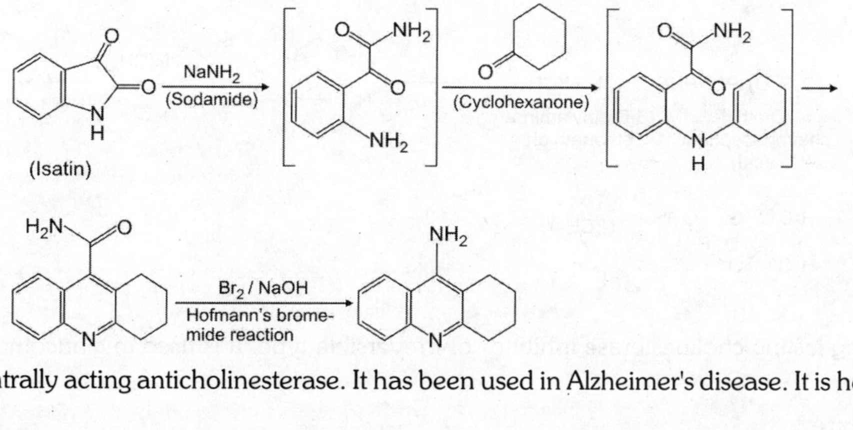

(Isatin)

NaNH$_2$ (Sodamide)

(Cyclohexanone)

Br$_2$ / NaOH Hofmann's brome- mide reaction

It is a centrally acting anticholinesterase. It has been used in Alzheimer's disease. It is hepatotoxic.

Donepezil

1-Benzyl-4-[(5, 6-dimethoxy-1-indanon-2-yl)methyl]piperidine

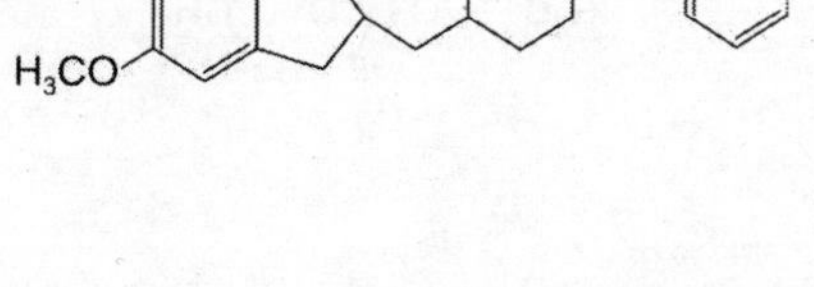

Synthesis

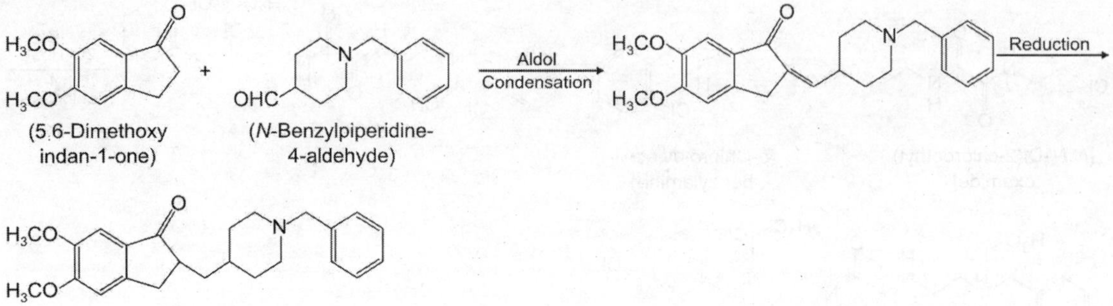

(5,6-Dimethoxy
indan-1-one) + (*N*-Benzylpiperidine-
4-aldehyde) → Aldol Condensation → → Reduction →

It is a non-competitive acetylcholinesterase inhibitor that has been recommended for Alzheimer's disease and dementia.

ACETYLCHOLINESTERASE INHIBITORS : IRREVERSIBLE

Echothiophate Iodide

2-Diethoxyphosphinylthioethyltrimethylammonium iodide

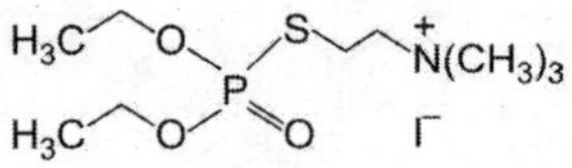

Synthesis

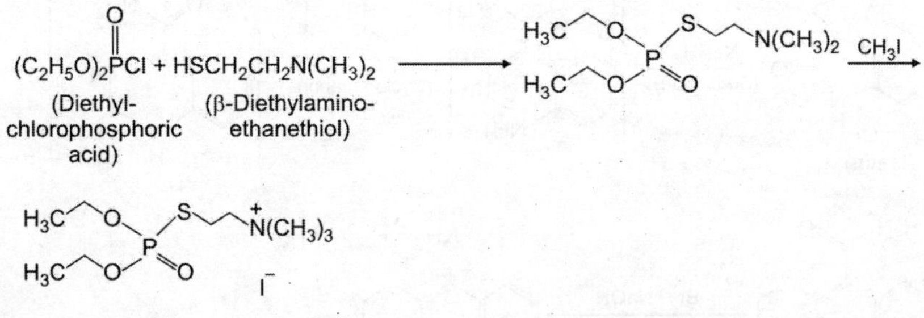

(Diethyl-
chlorophosphoric
acid) (β-Diethylamino-
ethanethiol)

It is a long lasting cholinesterase inhibitor of irreversible type. It is used in glaucoma.

Isoflurophate

Diisopropyl fluorophosphate

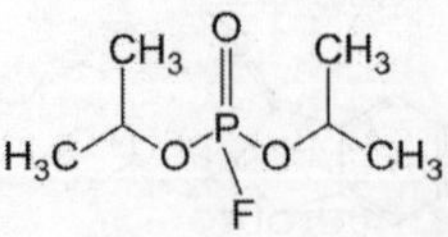

Synthesis

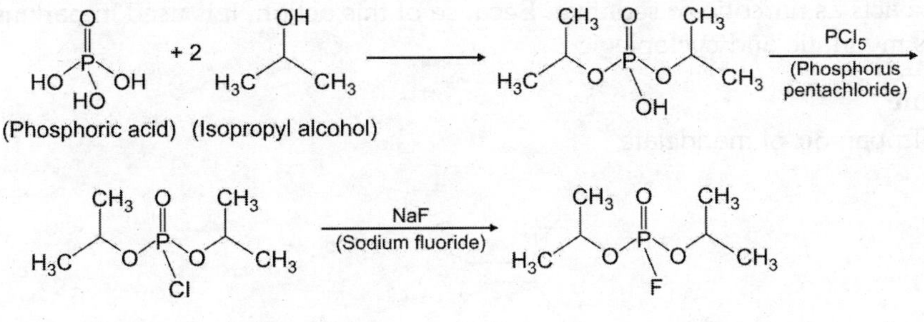

It is used for the treatment of glaucoma.

PARASYMPATHOLYTICS : SOLANACEOUS ALKALOIDS AND THEIR ANALOGS

Atropine

1 αH, 5αH-tropan-3α-ol (±)-tropate

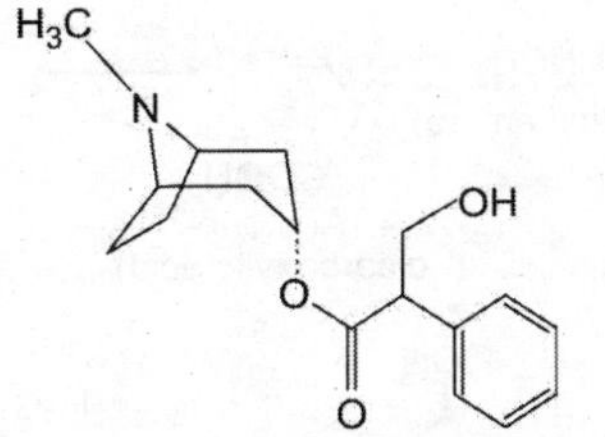

Atropine is a racemic mixture of *l*-hyoscyamine. It is used as methonitrate, methobromide, or as sulphate salt. Atropine and its salts are used as antispasmodic, mydriatics, and as preanesthetic medication to dry the oral and air secretions. It has also been used as antiarrhythmic, increasing the heart rate by blocking the effects of acetylcholine. It is also used as antidote for organophosphate anticholinesterases.

Scopolamine

6β, 7β-Epoxy-3α-tropanyl *S*-(–)-tropate

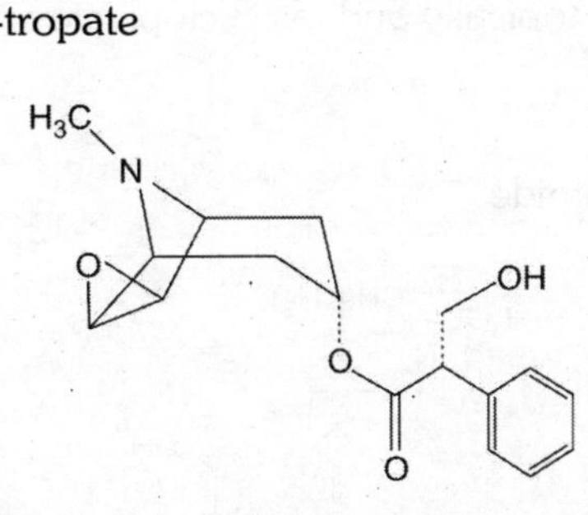

The alkaloid, scopolamine, is found in *Hyoscyamus niger, Duboisia myoporides, Scopola* species, and *Datura metel*. It is used as hydrobromide and butyl bromide salt. It has similar action as that of atropine. However, it differs in its action in central nervous system. While atropine (5) stimulates the central nervous system causing restlessness and talkativeness, scopolamine acts as narcotic or sedative. Because of this action, it is used in parkinsonism. It is also used as mydriatic and cycloplegic.

Homatropine

1α*H*, 5α*H*-Tropan-3α-ol mandelate

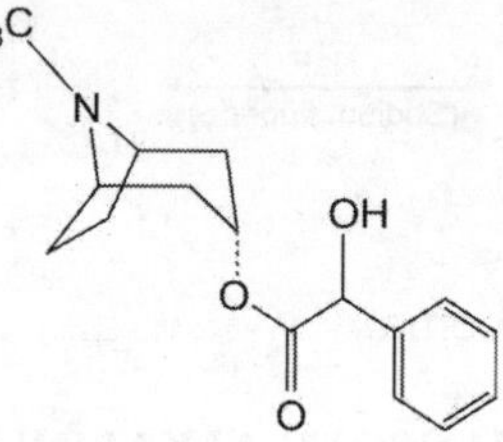

Synthesis

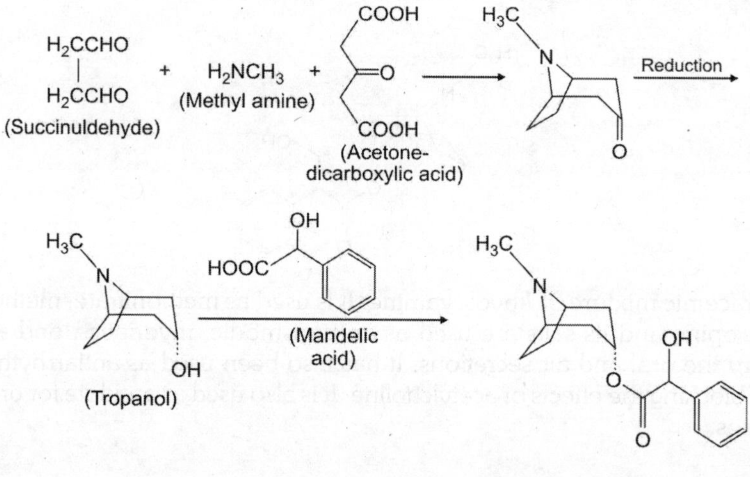

It is used as hydrobromide salt topically and as cycloplegic and mydriatic.

Ipratropium Bromide

8-Isopropylnoratropine methobromide

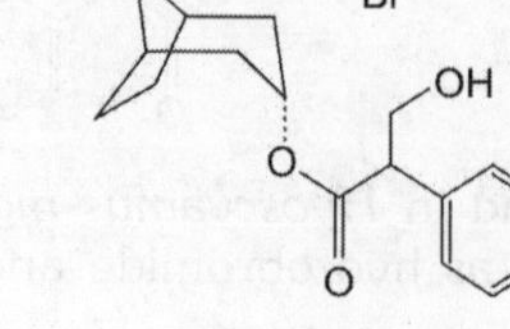

Synthesis

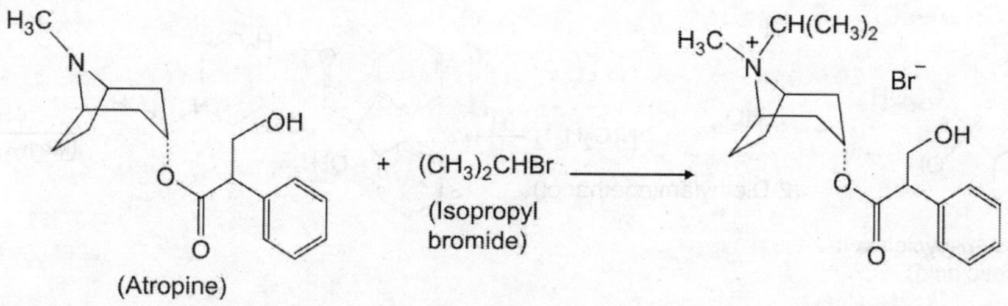

It is used as an inhalation for dilation of bronchial muscle in acute asthmatic attacks. It is also used as antiarrhythmic.

PARASYMPATHOLYTICS : AMINOALCOHOL ESTERS

Mebeverine

3, 4-Dimethoxybenzoic acid 4-[ethyl-[2-(4-methoxyphenyl)-1-methylethyl] amino] butyl-ester

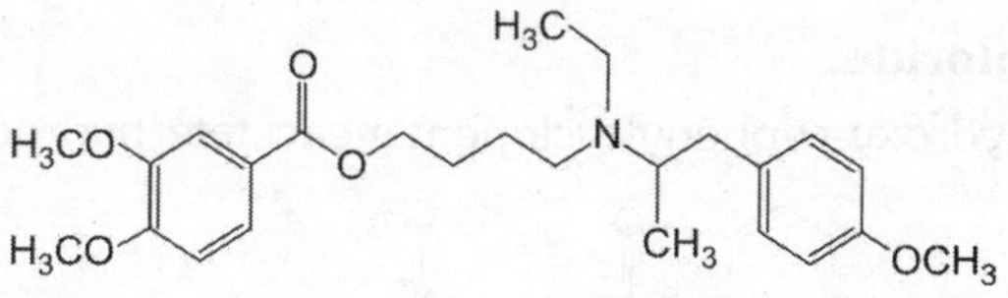

Synthesis

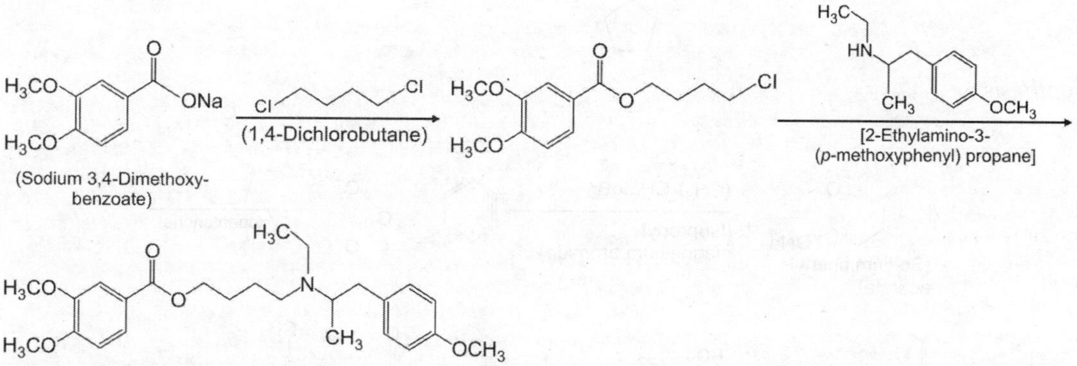

It is used as antispasmodic.

Oxyphenonium Bromide

2-Diethylaminoethyl α-cyclohexyl-α-phenylglycolate methobromide

Synthesis

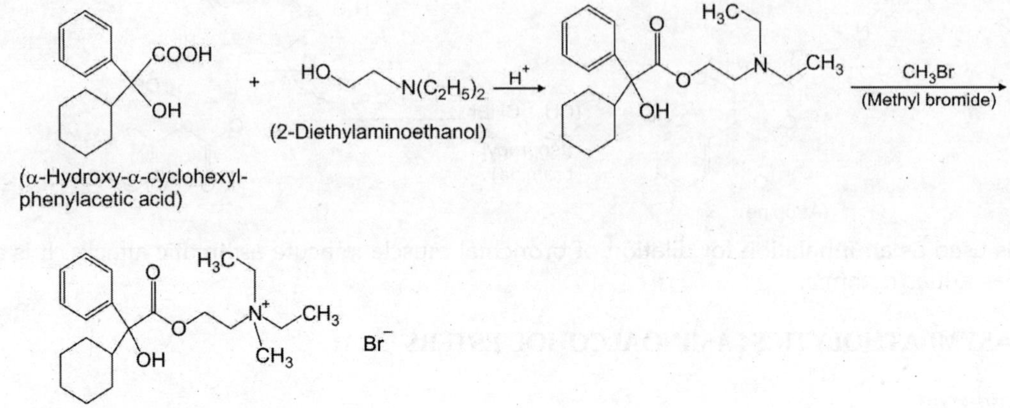

(α-Hydroxy-α-cyclohexyl-
phenylacetic acid)

(2-Diethylaminoethanol)

(Methyl bromide)

It is used as antispasmodic.

Cyclopentolate Hydrochloride

2-Dimethylaminoethyl-1-hydroxy-α-phenylcyclopentaneacetate hydrochloride

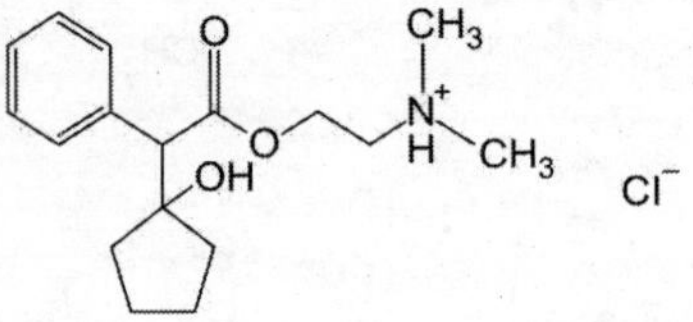

Synthesis

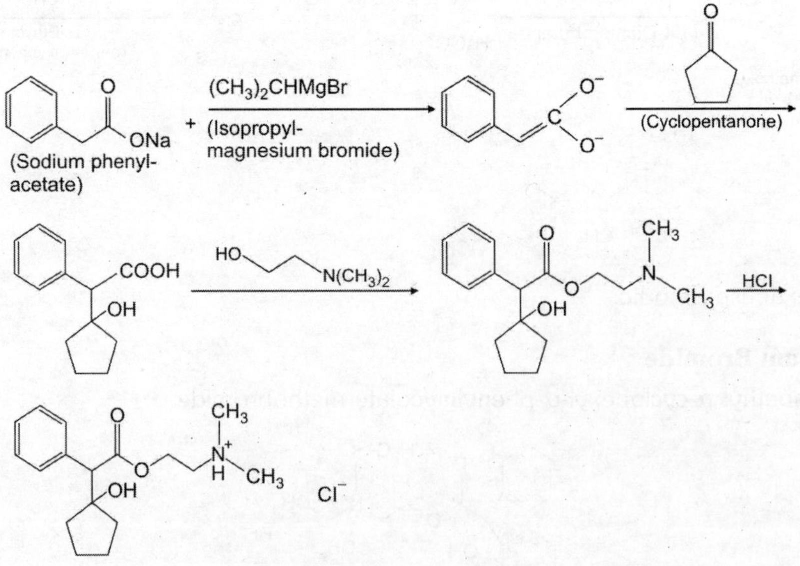

(Sodium phenyl-
acetate)

(Isopropyl-
magnesium bromide)

(Cyclopentanone)

It is used as cycloplegic and mydriatic.

Dicyclomine Hydrochloride

2-(Diethylamino)ethylbicyclohexyl-1-carboxylate hydrochloride.

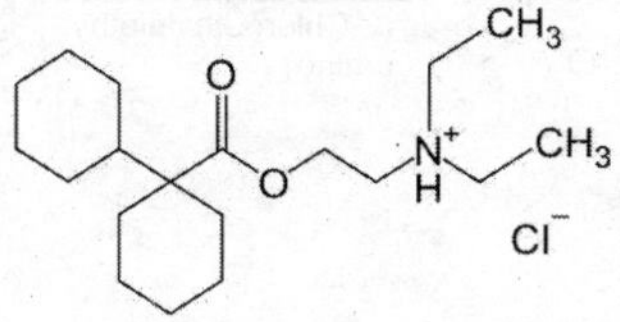

Synthesis

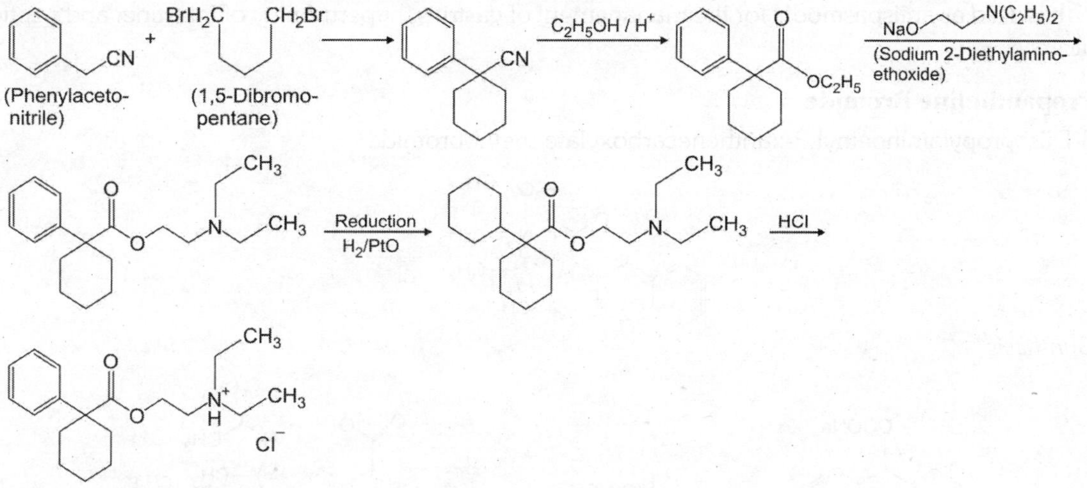

It is used as spasmolytic particularly for gastrointestinal tract.

Methantheline Bromide

Diethyl (2-hydroxyethyl) methylammonium-bromide xanthene-9-carboxylate

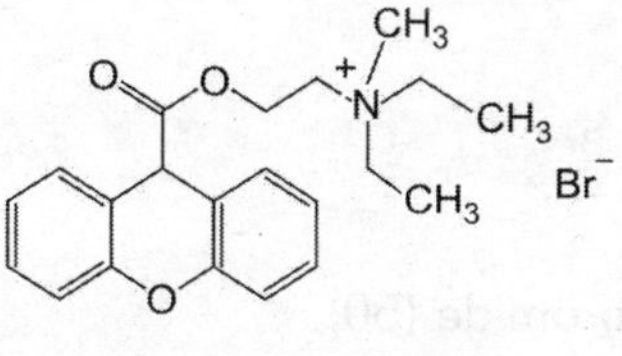

Synthesis

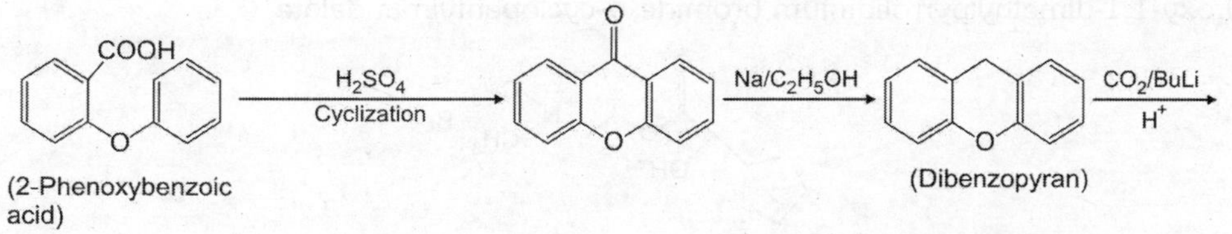

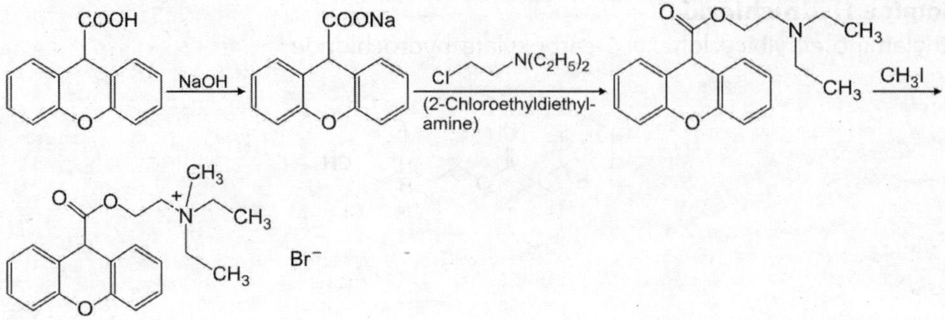

It is used as antispasmodic for the management of gastritis, hypermotility of intestine, and peptic ulcers.

Propantheline Bromide

β-Diisopropylaminoethyl 9-xanthenecarboxylate methobromide

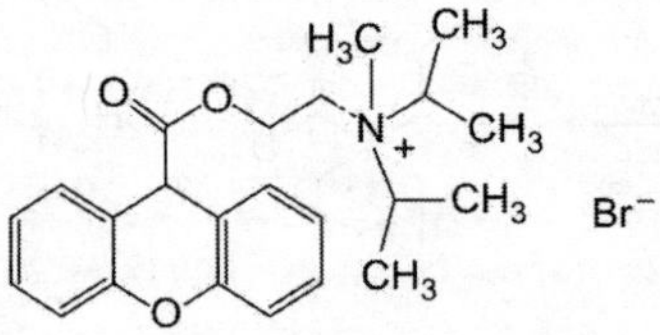

Synthesis

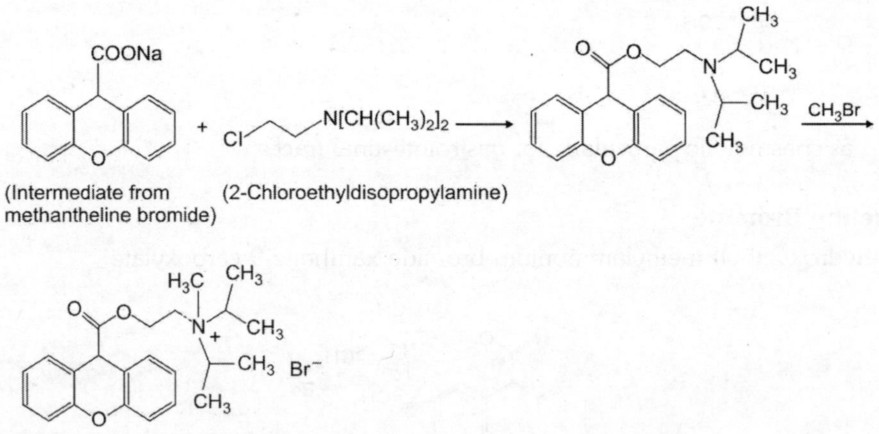

(Intermediate from   (2-Chloroethyldiisopropylamine)
methantheline bromide)

Same activity as methantheline bromide (50).

Glycopyrrolate

3-Hydroxy-1,1-dimethylpyrrolidinium bromide α-cyclopentylmandelate

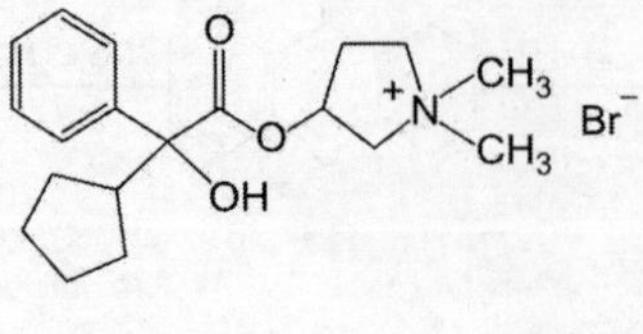

Synthesis

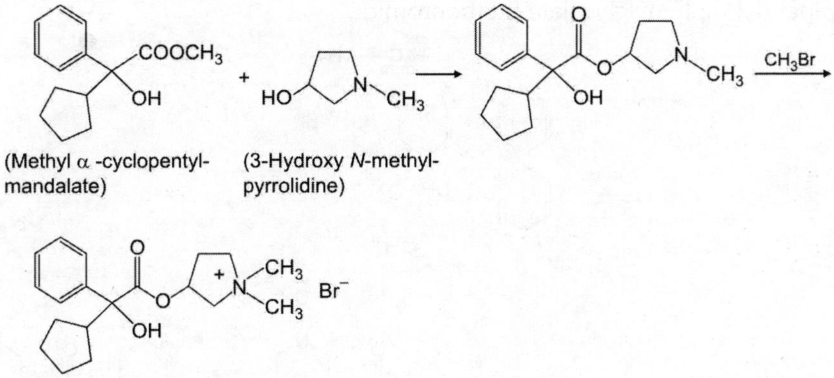

(Methyl α -cyclopentyl-mandalate)

(3-Hydroxy *N*-methyl-pyrrolidine)

It is used in gastrointestinal ailments particularly in peptic ulcers and in hyperacidity. It is a good antispasmodic and has fewer side effects. It rarely causes CNS disturbances because it cannot pass the blood-brain barrier.

Polidine Methylsulphate

2-Benziloyloxymethyl-1, 1-dimethylpyrrolidinium methyl sulphate

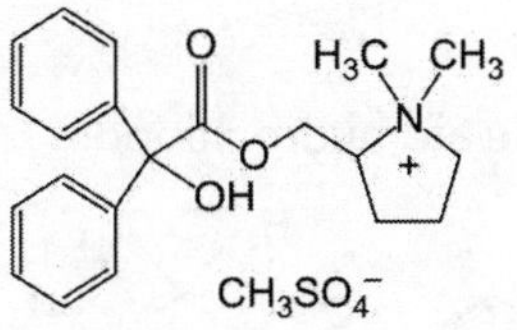

Synthesis

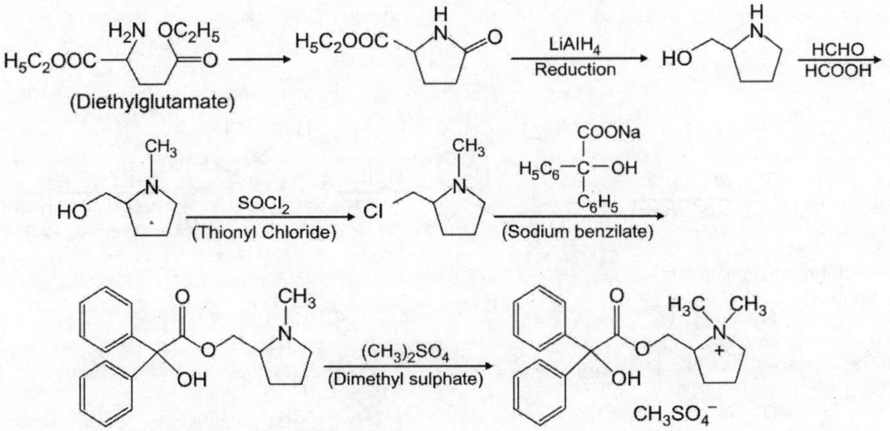

(Diethylglutamate)

(Thionyl Chloride)

(Sodium benzilate)

(Dimethyl sulphate)

It has similar activity as glycopyrrolate (52). It is used in gastrointestinal disorders and as an adjunct in management of peptic ulcers.

Mepenzolate Bromide

N-Methyl-3-piperidyl diphenylglycolate methobromide

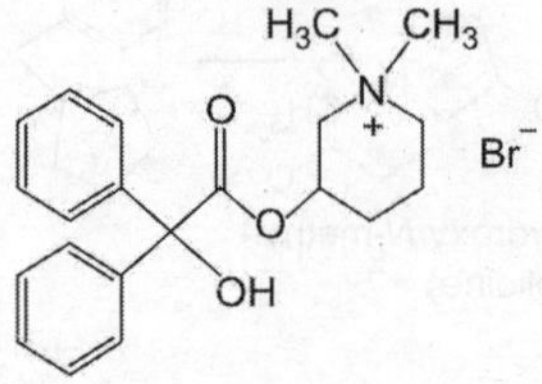

Synthesis

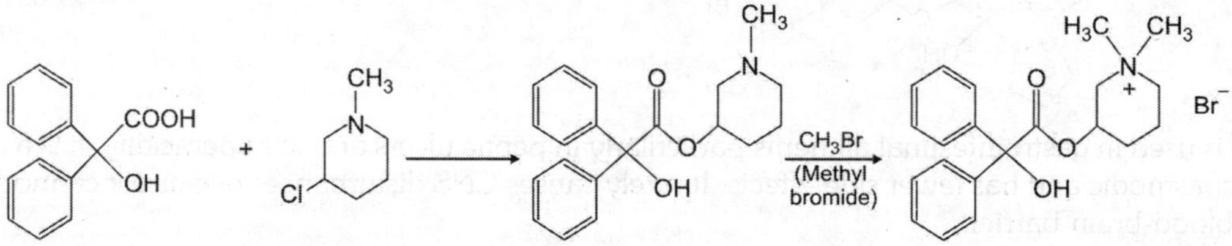

(Benzillic acid)   (1-Methyl-3-chl-
oropiperidine)

It is used for selective action in colonic hypermotility and as antispasmodic

Eucatropine Hydrochloride

1,2,2,6-Tetramethyl-4-piperidyl mandelate hydrochloride.

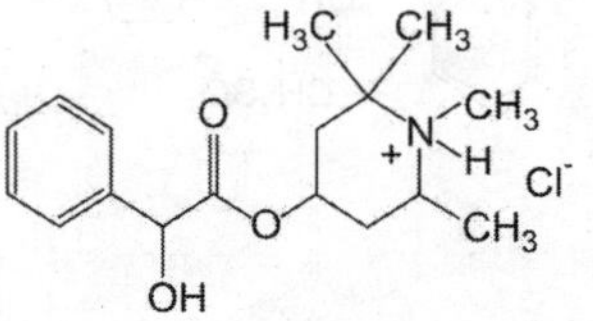

Synthesis

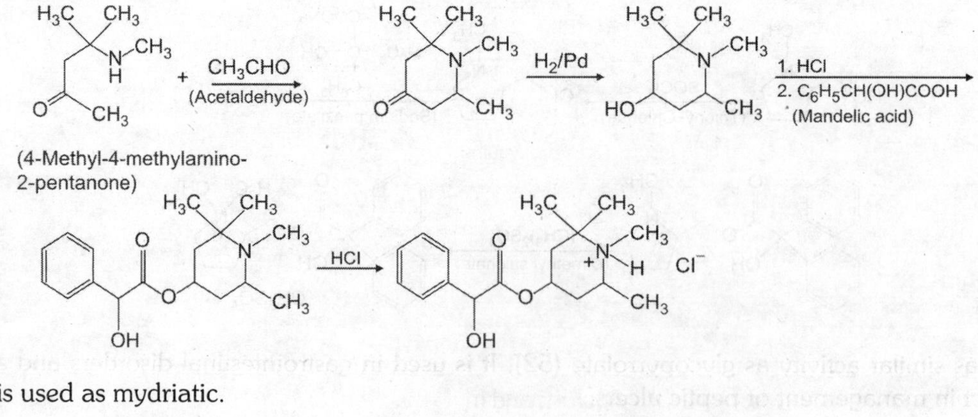

(4-Methyl-4-methylamino-
2-pentanone)

It is used as mydriatic.

Oxyphencyclimine Hydrochloride

1,4,5,6-Tetrahydro-1-methyl-2-pyrimidinylmethyl-α-phenylcyclohexaneglycolate mono-hydrochloride

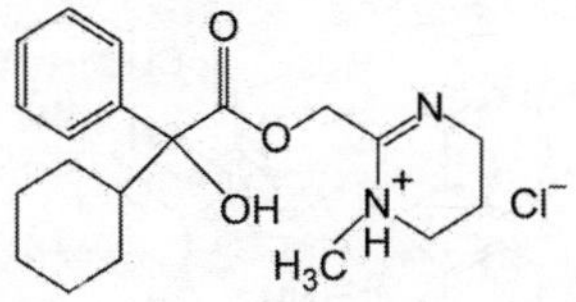

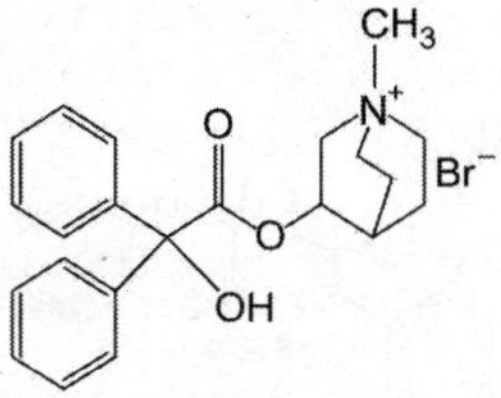

Synthesis

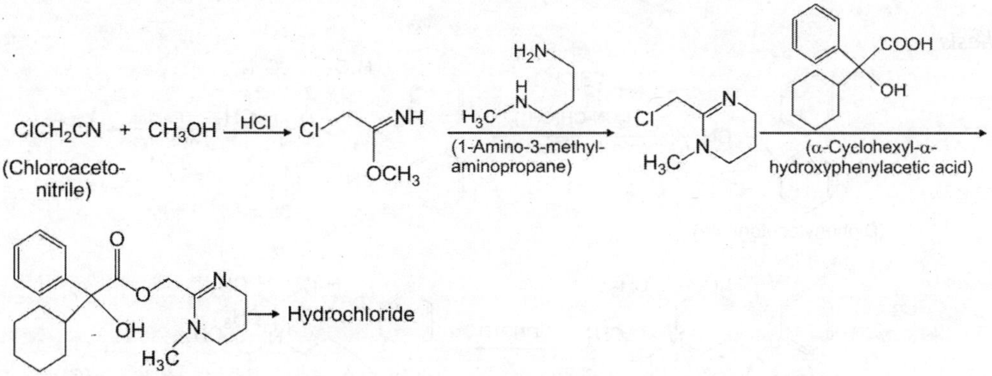

It is used in peptic ulcer. It reduces the volume and acid content of gastric juice.

Clidinium Bromide

3-Hydroxy-1-methylquinuclidinium bromide benzilate

Synthesis

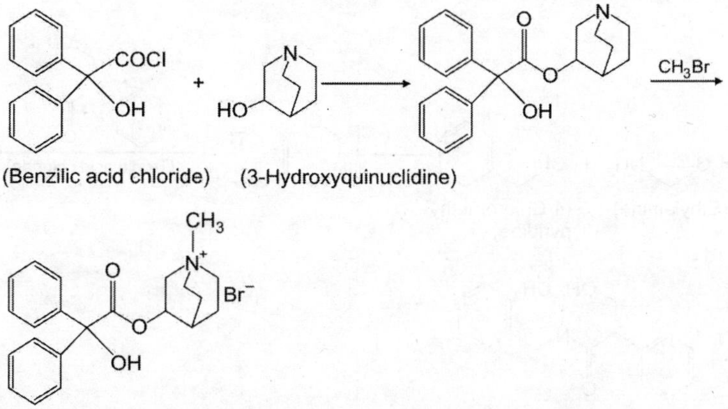

(Benzilic acid chloride) (3-Hydroxyquinuclidine)

It is used in peptic ulcers, ulcerative colon, and in irritable colon along with an antianxiety agent.

PARASYMPATHOLYTICS : AMINOAMIDES

Isopropamide Iodide

(3-Carbamoyl-3, 3-diphenylpropyl)diisopropylmethylammonium iodide

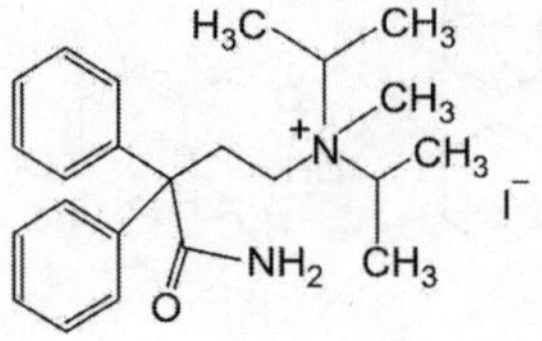

Synthesis

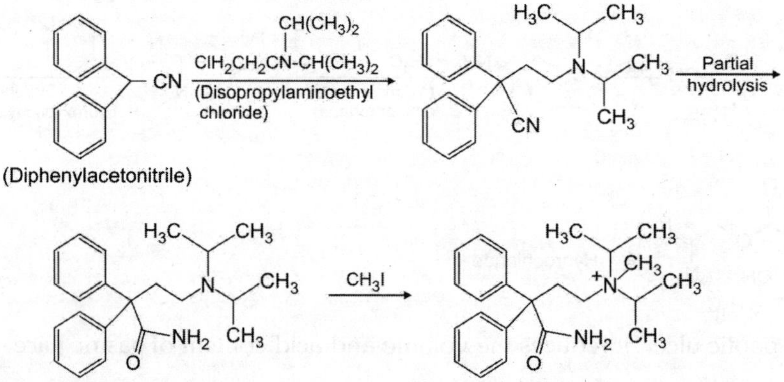

(Diphenylacetonitrile)

It is used in combination with other drugs for the treatment of peptic ulcers and in condition of gastrointestinal hypermotility.

Tropicamide

N-Ethyl-*N*-(4-pyridinylmethyl)-tropamide

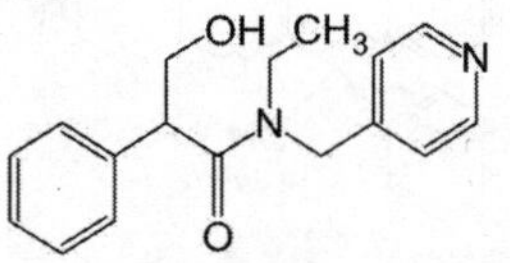

Synthesis

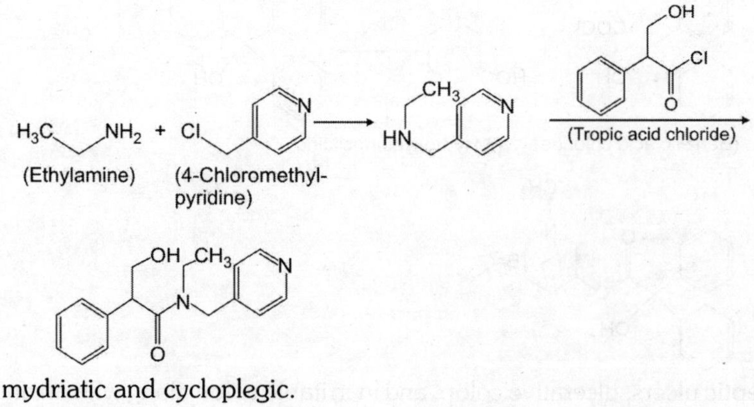

(Ethylamine)   (4-Chloromethyl-
                    pyridine)

It is used as mydriatic and cycloplegic.

Metoclopramide

4-Amino-5-chloro-*N*-[(2-diethylamino) ethyl]-2-methoxybenzamide

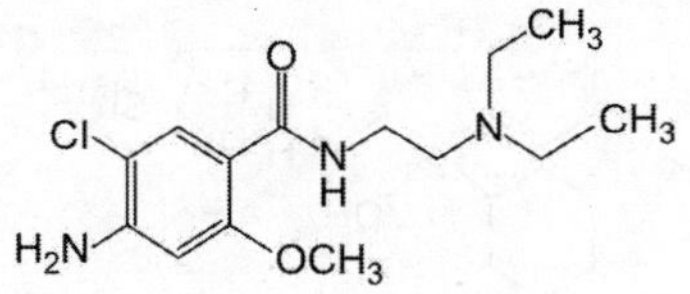

Synthesis

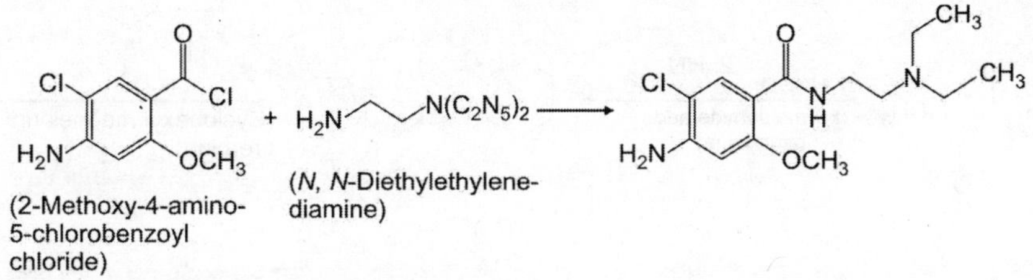

(2-Methoxy-4-amino-
5-chlorobenzoyl
chloride)

(*N, N*-Diethylethylene-
diamine)

It is used as antispasmodic and antiemetic

PARASYMPATHOLYTICS: AMINOALCOHOLS

Tridihexethyl Chloride

(3-Cyclohexyl-3-hydroxy-3-phenylpropyl)triethylammonium chloride

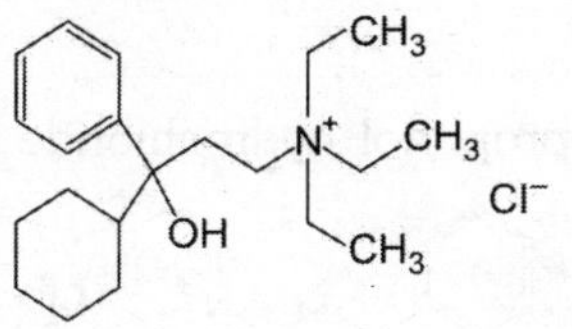

Synthesis

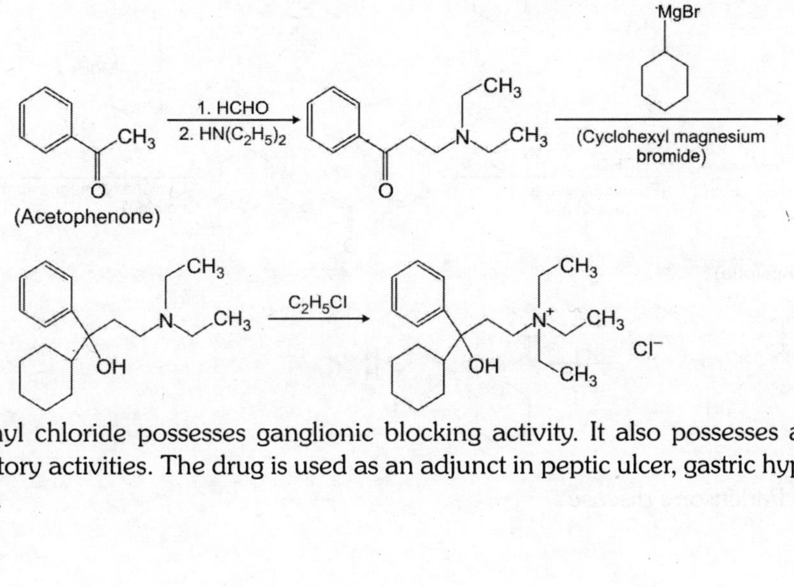

(Acetophenone)

1. HCHO
2. HN(C_2H_5)$_2$

(Cyclohexyl magnesium
bromide)

C_2H_5Cl

Tridihexethyl chloride possesses ganglionic blocking activity. It also possesses antispasmodic and antisecretory activities. The drug is used as an adjunct in peptic ulcer, gastric hyperacidity and hypermotility.

Procyclidine Hydrochloride

α-Cyclohexyl-α-phenyl-1-pyrrolidinepropanol hydrochloride

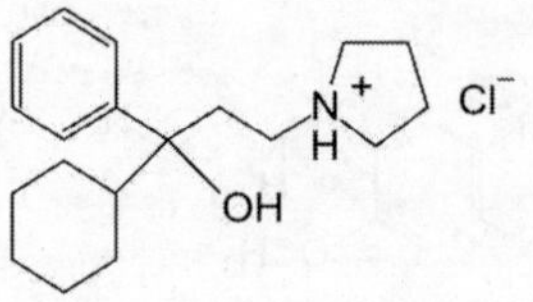

Synthesis

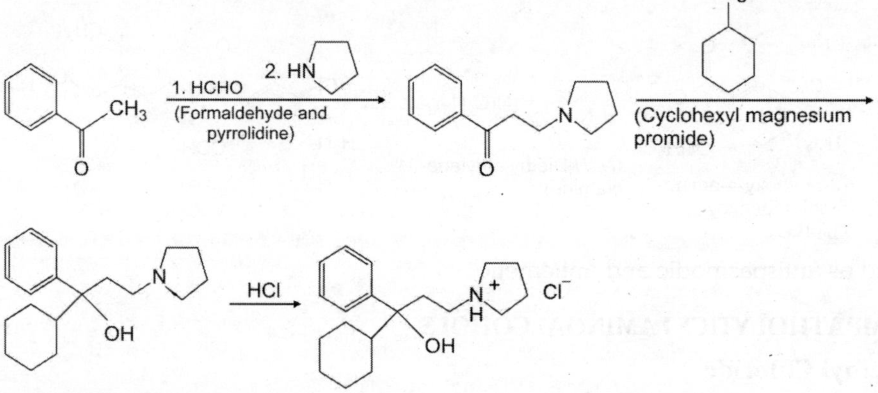

It is used in Parkinson's disease.

Trihexyphenidyl Hydrochloride

α-Cyclohexyl-α-phenyl-1-piperidinepropanol hydrochloride

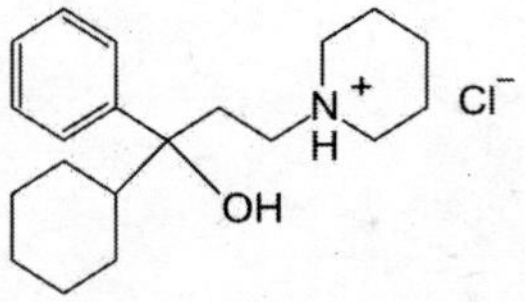

Synthesis

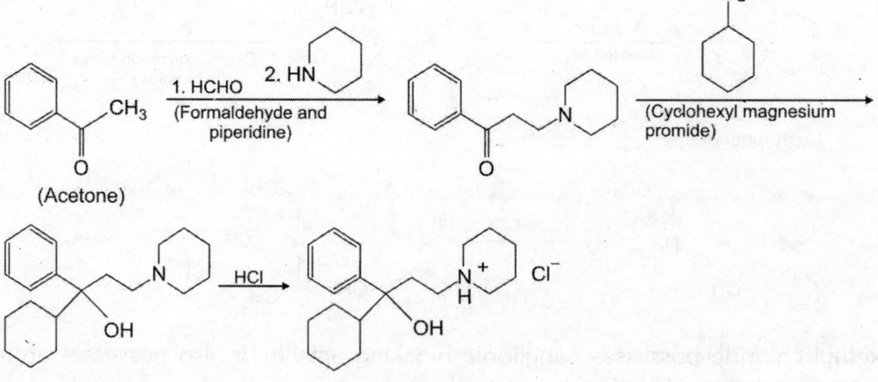

It is used in Parkinson's disease.

Biperiden

α–5-Norbornen-2yl-α-phenyl-1-piperidinepropanol

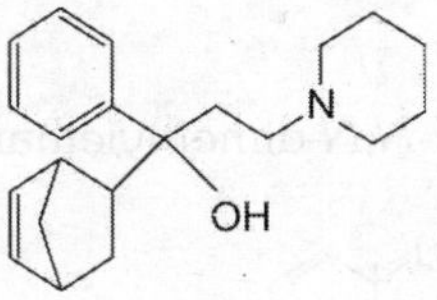
N
OH

Synthesis

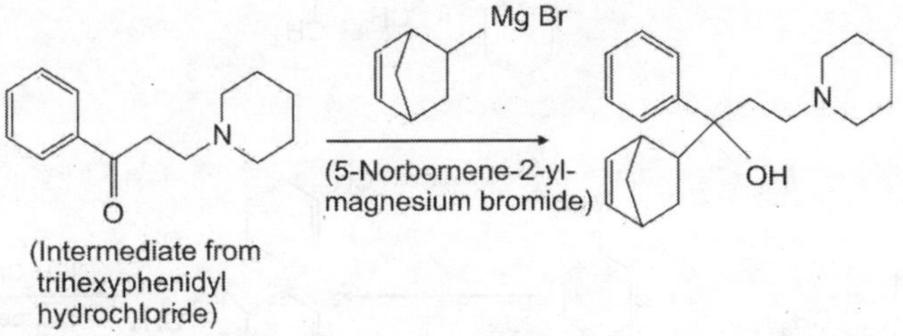
Mg Br
N
O
(Intermediate from trihexyphenidyl hydrochloride)
(5-Norbornene-2-yl-magnesium bromide)
N
OH

It has a strong musculotropic action which is nearly same as papaverine (73). It is used in Parkinson's disease.

PARASYMPATHOLYTICS : AMINOETHERS

Benztropine Mesylate

3α–(Diphenylmethoxy)-1α*H*,5α*H*-tropane methanesulphonate

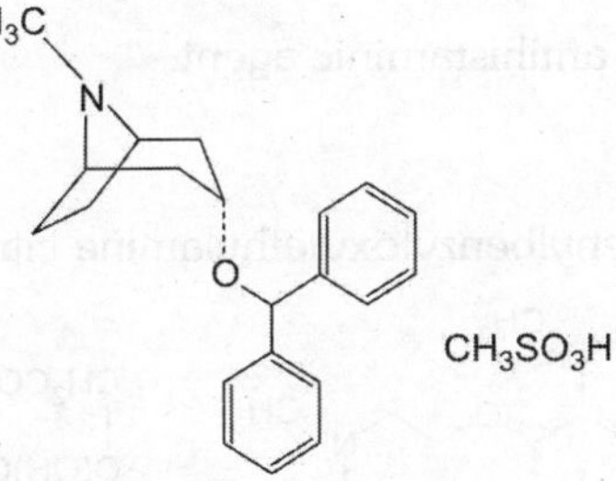
H3C
N
O
CH3SO3H

Synthesis

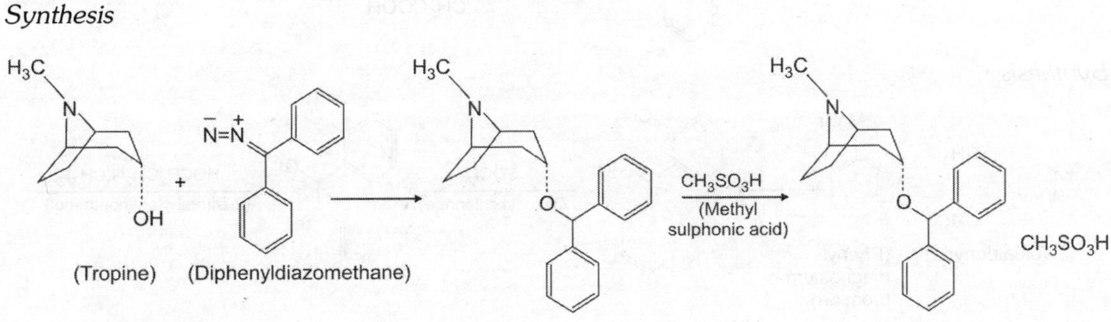
H3C
N
OH
(Tropine)
N=N
+
(Diphenyldiazomethane)
H3C
N
O
CH3SO3H
(Methyl sulphonic acid)
H3C
N
O
CH3SO3H

It possesses anticholinergic, antihistaminic, and local anesthetic activities. It is used in Parkinson's disease. It has sedative action because of its antihistaminic property.

Chlorphenoxamine

2[1-(4-Chlorophenyl)-1-phenylethoxy]-*N,N*-dimethylethanamine

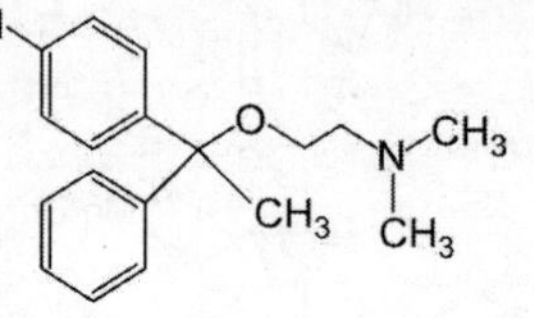

Synthesis

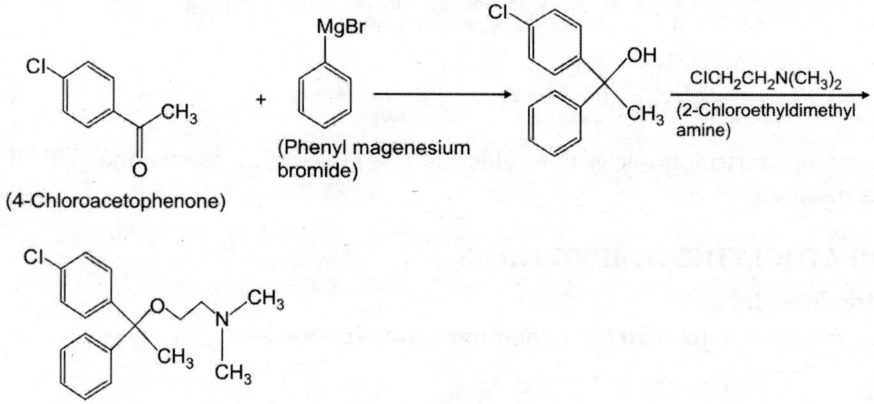

It has been found useful as an antihistaminic agent.

Orphenadrine Citrate

N, N-Dimethyl-2-(*o*-methyl-α phenylbenzyloxy)ethylamine citrate

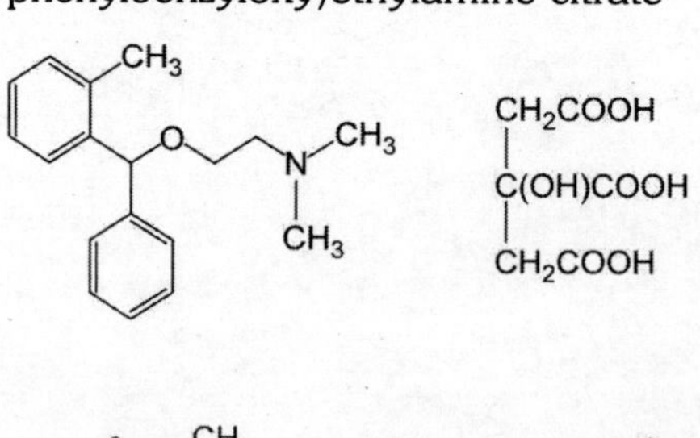

Synthesis

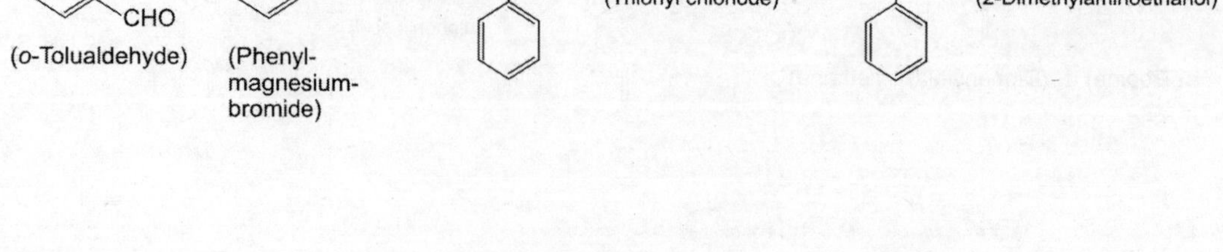

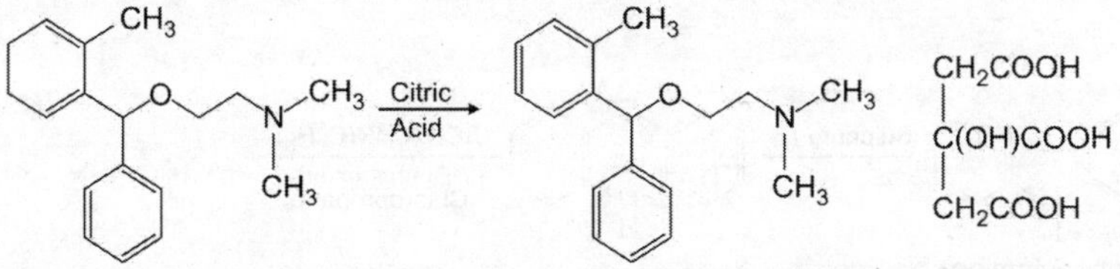

It is used in Parkinson's disease along with other drugs. It is also used to relieve the pain of muscle spasm.

PARASYMPATHOLYTICS : MISCELLANEOUS COMPOUNDS

Diphemanil Methylsulphate

4-(Diphenylmethylene)-1,1-dimethylpiperidinium methyl sulphate

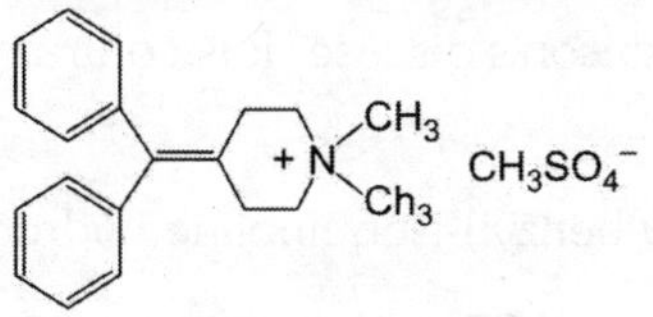

Synthesis

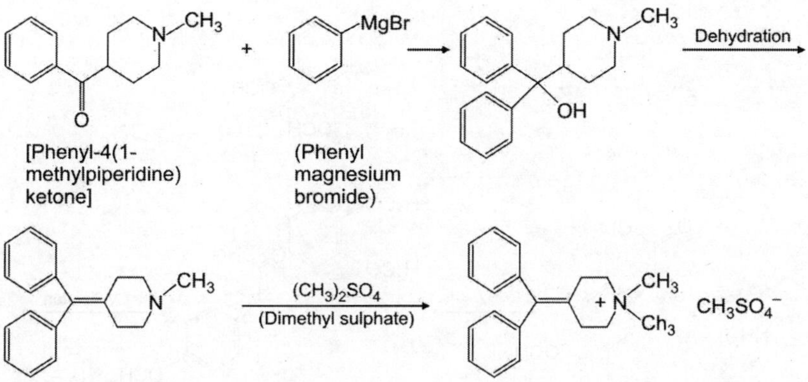

[Phenyl-4(1-methylpiperidine) ketone]

(Phenyl magnesium bromide)

(CH$_3$)$_2$SO$_4$
(Dimethyl sulphate)

It has a highly specific action on gastrointestinal tract and is used in peptic ulcer.

Ethopropazine Hydrochloride

10-(2-Diethylaminopropyl)phenothiazine hydrochloride

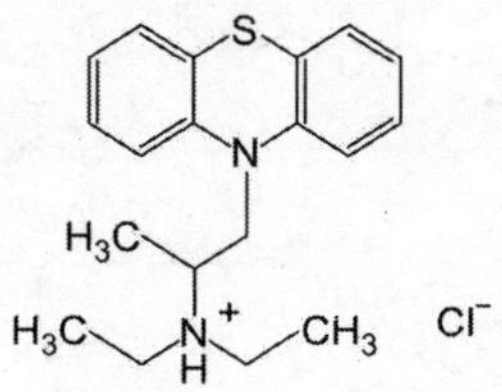

Synthesis

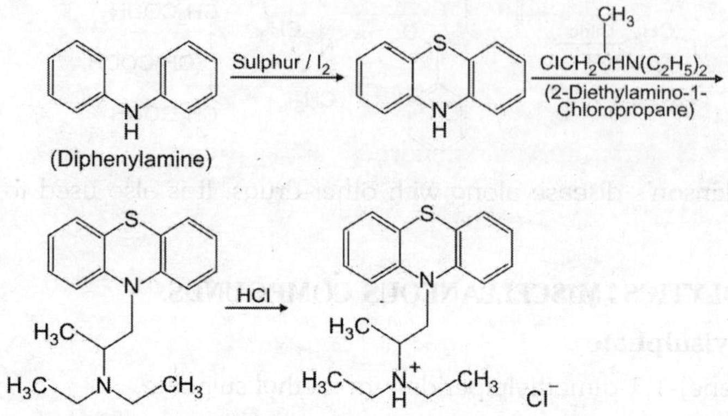

(Diphenylamine)

It has been found useful in Parkinson's disease. It is contraindicated in glaucoma.

Papaverine Hydrochloride

6, 7-Dimethoxy-1-(3, 4-dimethoxy benzyl)-isoquinoline hydrochloride

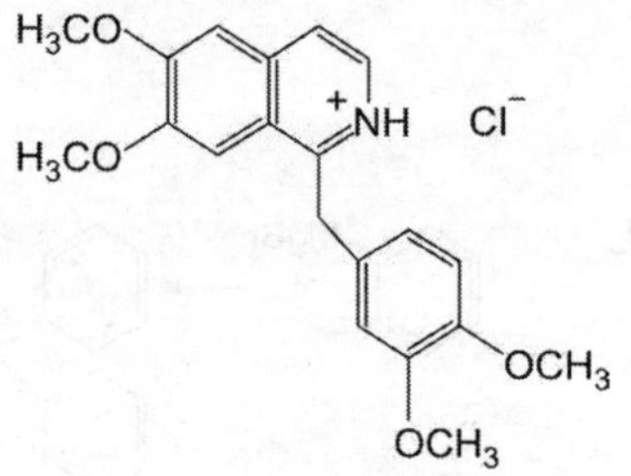

Synthesis

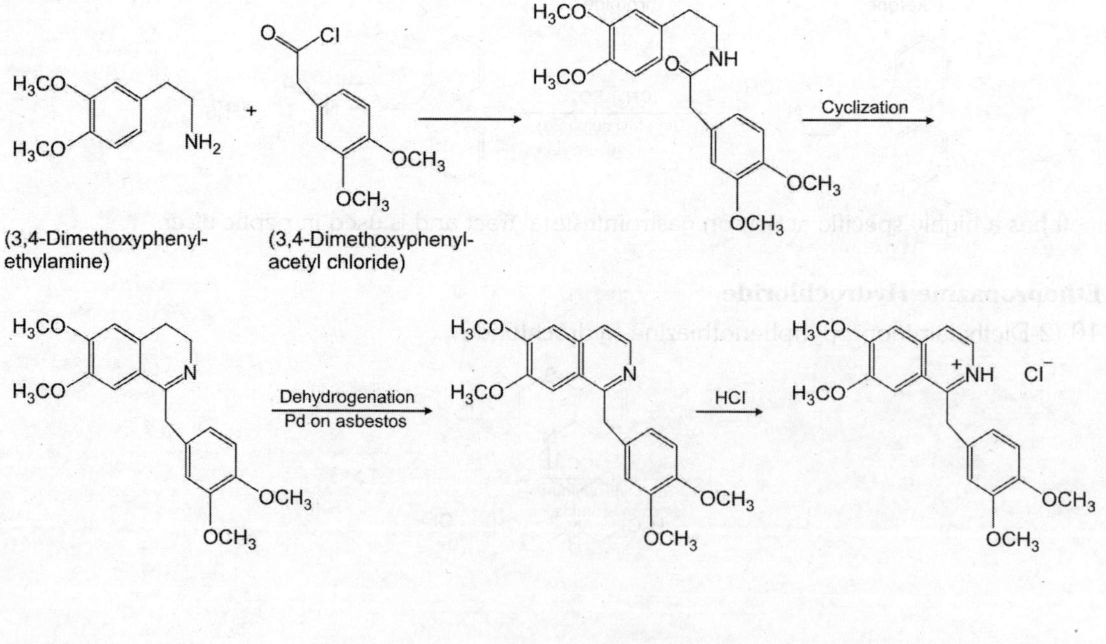

(3,4-Dimethoxyphenyl-ethylamine)

(3,4-Dimethoxyphenyl-acetyl chloride)

It has spasmolytic activity on gastrointestinal tract as well as on blood vessels. It is useful in relieving of arterial spasm and also in treatment of peripheral, coronary, and pulmonary occlusion.

GANGLIONIC BLOCKING AGENTS

Mecamylamine Hydrochloride

N, 2, 3, 3-Tetramethyl-2-norbornanamine hydrochloride

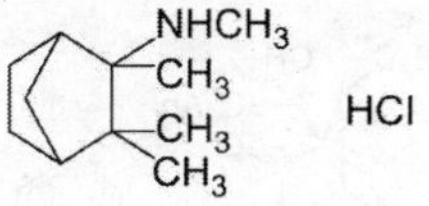

Synthesis

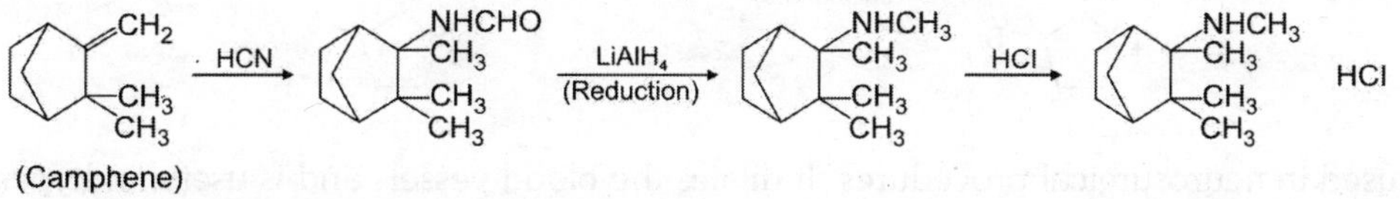

It is indicated in malignant hypertension.

Trimethaphan Camsylate

(+)–1, 3-Dibenzyldecahydro-2-oxoimidazo[4, 5-c]thieno[1, 2-α]-thiolium 2-oxo-10-bornane sulphonate

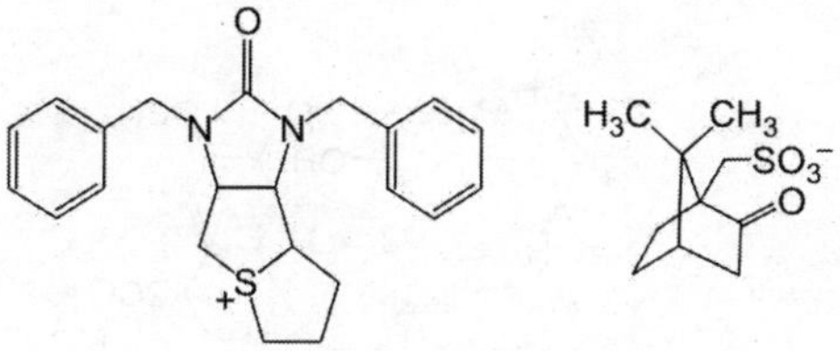

Synthesis

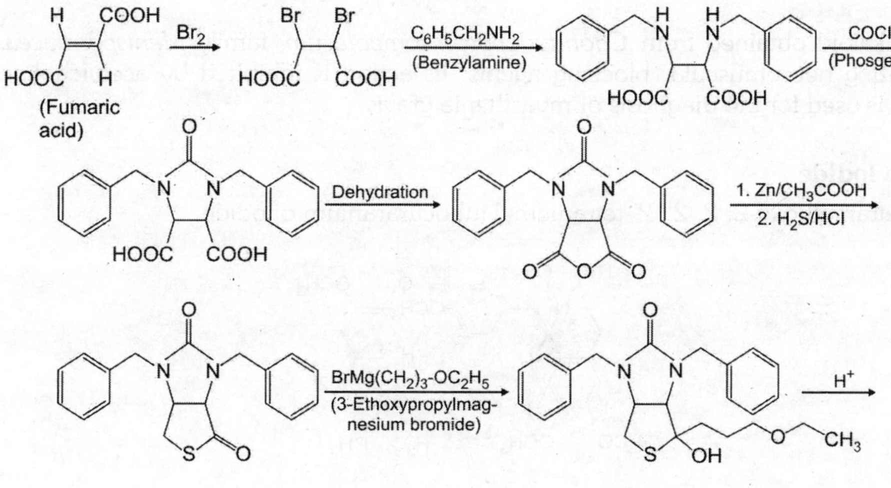

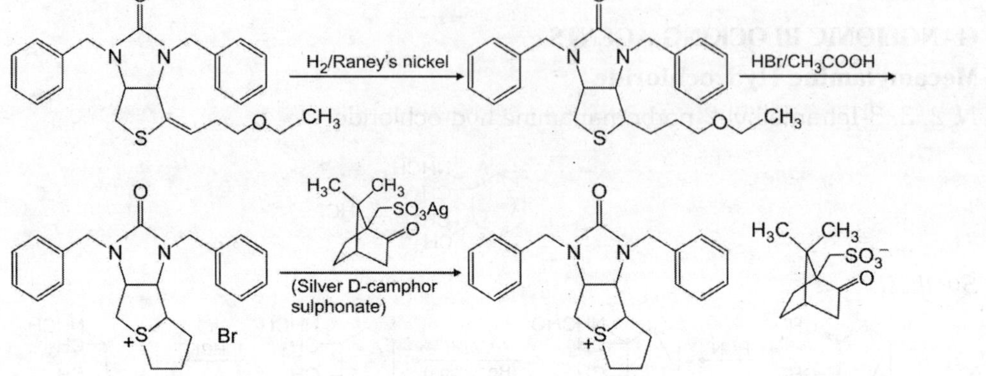

It is used in neurosurgical procedures. It dilates the blood vessels and is useful in hypertensive control.

NEUROMUSCULAR BLOCKING AGENTS : NONDEPOLARIZING

Tubocurarine Chloride

7', 12'-Dihydroxy-6, 6'-dimethoxy-2, 2', 2'-trimethyltubocurarinium chloride hydrochloride

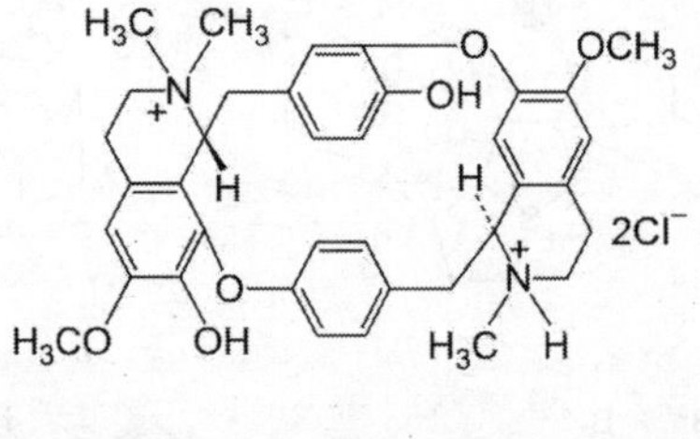

It is an alkaloid obtained from *Chondodendron tomentosum*, family *Menispermacea*. It is a nondepolarizing neuromuscular blocking agents. Its action is inhibited by acetylcholinesterase inhibitors. It is used for the diagnosis of myasthenia gravis.

Metocurine Iodide

6,6',7',12'-Tetramethoxy-2, 2, 2', 2'-tetramethyl tubocuraranium diiodide

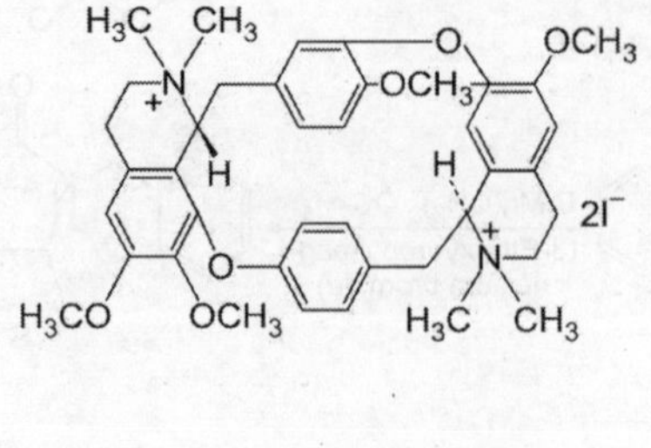

It has similar pharmacological action as tubocurarine chloride (80) but is much more potent than it,

Gallamine Triethiodide

1,2,3-Tris(2-triethylamonium ethoxy) benzene triiodide

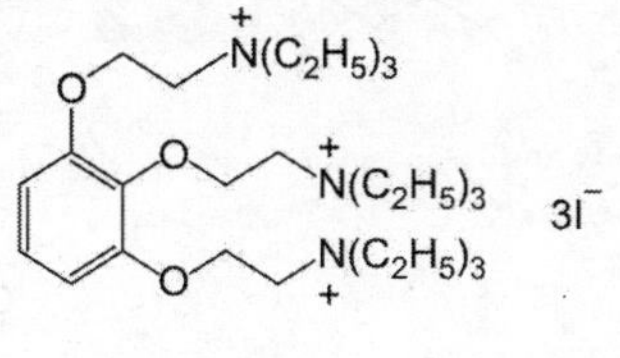

Synthesis

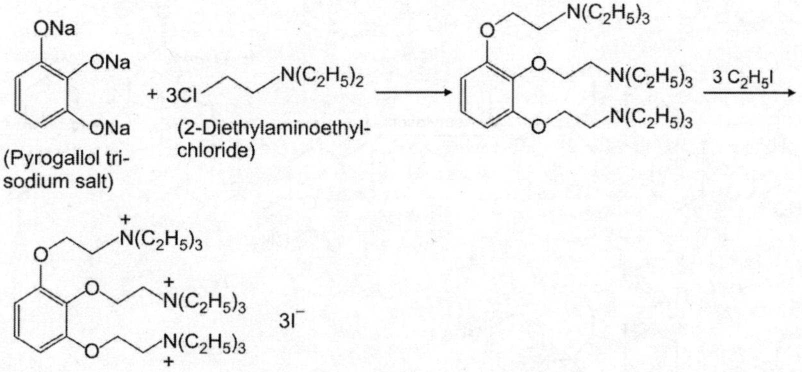

It is used as muscle relaxant for both surgical and non-surgical procedures. It has a little or no effect on autonomic ganglia. It is contraindicated in myasthenia gravis.

Pancuronium Bromide

1,1'-(3α, 17β-Dihydroxy-5α-androstan-2β, 16β-ylene)bis(1-methylpiperidinium) dibromide diacetate

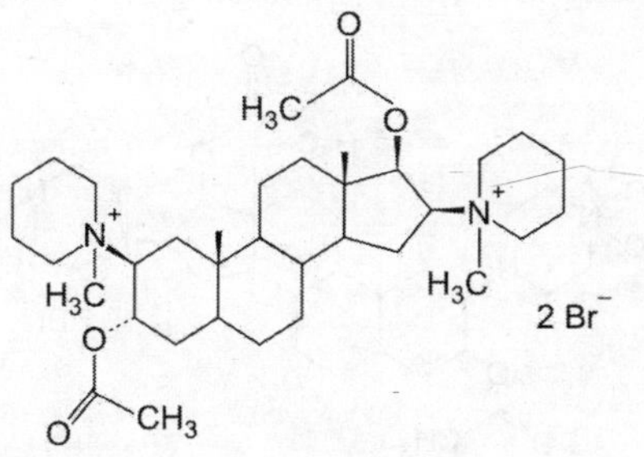

Synthesis

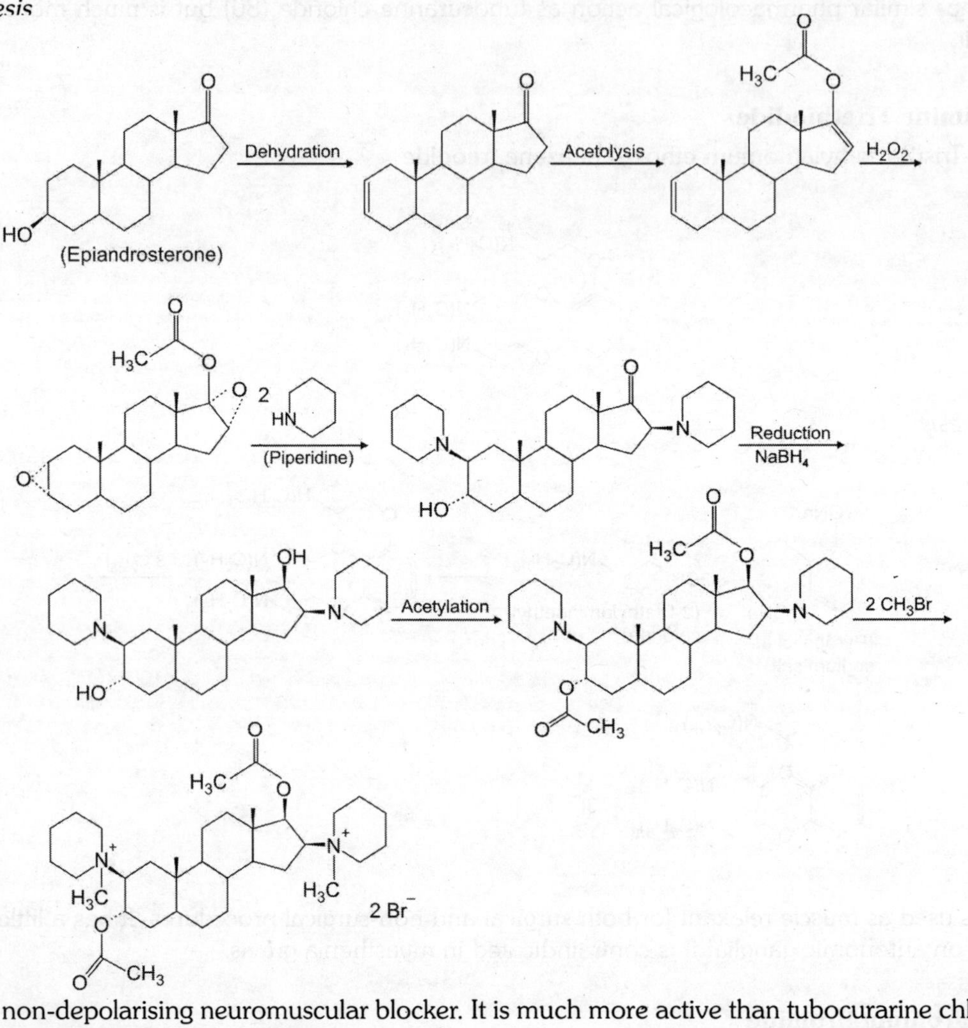

(Epiandrosterone)

Dehydration

Acetolysis

H_2O_2

2

HN

(Piperidine)

Reduction
$NaBH_4$

Acetylation

2 CH_3Br

2 Br⁻

It is non-depolarising neuromuscular blocker. It is much more active than tubocurarine chloride (80) with similar duration of action.

Pipecurium Bromide

4,4'-(3α, 17β-Dihydroxy-5α-androstan-2β, 16β-ylene) bis (1, 1-dimethyl piperazinium) dibromide diacetate

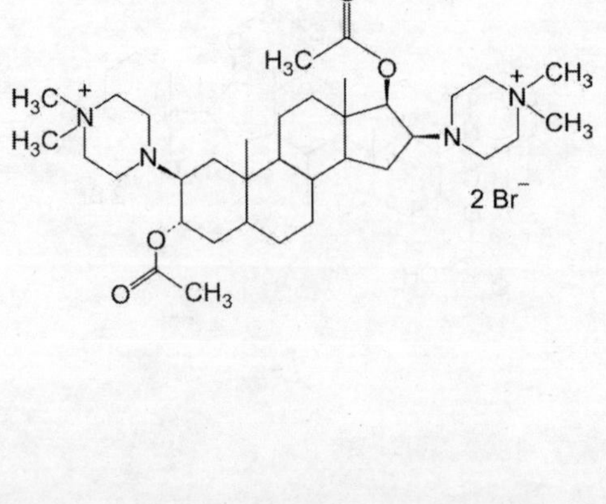

2 Br⁻

Synthesis

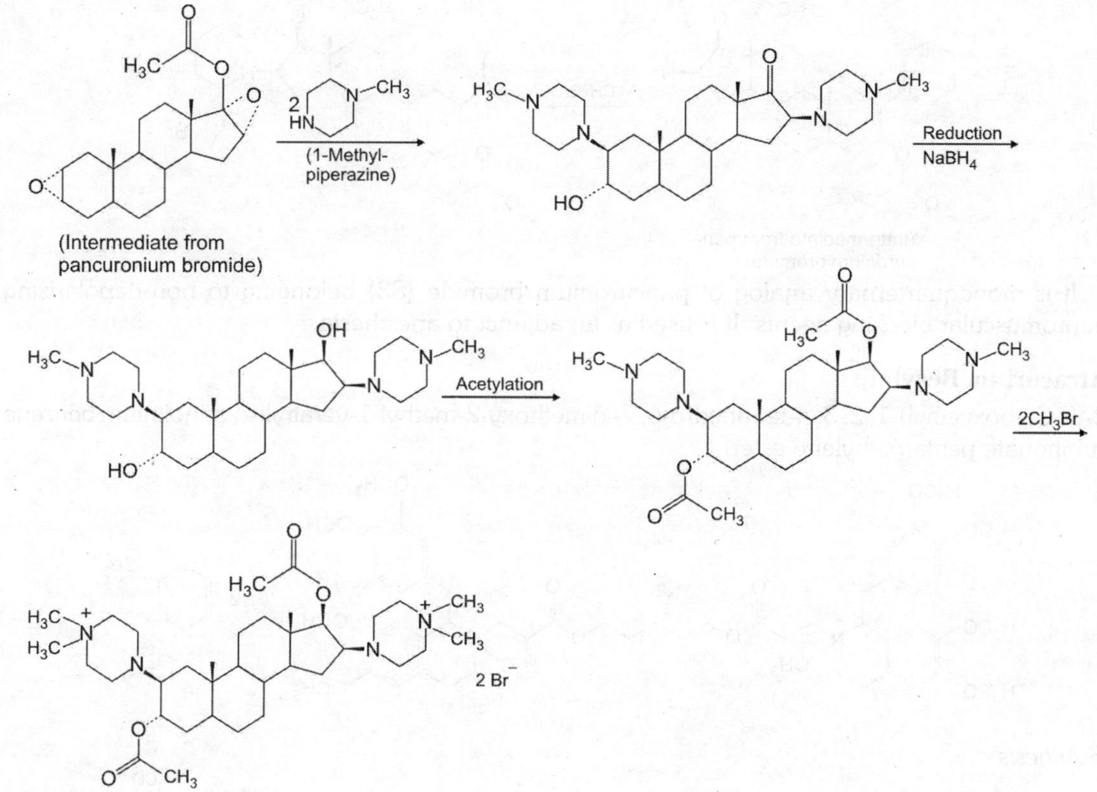

(Intermediate from
pancuronium bromide)

It is a long acting muscle relaxant and is used as an adjunct to anesthesia.

Vecuronium Bromide

1-[(2β,3α,5α,16β,17β)-3,17-bis(acetyloxy)-2-(1-piperdinyl)androstan-16-yl)-1-methylpiperidinium
bromide

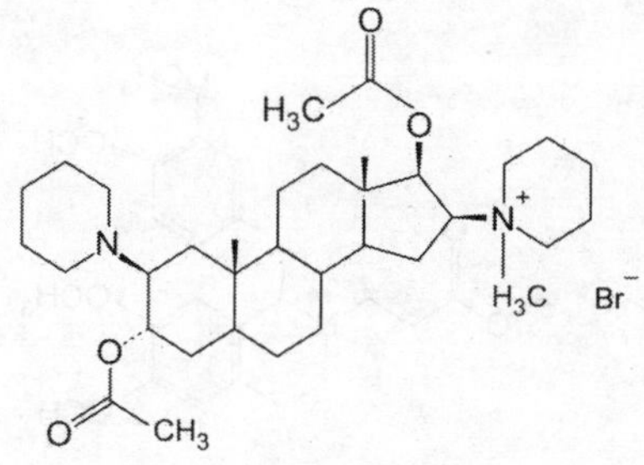

Synthesis

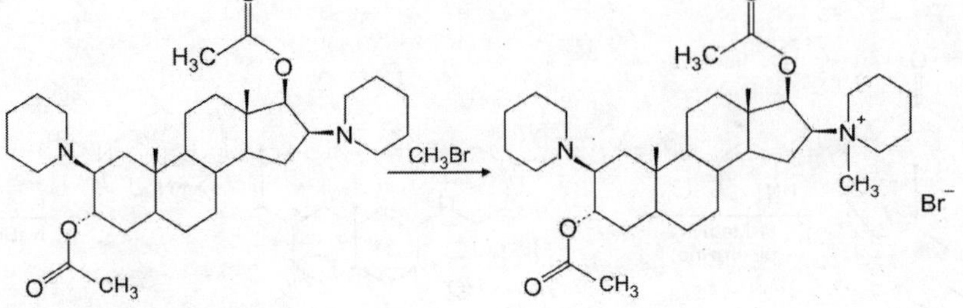
H3C
O
O
N
N
CH3Br
N+
CH3
Br−
O
CH3

(Inttermediate from pan-
curonium bromide)

It is monoquarternary analog of pancuronium bromide (83) belonging to non-depolarizing neuromuscular blocking agents. It is used as an adjunct to anesthesia.

Atracurium Besylate

2-(2-Carboxyethyl)-1, 2, 3, 4-tetrahydro-6, 7- dimethoxy-2-methyl-1-veratrylisoquinolinium benzene sulphonate pentamethylene ester

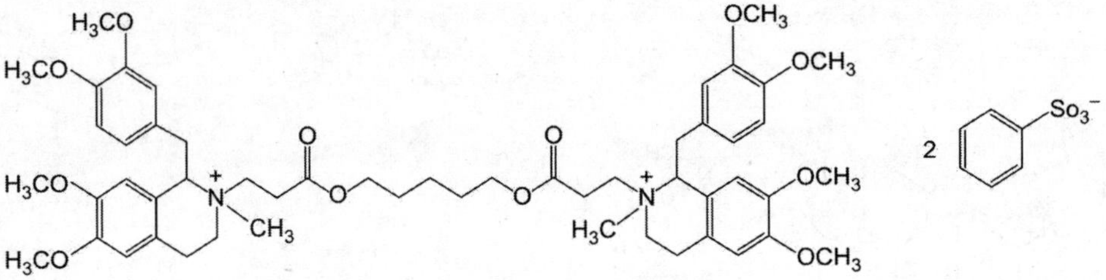
H3CO
OCH3
CH3
H3C
2
So3−

Synthesis

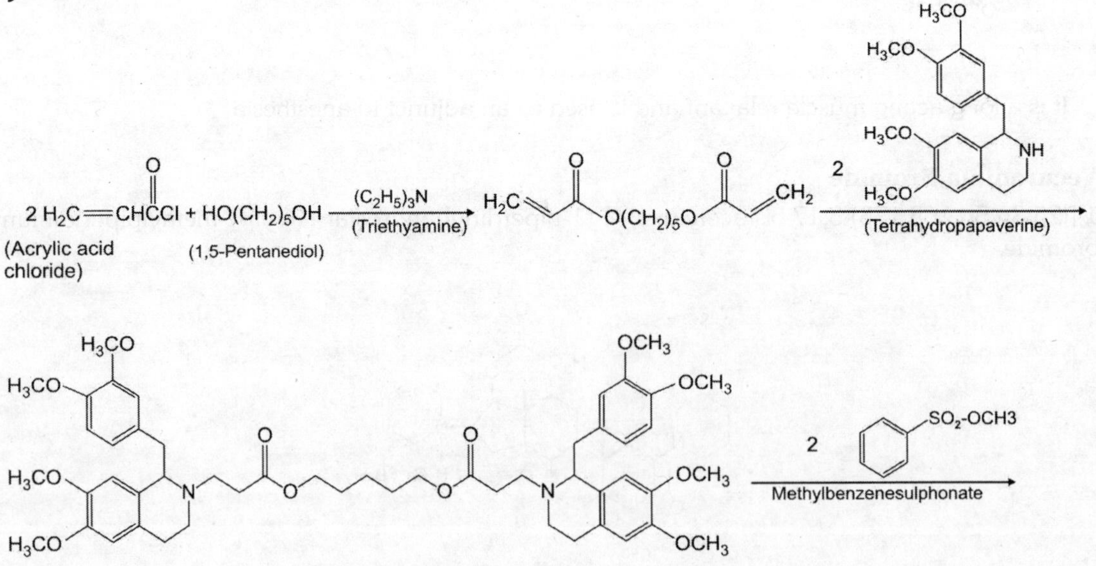
2 H2C=CHCCl + HO(CH2)5OH
(Acrylic acid
chloride)
(1,5-Pentanediol)
(C2H5)3N
(Triethyamine)
H2C
O(CH2)5O
CH2
2
(Tetrahydropapaverine)
NH
H3CO
OCH3
2
SO2-OCH3
Methylbenzenesulphonate

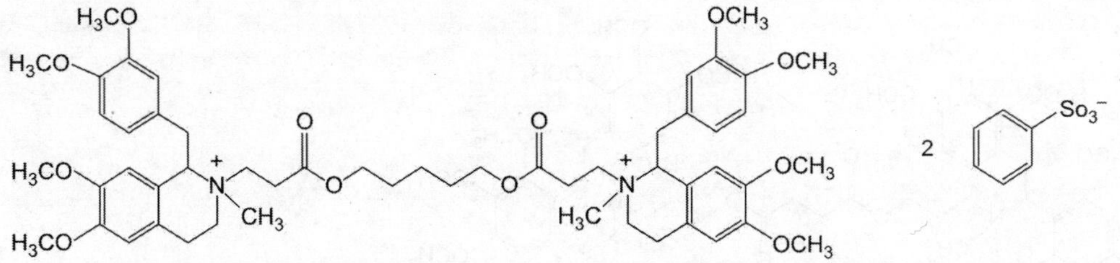

It is a non-depolarizing neuromuscular blocking agent. It is more potent than tubocurarine chloride (80).

Doxacurium Chloride

1,2,3,4-Tetrahydro-2-(3-hydroxypropyl)-6,7,8-trimethoxy-2-methyl-1-(3,4,5-trimethoxybenzyl) isoquinolinium chloride, succinate

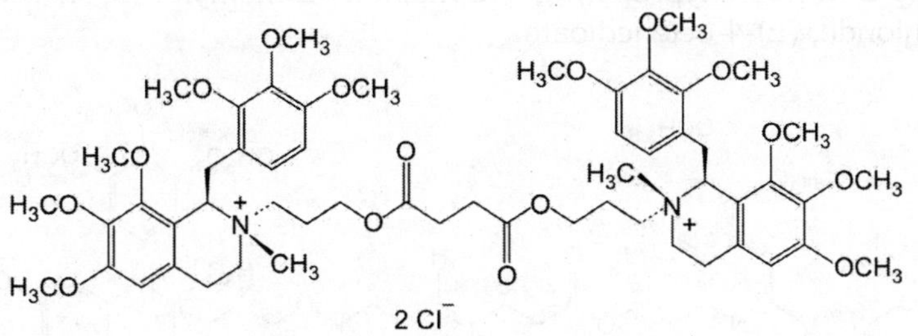

Synthesis

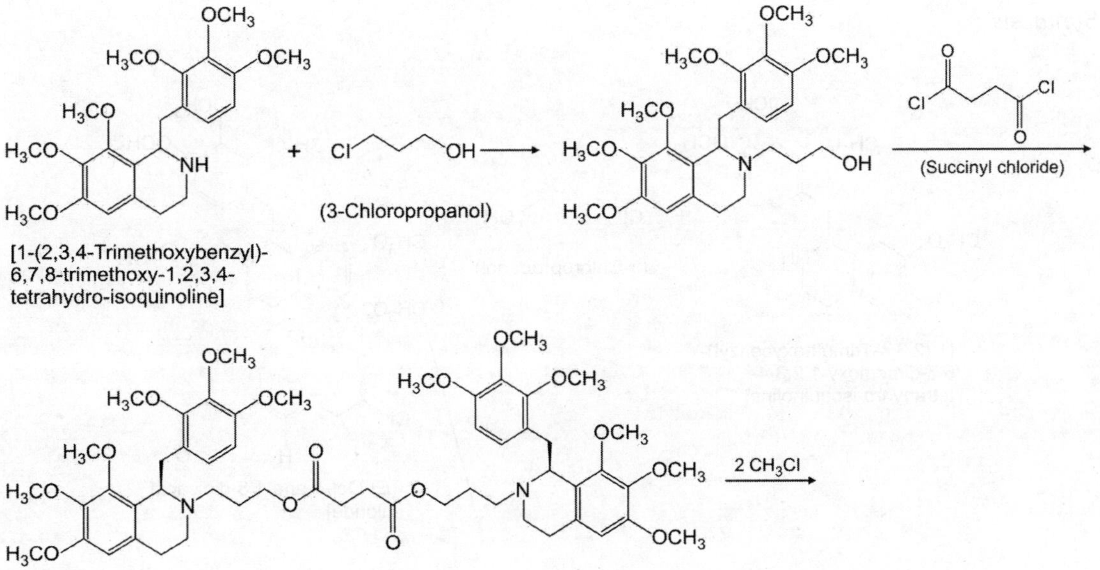

[1-(2,3,4-Trimethoxybenzyl)-
6,7,8-trimethoxy-1,2,3,4-
tetrahydro-isoquinoline]

(3-Chloropropanol)

(Succinyl chloride)

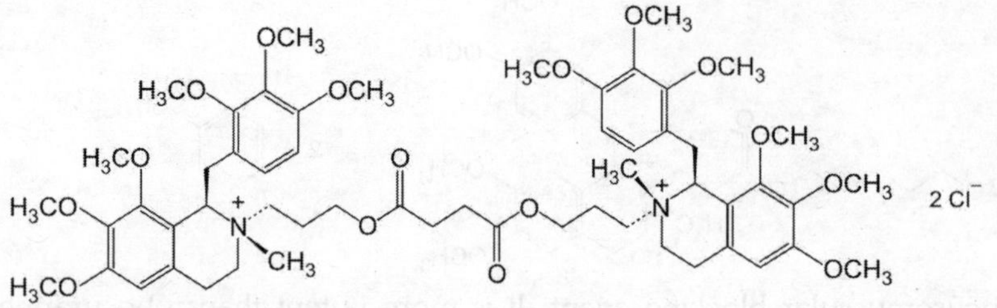

It is a long acting non-depolarizing neuromuscular blocking agent. It is used as skeletal muscle relaxant in surgical procedures.

Mivacurium Chloride

1,2,3,4-Tetrahydro-2-(3-hydroxypropyl)-6, 7-dimethoxy-2-methyl-1-(3, 4, 5-trimethoxybenzyl) isoquinolinium chloride, (*E*)-4-octenedioate

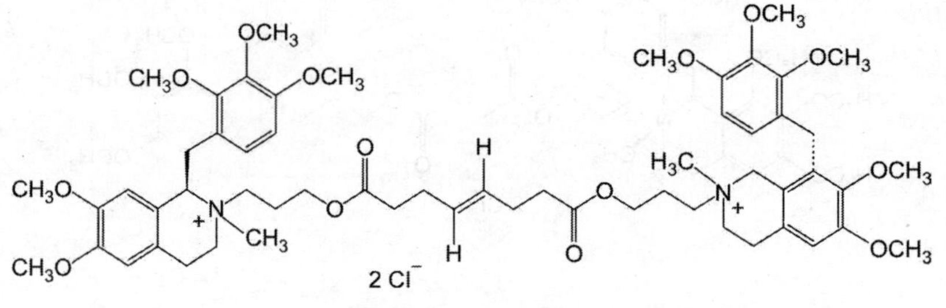

Synthesis

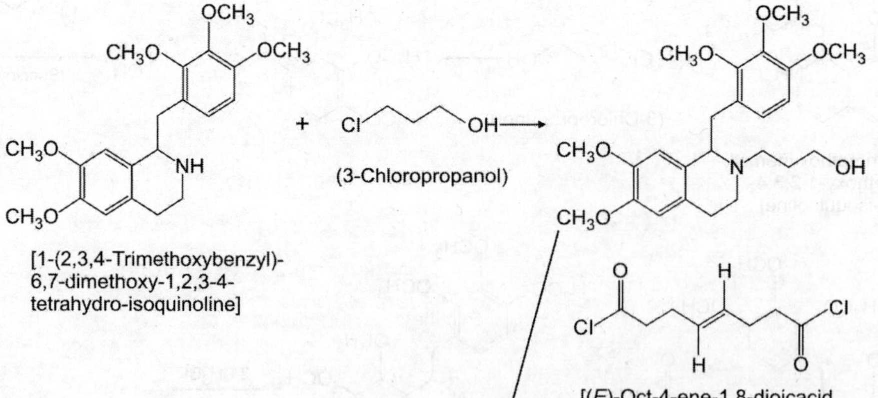

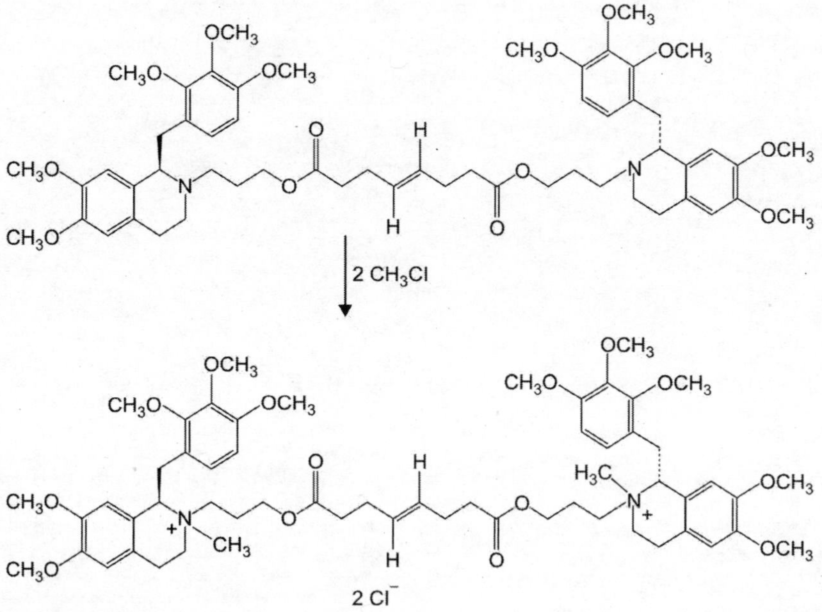

It is a short acting non-depolarizing drug used as an adjunct to anesthesia as a muscle relaxant.

NEUROMUSCULAR BLOCKING AGENTS : DEPOLARIZING

Suxamethonium Chloride

Succinylcholine chloride

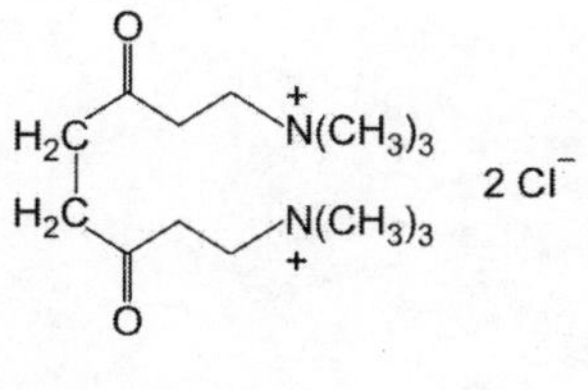

Synthesis

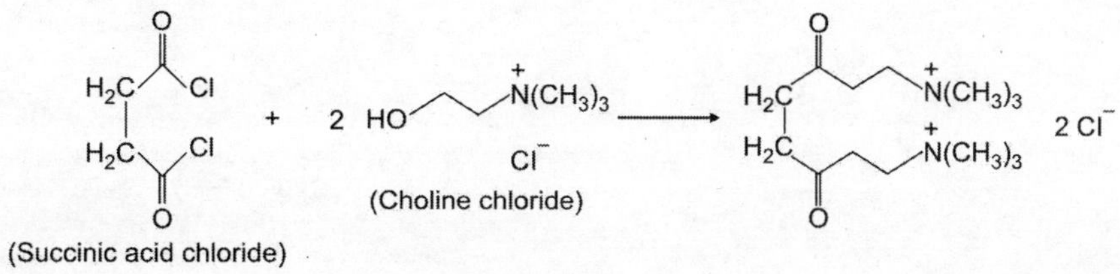

It has a short duration of action because of its hydrolysis by cholinesterases. It brings about typical muscular paralysis caused by blocking of nervous transmission at the myoneural junction. It is used as muscle relaxant for surgical procedures.

Section II
Drugs Affecting Central Nervous System

GENERAL ANESTHETICS

THE TERM "ANESTHESIA" is Greek word, literally meaning "insensitivity" or "without perception". "Narcosis", also Greek word, means a state of profound stupor (condition of insensibility) and indicates effects ranging from light sleep to unconsciousness.

Anesthetics are depressant drugs that affect vital functions of all types of cells especially those of nervous tissue. They depress central nervous system to such an extent that sensitivity to pain is abolished and the person suffers loss of consciousness. When applied to specific structures of central nervous system, particularly spinal cord, they block impulses transmitted by nerve fibers emanating from the region involved. Thus, they may be used as block anesthetics, to desensitise certain regions of the body. When peripheral endings are involved, local anesthetics are applied directly to a restricted area to abolish pain.

When used for surgical purposes general anesthetics produce analgesia, loss of consciousness, diminished reflex activity, and muscular relaxation with a minimal depression of vital functions of body.

General anesthetics may be classified as:

(a) Inhalation anesthetics also known as gaseous or volatile anesthetics, and

(b) intravenous anesthetics also known as fixed anesthetic.

Gaseous or volatile anesthetics are administered by respiratory route. They enter the bloodstream through lungs and quickly reach the central nervous system because of large amount of circulation. The rest of body is affected slowly because the tissues receive the required anesthetic concentration over a period of time. Therefore, the body serves as a buffer system, withdraws anesthetic slowly from the brains and retains it more consistently even after the brain tissue has given up the anesthetic.

The fixed or non-volatile anesthetics are administered parenterally or orally.

There are four stages of anesthesia and these are:

(a) Stage of analgesia,

(b) stage of delirium,

(c) stage of surgical anesthesia, and

(d) stage of medullary paralysis.

In the stage of analgesia, which constitutes the first stage, consciousness and sense of touch is retained. Loss of pain or analgesia is partial untill the second stage is reached.

In the second stage, there is loss of consciousness. It is characterized by excitement, irregular breathing, motor activity, susceptibility to external stimuli, and sympathetic discharge. It is terminated by relaxation.

The third stage is divided into four planes. In passing through these, there occurs progressive loss of reflexes, skeletal muscle relaxation, and depression of vital functions. This is the stage in which most of the operative procedures are carried out.

In the fourth stage which is overdosage, the vital function of the medulla and of brainstem are paralyzed. This stage may involve respiratory arrest and collapse of the vital motor functions and therefore, lead to death.

CHARACTERISTICS OF AN IDEAL ANESTHETIC

An ideal anesthetic should:

1. Cause pleasant induction without excitement or irritation. The patient should emerge from anesthesia without prolonged depression or other postoperative effects such as nausea and vomiting.
2. Have a pleasant odour, a wide margin of safety and low toxicity.
3. Be nonflammable, non-explosive, and stable so that it can be used in a closed system of an anesthetic machine with a carbon dioxide absorber.
4. Be devoid of adverse effects on vital functions such as respiration, cardiovascular system, liver, and kidney.
5. Be potent enough so that it can be used with high percentage of oxygen and should also be volatile enough so that it is exhaled immediately and excreted on removal of anesthetic mask.

INHALATION ANESTHETICS

INORGANIC
Nitrous Oxide
Dinitrogen monoxide

$$N_2O$$

Synthesis

$$NH_4NO_3 \longrightarrow N_2O + 2\,H_2O$$
(Ammonium nitrate)

Commonly known as laughing gas, it is obtained by heating ammonium nitrate to a temperature a little above its melting point. The reaction becomes explosive if the temperature is allowed to rise too high.

For surgical anesthesia, 80-85% is required with 15-20% oxygen for oxygenation of tissues.

HYDROCARBONS
Cyclopropane
Trimethylene

$$\triangle$$

Synthesis

$$\begin{array}{c} \text{CH}_2\text{Br} \\ \Big\langle \qquad\quad + \ \text{Zn} \longrightarrow \triangle \\ \text{CH}_2\text{Br} \end{array}$$
(Ethylene
bromide)

It is a colourless gas with an unpleasant odour. It is flammable and explodes when mixed with oxygen even in concentration as low as 3.8%. Surgical anesthesia is obtained following premedication with depressant drugs such as morphine or barbiturates with 15 volume percent cyclopropane and 85 volume percent oxygen. Induction of anesthesia is rapid requiring only 2 to 3 min. It is also eliminated rapidly.

Ethylene
Ethene

$$\text{H}_2\text{C} = \text{CH}_2$$

Synthesis

$$\text{C}_2\text{H}_5\,\text{OH} + \text{H}_2\text{SO}_4 \longrightarrow \text{H}_2\text{C} = \text{CH}_{2\,+}\,\text{H}_2\text{O}$$
(Ethanol)

Ethylene is highly flammable and forms explosive mixtures with air, nitrous oxide, and oxygen. It is slightly more potent than nitrous oxide. It produces surgical anesthesia in 80-85% which may cause anoxia necessitating use of high concentration of oxygen. This makes anesthetic mixture highly explosive. Because of this hazard it is seldom used.

HALOGENATED HYDROCARBONS
Chloroform
Trichloromethane

$$\text{CHCl}_3$$

Synthesis　　From ethanol

$$\text{CH}_3\text{CH}_2\text{OH} \ + \ \text{Ca(OCl)Cl} \longrightarrow \text{CH}_3\text{CHO} + \text{H}_2\text{O} + \text{CO}_2$$
　　　　　　(Ethanol)　　　(Calcium
　　　　　　　　　　　　chloride
　　　　　　　　　　　　hypochlorite)

$$\text{CH}_3\text{CHO} \ + 3\text{Cl}_2 \longrightarrow \text{CCl}_3\text{CHO} + 3\text{HCl}$$

$$\text{CCl}_3\text{CHO} + \text{Ca(OH)}_2 \longrightarrow \text{CHCl}_3 + (\text{HCOO})_2\text{Ca}$$

　　From acetone

$$\text{CH}_3\text{COCH}_3 + 3\text{Cl}_2 \longrightarrow \text{H}_3\text{CCOCCl}_3 + 3\text{HCl}$$
　　　　　(Acetone)

$$\text{H}_3\text{CCOCCl}_3 + \text{Ca(OH)}_2 \longrightarrow 2\text{CHCl}_3 + (\text{H}_3\text{CCOO})_2\text{Ca}$$

It is prepared by the action of bleaching powder on ethanol or acetone. Chloroform is a potent anesthetic that maintains surgical anesthesia at a concentration of 1.5% in the inspired air. Unlike some of the other general anesthetics, it is non-flamable. Some of the disadvantages associated with chloroform as anesthetic include its decomposition to phosgene (1), which is highly toxic. To neutralize the phosgene, the pharmacopoeia reccmmends addition of 1 to 2% ethyl alcohol. It has low margin of safety, undesirable and adverse effects on heart and kidney. It is seldom used excepting for obstetrical anesthesia.

$$2CHCl_3 + O_2 \longrightarrow 2COCl_2 + 2HCl$$

(1)

Ethyl Chloride

Chloroethane

$$C_2H_5Cl$$

Synthesis

$$C_2H_5OH + HCl \xrightarrow{ZnCl_2} C_2H_5Cl + H_2O$$

(Ethanol)

It is obtained by the passing dry hydrogen chloride gas into absolute ethyl alcohol in presence of zinc chloride. It is a gas at ordinary temperature and pressure, b.p. 12°.

Surgical anesthesia is obtained with 4 volume percent of vapour. It is, however, toxic to liver and causes cardiac arrhythmias and has limited application in anesthesia.

Halothane

2-Bromo-2-chloro-1,1,1-trifluoroethane

$$\begin{array}{c} CF_3 \\ | \\ CHClBr \end{array}$$

Synthesis

$$\begin{array}{c} CCl_2 \\ \| \\ CHCl \end{array} \xrightarrow{HCl} \begin{array}{c} CCl_3 \\ | \\ CH_2Cl \end{array} \xrightarrow{HF} \begin{array}{c} CF_3 \\ | \\ CH_2Cl \end{array} \xrightarrow{Br_2} \begin{array}{c} CF_3 \\ | \\ CHClBr \end{array}$$

(Trichloroethylene)

It is a potent, non-flammable, non-explosive and non-irritant general anesthetic. It has a potency 4- times that of ether and equal to that of chloroform, but possesses lower toxicity than chloroform. Further, the induction period is very rapid and surgical anesthesia is produced within 2–10 min. Recovery is also very rapid. Side effects include hypotension and bradycardia. Halothane forms an azeotropic mixture with diethylether which consists of 31.7% ether and 68.3% halothane, bp 51.5°. The anesthesia produced by azeotrope is similar to that of halothane. Because it is very potent, a precision vapourizer is used for its administration.

Trichloroethylene

1,1,2-Trichloroethene

$$\begin{array}{c} CCl_2 \\ \| \\ CHCl \end{array}$$

Synthesis

$$\begin{array}{c} CH \\ \||| \\ CH \end{array} + 2Cl_2 \longrightarrow \begin{array}{c} CHCl_2 \\ | \\ CHCl_2 \end{array} \xrightarrow[Ca(OH)_2]{CaO \ or} \begin{array}{c} CCl_2 \\ \| \\ CHCl \end{array}$$

(Acetylene)

It is obtained by the action of quicklime or lime on tetrachloroethylene. It is a heavy, volatile liquid. The official susbtance contains 0.01% w/w thymol as a preservative to prevent auto-oxidation to phosgene (1) and other toxic substances. Like chloroform, it is non-flammable but less toxic and less potent.

It should not be used in closed circuit with soda lime absorber, because it decomposes to dichloroacetylene which is toxic to cranial nerve. The other disadvantages include cardiac irregularity, tachypnea and sensitization of heart to catecholamines.

It has been recommended for use in obstertics for control of labour pain.

ETHERS
Diethyl Ether
Ethoxyethane

$$CH_3CH_2OCH_2CH_3$$

Synthesis

1. CH_3CH_2ONa + CH_3CH_2Br $\longrightarrow$ $CH_3CH_2OCH_2CH_3$
   (Sodium ethoxide)   (Ethyl bromide)

2. $CH_3CH_2OH + H_2SO_4$ $\longrightarrow$ $CH_3CH_2OSO_3H + H_2O$
   (Ethanol)

   $CH_3CHOSO_3H + C_2H_5OH$ $\longrightarrow$ $CH_3CH_2OCH_2CH_3 + H_2SO_4$

It is colourless liquid with a characteristic odour. It is flammable and forms explosive mixtures with air and oxygen. The pharmacopoeia recommends use of a an antioxidant (such as polyhydric phenols) in the concentration of not more than 0.02% w/v. These antioxidants prevent the formation of peroxides (2) and (3).

$$
\begin{array}{cc}
\underset{\underset{HO}{|}}{H_3CCH\cdot O\cdot O\cdot}\underset{\underset{OH}{|}}{CHCH_3} & \underset{\underset{CH_3}{|}}{H_3CCH_2-O-CH\cdot O\cdot OH} \\
(2) & (3)
\end{array}
$$

USP recommends addition of 4% alcohol and water to raise the boiling point in order to prevent frosting on the anesthetic mask.

Diethyl ether is a complete anesthetic. A concentration of 6-8% in inspired air is required for surgical anesthesia. It has a good margin of safety, causes excellent muscular relaxation without undue depression of CNS, stops respiration before causing heart arrest. Thus, the patient can be revived by means of artificial respirations.

Among disadvantages, it is flammable and forms explosive mixtures with air and oxygen. It also has a prolonged induction period which may be avoided by initial use of more rapidly acting anesthetic such as divinyl ether or nitrous oxide followed by gradual change to ether.

Methoxyflurane
2, 2-Dichloro-1, 1-difluoro-1-methoxyethane

Synthesis

$$Cl_2CHCF_2OCH_3$$

$$Cl_3CCF_2H \xrightarrow{KOH} \underset{Cl}{\overset{Cl}{>}}C=C\underset{F}{\overset{F}{<}} \xrightarrow{CH_3OH/KOH} Cl_2CHCF_2OCH_3$$

(1,1-Difluoro-2,2,2-trichloroethane)

It is a volatile liquid, bp, 101°. Its vapour produces general anesthesia with a slow onset and longer duration of action. It is non-flammable and produces anesthesia at concentration of 1.5 to 3%. It produces a profound muscular relaxation and analgesia. Among the disadvantages, it has a slow induction period and prolonged recovery due to low volatility and high solubility in body lipids. It does not sensitize heart to catecholamines to the same extent as chloroform or halothane.

Vinyl Ether
Divinyl oxide

$$O \begin{cases} CH=CH_2 \\ CH=CH_2 \end{cases}$$

Synthesis

$$2 \begin{vmatrix} CH_2OH \\ CH_2Cl \end{vmatrix} \xrightarrow[H_2SO_2]{140°} O \begin{cases} CH_2CH_2Cl \\ CH_2CH_2Cl \end{cases} \xrightarrow{alc.KOH} O \begin{cases} CH=CH_2 \\ CH=CH_2 \end{cases}$$

(2-Chloroethanol)

It is a colourless, flammable, highly volatile liquid, bp 28°. It is used for short duration anesthesia and as an induction anesthetic. The recovery is pleasant and rapid. There is minimal excitation, postoperative nausea and vomiting. Surgical anesthesia is maintained with 4 vol % of the drug.

It is somewhat more toxic than diethyl ether and is not safe for prolonged administration. Further, it is explosive, has tendency to polymerize, and possesses liver toxicity.

INTRAVENOUS ANESTHETICS

ULTRASHORT ACTING BARBITURATES
When injected intravenously, ultrashort acting barbiturates produce a rapid onset of unconsciousness and quick recovery after small doses. They are used for induction and for short surgical procedures. They are poor analgesics.

Methohexital Sodium
1-Methyl-5-allyl-5-(1-methyl-2-pentynyl) barbituric acid sodium salt

Synthesis

Step 1

(1-Butyne-1-magnesium bromide)   (Acetaldehyde)   (Phosphorus pentachloride)

(A)

Step 2

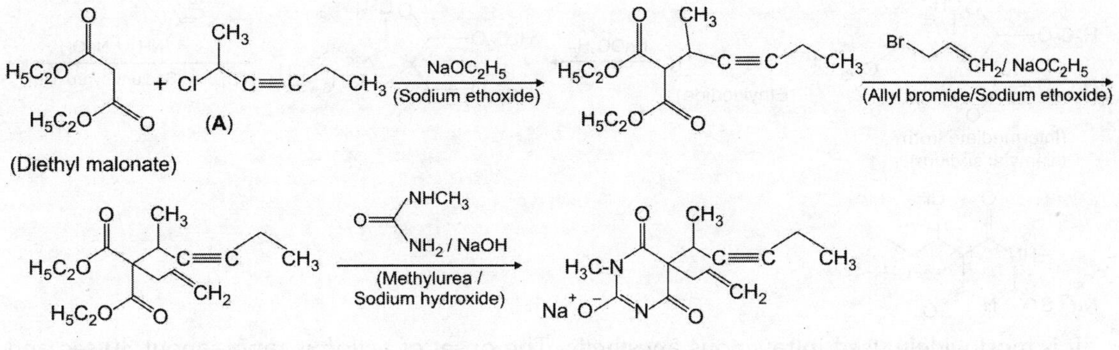

It is used for induction of anesthesia. It has a greater potency and its onset of action is rapid.

Thiamylal Sodium

5-Allyl-5-(1-methylbutyl)-2- thiobarbituric acid sodium salt

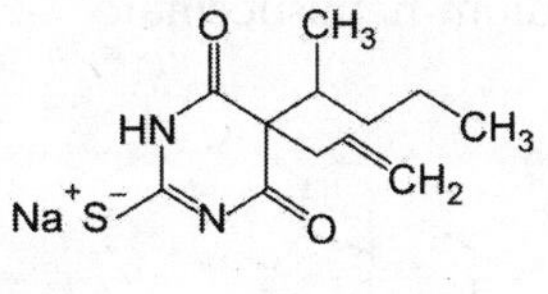

Synthesis

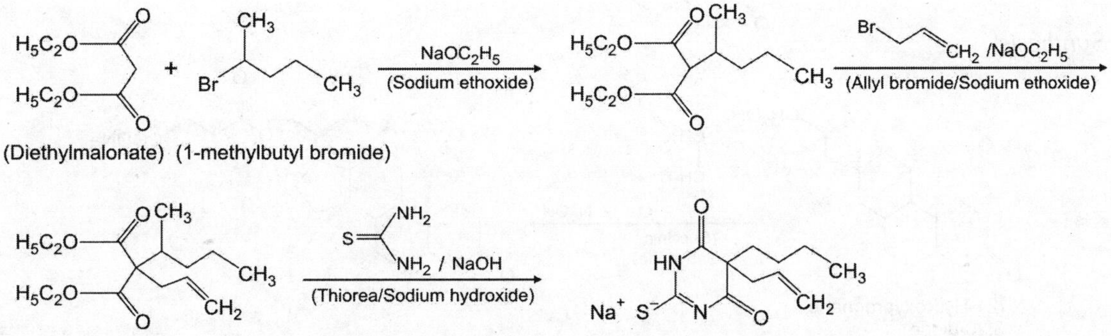

It is about 1.5 times as active as thiopental and is used in smaller doses. It is contraindicated in patients with liver dysfunction.

Thiopental Sodium

5-Ethyl-5-(1-methylbutyl)-2-thiobarbituric acid sodium salt

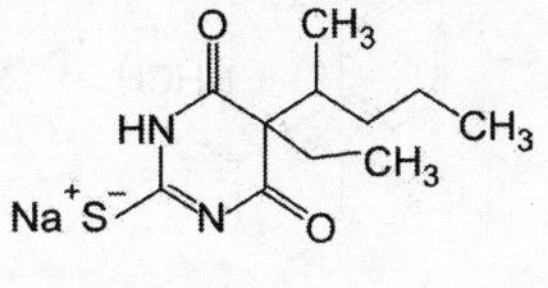

Synthesis

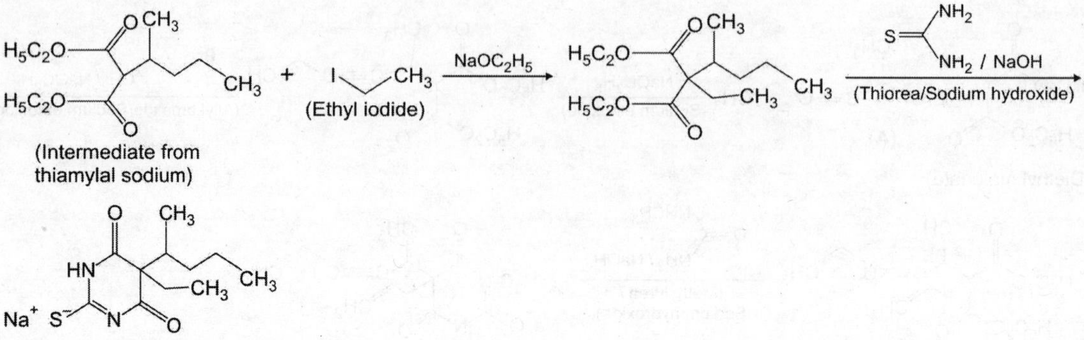

It is most widely used intravenous anesthetic. The onset of action is rapid, about 30 sec and duration short 10-30 min.

MISCELLANEOUS COMPOUNDS
Hydroxydione Sodium
21-Hydroxypregnane-3,20-dione sodium hemisuccinate

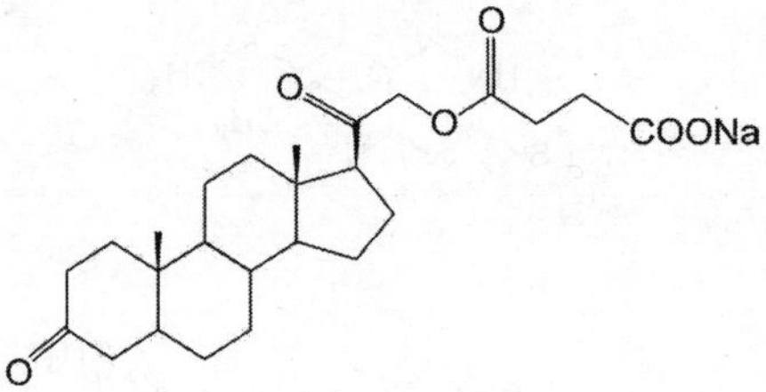

Synthesis

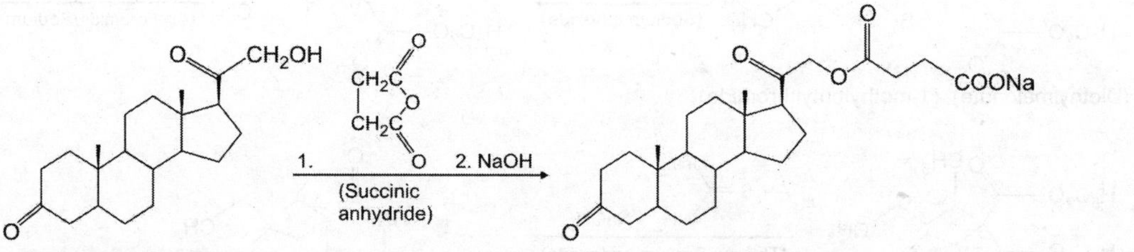

(21-Hydroxypregnane-
3,20-dione)

When administered intravenously it produces amnesia and unconsciousness. It has a weak analgesic and muscle relaxant property. The major drawback of this drug is its tendency to cause pain at the site of injection

Ketamine
2-(o-Chlorophenyl)-2-methylaminocyclohexanone

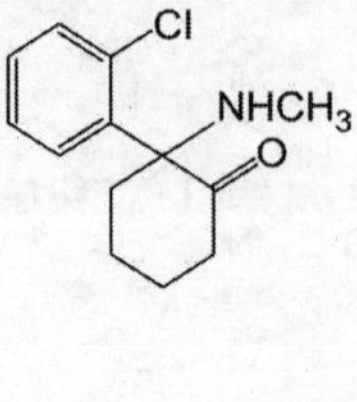

Synthesis

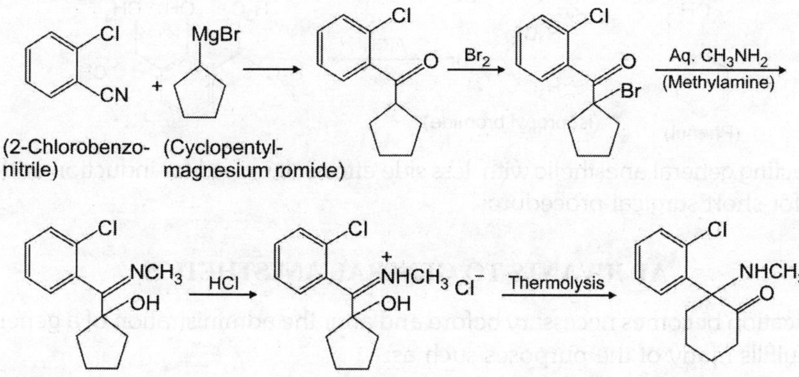

(2-Chlorobenzo-nitrile) (Cyclopentyl-magnesium romide)

It is a potent short acting anesthetic. It is used for short surgical procedures that do not require muscle relaxation.

Propanidid

Propyl [4-[(diethylcarbamoyl)methoxy]-3-methoxyphenyl]acetate

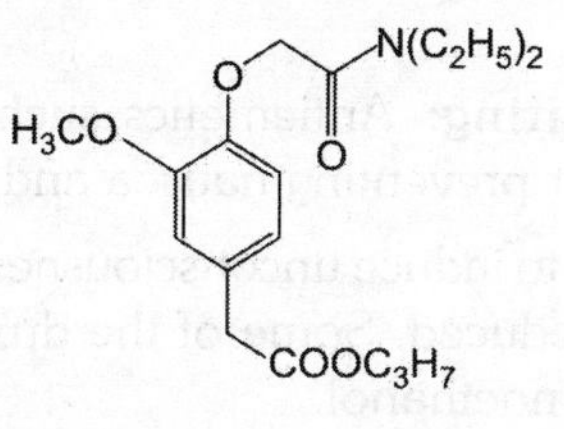

Synthesis

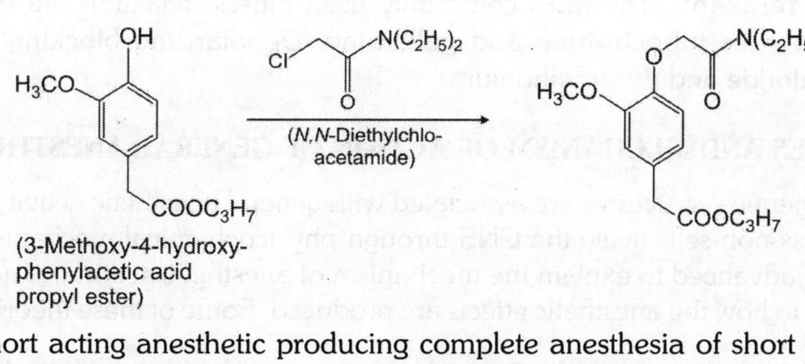

(3-Methoxy-4-hydroxy-phenylacetic acid propyl ester) (N,N-Diethylchlo-acetamide)

It is a ultrashort acting anesthetic producing complete anesthesia of short duration. It is also used for induction of anesthesia. It does not have muscle relaxant or analgesic activity.

Propofol

2, 6-Diisopropylphenol

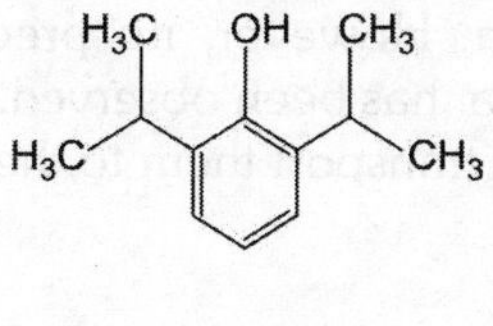

Synthesis

(Phenol)   (Isopropyl bromide)

It is a short acting general anesthetic with less side effects. It is used for induction and maintenance of anesthesia for short surgical procedures.

ADJUVANTS TO GENERAL ANESTHETICS

Auxiliary medication becomes necessary before and after the administration of a general anesthetic. This practice fulfills many of the purposes such as:

Reduction of anxiety: To overcome anxiety, antianxiety agents such as diazepam, lorazepam and midazolam are used.

Control of pain: Control of pain is achieved by using strong analgesics such as morphine, levorphanol, pentazocine, etc.

Inhibition of salivation: Inhibition of salivation is achieved by using anticholinergic agents such as atropine, scopolamine, etc.

Prevention of nausea and vomiting: Antiemetics such as promethazine, chlorpromazine, trimethobenzamide, etc. are used for preventing nausea and vomiting.

Basal anesthetics: These are used to induce unconsciousness. By use of these agents, the quantity of anesthetic used is considerably reduced. Some of the drugs used as basal anesthetics include fentanyl citrate, paraldehyde, tribromoethanol.

Skeletal muscle relaxant: The most commonly used muscle relaxants are non-depolarizing blocking agents such as tubocurarine and gallamine. Depolarizing blocking agents include suxamethonium chloride and decamethonium.

THEORIES AND MECHANISM OF ACTION OF GENERAL ANESTHETICS

A wide variety of chemical structures are associated with general anesthetic activity, indicating that these agents depress non-selectively the CNS through physicochemical mechanisms. Number of theories have been advanced to explain the mechanism of anesthetic action but none of these are able to elucidate as to how the anesthetic effects are produced. Some of these theories are discussed below.

Physical Theories

Colloid Theory

This was first proposed by Claud Bernard. He postulated that there is a casual relationship between anesthesia and protein precipitation. However, no precipitation by the chloroform, in the concentration that produces anesthesia, has been observed. They suggested that high protein and lipid solubility of anesthetics served to transport them to the sites where they could leave the lipid to combine with protoplasm.

Lipid Theory

Meyer and Overton found a relationship between the potency of the anesthetic and their relative solubilities in olive oil and water based on partition co-efficient in these solvents. The higher the partition co-efficient the greater the anesthetic activity of the substance. However, this generalization could not hold, because aromatic compounds which have higher oil/water distribution co-efficient do not produce anesthesia.

Permeability Theory

Lillie proposed that narcotics functioned by diminishing the permeability of cell membrane. However, this theory could be applied to a limited number of compounds.

Surface Tension or Adsorption Theory

In 1904, Traube proposed that anesthetic act by decreasing the surface tension. However, there are many substances, such as paraffins, which do not lower the surface tension but possess anesthetic activity.

Warburg suggested that accumulation of narcotics at the cell surfaces could change the metabolic processes and neural transmission and thus produce anesthesia. In case of inert gases, it is believed that nacrosis may be due to accumulation of sufficient amount of inert gases in lipids of a membrane so as to render the lipid phase more continuous. The membrane thus becomes more stabilized and transmission of impulses is inhibited.

Clathrate Theory

Linus Pauling has suggested that anesthetics act by causing the formation of submicroscopic crystals in aqueous component of brain tissue.

The atoms of rare gases may associate with other substances to form complexes which are called "clathrates". The "clathrates" may consist of two or more molecules held together by formation of cage-like structure of one component around other. The clathrates may be supported around by the molecules of water. The hydrated microcrystals thus formed with CNS can interfere with ionic mobility, electrical charges, chemical reactions, or enzymic activity.

Molecular Size Theory

Wulf and Featherstone advanced the hypothesis that anesthetic activity depends on the molecular volume of the compound. When the molecular volume is greater than water, oxygen and nitrogen, the substance occupies the space between the lipid and protein layer of cellular membrane. The molecular volumes of various substances are, water–3.05, oxygen–3.18, nitrogen– 3.91, nitrous oxide–4.4, xenon–5.1, ethylene–5.7, cyclopropane–7.5, chloroform–10.2, ethyl ether–13.4. By occupying the space, the general anesthetics could cause alteration in cellular structure with subsequent depression of function resulting in anesthesia.

Neurophysiological Theory

It has been reported that volatile anesthetics impair conduction along isolated nerve fibers, decreasing exciteability and depolarize nerve. The synapse is the primary point of attack. Ether and chloroform depress the synaptic transmission through a sympathetic ganglion in concentration similar to those known to exist in the blood during surgical anesthesia. The synaptic transmission is depresssed more readily than conduction along any type of axon.

Biochemical Theories

According to these theories, anesthetics exert a variety of effects on various brain enzymes. These include suppression of oxidation of glucose, lactate, pyruvate in the brain tissue. The anesthetics also affect the oxidative phosphorylation and cause suppression of ionic movement.

Currently, it is believed that presence of anesthetic molecules blocks or distorts neuronal membrane channels involved in sodium conductance. It has been suggested that as the anesthetics dissolve in neuronal membrane it results in disorganisation of lipid matrix with consequent expansion that distorts sodium channel. As a result there is blockade of sodium channel with consequent reduction in sodium conduction. This interference with sodium influx results in reduction in rate of rise of action potential.

Some of the anesthetics may act by enhancing the inhibitory neuronal activity. Thus, steroid anesthetics, barbiturates, and benzodiazepines bind on $GABA_A$ receptor/chloride channel complex that enhances GABA binding. When bound to its site, GABA causes chloride conducting channel to open resulting in the influx of chloride ions. This leads to hyperpolarization of postsynaptic membrane and inhibition of neuronal firing.

LOCAL ANESTHETICS

$\mathbf{A}$GENTS which are applied locally and block afferent nervous conduction from the periphery of the nerve path are called local anesthetics. They block the transmission of impulses in the peripheral pain conducting nerve endings. When applied near peripheral endings they prevent nervous reactions in the specific area. If applied to a part of CNS organ, they block transmission of impulses from and the impulses received by the organ without affecting the other parts of the nervous system. Like general anesthetics, they are not used to alleviate the symptoms of illness but are used by surgeons to carry out the surgical procedures on a patient without any resistance. However, unlike general anesthetics, the anesthesia produced by local anesthetics is without loss of consciousness. Further, local anesthetics act by blocking the sodium channels while as general anesthetics act through non-specific interaction with lipid layers which results in changes in membrane excitability through various mechanisms discussed under general anesthetics.

An ideal local anesthetic should produce a reversible blockade of sensory nerve fibers with a minimal effect on motor nerve fibers. It should have a rapid onset of action. It should also possess vasoconstriction properties which results in longer duration of action.

The various local anesthetics are discussed under:

1. Ester type local anesthetics,
2. amide type local anesthetics, and
3. miscellaneous compounds.

ESTER TYPE LOCAL ANESTHETICS

The development of local anesthetics started with cocaine (1), a naturally occurring alkaloid found in *Erythroxylon coca* and other species of *Erythroxylon*. Its structure and stereochemistry has been established and it is (-)-2β-carbomethoxy-3β-benzoyloxytropane.

(1)

117

As a local anesthetic, cocaine (1) exerts a strong local anesthetic activity. Moreover, it also possesses vasoconstriction properties because of which it has longer duration of action. However, it has number of disadvantages also and these include its higher toxicity, addiction liability, and cortical stimulation. Because of these properties and the legal restriction on its production and sale, search for newer non-habit forming, cheaper, and better local anesthetics was carried out. The search has yielded good local anesthetics which are used in clinical practice. However, cocaine (1) is still used in ophthalmology because of its mydriatic action.

Structure-Activity Relationship Studies

A study of structural analogs of cocaine (1) has shown that:

(a) Hydrolysis of carbomethoxyl group and benzoate group leading to ecgonine (2), results in loss of activity. However, decarbomethoxylated cocaine, tropacocaine (3), possessed local anesthetic activity.

(2)   (3)

(b) Synthesis and observance of local anesthetic activity in piperidine analogs, α-eucaine (4) and β-eucaine (5) showed that tropane moiety was not necessary for local anesthetic activity.

(4)   (5)

(c) Local anesthetic activity was also observed in ethyl p-aminobenzoate which is known under the name benzocaine (6). It is an effective local anesthetic and is retained in medicine being used as a dusting powder. The corresponding butyl analog, butesine (7), is used as picrate salt on denuded surfaces.

(6)   (7)

The data from structure-activity relationship studies of cocaine (1) and the activity of alkyl p-aminobenzoates led to a new series of local anesthetic called dialkylaminoalkyl esters of aromatic acids.

The anesthesophore group in cocaine (1) molecule, thus, consisted of aromatic acid esterified with a tertiary amino alcohol (8). Based on the above, a series of compounds belonging to dialkalyaminoalkyl esters of aromatic acids were synthesized. Of this procaine (9) had the most favourable therapeutic ratio. Its monohydrochloride is known as novocain.

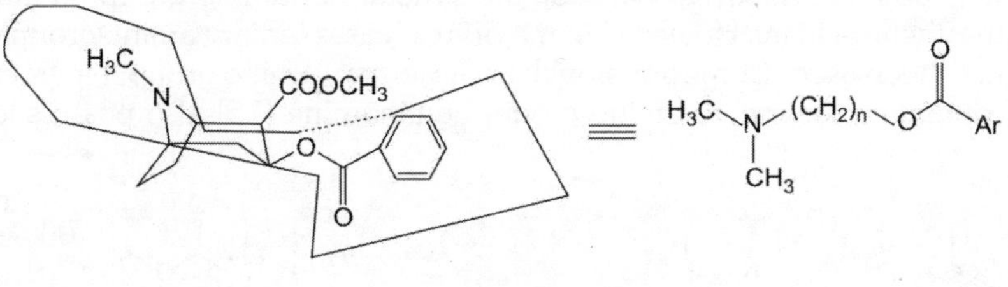

(8)

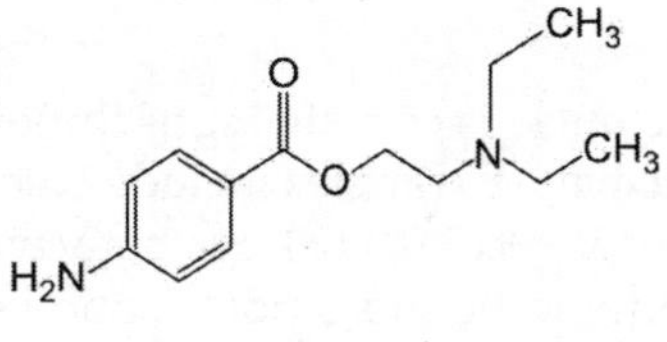

(9)

Procaine (9) has number of advantages and these include, low toxicity, low cost of its manufacture, and stability of its solutions. However, it has relatively weak local anesthetic action and the duration of its action is short. The short duration of action is overcome by giving it along with a vasoconstrictor such as epinephrine. Solution of procaine (9) in oil have been used as depot preparations for prolonged action. A combination of procaine (9) with benzocaine (6) in polyethylene glycol and propylene glycol has also been used for prolonged activity.

Structure-Activity Relationship Studies on Procaine

Studies on procaine (9) have shown that increase in the size of alkyl group on the amino nitrogen and increase in size of the chain leads to prolongation of duration of action. Thus butacaine (10) a surface anesthetic, has a more rapid onset of action which is of longer duration. Amethocaine (11), which has butyl group on nuclear amino group, is used for infiltration and surface anesthesia.

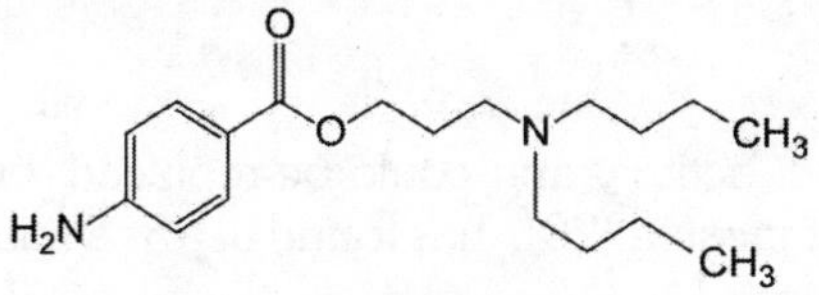

(10)

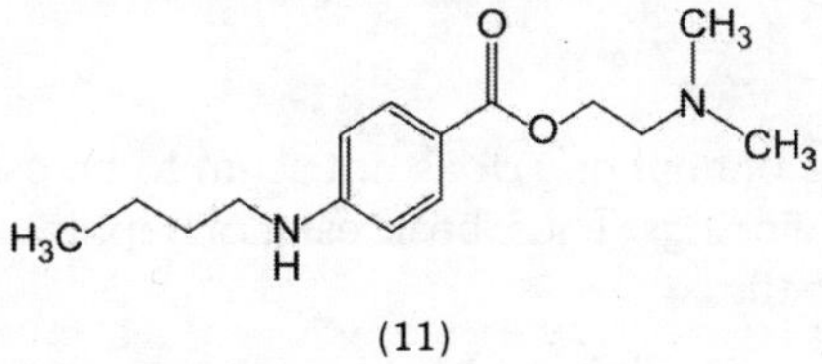

(11)

Branching of alkylene chain has also been successfully attempted. This has resulted in the synthesis of larocaine (12) an infiltration, long duration anesthetic, and butamin (13) a corneal infiltration anesthetic.

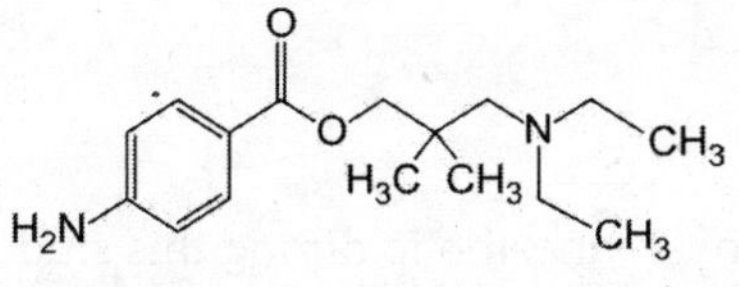

(12)

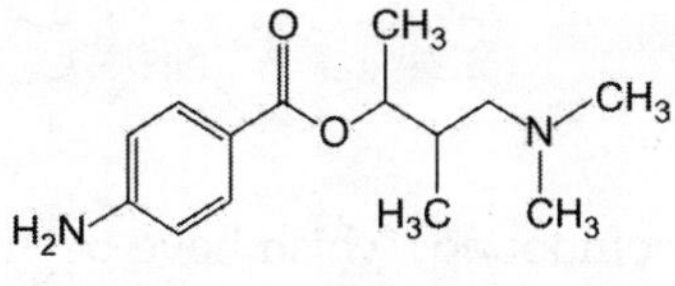

(13)

There seems to be no relationship between the structure of amino group on aminoalkyl chain and the local anesthetic activity. However, in majority of cases tertiary amino group with two equal alklyl groups have been used. Compounds with cyclic tertiary amino group, piperocaine (14), and a compound containing secondary amino group, butethamine (15) also possess local anesthetic activity.

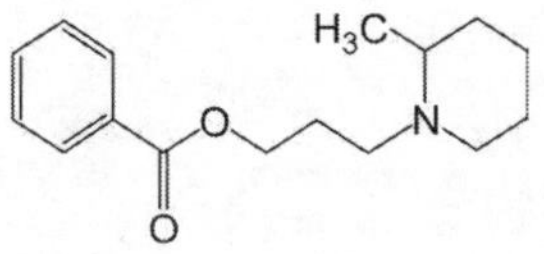

(14)

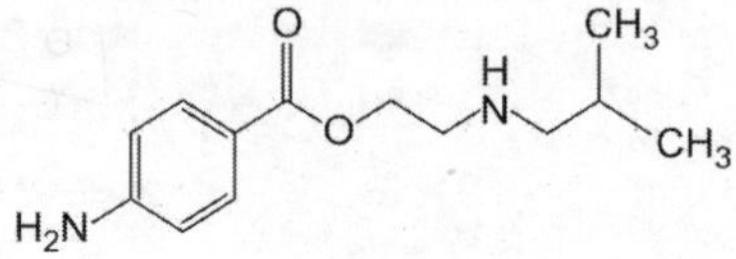

(15)

Compounds where the aromatic nucleus contains substitution at other positions have also been found to possess local anesthetic activity. Examples include chloroprocaine (16) used as infiltration anesthetic, benoxinate (17), and propoxycaine (18). Proparacaine (19) which is a structural isomer of propoxycaine (18) has been found to be more potent and less toxic than cocaine (1).

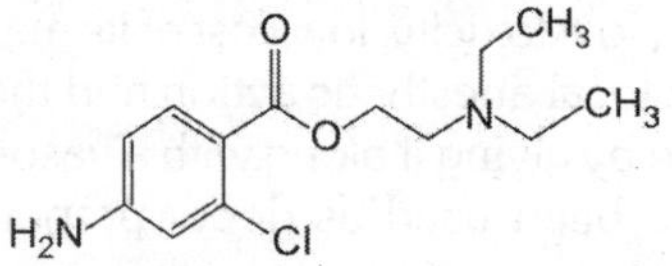

(16)

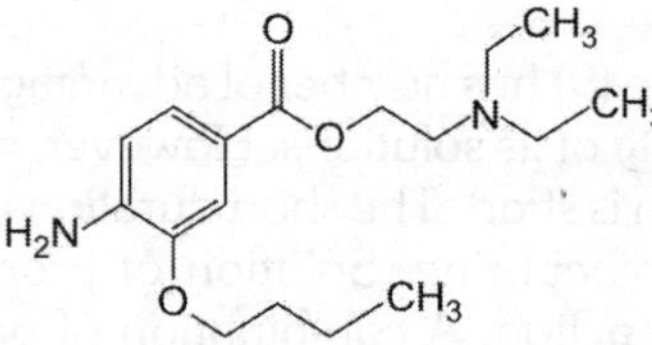

(17)

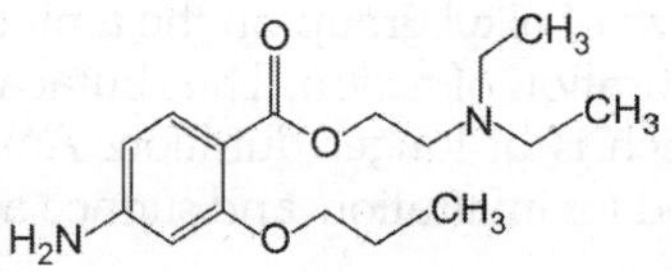

(18)

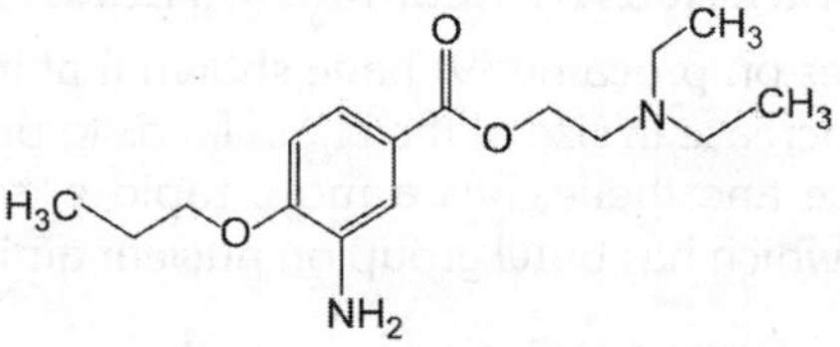

(19)

The phenyl ring does not seem to be essential for the activity and could be replaced by other aromatic rings. Thus, basic ester of naphthoic acid, naphthacaine (20), has found use as a infiltration anesthetic.

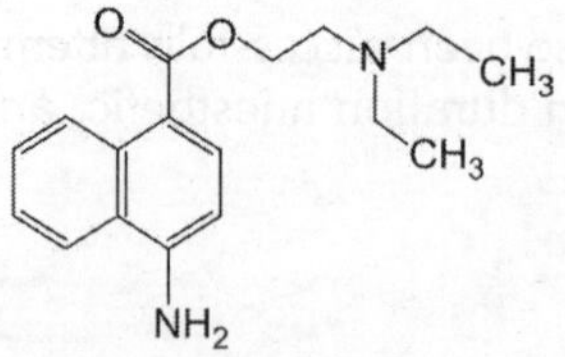

(20)

Other compounds which have been found useful as local anesthetic during this study include amylocaine (21), hexylcaine (22), isobucaine (23), meprylcaine (24), and cyclomethycaine (25).

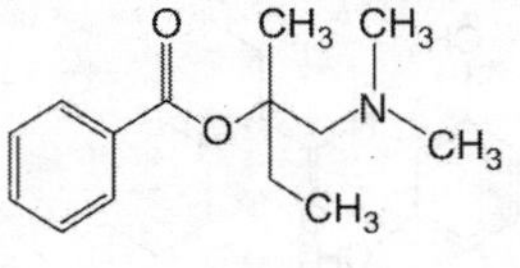

(21)

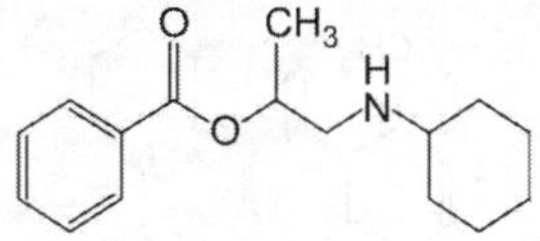

(22)

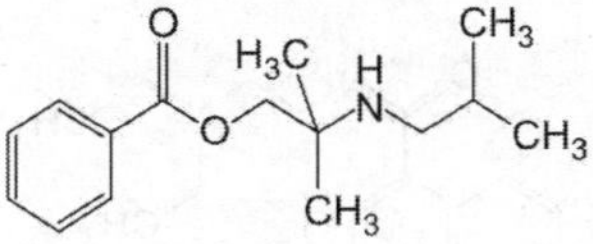

(23)

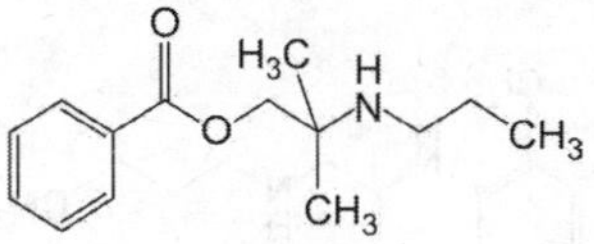

(24)

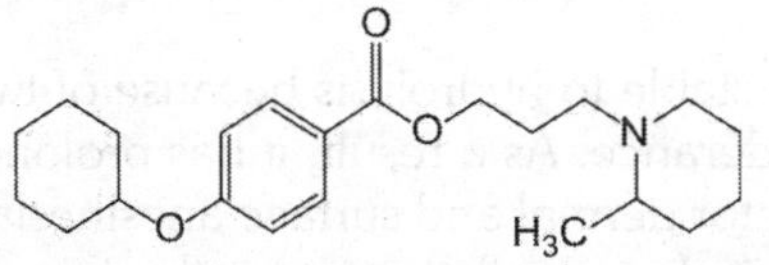

(25)

AMIDE TYPE LOCAL ANESTHETICS

Since amides are isosteric with esters, such compounds, therefore, would show similar biological activity. Moreover, since amides are difficult to hydrolyze as compared to esters, therefore, they would have longer duration of action as compared to esters. Based on this number of amides comparable to those of esters, were synthesized and tested for local anesthetic activity. Prominent among these are the amides such as prilocaine (26), lignocaine (27), pyrrocaine (28), etidocaine (29), mepivacaine (30), bupivacaine (31), and butanilicaine (32).

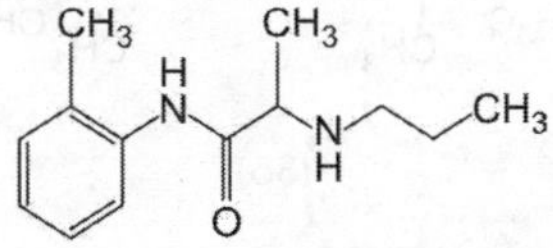

(26)

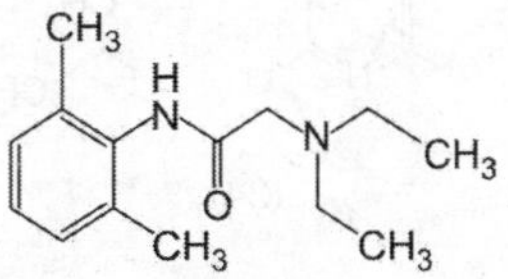

(27)

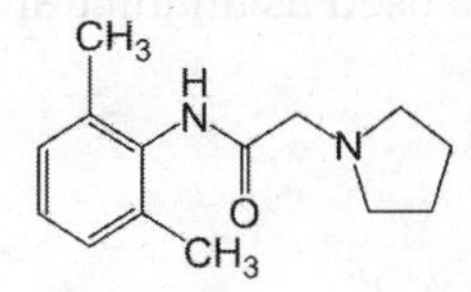

(28)

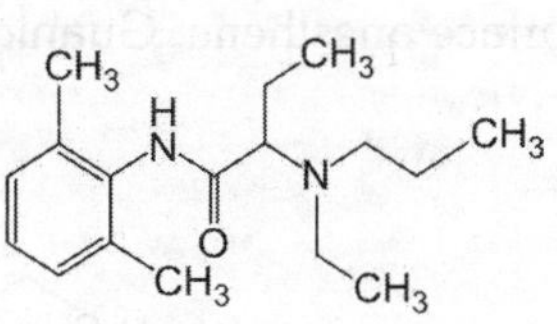

(29)

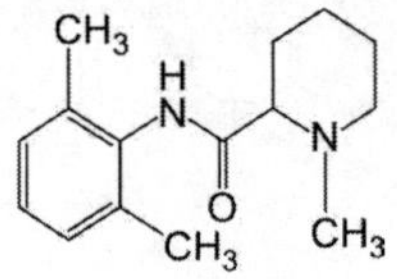

(30)

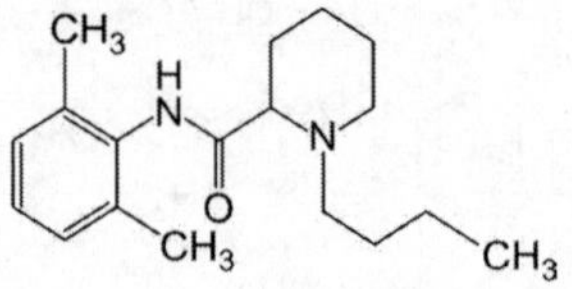

(31)

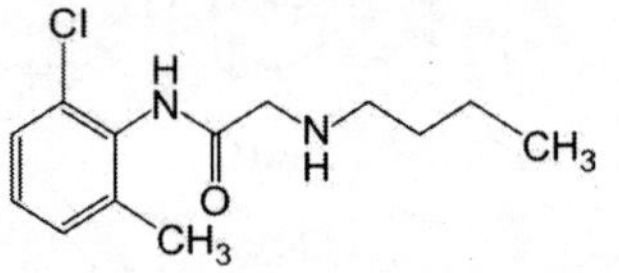

(32)

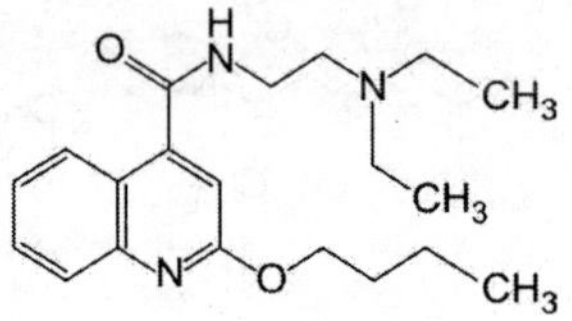

(33)

Lignocaine (27) is extremely stable to hydrolysis because of two methyl groups ortho to amide function which cause steric hindrance. As a result, it has prolonged duration of action. It is used intravenously for analgesia and for dermal and surface anesthesia with or without vasoconstrictor. Isomers of lignocaine (27) with only one alkyl group ortho to amide function have much shorter duration of action. It is not necessary that both the substituents ortho to the amide function should be alkyl groups. Butanilicaine (32) in which one of the ortho methyl group has been replaced with chloro, was found to be less toxic and more active than procaine (9).

Another amide discovered during search for antipyretics is dibucaine (33), an amide of cinchoninic acid. It has a potent local anesthetic activity. Reversed analog (34) of dibucaine (33) was found to be less active and more toxic than dibucaine (33). Among other amides having local anesthetic activity is oxethazaine (35). It has a prolonged and powerful surface anesthetic activity.

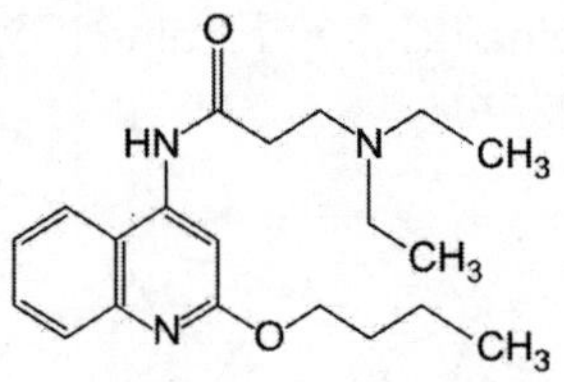

(34)

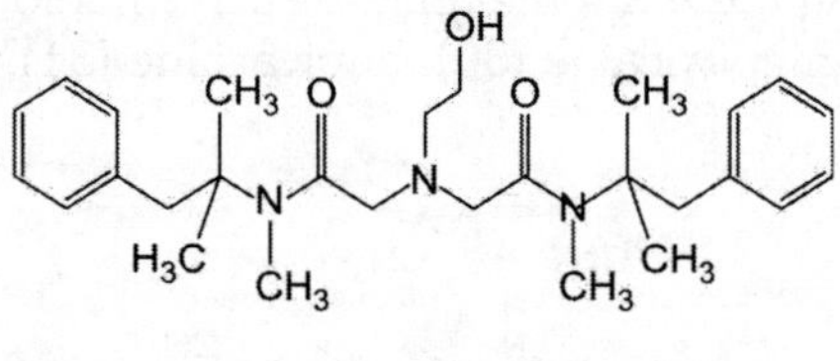

(35)

MISCELLANEOUS COMPOUNDS

Phenacaine (36), an amidine is one of the older drugs. It possesses systemic toxicity and is therefore used as a surface anesthetic. Guanidino derivative acoin (37) is used as an infiltration anesthetic.

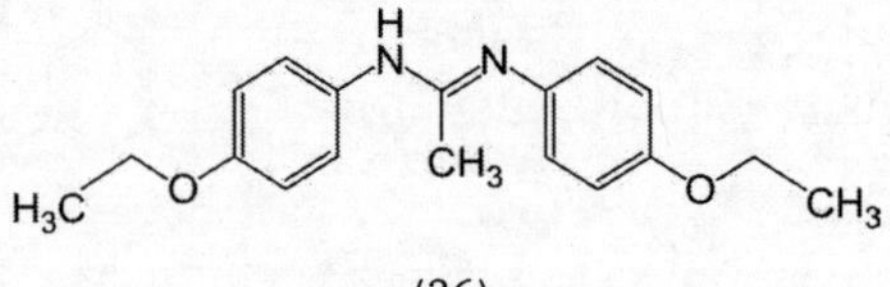

(36)

(37)

(38)

Among carbamates, which contain both ester and amide function, diperodon (38) has been found to possess longer duration of action.

Among aminoketones, propipocaine (39) and dyclonine (40) have been reported to possess local anesthetic activity.

(39), R = C_3H_7
(40), R = C_4H_9

Since ethers are much more difficult to hydrolyze as compared to amides, it was reasoned that aminoalkylethers should have longer duration of action than even aminoalkyl amides. Based on this, various aminoalkylethers were synthesized. Among these, two compounds namely pramoxine (41) and dimethisoquin (42) were found to possess prolonged activity with low toxicity. Dimethisoquin (42) is 1000 times more active than cocaine (1) when applied to rabbit cornea. It is used in dermatoses and other painful or irritating skin conditions.

(41)

(42)

Among nitrogen free local anesthetic, benzyl alcohol is the most important. It is used as tropical anesthetic. It produces local irritation which is due to its oxidation to benzoic acid.

MECHANISM OF ACTION

Local anesthetics act by decreasing the excitability of nerve cells. The excitability of nerve cells is associated with movement of sodium ions across the nerve membrane. They are believed to act by interfering with the movement of sodium ions by blocking the voltage sensitive sodium channels.

The transmembrane potential during resting phase is maintained at –90 to –60 mv. During excitation, the sodium channel open and fast inward current of sodium depolarizes the membrane raising the action potential from –70 to +40 mv. This results in closing of sodium channels and opening of potassium channels bringing the transmembrane potential to –90 mv.

Application of increasing concentrations of local anesthetic to nerve fiber results in increase in threshold for excitation and finally the ability to generate the action potential is abolished. This has been attributed to blockade of sodium channels by local anesthetics. The blockade of sodium channels by local anesthetics is both voltage and time dependent. The rested channels (which are in closed state and predominate in more negative potential) have lower affinity for the sodium ions than the activated channels (open state). The recovery of blocked sodium channels is slower and the nerve conducts fewer impulses.

ADMINSTRATION OF LOCAL ANESTHETICS

One of the clinical aspects of local anesthetics is selectivity in desensitization of a particular part of the body which ranges from a small local area in skin to specific region of the body. This is achieved through applying or injecting the local anesthetic in that area. Some of these are discussed below.

Topical Anesthesia

Local anesthetics when applied directly to mucous membrane or skin block the sensory nerve endings. The anesthetic can be applied as an aqueous solution, spray, cream, ointment or gel. For example in dental procedures topical anesthetic is used to prevent the pain on injection. Both water soluble salts of a local anesthetic and water insoluble bases are used. Since water insoluble bases are poorly absorbed their systemic toxicity is low. Some of the local anesthetics used topically include benzocaine (6) and lignocaine (27).

Infiltration Anesthesia

Infiltration anesthesia is used to desensitize an area of skin or mucosal surface. The local anesthetic is administered through intradermal or subcutaneous route. Some of the local anesthetics used for this purpose include procaine (9), lignocaine (27), and bupivacaine (31).

Field Block Anesthesia

It involves anesthetizing a larger area by injecting subcutaneously the local anesthetic at a point adjacent to the area to be anesthetized. This way the nerve transmission to the area is blocked. The drugs used in field block anesthesia are the same as in infiltration anesthesia.

Epidural Anesthesia

The drug in epidermal anesthesia is injected into the epidermal space between the vertebrae and spinal cord. This anesthetizes the nerve leading to uterus and pelvic region. This is useful for pain relief during labour. Local anesthesia used for this purpose is bupivacaine (31).

Block Anesthesia

Local anesthetics when injected into the subarachnoid space, block all the nerve impulses centred around the site of injection. Solutions with the same specific gravity as that of cerebrospinal fluid will remain at the site of injection, heavier or hyperbaric, lighter or hypobaric solutions when injected will either travel down or up the subarachnoid space, respectively. Thus, the specific regions may be anesthetized. The technique is useful for abdominal, pelvic and lower extremity surgery. Procaine (9) and amethocaine (11) along with a vasoconstrictor, such an epinephrine are usually used for this purpose.

INDIVIDUAL COMPOUNDS

ESTERS
Cocaine
2β-Carbomethoxy-3β-benzoyloxytropane

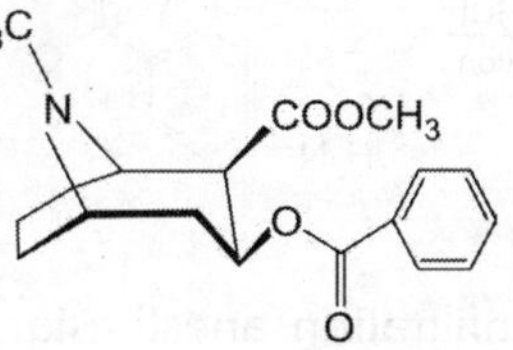

It is an alkaloid obtained from leaves of *Erythroxylon coca* Lam. and other species of *Erthroxylon*.

Cocaine occurs as a levo-rotatory, colorless crystals, or as white crystalline powder. Because of higher solubility in oil, it is used principally where oily solutions or ointments are indicated. It is also used as hydrochloride salt.

Benzocaine
Ethyl 4-aminobenzoate

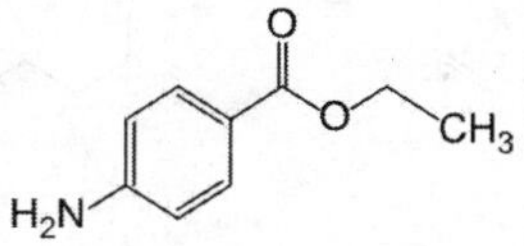

Synthesis

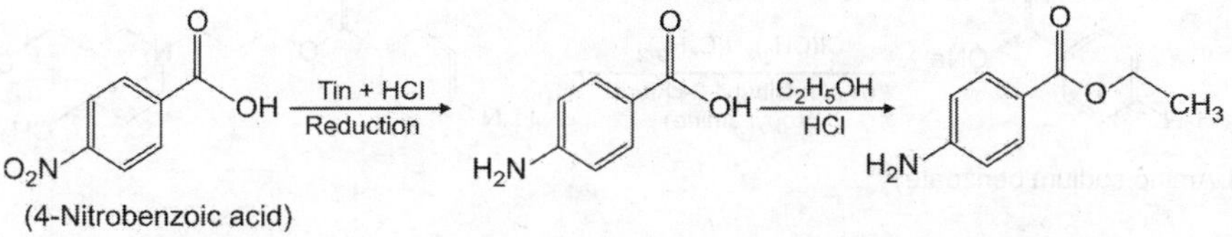

It is a white crystalline compound. It has low potency as well as low systemic toxicity. It is used as a topical anesthetic.

Procaine
2-Diethylaminoethyl 4-aminobenzoate

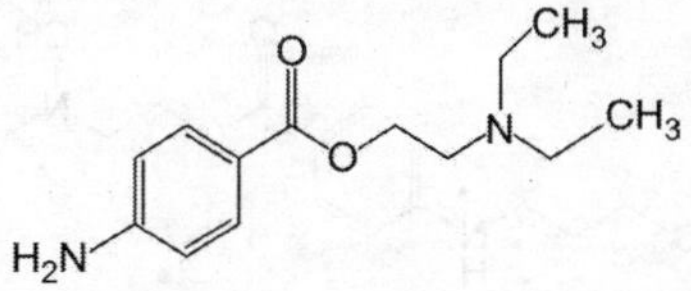

Synthesis

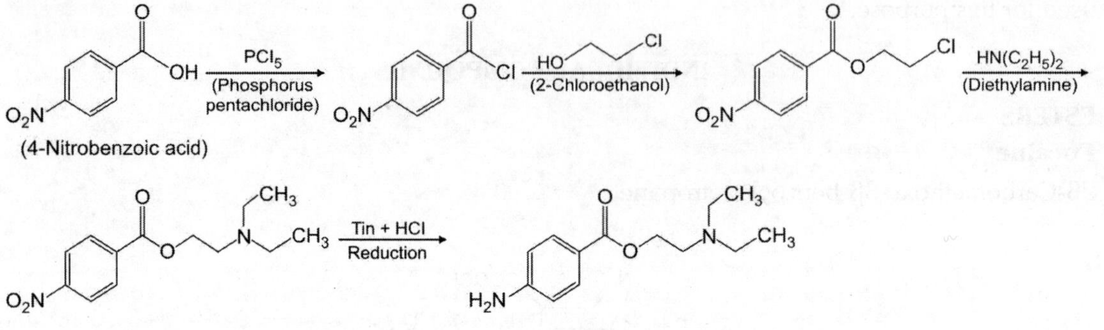

It is used as hydrochloride for infiltration anesthesia. Its action is prolonged by concurrent administration of epinephrine. Procaine forms an insoluble salt with penicillin G. The low solubility of this salt accounts for prolonged action of procaine penicillin G.

Butacaine

3-(Dibutylamino)-1-propanol 4-aminobenzoate

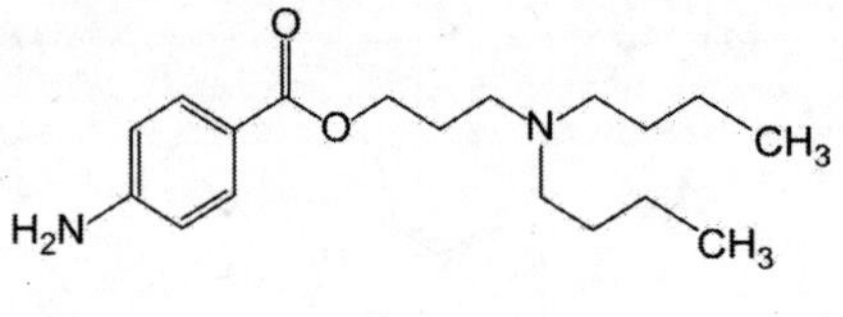

Synthesis

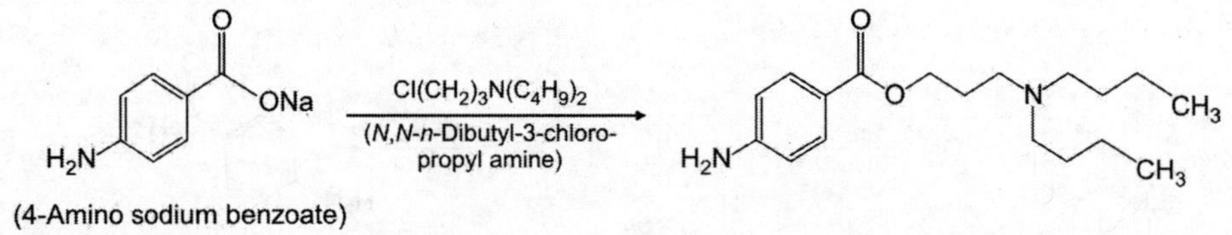

Butacaine is a liquid. It is used as a sulphate salt which is a white crystalline powder. Butacaine sulphate is used as topical anesthetic in dentistry. It is also used as nasal drops.

Amethocaine

2-Dimethylaminoethyl 4-*n*-butylaminobenzoate

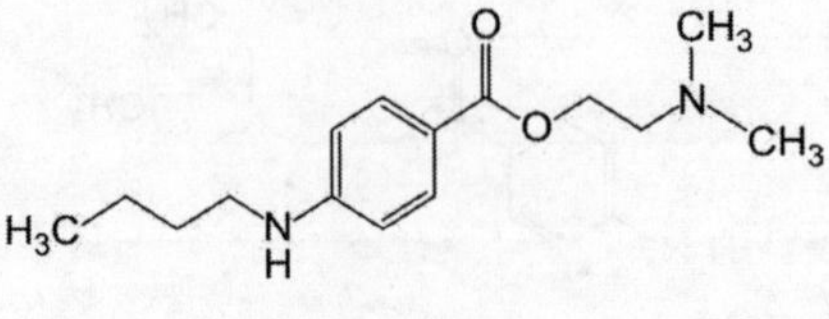

Synthesis

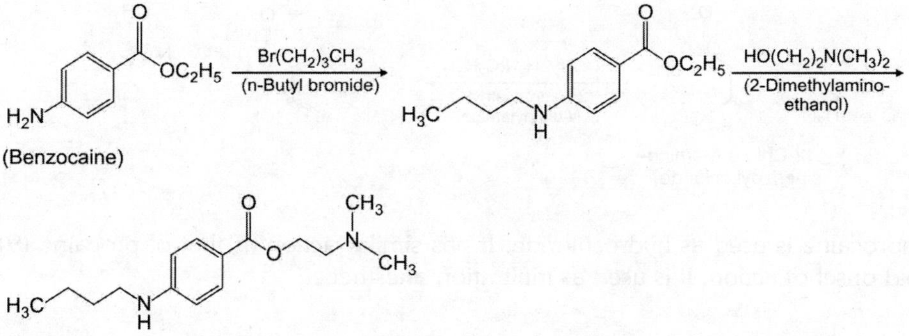

(Benzocaine)

Amethocaine is a white waxy solid. Its monohydrochloride, known as tetracaine hydrochloride, is a white hygroscopic, crystalline solid. It is mainly used as a topical anesthetic because of its higher toxicity. It is also used in spinal anesthesia.

Piperocaine
2-Methyl-1-piperidinepropanol benzoate

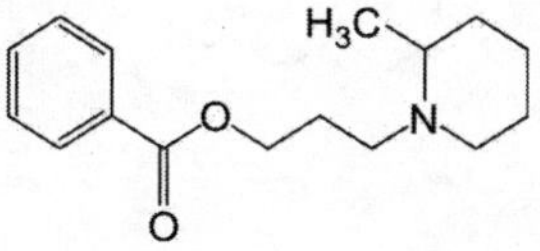

Synthesis

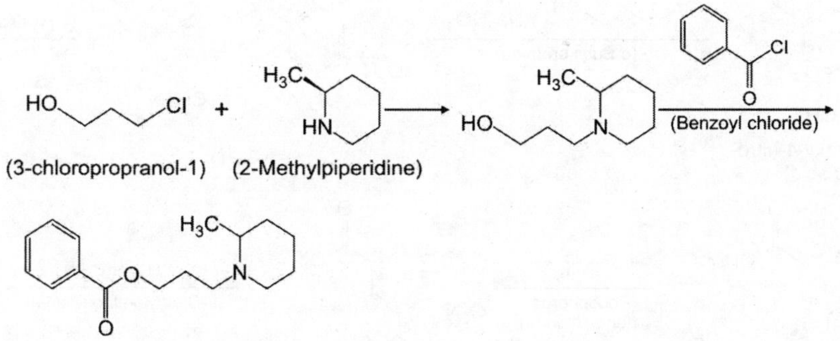

(3-chloropropranol-1)   (2-Methylpiperidine)

It is used as hydrochloride as a surface, infiltration, and regional nerve block anesthetic.

Chloroprocaine
2-Chloro-4-aminobenzoic acid diethylaminoethyl ester

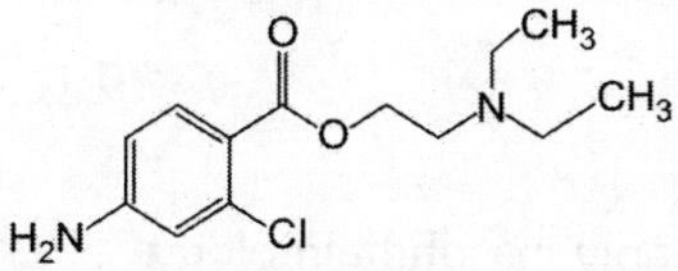

Synthesis

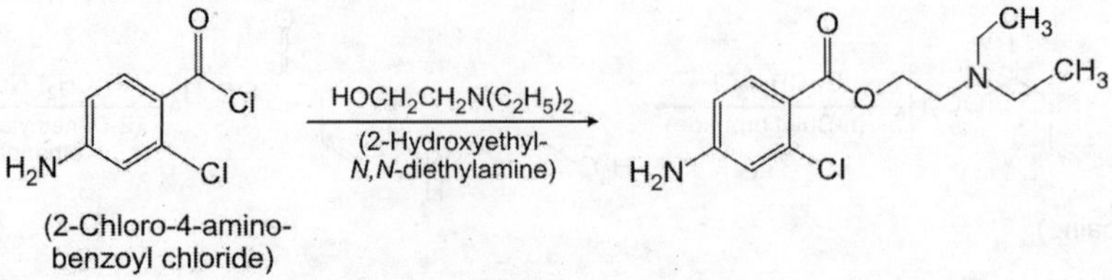

(2-Chloro-4-amino-
benzoyl chloride)

Chloroprocaine is used as hydrochloride. It has similar action as that of procaine (9) but has more rapid onset of action. It is used as infiltration anesthetic.

Benoxinate

2-(Diethylamino)ethyl 4-amino-3-*n*-butoxybenzoate

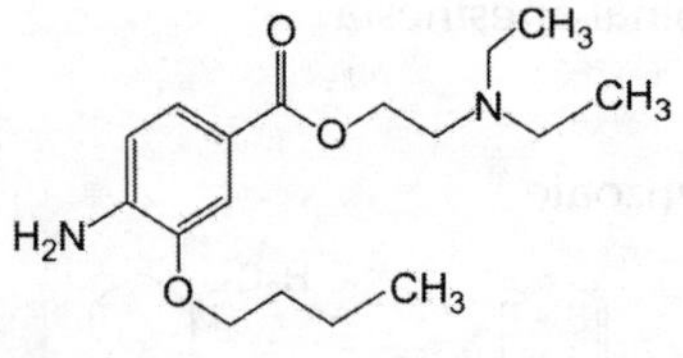

Synthesis

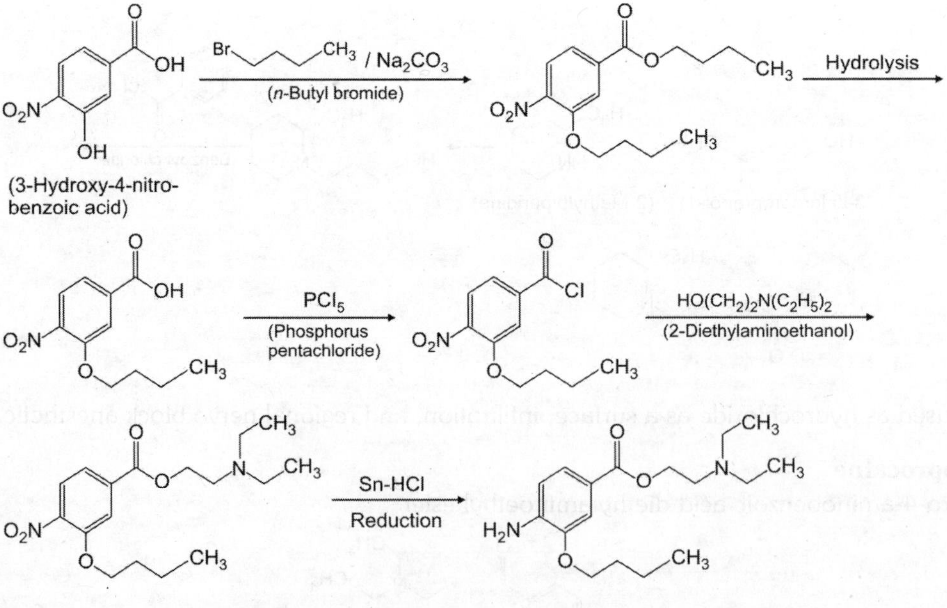

(3-Hydroxy-4-nitro-
benzoic acid)

It is used as hydrochloride primarily in ophthalmology.

Propoxycaine

2-Diethylaminoethyl 4-amino-2-propoxybenzoate

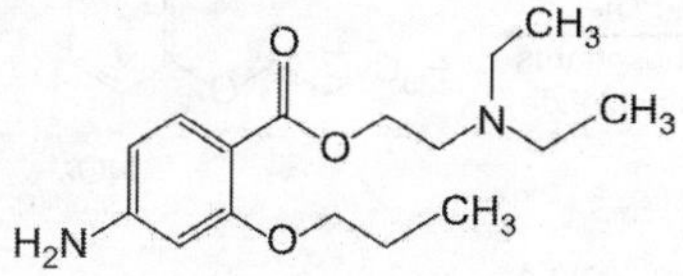

Synthesis

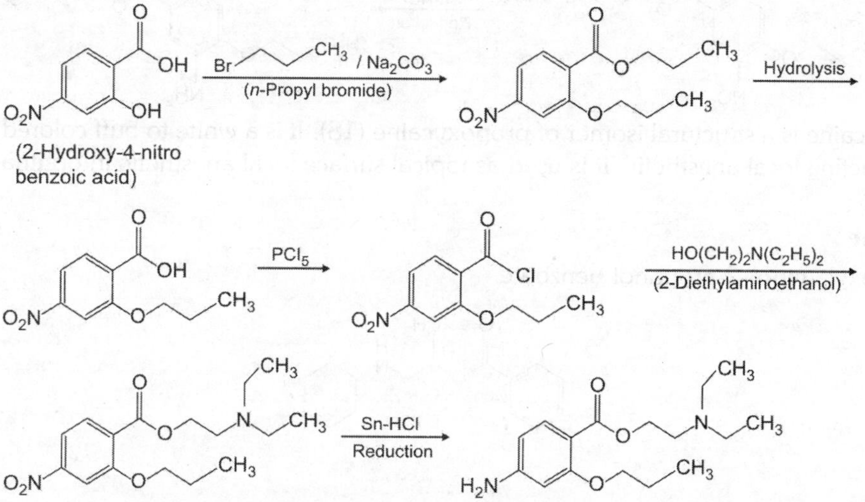

It is used as a hydrochloride as infiltration, nerve block anesthetic, and also as dental anesthetic.

Proparacaine

2-(Diethylamino)ethyl 3-amino-4-propoxybenzoate

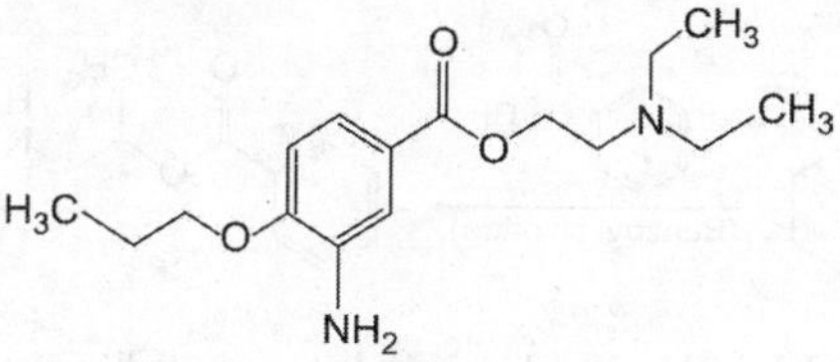

Synthesis

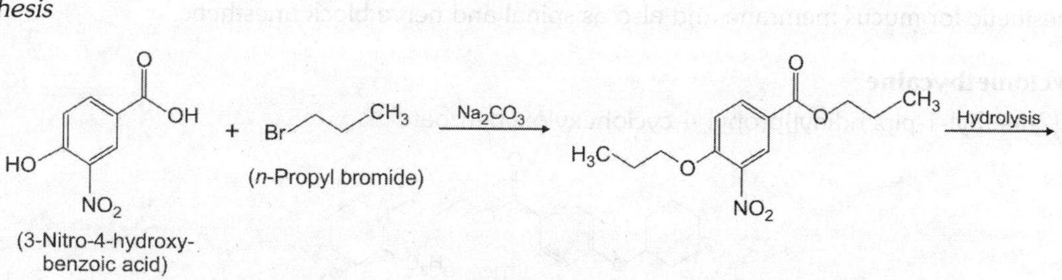

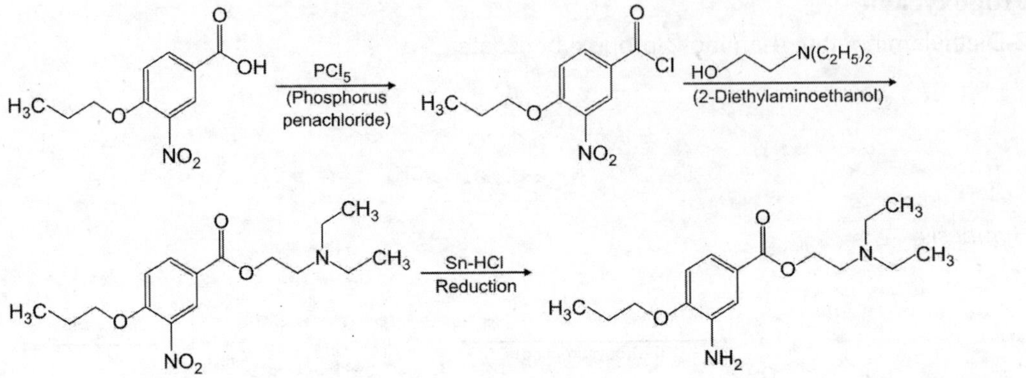

Proparacaine is a structural isomer of propoxycaine (18). It is a white to buff colored powder. It is a rapid acting local anesthetic. It is used as topical surface local anesthetic in ophthalmology.

Hexylcaine

1-(Cyclohexylamino)-2-propanol benzoate

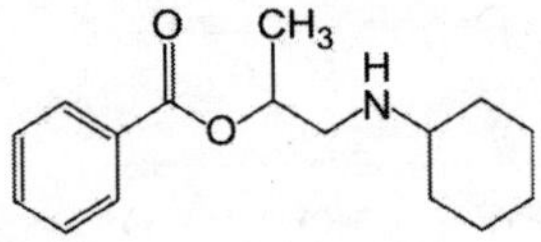

Synthesis

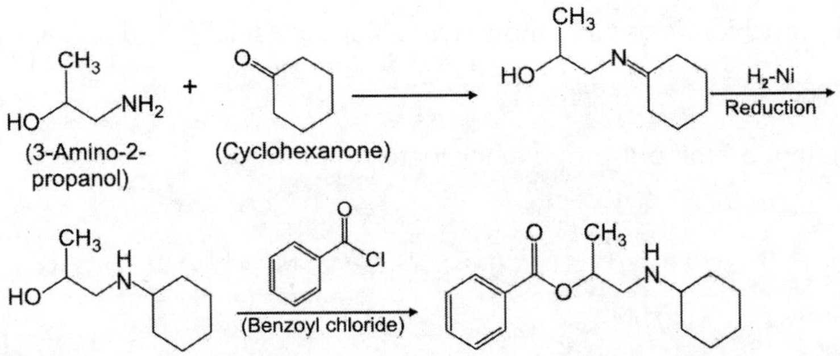

Hexylcaine is used as hydrochloride which is a white crystalline substance. It is used as a topical anesthetic for mucus memrane and also as spinal and nerve block anesthetic.

Cyclomethycaine

3-(2-Methyl-1-piperidinyl)propyl 4-cyclohexyloxybenzoate

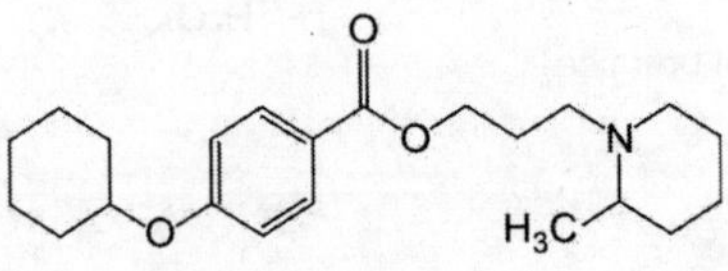

Synthesis

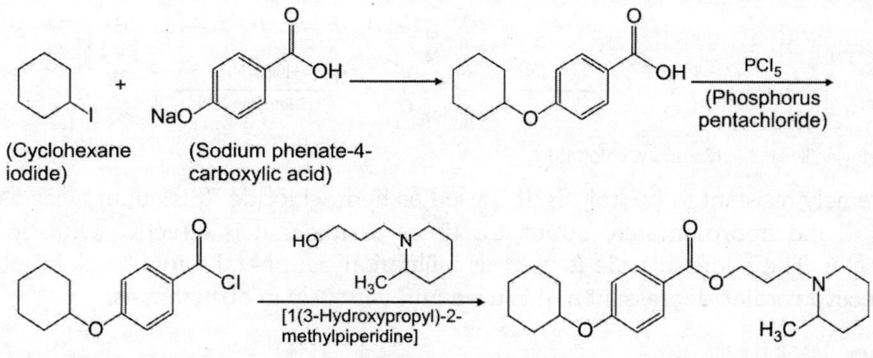

(Cyclohexane iodide) + (Sodium phenate-4-carboxylic acid) → → PCl₅ (Phosphorus pentachloride) →

[1(3-Hydroxypropyl)-2-methylpiperidine]

Cyclomethycaine is used as hydrogen sulphate salt. It is used topically on burns, abrasions and mucosa of rectum, and gentiourinary tract as ointment, jellies, creams and suppositores.

AMIDES

Prilocaine

N-(2-Methylphenyl)-2-(propylamino)propanamide

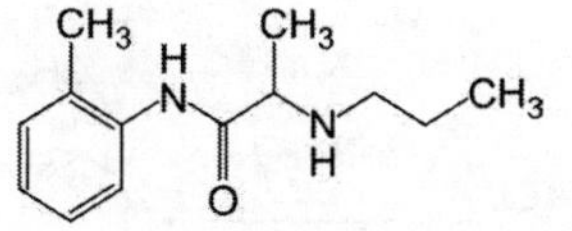

Synthesis

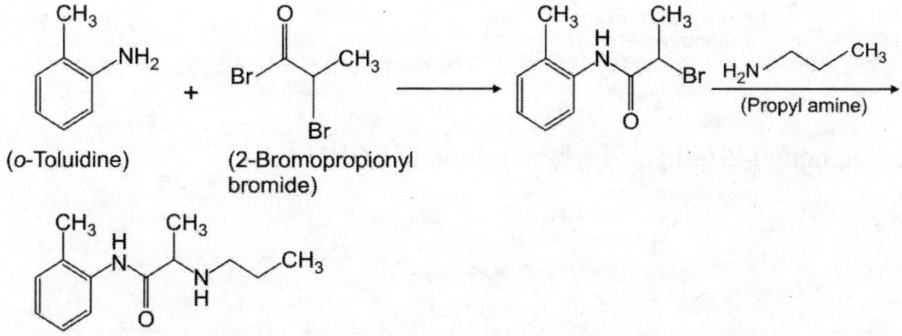

(o-Toluidine) + (2-Bromopropionyl bromide) → (Propyl amine) →

Prilocaine is used as hydrochloride which is a white powder. It is used as infiltration, intravenous, regional and nerve block anesthesia. Its potency as an anesthetic is similar to that of cocaine (1), but is less toxic than lignocaine (27).

Lignocaine

2-(Diethylamino)-N-(2, 6-dimethylphenyl)acetamide

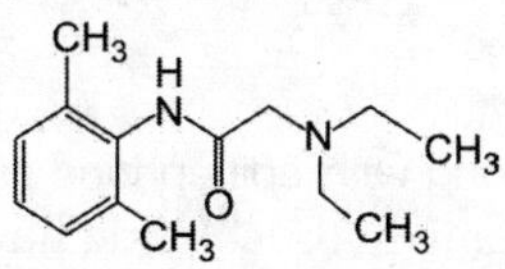

Synthesis

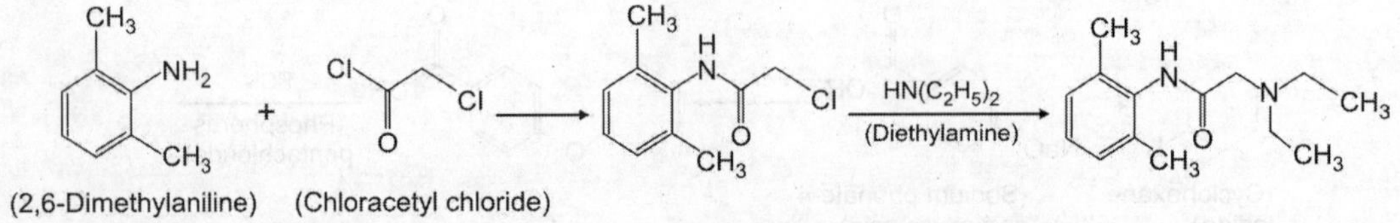

(2,6-Dimethylaniline)   (Chloracetyl chloride)

It is extremely resistant to hydrolysis. It is used as hydrochloride. It is about twice as potent as procaine (9) and approximately about 1.5 times as toxic. It is effective with or without a vasoconstrictor. The hydrochloride is used as infiltration peripheral nerve block anesthesia. It is also an effective cardiac depressant and is used intravenously in arrhythmias.

Pyrrocaine

N-(2,6-Dimethylphenyl)-1-pyrrolidineacetamide

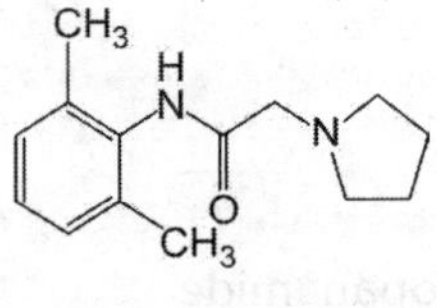

Synthesis

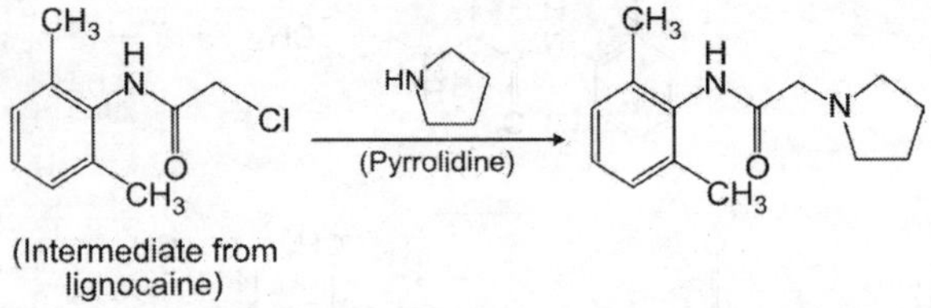

(Intermediate from
lignocaine)

Etidocaine

N-(2, 6-Dimethylphenyl)-2-(ethylpropylamino)butanamide

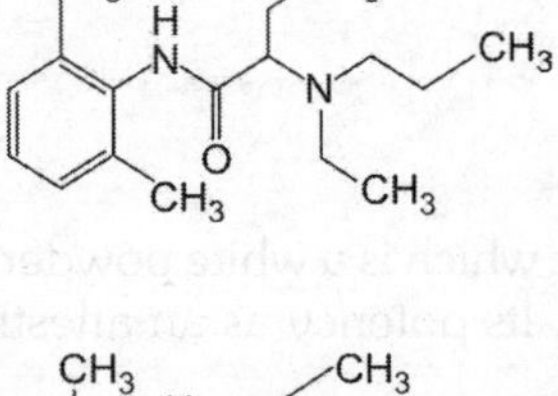

Synthesis

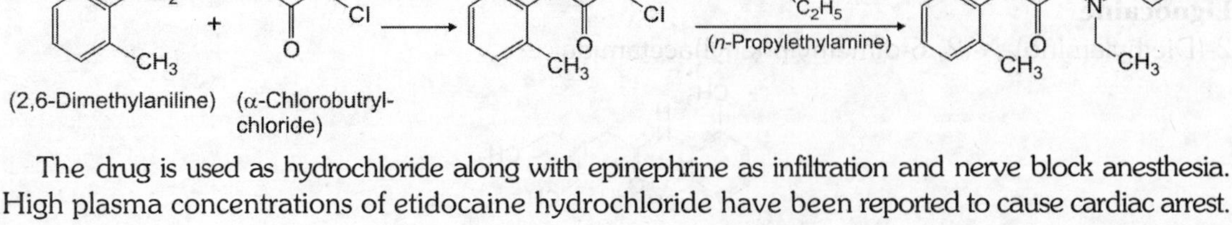

(2,6-Dimethylaniline)   (α-Chlorobutryl-
chloride)

The drug is used as hydrochloride along with epinephrine as infiltration and nerve block anesthesia. High plasma concentrations of etidocaine hydrochloride have been reported to cause cardiac arrest.

Mepivacaine

(*RS*)-*N*-(2, 6-Dimethylphenyl)-1-methyl-2-piperidinecarboxamide

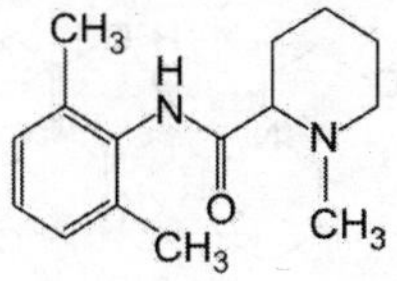

Synthesis

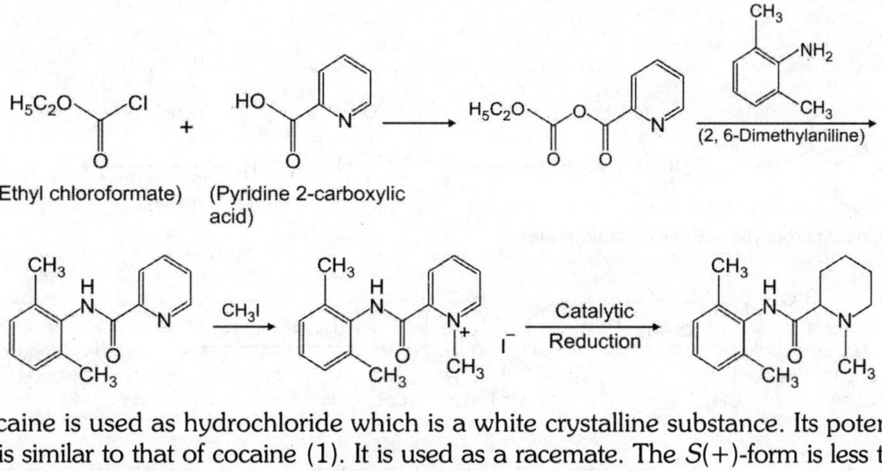

H_5C_2O
Cl
HO
N
H_5C_2O
O
CH_3
NH_2
(2, 6-Dimethylaniline)
(Ethyl chloroformate)
(Pyridine 2-carboxylic acid)
CH_3I
Catalytic Reduction

Mepivacaine is used as hydrochloride which is a white crystalline substance. Its potency as an anesthetic is similar to that of cocaine (1). It is used as a racemate. The *S*(+)-form is less toxic than *R*(–) form. It is used as infiltration and peripheral nerve anesthesia.

Bupivacaine

(*RS*)-1-Butyl-*N*-(2, 6-dimethylphenyl)-2-piperidinecarboxamide

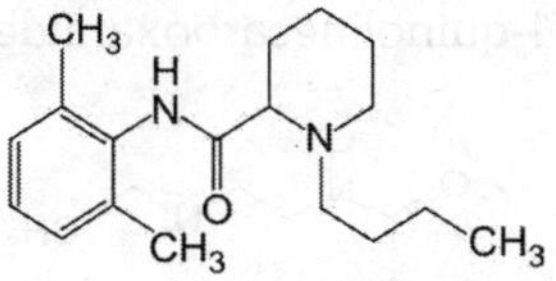

Synthesis

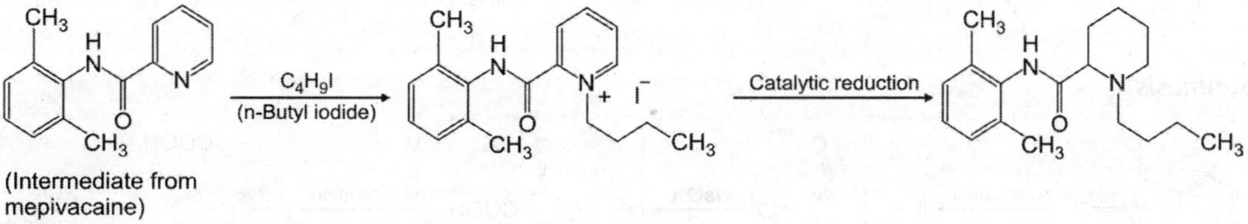

C_4H_9I
(n-Butyl iodide)
Catalytic reduction
(Intermediate from mepivacaine)

It is used in racemic form. The *S*(-)-isomer has a longer duration of action. Bupivacaine hydrochloride is used as infiltration and epidural anesthetic.

Ropivacaine

(2S)-N-(2,6-Dimethylphenyl)-1-propyl-2-piperidinecarboxamide

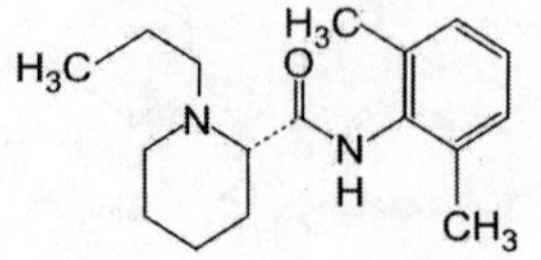

Synthesis

(Pyridine 2-carboxylic   (Ethyl chloroformate)
acid)

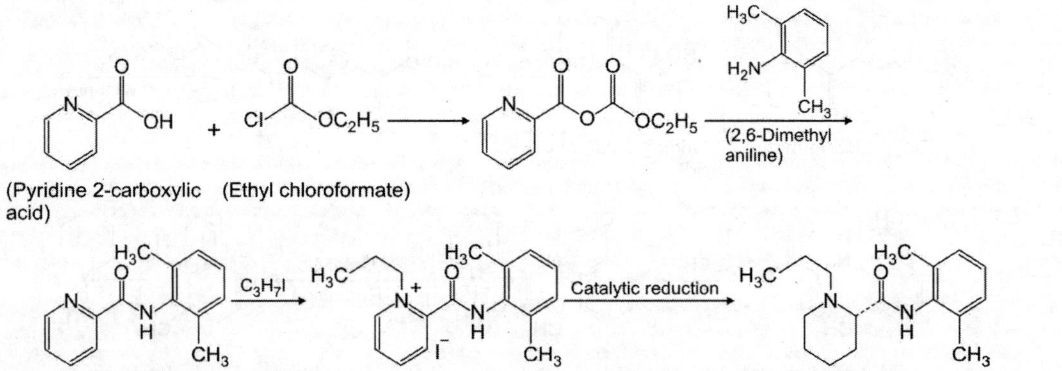

In clinical practice, hydrochloride of *S*-isomer is used. It is used as infiltration and peripheral nerve block anesthetic. It also possesses vasoconstrictor activity because of which it has a longer duration of action.

Dibucaine

2-Butoxy-N-[2-(diethylamino)ethyl]-4-quinolinecarboxamide

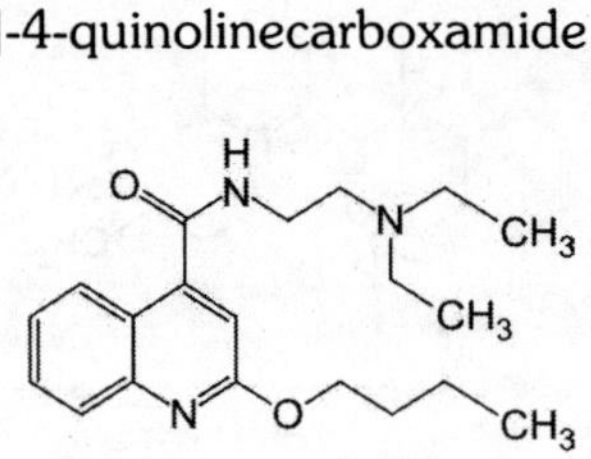

Synthesis

(Isatin)

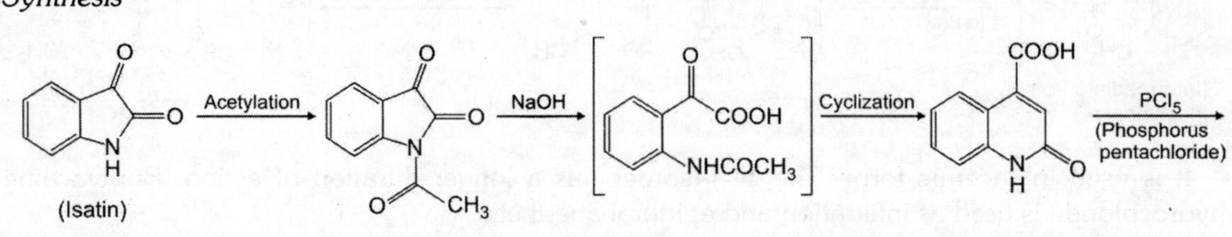

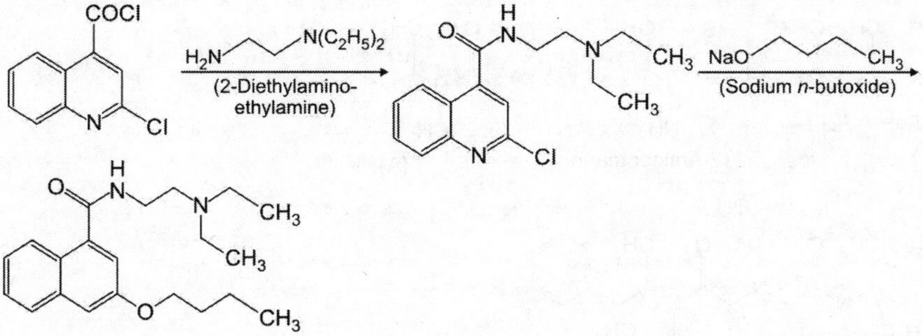

The base is used in ointments and rectal suppositories. The hydrochloride, which is more water soluble, is used in injectables. It is more potent and longer acting but more toxic.

Oxethazaine

N, *N*-Bis[*N*-methyl-*N*-phenyl-*tert*-butylacetamido]-β-hydroxyethylamine

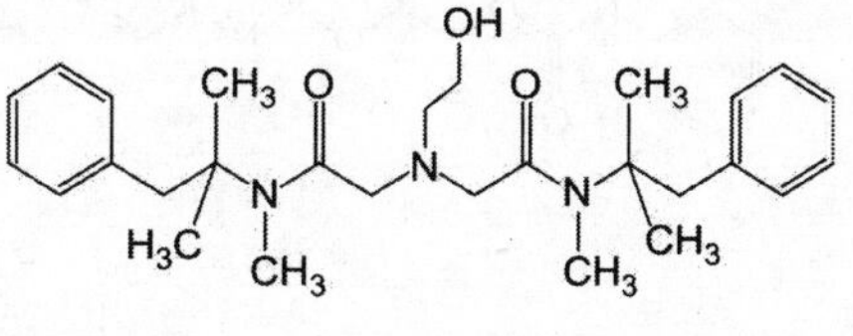

Synthesis

Step 1

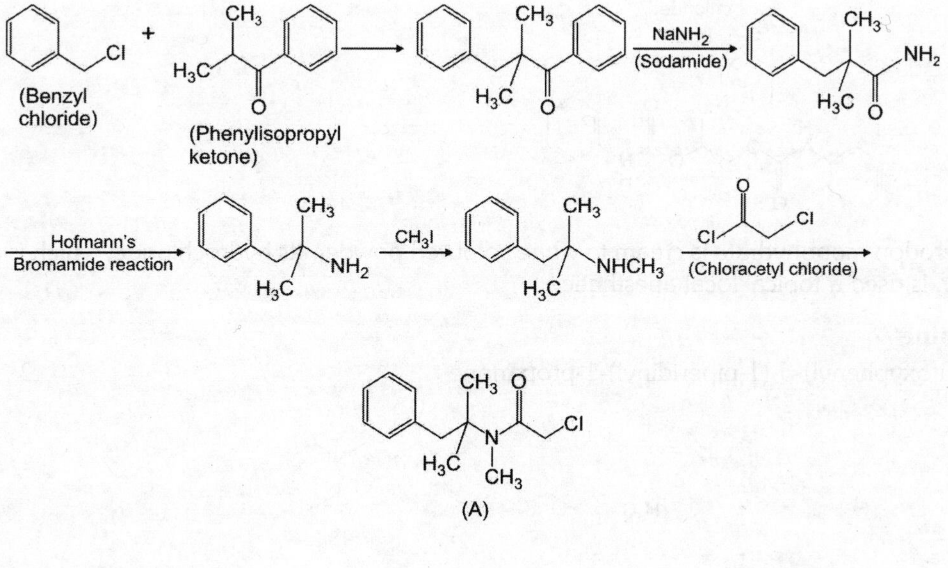

Step 2

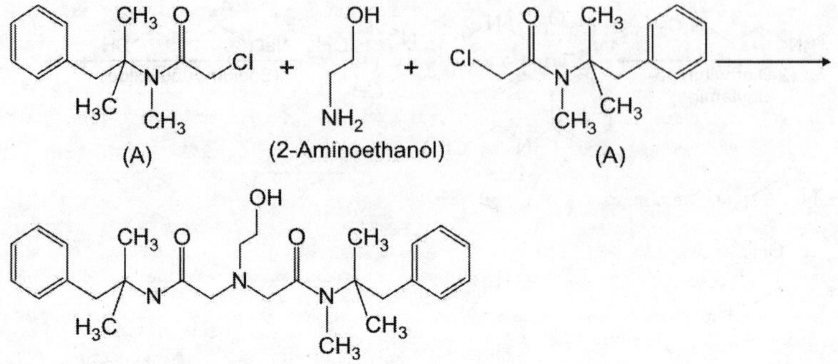

MISCELLANEOUS COMPOUNDS

Diperodon

3-(1-Piperidinyl)-1,2-propandiol bis(phenylcarbamate)

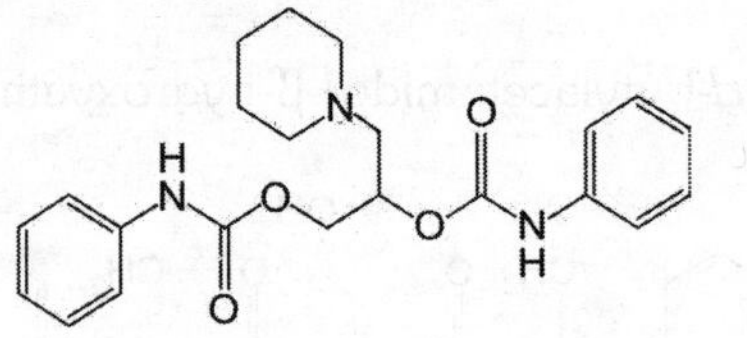

Synthesis

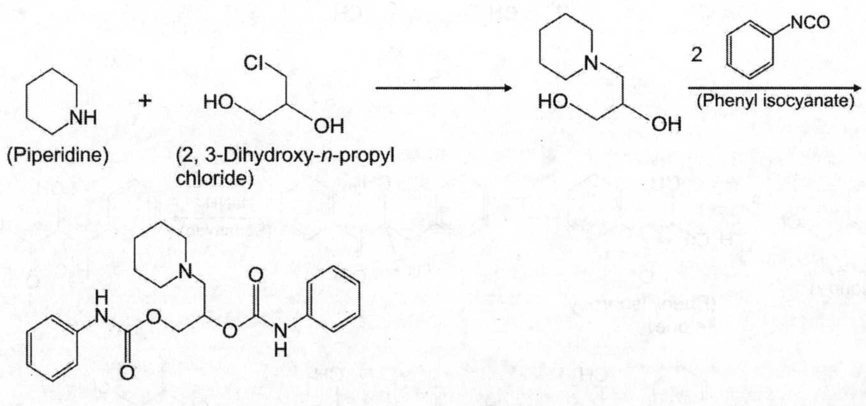

(Piperidine)   (2, 3-Dihydroxy-*n*-propyl chloride)   (Phenyl isocyanate)

Diperodon monohydrate is cream to white coloured powder. Its hydrochloride, which is a white powder, is used a topical local anesthetic.

Dyclonine

1-(4-Butoxyphenyl)-3-(1-piperidinyl)-1-propanone

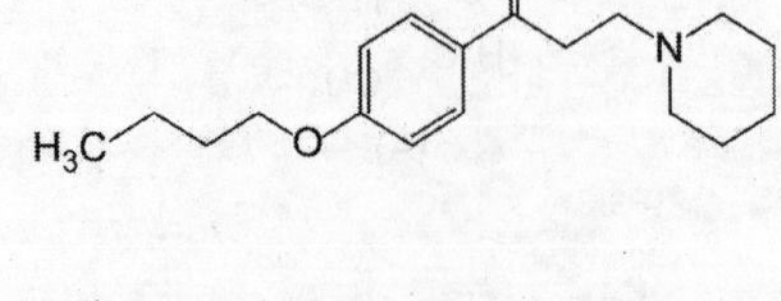

Synthesis

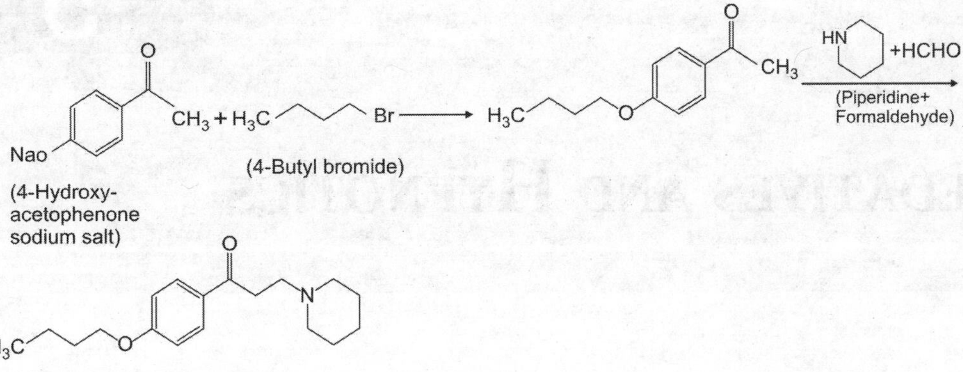

Dyclonine is used as hydrochloride. It is a white crystalline powder. It is used as mouthwash, and in gargles for sore throats.

Pramoxine

4-[3-(4-Butoxyphenoxy) propyl] morpholine

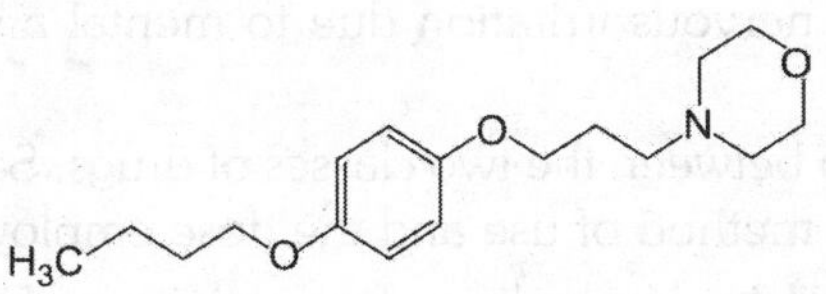

Synthesis

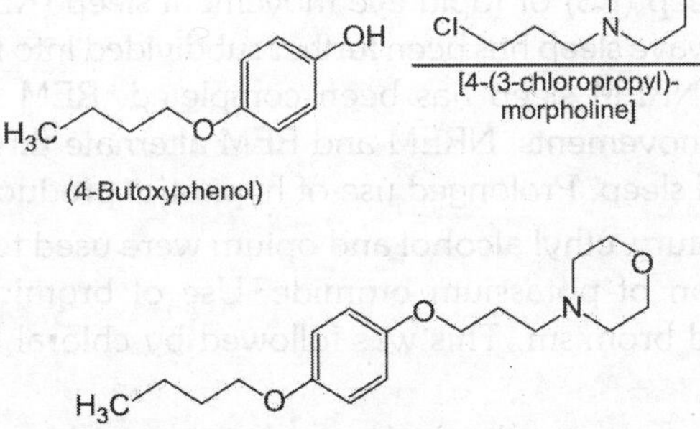

Pramoxine is used as hydrochloride which is a white powder. It is used as a topical anesthetic for the relief of insect bite and minor wounds.

SEDATIVES AND HYPNOTICS

SEDATIVES are depressant drugs which are used to remove inhibition and neurotic fears, allaying activity, and excitement. Hypnotics are also depressant drugs which induce a state resembling sleep from which the user can be aroused readily. Hypnotics are, therefore, used where natural sleep cannot be obtained. There are many situations where normal sleep cannot be obtained and these include, noise, journey, nervous irritation due to mental anguish, overwork, pain, and in maniacal states.

There is no sharp distinction between the two classes of drugs. Same drug may be used for both purposes depending upon the method of use and the dose employed.

Wakefulness is characterized by low-voltage fast activity of EEG, high muscle activity, and numerous rapid eye movements. Natural sleep, on the other hand, is composed of two alternating phases namely NREM—non-rapid eye movement sleep or slow wave sleep (SWS) which is non-dreaming, and paradoxic sleep (PS) or rapid eye movement sleep (REM sleep) in which most of dreaming takes place. Slow wave sleep has been further subdivided into four stages from drowsiness to intense sleep. After the NREM sleep has been completed, REM sleep takes over, which is characterized by rapid eye movements. NREM and REM alternate throughout the night. Most of the hypnotics suppress REM sleep. Prolonged use of hypnotics produces tolerance.

In early years of 19th century, ethyl alcohol and opium were used to induce sleep. These were followed by the introduction of potassium bromide. Use of bromides for prolonged periods produces intoxication called bromism. This was followed by chloral hydrate, paraldehyde and urethane.

The various classes of drugs presently used as sedatives and hypnotics include barbiturates, piperidinediones, benzodiazepines, non-benzodiazepine GABA$_A$ receptor agonists, and miscellaneous compounds.

BARBITURATES

Barbituric acid (1), a cyclic ureide, is obtained by condensation of urea with diethylmalonate. Number of clinically useful derivatives of barbituric acid (1), known as barbiturates, have been obtained by having substitution at position 1 or 5. In some derivatives, oxygen at position 2 has been replaced with sulphur.

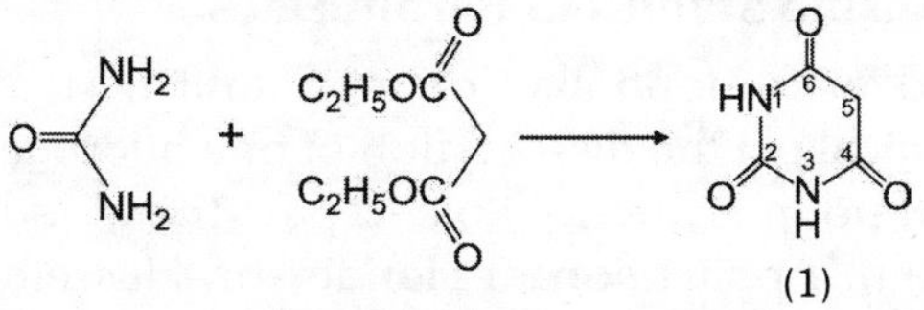

(1)

Depending upon the duration of action, barbiturates have been classified (Table 5.1) as:

1. Long acting (4-12 hr), 2. Intermediate acting (2-8 hr),
3. Short acting (2-4 hr), 4. Ultrashort acting (0.5-1 hr).

Table 5.1: Barbiturates

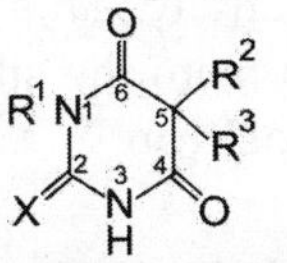

Name	R^1	X	R^2	R^3
Long acting				
Barbital	H	O	C_2H_5	C_2H_5
Metharbital	H_3C	O	C_2H_5	C_2H_5
Phenobarbital	H	O	C_2H_5	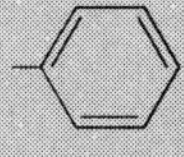 (phenyl ring)
Mephobarbital	H_3C	O	C_2H_5	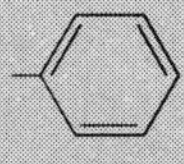 (phenyl ring)
Intermediate acting				
Allobarbital	H	O	$CH_2CH = CH_2$	$CH_2CH = CH_2$
Amobarbital	H	O	C_2H_5	$CH_2CH_2CH(CH_3)_2$
Butabarbital	H	O	$CH(CH_3)CH_2CH_3$	C_2H_5
Cyclobarbital	H	O	C_2H_5	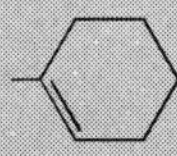 (cyclohexenyl ring)
Short acting				
Pentobarbital	H	O	C_2H_5	$CH(CH_3)CH_2CH_2CH_3$
Secobarbital	H	O	$CH_2CH = CH_2$	$CH(CH_3)CH_2CH_2CH_3$
Ultrashort acting				
Hexobarbital	H_3C	O	CH_3	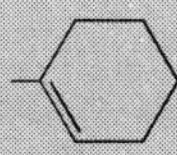 (cyclohexenyl ring)
Thiopental	H	S	C_2H_5	$CH(CH_3)CH_2CH_2CH_3$
Thiamylal	H	S	$CH_2CH = CH_2$	$CH(CH_3)CH_2CH_2CH_3$

Structure-Activity Relationship Studies in Barbiturates

1. The 5-unsubstituted or 5-monoalkyl or monoaryl derivatives are inactive. This is because at physiological pH the dissociation of one hydrogen at C_5 takes place readily. As a result, such compounds are not able to pass the blood-brain barrier to reach the site of action in brain. Application of Henderson-Hasselbalch equation (Eq. 1) has shown that at physiological pH, unsubstituted or monosubstituted brabituric acid derivatives are mostly present in dissociated form. 5, 5-Disubstituted derivatives such as 5-phenyl-5-ethyl barbituric acid (phenobarbital) on the other hand is present up to 43 % in undissociated form. Thus, it is able to penetrate the blood-brain barrier because of its higher lipid solubility. Disubstitution at position 5 increases the hypnotic activity till the total number of carbon atoms of both the substituents reaches 8. Further increase in carbon atoms leads to loss of activity. This could be due to loss of solubility in water which is necessary for its transport from the site of its absorption. Derivatives containing branched aliphatic groups at position 5 are more active and less toxic than the unbranched group.

$$pH = pKa + \log \frac{[A^-]}{[HA]} \qquad \text{(Eq. 1)}$$

2. The hypnotic activity of 5, 5-disubstituted brabiturates can be further increased by substitution on nitrogen. This is because such a substitution results in further decrease in ionization and increase in lipophilicity. Thus the pKa value of 5, 5-diethyl barbituric acid [barbital, (2)] is 7. 8. The pKa of its N-methyl derivatives [metharbital, (3)] is 8.2. According to Henderson-Hasselbalch equation, it is about 89% in undissociated form which results in its greater lipid solubility. Substitution on nitrogen also results in rapid onset of action. Introduction of an alkyl group on another nitrogen leads to compounds with convulsant action.

(2), R=H
(3), R=CH₃

(4), X=O
(5), X=S

3. Replacement of oxygen by sulphur at position 2 affects the depth and quality of the pharmacological response. Thus, secobarbital (4) is a short acting barbiturate on the other hand its sulfur isolog, thiamylal (5) is an ultrashort acting barbiturate with anesthetic activity.

Barbiturates have number of advantages such as:

1. They are not disagreeable to taste like chloral hydrate and paraldehyde.

2. Their use is not restricted to hypnosis alone, but by varying the dose, they can also be used as sedatives. Further, by suitable changes, they have also been used as anesthetics.
3. Various classes of barbiturates permit a gradation of sleep production according to needs.

Inspite of these advantages, the use of barbiturates is declining. This is because they have higher toxicity which is because of their ability to cause more CNS depression. They also cause tolerance and often dependence.

Mechanism of Action

Barbiturates markedly decrease the functional activity of brain. Like benzodiazepines, barbiturates enhance the action of GABA by binding to $GABA_A$ receptor/chloride channel at a site different from benzodiazepine. This binding results in potentiation of $GABA_A$-mediated chloride ion conductance. Increased chloride permeability results in hyperpolarization of cell, thereby, reducing its excitability.

PIPERIDINEDIONES

Among the piperidinediones, methyprylon (6), a 2, 4-piperidinedione and glutethimide (7), a 2, 6-piperidinedione analog, have been the most successful hypnotics. Both of these compounds possess good hypnotic activity but they cause habituation, tolerance, and addiction. They act in same way as barbiturates.

(6)

(7)

BENZODIAZEPINES

The discovery of sedative action in chlordiazepoxide (8) led to investigations of benzodiazepines as sedatives and hypnotics. Some of the benzodiazepines used clinically as sedatives and hypnotics include nitrazepam (9), nimetazepam (10), flunitrazepam (11), flurazepam (12), temazepam (13), and quazepam (14).

(8)

(9), $R_1 = R_2 = R_3 = H$, $X = O$, $R_4 = NO_2$ (10), $R_1 = CH_3$, $X = O$, $R_2 = R_3 = H$, $R_4 = NO_2$

(11), $R_1 = CH_3$, $X = O$, $R_2 = H$, $R_3 = F$, $R_4 = NO_2$ (12), $R_1 = CH_2CH_2N(C_2H_5)_2$, $X = O$, $R_2 = H$, $R_3 = F$, $R_4 = Cl$

(13), $R_1 = CH_3$, $X = O$, $R_2 = OH$, $R_3 = H$, $R_4 = Cl$ (14), $R_1 = CH_2 CF_3$, $X = S$, $R_2 = H$, R_3, $= F$, $R_4 = Cl$

Analogs in which hetrocyclic rings have been fused with benzodiazpine system include midazolam (15), loprazolam (16), estazolam (17), and triazolam (18).

(15)   (16)   (17), R = R' = H

(18), R = CH$_3$, R' = Cl

The onset of sleep with benzodiazepines is faster. They are active orally and also increase the duration of sleep. Benzodiazepines decrease anxiety and cause muscle relaxation. They have antiepileptic effect also. Like barbiturates, they have also been classified on the basis of duration of action.

Benzodiazepines increase the affinity of GABA for the receptor by binding at the regulatory site of $GABA_A$ receptors. This facilitates the binding of GABA to $GABA_A$ receptors and opening of chloride channel which results in hyperpolarization of cell thereby reducing its excitability.

NONBEZODIAZEPINE GABA$_A$ RECEPTOR AGONISTS

Some of the nonbenzodiazepine $GABA_A$ receptor agonists which have been introduced in clinical practice include zolpidem (19), zopiclone (20), and zaleplon (21). Both zolpidem (19) and zopiclone (20) have been reported to cause reduced physical dependence. Both of them are short acting hypnotics.

(19)   (20)   (21)

MISCELLANEOUS COMPOUNDS

Quinazolinones

Methaqualone (22), a quinazolinone, has been used where patients are unresponsive or intolerant to barbiturates. A close analog, mecloqualone (23), in which the *o*-tolyl residue has been replaced by *o*-chlorophenyl, has been found to be equally effective.

(22), R = CH$_3$

(23), R = Cl

Alcohols

Ethyl alcohol has been used as sedative and hypnotic ever since man learned to produce it. Alcohol is narcotic and depresses first the highest cerebral centres, then lower ones which include cerebellum and spinal cord.

The hypnotic activity of alcohols increases with molecular weight and maximum is reached with *n*-hexanol. However, the branching of alkyl chain as well as change from primary through secondary to tertiary alcohols raises the activity. Chlorobutanol (24) is a powerful hypnotic. It is now used more as preservative.

(24)

(25)

(26)

Introduction of acetylenic group at the carbinol carbon also produces hypnotic effect. Methylparafynol (25) is orally and parenterally active and has a short duration of action. Ethchlorvynol (26), which has both unsaturation as well as a halogen atom has a rapid onset of action. Habituation, tolerance and physical dependence seem to develop when it is used regularly.

Aldehydes

Aliphatic aldehydes are thought to exert their hypnotic effect by being converted to alcohol. Chloral hydrate (27), an adduct of chloral and water, is one of the oldest hypnotic. Its action is due to trichloroethanol (28) formed in body. It is a safe hypnotic but it has some disadvantages which include its undesirable taste, strong odour, and irritation to GI tract. To overcome this various derivatives of chloral hydrate (27) have been prepared. These analogs on hydrolysis yield chloral hydrate (27) or trichloroethanol (28). Some of these analogs are, triclofos (29) and pentaerythritol chloral (30).

(27)

(28)

(29)

(30)

Another aldehyde which has been used as hypnotic is paraldehyde (31), the cyclic polymer of acetaldehyde. It is usually given with iced beverages.

Carbamic acid analog ethinamate (32) has been reported to be useful in insomnia.

Some of the acyl ureas, namely monoureides, the open chain analogs of barbiturates which show sedative and hypnotic activity include carbromal (33) and bromisovalum (34).

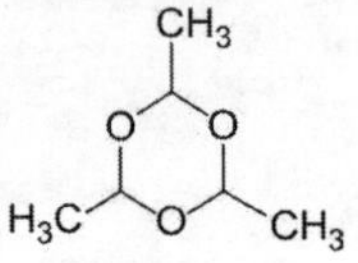

(31) 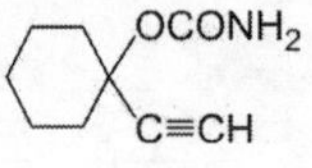   (32) 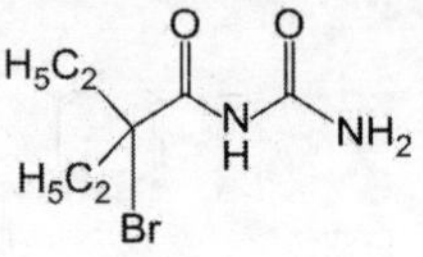   (33) 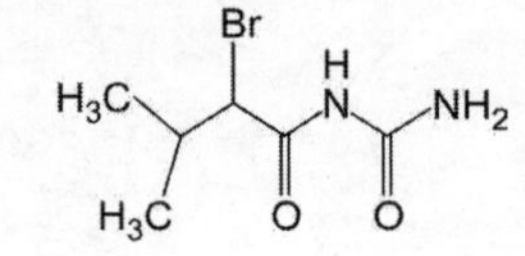   (34)

INDIVIDUAL COMPOUNDS

BARBITURATES
Barbital
5, 5-Diethylbarbituric acid

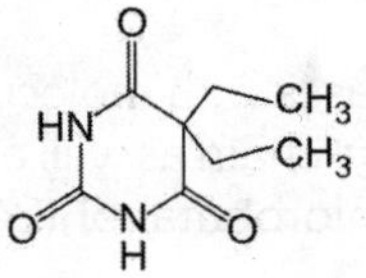

Synthesis

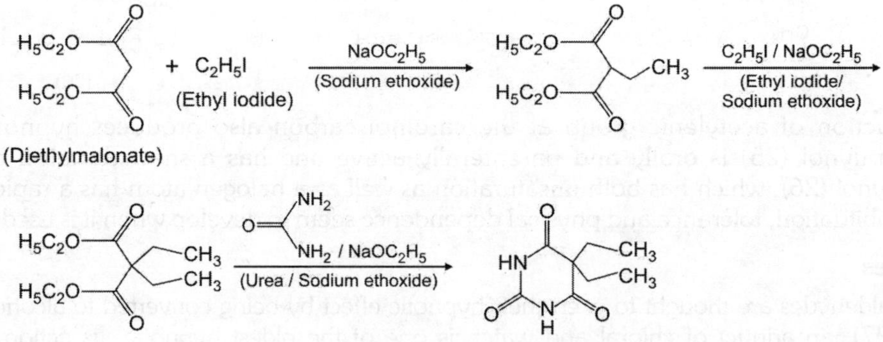

It is long acting sedative-hypnotic but not in use now. It is slowly eliminated through kidney.

Metharbital
5, 5-Diethyl-1-methylbarbituric acid

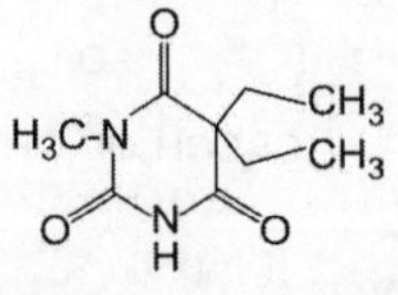

Synthesis

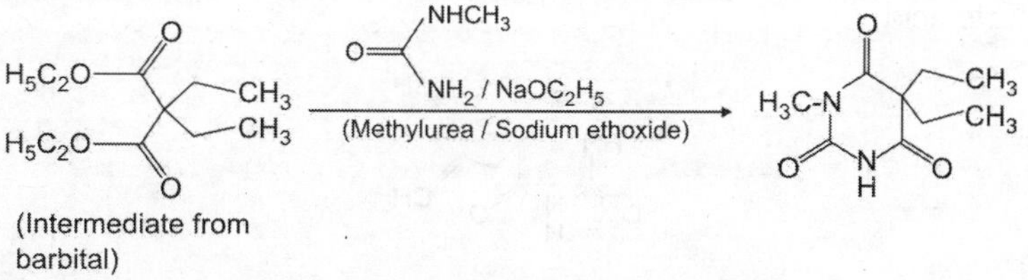

(Intermediate from barbital)

It is long acting barbiturate used in different types of epilepsies.

Phenobarbital

5-Ethyl-5-phenylbarbituric acid

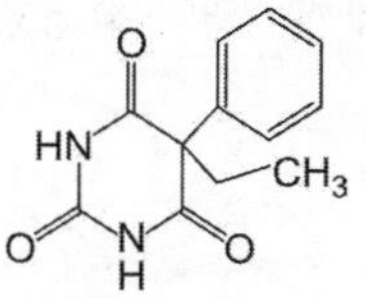

Synthesis

(Ethyl phenylacetate) (Diethyloxalate)

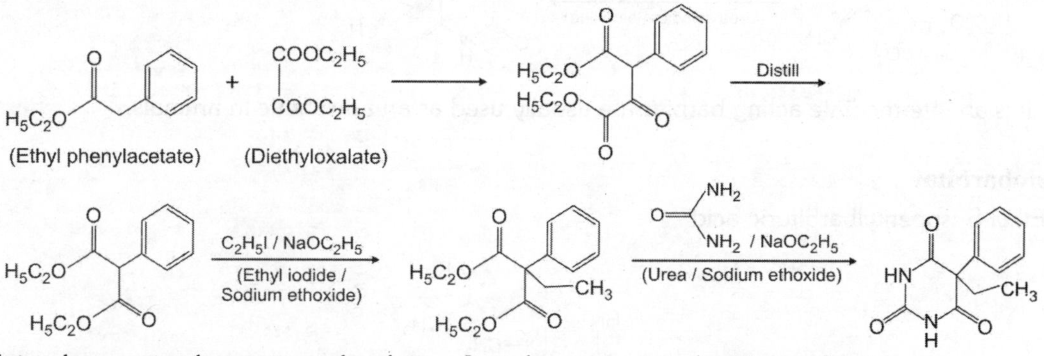

It is a long acting hypnotic and sedative. It is also a very good anticonvulsant.

Mephobarbital

5-Ethyl-5-phenyl-1-methylbarbituric acid

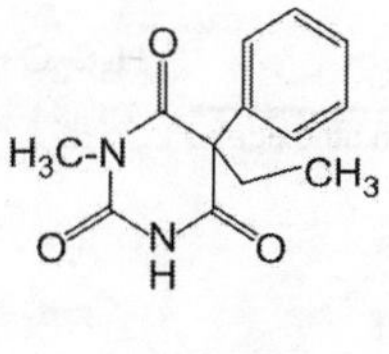

Synthesis

(Intermediate from phenobarbital)

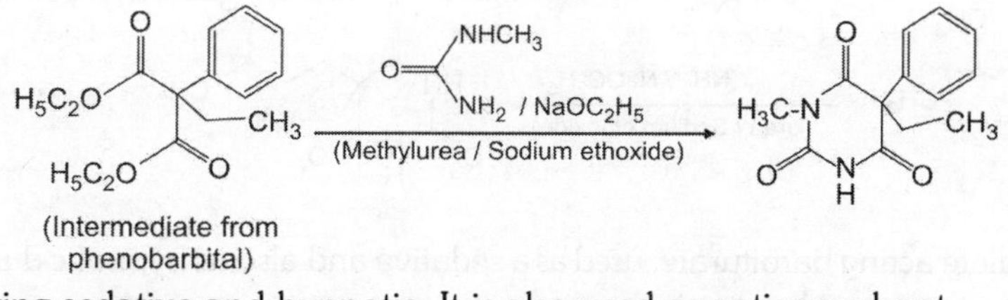

It is a long acting sedative and hypnotic. It is also used as anticonvulsant.

Allobarbital

5, 5-Diallylbarbituric acid

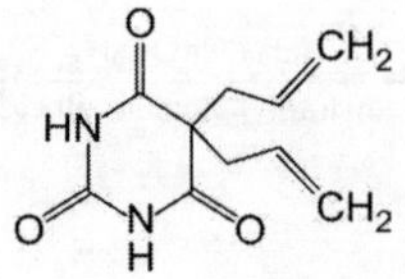

Synthesis

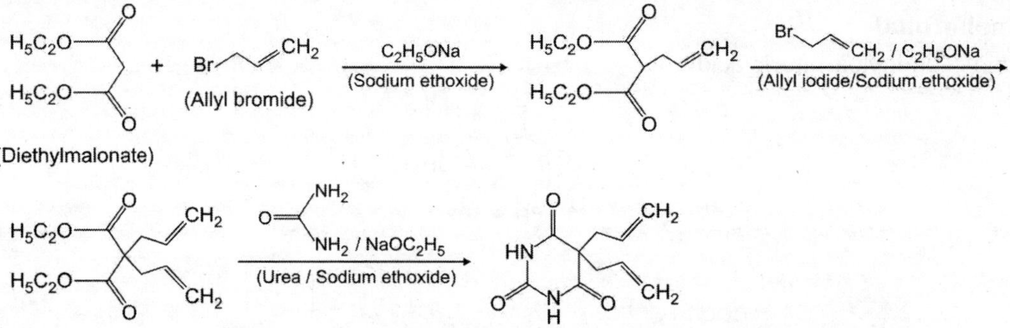

It is an intermediate acting barbiturate usually used as an anesthetic in animals.

Amobarbital

5-Ethyl-5-isopentylbarbituric acid

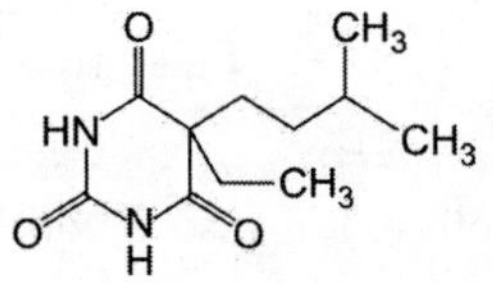

Synthesis

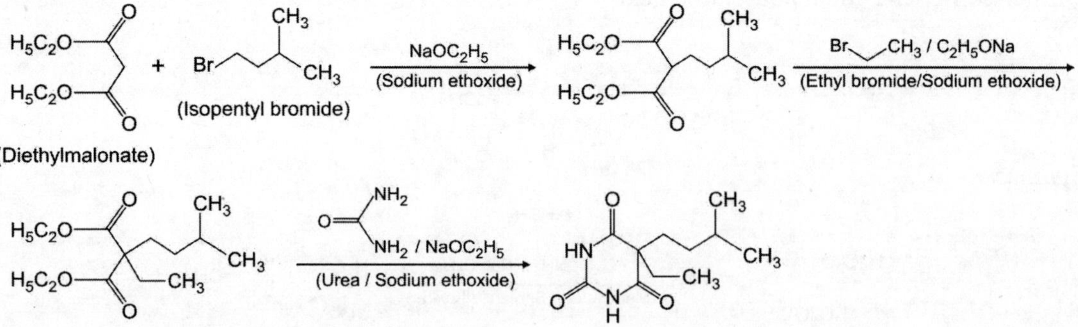

It is an intermediate acting barbiturate, used as a sedative and also as hypnotic during preanesthetic medication, and as anticonvulsant.

Butabarbital

5-Ethyl-5-(1-methylpropyl)barbituric acid

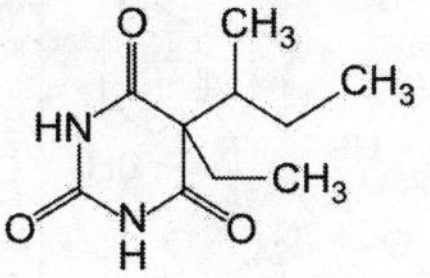

Synthesis

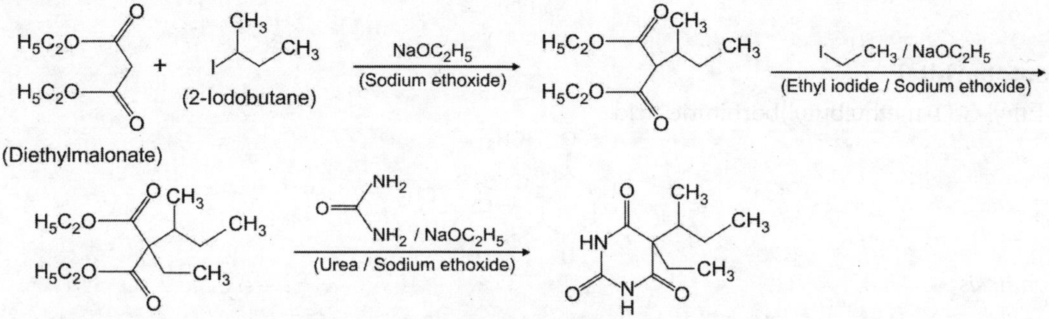

It is an intermediate acting barbiturate used as a hypnotic.

Cyclobarbital

5-(1-Cyclohexen-1-yl)-5-ethylbarbituric acid

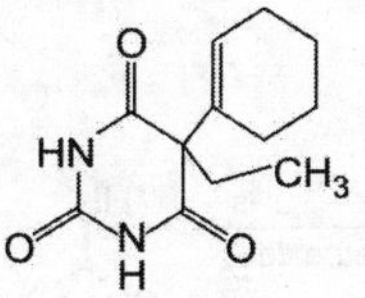

Synthesis

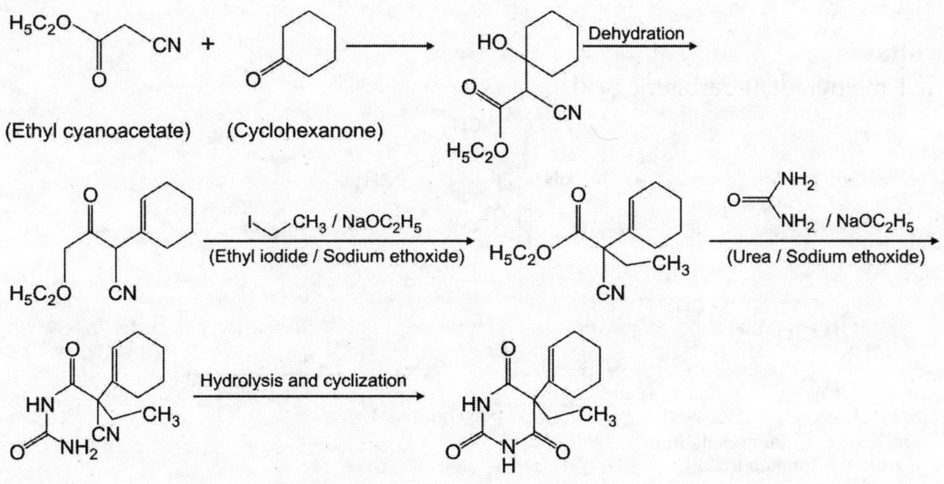

It is used as calcium salt (35) as hypnotic.

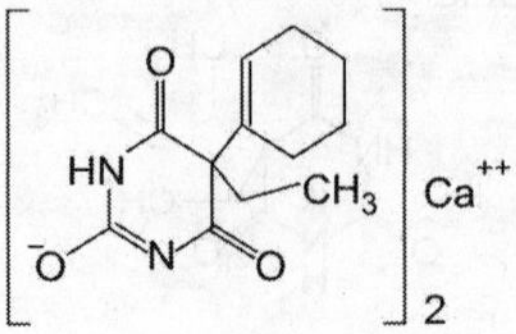

(35)

Pentobarbital

5-Ethyl-5-(1-methylbutyl)barbituric acid

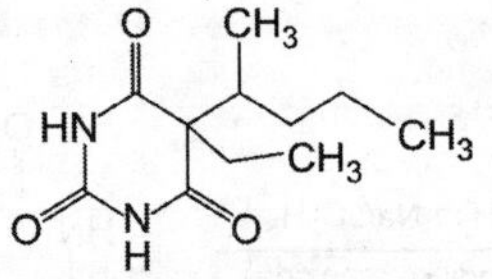

Synthesis

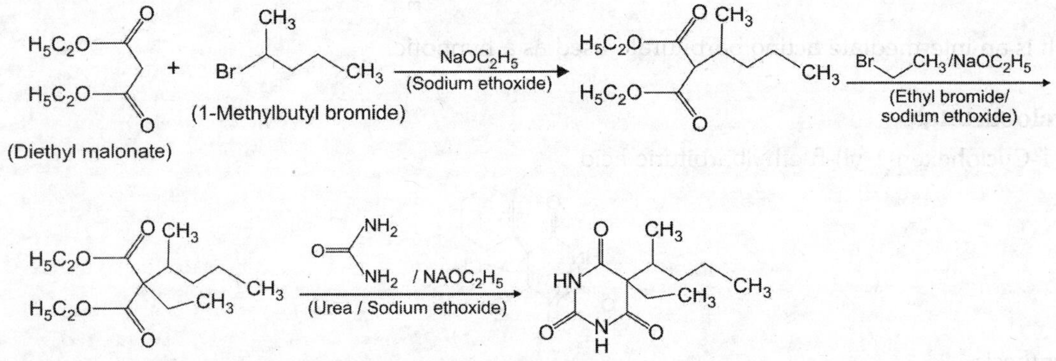

It is short acting barbiturate.

Secobarbital

5-Allyl-5-(1-methylbutyl) barbituric acid

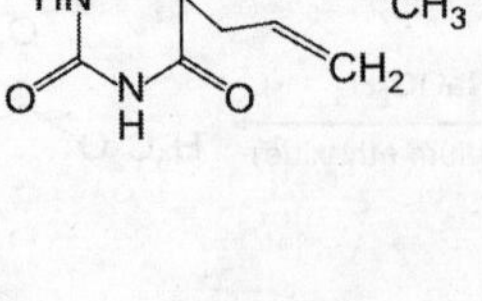

Synthesis

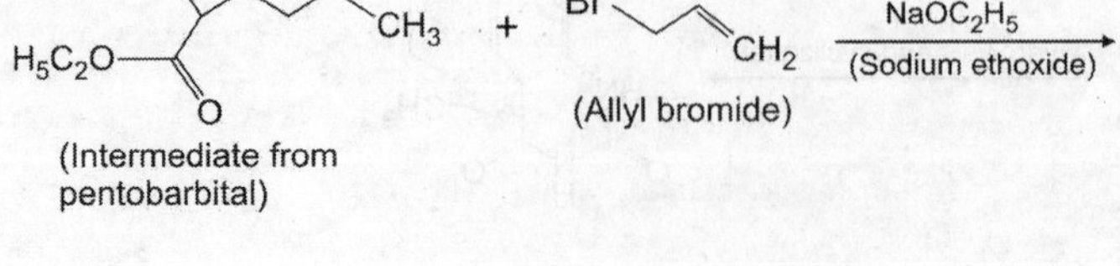

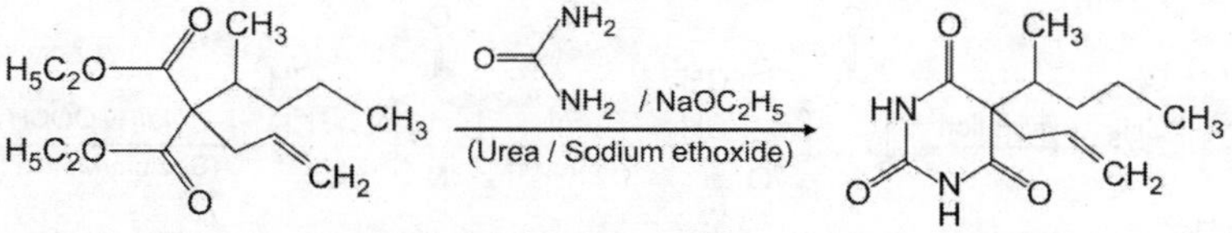

It is a short acting barbiturate used for hypnosis either orally or rectally.

Hexobarbital
5-(1-Cyclohexenyl-1-yl)-1, 5-dimethylbarbituric acid

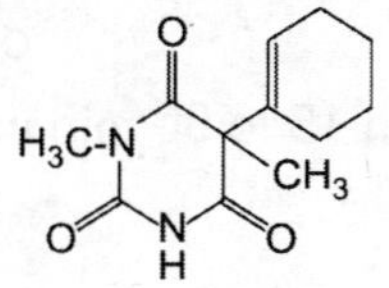

Synthesis

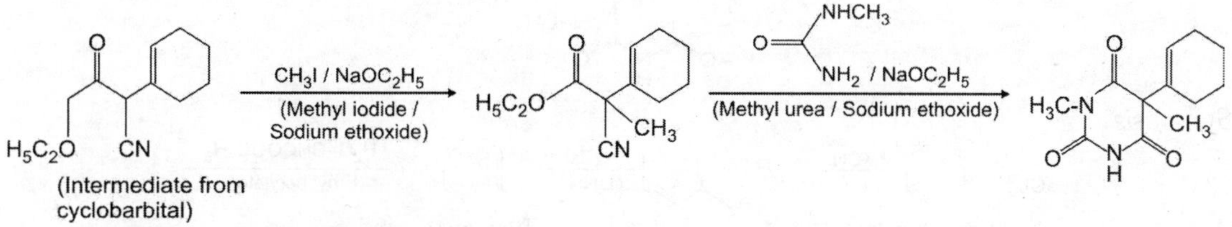

It is an ultrashort acting barbiturate

Thiopental Sodium and Thiamylal Sodium
See GENERAL ANESTHETICS

PIPERIDINEDIONES
Methyprylon
3, 3-Diethyl-5-methyl-2,4-piperidinedione

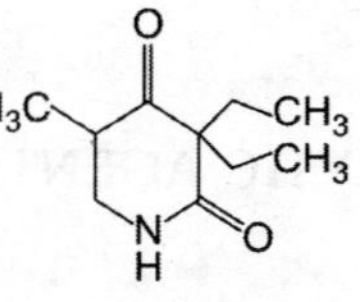

Synthesis

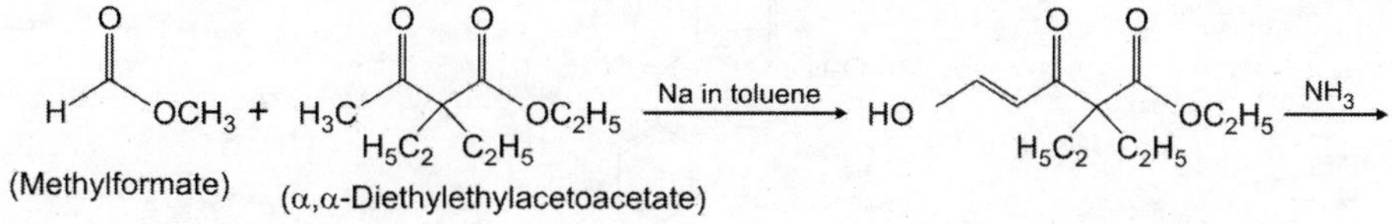

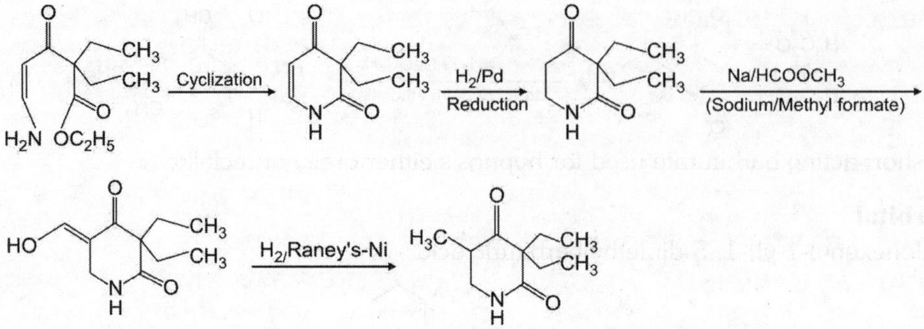

It is useful for induction of sleep within 15 to 30 min in patients suffering of insomnia.

Glutethimide

2-Ethyl-2-phenylglutarimide

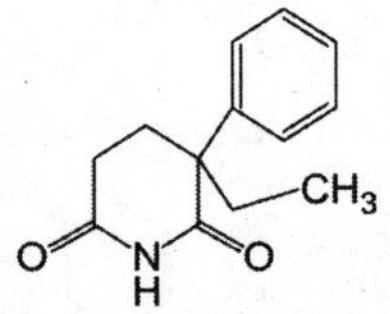

Synthesis

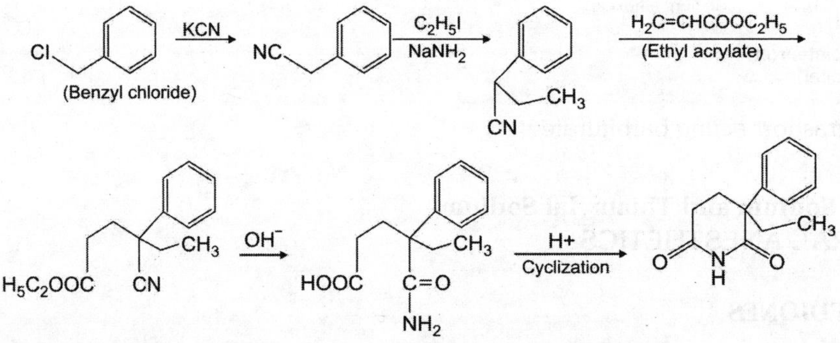

Its onset of hypnotic action is within 30 min which lasts for about 4-8 hours. It is an useful drug for insomnia and has been used as a day time sedative.

BENZODIAZEPINES

Chlordiazepoxide

See NEUROLEPTICS AND ANXIOLYTIC AGENTS

Nitrazepam

7-Nitro-1, 3-dihydro-5-phenyl-2*H*-1,4-benzodiazepin-2-one

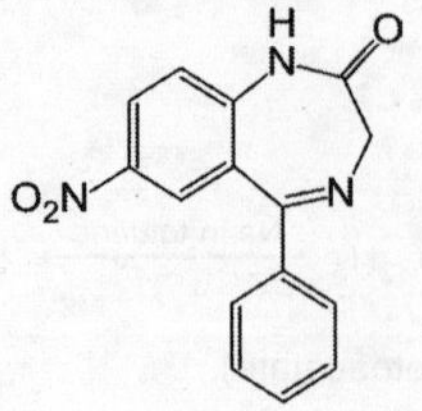

Synthesis

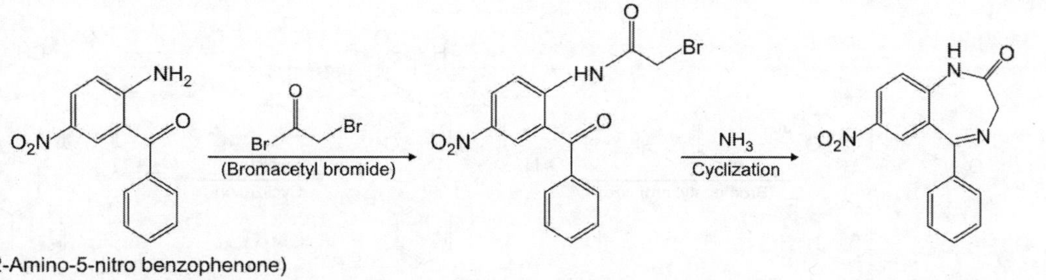

(2-Amino-5-nitro benzophenone)

It is used as hypnotic and anticonvulsant. The onset of its action is within 30-60 min with a duration of action of 6-8 hr.

Nimetazepam

1-Methyl-5-phenyl-7-nitro-1,3-dihydro-2*H*-1,4-benzodiazepin-2-one

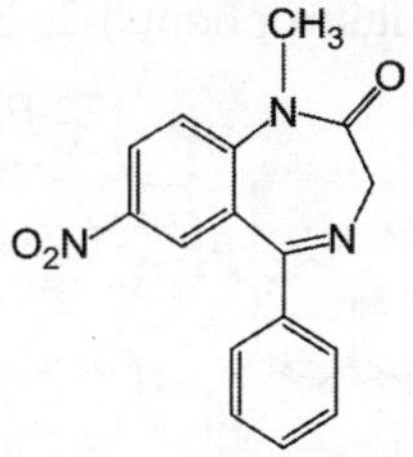

Synthesis

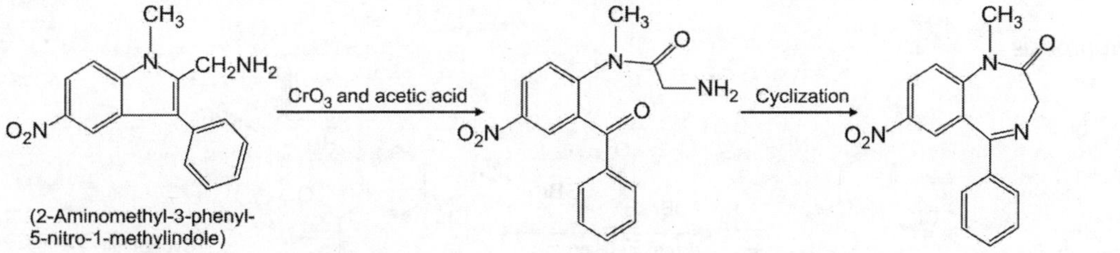

(2-Aminomethyl-3-phenyl-
5-nitro-1-methylindole)

It is used as sedative and hypnotic.

Flunitrazepam

7-Nitro-1, 3-dihydro-1-methyl-5-(2-fluorophenyl)-2*H*-1,4-benzodiazepin-2-one

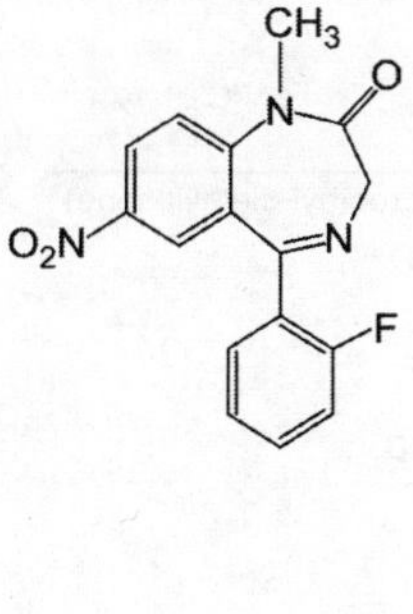

Synthesis

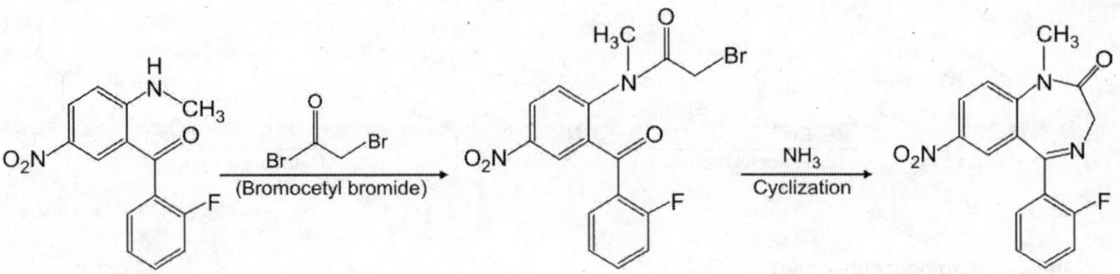

(2-methylamino-5-
nitro-2'-fluorobenzophenone)

It is used in insomnia and as premedication for anesthesia.

Flurazepam

7-Chloro-1-[2-(diethylamino)ethyl]-5-(2-fluorophenyl)-1, 3-dihydro-2*H*-1,4-benzodiazepin-2-one

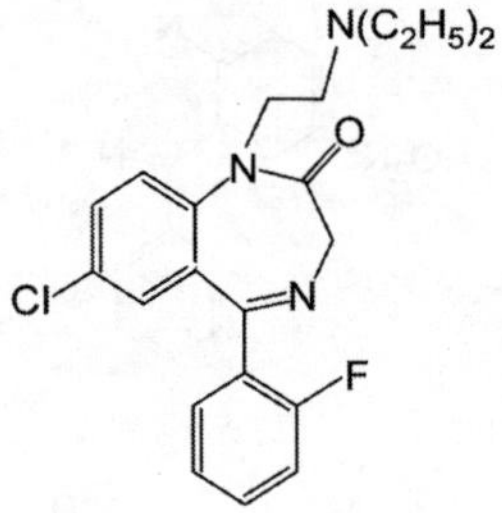

Synthesis

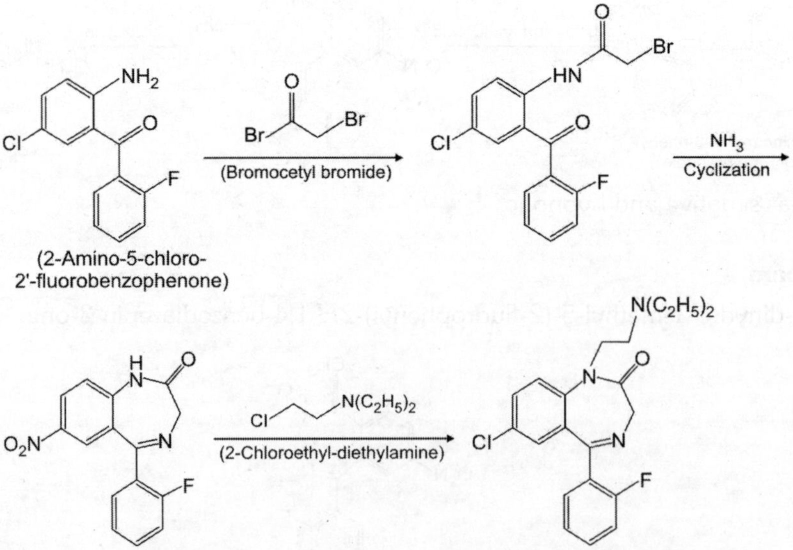

(2-Amino-5-chloro-
2'-fluorobenzophenone)

It is exclusively indicated in insomnia.

Temazepam

7-Chloro-1, 3-dihydro-3-hydroxy-1-methyl-5-phenyl-2*H*-1,4-benzodiazepin-2-one.

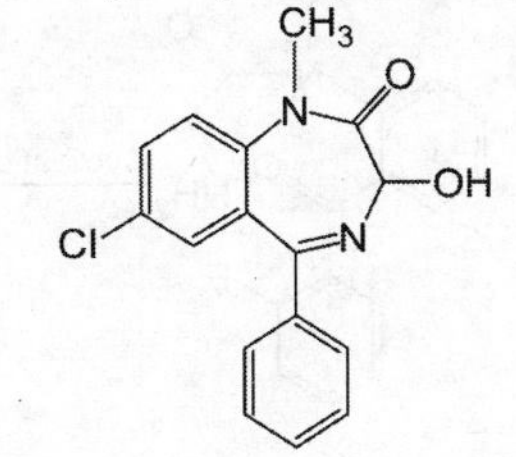

Synthesis

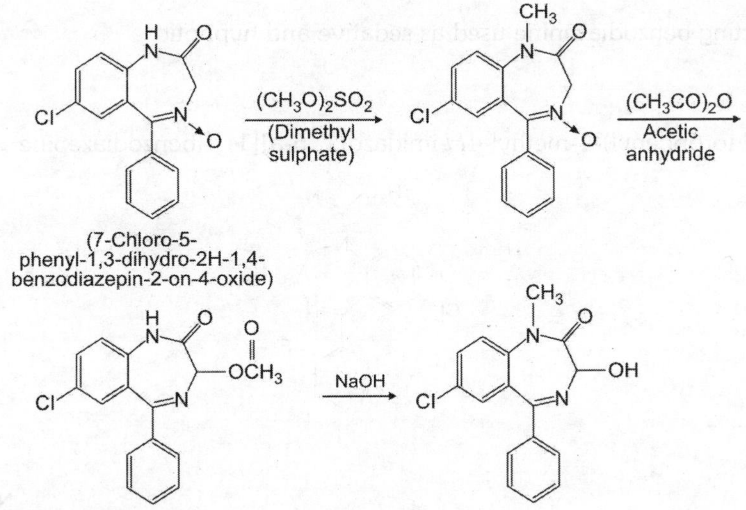

(7-Chloro-5-
phenyl-1,3-dihydro-2H-1,4-
benzodiazepin-2-on-4-oxide)

Used as sedative and hypnotic.

Quazepam

7-Chloro-5-(2-fluorophenyl)-1,3-dihydro-1(2,2,2,-trifluoroethyl)-2*H*-1,4-benzodiazepine-2-thione

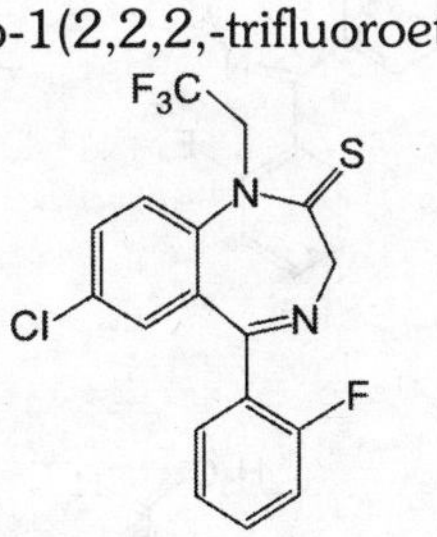

Synthesis

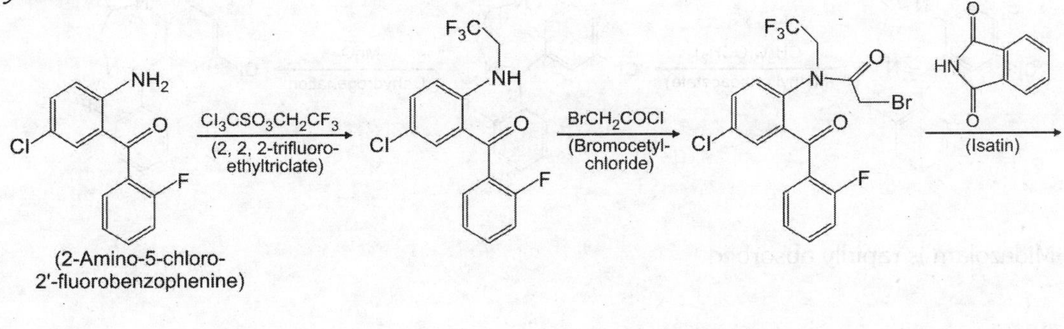

(2-Amino-5-chloro-
2'-fluorobenzophenine)

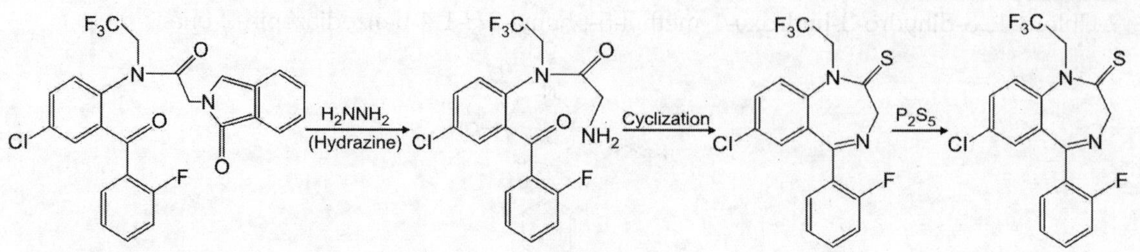

It is a long acting benzodiazepine used as sedative and hypnotic.

Midazolam

8-Chloro-6-(2-fluorophenyl)-1-methyl-4*H*-imidazo[1, 5-a][1, 4]benzodiazepine

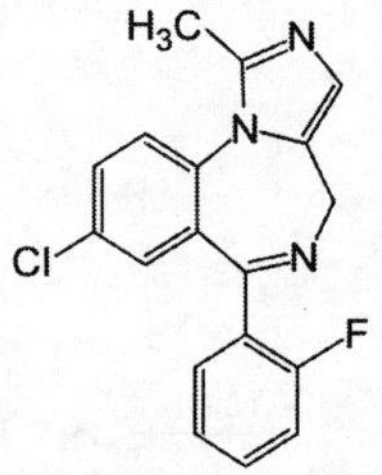

Synthesis

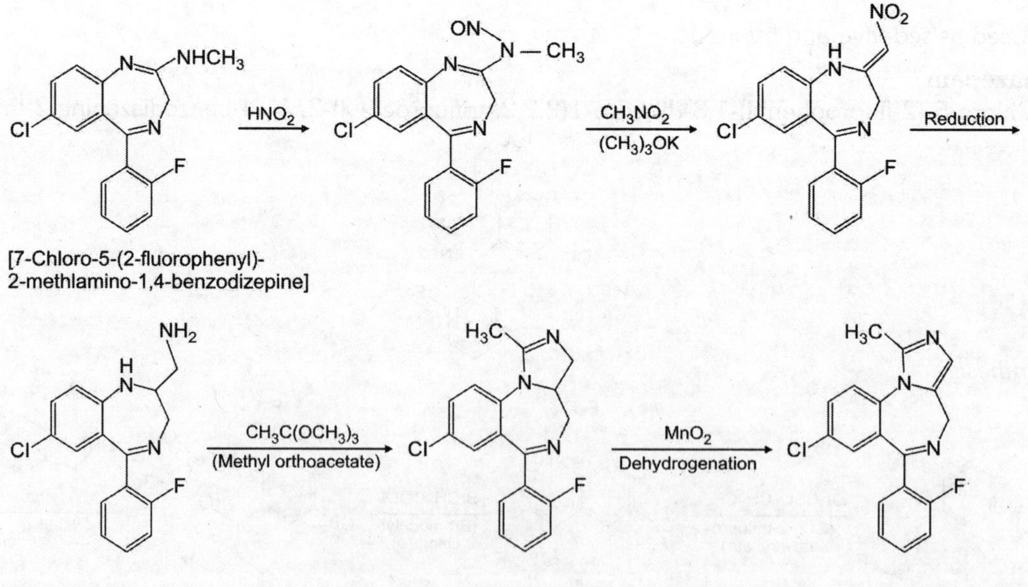

[7-Chloro-5-(2-fluorophenyl)-
2-methlamino-1,4-benzodizepine]

Midazolam is rapidly absorbed.

Loprazolam

(Z)-6-(2-Chlorophenyl)-2,4-dihydro-2-[(4-methyl-1-piperazinyl)methylene]-8-nitro-1H-imidazo-[1,2-a][1,4]benzodiazepine-1-one

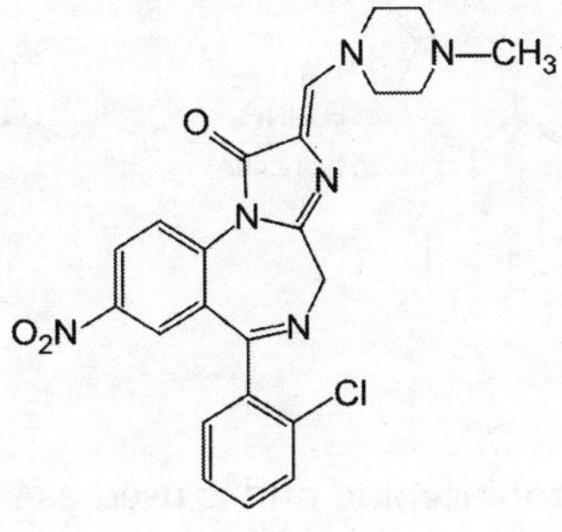

Synthesis

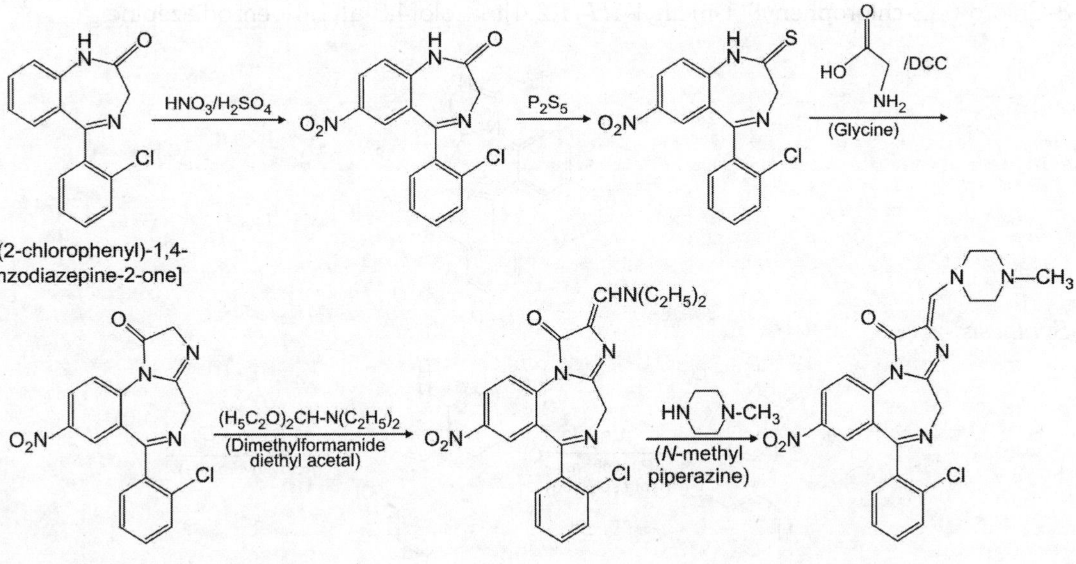

[5-(2-chlorophenyl)-1,4-benzodiazepine-2-one]

It is used as sedative, hypnotic.

Estazolam

8-Chloro-6-phenyl-4H[1,2,4]triazolo[4,3-a][1,4]benzodiazepine

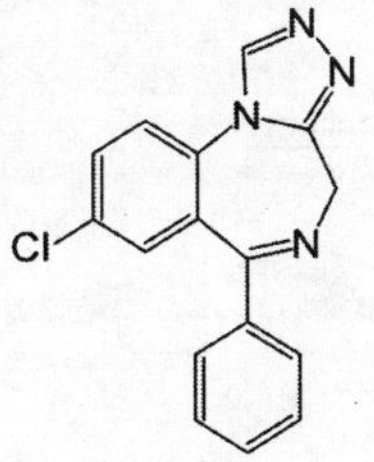

Synthesis

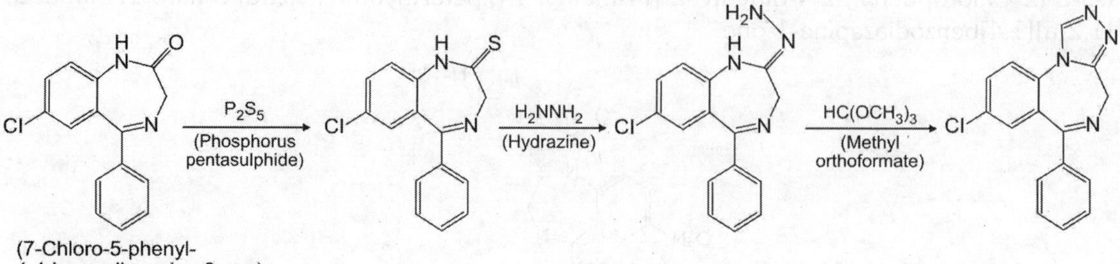

(7-Chloro-5-phenyl-
1,4-benzodiazepine-2-one)

It is an intermediate acting benzodiazepine and is used as sedative, hypnotic.

Triazolam

8-Chloro-6-(2-chlorophenyl)-1-methyl-4H-[1,2,4]triazolo[4,3-a][1,4]benzodiazepine

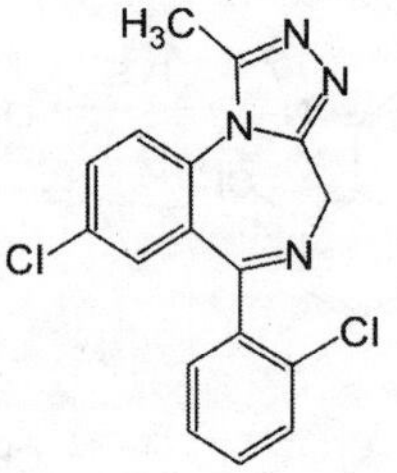

Synthesis

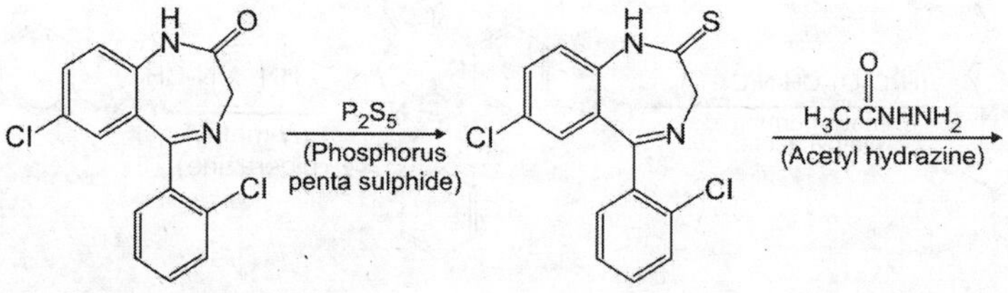

[7-Chloro-5- 2-(chlorophenyl)-
1, 4-denzodiazepine-2-one]

Used as sedative, hypnotic.

NON-BENZODIAZEPINE GABA$_A$ RECEPTOR AGONISTS

Zolpidem

N, N, 6-Trimethyl-2-(4-methylphenyl)imidazo[1,2-a]pyridine-3-acetamide

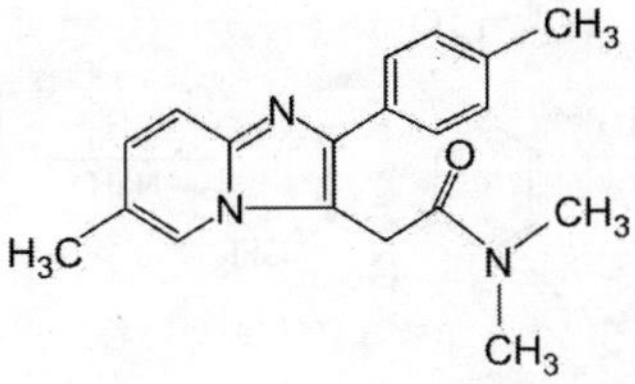

Synthesis

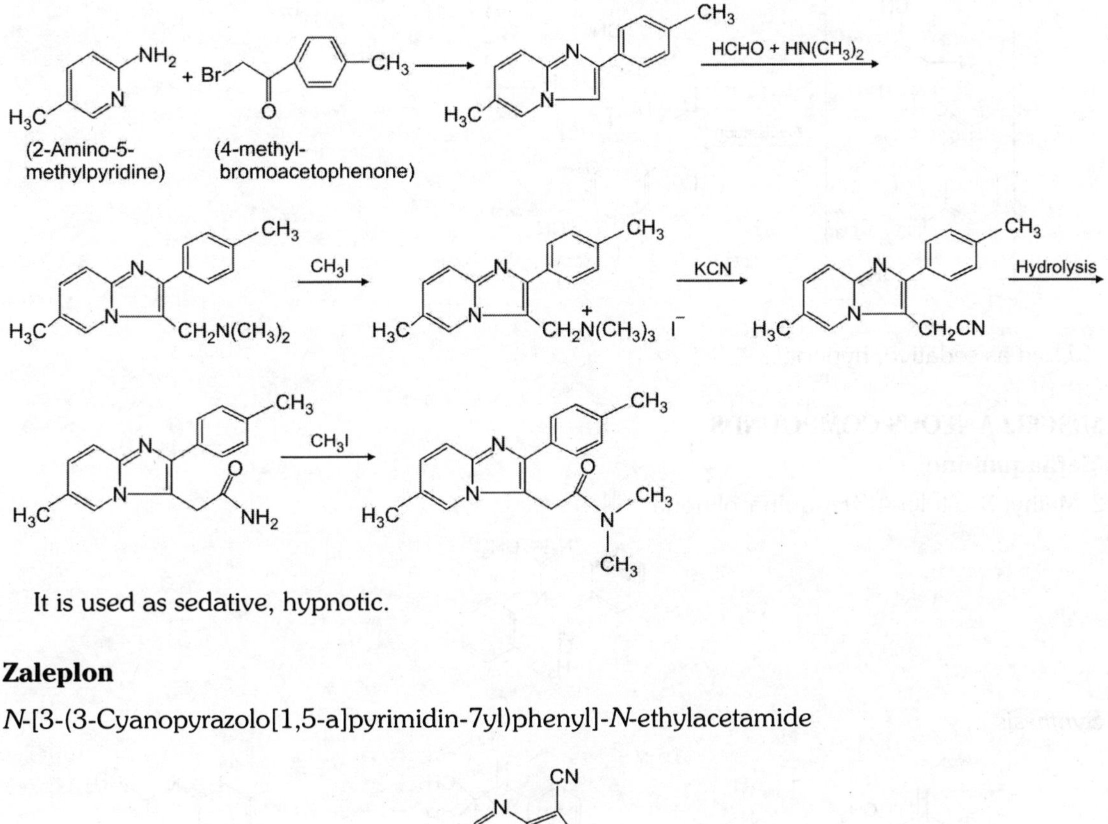

(2-Amino-5-methylpyridine)   (4-methyl-bromoacetophenone)

It is used as sedative, hypnotic.

Zaleplon

N-[3-(3-Cyanopyrazolo[1,5-a]pyrimidin-7yl)phenyl]-*N*-ethylacetamide

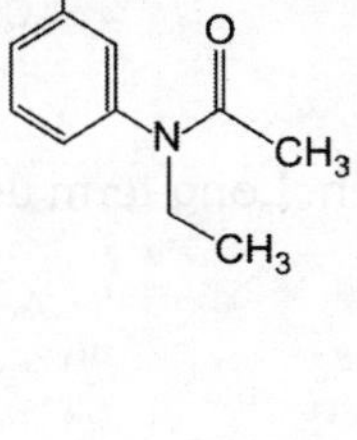

Synthesis

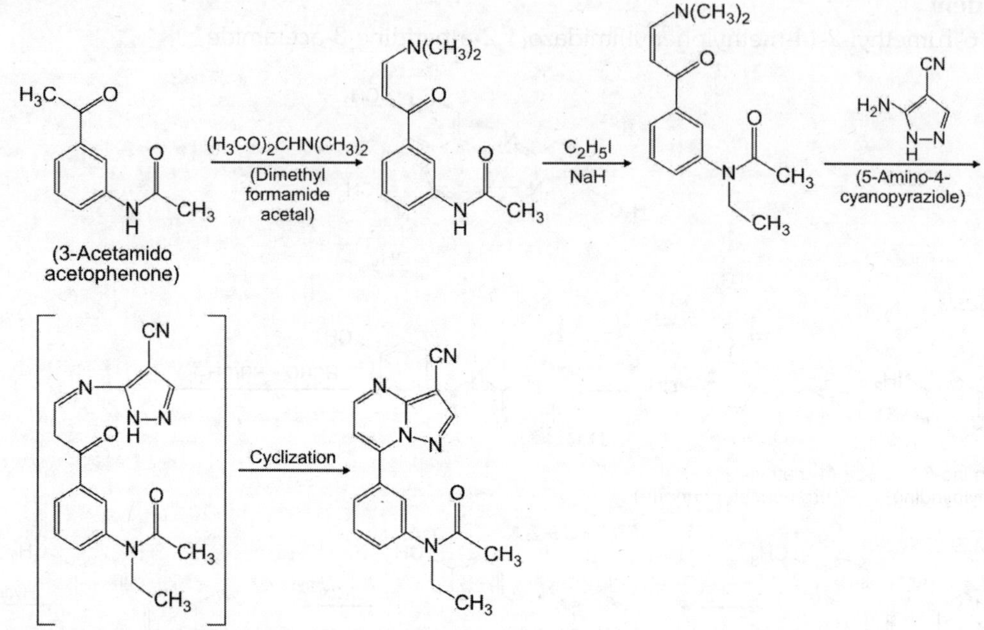
H3C
O
O
N
H
CH3
(3-Acetamido acetophenone)
(H3CO)2CHN(CH3)2
(Dimethyl formamide acetal)
N(CH3)2
C2H5I
NaH
CN
H2N
N–N
H
(5-Amino-4-cyanopyraziole)
Cyclization

Used as sedative, hypnotic.

MISCELLANEOUS COMPOUNDS

Methaqualone

2-Methyl-3-*o*-tolyl-4(3*H*)-quinazolinone

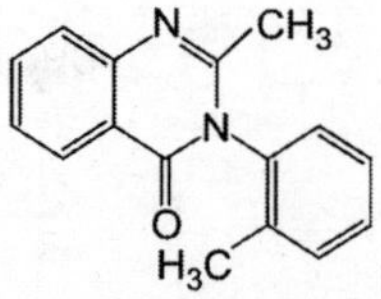
N
CH3
N
O
H3C

Synthesis

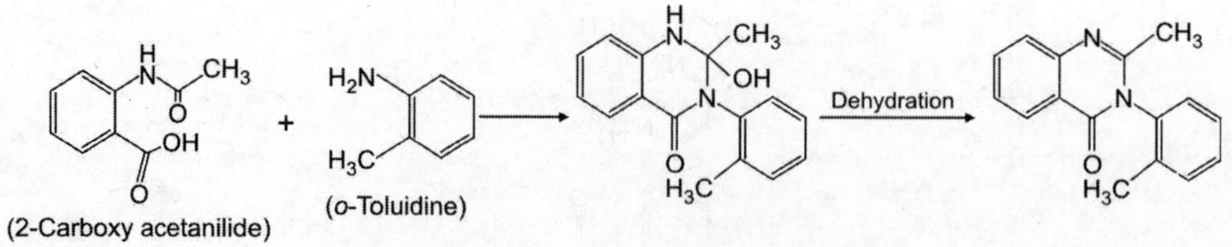
H
N
CH3
O
OH
O
(2-Carboxy acetanilide)
+
H2N
H3C
(o-Toluidine)
OH
Dehydration

It is contraindicated in pregnant women. Long-term use may lead to psychological and physical dependence.

Chloral Hydrate

2, 2, 2-Trichloroethane-1, 1-diol

$$Cl_3C-\overset{\displaystyle OH}{\underset{\displaystyle OH}{\diagdown}}$$

Synthesis

$$Cl_3C-CHO + H_2O \longrightarrow Cl_3C-\overset{\displaystyle OH}{\underset{\displaystyle OH}{\diagdown}}$$

(Chloral)

It is a safe and reliable hypnotic used in inducing sleep where insomnia is not due to pain. The sleep is light and patient can be aroused readily. It has disagreeable odour and taste.

Paraldehyde

2, 4, 6-Trimethyl-1, 3, 5-trioxane

Synthesis

$$\underset{\text{(Acetaldehyde)}}{H_3C-\overset{\displaystyle O}{\parallel}\,H} \xrightarrow{H_2SO_4}$$

It is less potent than chloral hydrate (27). The chief objection to its use is its disagreeable smell which is difficult to mask. It is mostly used in case of psychiatric patients.

Triclofos Sodium

Sodium 2, 2, 2-trichloroethylhydrogen orthophosphate

$$Cl_3C\diagdown\!\!\diagdown\!\!O-\overset{\displaystyle O}{\underset{\displaystyle OH}{\overset{\parallel}{P}}}-ONa$$

Synthesis

$$\underset{\text{(2, 2, 2-trichloroethanol)}}{Cl_3C\diagdown\!\!\diagdown\!\!OH} + HO-\overset{\displaystyle O}{\underset{\displaystyle OH}{\overset{\parallel}{P}}}-ONa \longrightarrow Cl_3C\diagdown\!\!\diagdown\!\!O-\overset{\displaystyle O}{\underset{\displaystyle OH}{\overset{\parallel}{P}}}-ONa$$

It is hydrolyzed in the body to the active sedative-hypnotic, trichloroethanol (28). It is free of unpleasant odour and taste of chloral hydrate (27).

Chlormethiazole

5-(2-Chloroethyl)-4-methylthiazole

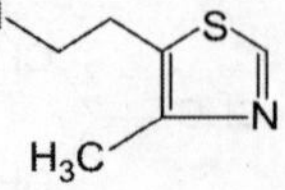

Synthesis

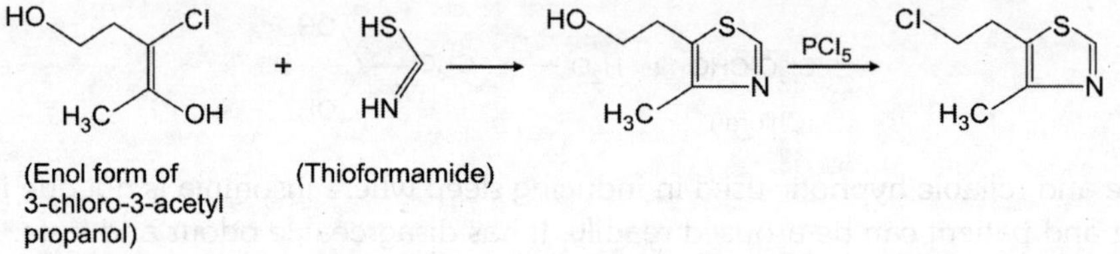

(Enol form of
3-chloro-3-acetyl
propanol)

(Thioformamide)

Its salt with ethanedisulphonate known as chlormethiazole edisylate is more stable. It is used as hypnotic, sedative, as well as anticonvulsant.

NEUROLEPTICS AND ANXIOLYTIC AGENTS

THE DRUGS used in mental diseases have been classified on their clinical usefulness and include:

(a) Neuroleptics or antipsychotic agents.
(b) Anti-anxiety or anxiolytics.
(c) Antidepressants or mood elevators.

In addition, certain drugs when given induce behavioural abnormalities which resemble psychosis. These drugs are called psychotogenic drugs and include LSD and mescaline.

Antidepressants or mood elevators will be discussed under Central Nervous System Stimulants.

NEUROLEPTICS

Neuroleptics or antipsychotics are used in major psychoses or schizophrenia. Schizophrenia is a particular kind of psychoses characterized by thought disorder, delusions, and social withdrawal. Schizophrenia has been linked with dopamine (1) hyperactivity. By blocking dopamine receptors by drugs, the metabolism of dopamine by MAO and COMT is increased and, thus, dopamine (1) is not available for binding to its receptors. Dopamine (1) is primarily involved in normal posture, muscle tone, coordination of movements, etc. Its role, biosynthesis, metabolism and dopamine receptors have been covered under Antiparkinsonian Drugs.

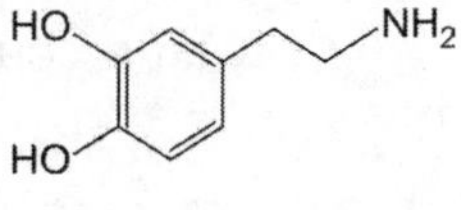

(1)

Antipsychotic drugs have been classified as:

(a) phenothiazines,
(b) thioxanthenes,
(c) dibenzoazepines,
(d) butyrophenones, and
(e) miscellaneous compounds.

Phenothiazines

Structure-activity relationship studies of number of phenothiazine (2) analogs have shown that:

(2)

(a) A three carbon chain at position 10 is optimal for the neuroleptic activity. Compounds with 2-carbon chain at position 10 show antihistaminic and anticholinergic activity.

(b) The substituent R^1 should be hydrogen for maximum neuroleptic activity. When R^1 is aromatic ring or it forms a part of ring the activity is either low or abolished.

(c) For optimum activity, the amino nitrogen at the end of 3-carbon chain should be tertiary. Maximum activity is found when R^2 and R^3 are methyl. Any deviation from this could result in decrease in activity. The nitrogen at the end of 3-carbon chain could also be a part of ring.

(d) For the substitution in the ring, position 2 is the best position. The substituent R^4 at position 2 should be electron withdrawing group or atom.

Several phenothiazine analogs have been synthesized and many of them have been accepted in clinical practice. Depending on the nature of the side chain. They have been further classified as:

(a) Phenothiazines with propyldialkylamino side chain,
(b) phenothiazines with alkylpiperidyl side chain, and
(c) phenothiazines with alkylpiperazine side chain.

Phenothiazines with propyldialkylamino side chain include promazine (3a), chlorpromazine (3b), and triflupromazine (3c). Clinically useful phenothiazines with alkylpiperidyl side chain include piperacetazine (4a), thioridazine (4b), and mesoridazine (4c). Phenothiazines with alkylpiperazine side chain at position 10 include prochlorperazine (5a), trifluoperazine (5b), thiethylperazine (5c), perphenazine (5d), fluphenazine (5e), and acetophenazine (5f).

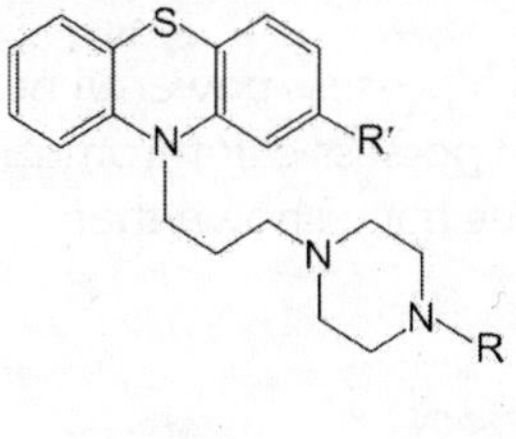

(a), R = CH$_3$, R' = Cl
(b), R = CH$_3$, R' = CF$_3$
(c), R = CH$_3$, R' = S CH$_2$CH$_3$
(d), R = CH$_2$CH$_2$OH, R'=Cl
(e), R = CH$_2$CH$_2$OH, R'=CF$_3$
(f), R = CH$_2$CH$_2$OH, R'=COCH$_3$

(5)

Thioxanthenes

Another group of tricyclic compounds used as neuroleptics include thioxanthenes (6). The clinically useful compounds in this class include chlorprothixene (6a) and thiothixene (6b).

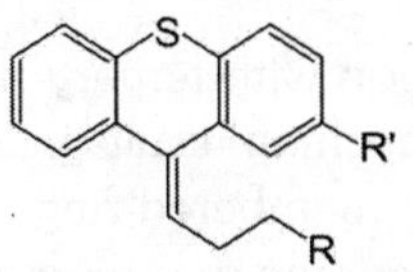

(a), R = N(CH$_3$)$_2$, R' = Cl

(b), R = [piperazine structure], R' = SO$_2$N(CH$_3$)$_2$

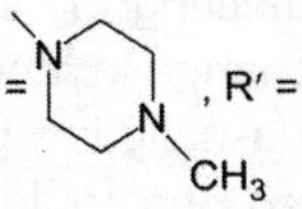

(6)

Dibenzoazepines

The Dibenzoazepines used as antipsychotic constitute the analogs of dibenzodiazepines (7, X = NH), dibenzoxazepines (7, X = O), and dibenzothiazepines (7, X = S)

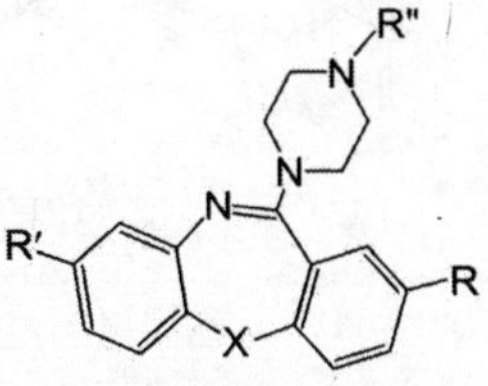

(a), x = NH, R = H, R' = Cl, R" = CH$_3$
(b), x = O, R = Cl, R' = R" = H
(c), x = O, R = Cl, R' = H, R" = CH$_3$
(d), x = S, R = Cl, R' = H, R" = CH$_3$
(e), x = S, R = CH$_3$, R' = H, R" = CH$_3$

(7)

Among the dibenzodiazepines the clinically useful compound is clozapine (7a). The clinically useful dibenzoxazepines include amoxapine (7b) and loxapine (7c). Clothiapine (7d) and metiapine (7e) represent the dibenzothiazepine analog. Some of the newer analogs in this series include, the dibenzthiazepine analog, quetiapine (8) and thienobenzodiazepine analog, olanzapine (9). Clozapine (7a), loxapine (7c) quetiapine (8) and olanzapine (9) have lower extrapyramidal side effects. However they do cause agranulocytosis which is the major drawback.

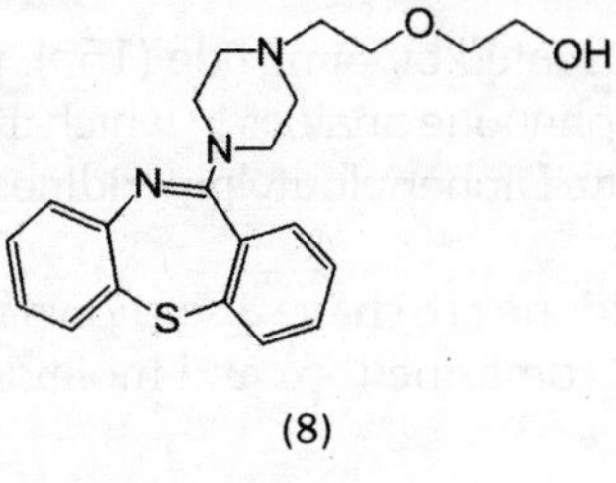

(8)

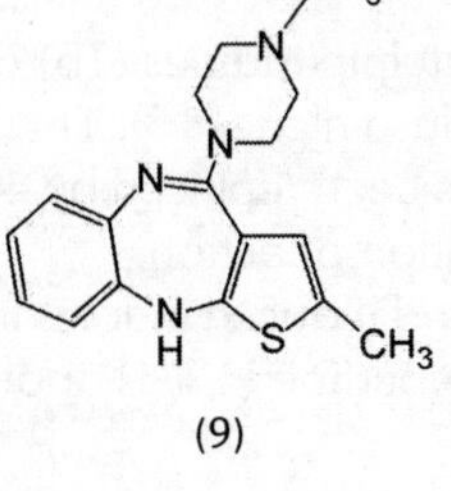

(9)

Butyrophenones

Butyrophenones (10) are a class of compounds which possess powerful neuroleptic activity. They are analogs of meperidine, a powerful analgesic, and possess chlorpromazine-like activity without analgesic action. Structure-activity relationship studies have shown that:

(10)

1. All potent butyrophenones have fluorine at *p*-position of aromatic ring (R).
2. Carbonyl function is must for neuroleptic activity and any change in this results in either less activity or complete loss of neuroleptic activity.
3. The three cabon chain connecting the keto function with tertiary nitrogen is the optimum length for the activity. Any change in length or branching results in loss of activity.
4. The tertiary amino nitrogen usually is a part of six-membered ring carrying a substituent at position 4. The six membered ring could be a piperidine or a piperazine moiety.

Some of the clinically useful butyrophenones include haloperidol (11), trifluperidol (12), spiperone (13), and droperidol (14).

(11)

(12)

(13)

(14)

Miscellaneous Compounds

Diphenylbutylpiperidines (15) class of neuroleptics are represented by pimozide (15a), penfluridol (15b), and fluspirilene (16). They can be considered as butyrophenone analogs in which the carbonyl function has been replaced by 4-fluorophenylmethane moiety. Diphenylbutylpiperidines (15) have longer duration of action.

Indoles and reduced indoles like oxypertine (17) and molindone (18) have also shown neuroleptic activity. Oxypertine (17) is about 3-times as potent as chlorpromazine (36) and molindone (18) is less active.

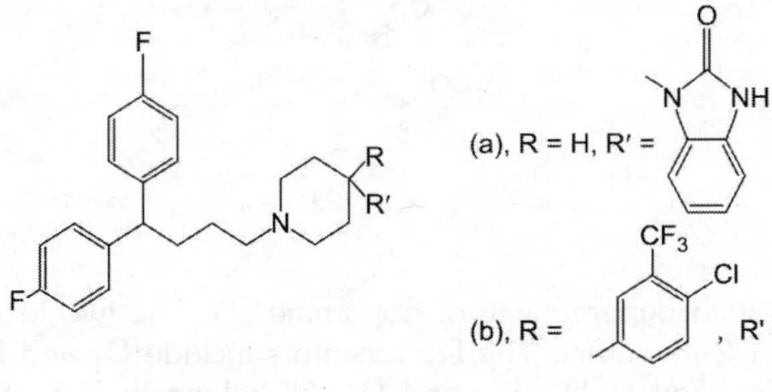

(a), R = H, R' = [benzimidazolone structure]

(b), R = [CF₃/Cl substituted phenyl], R' = OH

(15)

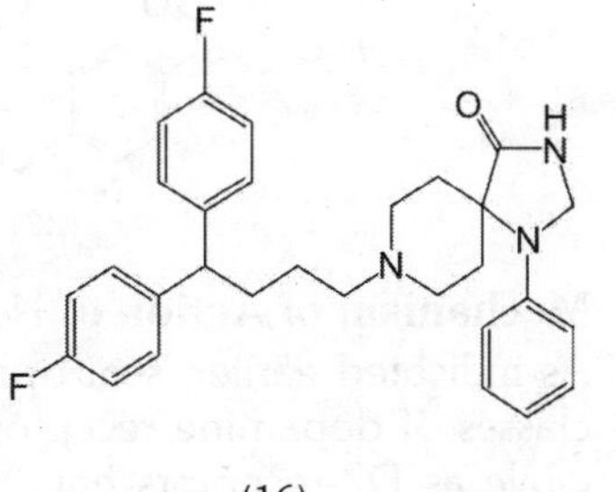

(16)

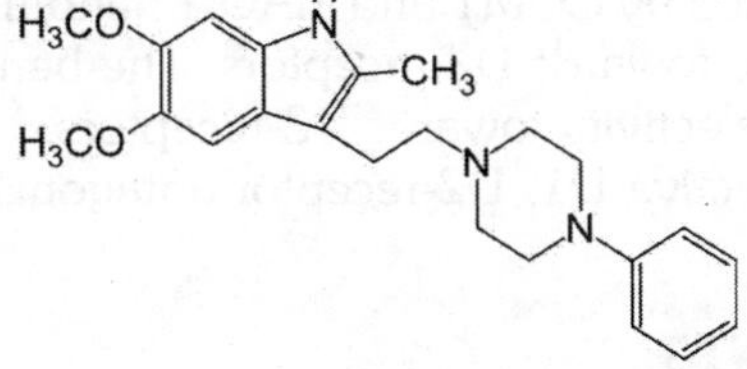

(17)

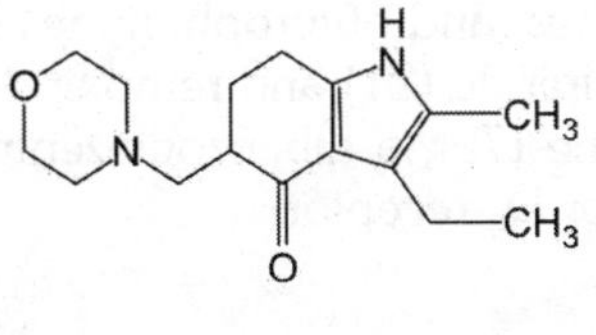

(18)

Reserpine (19), the principal alkaloid of *Rauwolfia* genus was used earlier as neuroleptic. It has number of side effects which include depression, hypotension, and diarrhea. It is no more used nowadays.

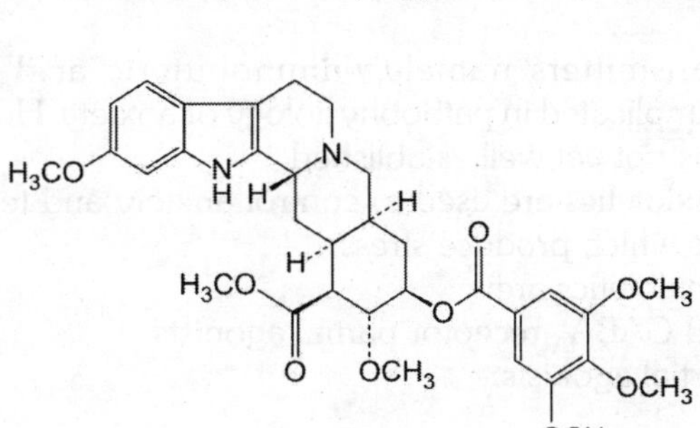

(19)

Metoclopramide (20), a benzamide, possesses dopamine antagonistic activity and has been shown to possess good neuroleptic activity. Other benzamide analogs include sulpiride (21), sultopride (22), and remoxipride (23).

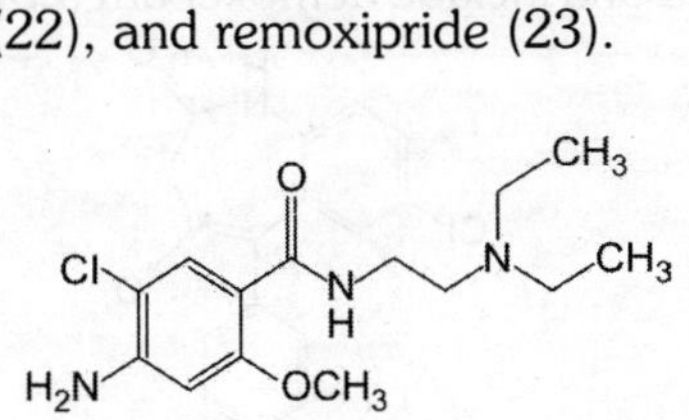

(20)

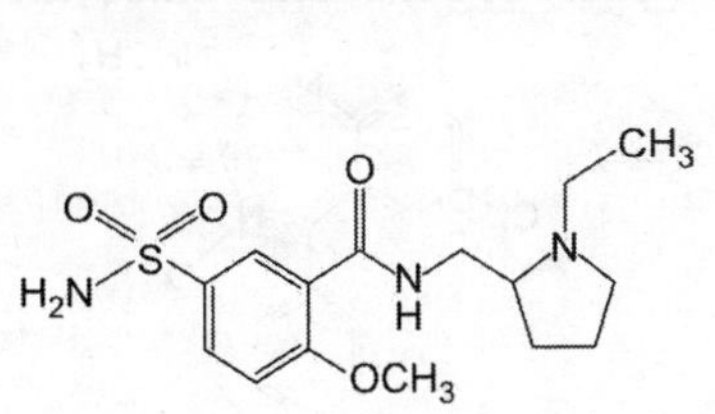

(21)

(22)   (23)

Mechanism of Action of Neuroleptics

As indicated earlier, schizophrenia is linked with hyperactivity of dopamine (1). The two broad classes of dopamine receptors are D1- and D2-receptors. The D1 receptors include D_1 and D_5, while as D2-receptors have been further classified as D_2, D_3, and D_4. All belong to G-protein coupled receptors. D1-receptors increase the adenylate cyclase activity while as D2-receptors mediate the pre- and postsynaptic inhibitory action of dopamine (1). The neuroleptic agents act by blocking the D2-receptors. The free dopamine (1) is then metabolized by COMT and MAO. Phenothiazines, thioxanthines, and butyrophenones have some selectivity towards D2-receptors. The benzamide analogs sulpiride (21) and remoxipride (23) show high selectivity towards D2-receptors.

Clozapine (7a), a dibenzodiazepine analog is non-selective D1, D2-receptor antagonist but is selective for D_4-receptor.

ANXIOLYTIC AGENTS

Anxiety is a state of apprehension and fear. It is accompanied by restlessness and uncertainty. The symptoms commonly associated with anxiety include chronic neurotic depression, restlessness, agitation, sweating, weeping, and gastrointestinal disturbances. There is also interference with the normal activities.

A number of neurotransmitters namely,γ-aminobutyric acid (GABA), serotonin, and norepinephrine have been implicated in pathophysiology of anxiety. However, the interrelationship of these neurotransmitters is not yet well established.

Antianxiety agents or anxiolytics are used to control anxiety and tension in patients. They are also indicated during illness which produce stress.

The various classes of anxiolytics are:
1. Benzodiazepines and $GABA_A$ receptor partial agonists.
2. 5-HT$_{1A}$ Receptor partial agonists.
3. Barbiturates.
4. β-Adrenoreceptor antagonists.
5. Miscellaneous agents.

Benzodiazepine and GABA$_A$ Receptor Partial Agonists

Chlordiazepoxide (24) was the first benzodiazepine which was used in clinical practice in 1960. Since then many of benzodiazepines have been introduced and include demoxepam (25), diazepam

(24)   (25)

(26), halazepam (27), pinazepam (28), prazepam (29), oxazepam (30), lorazepam (31), clorazepate potassium (32), alprazolam (33), and clobazam (34).

(26), $R_1 = CH_3$, $R_2 = R_3 = H$
(27), $R_1 = CH_2CF_3$, $R_2 = R_3 = H$
(28), $R_1 = CH_2C \equiv CH$, $R_2 = R_3 = H$
(29), $R_1 = CH_2$–◁, $R_2 = R_3 = H$
(30), $R_1 = R_3 = H$, $R_2 = OH$
(31), $R_1 = H$, $= R_2 = OH$, $R_3 = Cl$
(32), $R_1 = R_3 = H$, $R_2 = COOK$

(33)

(34)

Pharmacological Activity

Benzodiazepines are active orally and they cause reduction in anxiety, sedation, and muscle relaxation. Different members differ in duration of action. The side effects of benzodiazepines are drowsiness, confusion, amnesia, and impaired coordination. They interact with alcohol which results in long lasting hangover and development of dependence.

Mechanism of Action

Benzodiazepine receptor which is a regulatory site, is an integral part of GABA-receptor-chloride channel complex. By binding to its receptor, benzodiazepines facilitate the binding of GABA to $GABA_A$ receptor which results in opening of chloride channel. The opening of chloride channel leads to flow of chloride ion leading to anticonvulsant/anxiolytic effects.

The agonist, partial agonist and antagonist action has been explained on the basis of three conformational states of benzodiazepine $GABA_A$ receptor. These have been described as "active" or agonist, "neutral" or resting, and "inactive" or antagonist or inverse agonist. The benzodiazepine agonists or partial agonists stabilize the "active" state in which the chloride channels are opened. The benzodiazepine competitive antagonists stablize the "neutral" state by binding equally to both states which results in no change in GABA receptor function or chloride conductance. The antagonists on the other hand bind to stabilize the "inactive" state, as a result the binding of GABA to $GABA_A$ receptor does not take place and the chloride channels remain closed.

Structure-Activity Relationship Studies in Benzodiazepines

Number of 5-phenyl-1, 4-benzodiazepin-2-ones (35) have been synthesized and pharmacological activity studied. Some of the important observations of these studies are:

(35)

1. For binding to the receptor, ring A should be aromatic or hetero-aromatic. An electro-negative group at position 7 of the aromatic ring enhances anxiolytic activity. Similar substitution at 6, 8, or 9 decreases the anxiolytic activity.

2. The carbonyl function at position 2 seems to be necessary for binding to the receptor. The double bond between 4 and 5 does not seem to be essential. Compounds in which double bond at position 4 is reduced get oxidized back to C = N.

3. Annelation of 1, 2-bond of ring B with electron rich rings enhances the anxiolytic activity, examples include 5-triazolobenzodiazepines, alprazolam (33).

4. Hydroxy analogs in which the hydroxyl group is at position 3, have been found to possess anxiolytic activity comparable to non-hydroxylated compounds. Many of the clinically useful benzodiazepines do not have chiral centre. The 3-hydroxylated analogs like oxazepam (30) and lorazepam (31) are available in racemic form. However, studies on 3-methyldiazepam (36) have shown that most of the activity lies in the *S*-isomer indicating that enantiomeric differences in activity do exist.

5. Ring C does not seem to be necessary for binding to receptor. However, it contributes favourably to the receptor binding of other parts of the molecule. Substitution in the phenyl ring should be at position 2'. Substitution at other positions usually results in unfavourable activity.

    Among GABA$_A$ partial agonists, imidazenil (37), bretazenil (38), and a β-carboline analog abecarnil (39) are being investigated. Partial agonists possess lower side effects such as sedation and incoordination of muscles, an advantage over full agonists.

(36)

(37)

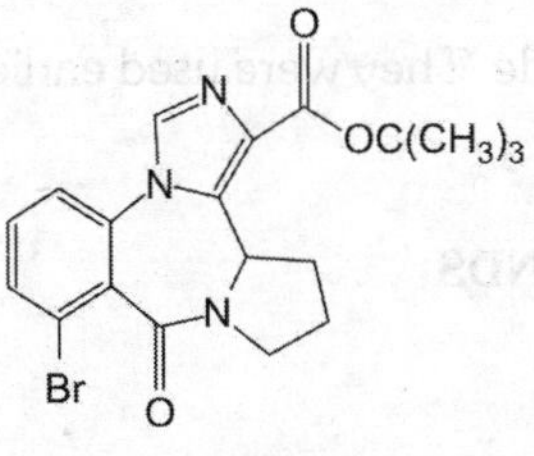

(38)

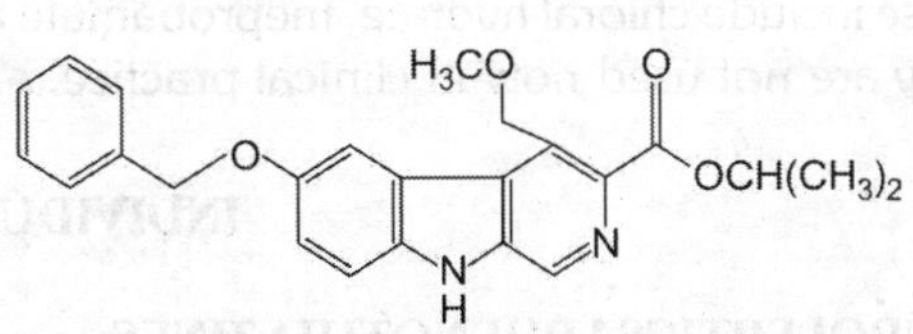

(39)

5-HT$_{1A}$ Receptor Partial Agonists

Serotonin [5-hydroxytryptamine (40)] has also been implicated in anxiety and panic disorders. Buspirone (41), ipsapirone (42), and gepirone (43) are some of the 5-HT$_{1A}$ receptor agonists which have shown anxiolytic activity. However, the anxiolytic effect takes days to develop. Further, the side effects found with benzodiazepines are much less intense and include dizziness and headache but not sedation and loss of co-ordination. The mechanism of their action is not yet known.

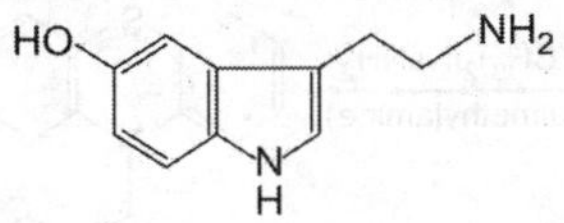

(40)

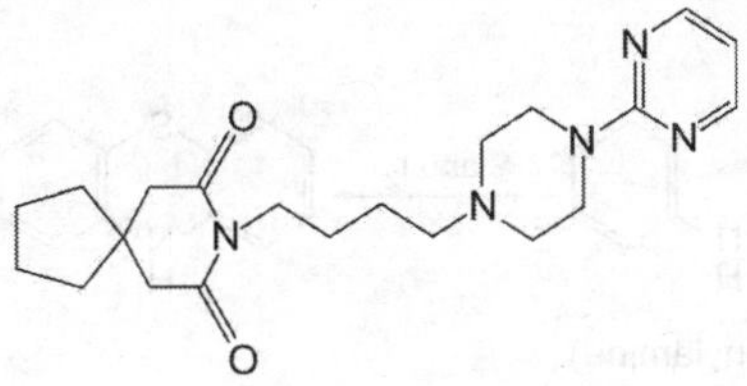

(41)

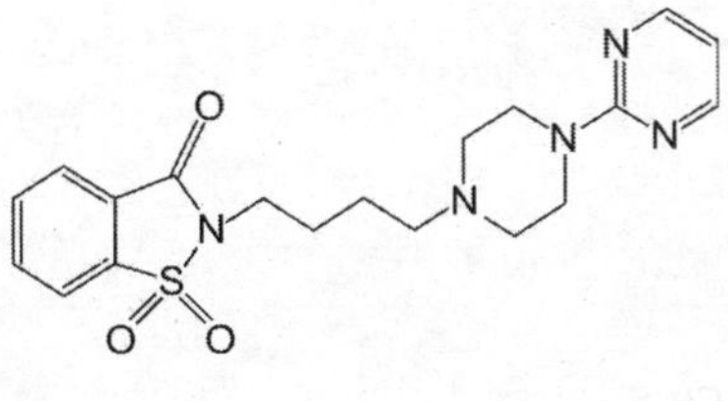

(42)

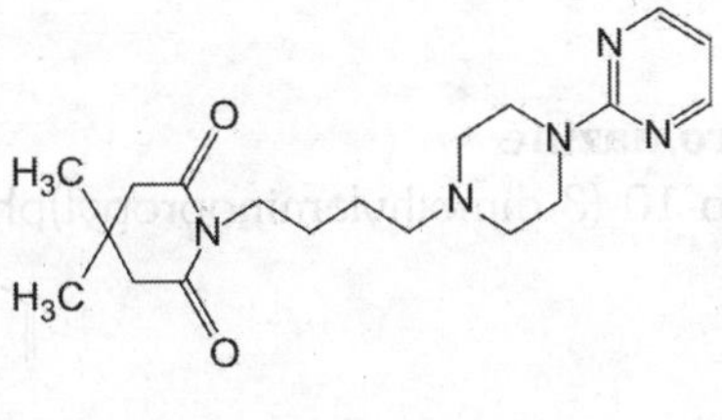

(43)

Barbiturates

Barbiturates have already been discussed under hypnotics and sedatives. Although barbiturates were used till 1960's now they have been replaced with much safer drugs. Some of the barbiturates which have specific use are phenobarbital as anticonvulsants and thiopental as anesthetic agents.

Barbiturates enhance the action of GABA by binding to a site which is different from the site where benzodiazepines bind.

β-Adrenoreceptor Antagonists

They have been discussed under drugs acting on adrenergic receptors. They are used when certain conditions such as sweating, tremors, and tachycardia are the cause of anxiety.

Miscellaneous Agents

These include chloral hydrate, meprobamate and paraldehyde. They were used earlier as hypnotics. They are not used now in clinical practice.

INDIVIDUAL COMPOUNDS

NEUROLEPTICS : PHENOTHIAZINES

Promazine

10-(3-Dimethylaminopropyl)phenothiazine

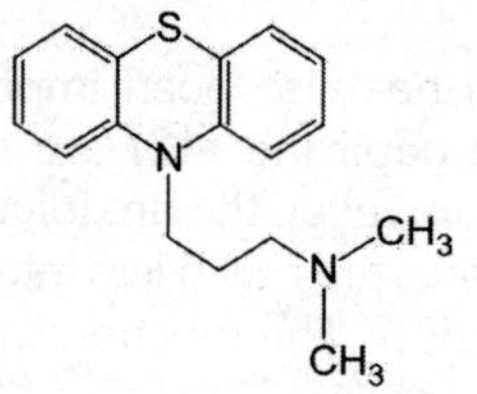

Synthesis

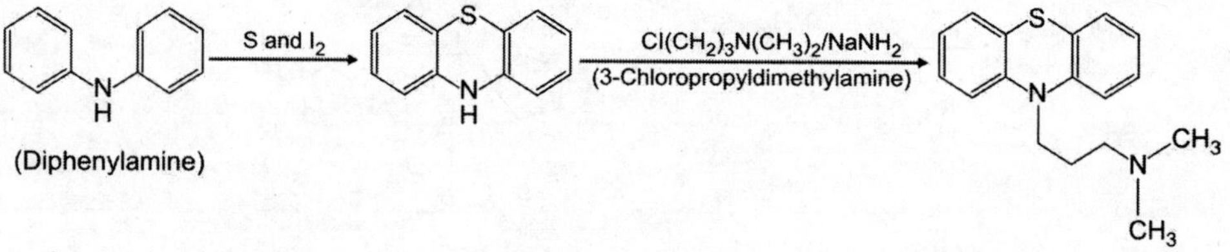

　　It is used as hydrochloride in acute neuropsychiatric agitation but is less potent than chlorpromazine (3b).

Chlorpromazine

2-Chloro-10-(3-dimethylaminopropyl)phenothiazine

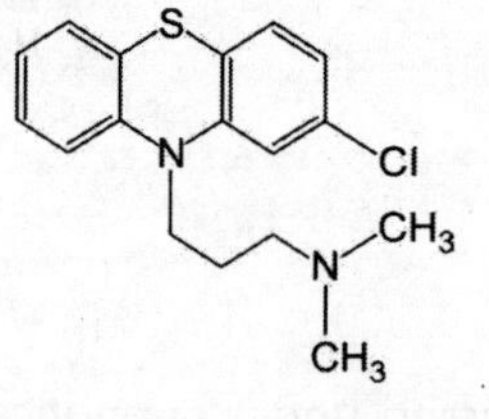

Synthesis

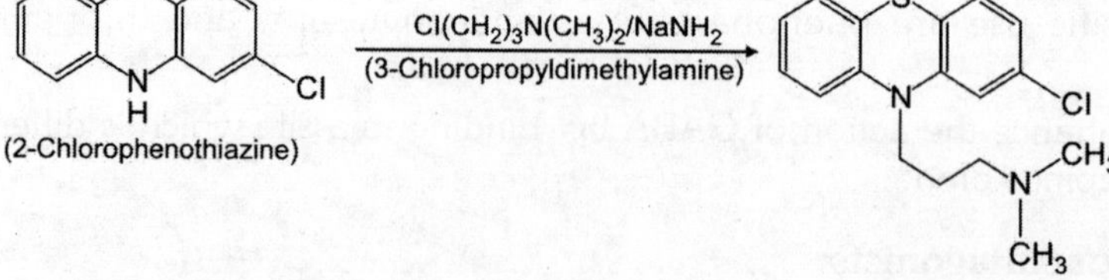

　　It is used as hydrochloride for the treatment of nausea and vomiting. It has significant sedative and hypotensive activity.

Triflupromazine

2-Trifluromethyl-10-(3-dimethylaminopropyl)phenothiazine

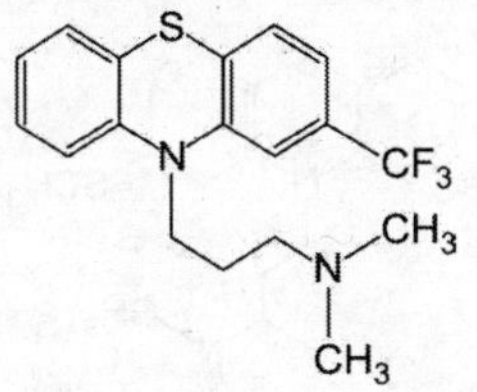

Synthesis

$$Cl(CH_2)_3N(CH_3)_2/NaNH_2$$
(3-Chloropropyldimethylamine)

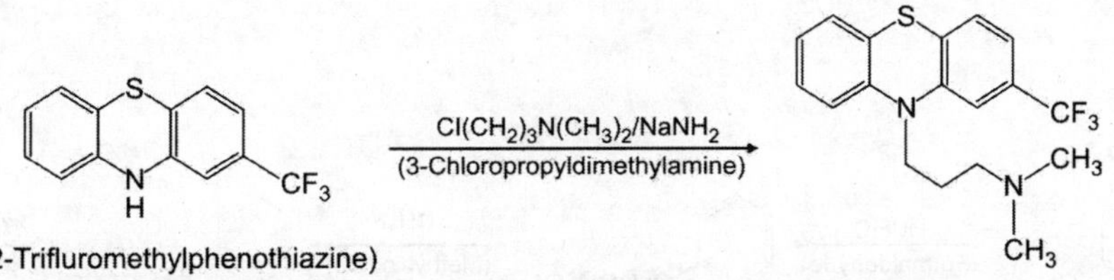

(2-Trifluromethylphenothiazine)

It is employed as hydrochloride for the management of psychotic disorders and in the treatment of anxiety and tension. It is also used for the control of nausea and vomiting.

Piperacetazine

2-Acetyl-10-[3-[4-(β-hydroxyethyl)piperidino]propyl]phenothiazine

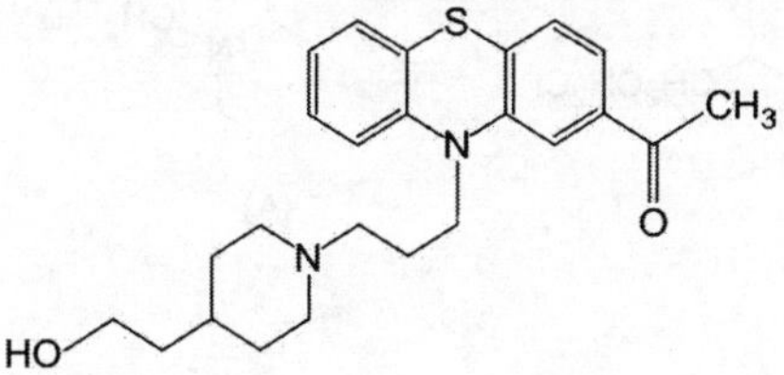

Synthesis

(2-Chlorobenzoic acid)

(3-Aminoacetophenone)

Decarboxylation

$$S + I_2$$

$$Cl(CH_2)_3Cl$$
(1, 3-Dichloropropane)

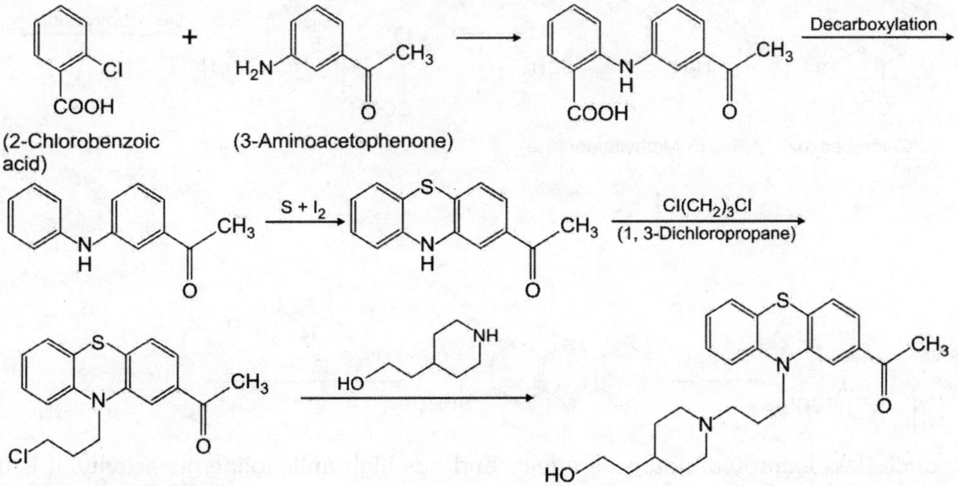

It has a moderate activity.

Thioridazine

2-Methylmercapto-10[2-(*N*-methyl-2-piperidyl)ethyl]phenothiazine

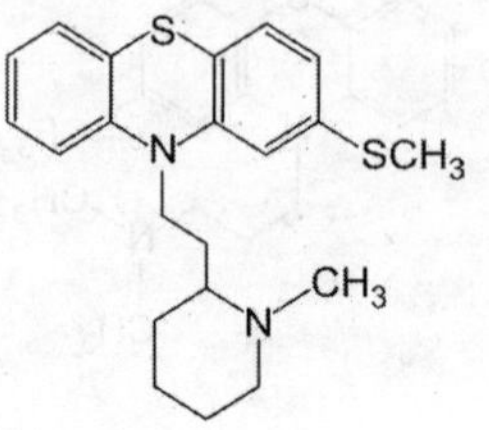

Synthesis

Step 1

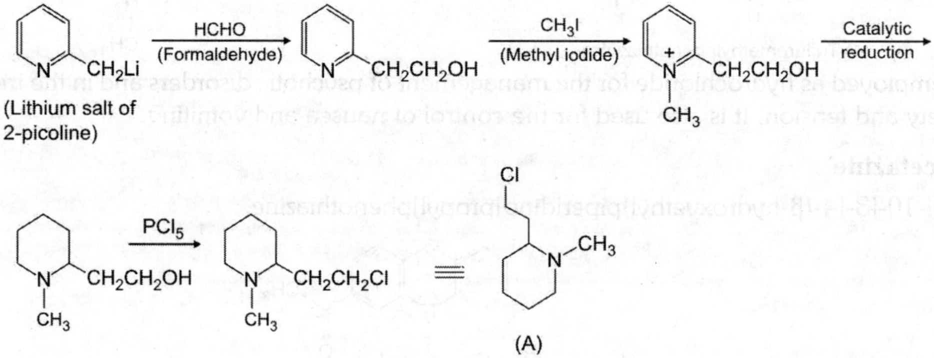

(Lithium salt of
2-picoline)

Step 2

(2-Chlorobenzoic
acid)

(3-Methylthioaniline)

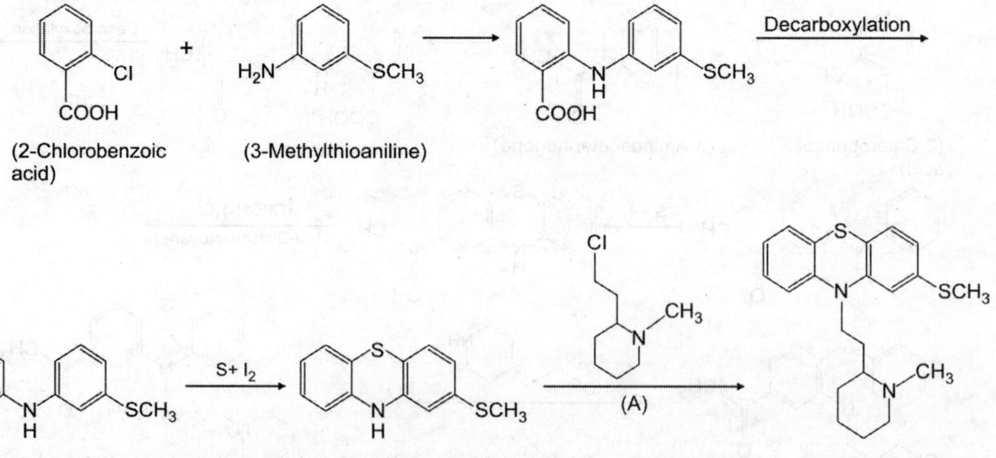

It produces less extrapyramidal side effects and has high anticholinergic activity. It is used as hydrochloride. Its metabolite is mesoridazine (4c).

Mesoridazine

10-[2-(1-Methyl-2-piperidinyl)ethyl]-2-(methylsulfinyl)-10*H*-phenothiazine

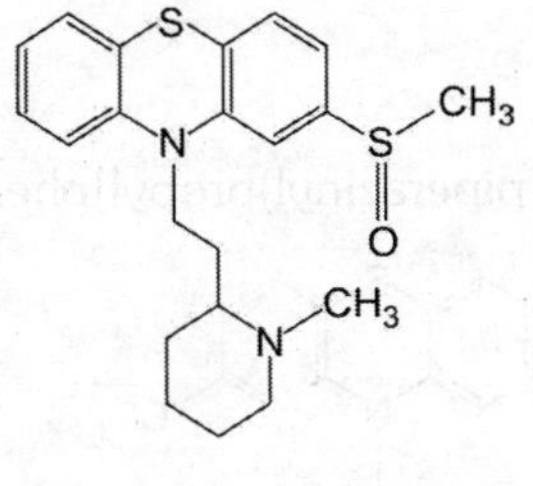

Synthesis

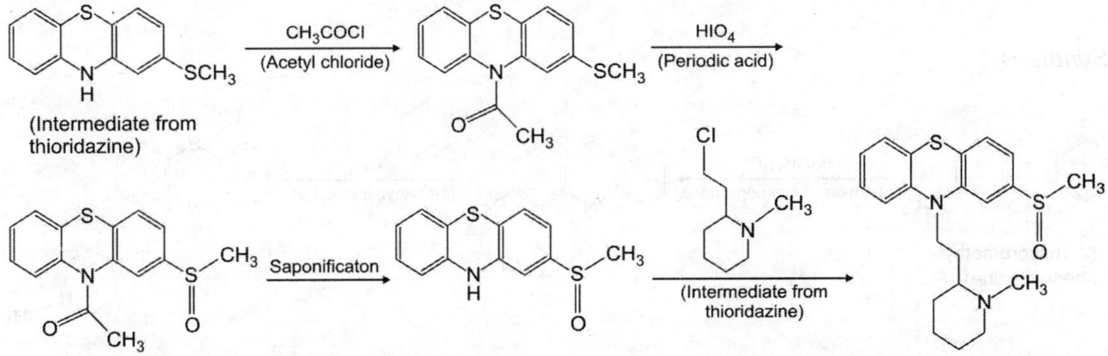

It has similar activity as thioridazine (4b) and is used as benzenesulphonate (besylate) salt.

Prochlorperazine

2-Chloro-10-[3-(1-methyl-4-piperazinyl) propyl]phenothiazine

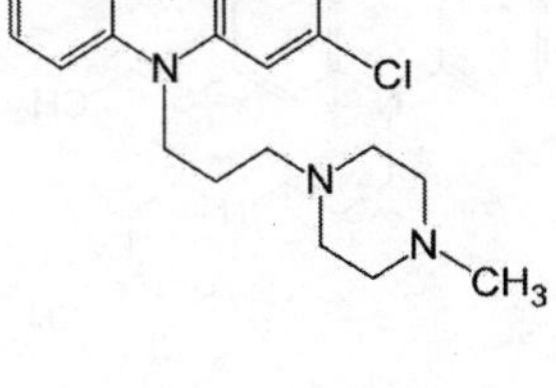

Synthesis

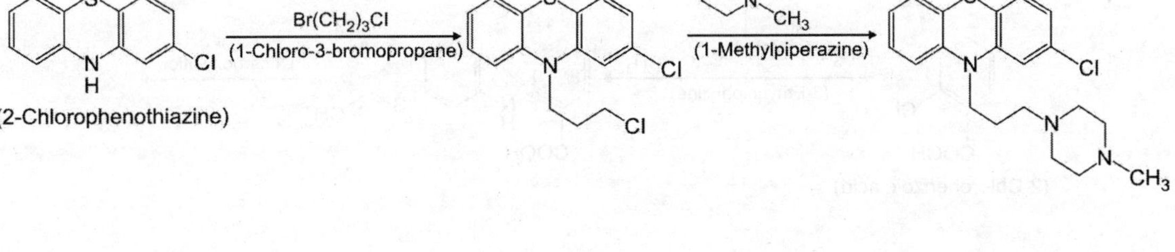

It is used as maleate and methanesulphonate (mesylate) salts. The maleate salt is insoluble and is used orally while mesylate salt is used both orally as well as parenterally. It has similar activity as chlorpromazine (3b).

Trifluoperazine

2-Trifluoromethyl-10-[3'-(1-methyl-4-piperazinyl)propyl]phenothiazine

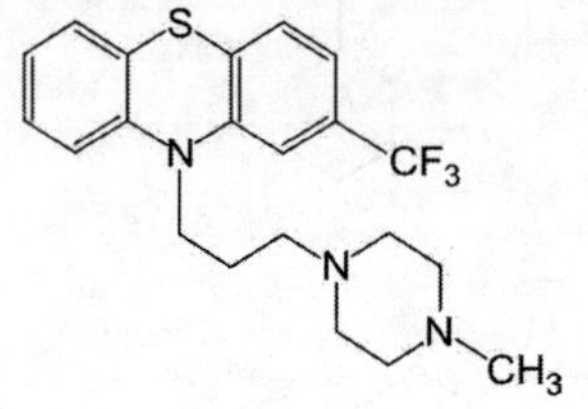

Synthesis

(2-Trifluoromethyl-phenothiazine)

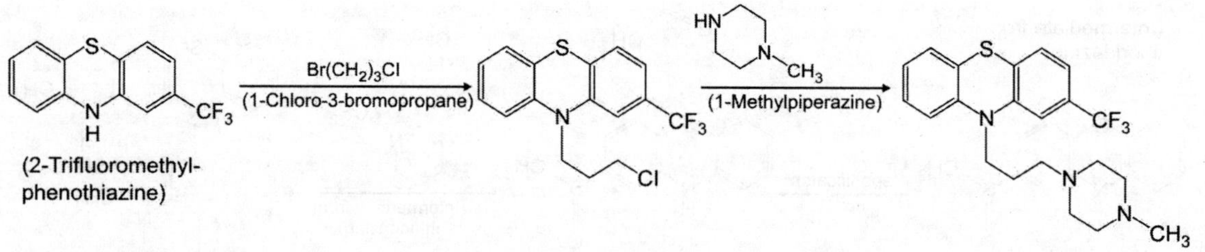

It is relatively potent drug and is used in the control of acute and chronic psychoses marked by hyperactivity.

Thiethylperazine

2-(Ethylthio)-10-[3-(4-methyl-1-piperazinyl)propyl]phenothiazine

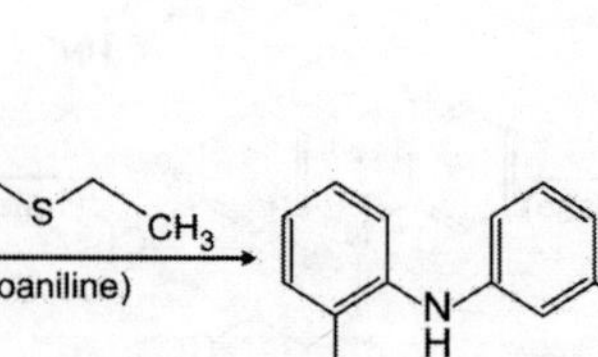

Synthesis

(2-Chlorobenzoic acid)

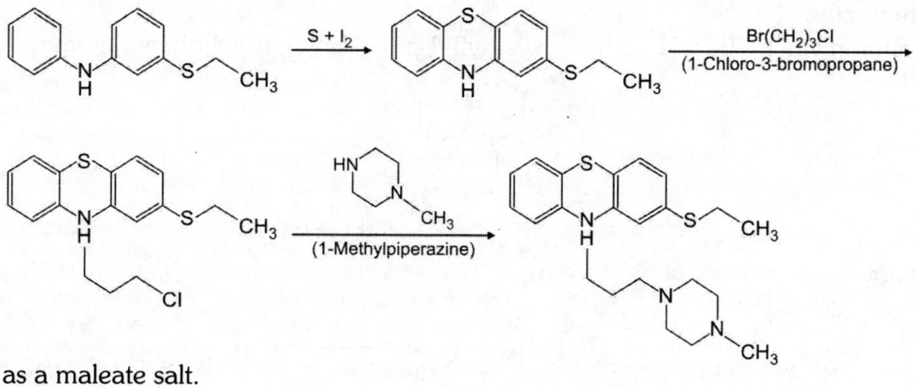

It is used as a maleate salt.

Perphenazine
2-Chloro-10-[3-[1-(2-hydroxyethyl)-4-piperazinyl]propyl]phenothiazine

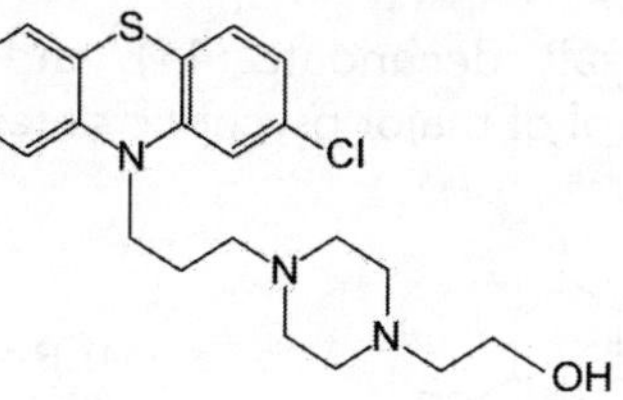

Synthesis

Step 1

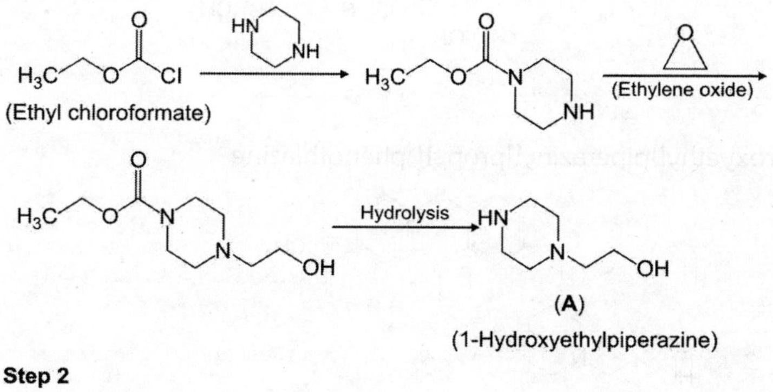

(A)
(1-Hydroxyethylpiperazine)

Step 2

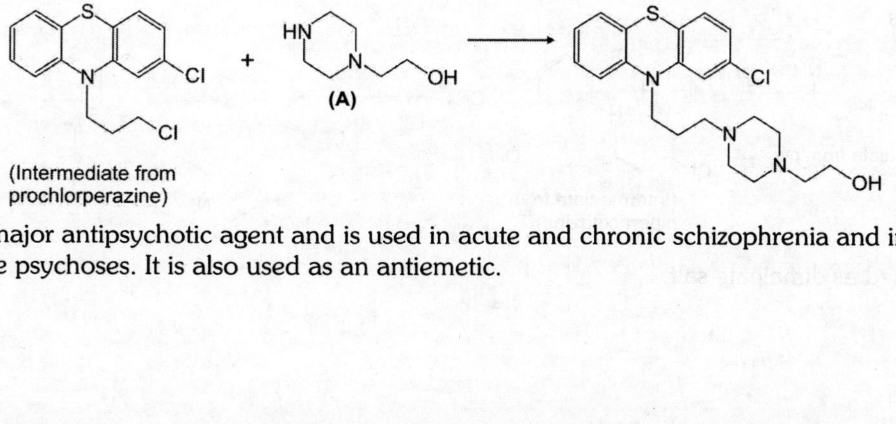

(Intermediate from prochlorperazine)

It is a major antipsychotic agent and is used in acute and chronic schizophrenia and in manic-depressive psychoses. It is also used as an antiemetic.

Fluphenazine

2-(Trifluoromethyl)-10-[3-[1-(β-hydroxyethyl)-4-piperazinyl]propyl]phenothiazine

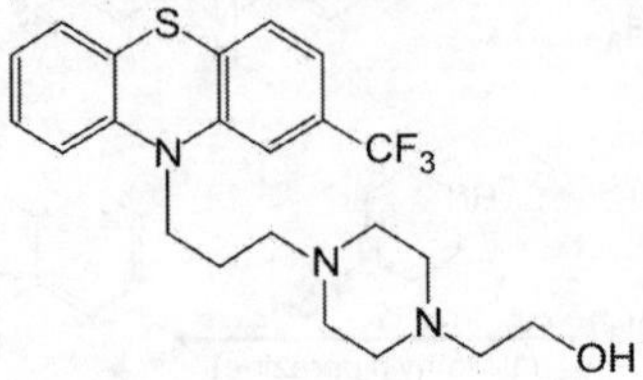

Synthesis

(Intermediate from
trifluperazine)

+

(Intermediate from
perphenazine)

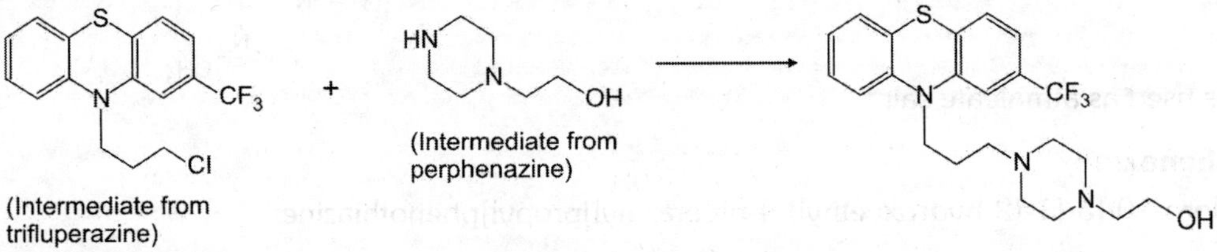

It is used as dihydrochloride salt, decanoate (44), and enanthate (45) ester. It is potent phenothiazine and is used in control of major psychotic states. Its action is accompanied by high extrapyramidal side effects.

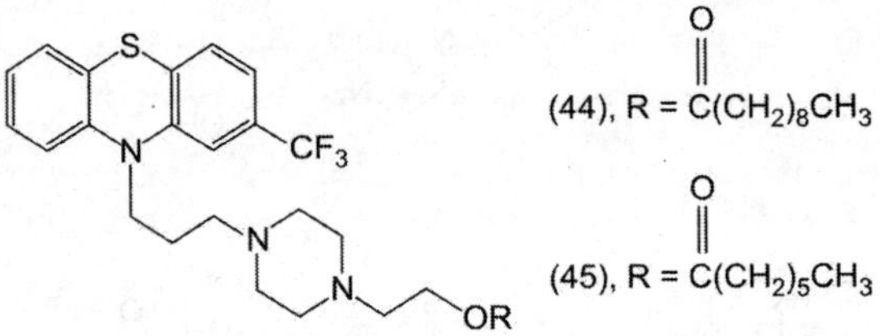

$$(44), R = \overset{\overset{\textstyle O}{\|}}{C}(CH_2)_8CH_3$$

$$(45), R = \overset{\overset{\textstyle O}{\|}}{C}(CH_2)_5CH_3$$

Acetophenazine

2-Acetyl-10-[3-[4-(β-hydroxyethyl)piperazinyl]propyl] phenothiazine

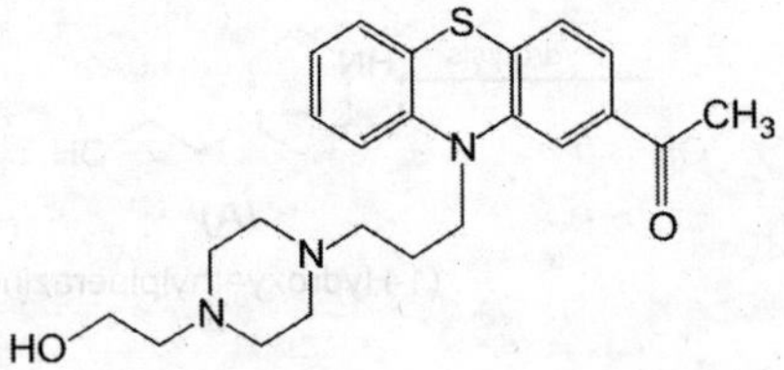

Synthesis

(Intermediate from per-
phenazine)

+

(Intermediate from
piperacetazine)

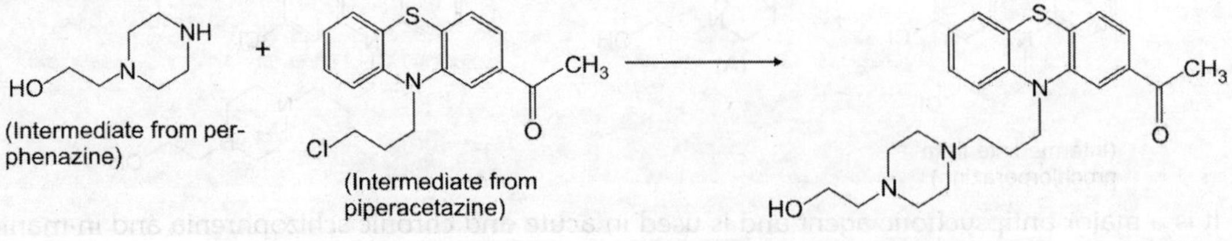

It is used as dimaleate salt.

NEUROLEPTICS : THIOXANTHENES

Chlorprothixene

(Z)-3-(2-Chloro-9H-thioxanthen-9-ylidene)-N,N-dimethyl-1-propanamine

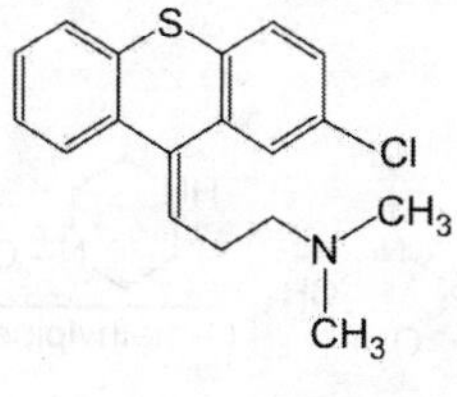

Synthesis

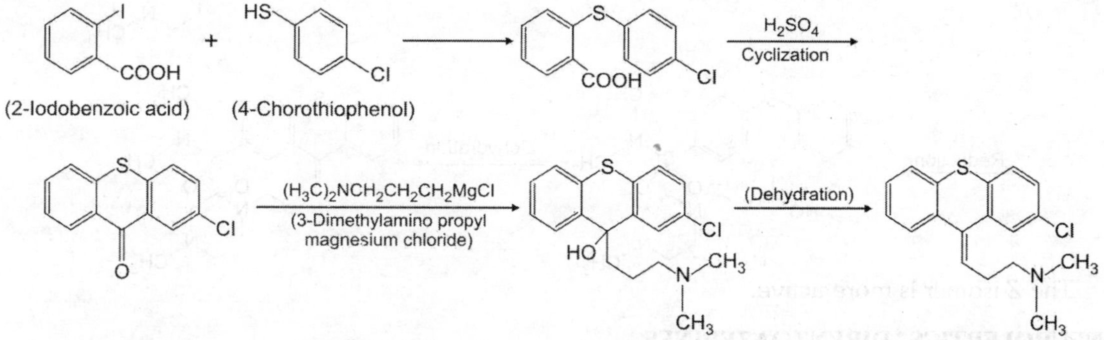

(2-Iodobenzoic acid)   (4-Chorothiophenol)

(3-Dimethylamino propyl magnesium chloride)

It exists in two isomers Z and E. The Z-isomer is more active. It has similar pharmacological action as chlorpromazine (3b).

Thiothixene

cis-9-[3-(4-Methyl-1-piperazinyl)propylidene]-2-(dimethylsulphonamido)thioxanthene

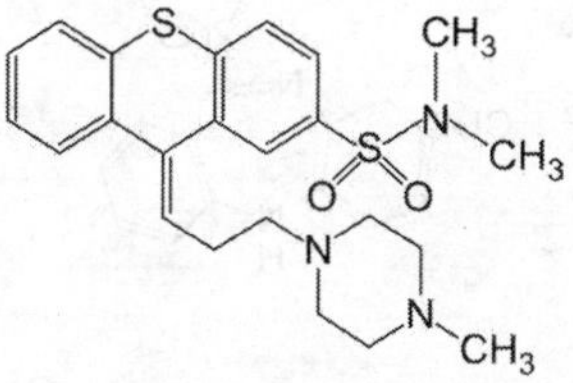

Synthesis

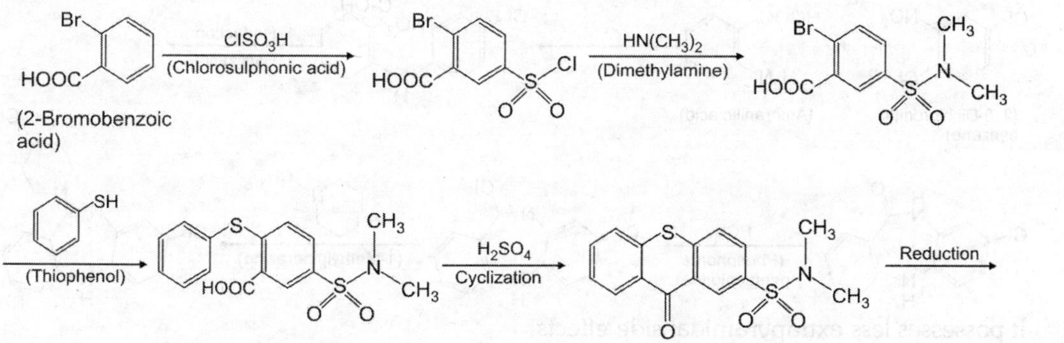

(2-Bromobenzoic acid)

(Thiophenol)

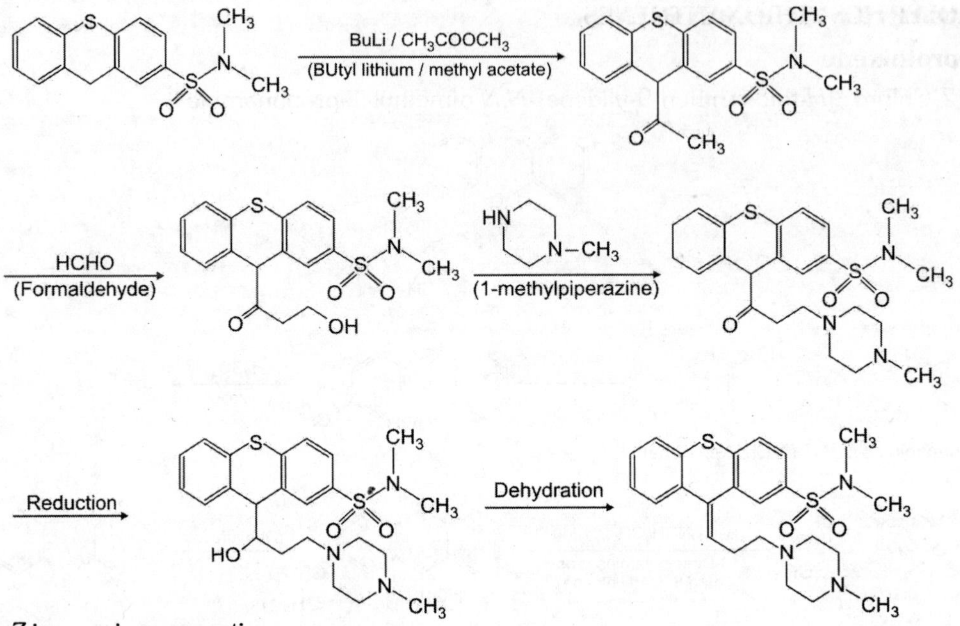

The *Z*-isomer is more active.

NEUROLEPTICS : DIBENZOAZEPINES

Clozapine

8-Chloro-11-(4-methyl-1-piperazinyl)-5*H*-dibenzo[*b*, *e*][1, 4]diazepine

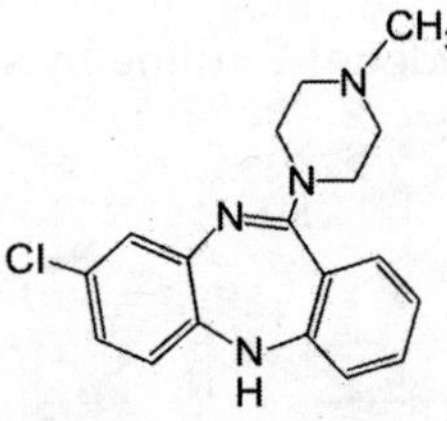

Synthesis

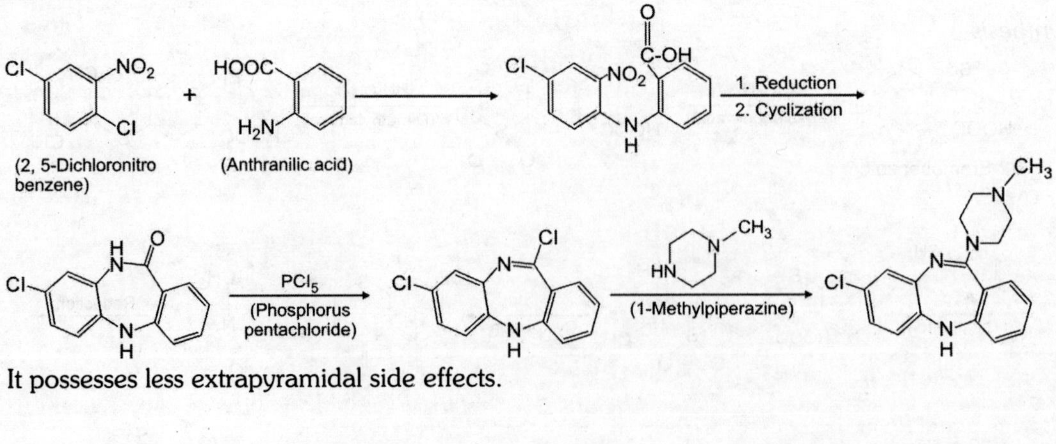

(2, 5-Dichloronitro benzene)   (Anthranilic acid)

It possesses less extrapyramidal side effects.

Amoxapine

2-Chloro-11-(1-piperazinyl)dibenz[b, f][1,4]oxazepine

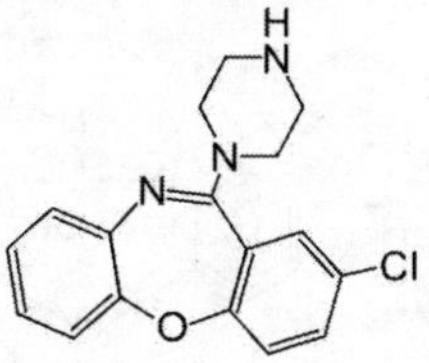

Synthesis

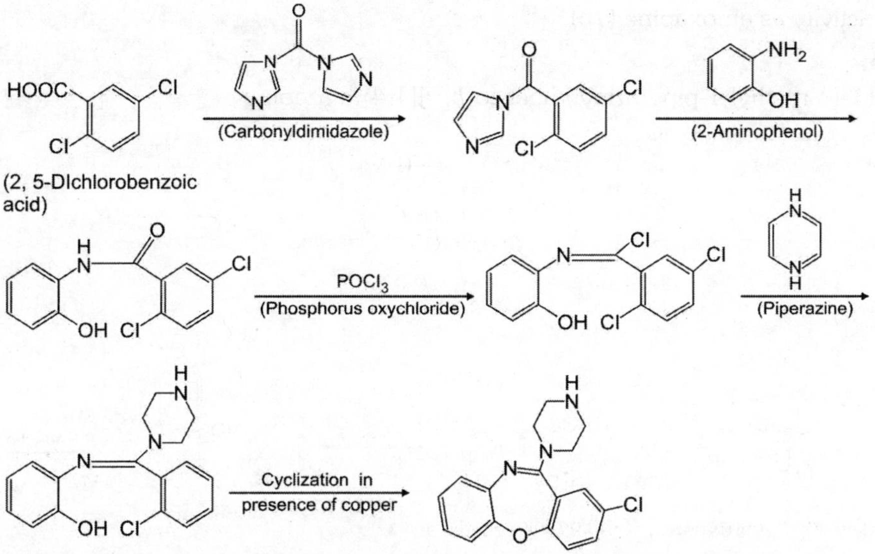

It is an effective neuroleptic and antidepressant. It is a metabolite of loxapine (7c) and used more as antidepressant rather than neuroleptic

Loxapine

2-Chloro-11-(4-methyl-1-piperazinyl)dibenz[b, f][1, 4]oxazepine

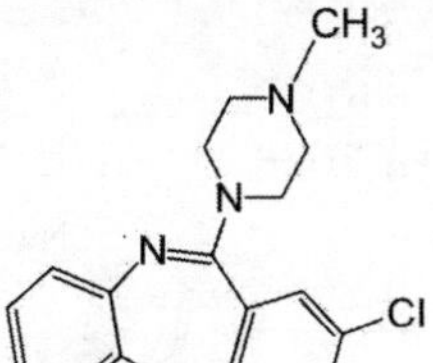

Synthesis

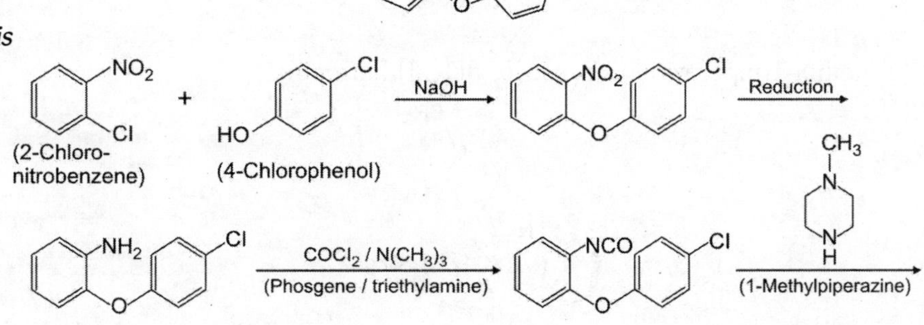

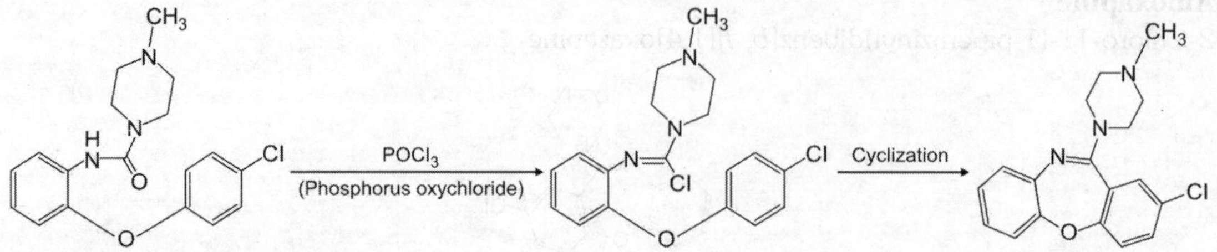

Similar activity as amoxapine (7b).

Clothiapine
2-Chloro-11-(4-methyl-1-piperazinyl)dibenzo[b, f][1,4]thiazepine

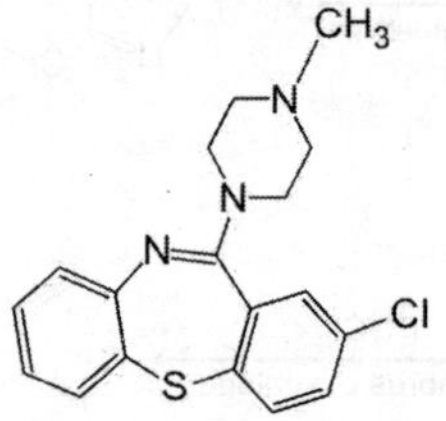

Synthesis

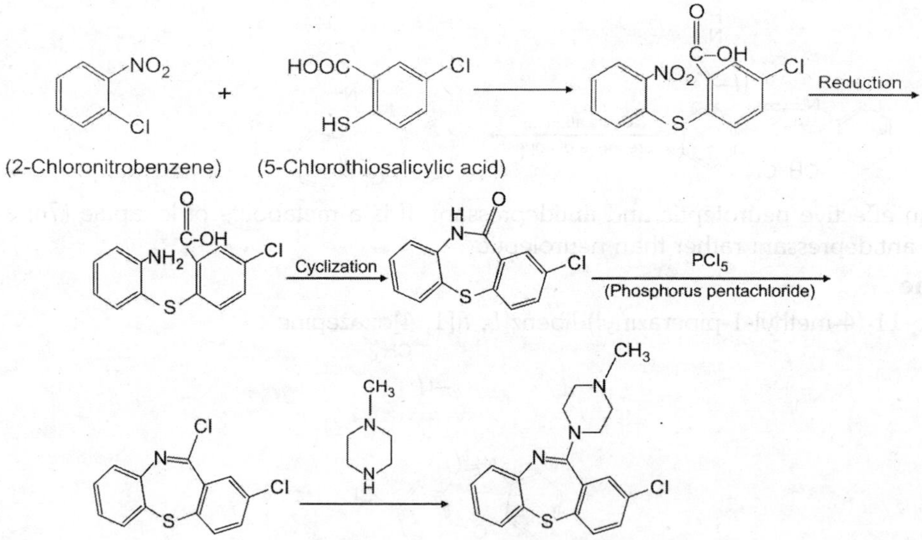

(2-Chloronitrobenzene)   (5-Chlorothiosalicylic acid)

Metiapine
2-Methyl-11-(4-methyl-1-piperazinyl)dibenzo[b, f][1, 4]thiazepine

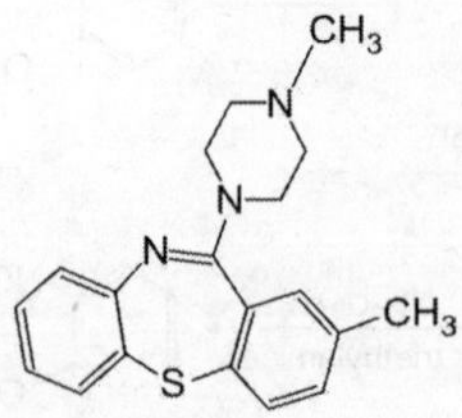

Synthesi

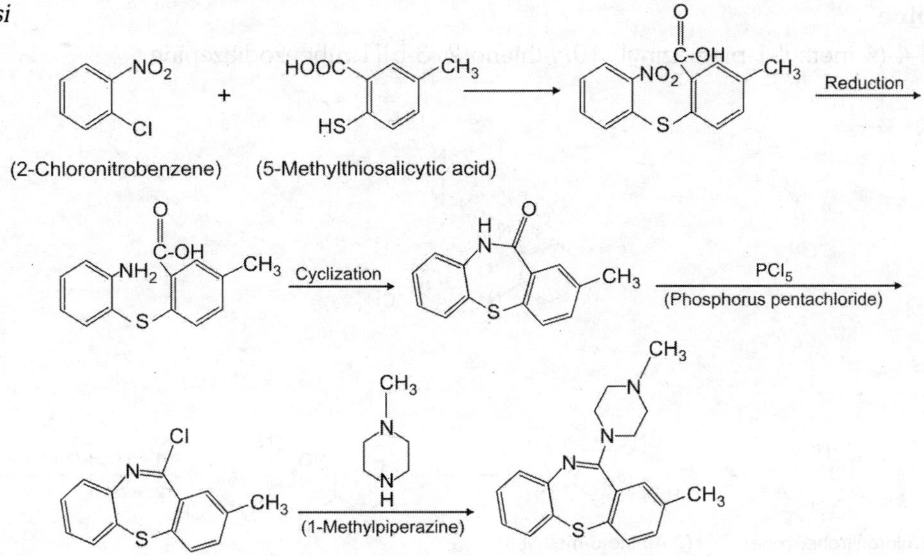
(2-Chloronitrobenzene)
(5-Methylthiosalicytic acid)
Reduction
Cyclization
PCl5
(Phosphorus pentachloride)
(1-Methylpiperazine)

Quetiapine

2-[2-(4-Dibenzo[b,f][1,4]thiazepin-11-yl-1-piperazinyl)ethoxy]ethanol

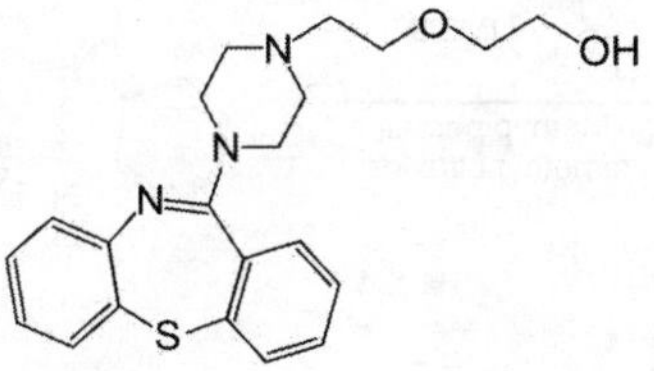

Synthesis

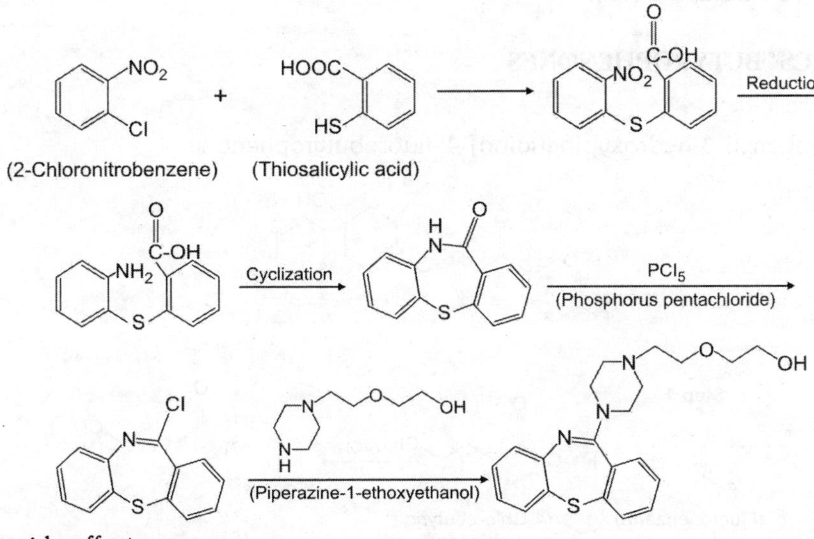
(2-Chloronitrobenzene)
(Thiosalicylic acid)
Reduction
Cyclization
PCl5
(Phosphorus pentachloride)
(Piperazine-1-ethoxyethanol)

It has less side effects.

Olanzapine

2-Methyl-4-(4-methyl-1-piperazinyl)-10*H*-thieno[2, 3-b][1,5]benzodiazepine

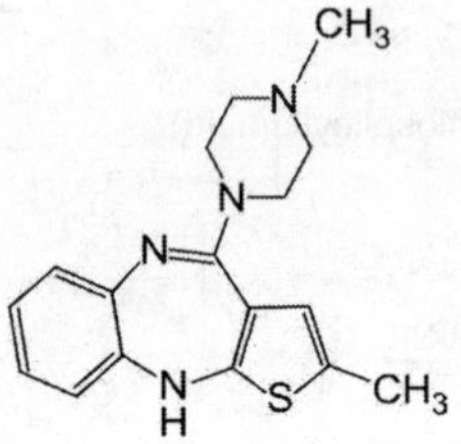

Synthesis

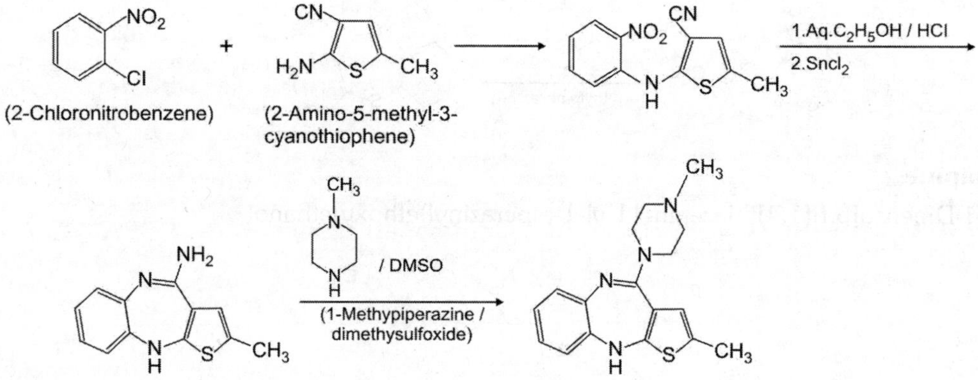
(2-Chloronitrobenzene)
(2-Amino-5-methyl-3-cyanothiophene)
1.Aq.C2H5OH / HCl
2.Sncl2
/ DMSO
(1-Methypiperazine / dimethysulfoxide)

Same activity as clozapine (7a).

NEUROLEPTICS : BUTYROPHENONES

Haloperidol

4-[4-(*p*-Chlorophenyl)-4-hydroxypiperidino]-4'-fluorobutyrophenone

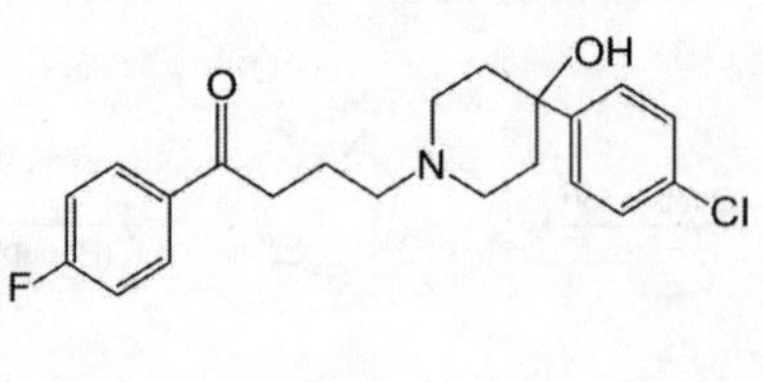

Synthesis

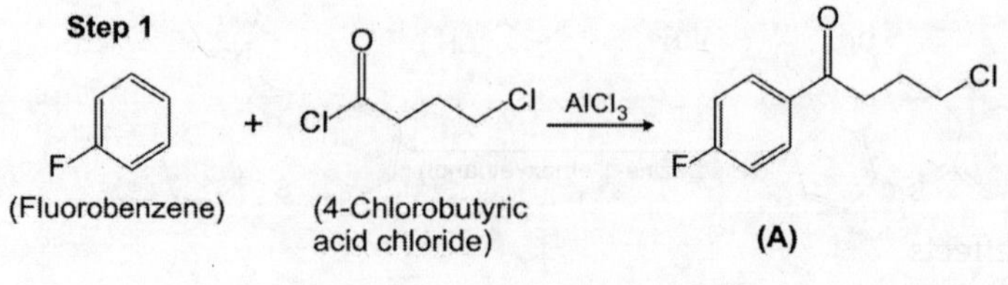
Step 1
AlCl3
(Fluorobenzene)
(4-Chlorobutyric acid chloride)
(A)

Step 2

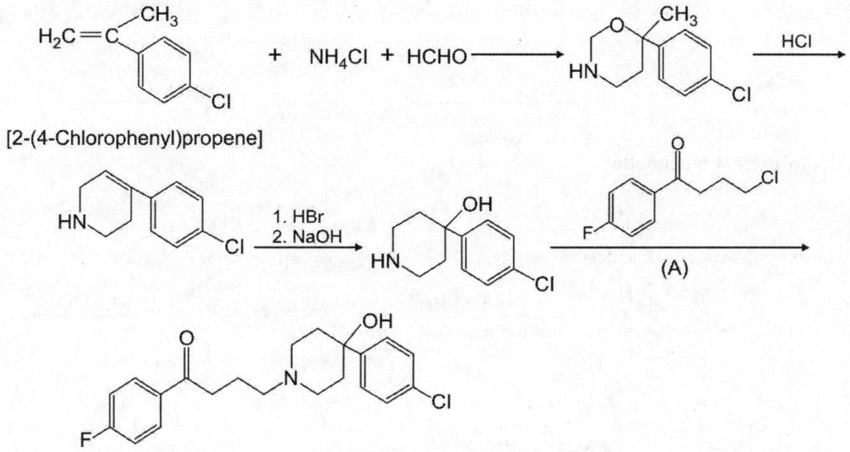

[2-(4-Chlorophenyl)propene]

The compound is used in schizophrenia and in psychosis caused by brain damage.

Trifluperidol

1-(4-Fluorophenyl)-4-[4-hydroxy-4-[3-(trifluoromethyl)-phenyl]-1-piperidinyl-1-butanone

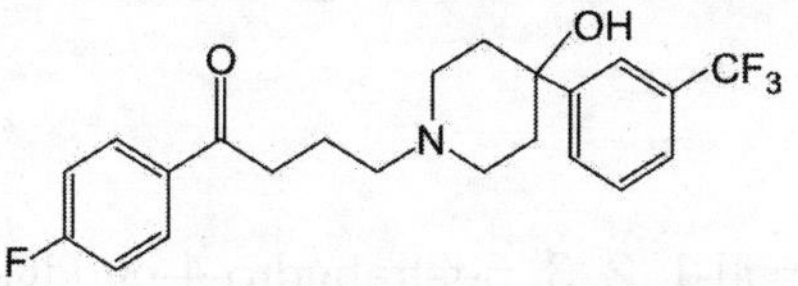

Synthesis

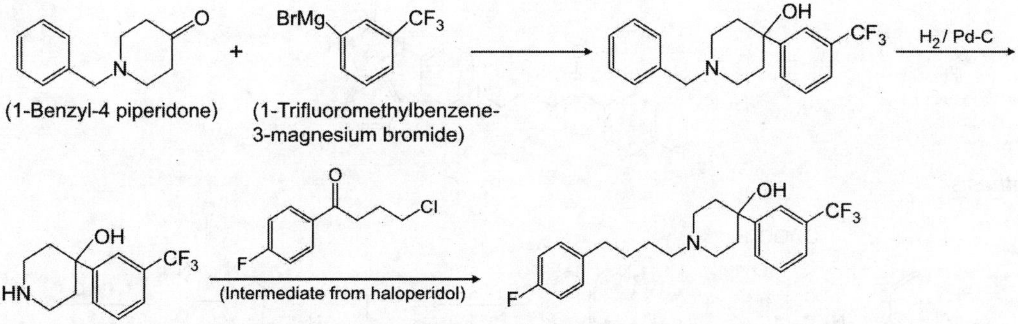

(1-Benzyl-4 piperidone)   (1-Trifluoromethylbenzene-
3-magnesium bromide)

(Intermediate from haloperidol)

It is a powerful antipsychotic drug. It also possesses anticonvulsant and antiemetic actions.

Spiperone

8-[4-(4-Fluorophenyl)-4-oxobutyl]-1-phenyl-1, 3, 8-triazaspiro[4, 5]decan-4-one

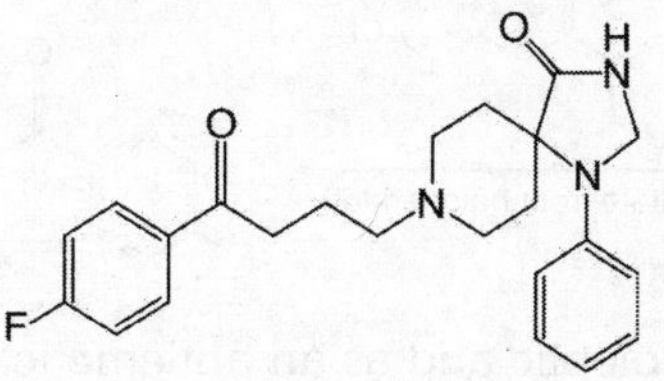

Synthesis

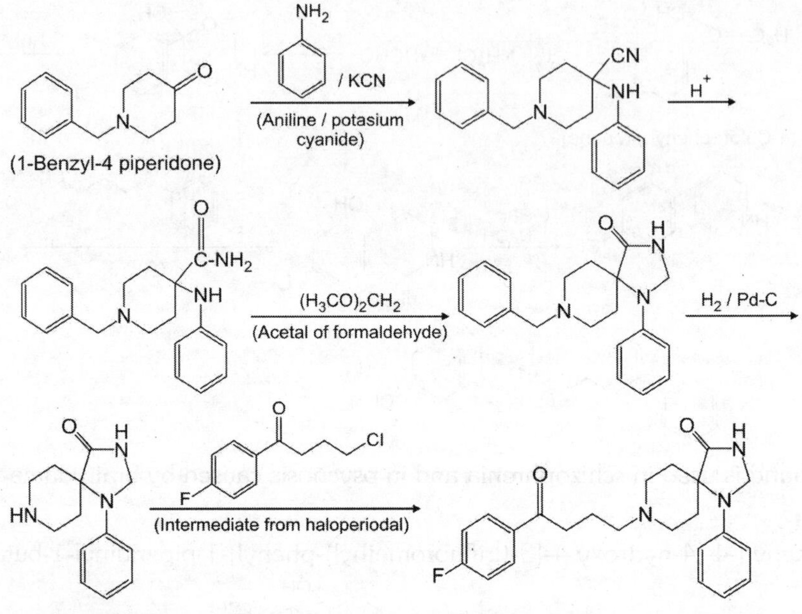

(1-Benzyl-4 piperidone)

(Aniline / potasium cyanide)

H⁺ →

(H₃CO)₂CH₂ (Acetal of formaldehyde)

H₂ / Pd-C →

(Intermediate from haloperiodal)

It is used as antipsychotic.

Droperidol

1-[1-[3-(*p*- Fluorobenzoyl) propyl]-1, 2, 3, 6-tetrahydro-4-pyridyl]-2-benzimidazolinone

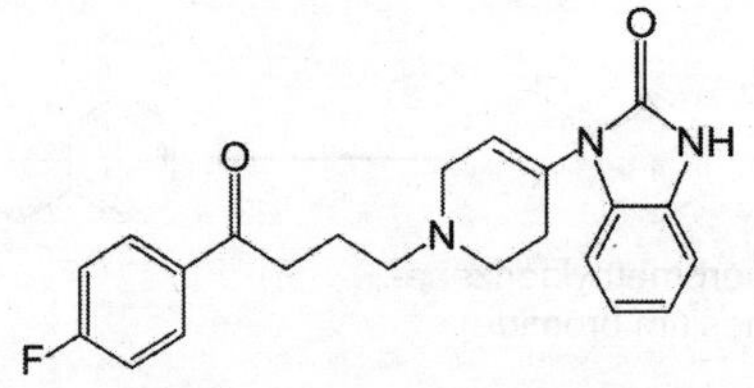

Synthesis

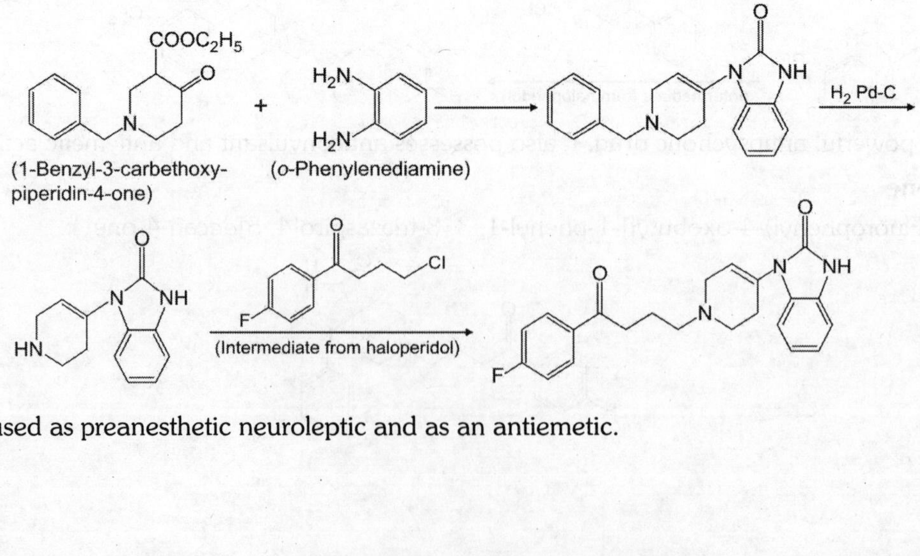

(1-Benzyl-3-carbethoxy-piperidin-4-one)

+

(*o*-Phenylenediamine)

H₂ Pd-C →

(Intermediate from haloperidol)

It is used as preanesthetic neuroleptic and as an antiemetic.

NEUROLEPTICS: MISCELLANEOUS COMPOUNDS

Pimozide

1-[1-[4, 4-Bis (4-fluorophenyl)butyl]-4-piperidinyl]-1, 3-dihydro-2*H*-benzimidazol-2-one

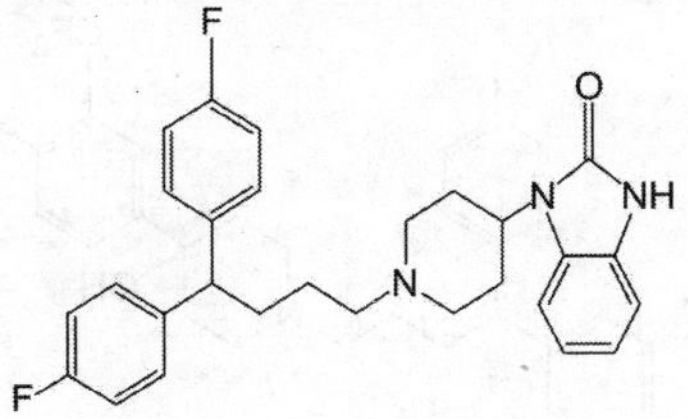
F
O
N
NH
N
F

Synthesis

Step 1

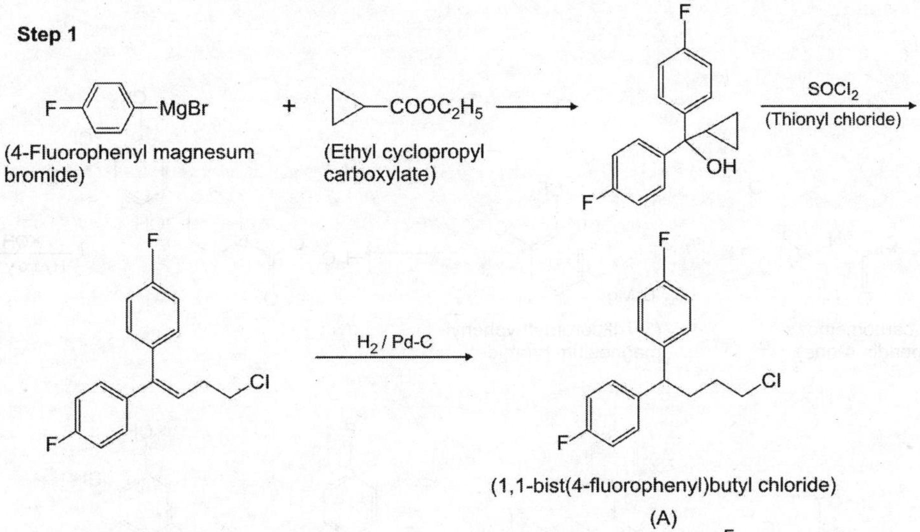
F—⟨⟩—MgBr
+
—COOC$_2$H$_5$
(4-Fluorophenyl magnesum bromide)
(Ethyl cyclopropyl carboxylate)
F
OH
F
SOCl$_2$
(Thionyl chloride)
F
Cl
F
H$_2$ / Pd-C
F
Cl
F
(1,1-bist(4-fluorophenyl)butyl chloride)
(A)

Step 2

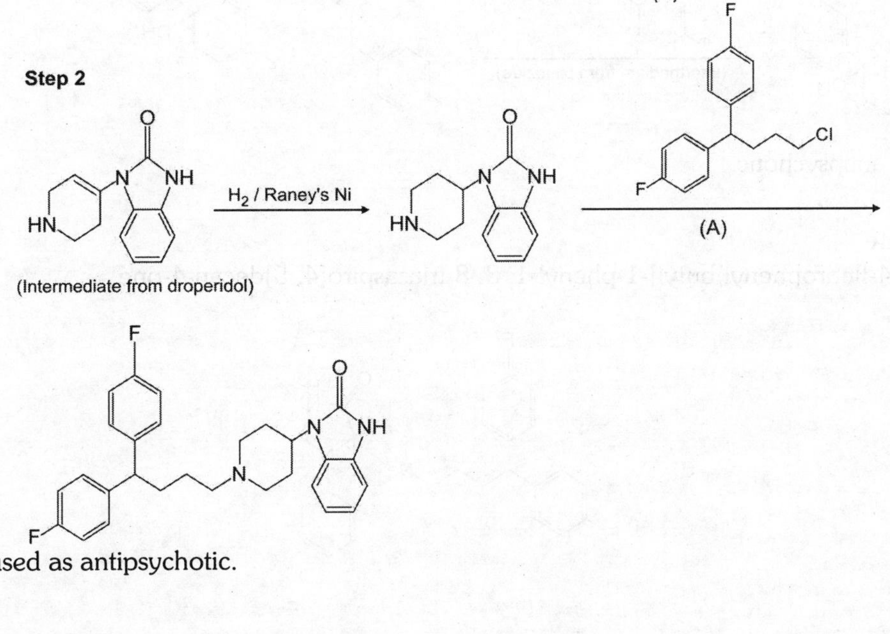
O
N
NH
HN
(Intermediate from droperidol)
H$_2$ / Raney's Ni
O
N
NH
HN
F
Cl
F
(A)
F
O
N
NH
N
F

It is used as antipsychotic.

Penfluoridol

1-[4,4-Bis(4-fluorophenyl)butyl]-4-[4-chloro-3-(trifluoromethyl)phenyl]-4-piperidinol

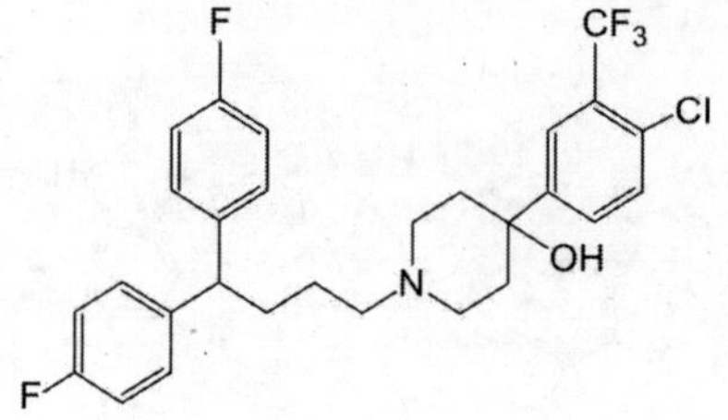

Synthesis

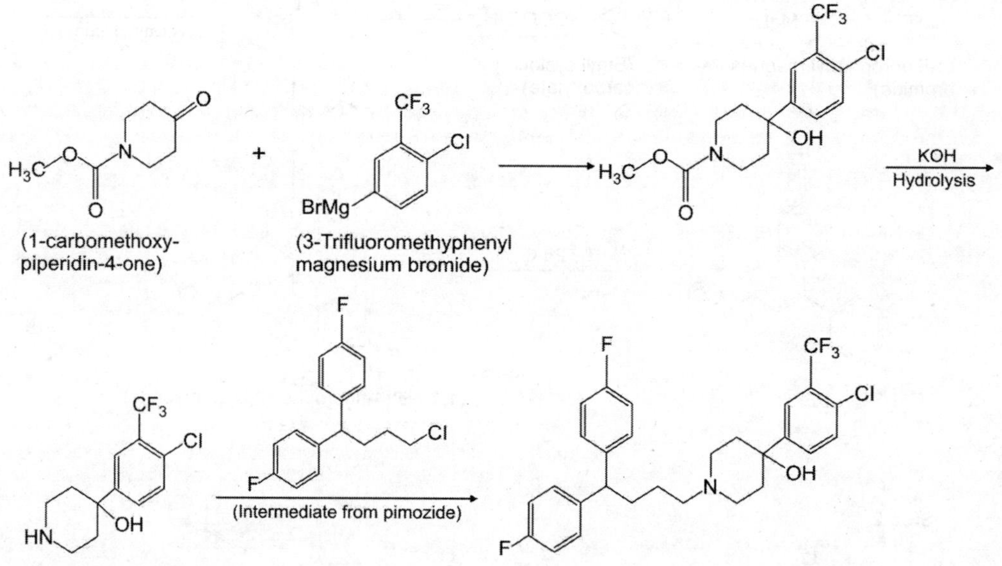

(1-carbomethoxy-
piperidin-4-one)

(3-Trifluoromethyphenyl
magnesium bromide)

KOH
Hydrolysis

(Intermediate from pimozide)

Used as antipsychotic.

Fluspirilene

8-[4,4-Bis(4-fluorophenyl)butyl]-1-phenyl-1, 3, 8-triazaspiro[4, 5]decan-4-one

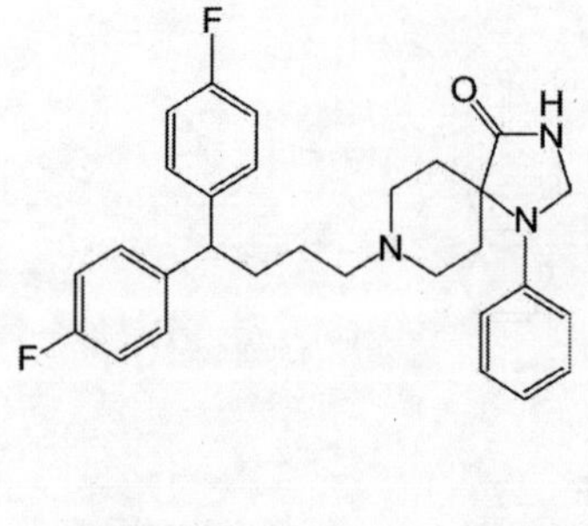

Synthesis

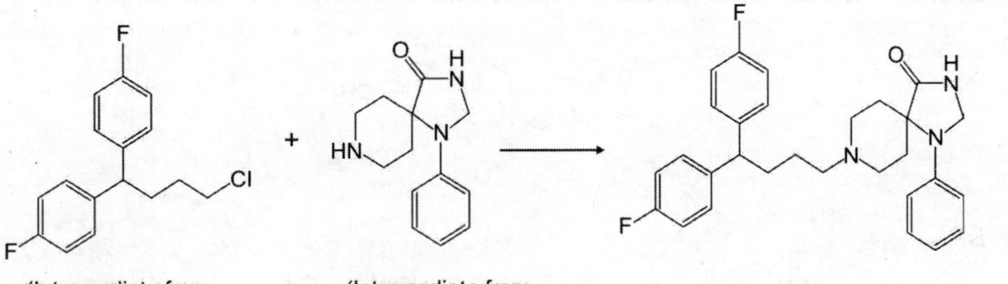

(Intermediate from pimozide) + (Intermediate from spiperone) →

Used as antipsychotic.

Oxypertine

5,6-Dimethoxy-2-methyl-3-[2-(4-phenyl-1-piperazinyl)ethyl]-1*H*-indole

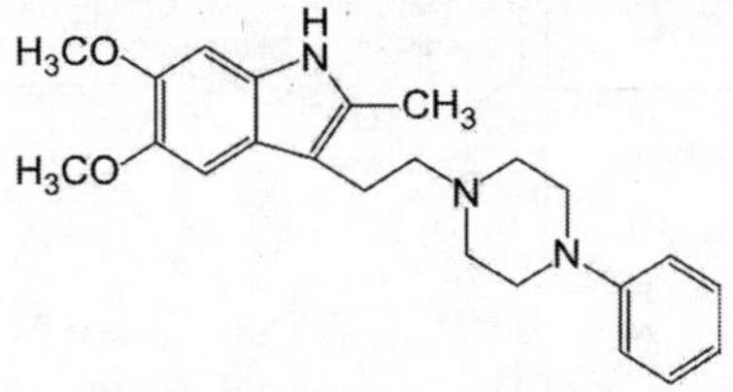

Synthesis

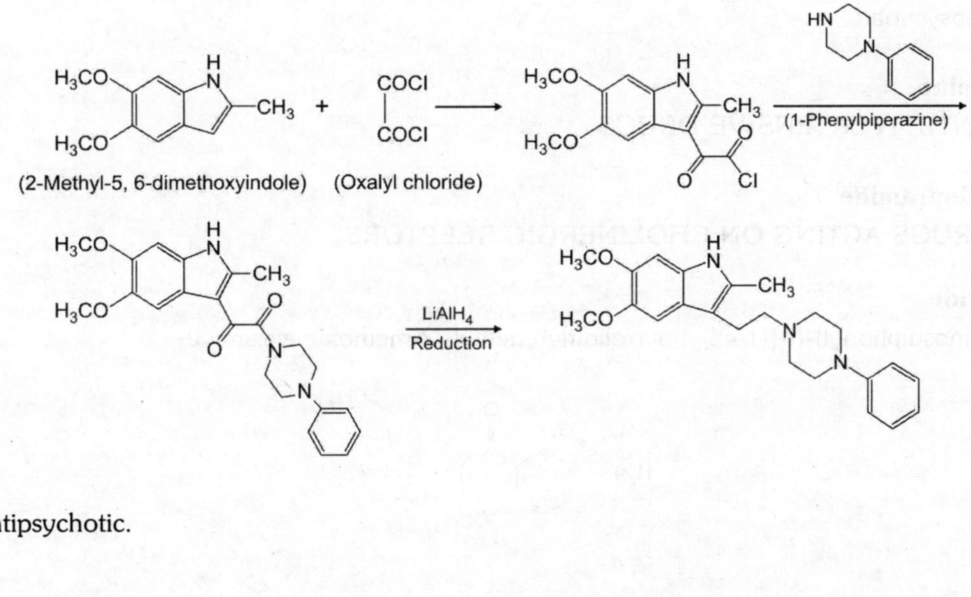

(2-Methyl-5, 6-dimethoxyindole) (Oxalyl chloride) (1-Phenylpiperazine)

$LiAlH_4$ Reduction

Antipsychotic.

Molindone

3-Ethyl-1, 5, 6, 7-tetrahydro-2-methyl-5-(4-morpholinylmethyl)-4-*H*-indol-4-one

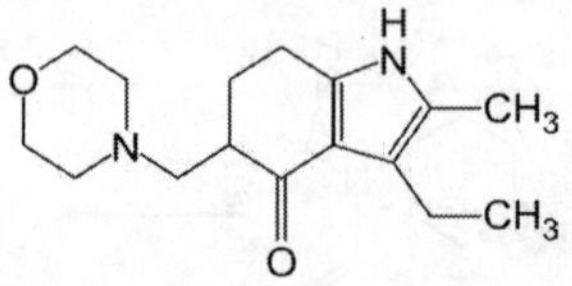

Synthesis

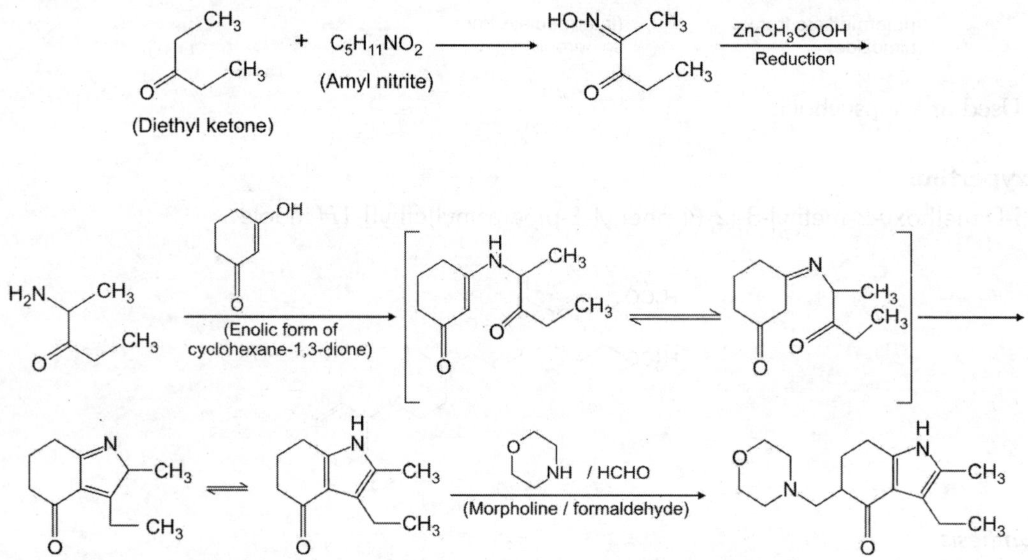

Antipsychotic.

Reserpine

See ANTIHYPERTENSIVE DRUGS

Metoclopramide

See DRUGS ACTING ON CHOLINERGIC REEPTORS

Sulpiride

5-(Aminosulphonyl)-*N*-[(1-ethyl-pyrrolidinyl)methyl]-2-methoxybenzamide

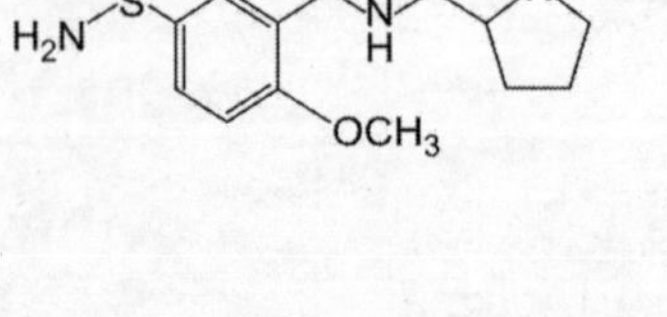

Synthesis

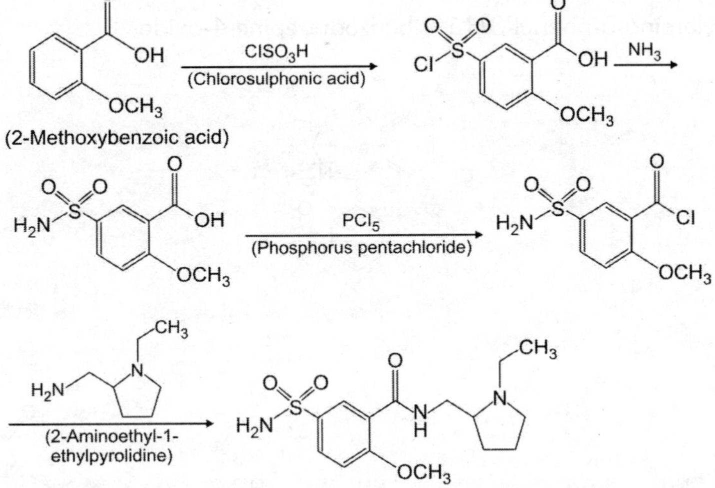

It has a moderate neuroleptic activity along with some stimulating and antidepressant activity.

Remoxipride

(*S*)-3-Bromo-*N*-[(1-ethyl-2-pyrrolidinyl)methyl]-2, 6-dimethoxybenzamide

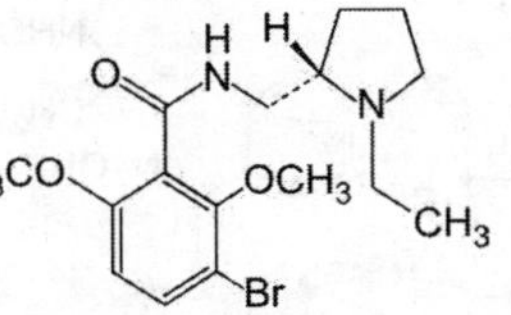

Synthesis

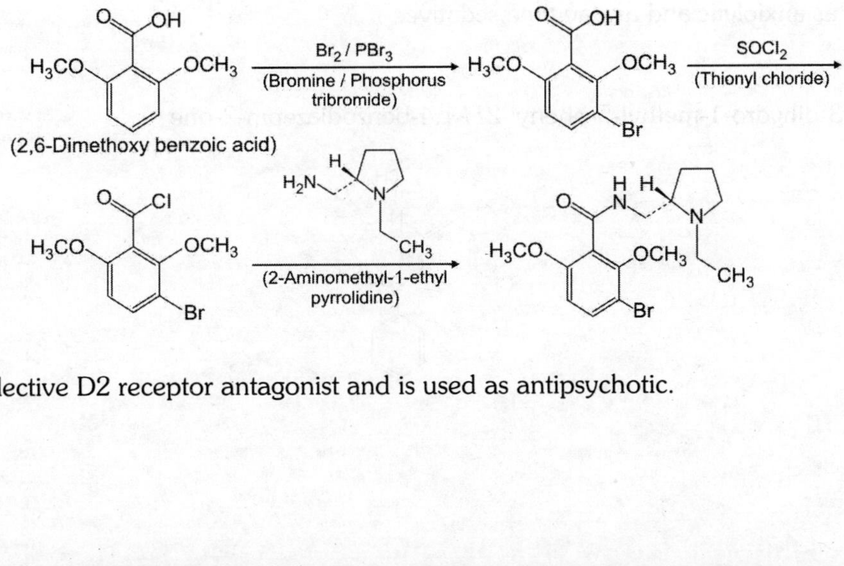

It is a selective D2 receptor antagonist and is used as antipsychotic.

ANXIOLYTICS : BENZODIAZEPINES AND GABA$_A$ RECEPTOR PARTIAL AGONISTS

Chlordiazepoxide

7-Chloro-2-methylamino-5-phenyl-3*H*-1,4-benzodiazepine-4-oxide

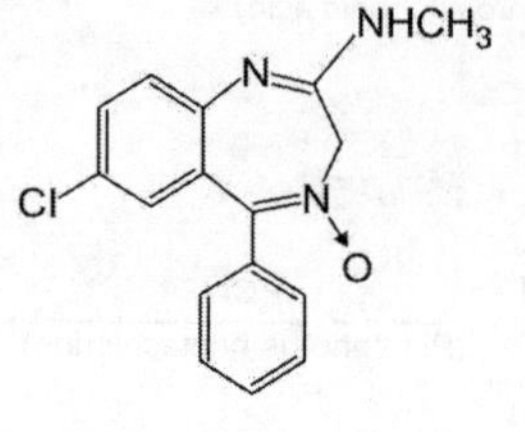

Synthesis

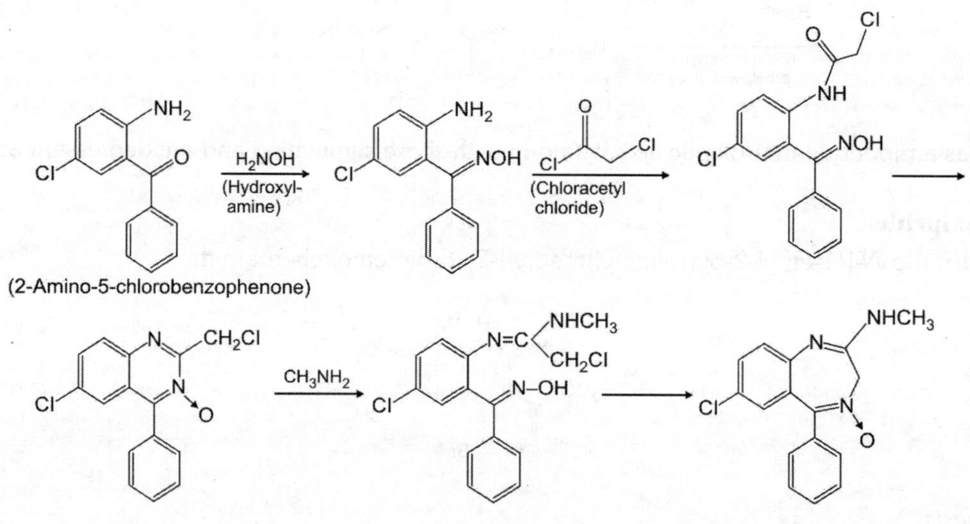

(2-Amino-5-chlorobenzophenone)

It is used as anxiolytic and as day time sedative

Diazepam

7-Chloro-1,3-dihydro-1-methyl-5-phenyl-2*H*-1,4-benzodiazepin-2-one

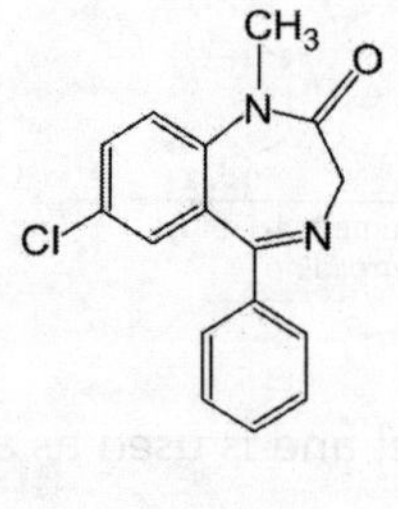

Synthesis

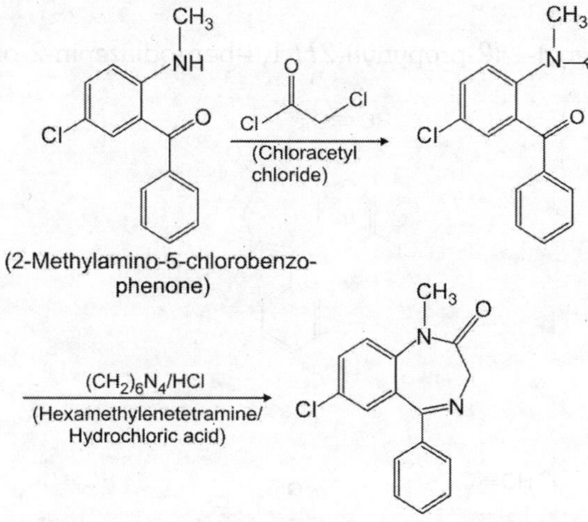

(2-Methylamino-5-chlorobenzo-
phenone)

$$\xrightarrow[\text{(Hexamethylenetetramine/}]{\text{(CH}_2)_6\text{N}_4\text{/HCl}}$$
Hydrochloric acid)

Diazepam is used for control of anxiety relief of muscular spasm and as anticonvulsant.

Halazepam

7-Chloro-1,3-dihydro-5-phenyl-1-(2,2,2-trifluoroethyl)-2*H*-1,4-benzodiazepin-2-one

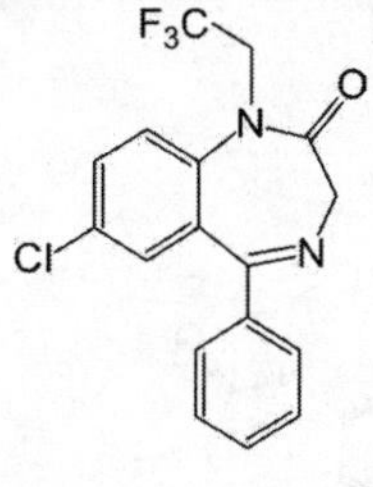

Synthesis

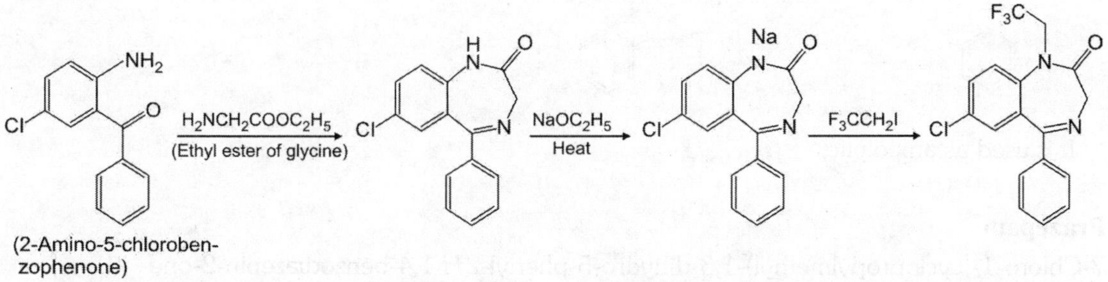

(2-Amino-5-chloroben-
zophenone)

It is used as anxiolytic. Its activity is due to its metabolites oxazepam (30) and nordazepam (46).

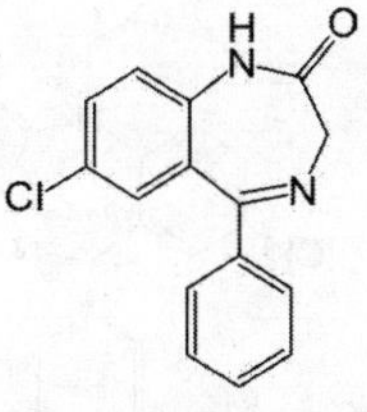

(46)

Pinazepam

7-Chloro-1,3-dihydro-5-phenyl-1-(2-propynyl)-2*H*-1,4-benzodiazepin-2-one

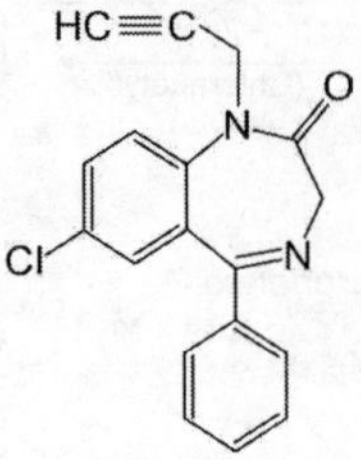

Synthesis

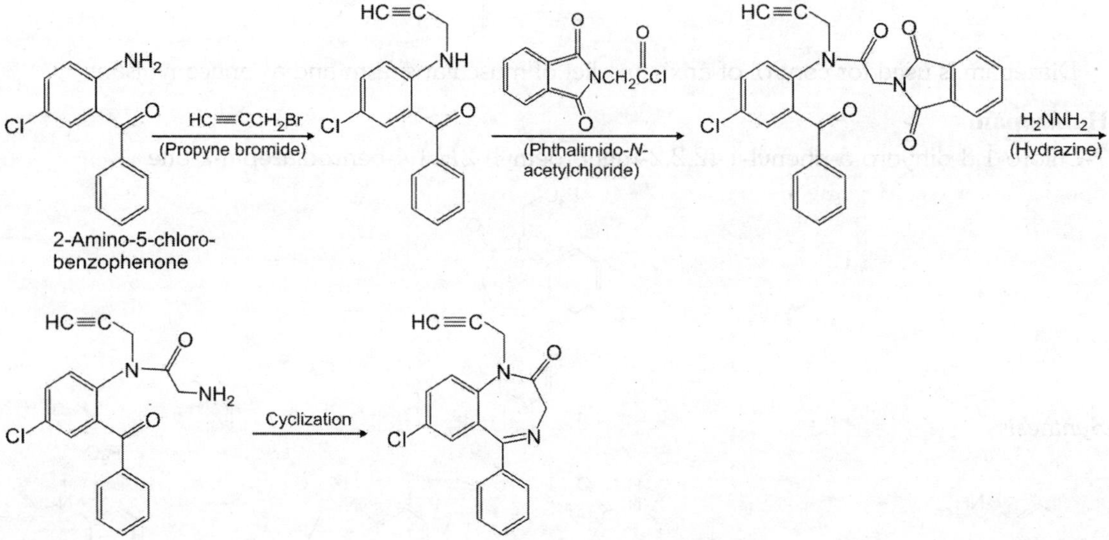

2-Amino-5-chloro-
benzophenone

It is used as anxiolytic.

Prazepam

7-Chloro-1-(cyclopropylmethyl)-1,3-dihydro-5-phenyl-2*H*-1,4-benzodiazepin-2-one

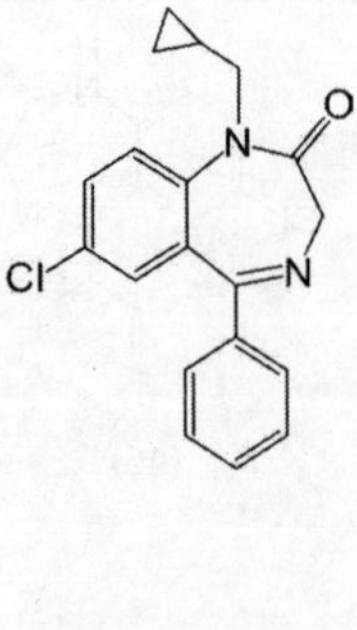

Synthesis

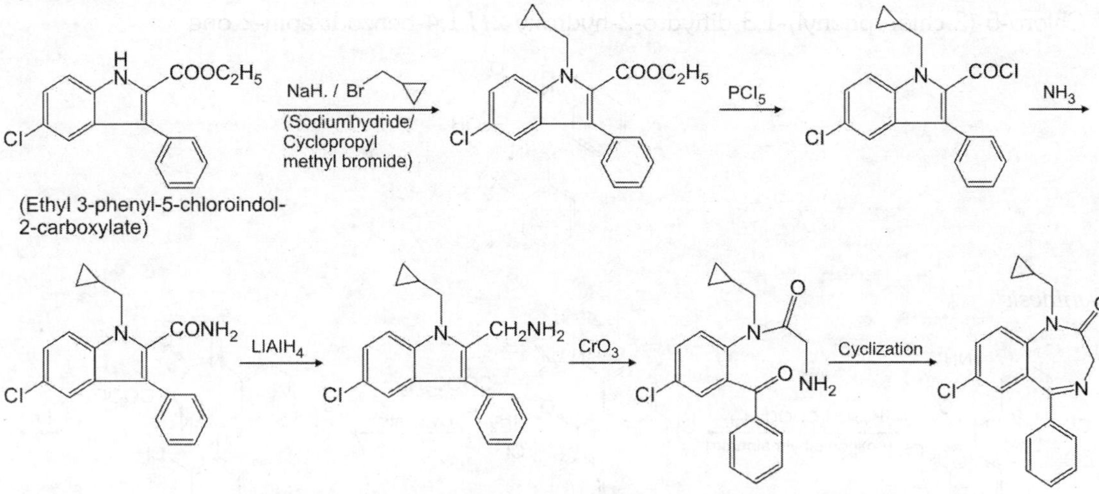

(Ethyl 3-phenyl-5-chloroindol-
2-carboxylate)

Its anxiolytic activity is due to its metabolism to oxazepam (30).

Oxazepam
7-Chloro-1,3-dihydro-3-hydroxy-5-phenyl-2*H*-1,4-benzodiazepin-2-one

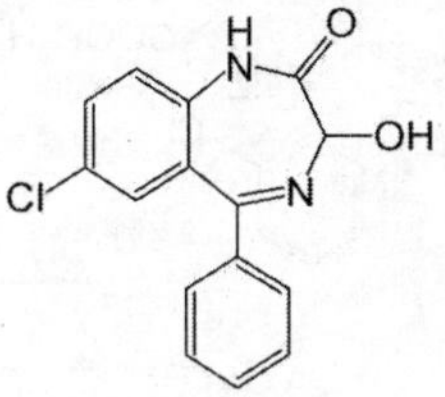

Synthesis

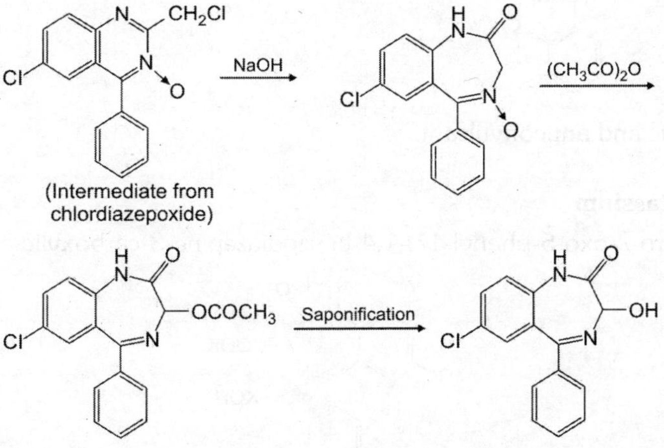

(Intermediate from
chlordiazepoxide)

Used as anxiolytic.

Lorazepam

7-Chloro-5-(2-chlorophenyl)-1,3-dihydro-2-hydroxy-2H-1,4-benzodizepin-2-one

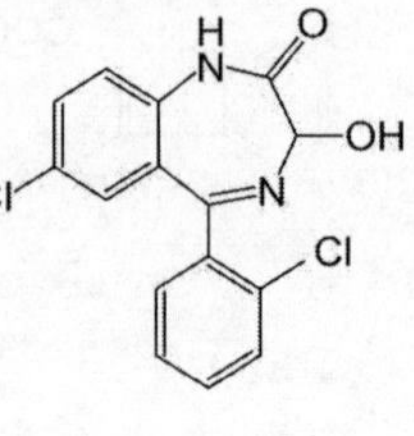

Synthesis

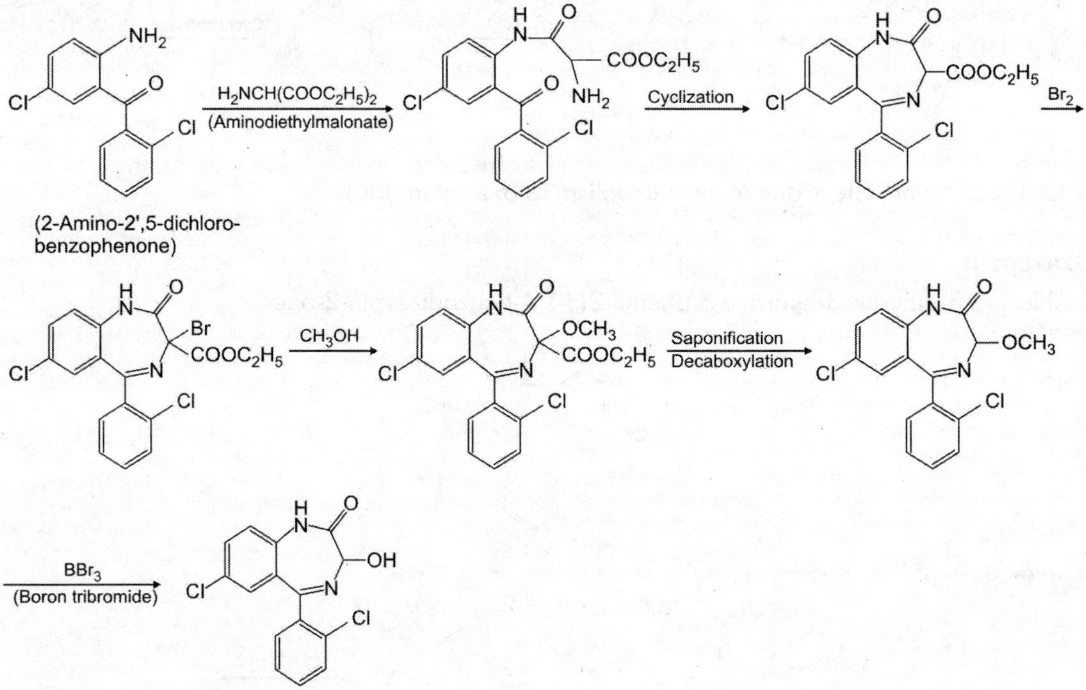

(2-Amino-2',5-dichloro-
benzophenone)

Used as anxiolytic and anticonvulsant.

Clorazepate Dipotassium

7-Chloro-2,3-dihydro-2-oxo-5-phenyl-1H-1,4-benzodiazepine-3-carboxylic acid dipotassium

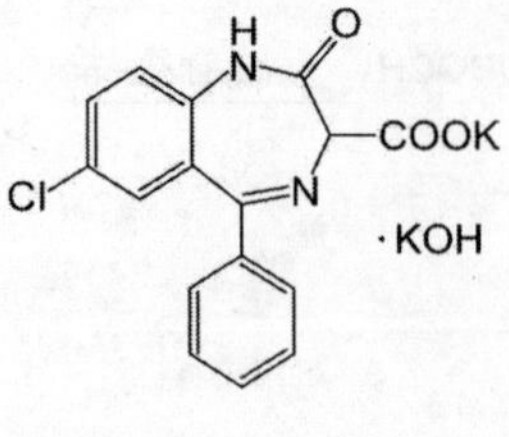

Synthesis

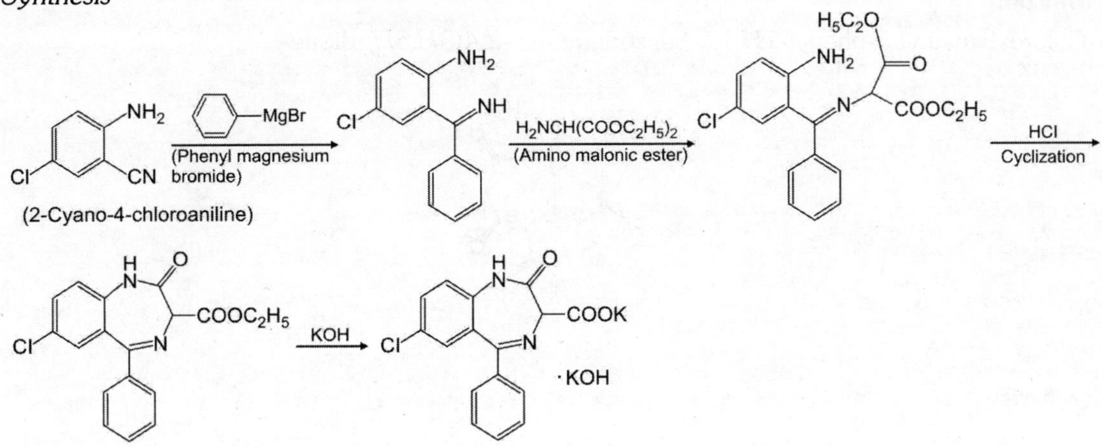

(2-Cyano-4-chloroaniline)

It is used as anxiolytic and anticonvulsant.

Alprazolam

8-Chloro-1-methyl-6-phenyl-4H-[1, 2, 4]triazolo[4, 3-a][1, 4]benzodiazepine

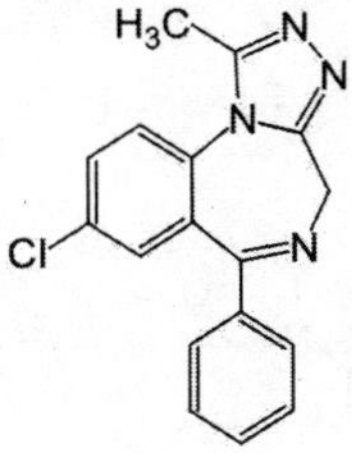

Synthesis

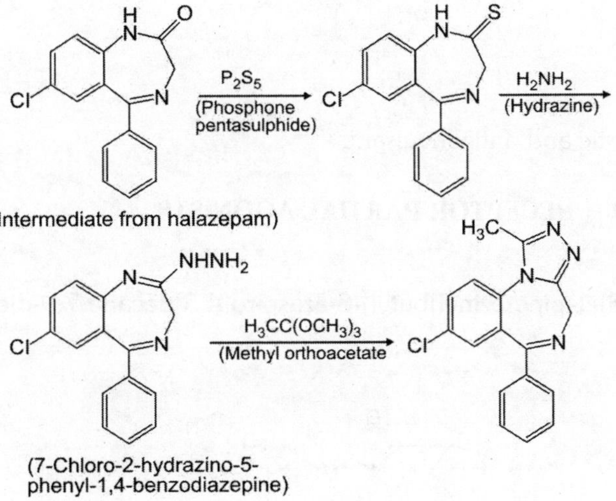

(Intermediate from halazepam)

(7-Chloro-2-hydrazino-5-
phenyl-1,4-benzodiazepine)

The drug is a potent anxiolytic.

Clobazam

7-Chloro-1-methyl-5-phenyl-1*H*-1,5-benzodiazepine-2,4(3*H*,5*H*)-dione

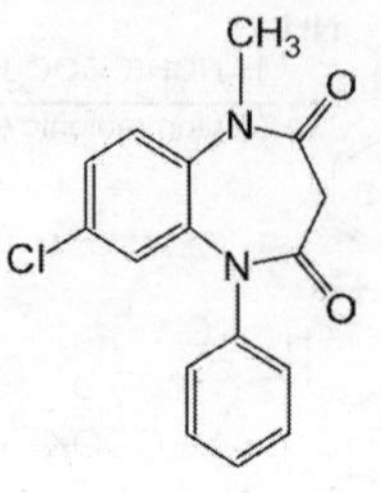

Synthesis

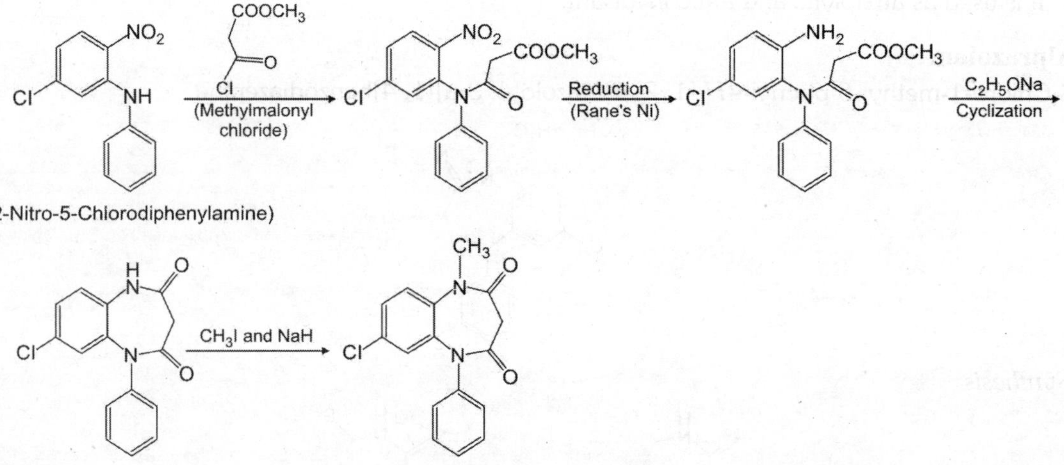

(2-Nitro-5-Chlorodiphenylamine)

It is used as anxiolytic and anticonvulsant.

ANXIOLYTICS : 5-HT$_{1A}$ RECEPTOR PARTIAL AGONISTS

Buspirone

8-[4-[4-(2-Pyrimidinyl)-1-piperazinyl]butyl]-8-azaspiro[4.5]decane-7,9-dione

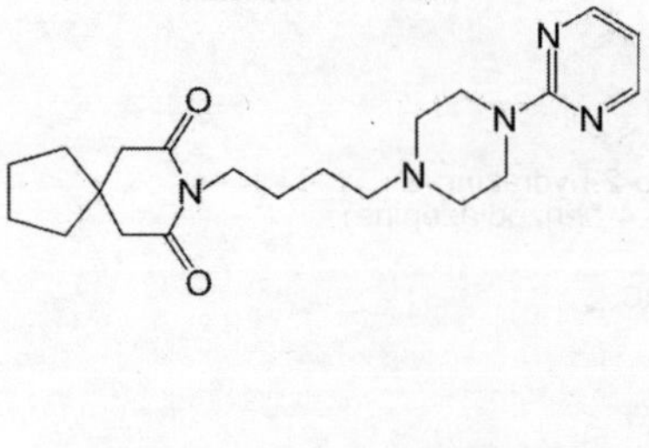

Synthesis

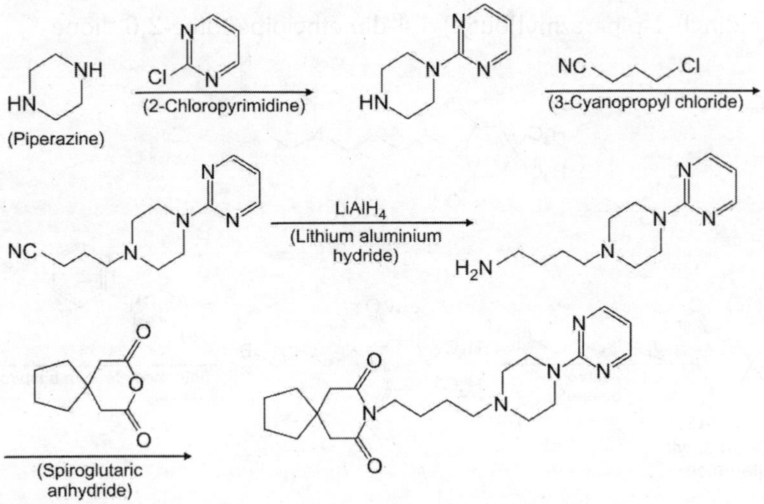

It is a non-sedating with moderate anxiolytic properties. It is not as effective as benzodiazepines. But it is non-addictive.

Ipsapirone

2-[4-[4-(2-Pyrimidinyl)-1-piperazinyl]buty]-1,2-benzisothiazolin-3(2*H*)-one

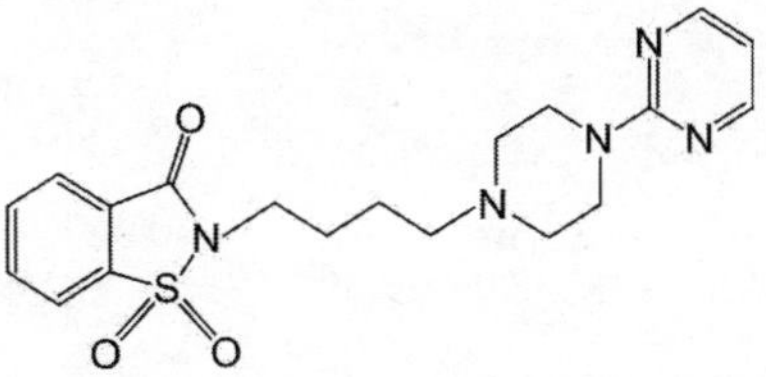

Synthesis

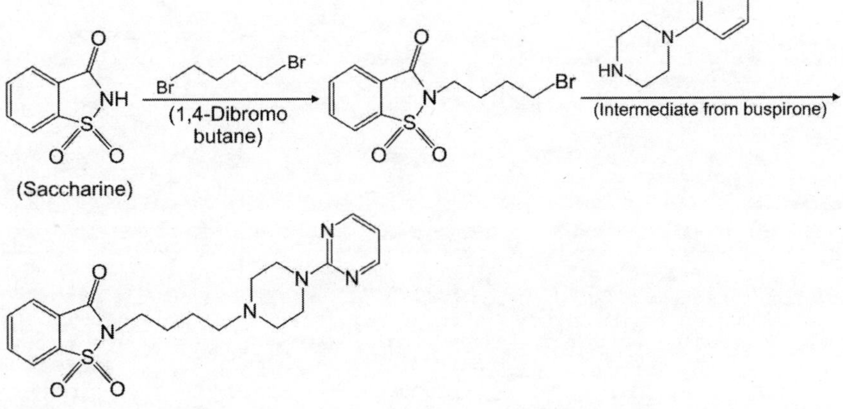

Similar activity as buspirone (41).

Gepirone

1-[4-[4-(2-Pyrimidinyl)-1-piperazinyl]butyl]-4,4-dimethylpiperidine-2,6-dione

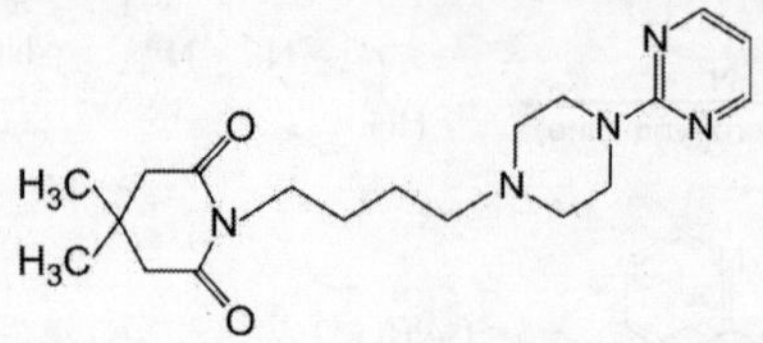

Synthesis

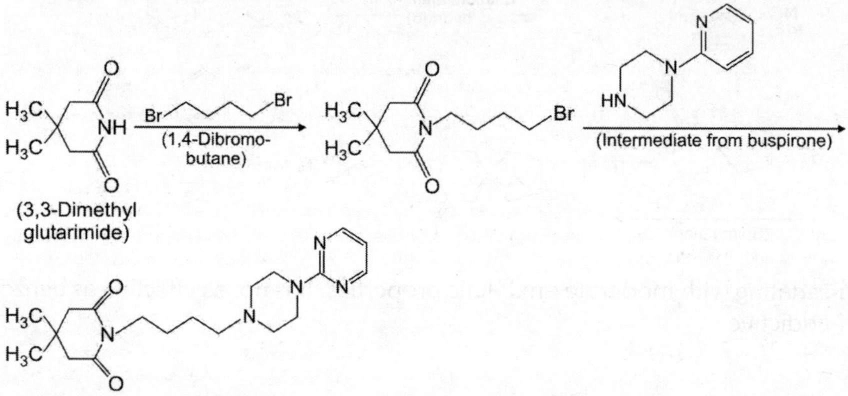

(3,3-Dimethyl glutarimide)

(1,4-Dibromo-butane)

(Intermediate from buspirone)

Same activity as buspirone (41).

ANTIEPILEPTIC DRUGS

Epilepsy is actually CNS malfunction. During epileptic seizures, there is excessive discharge of electricity by a group of neurons in brain which may then spread to other areas of brain. The function and the part of brain that is affected determines the symptoms. Thus, convulsions result when motor cortex is involved. Peripheral autonomic discharge is produced as a result of involvement of hypothalamus and involvement of reticular formation in upper brainstem results in loss of consciousness.

Clinically, epilepsy has been classified into two broad classes, i.e. partial and generalized type seizures. Partial epilepsy has been further subdivided in cortical or Jacksonian seizures. It involves partial epilepsy in the form of localized convulsions that may occur without the loss of consciousness. This disorder is as a result of localized organic brain lesions that can promote extremely rapid discharges in local neurons. Another type of partial epilepsy is known as psychomotor seizures. It is characterized by short period of amnesia, an attack of abnormal rage, sudden anxiety, and a moment of incoherent speech.

The generalized types include grand mal and petit mal. The grand mal type involves generalized seizures, chewing motion, and loss of consciousness. It is characterised by fast brain waves, neuronal discharges originating in mesencephalic portion of reticular activating system. These then spread through CNS including cortex, lower portion of brain, and spinal cord resulting in tonic and clonic convulsions. The petit mal type of epilepsy is characterised by hyperactivity of all parts of brain. It can be of two types myoclonic form and absence form. In myoclonic form, there is a burst of neuronal discharge lasting a fraction of a second throughout the nervous system. The entire process stops before consciousness is lost. In absence form, there is unconsciousness for about 5-20 sec. and some symmetrical clonic motor activity.

Some of the factors responsible for epileptic seizures could be congenital, head trauma, fracture of skull, abscess, neoplasm, inflammatory vascular diseases, and certain psychotropic agents.

CHARACTERISTICS OF AN IDEAL ANTIEPILEPTIC DRUG

1. It should have minimal sedative-hypnotic effect.
2. Since antiepileptic drugs may have to be used throughout life, it should have least long-term toxicity.

Many of the antiepileptics produce side effects such as damage to bone marrow, liver, kidney, gastrointestinal disturbances, and neuropathies. Further, antiepileptics used for one type of epilepsy may aggravate or precipitate seizures of other type.

ANTIEPILEPTIC DRUGS

Bromides

Bromides of sodium and potassium were the drugs used earlier for grand mal type of epilepsy. With the advent of newer drugs these salts are no more used. Further, continued use of bromides results in bromism which is characterised by headache, sleepiness, loss of strength, and sexual drive.

Barbiturates

The barbiturates used clinically as antiepileptics include phenobarbital (1), metharbital (2), and mephobarbital (3). Barbiturates are effective in generalized tonic-clonic and parial seizures. The exact mechanism of action of barbiturates is not known. It probably involves binding of barbiturates at the allosteric site of $GABA_A$ receptor and potentiation of the action of endogenous GABA by increasing the duration of Cl^- channel opening. The mechanism may also involve blockade of sodium channel.

(1), R=H, R'=C_2H_5,R"=

(2), R=CH_3,R'=R"=C_2H_5

(3), R=CH_3,R'=C_2H_5,R"=

Hydantoins

Hydantoins can be considered barbiturates in which the -CONH moiety has been replaced by -NH- group. Some of the hydantoins used in clinical practice include phenylethylhydantoin (4), phenytoin (5), phethenylate (6), mephenytoin (7), ethotoin (8), fosphenytoin (9), and albutoin (10). Phenytoin (5) and other hydantoins act by binding to Na^+ channel thus slowing the recovery of inactivated Na^+ channel to the closed state. This results in increased threshold for action potential and prevention of repetitive firing.

Hydantoins are effective in partial and generalized toinc-clonic seizures.

(4), X=O, R=H, R'=C_2H_5, R"=

(5), X=O, R=H, R'= R"=

(6), X=O, R=H, R'= , R"=

(7), X=O, R=CH_3, R'= C_2H_5, R"=

(8), X=O, R=C_2H_5, R'= H, R"=

(9), X=O, R=$CH_2OPO_3H_2$, R'= R"=

(10) X=S, R=$CH_2CH=CH_2$, R'= H, R"=$CH_2CH(CH_3)_2$

2, 4-Oxazolidinediones

2, 4-Oxazolidinediones are close analogs of hydantoins in which -NH- has been replaced by -O-. Some of the analogs include trimethadione (11), paramethadione (12), and ethadione (13). Out of these only trimethadione (11) is used now. Its active metabolite is the *N*-demethylated analog, dimethadione (14) which acts by blocking the calcium T channels. It is effective against absence seizures.

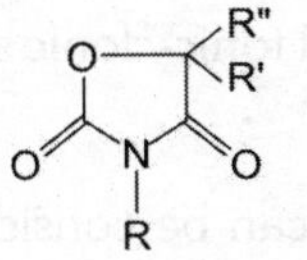

(11), R= R'= R"=CH₃

(12), R= R'= CH₃, R"=C₂H₅

(13), R=C₂H₅, R'= R"=CH₃

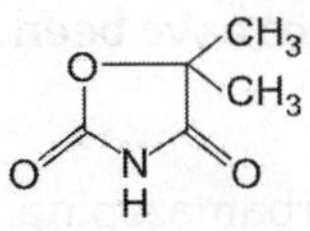

(14)

Imides

Substitution of oxygen in 2,4-oxazolidinediones by -CH₂- leads to succinimdes. Substituted succinimides have shown significant antiepiletic activity. Some of the clinically useful compounds in this series include phensuximide (15), methsuximides (16), and ethosuximide (17). Their mechanism of action involves reduction in activity of calcium T channel. Succinimides are effective against absence seizures.

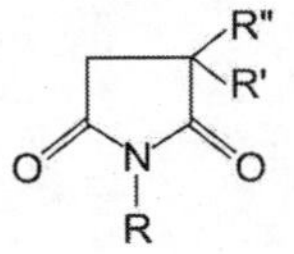

(15), R= CH₃,R'=H,R"=

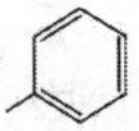

(16), R= R'=CH₃, R"=

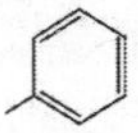

(17), R= H,=R'=C₂H₅,R"=CH₃

Benzodiazepines

Benzodiazepines are useful sedatives, hypnotics, and antianxiety agents. Some of these prossess useful antiseizure activity also. The benzodiazepines useful as antiepileptics include diazepam (18), nitrazepam (19), clonazepam (20), clorazepate potassium (21), lorazepam (22), midazolam (23), and clobazam (24).

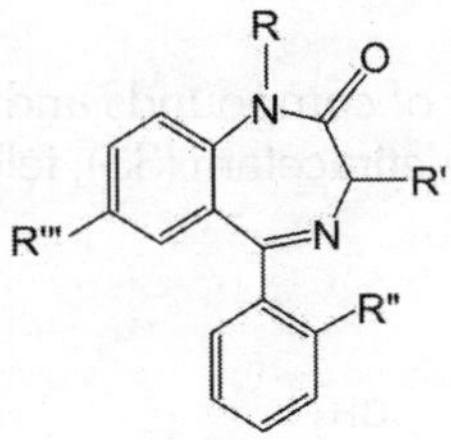

(18), R = CH₃, R'=R"=H, R'''=Cl
(19), R = R'=R"=H, R'''=NO₂
(20), R = R'=H, R"=Cl,R'''=NO₂
(21), R = R"=H, R'=COOK, R'''=Cl
(22), R = H, R'=OH, R"=R'''=Cl

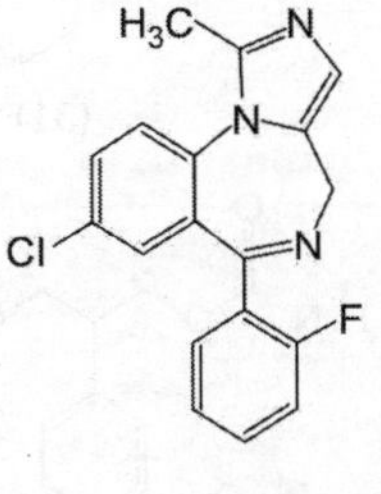

(23)

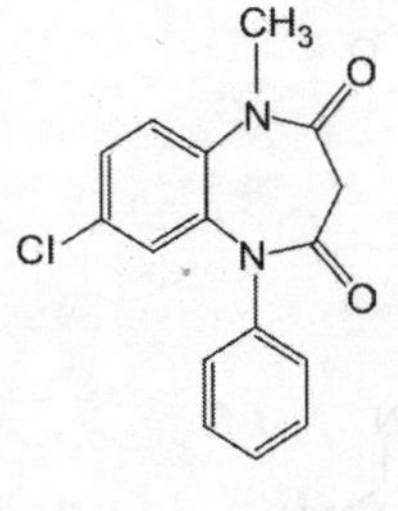

(24)

Benzodiazepines enhance the affinity of inhibitory neurotransmitter GABA to $GABA_A$ receptor thereby increase the influx of Cl^- through the chloride channel. Additional evidence also suggests that benzodiazepines may also be involved in diminishing the Na^+, K^+ and Ca^{2+} currents which is independent of the effect due to complexation with $GABA_A$ receptor.

Benzodiazepines have been found to be effective in partial and generalized tonic-clonic seizures.

Iminostilbenes

These include carbamazepine (25) and oxcarbazepine (26). Both of these can be considered as 1,1-diphenyl ureas, in which the phenyl rings have been bridged by a two carbon unit. Both of these act by blocking the voltage dependent sodium channels thereby decreasing the repetitive firing and spread of electrical activity. The active metabolite of carbamazepine (25) is 2-hydroxyiminostilbene (27), while 10-hydroxycarbazepine (28) is the active metabolite of oxcarbazepine (26). Both of these compounds are used in partial and generalized tonic-clonic seizures.

(25)

(26)

(27)

(28)

Miscellaneous Agents

This class of anticonvulsants comprises of diverse type of compounds and include primidone (29), valproic acid (30), gabapentin (31), lamotrigine (32), levetiracetam (33), felbamate (34), zonisamide (35), and tiagabine (36).

(29)

(30)

(31)

(32)

(33)

(34)

(35)

(36)

Primidone (29), a pyrimidinedione, is 2-desoxyphenylbarbital. Excepting in absence type of seizures it has been found to be effective in all types of seizures. Its activity is due to its conversion to phenobarbital (1).

Valproic acid (30) or 2-propylpentanoic acid shows good activity in several types of seizures. It is particularly effective in absence type of seizures. It acts by slowing down the rate of recovery of Na^+ channels from the inactivated state. In vitro studies have shown that it increases the activity of glutamic acid decarboxylase, an enzyme responsible for GABA synthesis. This results in increased concentration of GABA which ultimately results in increased GABA mediated inhibition.

Gabapentin (31), an analog of GABA increases the concentration of GABA in neurons. Its main effect is through inhibition of high voltage activated Ca^{++} channels. It is used as an adjunct for the treatment of partial seizures.

Lamotrigine (32) is a triazine derivative and is used as an adjunct for partial seizures in adults. It slows down the Na^+ channel recovery from its inactivated state. It is useful alternative to carbamazepine (25), as a treatment for partial and tonic-clonic seizures.

Levetiracetam (33), has been used in partial and tonic-clonic seizures.

Felbamate (34), a biscarbamate ester, has been found effective against partial seizures. It antagonizes the NMDA receptor by binding to glycine recognition site, thus preventing the glycine induced increase in calcium channel opening.

Zonisamide (35), acts by blocking both sodium and T-type calcium channels and is used as adjunct for partial seizures.

Tiagabine (36), has been found to be effective in refractory partial seizures. It inhibits GABA transporter GAT-1 and thus reduces the uptake of GABA into storage sites which results in increased GABA mediated inhibition.

A comparision of structures of barbiturates, hydantoins, oxazolidinediones, and succinimides shows that segment (37) forms a common feature of these compounds. Structure-activity relationship

Barbitrates   Hydantoins   Oxazolidinedione   Succinimides

(37)

studies have shown that the R and R´ should be hydrocarbons. If R and R´ are lower alkyl groups, the compounds are active against absence type of seizures. On the otherhand, if one of the groups is aromatic, the compounds are active against generalized tonic-clonic and partial type of seizures.

INDIVIDUAL COMPOUNDS

BARBITURATES
Phenobarbital, Metharbital, and Mephobarbital
See **SEDATIVES AND HYPNOTICS**

HYDANTOINS
Phenylethylhydantoin
5-Ethyl-5-phenylhydantoin

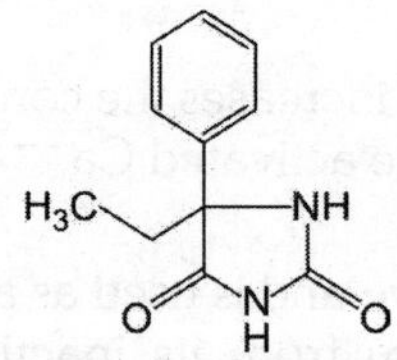

Synthesis

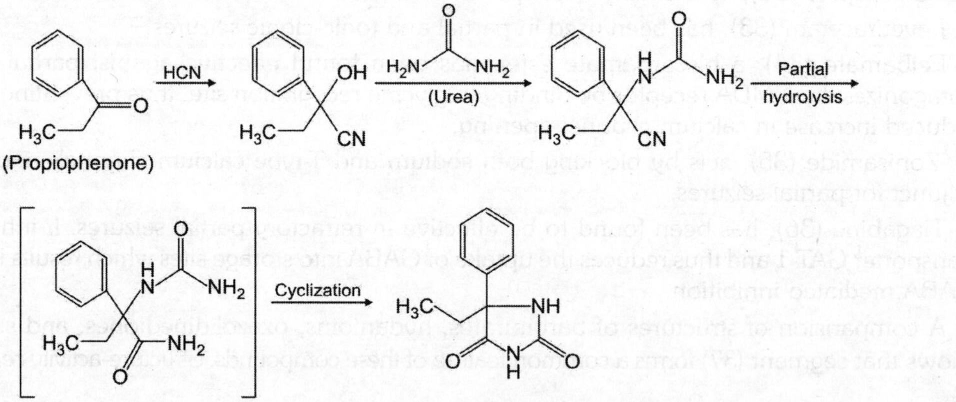

Its structure is analogous to phenobarbital (1). It is used in partial and generalized tonic-clonic seizures.

Phenytoin
5,5-Diphenylhydantoin

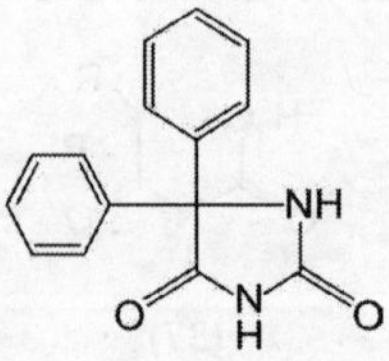

Synthesis

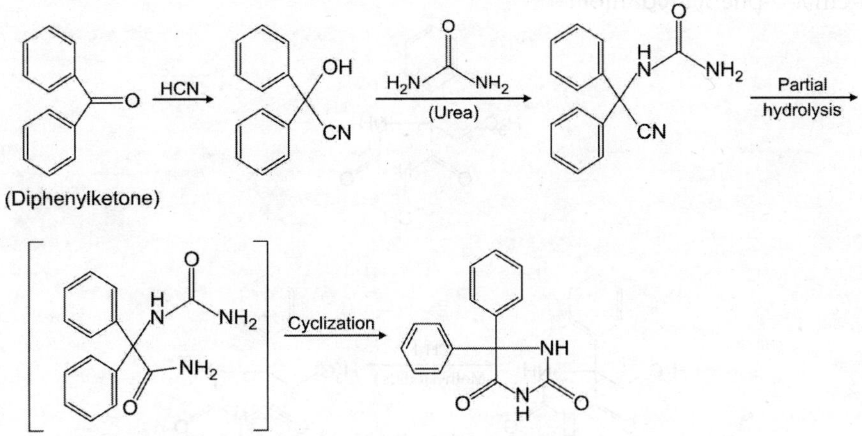

(Diphenylketone)

It is also used as sodium salt. It acts by binding to sodium channels to prevent the spread of seizure. It also causes decreased permeability to Ca^{2+}.

Phethenylate Sodium

5-Phenyl-5(2-thienyl)-2,4-imidazolidinedione monosodium salt

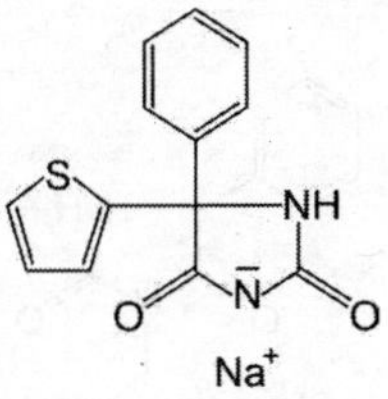

Synthesis

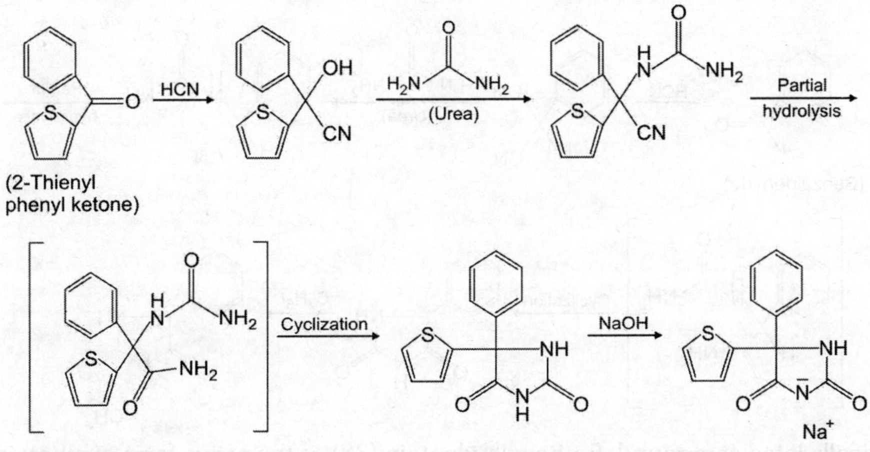

(2-Thienyl
phenyl ketone)

Same use as phenytoin (5).

Mephenytoin

3-Methyl-5-ethyl-5-phenylhydantoin

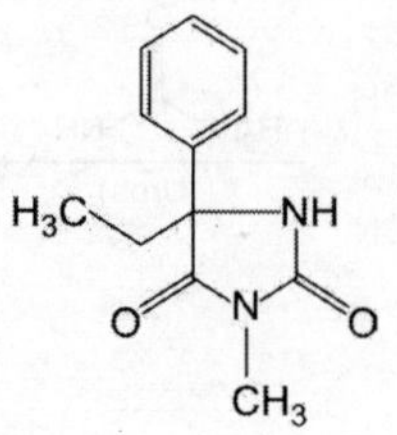

Synthesis

(Phenylethylhydanition)

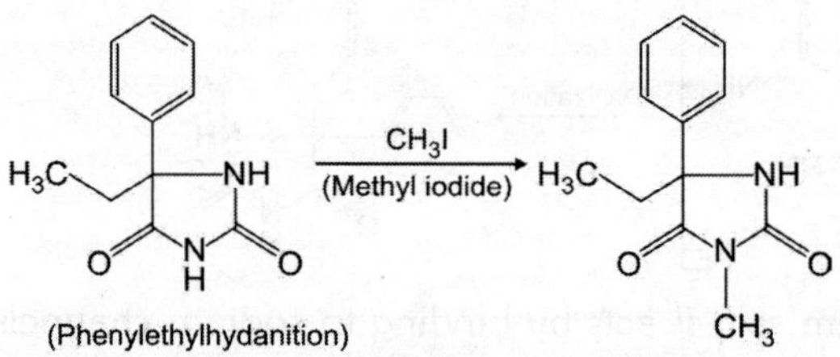

The active form of mephenytoin is phenylethylhydantoin (4). Similar action as phenytoin (5).

Ethotoin

3-Ethyl-5-phenylhydantoin

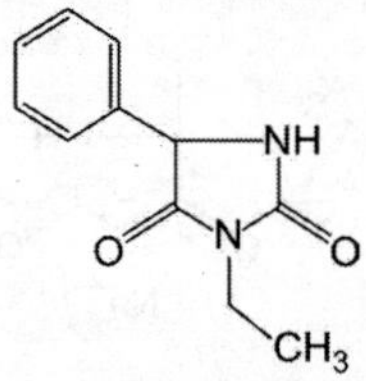

Synthesis

(Benzaldehyde)

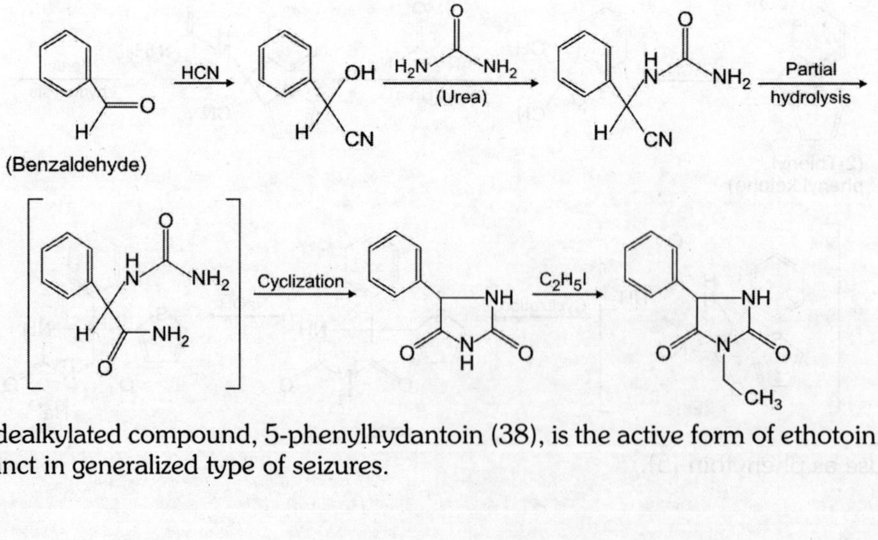

The N-dealkylated compound, 5-phenylhydantoin (38), is the active form of ethotoin. It is used as an adjunct in generalized type of seizures.

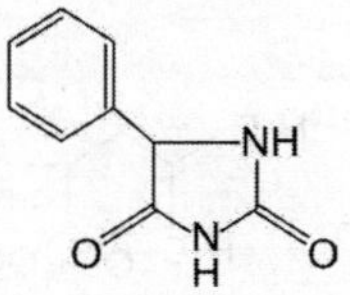

(38)

Fosphenytoin

5,5-Disphenyl-3-[(phosphonooxy)methyl]-2,4-imidazolidinedione

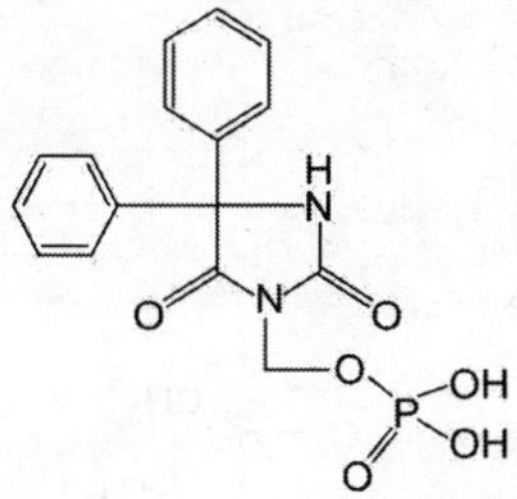

Synthesis

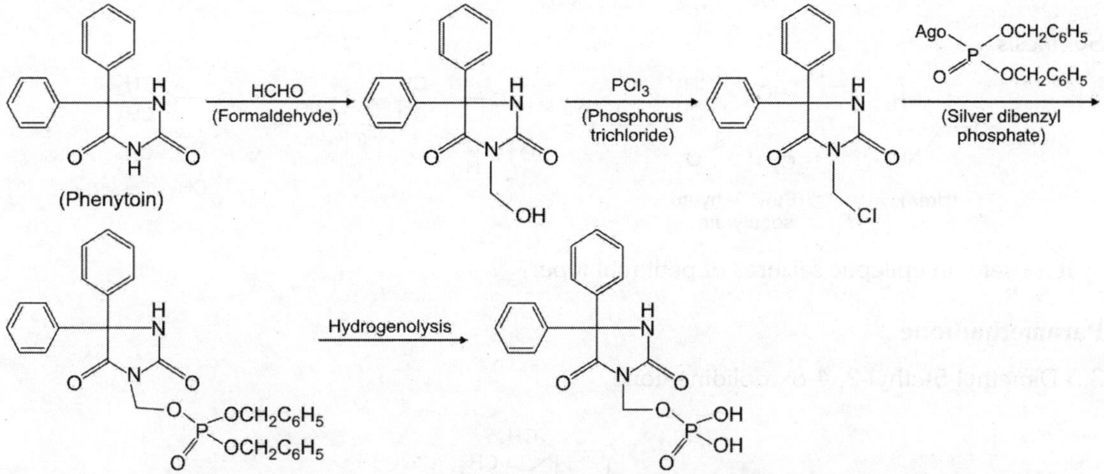

(Phenytoin)

Because of poor solubility of phenytoin (5) in water, its oral administration gives variable blood levels of phenytoin (5). In order to overcome this problem, phenytoin (5) has been converted to a water soluble prodrug, fosphenytoin. It is administered parentrally and it gives consistent blood levels.

Albutoin

5-(2-Methylpropyl)-3-(2-propenyl)-2-thioxo-4-imidazolidinone

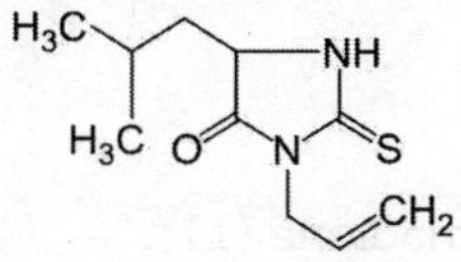

Synthesis

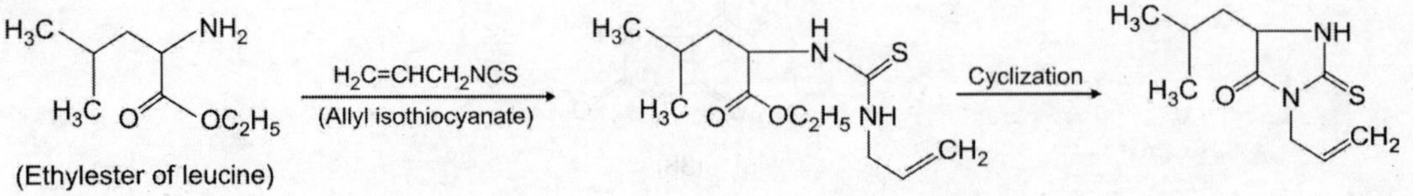
H₃C
NH₂
H₃C
O
OC₂H₅
(Ethylester of leucine)
H₂C=CHCH₂NCS
(Allyl isothiocyanate)
H
N
S
OC₂H₅
NH
CH₂
Cyclization
NH
N
S

Replacement of one of the carbonyl group with thiocarbonyl group gives better anticonvulsant activity.

2, 4-OXAZOLIDINEDIONES

Trimethadione

3,5,5-Trimethyl-2, 4-oxazolidinedione

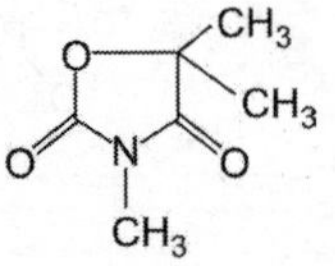
CH₃
O
CH₃
O
N
O
CH₃

Synthesis

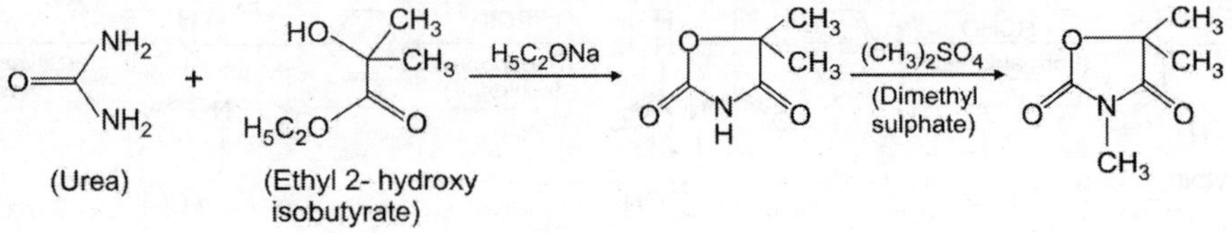
NH₂
O
NH₂
(Urea)
+
HO
CH₃
CH₃
H₅C₂O
O
(Ethyl 2- hydroxy isobutyrate)
H₅C₂ONa
N
H
(CH₃)₂SO₄
(Dimethyl sulphate)
CH₃

It is useful in epileptic seizures of petit mal type.

Paramethadione

3,5-Dimethyl-5-ethyl-2, 4-oxazolidinedione

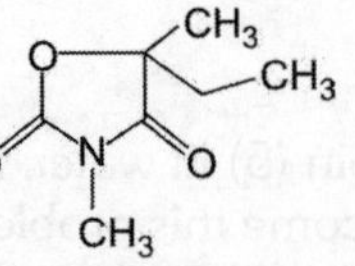
CH₃
CH₃
O
N
O
CH₃

Synthesis

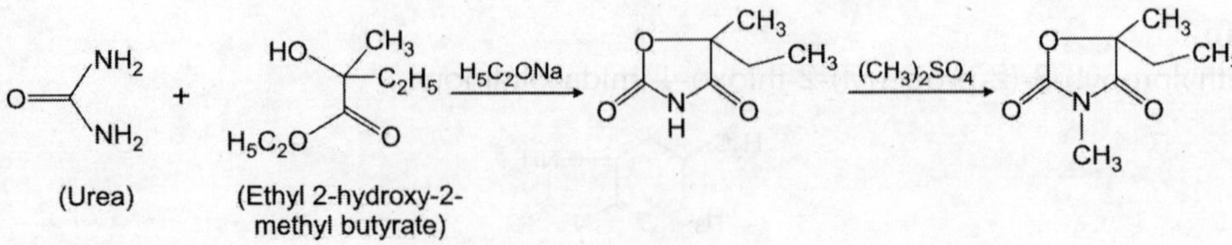
NH₂
O
NH₂
(Urea)
+
HO
CH₃
C₂H₅
H₅C₂O
O
(Ethyl 2-hydroxy-2-methyl butyrate)
H₅C₂ONa
N
H
(CH₃)₂SO₄
CH₃

It has similar action as that of trimethadione (11).

Ethadione

3-Ethyl-5, 5-dimethyl-2, 4-oxazolidinedione

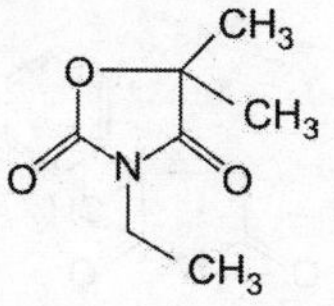

Synthesis

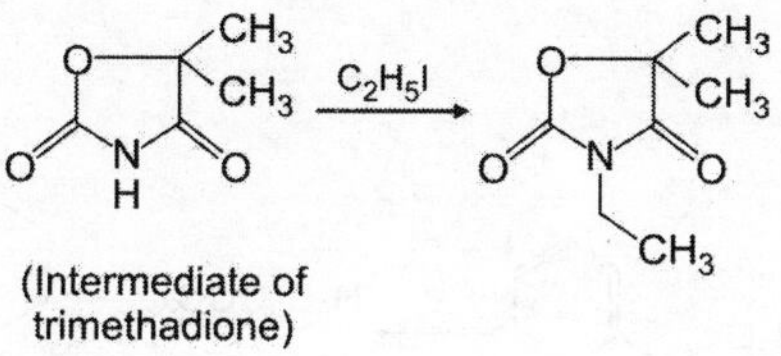

(Intermediate of
trimethadione)

IMIDES

Phensuximide

N-Methyl-2-phenylsuccinimide

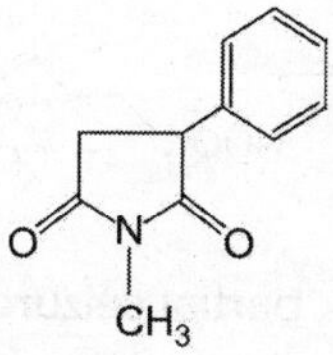

Synthesis

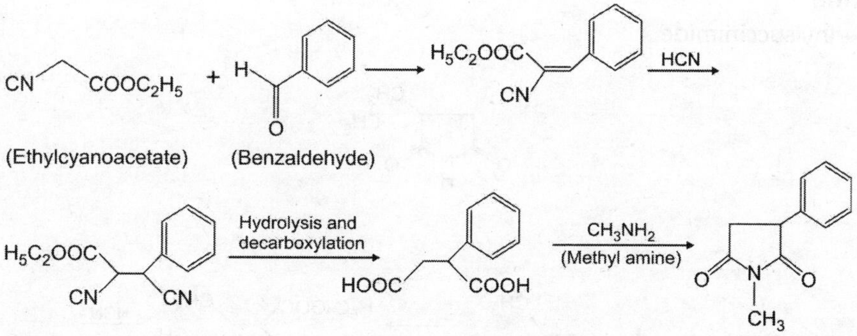

(Ethylcyanoacetate)   (Benzaldehyde)

Phensuximide is metabolized to *N*-demethylated compound (39) which is the active form.

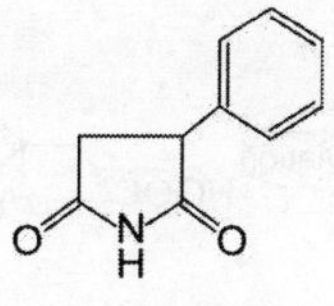

(39)

Methsuximide
N,2-Dimethyl-2-phenylsuccinimide

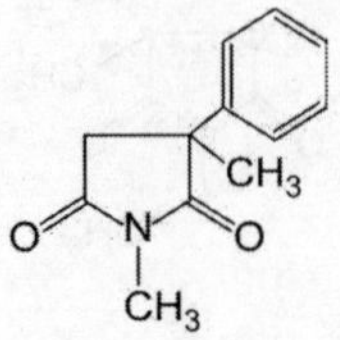

Synthesis

(Ethylcyanoacetate)   (Acetophenone)

1. Hydrolysis
2. Decarboxylation

CH$_3$NH$_2$
(Methyl amine)

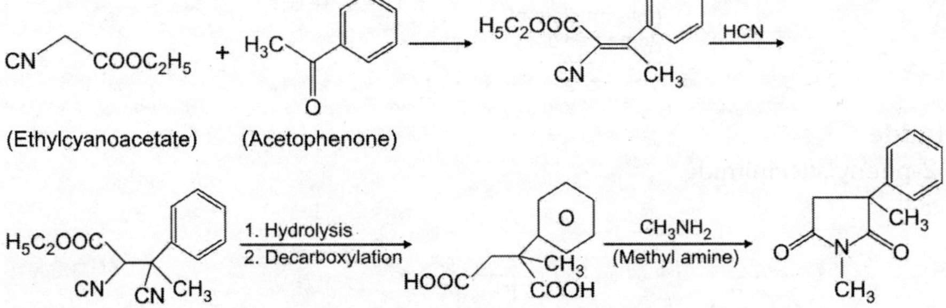

It is used against absence and complex partial seizures.

Ethosuximide
2-Methyl-2-ethylsuccinimide

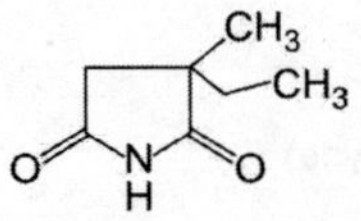

Synthesis

(Ethyl cyanoacetate)   (Ethyl methyl ketone)

1. Hydrolysis
2. Decarboxylation

NH$_3$

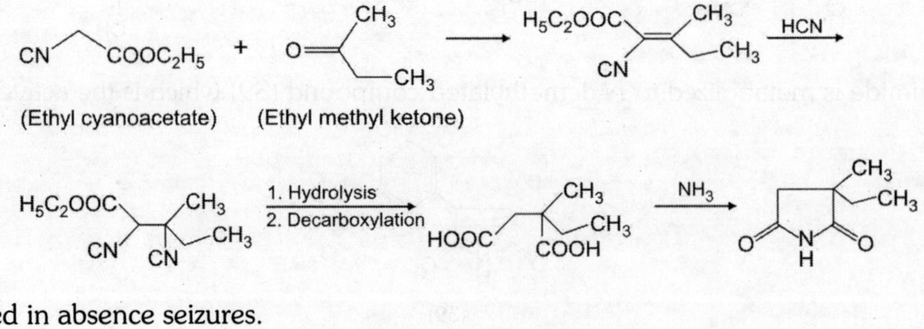

It is used in absence seizures.

BENZODIAZEPINES

Nitrazepam and Midazolam

See SEDATIVES AND HYPNOTICS

Diazepam, Clorazepate Dipotassium, Lorazepam, and Clobazam

See NEUROLEPTICS AND ANXIOLYTICS

Clonazepam

5-(2-Chlorophenyl)-1, 3-dihydro-7-nitro-2*H*-1, 4-benzodiazepin-2-one

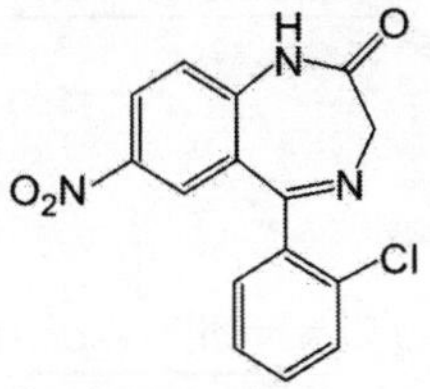

Synthesis

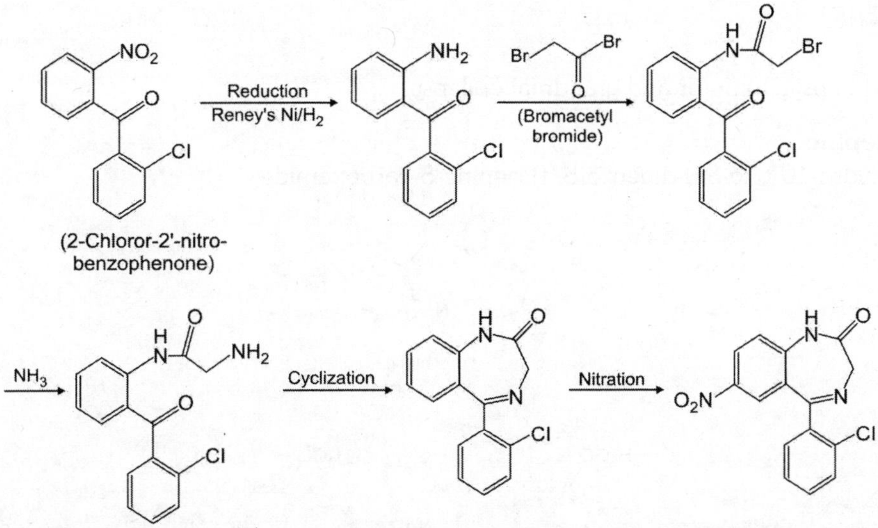

(2-Chloror-2'-nitro-
benzophenone)

It has been found useful in absence seizures and myoclonic seizures. One of the drawbacks of this compound is development of tolerance.

IMINOSTILBENES

Carbamazepine

5-Carbamoyl-5*H*-dibenzo[b.f.]azepine

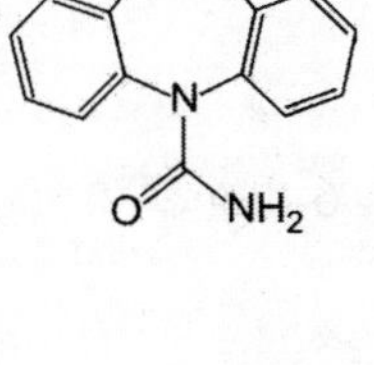

Synthesis

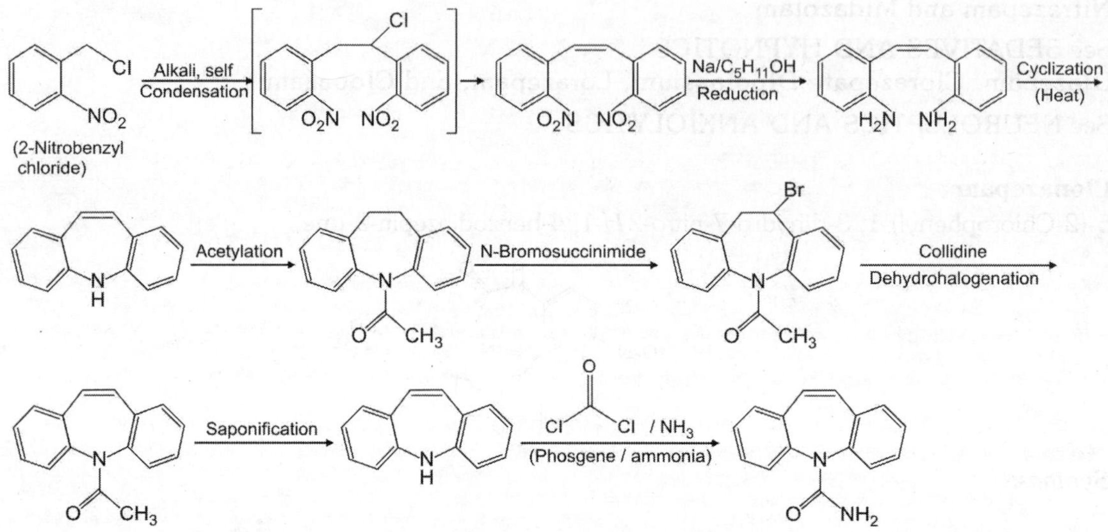

It is used in psychomotor and grandmal epilepsy.

Oxcarbazepine

10, 11-Dihydro-10-oxo-5*H*-dibenzo[b, f]azepine-5-carboxamide

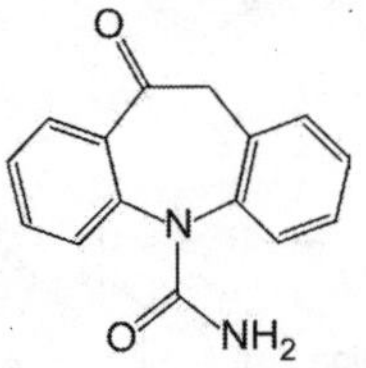

Synthesis

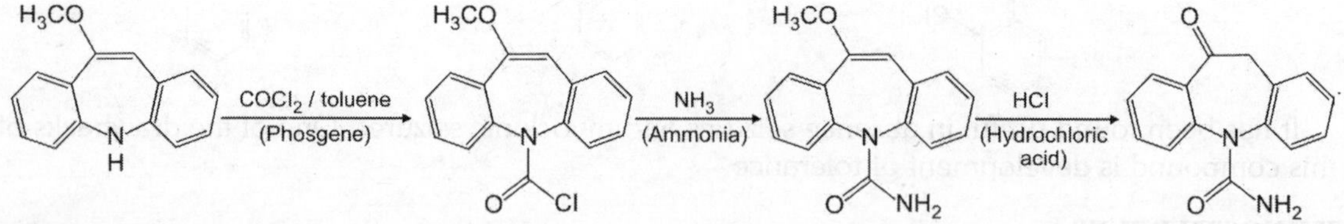

(10-Methoxy-5*H*-dibenz-[b,f]azepine)

It is used in partial and generalized tonic-clonic convulsions.

MISCELLANEOUS AGENTS

Primidone

5-Ethyl-5-phenylhexahydropyrimidine-4, 6-dione

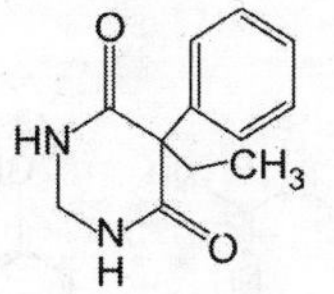

Synthesis

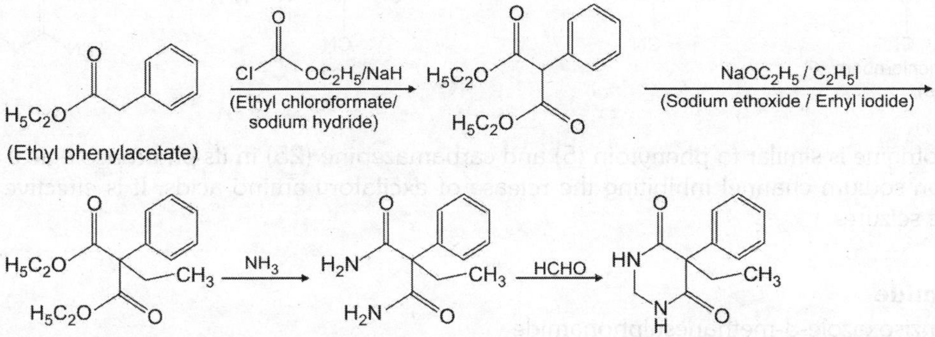

It is a deoxy analog of phenobarbital (1) and is used for grand mal and psychomotor epilepsy. Its activity is due to its oxidation to phenobarbital (1).

Valproic acid

2-Propylpentanoic acid

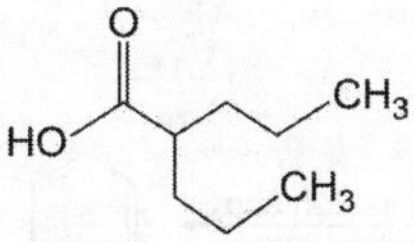

Synthesis

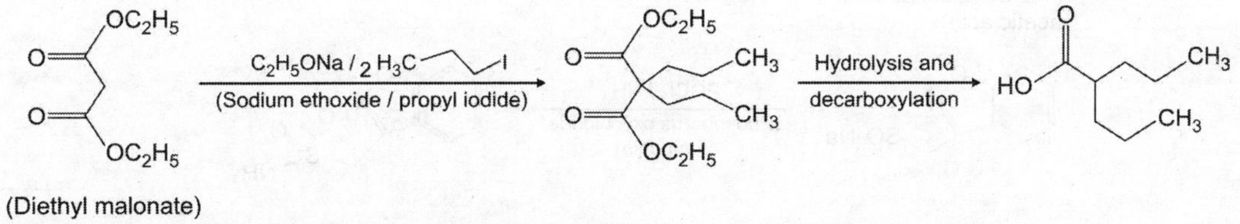

(Diethyl malonate)

It is used as sodium salt in petit mal and absence form of seizures. Its anticonvulsant activity may be due to increased GABA levels in brain.

Lamotrigine

6-(2, 3-Dichlorophenyl)-1,2,4-triazine-3, 5-diamine

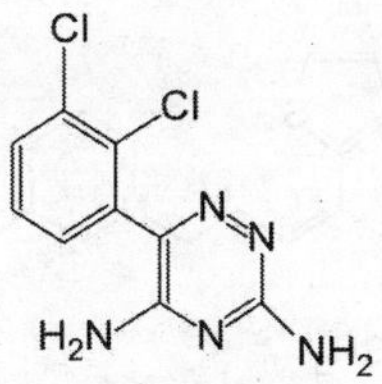

Synthesis

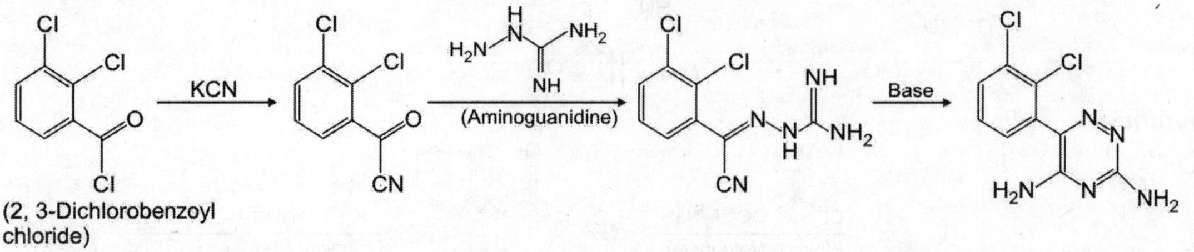
Cl
Cl
O
Cl
(2, 3-Dichlorobenzoyl chloride)
KCN
CN
H2N
NH2
NH
(Aminoguanidine)
N
NH
NH2
Base
N
H2N
NH2

Lamotrigine is similar to phenytoin (5) and carbamazepine (25) in its pharmacological actions. It acts on sodium channel inhibiting the release of excitatory amino acids. It is effective against absence seizures.

Zonisamide

1, 2-Benzisoxazole-3-methanesulphonamide

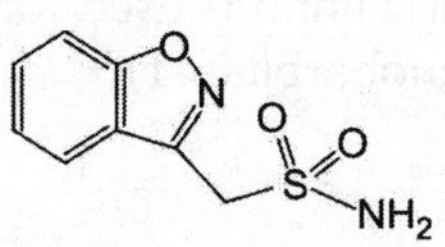

Synthesis

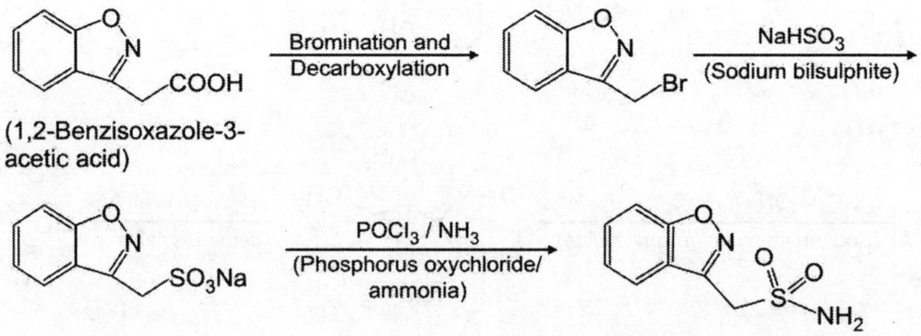
COOH
(1,2-Benzisoxazole-3-acetic acid)
Bromination and Decarboxylation
Br
NaHSO3
(Sodium bilsulphite)
SO3Na
POCl3 / NH3
(Phosphorus oxychloride/ ammonia)
NH2

It is used as an adjunct for partial seizures. It probably acts through sodium and calcium channel blockade.

Tiagabine

(-)-(R)-1-[4,4-bis(3-Methyl-2-thienyl)-3-butenyl]nipecotic acid

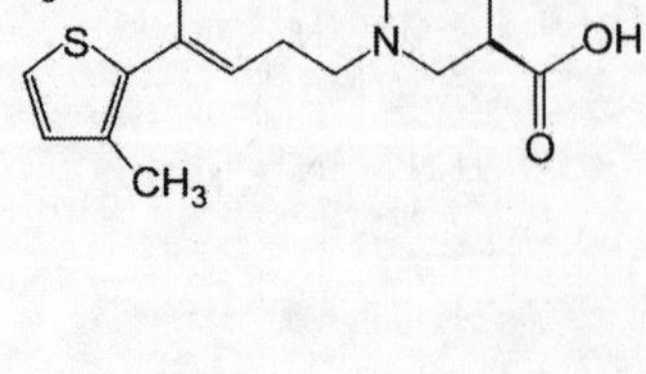
H3C
S
S
N
OH
O
CH3

Synthesis

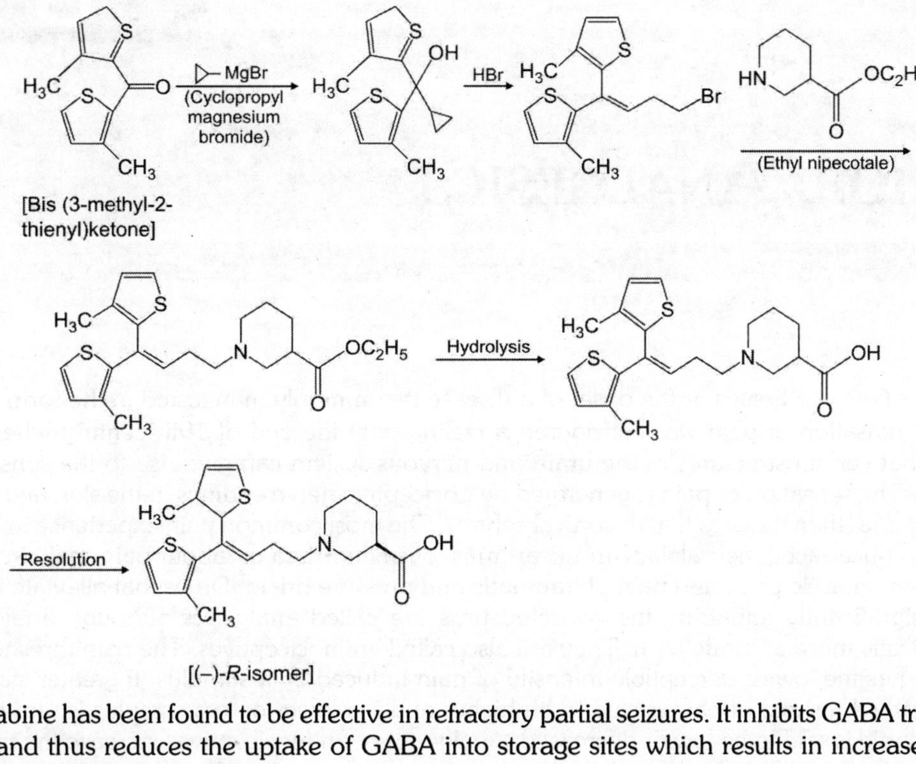

H3C
O
S
CH3
MgBr
(Cyclopropyl magnesium bromide)
OH
HBr
Br
HN
OC2H5
(Ethyl nipecotale)
[Bis (3-methyl-2-thienyl)ketone]
N
Hydrolysis
Resolution

[(–)-*R*-isomer]

Tiagabine has been found to be effective in refractory partial seizures. It inhibits GABA transporter GAT-1 and thus reduces the uptake of GABA into storage sites which results in increased GABA mediated inhibition.

OPIOID ANALGESICS

A SIMPLE INJURY to tissues or the onset of a disease is commonly manifested in the form of pain. The sensation of pain was considered a feeling until the end of 19th century when it was realized that certain structures in the brain and nervous system can give rise to the sensation of pain only. The sensation of pain is generated by nociceptive nerve endings in the skin and viscera. These impulses then travel to higher cortical centres. The most common pain experience in humans are those of headache, neuralgia, chronic arthritis, dysmenorrhea or labour pain, pain in viscera, cardiac pain, muscle pain, and pain of traumatic and pressure origin. Drugs that alleviate the pain without significantly impairing the consciousness are called analgesics although analgetics is grammatically more accurate term. They are also called antinociceptives. The pain threshold may be defined as the lowest perceptible intensity of pain induced by a stimulus. If greater stimulus is required, the threshold of pain is said to be higher and if a lower or less stimulus is required, the pain threshold is said to be low or decreased. Analgesics or antinociceptives increase the threshold of pain.

Analgesics have been classified according to the site of action and include centrally acting analgesics which may be narcotic or non-narcotic. Peripherally acting analgesics include non-steroidal anti-inflammatory analgesics and antipyretics. Narcotic analgesics are analgesics which cause sleep or loss of consciousness along with analgesia. Since opium possesses such a property, all the natural products, synthetic analogs, and peptides which possess pharmacological actions similar to that of opium are known as "opioids". The term "opiate", on the other hand, refers to compounds which are structurally similar to morphine.

In this chapter, centrally acting analgesics will be discussed.

OPIUM AND MORPHINE ANALOGS

Opium is the dried milky exudate obtained from the unripe fruits of poppy, *Papaver somniferum*, family *Papaveraceae*. About 23 alkaloids have been isolated from opium and these alkaloids constitute about 20% of the weight of opium. The alkaloids of opium are of two types, one containing partially hydrogenated phenanthrene nucleus and the other containing 1-benzylisoquinoline system. Alkaloids with partially hydrogenated phenanthrene nucleus include morphine [10% (1)], codeine [0.5% (2)], and thebaine [0.2% (3)]. The benzylisoquinoline type of alkaloids include papaverine [1% (4)] and narcotine [6% (5)].

The action of opium is mainly due to morphine (1). In addition to its excellent analgesic properties it also possesses undesirable side effects such as euphoria which is responsible for its addiction liability, gastrointestinal disturbances, respiratory, and circulatory depression.

Codeine (2) which has excellent cough suppressant properties has weak analgesic activity. It is usually used as an antidiarrheal and cough suppressant.

Thebaine (3) does not possess any analgesic activity but is a convulsant. Papaverine (4) possesses smooth muscle relaxant properties and narcotine (5) is used as antitussive.

The structure of morphine (1), as proposed by Gulland and Robinson, was confirmed by its synthesis by Gates and Tschudi. Its stereochemistry is completely known. The hydrogens at 5, 6, and 14 are *cis*-oriented with respect to iminoethano-system which is *cis*-fused at carbon 9 and 13.

(1)   (2)   (3)

(4)   (5)   (6)

Structure-Activity Relationship Studies in Morphine

To overcome its undesirable property of addiction, structure-activity studies were carried out on morphine (1).

Alteration of phenolic hydroxyl group in morphine (1) by etherification or esterification decreases morphine-like action, e.g. codeine (2), which is the methyl ether of morphine has 1/7 th the potency of morphine (1). Dionin (6), the ethyl ether, and peronin (7), the benzyl ether, have analgesic activities lying between morphine and codeine (2).

Etherification or acylation of hydroxyl group at position 6, leads to compounds which are much more active than morphine. Thus, heterocodeine (8), the 6-methyl ether analog is 5-times more active than morphine while as the 6-acetyl analog, 6-acetylmorphine (9) is 4-times more active. Since 6-acetylmorphine is 4-times as active as morphine, the increased activity of diacetylmorphine [heroin; (10)] is because of acetyl group at position 6.

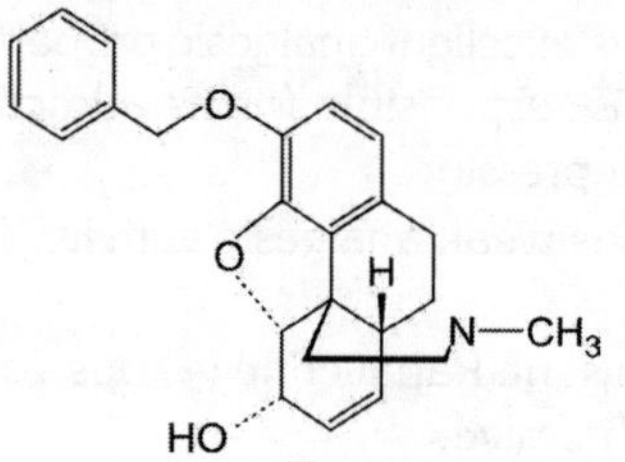

(7)

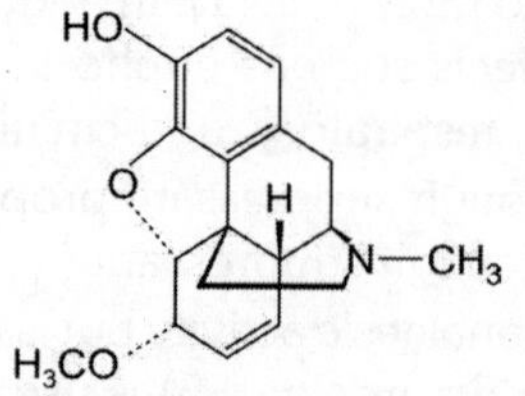

(8)

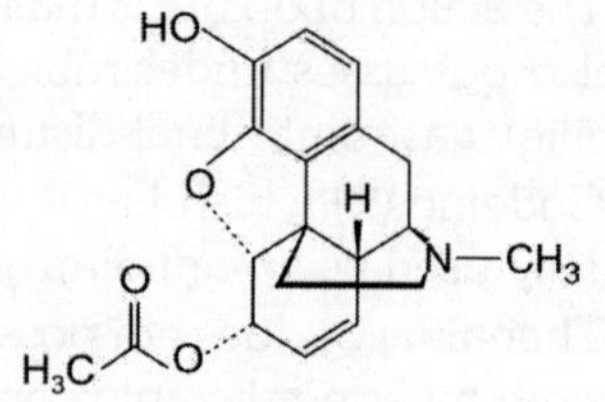

(9)

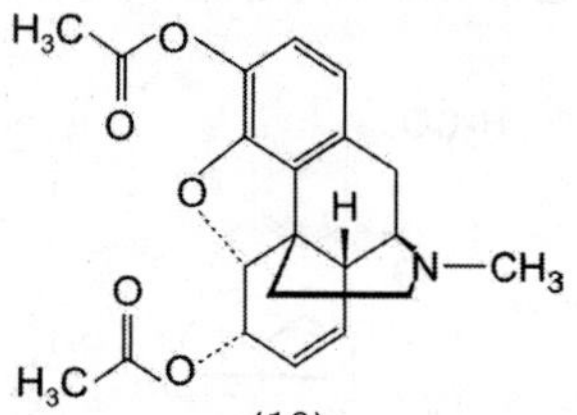

(10)

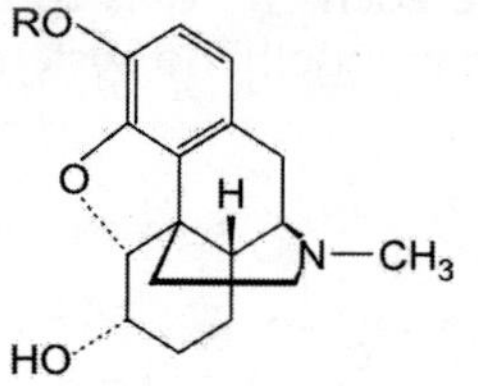

(11), R = H
(12), R = CH₃

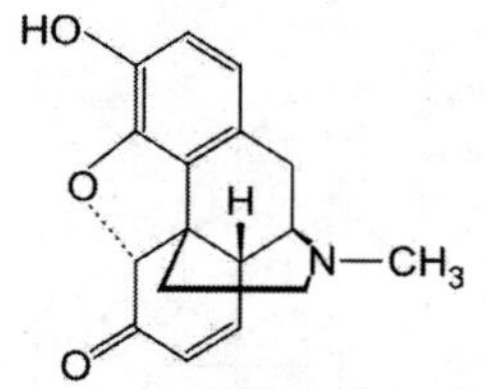

(13)

The double bond at position 7 does not seem to be essential for activity as both dihydromorphine (11) and dihydrocodeine (12) are active.

Oxidation of secondary hydroxyl group at position 6 in morphine (1) leads to morphinone(13), which is an active analgesic.

Dihydromorphinone (14), in which the secondary hydroxyl group has been oxidized to keto group and the double bond reduced, is about 10 times more potent than morphine (1). Similarly, its methyl ether analog, dihydrocodeinone (15), is also a potent analgesic.

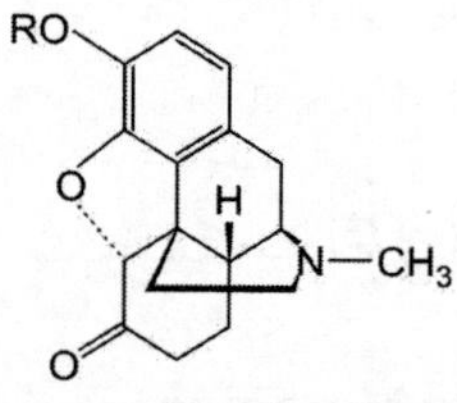

(14), R=H
(15), R= CH₃

Introduction of an additional substituent in either aromatic nucleus or the alicyclic ring results in reduction of activity. However, introduction of methyl group at position 5 in dihydromorphinone (14) results in metopon (16) which is as potent as morphine (1) with less withdrawal symptoms.

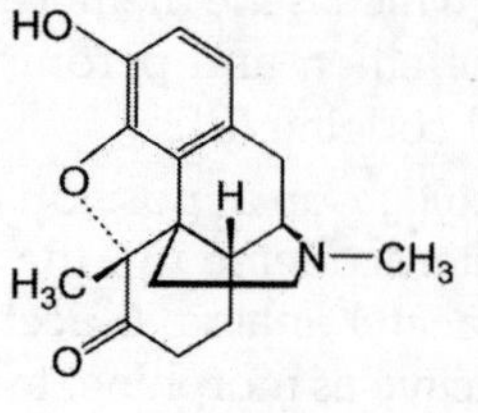

(16)

Substitution of methyl group on tertiary nitrogen by phenylethyl group leads to *N*-phenyl-ethylnormorphine (17) which is a potent analgesic. Substitution by allyl group, leading to nalorphine [*N*-allylnormorphine (18)], on the other hand is a potent antagonist of morphine (1). It antagonizes most of the pharmacological actions of morphine and also possesses postoperative analgesic properties.

(17), R=CH$_2$CH$_2$C$_6$H$_5$
(18), R= CH$_2$–CH=CH$_2$

SYNTHETIC OPIOIDS

Attempts have been made to design compounds that would have the useful analgesic activity of morphine (1) without its unwanted side effects. A close look at structure of morphine (1) shows that it is a derivative of various ring systems namely, partially hydrogenated phenanthrene, morphinan, 4-phenylpiperidine, benzomorphan, isoquinoline etc. Accordingly, compounds containing these ring systems were synthesized and tested for analgesic activities.

Morphinans

Morphinans (19) represent a structure which closely resemble morphine (1). The first compound in this series was *N*-methylmorphinan (20) which is 1/5th as potent as morphine. This proved that the 4, 5-oxide bridge of morphine was not necessary for its analgesic action. In *N*-methylmorphinan (20) rings, B and C are *cis*-fused as in morphine(1), its *trans*-analog *N*-methyl isomorphinan was devoid of any activity. This indicated physiological significance of *cis*-fusion.

(19), R=H
(20), R= CH$_3$

Introduction of hydroxyl group at position 3 resulted in 3-hydroxy-*N*-methylmorphinan (21) the racemic form of which is known as racemorphan. The analgesic activity as well as the addiction liability of racemorphan lies in the *levo*-enantiomer (levorphanol) which is 4 times as potent as morphine (1).

Substitution of methyl group on nitrogen by allyl group leads to levallorphan (22) which is a potent narcotic antagonist and a useful drug, will be discussed under narcotic antagonist as analgesic. Other compounds in this series include 14-hydroxy derivatives of morphinan such as butorphanol (23) and oxilorphan (24).

(21)

(22)

(23), R = H$_2$C

(24), R = H$_2$C

6, 7-Benzomorphans

Simplification of morphinans further by scissoring of ring C results in 6,7-benzomorphan (25). Compounds in this series show definite separation of analgesic activity from that of addiction liability. This structure has the features of morphine (1) which are associated with its analgesic activity and include a benzene ring, a quaternary carbon (C$_5$), and tertiary nitrogen. Further, it has been also observed that benzomorphans which possess analgesic activity have two alkyl substituents at C$_5$ and C$_9$ *cis* to each other as in case of morphine where ring B/C fusion is *cis*. Moreover, out of the two isomers the levo-form in *cis*-isomer is more active. They show analgesic and narcotic antagonist activity. Some of the clinically useful compounds in this series include, metazocine (26), phenazocine (27), which are potent analgesics with lower narcotic properties, *N*-dimethylallyl analog, pentazocine, (28), and *N*-cyclopropylmethyl analog, cyclazocine, (29) are analgesic with either weak narcotic or narcotic antagonistic properties. The most potent compound in this series is β-(±)-5-ethyl-2, 9-dimethyl-2'-hydroxy-6, 7-benzomorphan (30) which is about 30 times as potent as morphine with intermediate dependence liability.

(25)

(26), R = CH$_3$

(27), R = CH$_2$CH$_2$—⟨⟩

(28), R = CH$_2$CH = C(CH$_3$)$_2$

(29), R = CH$_2$ —◁

(30)

4-Phenylpiperidine Analogs

A large number of piperidine analogs were prepared with the intention of testing them for spasmolytic activity. However, several of these compounds exhibited marked analgesic activity in addition to spasmolytic activity. The most important compound in this series was meperidine [pethidine, (31)] which is 1-methyl-4-carbethoxy-4-phenylpiperidine. A close examination of morphine (1) structure reveals that such moiety is present in morphine (1). Meperidine (31), thus is further simplification of morphine (1) structure. Meperidine (31) is the the most accepted substitute of morphine (1). It has 1/8th potency of morphine (1) in man and has been found valuable in obstetrical, preoperative and, postsurgical procedures. It has dependence liability and is respiratory depressant. Further modifications of meperidine (31) structure have been carried out. Some of *N*-substituted analogs which have been found useful clinically include, *N-p*-aminophenylethyl derivative, anileridine (32), which is about 2 to 3 times more potent than meperidine (31). Diphenoxylate (33) and loperamide (34) which are devoid of analgesic activity, but are very good spasmolytics and are used in diarrhea. Substitution of phenyl ring at para-position in meperidine (31) results in loss of activity. Replacement of phenyl ring by naphthalene also results in loss of activity.

(31)   (1)

(32)   (33)   (34)

Introduction of hydroxyl group at *meta*-postion of the phenyl nucleus in meperidine (31) gives bemidone (35) which has analgesic activity comparable to that of meperidine (31). Further, replacement of carbethoxy groups in bemidone (35) with propanone group results in ketobemidone (36) which is 20 times more potent than meperidine(31). Both bemidone (35) and ketobemidone (36) have addiction liability.

(35)   (36)

Reversed esters of 4-piperdinols have also yielded compounds with analgesic activity. Thus, 1-methyl-4-phenyl-4-propionoxypiperidine (37) was found to be 5-times more effective than meperidine (31). Introduction of a methyl group at position 3 of (37) yields racemates of α-prodine (38) and β-prodine (39). α-Prodine (38), a mixture of cis-isomers is about 3-5 times and β-prodine (39), a mixture of *trans*-isomers is about 2-4 times, as actve as meperidine (31).

(37)   (38)   (39)

Anilino analogs, in which phenyl ring has been replaced by aniline moiety, include fentanyl (40). It is about 80 times more active than morphine (1). It is fast acting analgesic with short duration of action. Alfentanil (41), a close analog of fantanyl (40), also has rapid onset of action with a short duration. Sufentanil (42), another anilino analog, is more active than fantanyl (40). Remifentanil (43), also an anilino analog, has been found to be 20 times more active than alfentanil (41), with rapid onset of action.

(40)   (41)

(42)   (43)

Modification of piperidine ring in terms of size of the ring has also been tried. Thus, substitution of piperidine ring by seven membered nitrogen ring in meperidine (31) gives ethoheptazine (44), which has low analgesic activity with no addiction liability.

(44)

Methadone and Related Analogs

During World War II, search for analgesics led to the synthesis and testing of hundreds of compounds. Of these methadone [6-dimethylamino-4, 4-diphenyl-3-heptanone (45)] was the most active. Although it is an acyclic compound but its favourable conformation is that in which the free electron pair of amino nitrogen can interact with positive carbonyl carbon, thus showing a close resemblance to meperidine (31) and morphine (1). Racemic methadone resembles morphine (1) in its pharmacological activities. It has less severe withdrawal symptoms and is used as a substitute for morphine (1). The levo-isomer is twice as potent as morphine (1), while as dextro-isomer is 1/10th as active as morphine (1). Isomethadone (46), the *levo*-isomer of which is as potent as methadone (45) has not gained acceptance in clinical practice.

(45)   (46)

Substitution in either or both phenyl rings of methadone (45) or isomethadone (46) either decreases markedly or abolishes the analgesic activity.

Analogs of methadone in which dimethylamino group has been substituted by other moieties include phenadoxone (47) and dipipanone (48). Both of these have moderate analgesic activity with lower addiction liability.

(47), R =

(48), R =

Isomethadone (46) related analogs include dextromoramide (49) and dextropropoxyphene (50). Dextromoramide (49) has an amide function instead of keto function on the quarternary carbon. It is slightly more active than morphine (1), while dextropropoxyphene (50) has an ester function instead of keto group and a benzyl group instead of a phenyl group on the quarternary carbon. It has four stereoisomers and analgesic activity is in *dextro*-isomer. Dextropropoxyphene (50) is 1/2 as potent as codeine (2). The *levo*- isomer possesses antitussive activity.

(49)   (50)   (51)

Reduction of keto function of methadone (45) gives α- and β-methadols (51) which are much less active. Acylation of hydroxyl group increases the activity. Similar results have been obtained with isomethadone (46).

NARCOTIC ANTAGONISTS AS ANALGESICS

Narcotic antagonists are agents that reverse or cancel most of the pharmacological effects of morphine-like substances. One of the prominent narcotic antagonists is nalorphine (18). Its analgesic potency is comparable to morphine (1) and is free from addiction liability, but it possesses hallucinogenic and psychomimetic properties, therefore, is not used clinically.

Among 14-hydroxymorphone, naloxone (52) and naltrexone (53) are the two narcotic antagonists.

(52), R = CH$_2$CH=CH$_2$

(53), R = H$_2$C

(54)

Levallorphan (22) and cyclorphan (54) are the analogs of 3-hydroxymorphinan possessing agonist-antagonist activity and are used as non-addicting analgesics in clinical practice.

Among the benzomorphan series, pentazocine (28) and cyclazocine (29) are two useful agonist-antagonists.

ENDOGENOUS OPIOID PEPTIDES

Isolation of two pentapeptides by Hughes and Kosterlitz from pig brain was reported in 1975. These substances had opioid-like activity and were called enkephalins. They include met-enkephalin (55) and leu-enkephalin (56), the methionine and leucine being the carboxyl terminals. These peptides compete strongly with morphine-like drugs for binding to the receptors. They have been shown to be present in all animals and also in humans.

Tyr — Gly — Gly — Phe — Met — OH   Tyr — Gly — Gly — Phe — Leu — OH

(55)   (56)

Other endogenous opioid peptides isolated include, β-endorphin (57) which has been isolated from piuitary gland. Dynorphin (58) is another endogenous peptide isolated from posterior pituitary.

Recently another class of opioid peptide, nociceptin (59), has been reported.

Tyr — Gly — Gly — Phe — Met — Thr — Ser — Glu — Lys — Ser

Asn — Lys — Phe — Leu — Thr — Val — Leu — Pro — Thr — Gln

Ala — Ile — Ile — Lys — Asn — Ala — Tyr — Lys — Lys — Gly — Glu — OH

(57)

Tyr — Gly — Gly — Phe — Leu — Arg — Arg — Ile — Arg — Pro — Lys

Gln — Asn — Asp — Trp — Lys — Leu

(58)

Phe — Gly — Gly — Phe — Thr — Gly — Ala — Arg — Lys

Gln — Asn — Ala — Leu — Lys — Arg — Ala — Ser

(59)

Endogenous opioid peptides exert analgesic action by binding to analgesic receptors. In CNS, they exert an inhibitory neurotransmitter or neuromodulator action on afferent pain signalling neurons. Analgesia which results from acupuncture is caused by release of endogenous endorphins.

In addition to opioid peptides, tachykinins have also been associated with nociceptive pathway. Nociceptive transmission and neurogenic inflammation is mediated through binding of tachykinins to their receptors.

OPIOID RECEPTORS

Three types of opioid receptors have been identified and these include mu (μ), delta (δ), and kappa (κ) receptors. There is evidence that there are further subdivisions of these three types of receptors. Most of the pharmacological effects of morphine (1) are mediated through binding to mu-receptor.

Receptor Topography

One of the common features of opioid analgesics is N-Methyl-γ-phenylpiperidine moiety. Based on this, Beckett and Casey proposed the topography of opioid receptor (60). According to them, there are essentially three sites.

1. A flat structure, where the aromatic ring is bound through Van der Waal forces.
2. An anionic site which is able to associate positively charged nitrogen.
3. A cavity to accommodate the CH_2–CH_2 portion relative to carbon 15 and 16 projecting from piperidine ring that lies in front of the plane containing the aromatic ring and the basic centre.

The topography of Beckett and Casey model was not complementary to certain compounds which possessed high analgesic activity. To overcome this, Portoghese proposed an alternative hypothesis. This hypothesis is based on the observation that macromolecules undergo conformational changes on interaction with small molecules. According to Portoghese, the interaction of analgetics, 3S: 6S-methadol and 6R-methadone with receptors, could occur as represented in (61). The dipole that these analgetics develop may attach to the receptor by hydrogen bonding, either donating a proton (X) or accepting the proton (Y).

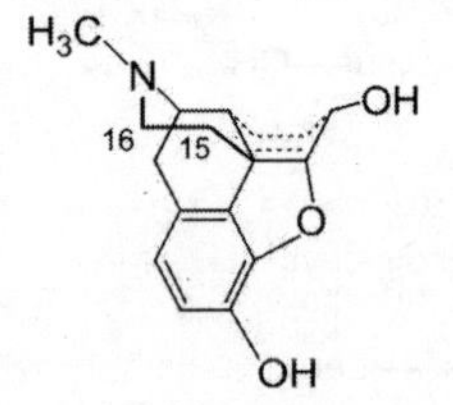

(1)

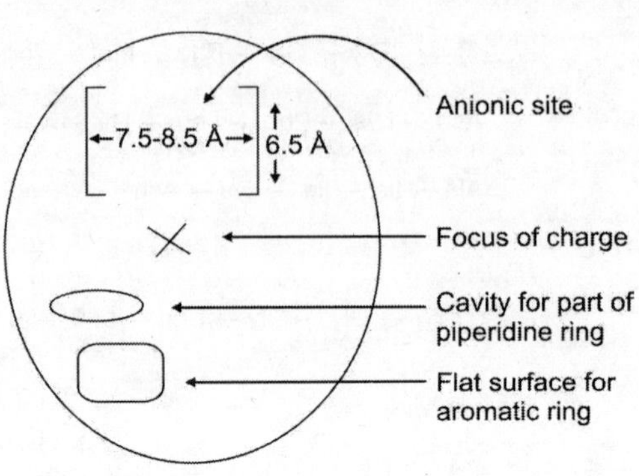

(60)

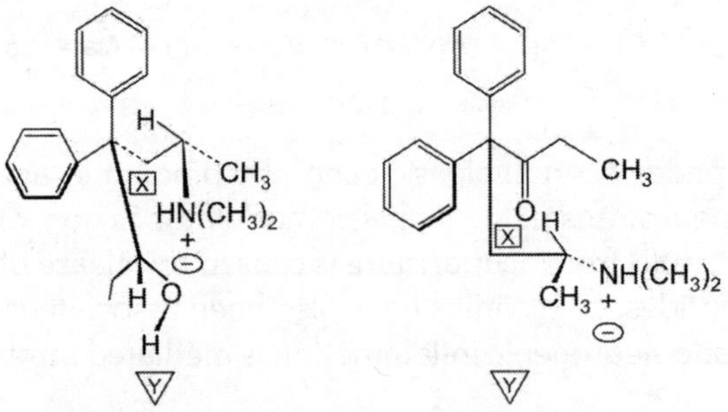

Anionic site

Focus of charge

Cavity for part of piperidine ring

Flat surface for aromatic ring

3S:6S-Methadol   7R-Methadone

6R-Methadone

(61)

Mechanism of Action of Opioids

Opioid receptors are G-protein coupled receptors. Binding of agonist to these receptors results in inhibiting of adenylyl cyclase. This in turn reduces c-AMP content at cellular level. The binding to receptors also exerts effect on ion channels, promoting the opening of potassium channels and inhibition of the voltage gated calcium channels. Opening of potassium channels results in hyperpolarisation and consequent reduction in neuronal excitability. The inhibition of voltage-gated calcium channels results in inhibition of transmitter release. The overal effect is inhibitory at cellular level.

INDIVIDUAL COMPOUNDS

MORPHINE, CODEINE, AND THEIR ANALOGS
Morphine

(5α, 6α)-7,8-Didehydro-4,5-epoxy-17-methylmorphinan-3,6-diol

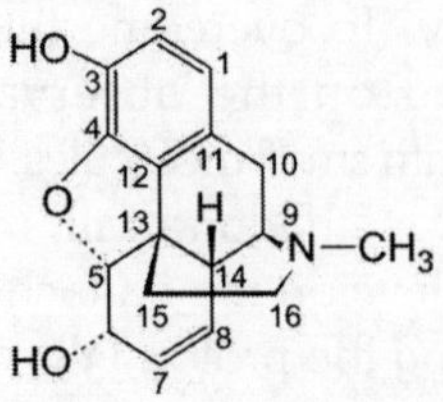

The alkaloid morphine is obtained from opium, which is dried milky exudates obtained from unripe fruits of *Pappaver somniferrum*, family *Pappaveracea*. It has got 5 asymmetric centers at 5,6,9,13, and 14. Naturally occurring morphine is levorotatory and is obtained as odorless white needle-like crystals. It is almost insoluble in water. It is a monoacidic base. Because of its addiction liability, morphine is used only when other analgesics prove inadequate. It is used as hydrochloride and sulphate.

Codeine

(5α, 6α)-7,8-Didehydro-4,5-epoxy-3-methoxy-17-methylmorphinan-6-ol

Codeine occurs naturally in opium. It is 3-methyl ether of morphine (1). It is obtained synthetically from morphine (1) by methylating the phenolic hydroxyl group with diazomethane,, dimethyl sulphate or methyl iodide. It has weak analgesic property. It is mainly used as an antidiarrheal and cough suppressant. It is used as sulphate and phosphate salts.

Dionin

7,8-Didehydro-4,5-epoxy-3-ethoxy-17-methyl-morphinan-6-ol

It is prepared by ethylation of morphine (1). It is as effective as codeine (2) in suppressing the cough. Its chief use is in ophthalmology where because of its irritant dilating action it is used to stimulate the vascular and lymphatic circulation of eye. Because of this action it is useful in chemosis which is characterised by excessive edema of ocular conjunctiva.

Diacetylmorphine

(5α,6α)-7,8-Didehydro-4, 5-epoxy-17-methylmorphinan-3, 6-diol diacetate

It is obtained by acylation of morphine (1). It is 2-3 times more potent than morphine (1) but its sale and use is banned in many countries because of its intense addiction liability.

Dihydrocodeine Acid Tartrate

(5α, 6α)-4,5-Epoxy-3-methoxy-17-methylmorphinan-6-ol hydrogen tartrate

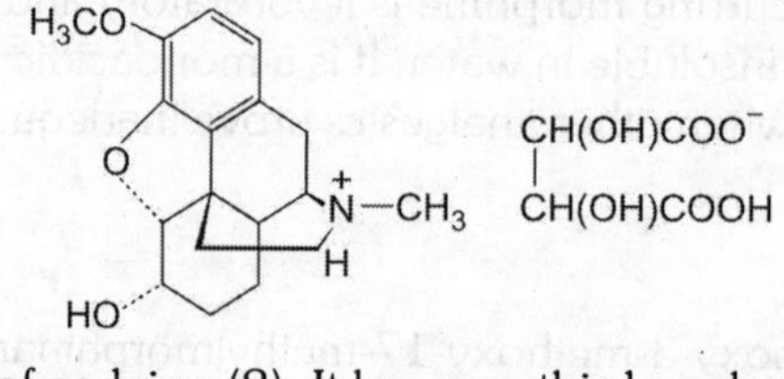

It is prepared by reduction of codeine (2). It has one-third analgesic activity of that of morphine (1). It has addiction liability and is used as a component in cough mixtures.

Nalorphine

17-Allyl-7,8-didehydro-4, 5α-epoxymorphinan-3,6α-diol

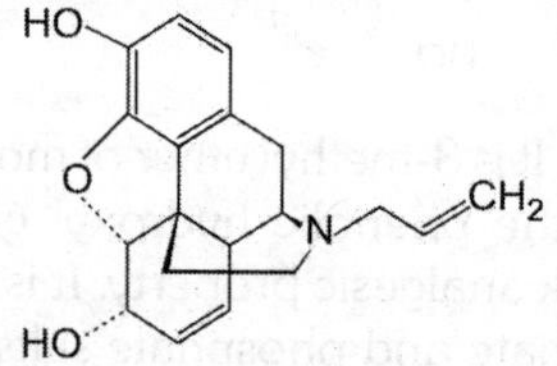

Synthesis

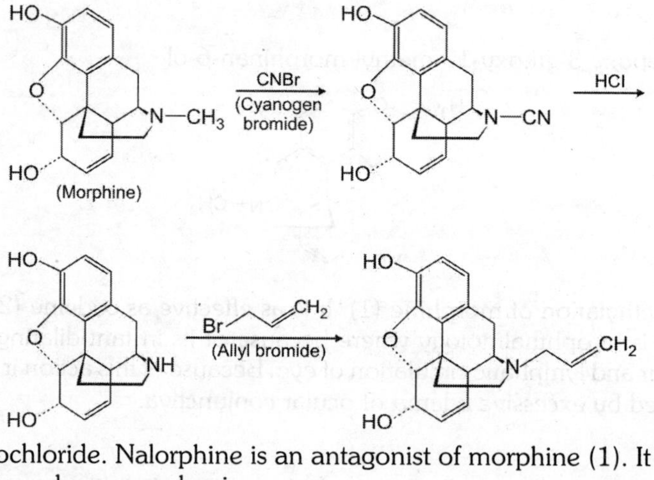

It is used as hydrochloride. Nalorphine is an antagonist of morphine (1). It has some analgesic properties but is not used as an analgesic.

Naloxone

17-Allyl-4, 5α-epoxy-3,14-dihydroxy-morphinan-6-one

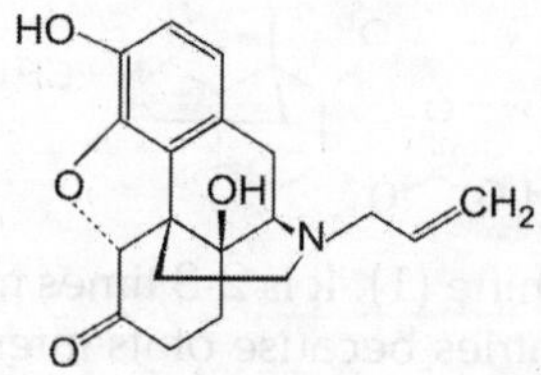

Synthesis

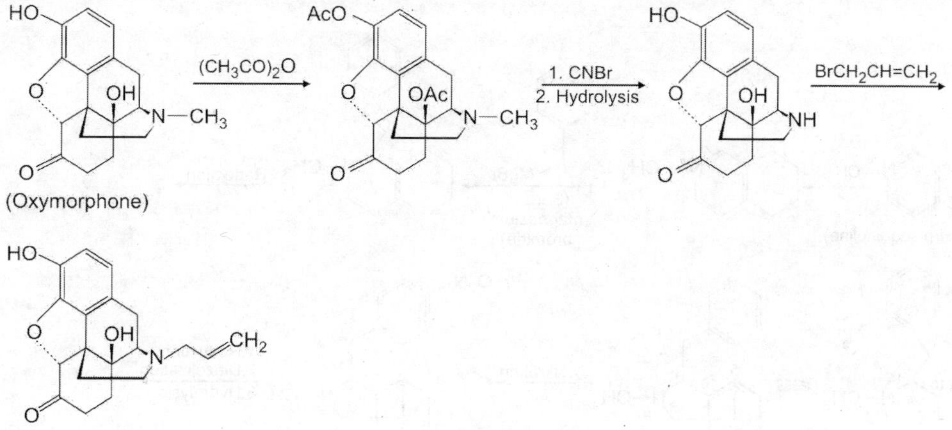

(Oxymorphone)

It is used as a hydrochloride. Unlike nalorphine (18), it is a pure antagonist.

Naltrexone

(5α)-17-(Cyclopropylmethyl)-4,5-epoxy-3,14-dihydroxymorphinan-6-one

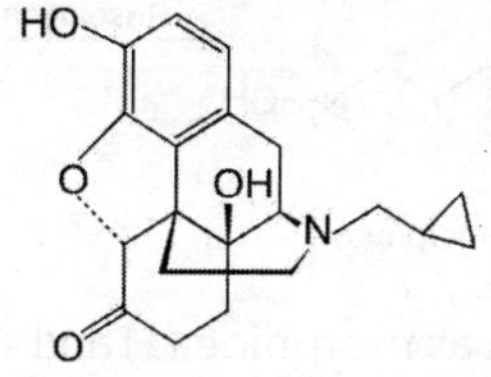

Synthesis

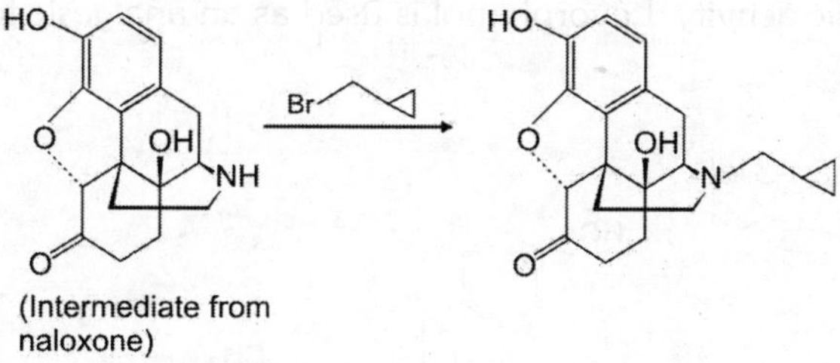

(Intermediate from
naloxone)

Narcotic antagonist

SYNTHETIC OPIOID : MORPHINANS

Levorphanol Tartrate

(-)-3- Hydroxy-N-methylmorphinan hydrogen tartrate

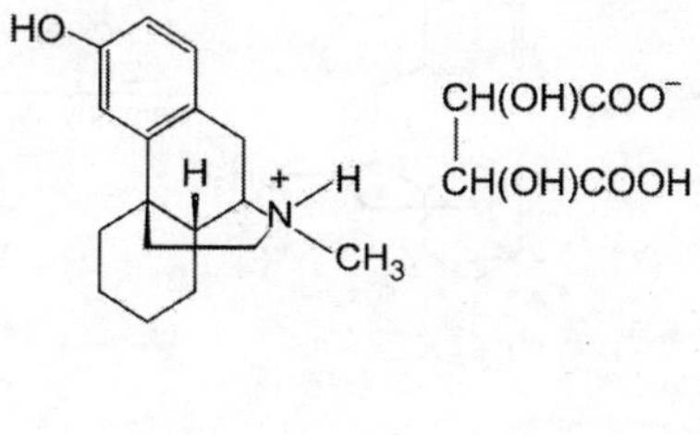

Synthesis

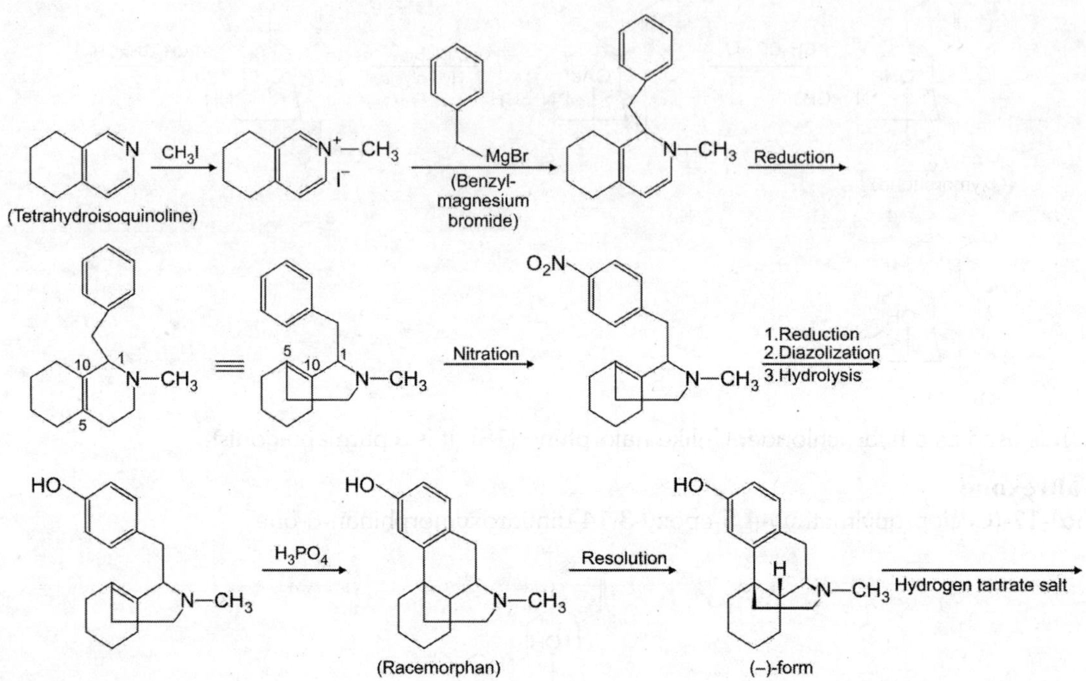
N
CH_3I
N^+-CH_3
I^-
MgBr
(Benzyl-
magnesium
bromide)
$N-CH_3$
Reduction
(Tetrahydroisoquinoline)
$N-CH_3$
Nitration
O_2N
1.Reduction
2.Diazolization
3.Hydrolysis
HO
H_3PO_4
Resolution
H
Hydrogen tartrate salt
(Racemorphan)
(–)-form

Levorphanol is 6 to 8 times as potent as morphine (1) and shows similar pharmacological activities as that of mrophine (1). The addiction liability is also higher than morphine (1). The dextro-isomer is devoid of any analgesic activity. Levorphanol is used as an analgesic for severe pain.

Levallorphan

17-(2-Propenyl)morphinan-3-ol

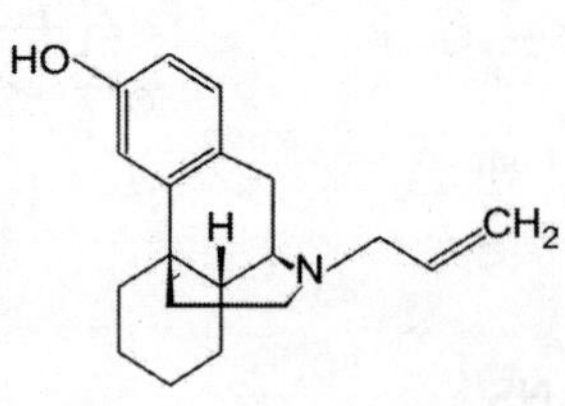
HO
H
N
CH_2

Synthesis

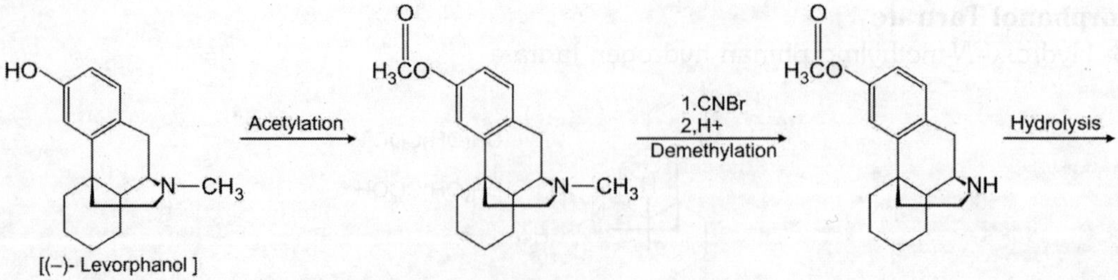
HO
$N-CH_3$
[(–)- Levorphanol]
Acetylation
H_3CO
O
1.CNBr
2,H+
Demethylation
NH
Hydrolysis

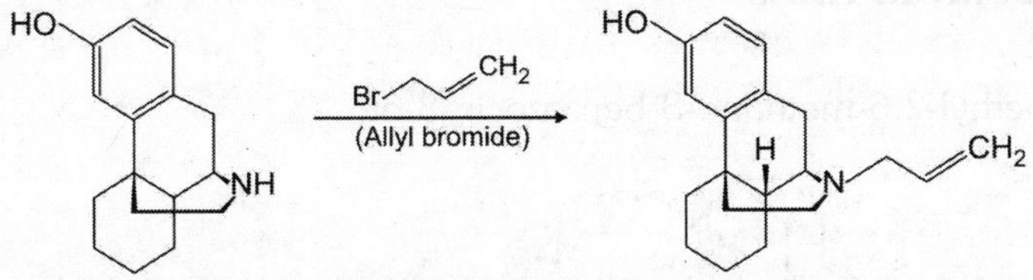

It is a narcotic antagonist and a potent analgesic.

Butorphanol Tartrate

17-(Cyclobutylmethyl)-morphinan-3,14-diol hydrogen tartrate.

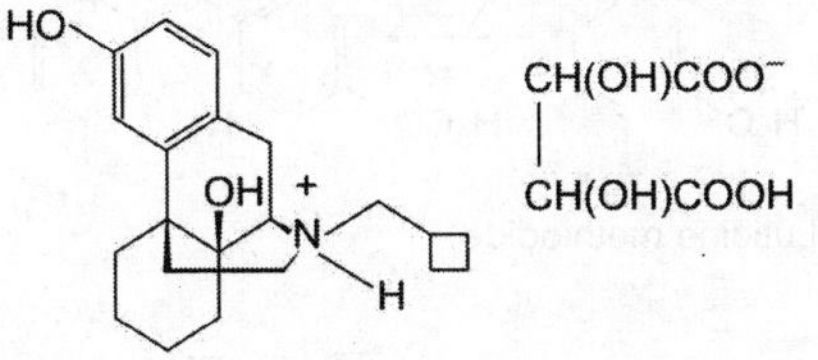

Synthesis

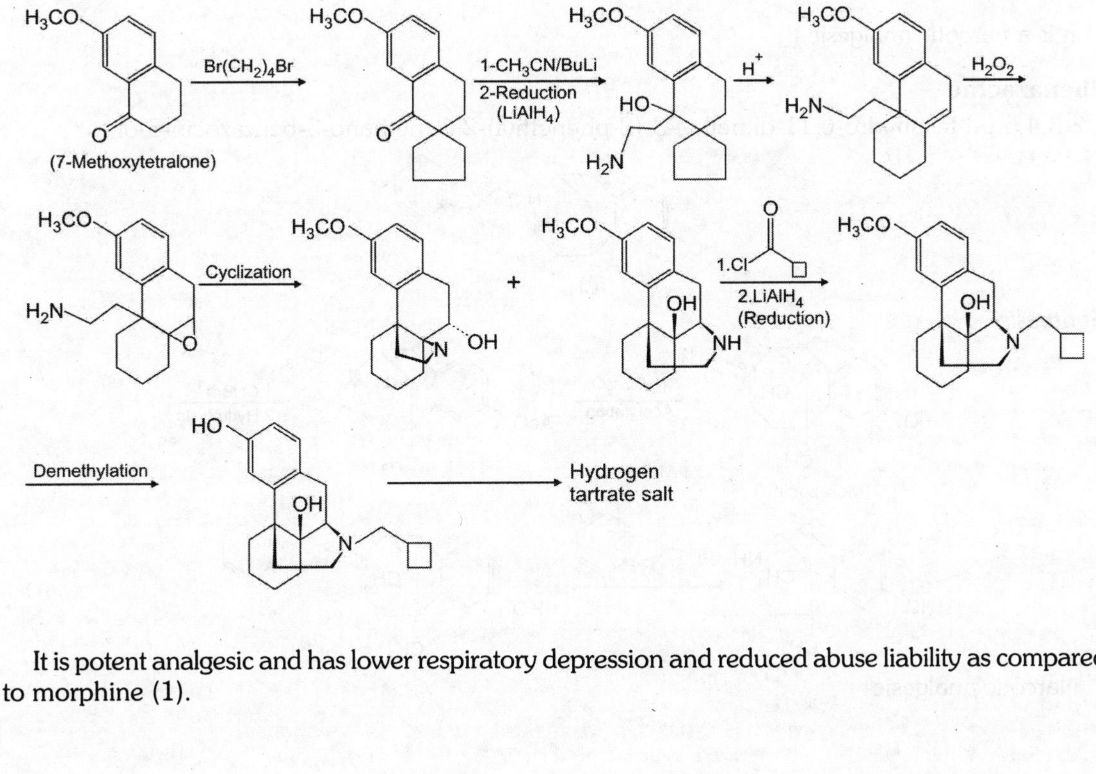

It is potent analgesic and has lower respiratory depression and reduced abuse liability as compared to morphine (1).

SYNTHETIC OPIOIDS : 6, 7-BENZOMORPHANS
Metazocine

1,2,3,4,5,6-Hexahydro-3,6,11-trimethyl-2,6-methano-3-benzazocin-8-ol

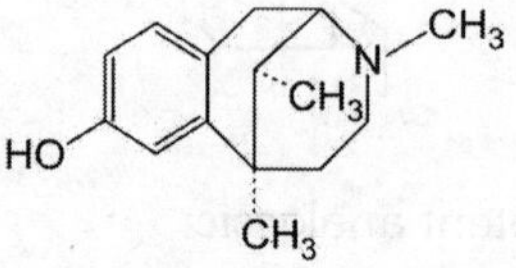

Synthesis

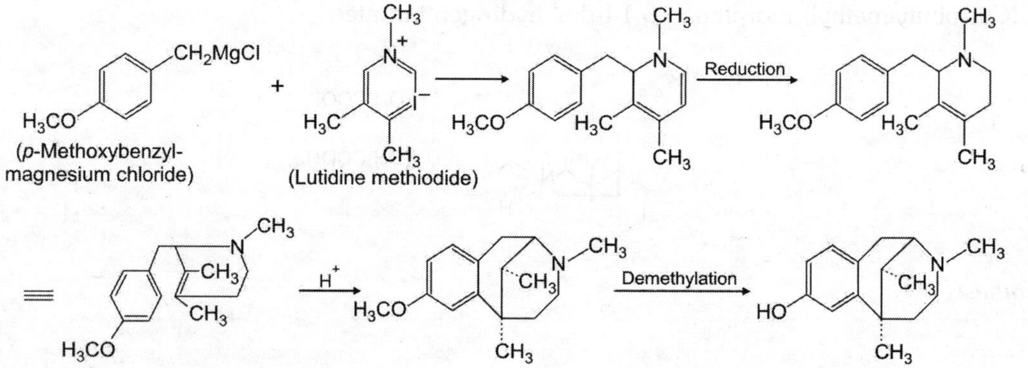

It is a narcotic analgesic

Phenazocine

1,2,3,4,5,6-Hexahydro-6,11-dimethyl-3-(2-phenethyl)-2,6-methano-3-benzazocin-8-ol

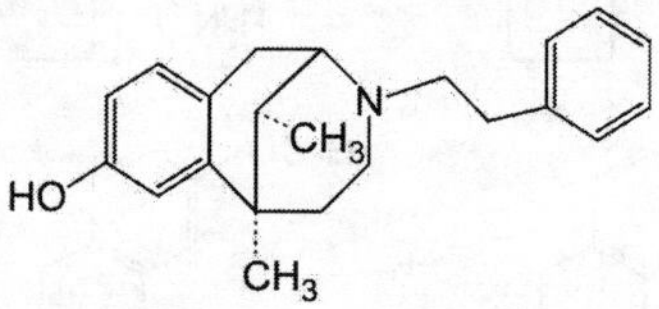

Synthesis

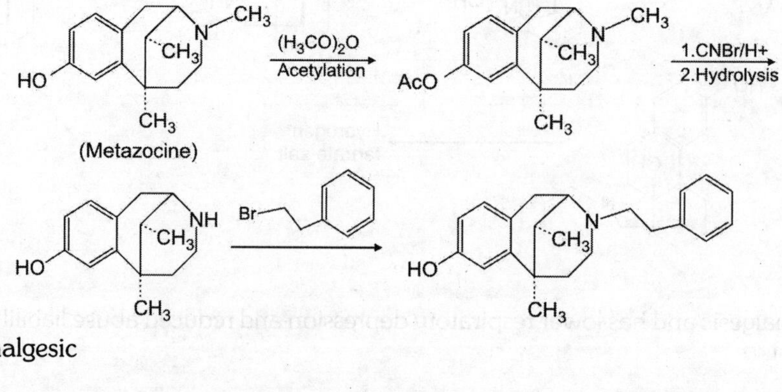

Narcotic analgesic

Pentazocine
(2*R*,6*R*,11*R*)-1,2,3,4,5,6-Hexahydro-6,11-dimethyl-3-(3-methyl-2-butenyl)-2,6-methano-3-benzazocin-8-ol

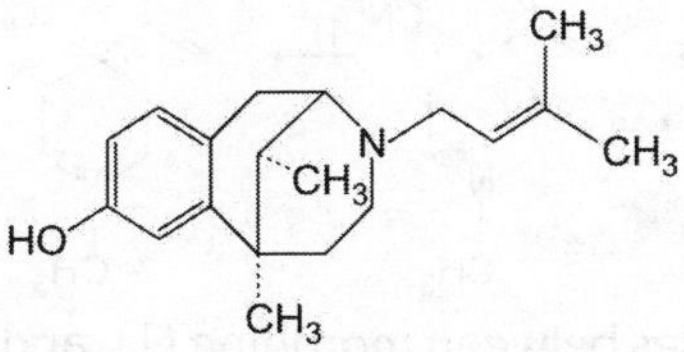

Synthesis

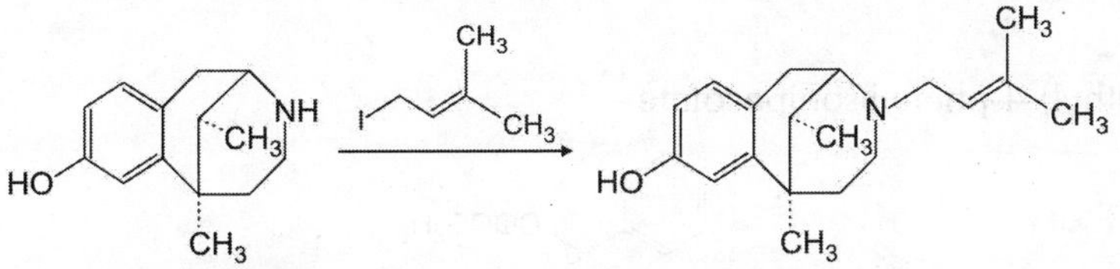

The levo-isomer is active as analgesic. It has morphine-like side effects with greater respiratory depressant effect.

Cyclazocine
3-(Cyclopropylmethyl)-1,2,3,4,5,6-hexahydro-6,11-dimethyl-2,6-methano-3-benzazocin-8-ol

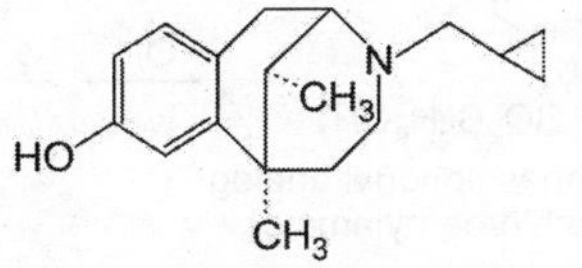

Synthesis

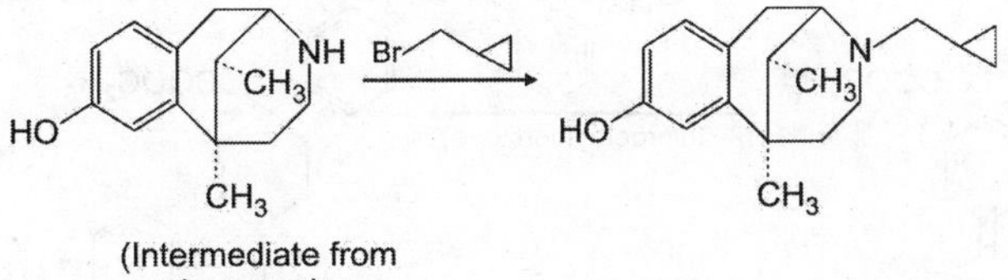

Narcotic antagonist

SYNTHETIC OPIOIDS : 4-PHENYLPIPERIDINE ANALOGS
Meperidine
Ethyl 1-methyl-4-phenylisonipecotate

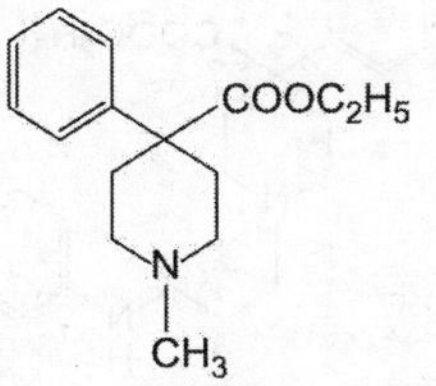

Synthesis

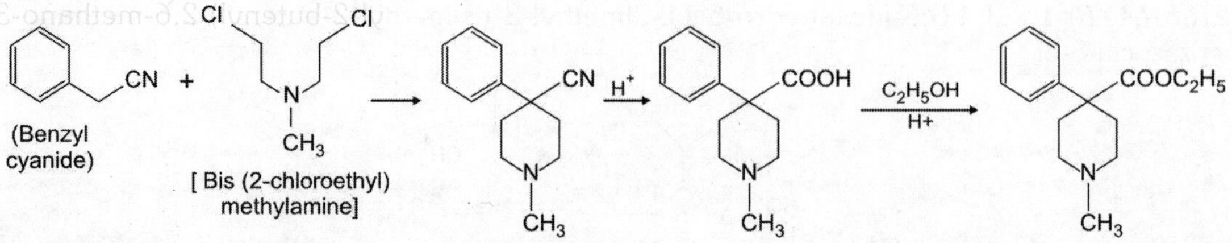

It has analgesic activity which lies between morphine (1), and codeine (2). It possesses addiction liability.

Pheneridine

Ethyl 1(2-phenethyl)-4-phenylisonipecotate

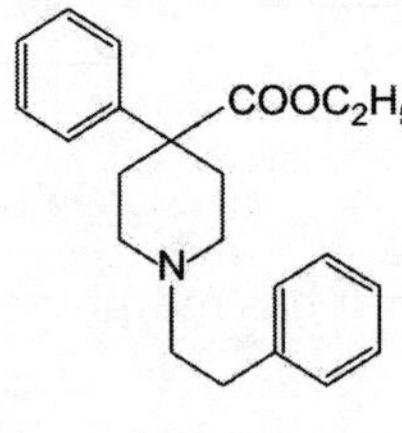

Synthesis

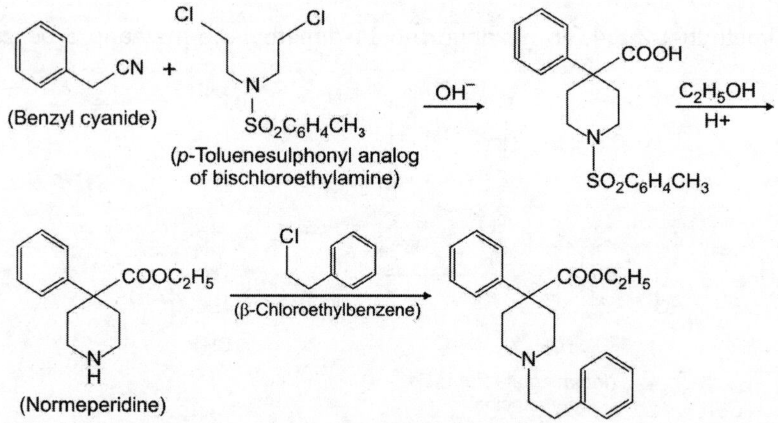

Pheneridine is about 2.5 times as active as meperidine (31).

Piminodine

1-(3-Anilinopropyl)-4-phenylisonipecotic acid ethyl ester

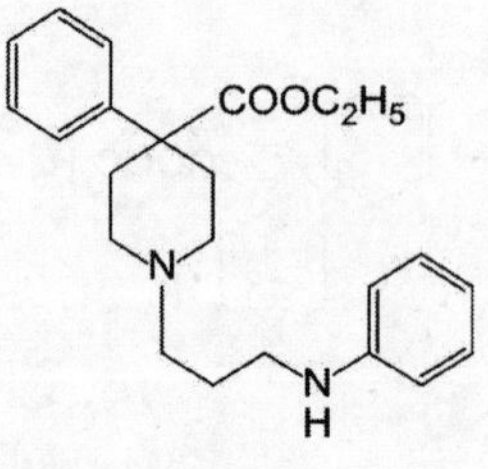

Synthesis

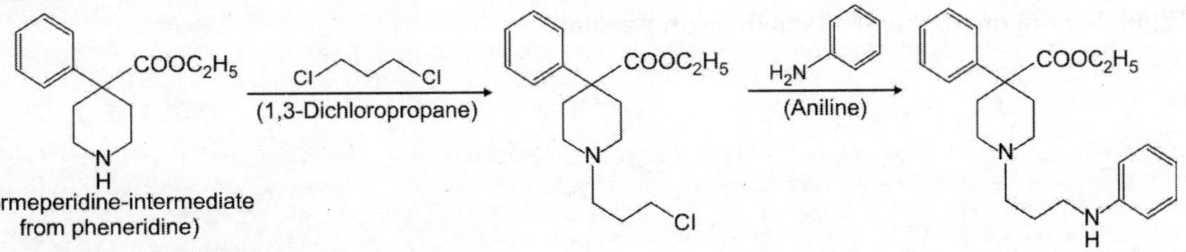

(Normeperidine-intermediate
from pheneridine)

(1,3-Dichloropropane)

(Aniline)

It is highly active analgesic.

Anileridine

Ethyl 1-(*p*-aminophenethyl)-4-phenylisonipecotate

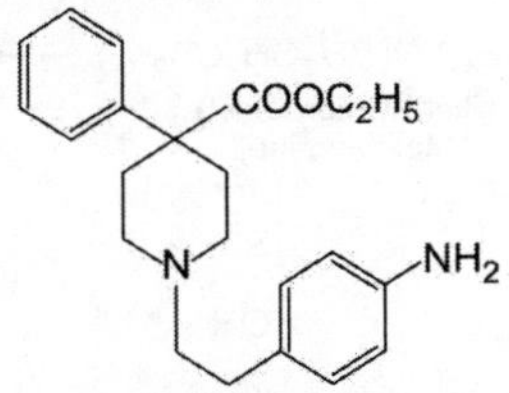

Synthesis

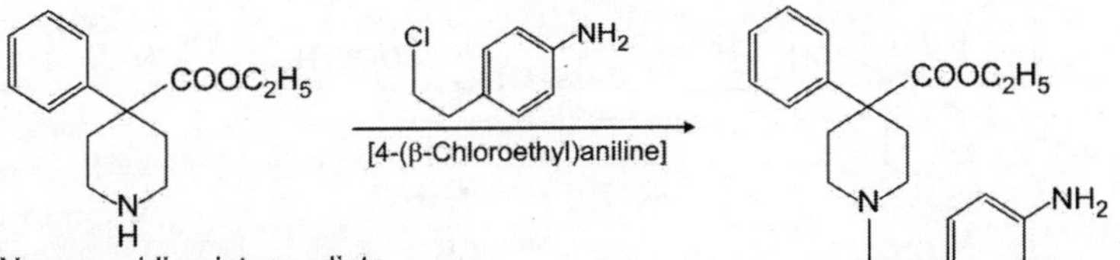

(Normeperidine-intermediate
from pheneridine)

[4-(β-Chloroethyl)aniline]

It is about 3.5-times as active as meperidine (31). It has less dependence liability and is used as a substitute for meperidine (31).

Properidine

Isopropyl 1-methyl-4-phenylisonipecotate

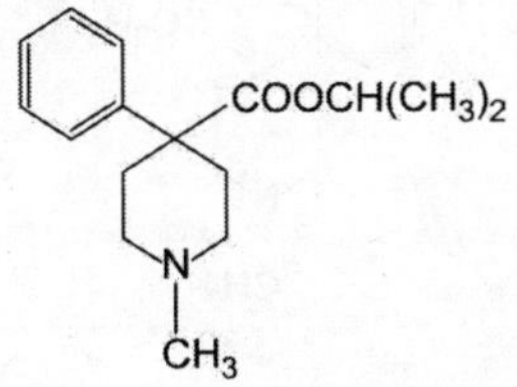

Synthesis

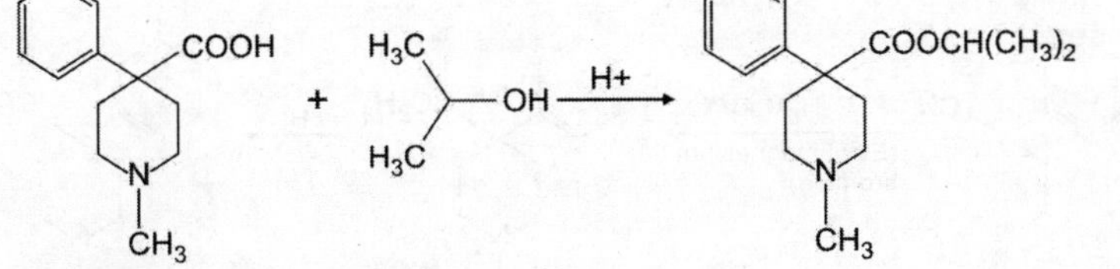

(Intermediate from
meperidine)

(Isopropanol)

It is about 15-times as active as meperidine (31).

Bemidone

Ethyl-4-(*m*-hydroxyphenyl)-1-methylisonipecotate

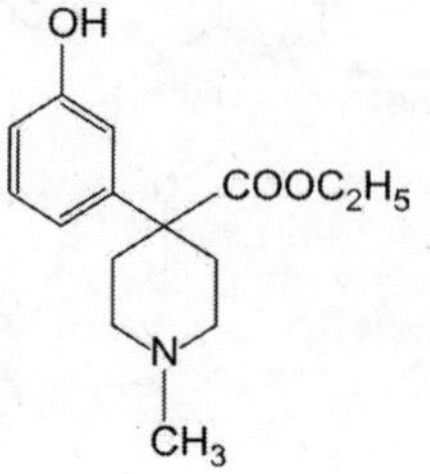

Synthesis

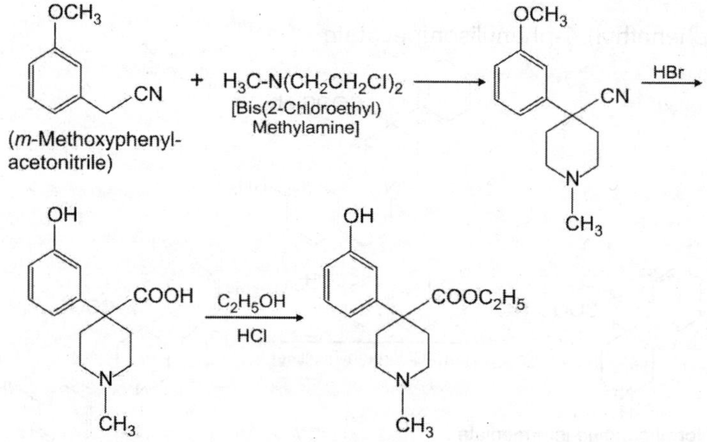

It is about 1.5-times as active as meperidine (31).

Ketobemidone

4-(*m*- Hydroxyphenyl)-1-methyl-4-piperidyl ethyl ketone

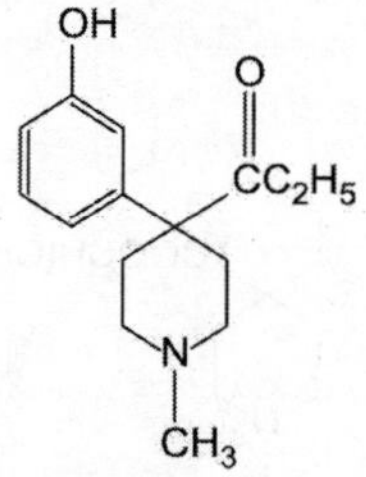

Synthesis

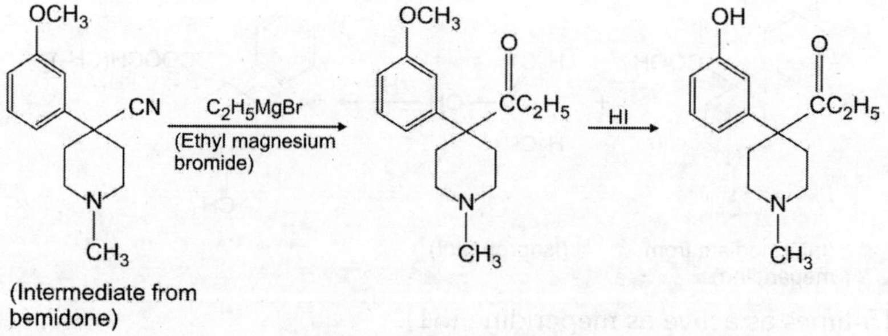

It is an effective analgesic with about 6-times the activity as that of mepridine (31).

α-Prodine

dl-α-1, 3-Dimethyl-4-phenyl-4-propionoxypiperidine

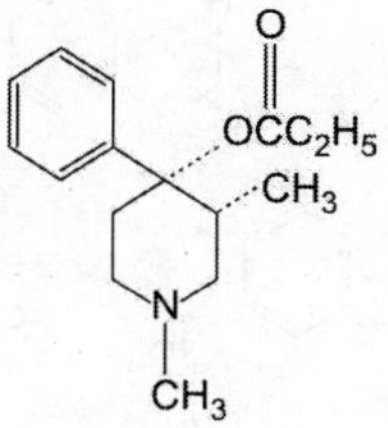

Synthesis

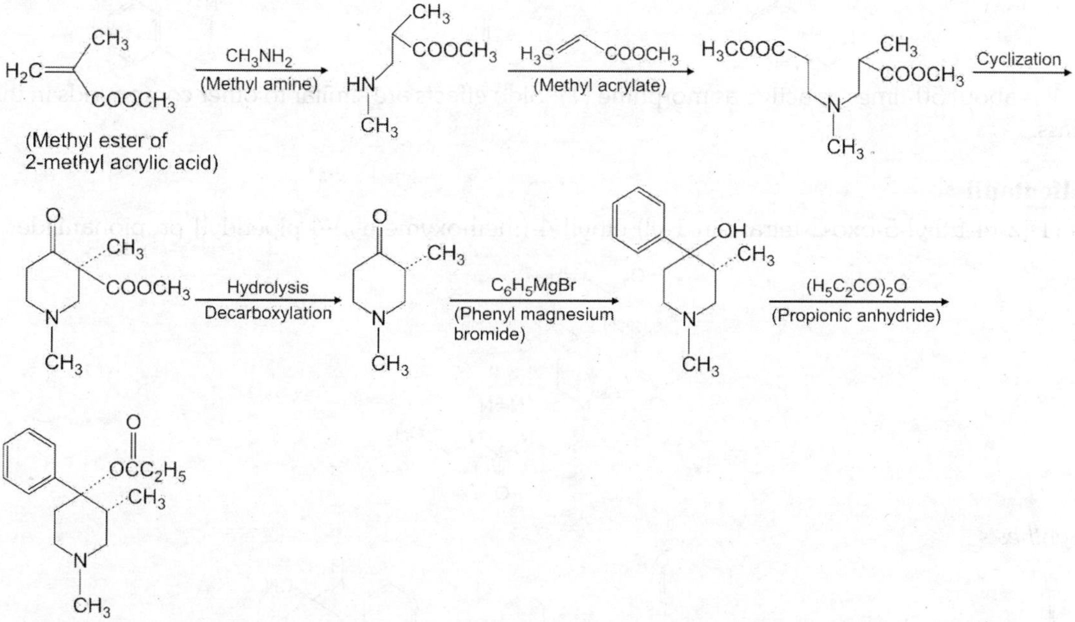

It is about 5 times as active as meperidine (31) and is used as analgesic in obstetrics. It has a rapid onset and short duration of action.

Fentanyl

N-(1-Phenethyl-4-piperidyl)propionanilide

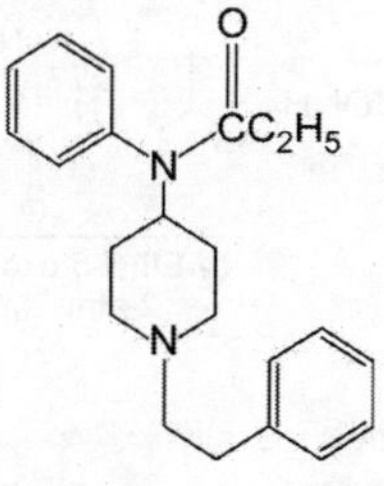

Synthesis

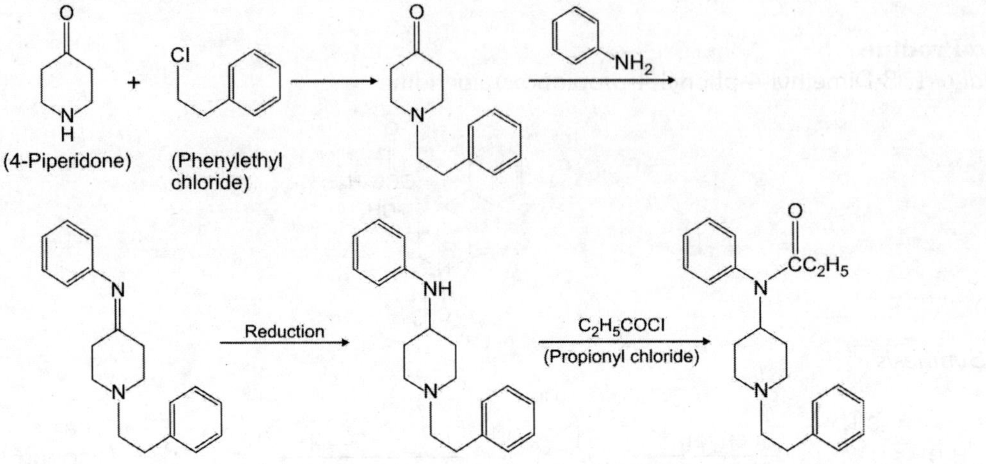

(4-Piperidone)   (Phenylethyl chloride)

Reduction

C_2H_5COCl
(Propionyl chloride)

It is about 50-times as active as morphine (1). Side effects are similar to other compounds in this class.

Alfentanil

N-[1-[2-(4-Ethyl-5-oxo-2-tetrazolin-1-yl) ethyl]-4-(methoxymethyl)-4 piperidyl] propionanilide

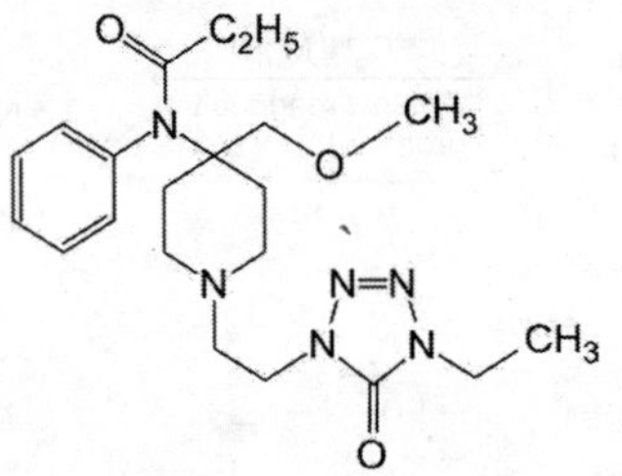

Synthesis

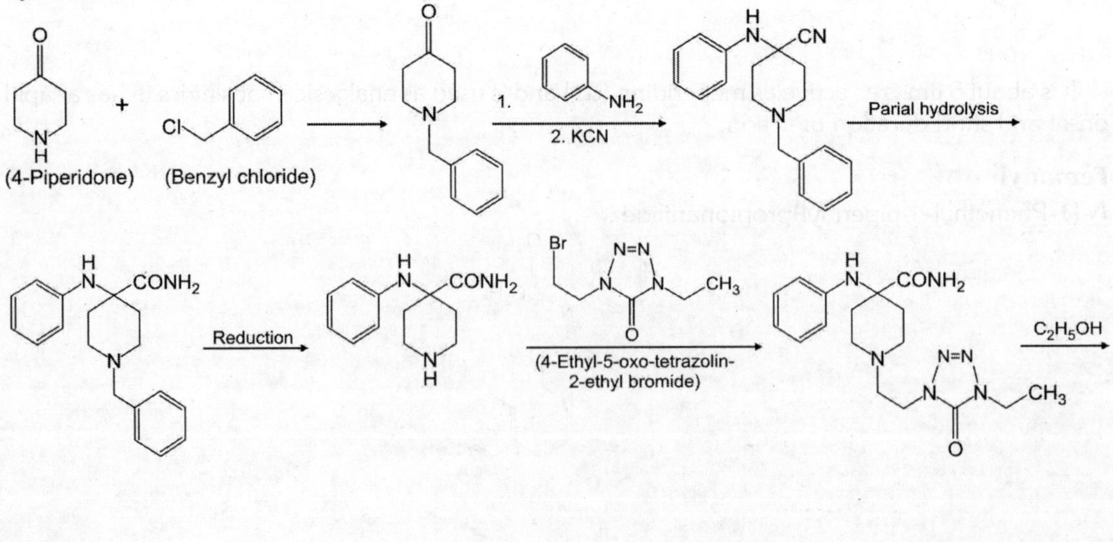

(4-Piperidone)   (Benzyl chloride)

1. NH_2
2. KCN

Parial hydrolysis

Reduction

(4-Ethyl-5-oxo-tetrazolin-2-ethyl bromide)

C_2H_5OH

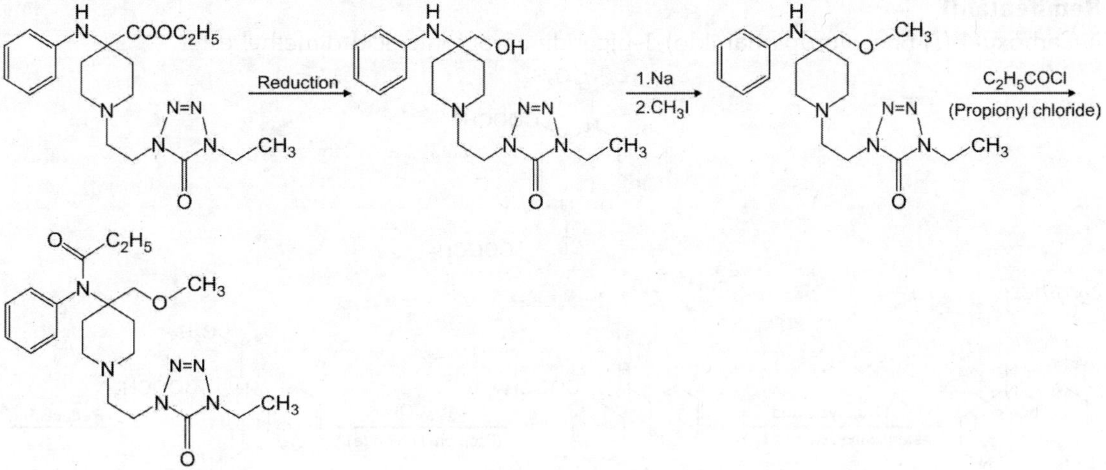

It is a potent analgesic and is also used as an adjunct in the maintenance of anesthesia.

Sufentanil

N-[4-(Methoxymethyl)-1-[2-(2-thienyl)ethyl]-4-piperidinyl]-*N*-phenylpropanamide

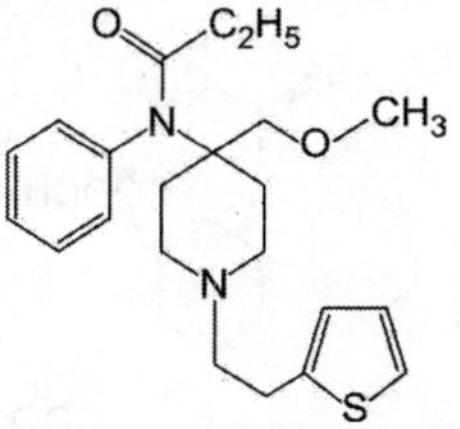

Synthesis

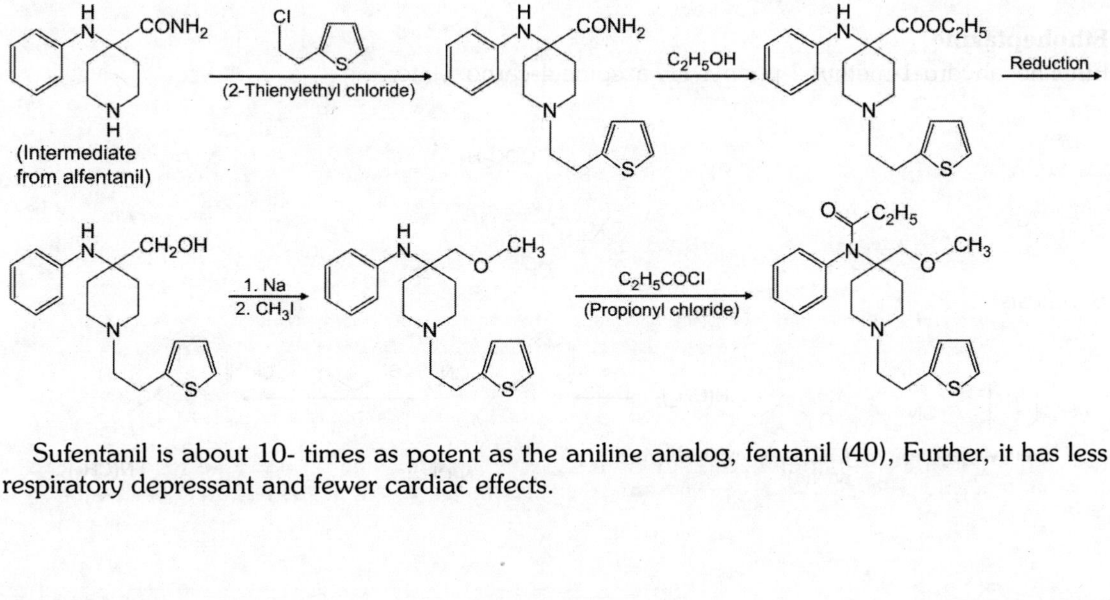

Sufentanil is about 10- times as potent as the aniline analog, fentanil (40), Further, it has less respiratory depressant and fewer cardiac effects.

Remifentanil
4-Carboxy-4-(N-phenylpropionamido)-1-piperidinepropionic acid dimethyl ester

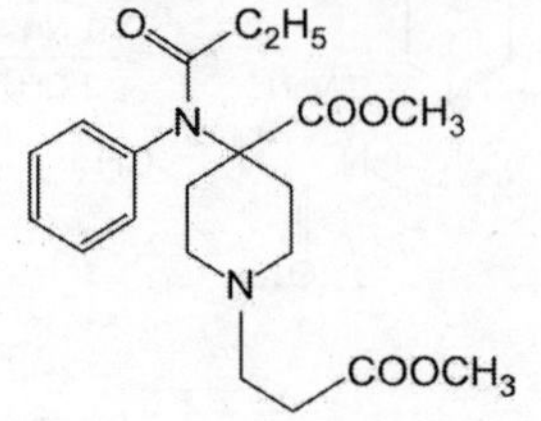

Synthesis

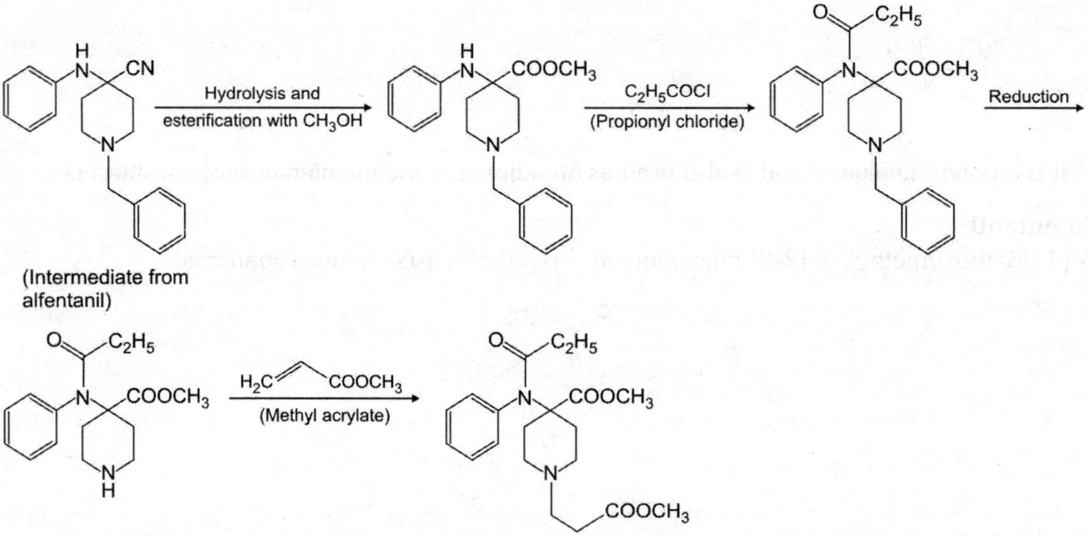

(Intermediate from alfentanil)

(Methyl acrylate)

Narcotic analgesic

Ethoheptazine
Ethyl hexahydro-1-methyl-4-phenyl-1H-azepine 4-carboxylate.

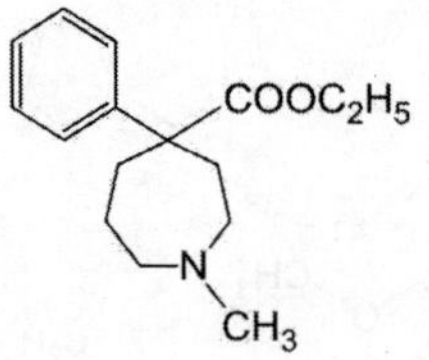

Synthesis

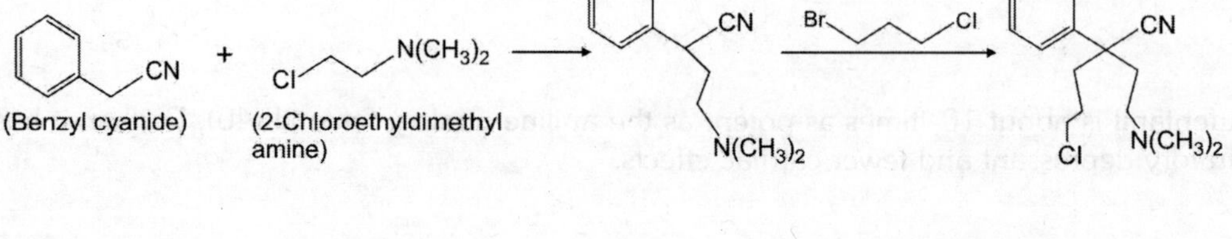

(Benzyl cyanide)   +   (2-Chloroethyldimethyl amine)

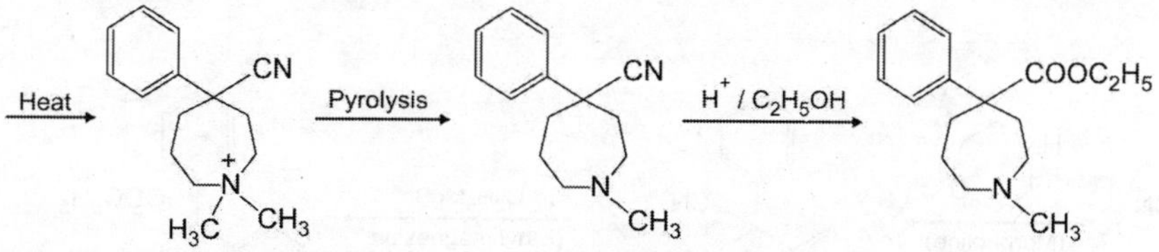

It is an orally effective analgesic with no addiction liability.

SYNTHETIC OPIOIDS : METHADONE AND RELATED ANALOGS

Methadone

(*RS*)-6-Dimethylamino-4,4-diphenyl-3-heptanone

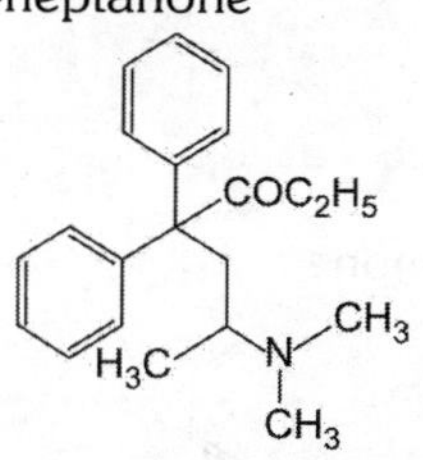

Synthesis

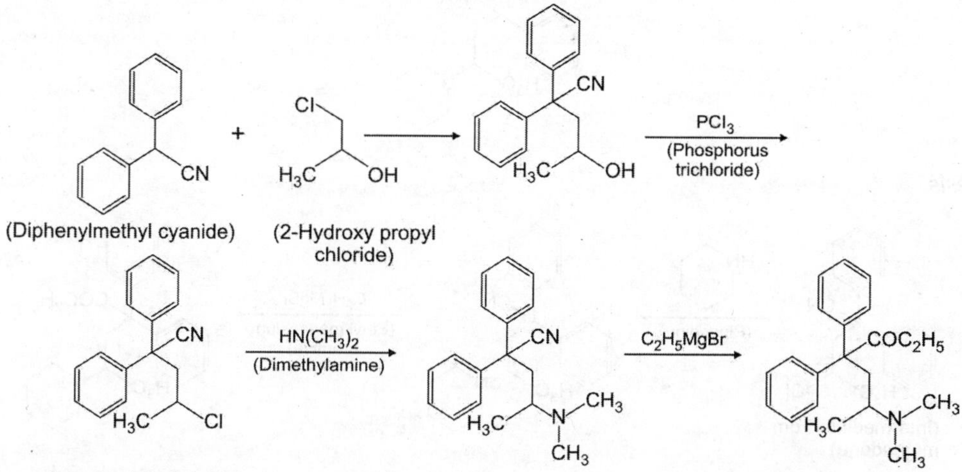

(Diphenylmethyl cyanide)   (2-Hydroxy propyl chloride)

It is used as hydrochloride in racemic form. It is twice as active as morphine (1) and 10 times as active as meperidine (31).

Phenadoxone

6-(4-Morpholinyl)-4,4-diphenyl-3-heptanone

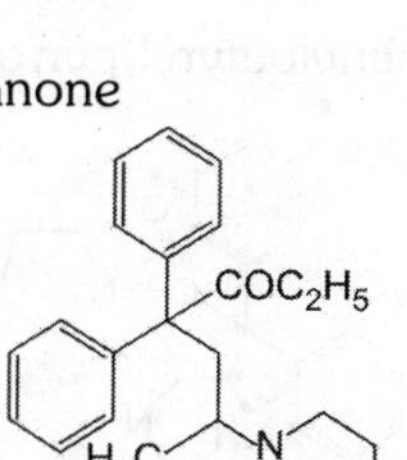

Synthesis

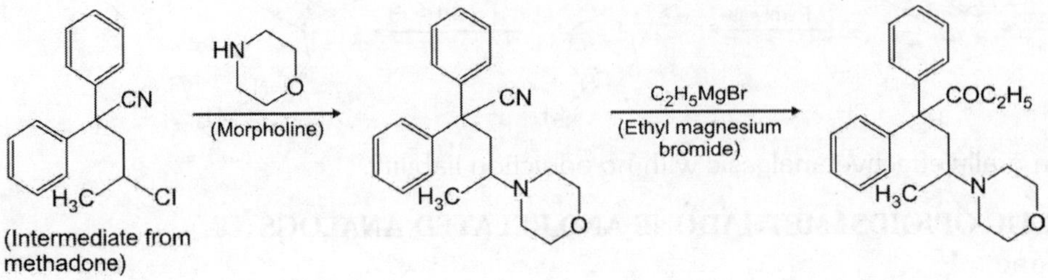

(Intermediate from methadone) → (Morpholine) → → C₂H₅MgBr (Ethyl magnesium bromide) →

It is a narcotic analgesic.

Dipipanone

4,4-Diphenyl-6-(-1-piperidinyl)-3-heptanone

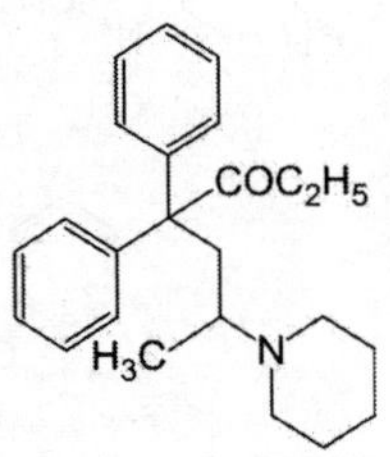

Synthesis

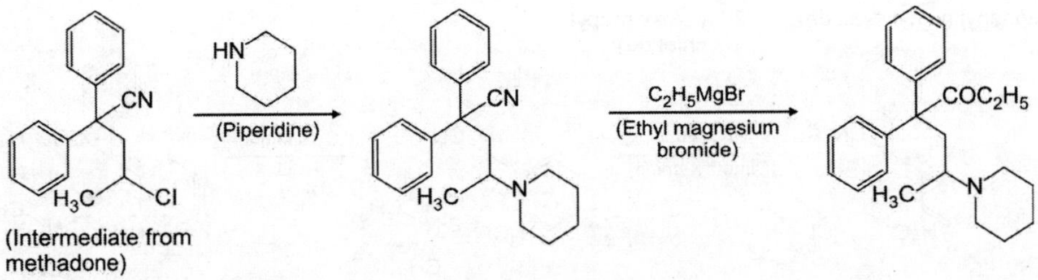

(Intermediate from methadone) → (Piperidine) → → C₂H₅MgBr (Ethyl magnesium bromide) →

It is less active than methadone (45) and is used for the treatment of moderate to severe pain.

Dextromoramide

(+)-1-(3-Methyl-4-morpholino-2,2-diphenylbutyryl)pyrrolidine

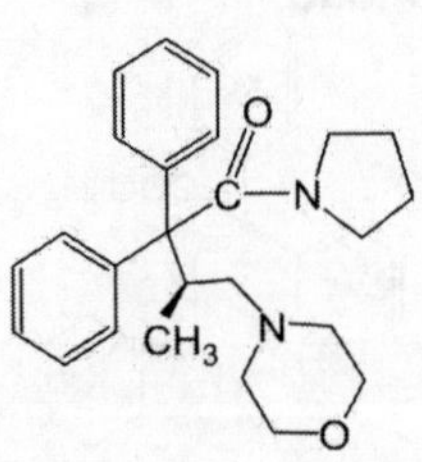

Synthesis

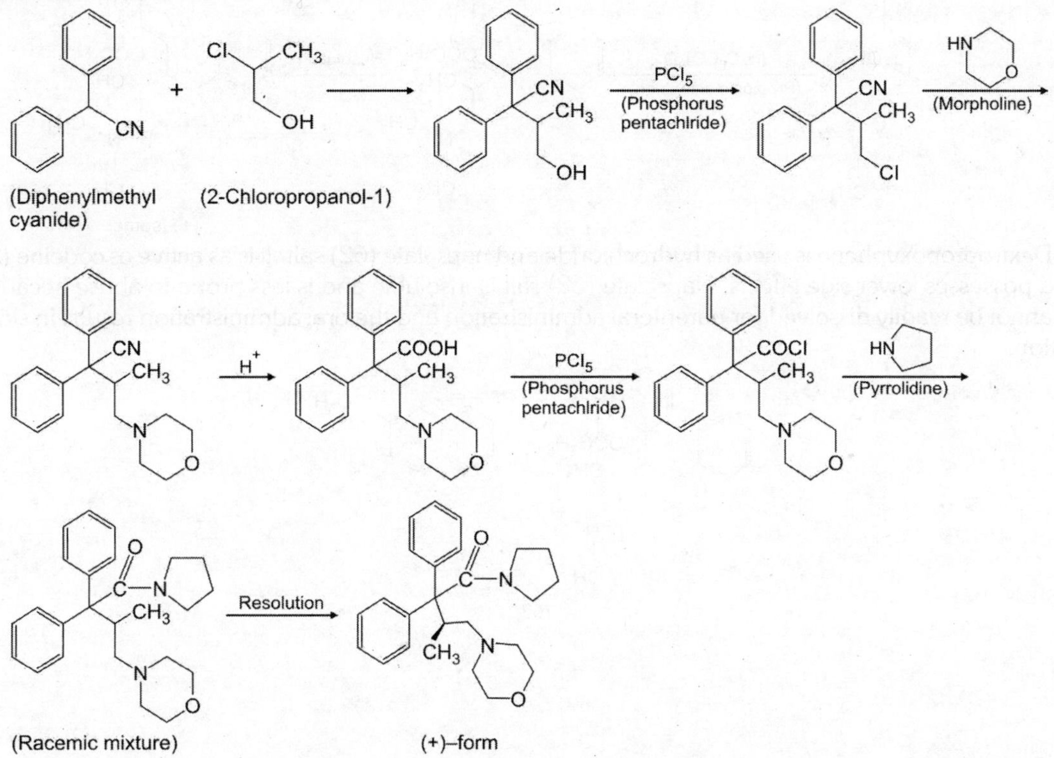

(Diphenylmethyl cyanide)   (2-Chloropropanol-1)

Dextromoramide is used as hydrogen tartrate salt. It is about 13 times as active as methadone (45).

Dextropropoxyphene

(1S,2R)-1-Benzyl-3-dimethylamino-2-methyl-1-phenylpropyl propionate

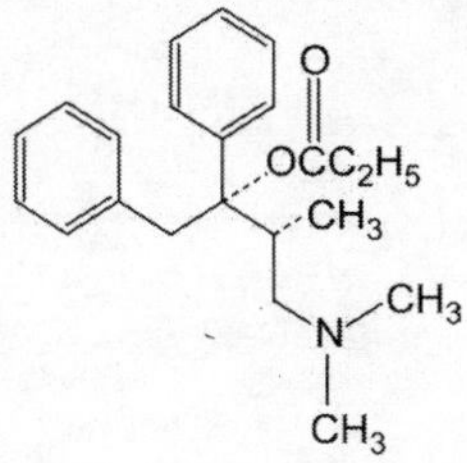

Synthesis

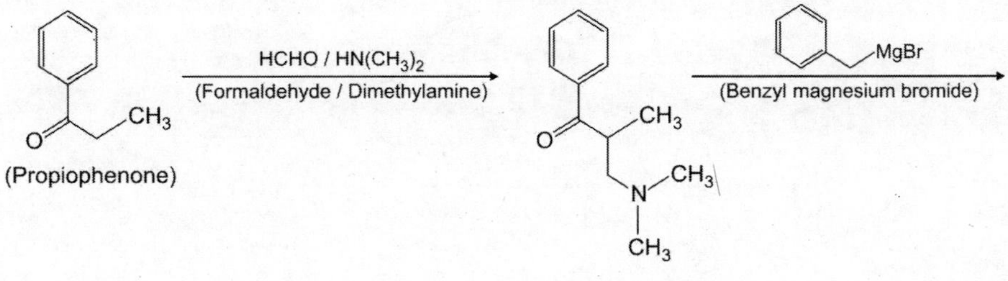

(Propiophenone)

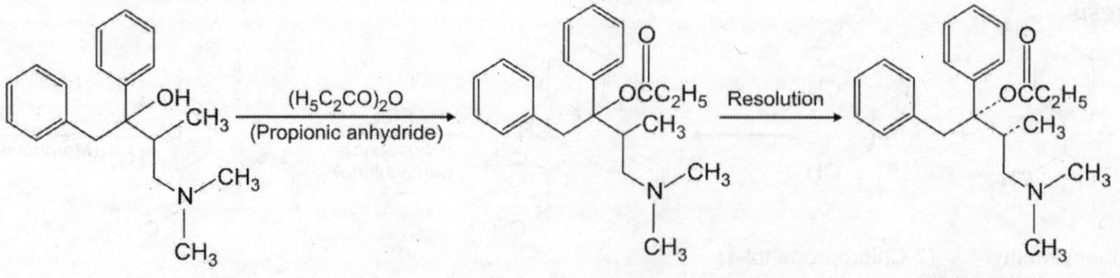

(+)-isomer

Dextropropoxyphene is used as hydrochloride and napsylate (62) salt. It is as active as codeine (2) and possesses lower side effects. Napsylate (62) salt is insoluble and is less prone to abuse because it cannot be readily dissolved for parenteral administration and the oral administration results in slow action.

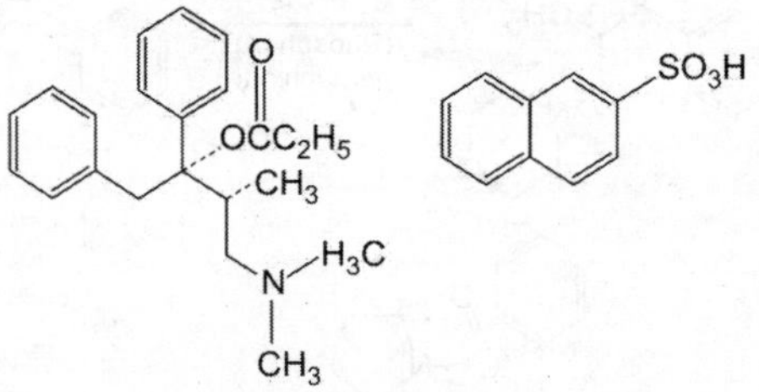

(62)

CHAPTER
9

ANTIPARKINSONIAN DRUGS

PARKINSONISM AND DOPAMINE

PARKINSONISM is a degenerative disease characterized by slowness of movement (bradykinesia), muscular rigidity, resting tremors, and impairment of postural balance. It occurs mainly in elderly people.

In parkinsonism, there is deficiency of neurotransmitter dopamine (1). Dopamine (1) is synthesized by the pigmented cells in substantia nigra of the mid-brain. Loss of these pigmented cells results in deficiency of dopamine (1). Dopamine (1) is an inhibitory neurotransmitter and it maintains the balance with the excitatory neurotransmitter acetylcholine. Any disturbance in this results in the symptoms of Parkinson's disease.

(1)

The dopamine (1) deficiency can also be induced by drugs such as reserpine which reduces the amount of dopamine in the brain or by antipsychotic drugs which block the dopamine receptors. Similarly, administration of neurotoxin such as N-methyl-4-phenyl-1, 2, 3, 6-tetrahydropyridine (MPTP), which causes irreversible damage of nigrostriatal dopaminergic neurons, also causes Parkinson's disease.

Dopamine (1) is synthesized in terminals of dopaminergic neurons from tyrosine (2). Tyrosine hydroxylase converts tyrosine (2) to dopa (3) which is then decarboxylated by dopa decarboxylase to give dopamine. It is then transported to storage sites by transporter protein. The release of the dopamine (1) from its storage sites takes place by depolarization and entry of Ca^{2+}. The released dopamine (1) then binds to postsynaptic dopamine receptors.

Dopamine receptors through which the action of dopamine is mediated have been identified. They are proteins and possess seven α-helical segments. Two types of receptors, D1 and D2, were originally distinguished. However, gene cloning has revealed further subgroups, D_1 to D_5.The original D1-family constitutes of D_1 and D_5, while D_2, D_3, and D_4 constitute D2-receptor family. The D1-receptor stimulates c-AMP synthesis and phosphatidyl inositol hydrolysis. The D2-receptors decrease c-AMP formation and modulate the K^+ and Ca^{2+} currents.

The action of dopamine (1) is terminated in several ways. After getting bound to the receptors and stimulating the dopamine receptors, most of the remaining dopamine (1) is transported back into presynaptic cell by dopamine transporter. The dopamine (1) in presynaptic cell is either recycled into storage vesicles for further use or is metabolized by the enzymes monoamine oxidase (MAO) and catechol o-methyl transferase (COMT) (Fig. 9.1). The remaining dopamine (1) in synaptic cleft is also metabolized by these enzymes.

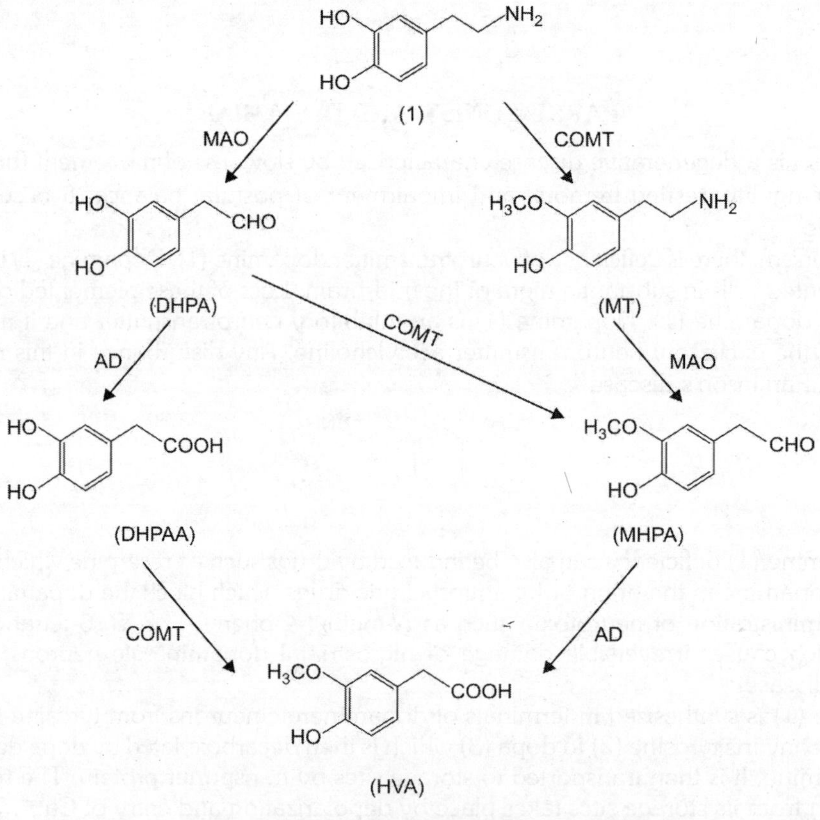

Fig. 9.1: Metabolism of dopamine (1)

(AD-aldehyde dehydrogenase; COMT-catechol o-methyltransferase; MAO-monoamine oxidase; DHPAA-dihydroxyphenylacetic acid; DHPA-dihydroxyphenylacetaldhyde; HVA-homovanillic acid; MHPA-3-methoxy-4-hydroxyphenylacetaldehyde; MT-3-methoxytyramine.)

Since Parkinson's disease has been associated with deficiency of dopamine and disturbances of acetylcholine-dopamine balance, the approaches towards treatment of Parkinson's disease include:

1. Increasing the levels of dopamine (1), through:
   (a) augmentation of dopamine (1) levels in brain,
   (b) decreasing the dopamine (1) catabolism, and
   (c) stimulation of dopamine release from presynaptic site.
2. Use of dopamine receptor agonists.
3. Use of anticholinergic drugs.

Marked improvement in clinical symptoms has been observed when large doses of dopamine (1) are administered. One of the problems with dopamine (1) is that it cannot pass blood-brain barrier because it remains in ionic form. Its precursor, the levo-isomer of dopa, levodopa (3), which is less basic, can pass the blood-brain barrier and reach brain faster. Levodopa (3) is usually administered along with carbidopa (4) or benserazide (5), which are inhibitors of peripheral dopa decarboxylase. The dose needed after co-administration of these agents is reduced to a large extent and side effects are also reduced. After levodopa (3) reaches brain, it is decarboxylated to dopamine (1).

(4)

(5)

The brain dopamine (1) levels can also be increased by decreasing its degradation. MAO inhibitor selegiline (6) is a selective inhibitor of MAO-B, which inactivates dopamine (1). Use of selegiline (6) results in decreased metabolism and increased levels of dopamine (1).

The COMT inhibitors namely tolcapone (7) and entacapone (8) act by inhibiting the methylation and subsequent inactivation of dopamine (1).

(6)

(7)

(8)

Dopamine (1) levels can also be increased by stimulation of dopamine release from its neuronal storage sites. Amantadine (9), an antiviral agent, has been found clinically useful in Parkinson's disease.

(9)

It increases the release of dopamine (1) which results in its increased levels in brain. When used in combination with levodopa (3), the results are still better. Although amantadine (9) is more basic than dopamine (1) [amantadine (9) pKa 10.8 and dopamine (1) pKa 10.6], yet it crosses blood-brain barrier in sufficient concentration. This is because it has a cage-like structure which is much more lipophilic. Further, because of this, its oxidative metabolism is almost nil.

Stimulation of dopamine receptors by agonists is another line of treatment for Parkinson's disease. Among the drugs which act as dopamine receptor agonists include bromocriptine (10), pergolide (11), pramipexole (12), and ropinirole (13). Bromocriptine (10) and pergolide (11) are ergot alkaloid derivatives. While bromocriptine (10) is a D_2 receptor agonist, pergolide (11) is D_1 and D_2 receptor agonist. The non-ergot alkaloid agonists, pramipexole (12) and ropinirole (13), are D_2 and D_3 receptor agonists. All the dopamine receptor agonists are used along with levodopa (3) in therapy.

Both bromocriptine (10) and pergolide (11) cause significant nausea, peripheral edema, and hypotension. Pramipexole (12) and ropinirole (13) are free of these side effects.

(10)

(11)

(12)

(13)

Earlier the treatment of Parkinson's disease was by the use of atropine (14). Suppression of excitatory effects of muscarinic receptors can restore, to a large extent, the disturbances in the acetylcholine-dopamine balance. The use of antimuscarinic agents results in diminishing of tremors only. Their use also results in other side effects such as dryness of mouth, constipation, impaired vision, and urinary retention. Some of the other antimuscarinic agents used include procyclidine (15), trihexyphenidyl (16), biperiden (17), and benztropine (18). Ethopropazine (19) a phenothiazine derivative which possesses central anicholinergic activity has also been found to improve the symptoms of Parkinson' disease.

(14)

(15)

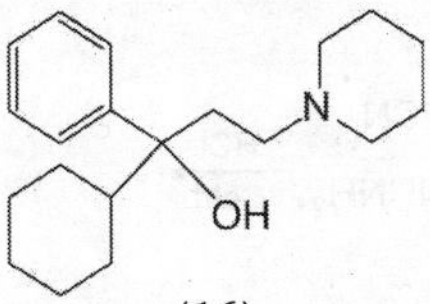

(16)

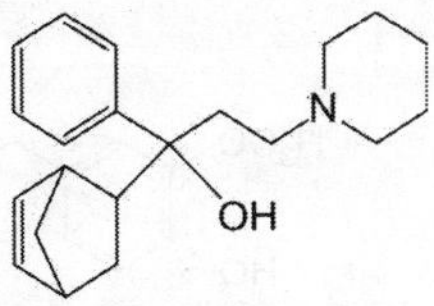

(17)

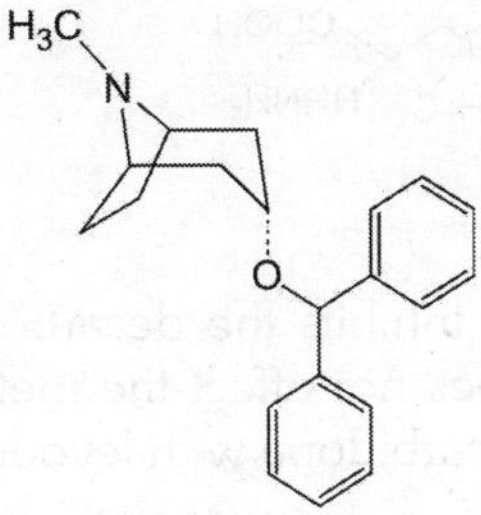

(18)

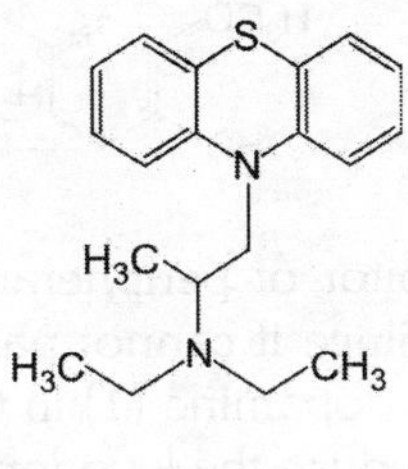

(19)

INDIVIDUAL COMPOUNDS

DOPAMINE PRECURSORS

Levodopa

(–)-3-Hydroxy-L-tyrosine

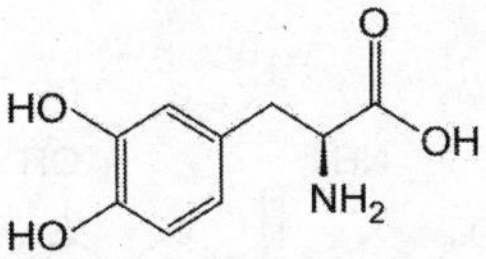

Synthesis

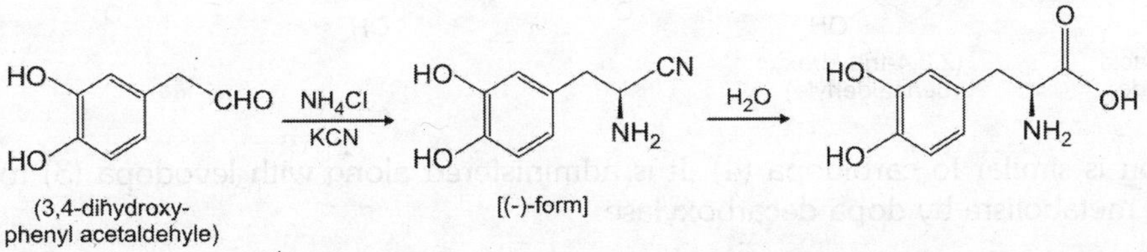

(3,4-dihydroxy-phenyl acetaldehyle)
NH4Cl
KCN
[(-)-form]
H2O

Levodopa is precursor of dopamine (1) and has been found to be effective in Parkinson's disease. Levodopa crosses blood-brain barrier and is then metabolized to dopamine (1) in brain.

PERIPHERAL DOPA DECARBOXYLASE INHIBITORS

Carbidopa

(*S*)-2-(3, 4-Dihydroxybenzyl)-2-hydrazinopropionic acid

Synthesis

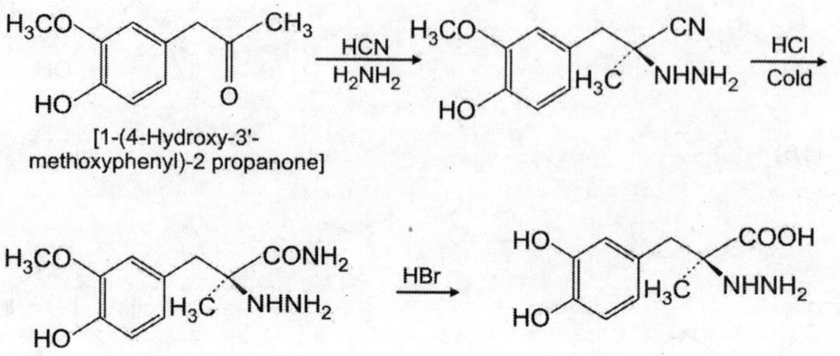

[1-(4-Hydroxy-3'-
methoxyphenyl)-2 propanone]

It is an inhibitor of peripheral dopa decarboxylase and thus inhibits the decarboxylation of levodopa (3). Since it cannot pass the blood-brain barrier, it does not affect the metabolism of levodopa (3) to dopamine (1) in the brain. Co-administration of carbidopa with levodopa (3) has been found to reduce the levodopa (3) requirement by 75%.

Benserazide

N-(DL-Seryl)-*N'*-(2, 3, 4-trihydroxybenzyl)hydrazine

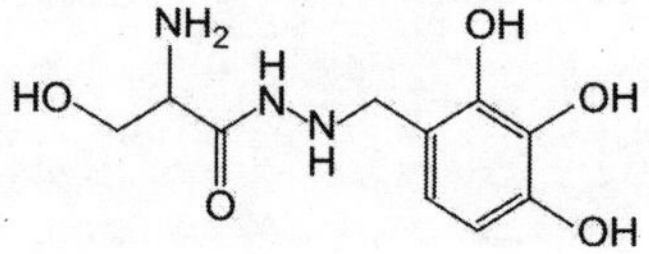

Synthesis

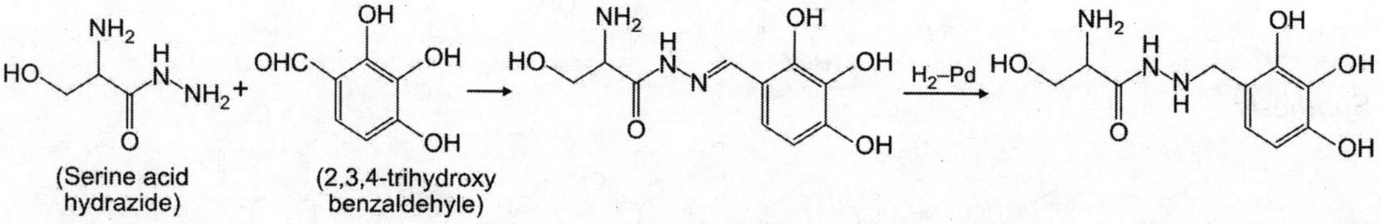

(Serine acid   (2,3,4-trihydroxy
hydrazide)   benzaldehyle)

Its action is similar to carbidopa (4). It is administered along with levodopa (3) to inhibit its peripheral metabolism by dopa decarboxylase.

INHIBITORS OF DOPAMINE METABOLISM

Tolcapone

3,4-Dihydroxy-4'-methyl-5-nitrobenzophenone

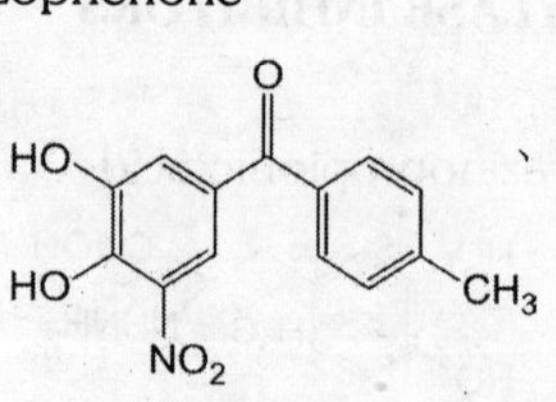

Synthesis

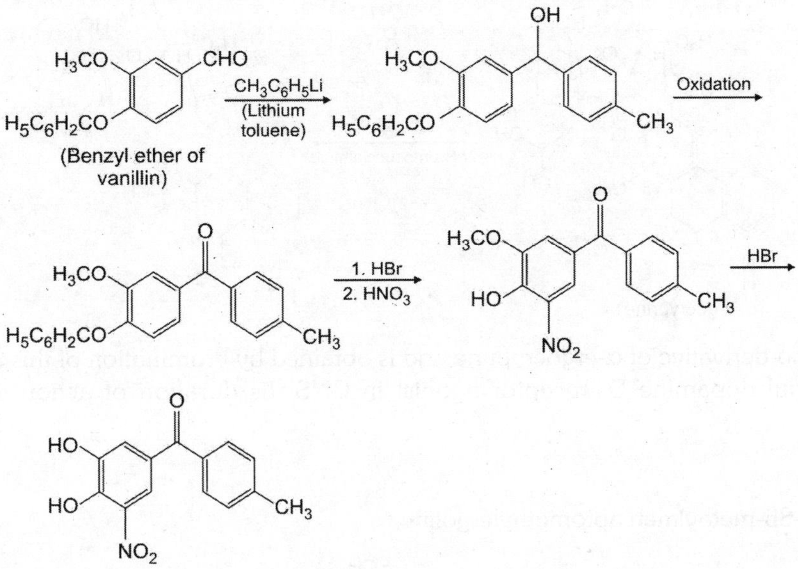

It inhibits the enzyme COMT which is responsible for methylation and subsequent inactivation of levodopa (3). It is used along with levodopa (3).

DOPAMINE RELEASE STIMULANTS

Amantadine

It is used as hydrochloride. It acts by increasing the release of dopamine (1). However, it is less effective than levodopa (3) or bromocriptine (10).

See ANTIVIRAL AGENTS

DOPAMINE RECEPTOR AGONISTS

Bromocriptine

(5′α)-2-Bromo-12′-hydroxy-2′-(1-methylethyl)-5′-(2-methylpropyl)-ergotaman-3′,6′,18-trione

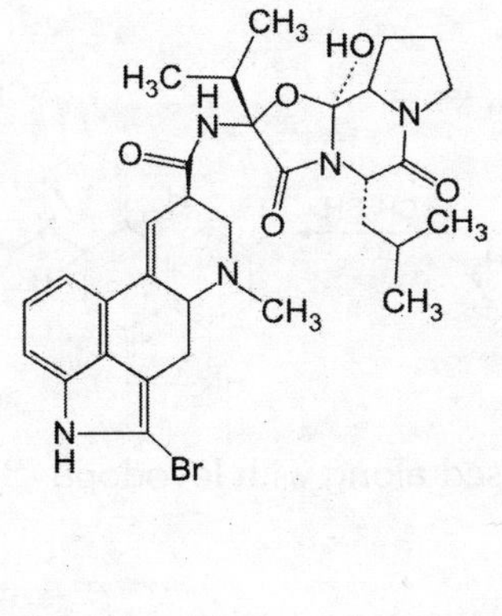

Synthesis

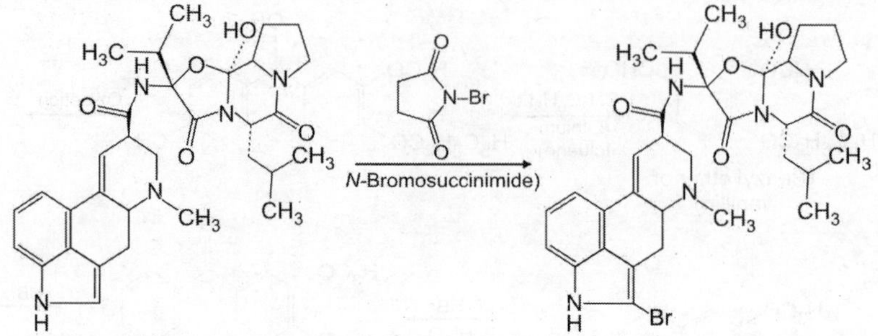

(α-Ergocryprine)

It is a bromo-derivative of α-ergocryptine and is obtained by bromination of this ergot alkaloid. It is a powerful dopamine D_2 receptor agonist in CNS. Its duration of action is longer than levodopa (3).

Pergolide

D-6-*n*-Propyl-8β-methylmercaptomethylergoline

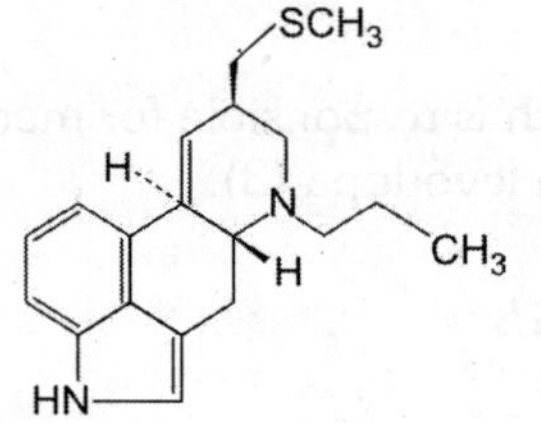

Synthesis

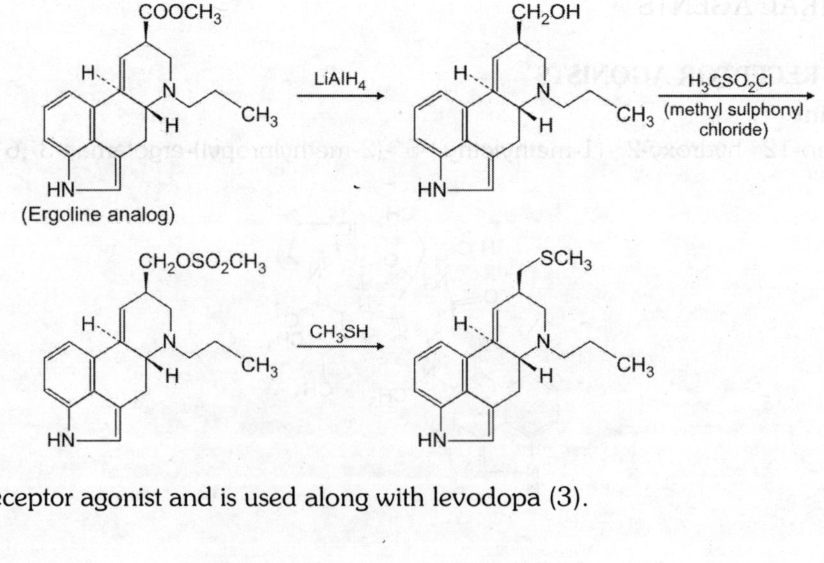

(Ergoline analog)

It is D_2 receptor agonist and is used along with levodopa (3).

Pramipexole

(*S*)-2-Amino-4,5,6,7-tetrahydro-6-(propylamino)benzothiazole

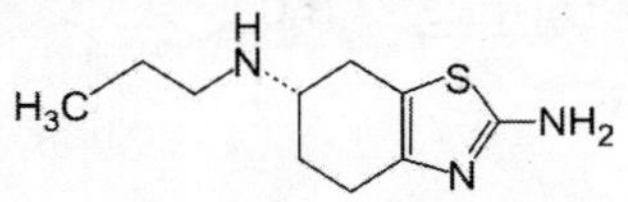

Synthesis

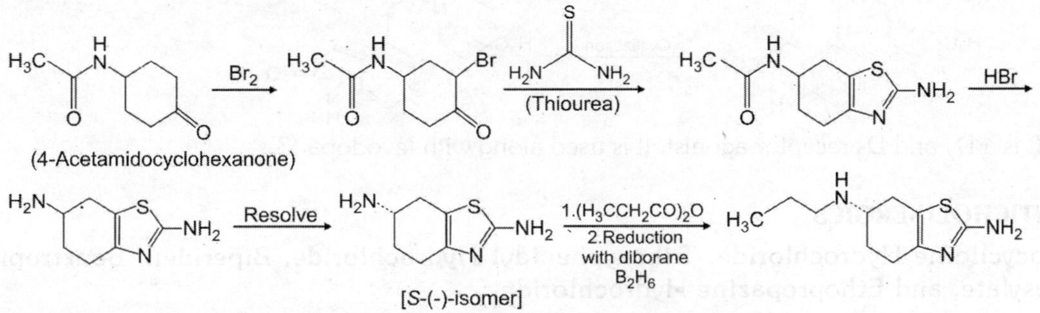
Br2
H2N NH2
(Thiourea)
HBr
(4-Acetamidocyclohexanone)
Resolve
1.(H3CCH2CO)2O
2.Reduction with diborane B2H6
[S-(-)-isomer]

It is a D_2 and D_3 receptor agonist. It is used along with levodopa (3).

Ropinirole

4-[2-Di-*n*-propylamino)ethyl]-2(3*H*)-indolone

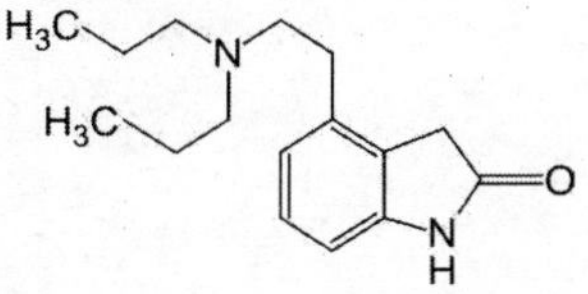

Synthesis

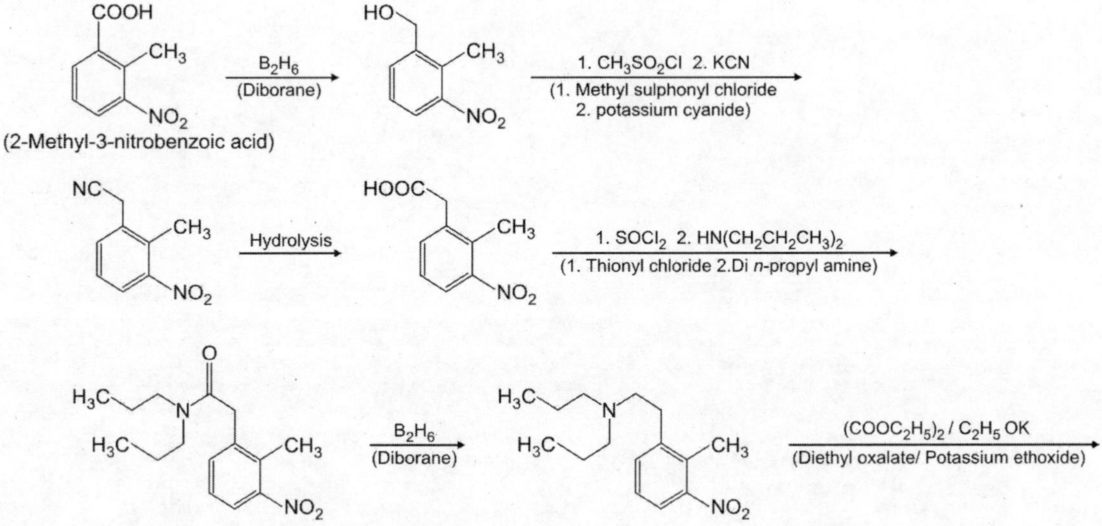
B2H6
(Diborane)
(2-Methyl-3-nitrobenzoic acid)
1. CH3SO2Cl 2. KCN
(1. Methyl sulphonyl chloride
2. potassium cyanide)
Hydrolysis
1. SOCl2 2. HN(CH2CH2CH3)2
(1. Thionyl chloride 2.Di n-propyl amine)
B2H6
(Diborane)
(COOC2H5)2 / C2H5 OK
(Diethyl oxalate/ Potassium ethoxide)

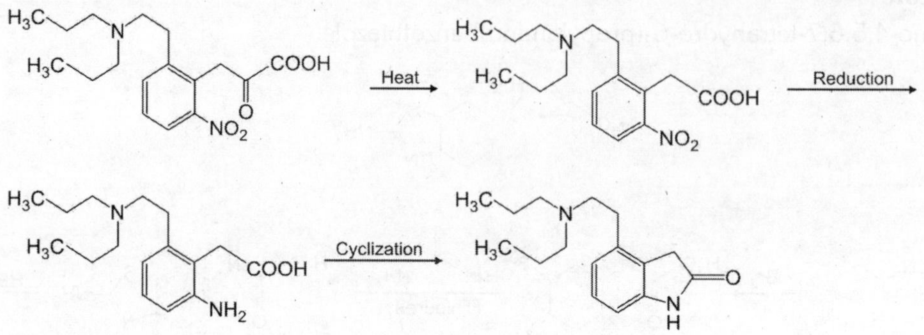

It is a D_2 and D_3 receptor agonist. It is used along with levodopa (3).

ANTICHOLINERGICS

Procyclidine Hydrochloride, Trihexyphenidyl Hydrochloride, Biperiden, Benztropine Mesylate, and Ethopropazine Hydrochloride

See **DRUGS ACTING ON CHOLINERGIC RECEPTORS**

CENTRAL NERVOUS SYSTEM STIMULANTS

DRUGS UNDER THIS CATEGORY include analeptics, psychomotor stimulants, antidepressant drugs, and psychotomimetics or hallucinogens.

ANALEPTICS

Analeptics are drugs which stimulate central nervous system. They act by stimulating the medullary center. These drugs were used earlier as respiratory stimulants. Some of these drugs are used now in chronic obstructive pulmonary diseases. Various analeptics include strychnine (1), picrotoxinin (2), amiphenazole (3), doxapram (4), pentylenetetrazole (5), nikethamide (6), and bicuculline (7).

Strychnine (1) is an alkaloid found in the seeds of *Strychnos nux-vomica*. It is a powerful convulsant. It acts by blocking the receptors of inhibitor transmitter, glycine. In small doses, it causes improvement in vision and hearing.

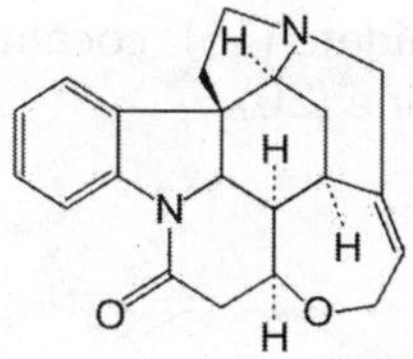

(1)

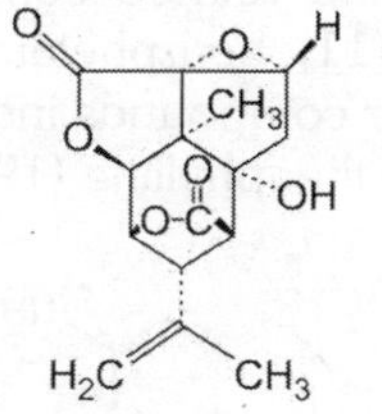

(2)

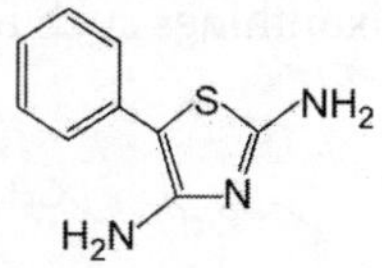

(3)

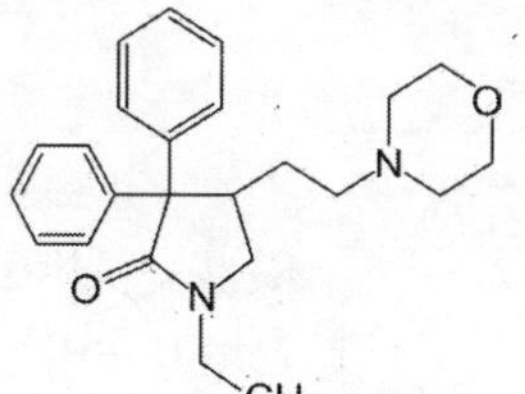

(4)

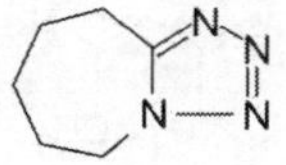

(5)

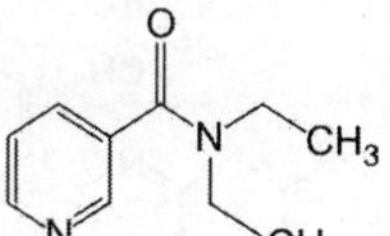

(6)

(7)   (8)

Picrotoxin, which is a mixture of picrotoxinin (2) and picrotin (8), has been isolated from *Anamirta cocculus*. Picrotoxinin (2) is the active principle. It blocks the action of GABA on chloride channels. It causes convulsions and has no therapeutic significance.

Amiphenazole (3) is occasionally used as respiratory stimulant. Its mechanism of action is not known.

Doxapram (4) is also used in clinical practice as a respiratory stimulant. It is used as hydrochloride. Like amiphenazole (3), its mechanism of action is not known.

Pentylenetetrazole (5), a tetrazole has been used as an experimental tool. The mechanism of its action is not established. It probably acts by reducing GABA-ergic inhibition.

Nikethamide (6) is diethylamide of nicotinic acid. It has been used as respiratory stimulant. Its mechanism of action is not known.

Bicuculline (7), an alkaloid, is obtained from *Dicentra curcullaria*. It acts by blocking the receptors of GABA and its action is confined to $GABA_A$-receptors. It has no clinical significance but is used in experimental pharmacology.

PSYCHOMOTOR STIMULANTS

This class includes amphetamines and related compounds such as dexamphetamine (9), methamphetamine (10), phentermine (11), benzphetamine (12), fenfluramine (13), chlorphentermine (14), and clortermine (15). Other compounds include methylphenidate (16), cocaine (17), methylxanthines such as caffeine (18), theophylline (19), and theobromine (20).

(9)   (10)   (11)

(12)   (13)   (14)

(15)   (16)   (17)

(18)   (19)   (20)

Amphetamines and related compounds (9-16) cause locomotor stimulation, euphoria, excitement, and anorexia. All of these act by releasing norepinephrine, dopamine, and serotonin from the nerve terminals. The stimulant effect which lasts for few hours is followed by depression. Some of these are used as appetite suppressants.

Cocaine (17) an alkaloid is obtained from leaves of *Erythroxylan coca.* Its action is similar to that of amphetamines. It acts by inhibiting catecholamine uptake. Cocaine (17), like amphetamines is a drug of abuse and causes severe adverse reactions.

The central stimulant effects of tea and coffee are due to methylxanthines. The compounds responsible for these effects are caffeine (18), theophylline (19), and theobromine (20). The main pharmacological effects of caffeine (18) and theophylline (19) are locomotor stimulation, euphoria, excitement, and anorexia. Methylxanthines act by antagonism at A_2-purine receptors and inhibition of phosphodiesterase. This results in effects similar to those of β-adrenoreceptor agonists. They also cause diuresis.

Theophylline (19) is used clinically as bronchodilator in form of salts such as aminophylline, a salt of theophylline and ethylenediamine, and choline theophyllinate, a salt of choline and theophylline.

Analogs of methylxanthine such as diprophylline (21), etamiphyllin (22), etofylline (23), proxyphylline (24), doxofylline (25), and pentoxifylline (26) have been used as bronchodilators.

(21), R= $CH_2CH(OH)CH_2OH$
(22), R= $CH_2CH_2N(C_2H_5)_2$
(23), R= CH_2CH_2OH
(24), R= $CH_2CH(OH)CH_3$
(25) R= CH_2

(26)

ANTIDEPRESSANT DRUGS

Emotional disturbances usually lead to changes in mood resulting in depression or mania. The characteristics of depression include feeling of sadness and guilt, low self-esteem, indecisiveness, and loss of motivation. In addition to these emotional symptoms, biological symptoms like loss of sleep, retardation of thought and action are also observed in depressed state.

In mania, there is excessive enthusiasm or excitement, over-confidence, impulsive action marked by irritability, impatience, and aggression.

Depression is of two types—unipolar and bipolar. In unipolar depression, the mood swings always in the same direction while as in bipolar, the mood alternates between depression and mania. Unipolar depression is common.

Depression results from deficiency of serotonin [5-hydroxytryptamine (27)] transmission in CNS. This theory is based on the effectiveness of monoamine oxidase inhibitors and tricyclic antidepressants in depression.

The different types of antidepressant drugs include:

1. Monoamine oxidase inhibitors.
2. Tricyclic antidepressants.
3. Selective serotonin reuptake inhibitors.
4. Miscellaneous compounds.

Monoamine Oxidase Inhibitors

Monoamine oxidases, the flavin containing enzymes, are responsible for metabolism of various biogenic amines such as serotonin [(27), Fig. 10.1], norepinephrine [(28), for metabolism see Adrenergic Drugs], dopamine [(29), for metabolism see Antiparkinsonian Drugs] and tryptamine [(30), Fig. 10.2].

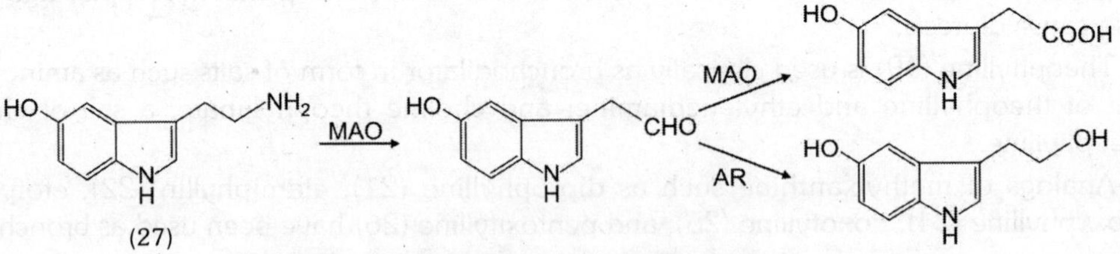

Fig. 10.1: Metabolism of serotonin (27).

(MAO- Monoamine oxidase; AR- Aldehyde reductase.)

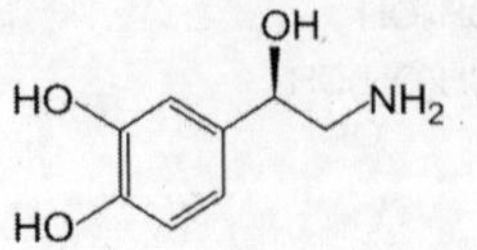

(28)

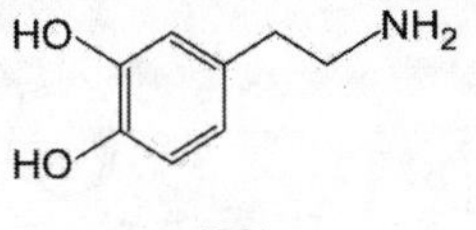

(29)

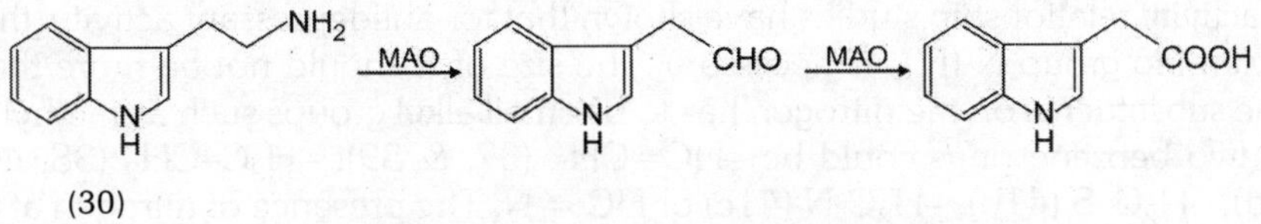

(30)

Fig. 10.2: Metabolism of tryptamine (30).

(MAO – Monoamine oxidase.)

Some of the MAO inhibitors include hydrazine derivatives such as phenelzine (31), isocarboxazid (32), and pheniprazine (33). The non-hydrazine analogs include tranylcypromine (34), moclobemide (35), and selegiline (36).

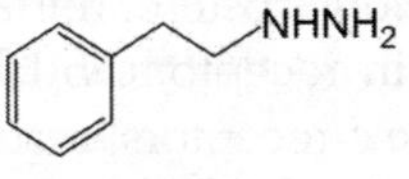

(31)

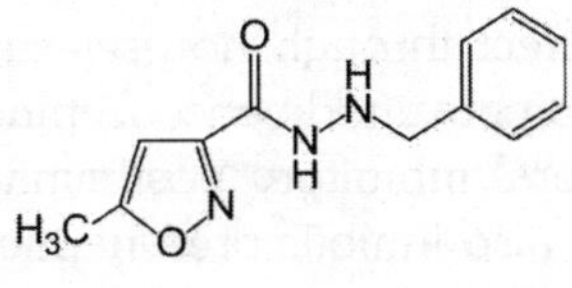

(32)

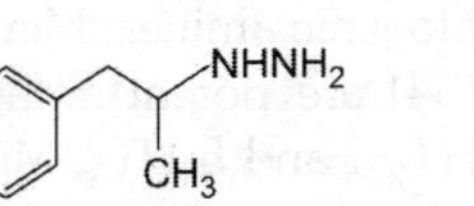

(33)

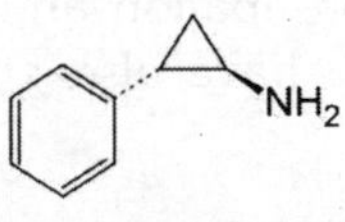

(34)

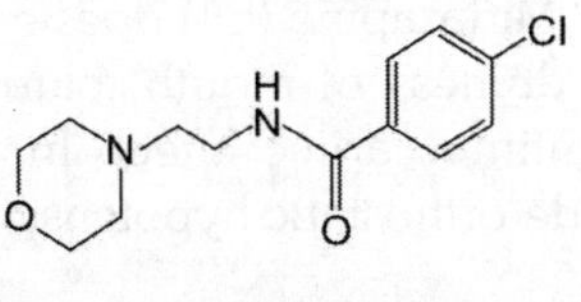

(35)

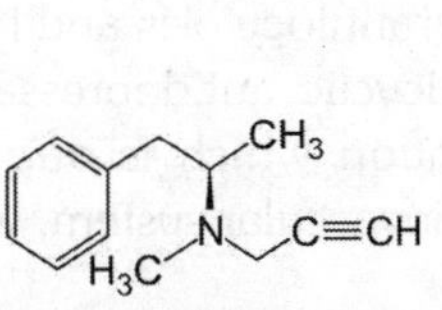

(36)

Monoamine oxidase inhibitors act by inhibiting one or both types of MAO, thus increasing concentration of amines such as serotonin (27), norepinephrine (28), and dopamine (29).

Tricyclic Antidepressants

Some of these systems include 5*H*-dibenzocycloheptene (37), 10, 11-dihydro-5*H*-dibenzo-cycloheptene (38), 5*H*-dibenzazepine (39), 10, 11-dihydro-5*H*-dibenzazepine (40), 10, 11-dihydro-5*H*-dibenzocycloheptene with one hetero-atom such as oxygen (41a), sulphur (41b) or nitrogen (41c) or with two hetero-atoms such as oxygen and nitrogen (41d).

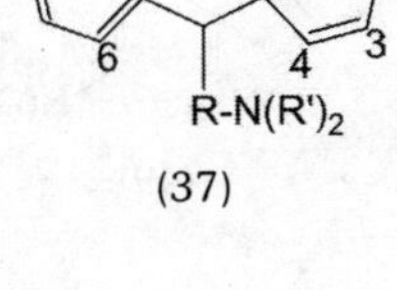

(37)

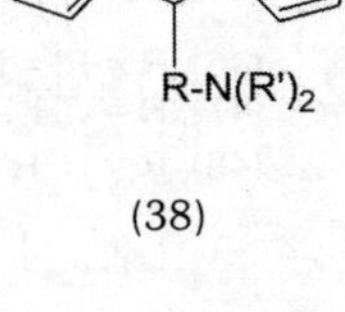

(38)

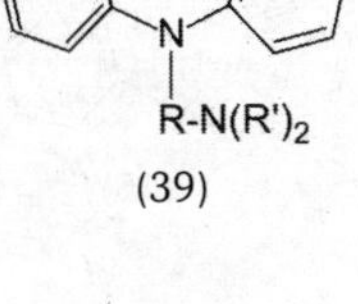

(39)

(a), x = O, Y = CH$_2$
(b), x = S, Y = CH$_2$
(c), x = N, Y = CH$_2$
(d), x = O, Y = N

(40)   (41)

Structure-activity relationship studies have shown that for antidepressant activity, the side chain R with dialkylamino group N (R')$_2$ is necessary. The size of R should not be more than 3-carbon atoms and the substituents on the nitrogen has to be small alkyl groups such as methyl. The bridge between the two benzene rings could be –HC=CH– (37, & 39), –H$_2$C–CH$_2$ (38, 40) –H$_2$C-O- (41a and 41d), –H$_2$C-S (41b), –H$_2$C-N (41c) or HC = N. The presence of nitrogen at position 5 is not necessary as compounds like cycloheptenes (37), dihydrocycloheptenes (38), dibenzoxepin (41a), and dibenzothiepin (41b) have shown activity.

The tricyclic antidepressants show their effect through various mechanisms. One of the mechanisms involves inhibition of norepinephrine (28) reuptake. Some of the clinically useful compounds belonging to this class include protriptyline (42), nortiptyline (43), desipramine (44), and amoxapine (45). Imipramine (46), trimipramine (47), clomipramine (48), amitriptyline (49), lofepramine (50), doxepin (51), and dothiepin (52) are some of the clinically useful compounds which show their antidepressant effect through non-selective inhibition of reuptake of various biogenic amines. Mianserin (53), a piperazinodibenzoazepine and its pyridyl isostere, mirtazapine (54) are potent antagonists at several inhibitory post synaptic serotonin receptors, 5-HT$_{2A}$, 5-HT$_{2C}$, and 5-HT$_3$. Mirtazapine (54) also inhibits presynaptic α_2-adrenergic receptors, resulting in increased release of norepinephrine (28) in synapse. Further, mirtazapine (54) is also a potent histamine H$_1$-receptor antagonist which results in sedation. Administration of mianserin (53) results in agranulocytosis and leukopenia. Mirtazapine (54) does not possess these side effects.

Tricyclic antidepressants cause dryness of mouth, blurred vision, constipation and urinary retention which is due to their antimuscarinic effect. In addition, they have also effects on cardiovascular system, which include orthostatic hypotension.

(42)   (43)   (44)

(45)

(46), R = R' = H
(47), R = CH$_3$, R' = H
(48), R = H, R' = Cl

(49)

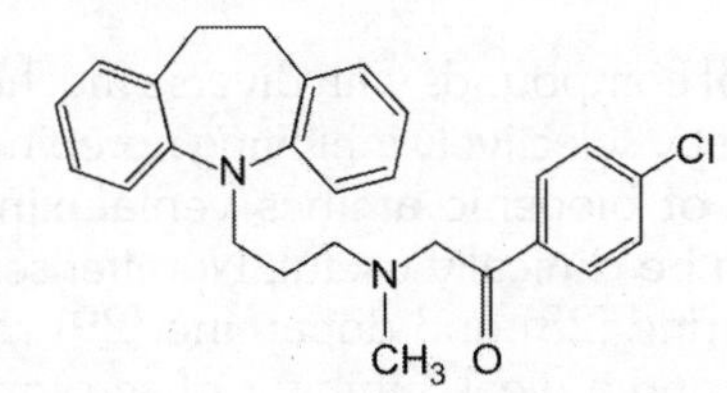

(50)

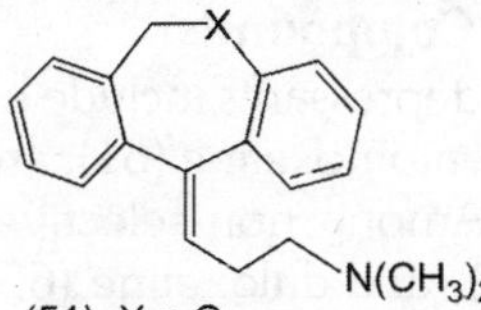

(51), X = O
(52), X = S

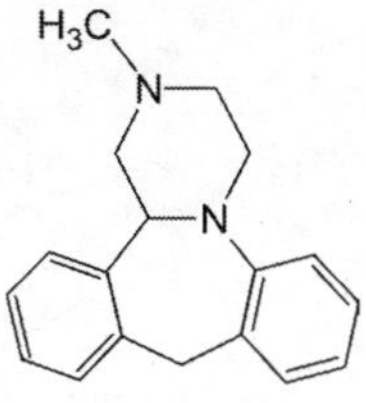

(53)

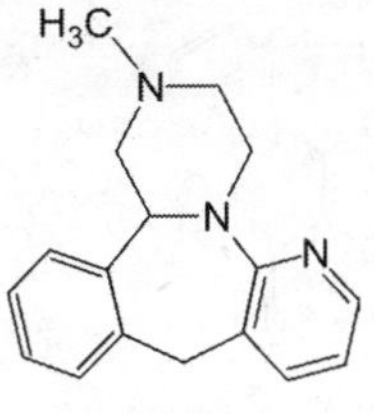

(54)

Selective Serotonin Reuptake Inhibitors

Serotonin (27) uptake inhibitors are also commonly known as Selective Serotonin Reuptake Inhibitors (SSRI's). These compounds selectively inhibit the SERT, the reuptake transporter for serotonin (27). As a result of this inhibition more of serotonin (27) is available in synapse for interaction with postsynaptic receptors. The clinically useful antidepressants in this category include fluoxetine (55), fluvoxamine (56), paroxetine (57), sertraline (58), and citalopram (59). These compounds have very little or no affinity for norepinephrine (28) or dopamine (29) transporters. The SSRI's have very few side effects as compared to tricyclic antidepressants.

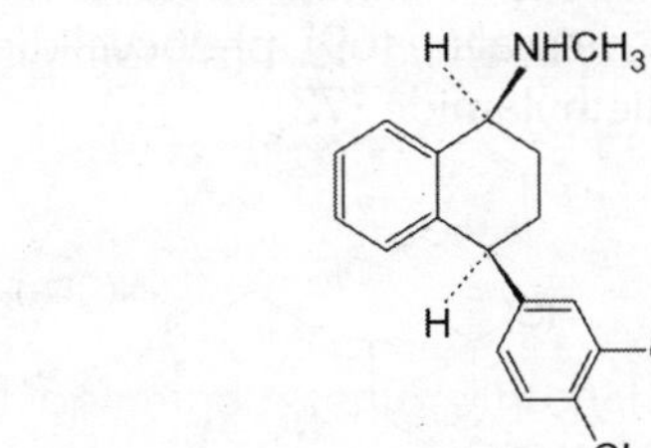

(55)

(56)

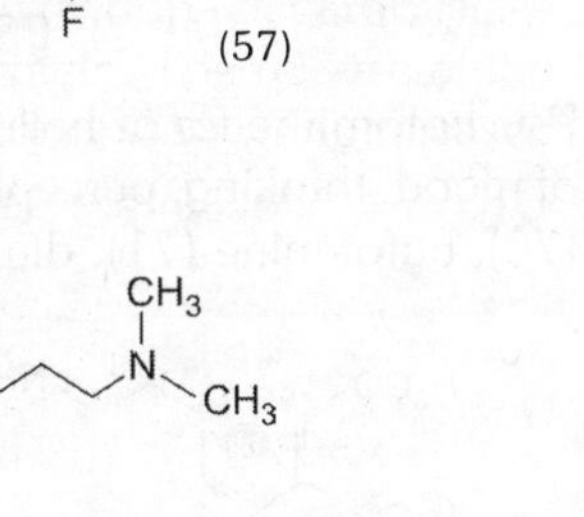

(57)

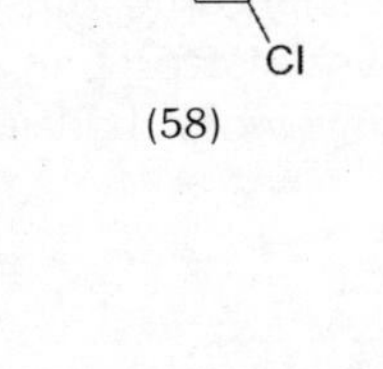

(58)

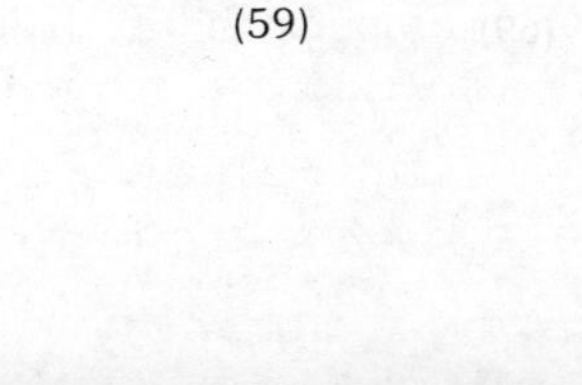

(59)

Miscellaneous Compounds

This class of antidepressants include heterogenous groups of compounds with diverse mechanisms. Reboxetine (60), atomoxetine (61), and maprotiline (62) act by selectively inhibiting norepinephrine (28) reuptake. Among non-selective reuptake inhibitors of biogenic amines venlafaxine (63), milnacipran (64), and duloxetine (65) have been found to be clinically useful. Nomifensene (66) and bupropion (67) are selective inhibitors of norepinephrine (28) and dopamine (29) reuptake while trazodone (68) is an antagonist at $5HT_{2A}$ receptors and a weak inhibitor of serotonin (27) reuptake at presynaptic neuronal membrane.

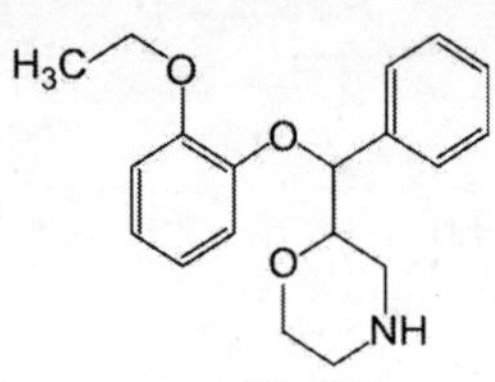

(60) 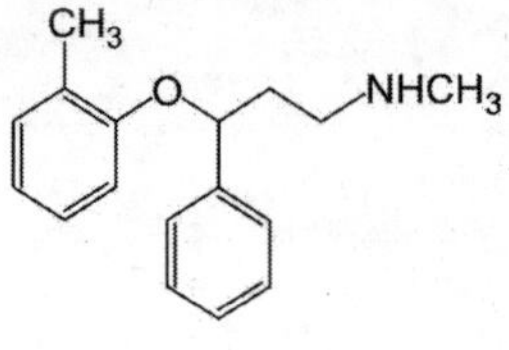   (61) 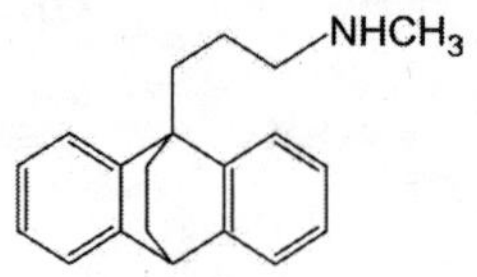   (62)

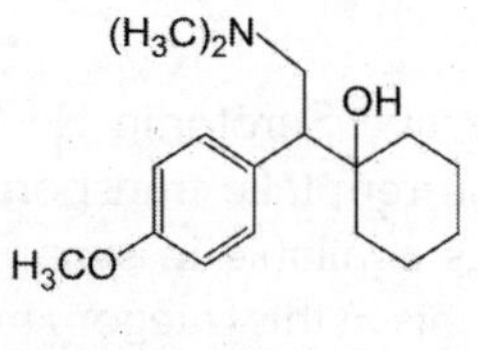

(63) 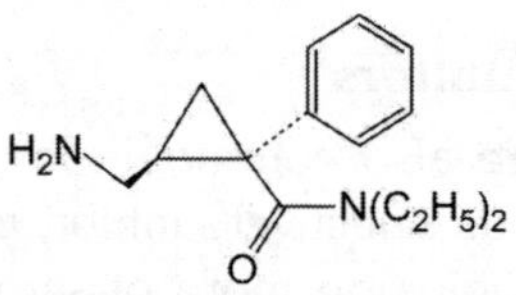   (64) 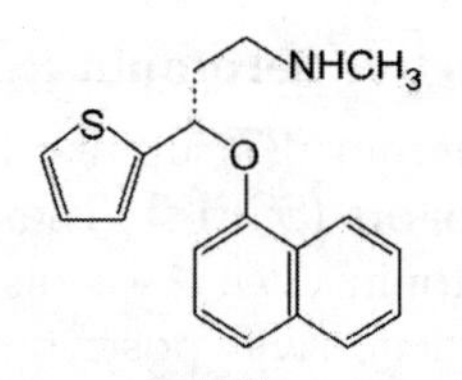   (65)

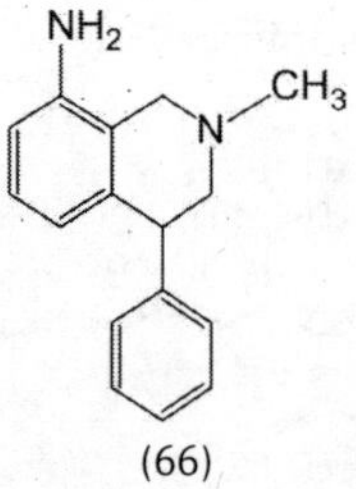

(66) 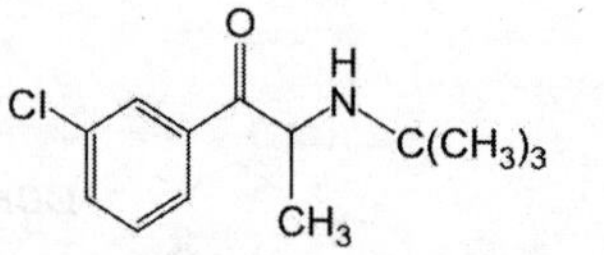   (67) 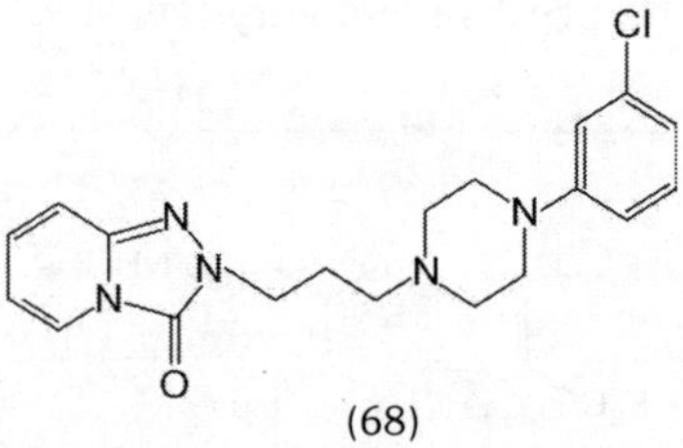   (68)

PSYCHOTOMIMETICS AND HALLUCINOGENS

Psychotomimetics or hallucinogens are the drugs of abuse. They produce in humans altered state of mood, thinking, perception and behaviour. Some of these include mescaline (69), phencyclidine (70), bufotenine (71), dimethyltryptamine (72), and lysergic acid diethylamide (73).

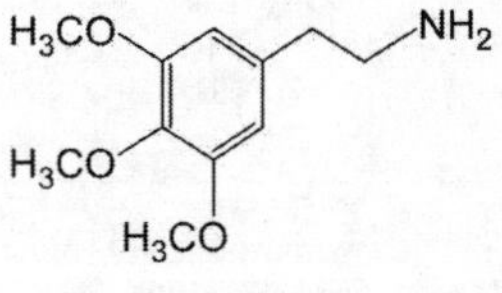

(69) 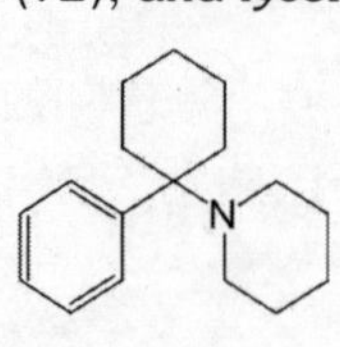   (70) 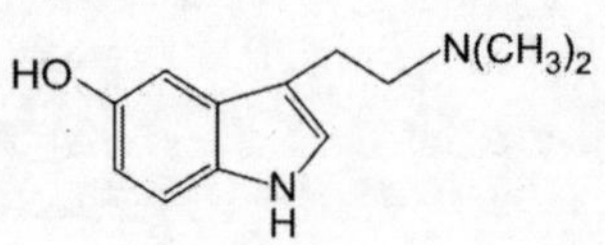   (71)

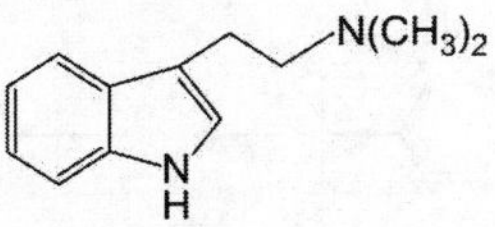

(72)

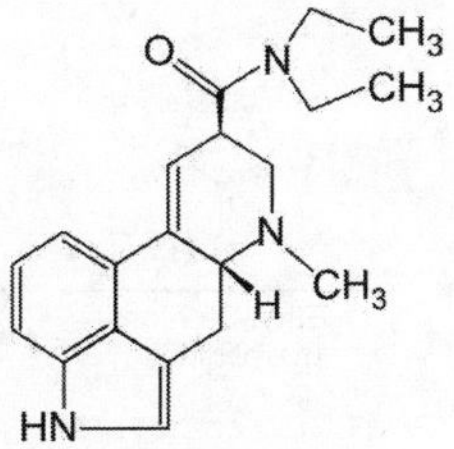

(73)

INDIVIDUAL COMPOUNDS

ANALEPTICS
Strychnine
Strychnidin-10-one

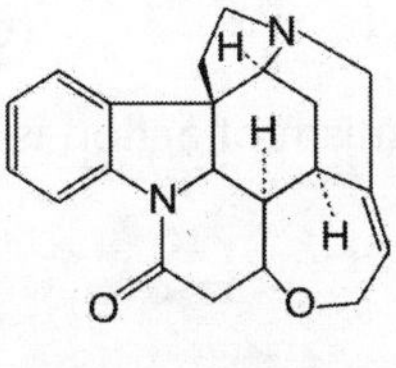

It is an alkaloid obtained from the seeds of *Strychnos nux-vomica* belonging to the family *Loganiaceae*. It is a powerful convulsant and is not used in therapy.

Picrotoxinin
[1a*R*-(1aα,2aβ,3β,6β,6aβ,8a*S**,8bβ,9*R**)-Hexahydro-2a-hydroxy-8b-methyl-9-(1-methylethenyl)-3, 6-methano-8*H*-1, 5, 7-trioxacyclpenta[ij]cycloprop[a]azulene-4, 8(3*H*)-dione

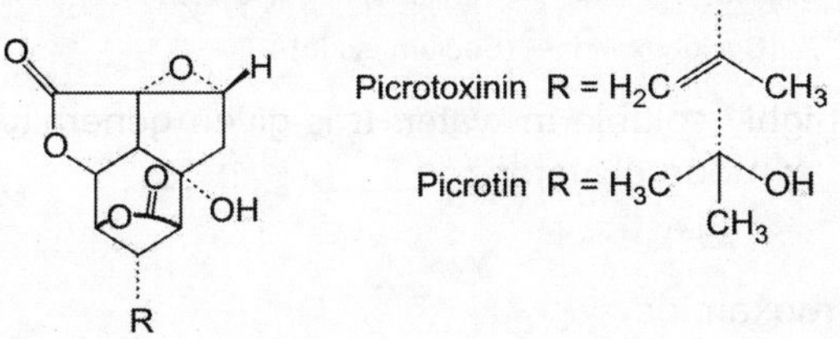

Picrotoxinin R = H_2C―CH_3

Picrotin R = H_3C―OH, CH_3

Picrotoxin, a mixture of picrotoxinin and picrotin, is obtained from *Anamirta cocculus*. Picrotoxinin is the active principle. It is a non-competitive antagonist of GABA.

Doxapram
1-Ethyl-4 [2-(4-morpholinyl) ethyl]-3, 3-diphenyl-2-pyrrolidinone

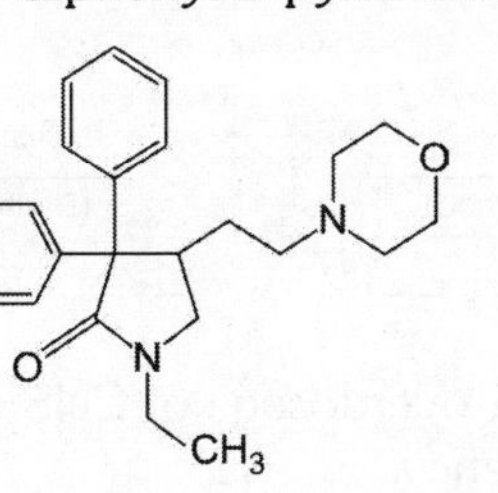

Synthesis

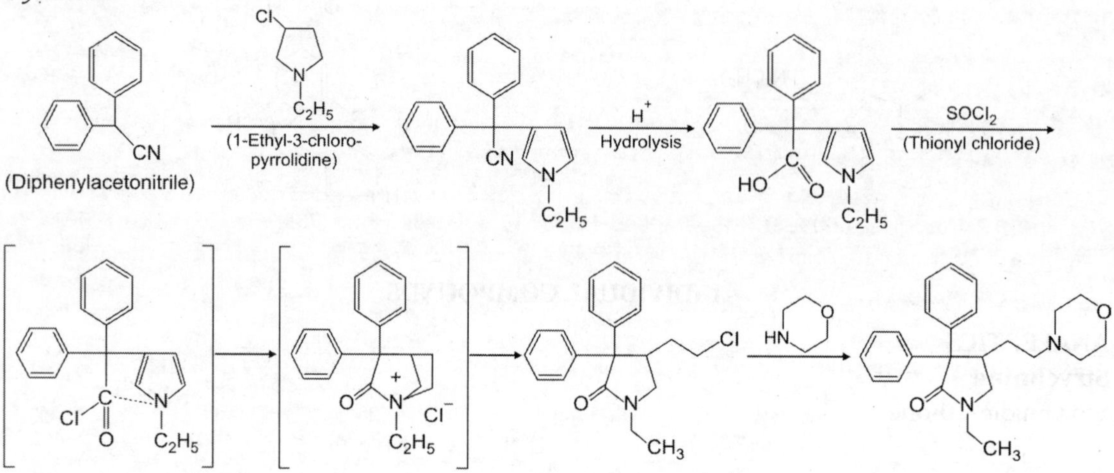

It is a respiratory stimulant. Its mechanism of action is not known.

Pentylenetetrazole
1,5-pentamethylenetetrazole

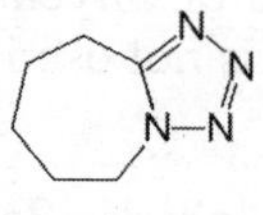

Synthesis

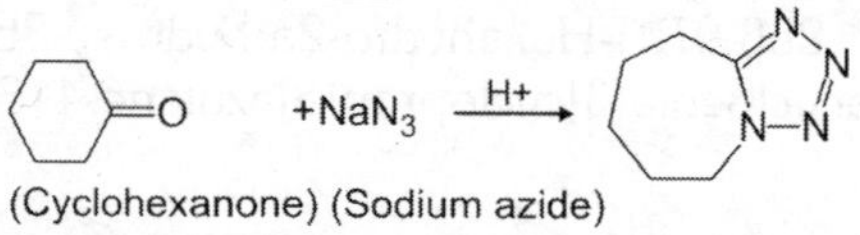

(Cyclohexanone) (Sodium azide)

It is a crystalline solid highly soluble in water. It is given generally by injection. It is used in barbiturate poisoning and as mood elevator.

Nikethamide
N, N-Diethyl-3-pyridinecarboxamide

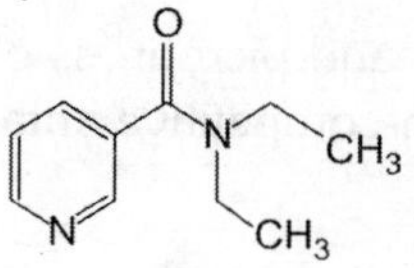

Synthesis

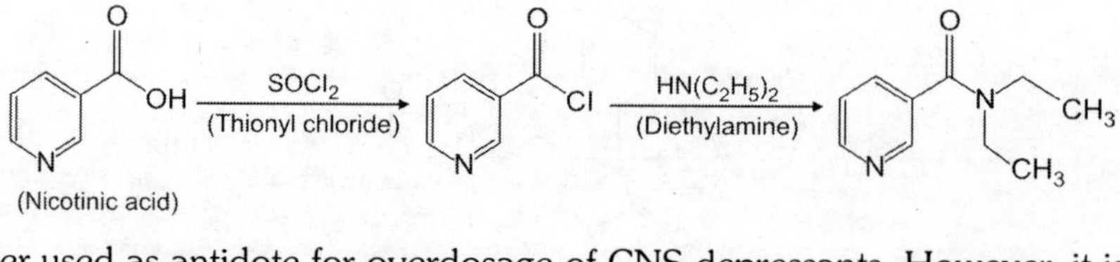

(Nicotinic acid)

It was earlier used as antidote for overdosage of CNS depressants. However, it is now used as respiratory stimulant only in emergency.

PSYCHOMOTOR STIMULANTS
Dexamphetamine
(+)-(S)-α-Methylphenethylamine

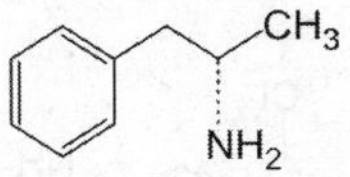

Synthesis

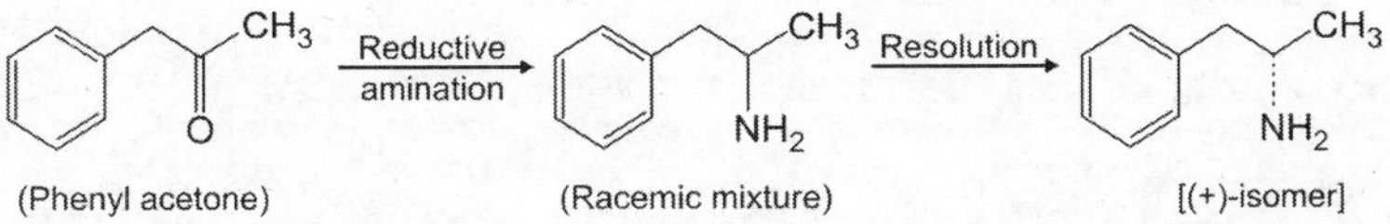

(Phenyl acetone)   (Racemic mixture)   [(+)-isomer]

Dexamphetamine, the (+)-isomer, is the active form of the racemic amphetamine. It is usually used as sulphate or phosphate salt. It acts by releasing norepinephrine (28), dopamine (29), and serotonin (27) from nerve terminals.

Methamphetamine, Phentermine, and Benzphetamine
See DRUGS ACTING ON ADRENERGIC RECEPTORS

Fenfluramine
N-Ethyl-α-methyl-3-(trifluoromethyl)phenylethylamine

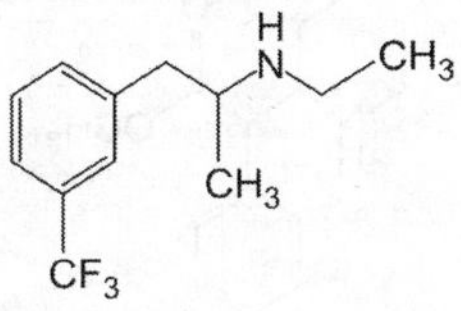

Synthesis

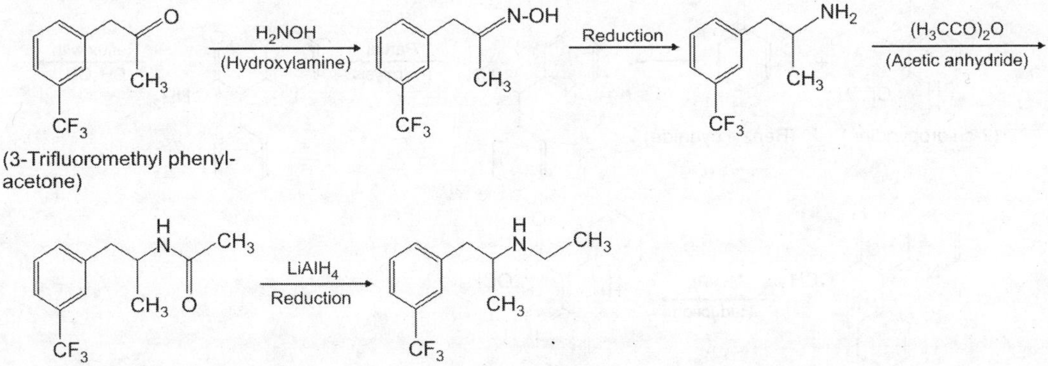

(3-Trifluoromethyl phenylacetone)

It is also used as appetite suppressant. It has sedative effect rather than CNS stimulatory effect. This action may be due to release of serotonin (27) rather than norepinephrine (28) and dopamine (29). It is used as hydrochloride salt. Its (+)-isomer is used clinically.

Chlorphentermine

See DRUGS ACTING ON ADRENERGIC RECEPTORS

Clortermine

2-Chloro-α,α-dimethylphenethylamine

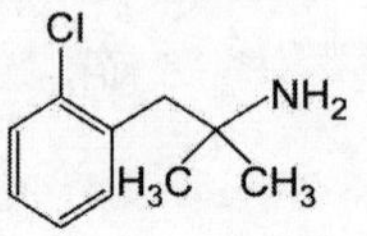

Synthesis

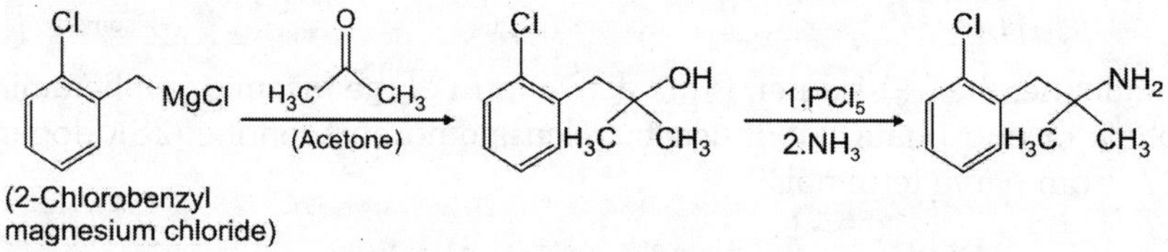

(2-Chlorobenzyl
magnesium chloride)

It is the *o*-isomer of chlorphentermine (14) and is used as hydrochloride as appetite suppressant.

Methylphenidate

α-Phenyl-2-piperidineacetic acid methyl ester

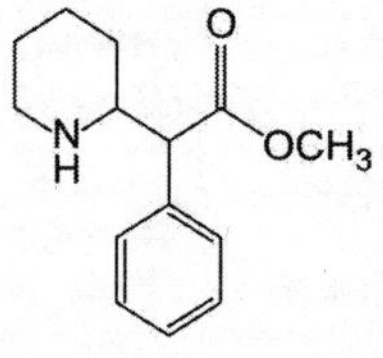

Synthesis

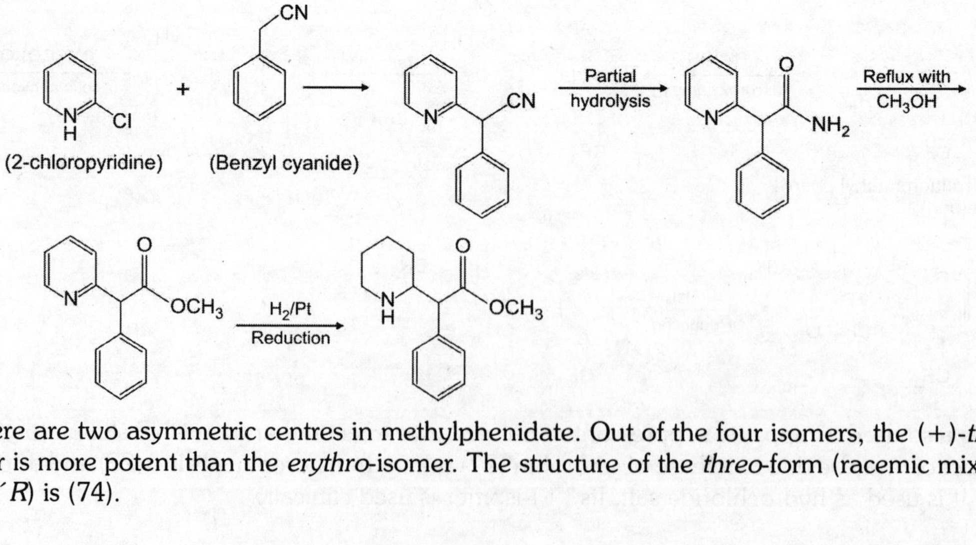

(2-chloropyridine)   (Benzyl cyanide)

There are two asymmetric centres in methylphenidate. Out of the four isomers, the (+)-*threo*-isomer is more potent than the *erythro*-isomer. The structure of the *threo*-form (racemic mixture) (2R, 2′R) is (74).

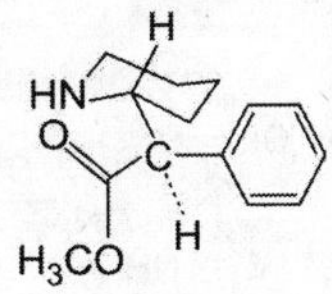

(74)

Methylphenidate and its *p*-hydroxy metabolite block the uptake of norepinephrine (28), and act as postsynaptic agonist. It also blocks the dopamine (29) uptake. It is used as hydrochloride.

Caffeine

1,3,7-Trimethylxanthine

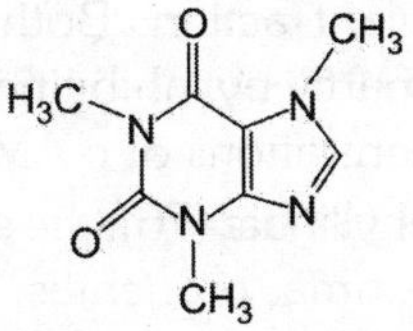

Synthesis

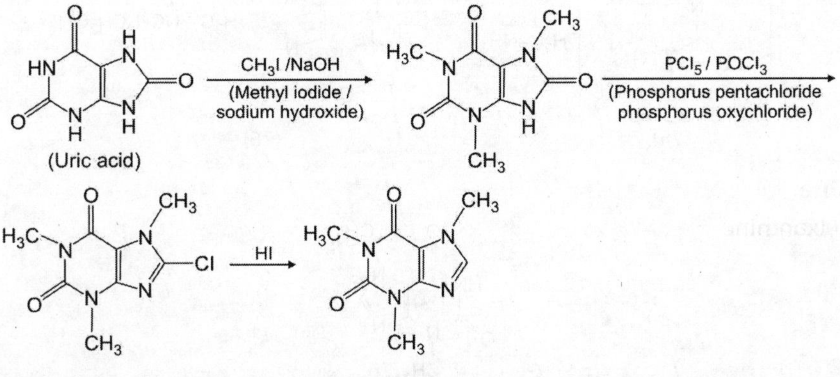

Caffeine, is a constituent of coffee, tea, and cola beverages. It is used as a CNS stimulant facilitating clear thinking and ability to concentrate. In higher doses, it causes restlessness, nervousness, and anxiety. It is not used clinically.

Theophylline

1,3-Dimethylxanthine

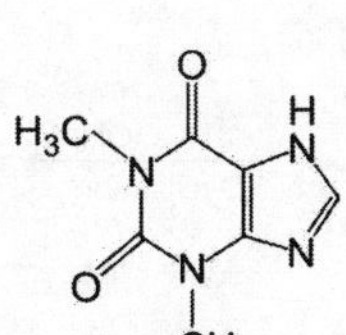

Synthesis

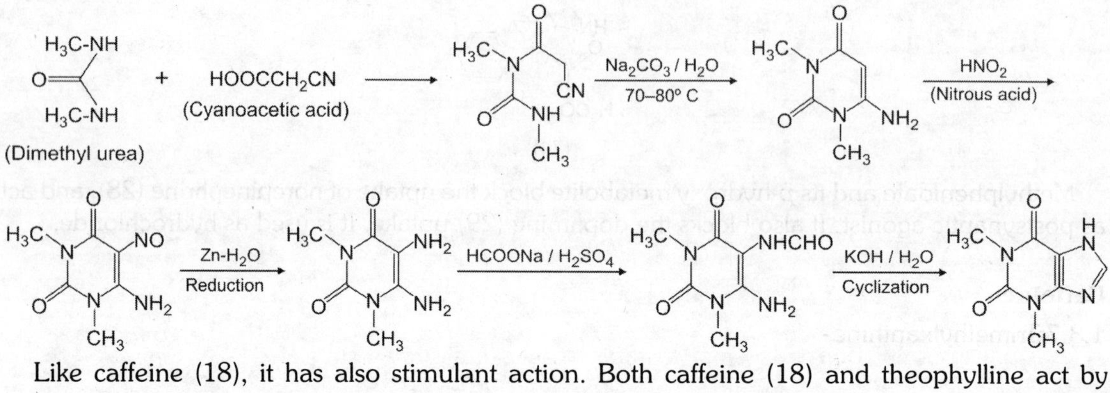

Like caffeine (18), it has also stimulant action. Both caffeine (18) and theophylline act by antagonism at A_2-purine receptors and partly by inhibiting phosphodiesterase which is responsible for hydrolysis of c-AMP. Increased concentrations of c-AMP lead to smooth muscle relaxation.

Aminophylline (75) and choline theophyllinate (76), the salts of theophylline with ethylenediamine and choline, respectively, are used in asthma, bronchitis, and in respiratory diseases.

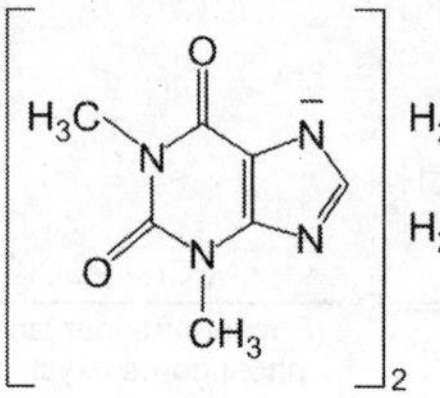

(75) 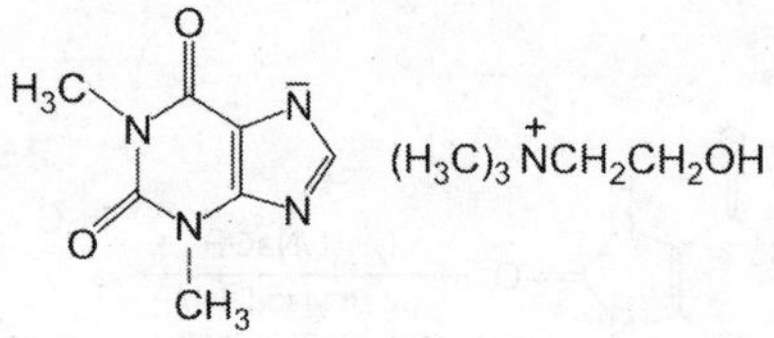   (76)

Theobromine
3,7-Dimethylxanthine

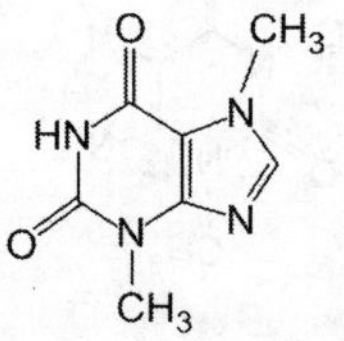

Synthesis

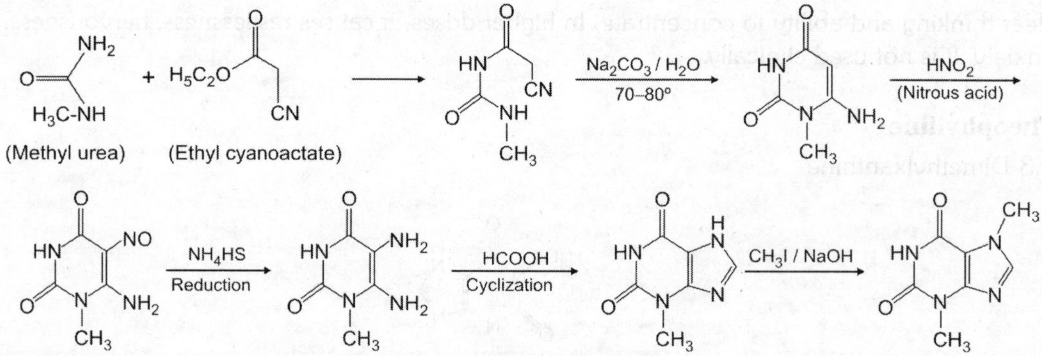

Theobromine was used earlier as a diuretic and in hypertension.

Diprophylline
7-(2,3-Dihydroxypropyl)theophylline

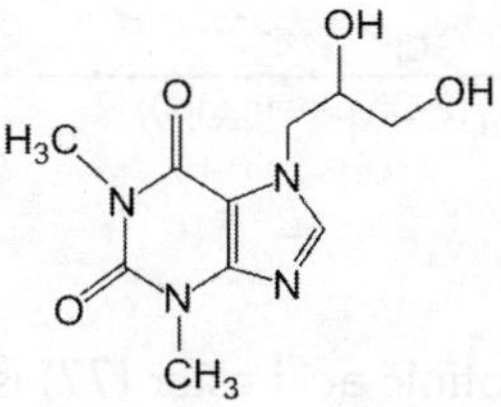

Synthesis

(Theophylline)

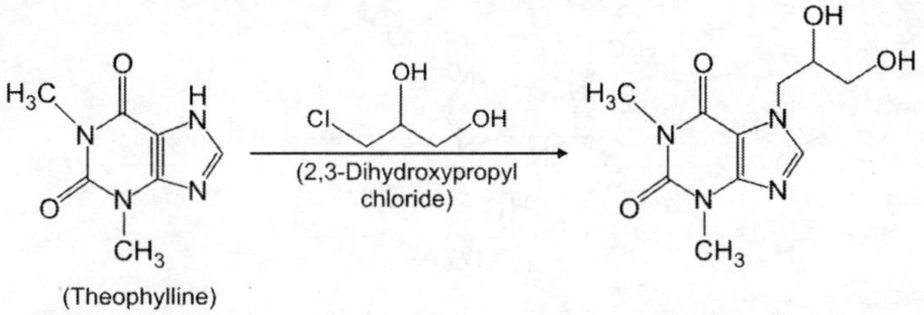

It is used as a bronchodilator.

Etamiphyllin
7-(2-Diethylaminoethyl)theophylline

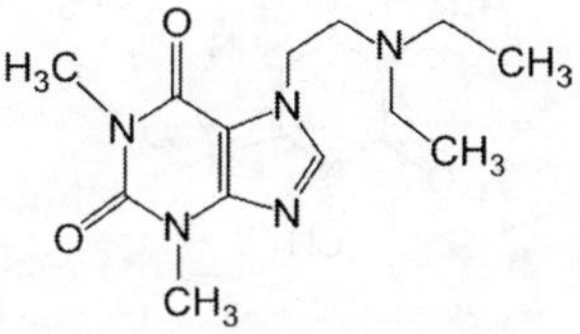

Synthesis

(Theophyline)

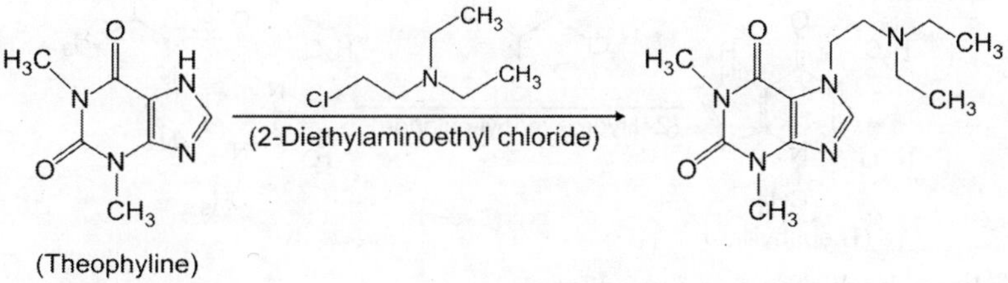

It is used as bronchodilator.

Etofylline
7-(2-Hydroxyethyl)theophylline

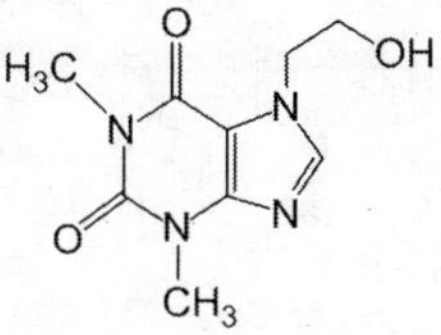

Synthesis

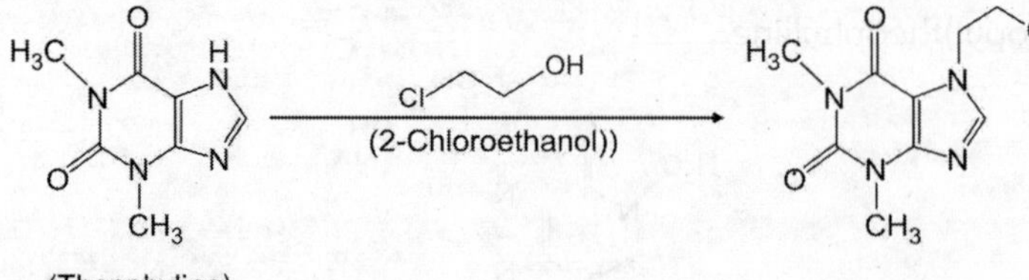

(Theophyline)   (2-Chloroethanol))

It is used as a bronchodilator. Its nicotinic acid ester (77) is used as vasodilator.

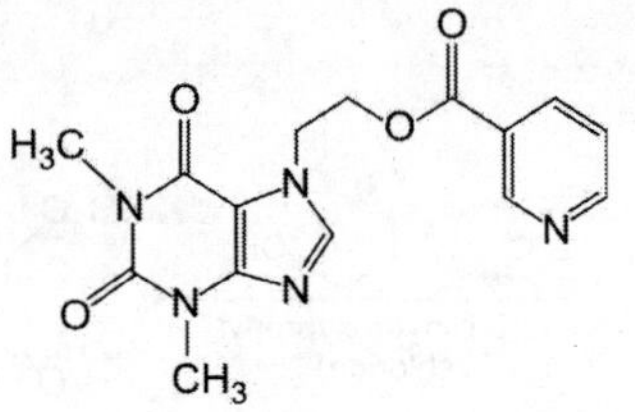

(77)

Proxyphylline
7-(2-Hydroxypropyl)theophylline

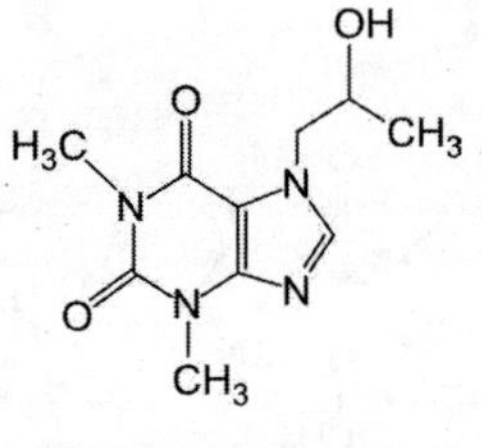

Synthesis

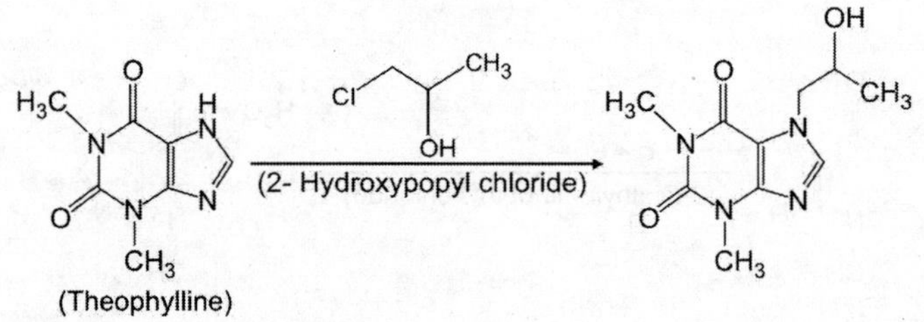

(Theophyllline)   (2- Hydroxypopyl chloride)

It is used as bronchodilator and vasodilator.

Doxofylline
7-(1,3-Dioxolan-2-yl-methyl)theophylline

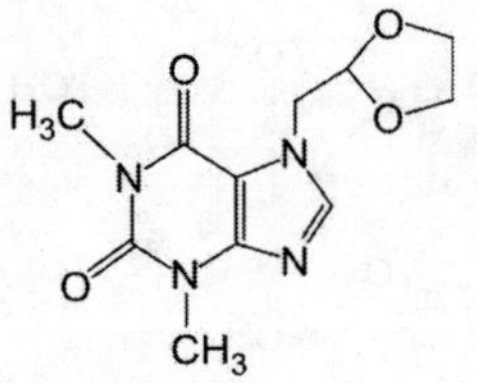

Synthesis

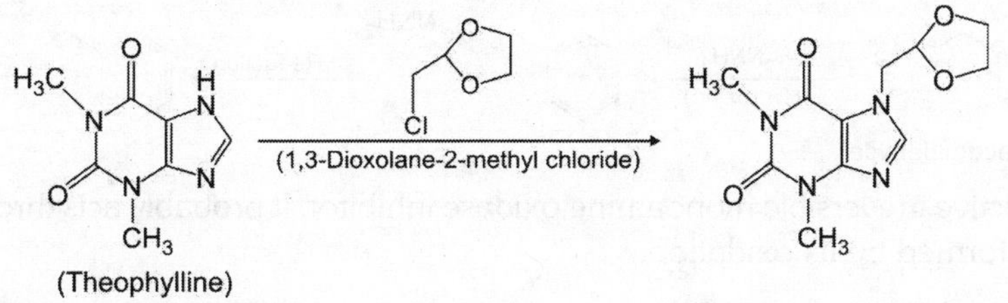

(Theophylline)

It is used as bronchodilator.

Pentoxifylline
1-(5-Oxohexyl)theobromine

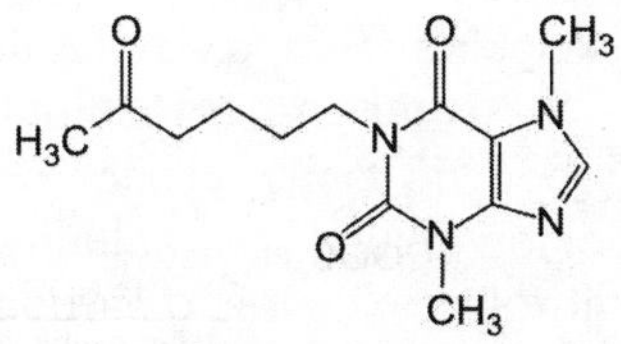

Synthesis

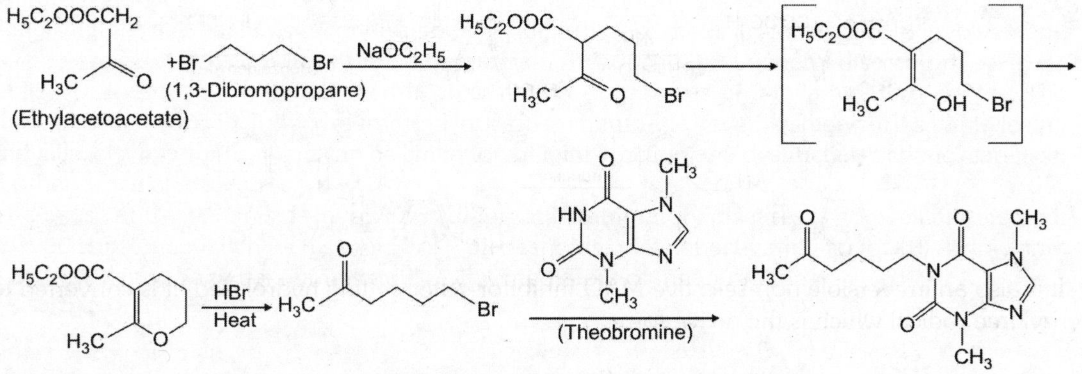

It has a greater selectivity for vascular smooth muscle.

ANTIDEPRESSANTS : MONOAMINE OXIDASE INHIBITORS
Phenelzine
(2-Phenylethyl) hydrazine

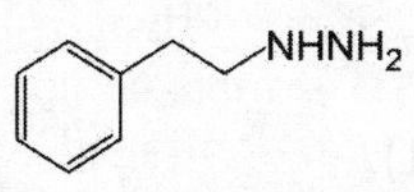

Synthesis

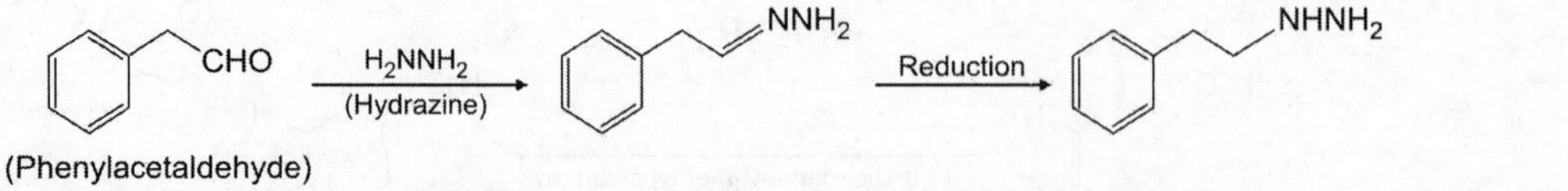

(Phenylacetaldehyde)

It is a non-selective irreversible monoamine oxidase inhibitor. It probably acts through phenylethyl radical which is formed by its oxidation.

Isocarboxazid
5-Methyl-3-isoxazolecarboxylic acid 2-benzylhydrazide

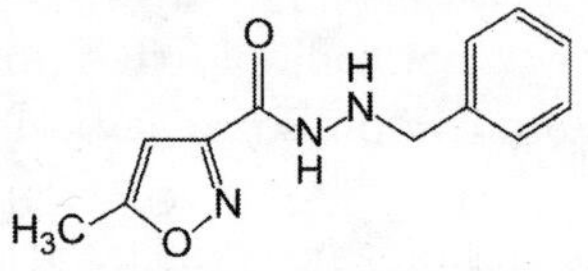

Synthesis

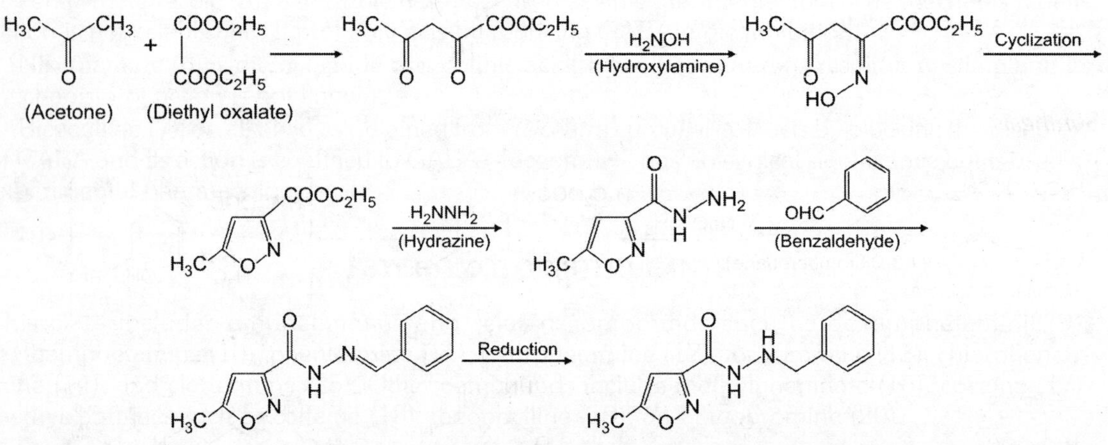

(Acetone)   (Diethyl oxalate)

It is also an irreversible non-selective MAO inhibitor. After getting hydrolyzed, it is converted to benzyl free radical which is the active form.

Pheniprazine
(1-Methyl-2-phenethyl)hydrazine

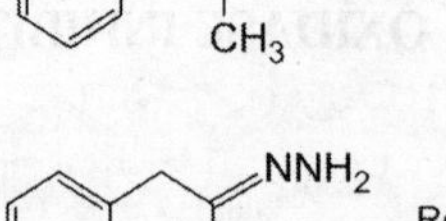

Synthesis

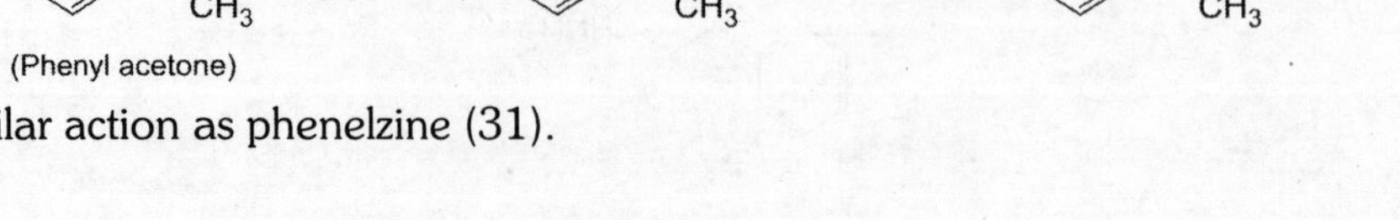

(Phenyl acetone)

It has similar action as phenelzine (31).

Tranylcypromine

trans-(±)-2-Phenylcyclopropanamine

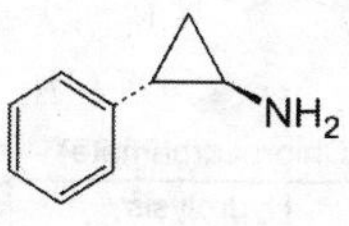

Synthesis

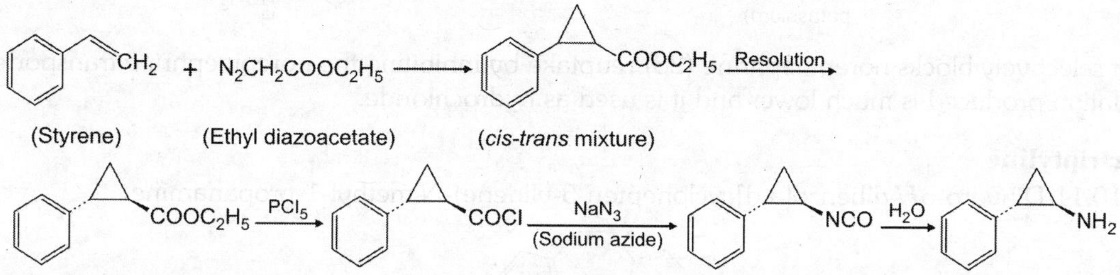

(Styrene)   (Ethyl diazoacetate)   (*cis-trans* mixture)

It is used as a sulphate salt. It acts by inhibiting MAO through its free radical formed after opening of the cyclopropyl ring.

Moclobemide

4-Chloro-*N*-[2-(4-morpholinoethyl)]benzamide

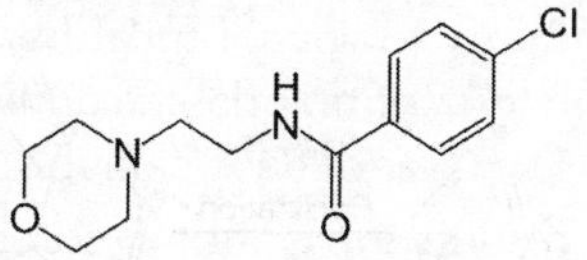

Synthesis

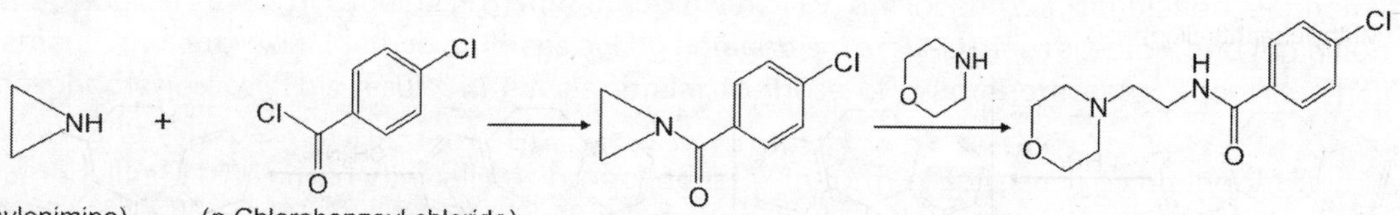

(Ethylenimine)   (*p*-Chlorobenzoyl chloride)

It is a non-hydrazine MAO inhibitor antidepressant and is specific for MAO-A type enzyme which has substrate preference for serotonin (27).

ANTIDEPRESSANTS : TRICYCLIC ANTIDEPRESSANTS

Protriptyline

N-Methyl-5*H*-dibenzo[a,d]cycloheptene-5-propanamine

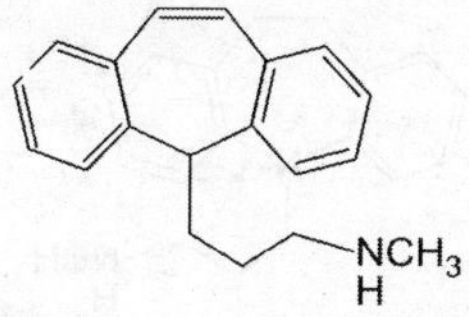

Synthesis

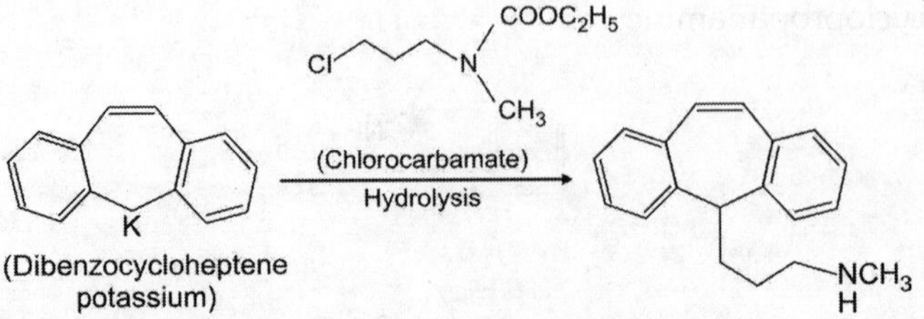

It selectively blocks norepinephrine (28) reuptake by inhibiting the norepinephrine transporter. Sedation produced is much lower and it is used as hydrochloride.

Nortriptyline

3-(10,11-Dihydro-5*H*-dibenzo[a,d]cyclohepten-5-ylidene)-*N*-methyl-1-propanamine

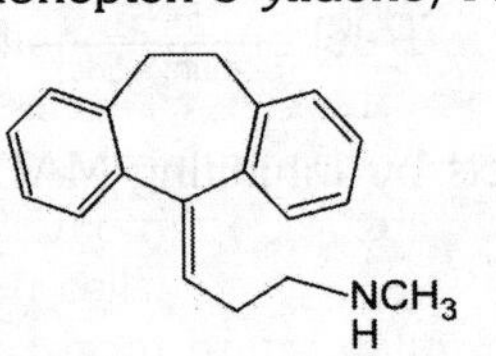

Synthesis

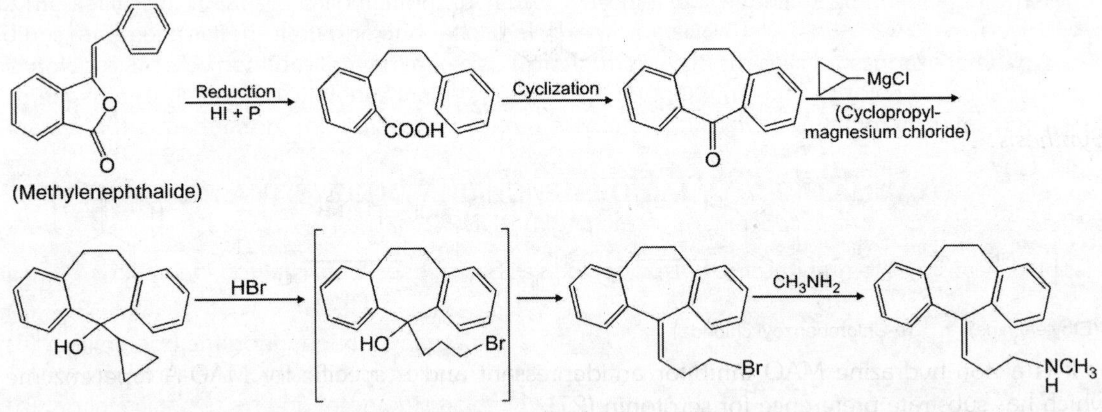

Activity and mechanism similar to protriptyline (42).

Desipramine

10, 11-Dihydro-*N*-methyl-5*H*-dibenz[b,f]azepine-5-propanamine

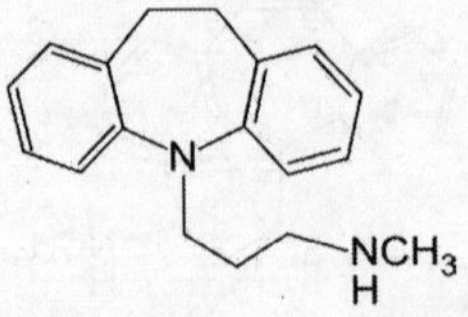

Synthesis

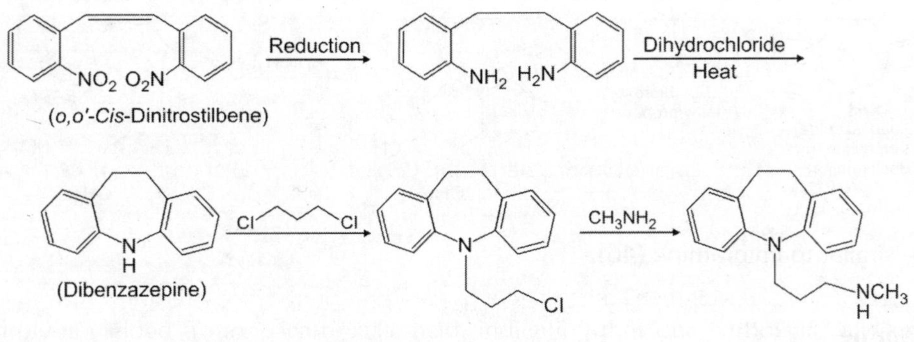

(*o,o'-Cis*-Dinitrostilbene)

(Dibenzazepine)

Activity and mechanism similar to protriptyline (42).

Amoxapine
See NEUROLEPTICS AND ANXIOLYTIC AGENTS

Imipramine
10,11-Dihydro-N, N-dimethyl-5H-dibenz[b,f]azepine-5-propanamine

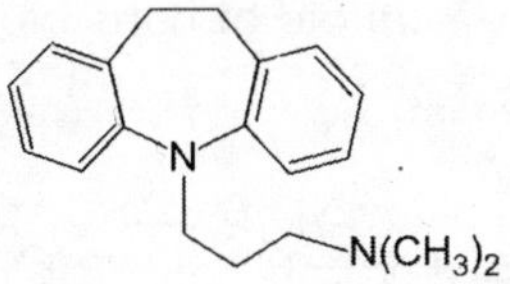

Synthesis

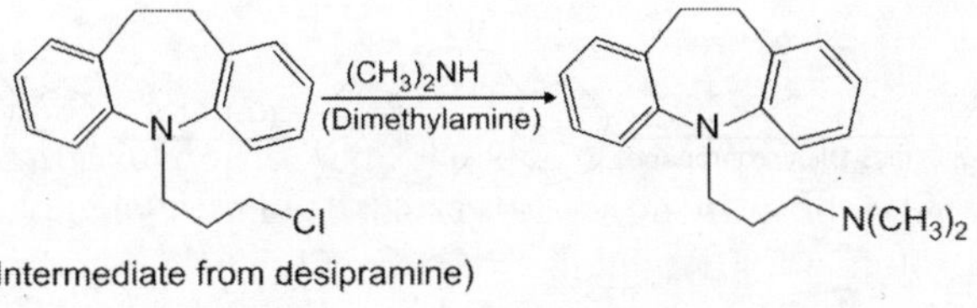

(Intermediate from desipramine)

It is non-selective inhibitor of reuptake of various biogenic amines. It is used as hydrochloride.

Trimipramine
10,11-Dihydro-N,N, β-trimethyl-5H-dibenz[b,f]azepine-5-propanamine

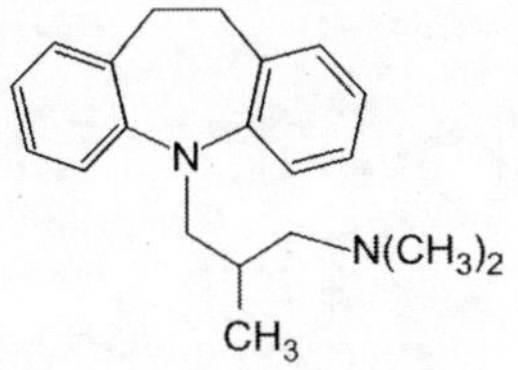

Synthesis

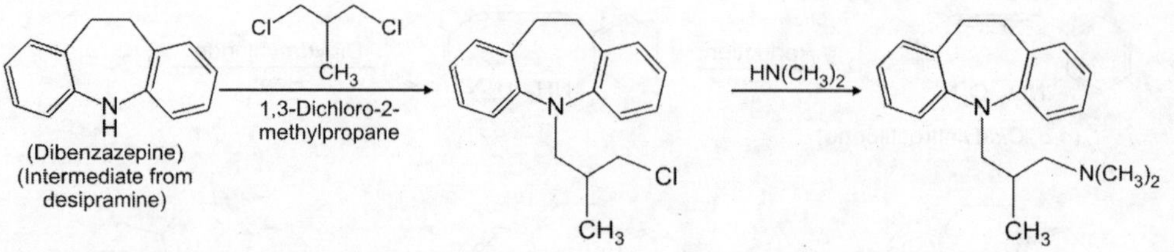

Activity similar to imipramine (46).

Clomipramine

3-Chloro-10,11-dihydro-*N*,*N*-dimethyl-5*H*-dibenz[b,f]azepine-5-propanamine

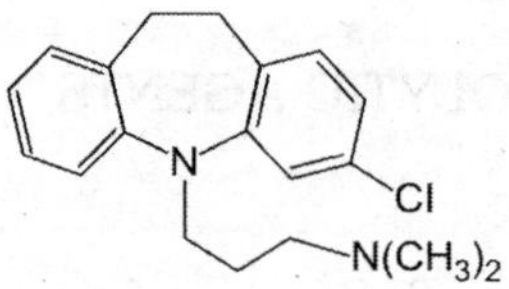

Synthesis

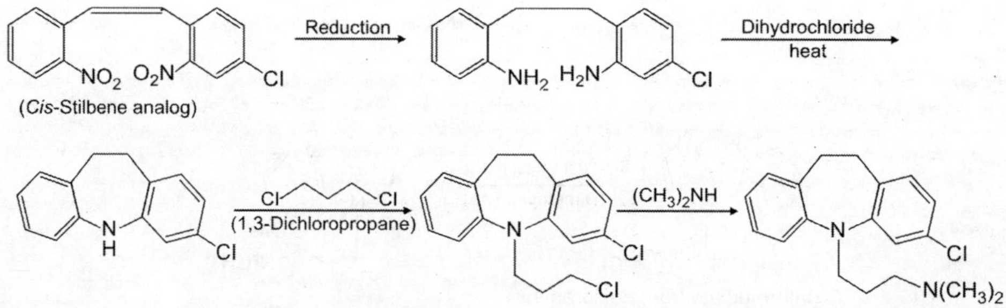

It is about 50 times as potent as imipramine (46). Mechanism similar to that of imipramine (46).

Amitriptyline

3-(10,11-Dihydro-5*H*-dibenzo[a,d]cyclohepten-5-ylidene)-*N*, *N*-dimethyl-1-propanamine

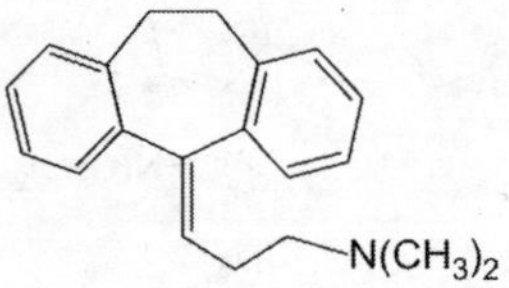

Synthesis

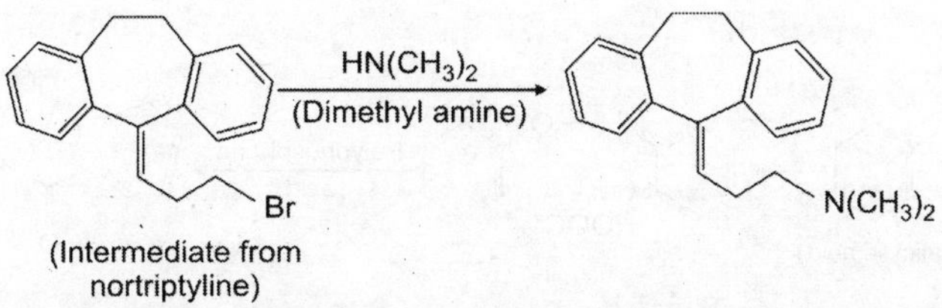

(Intermediate from nortriptyline)

It is used as hydrochloride and embonate salt. The side effects include anticholinergic actions such as dryness of mouth, blurred vision, tachycardia and urinary retention. Its *N*-oxide (78) analog is also used as antidepressant.

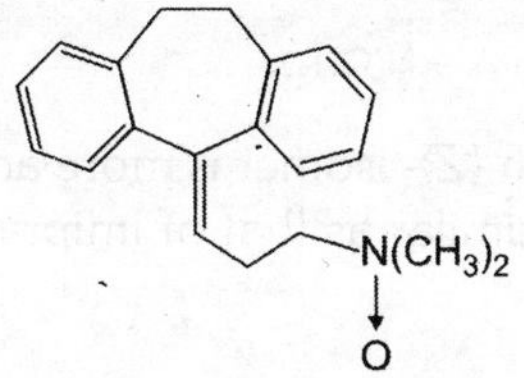

(78)

Lofepramine

1-(4-Chlorophenyl)-2[[3-(10, 11-dihydro-5*H*-dibenz[b, f]azepin-5-yl)propyl]methylamino]ethanone

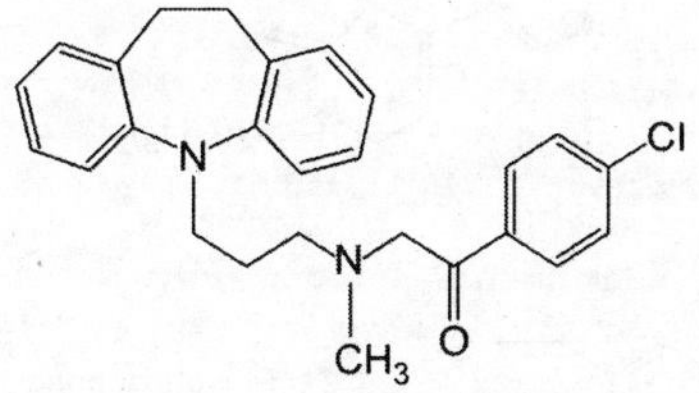

Synthesis

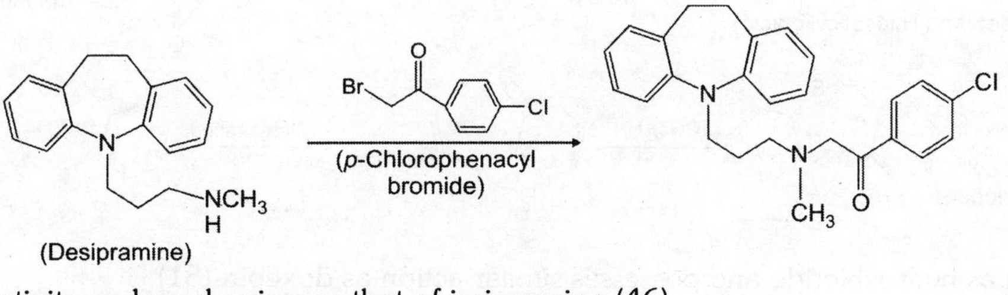

(Desipramine)

(*p*-Chlorophenacyl bromide)

Similar activity and mechanism as that of imipramine (46).

Doxepin

11-(3-Dimethylaminopropylidene)-6,11-dihydrodibenz[b,e]oxepin

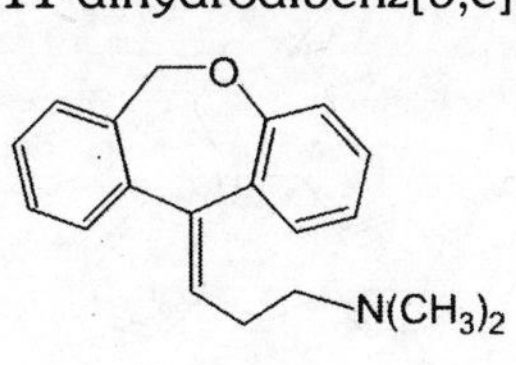

Synthesis

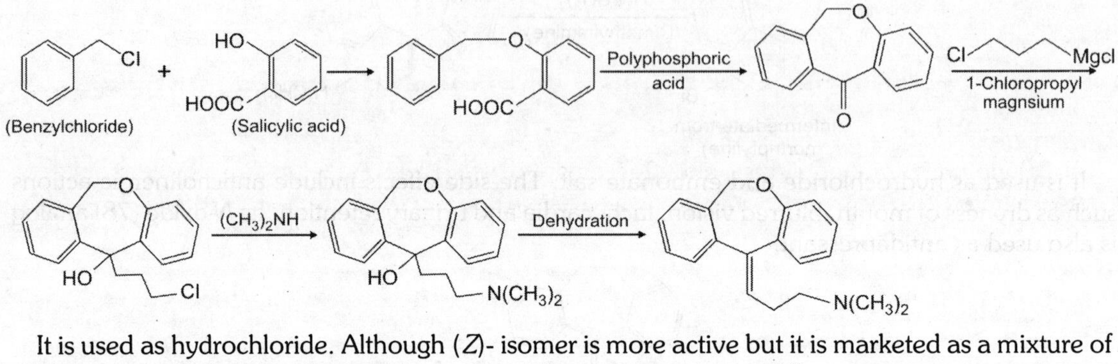

It is used as hydrochloride. Although (*Z*)- isomer is more active but it is marketed as a mixture of two isomers. Mechanism of action is similar as that of imipramine (46).

Dothiepin

3-Dibenzo[b,e]thiepin-11(6*H*)-ylidene-*N*, *N*-dimethyl-1-propanamine

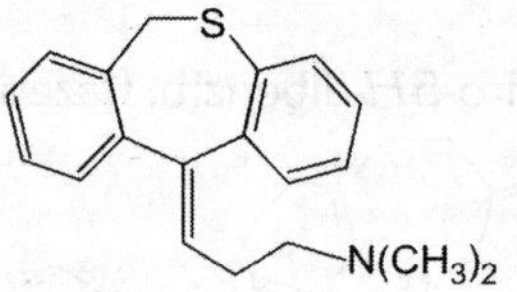

Synthesis

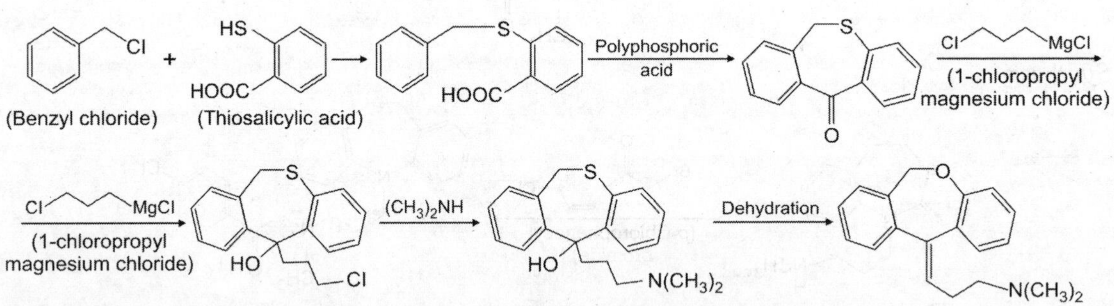

It is used as hydrochloride and possesses similar action as doxepin (51).

Mianserin

1,2,3,4,10,14b-Hexahydro-2-methyldibenzo[c.f]pyrazino[1,2-a]azepine

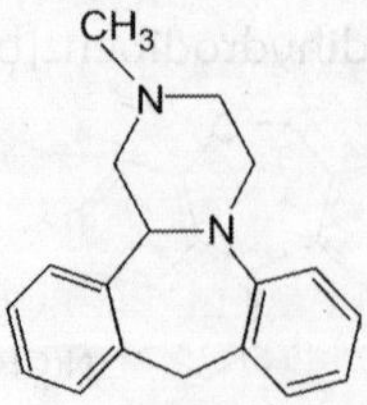

Synthesis

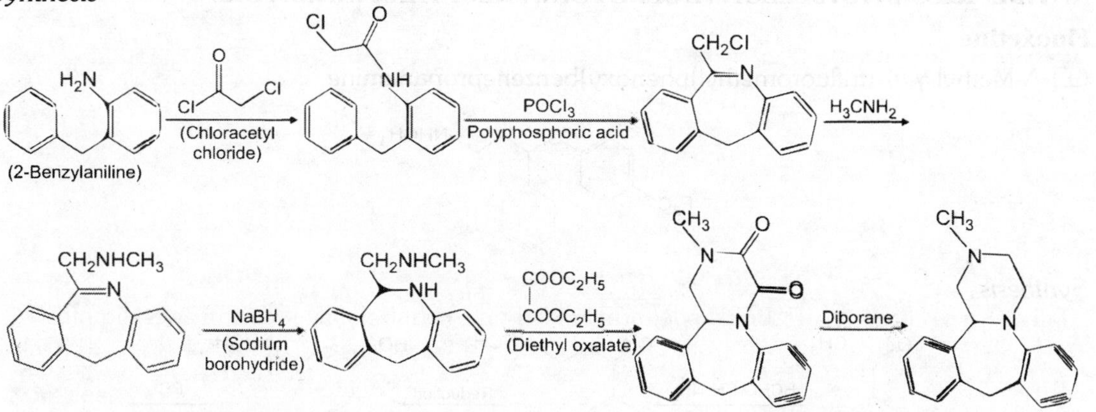

It is a potent antagonist at several post synaptic serotonin receptors. Side effects include agraulocytosis and leukepenia.

Mirtazapine

2-Methyl-1,2,3,4,10,14b- hexahydrobenzo[c]pyrazino[1,2-a]pyrido[3,2-f]azepine

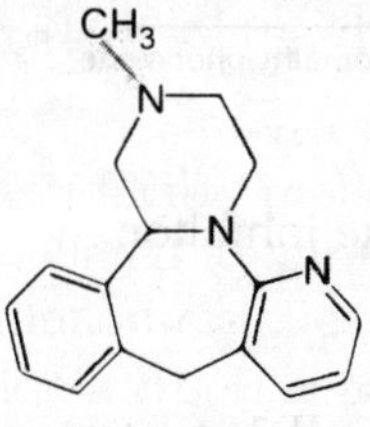

Synthesis

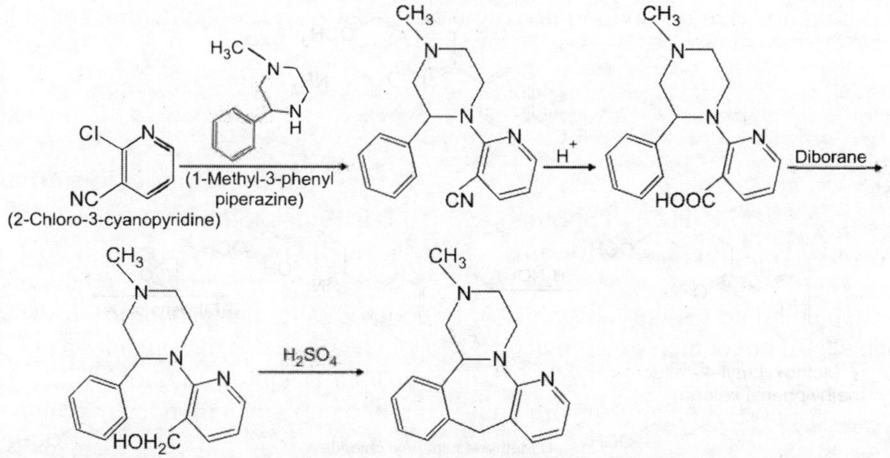

It is an isostere of mianserin (53) in which one of the benzene ring of mianserin (53) has been replaced by its isostere pyridine. It is antagonist at several post synaptic serotonin receptors as well as inhibitor of presynaptic a₂-adrenergic receptors. It is also a potent H_1-receptor antagonist, which results in sedative action.

ANTIDEPRESSANTS : SELECTIVE SEROTONIN REUPTAKE INHIBITORS

Fluoxetine

(±)-N-Methyl-γ-[4-(trifluoromethyl)phenoxy]benzenepropanamine

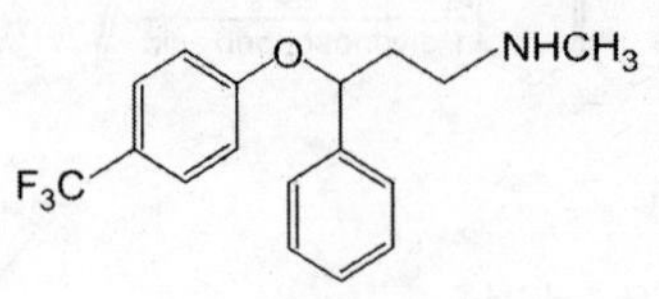

Synthesis

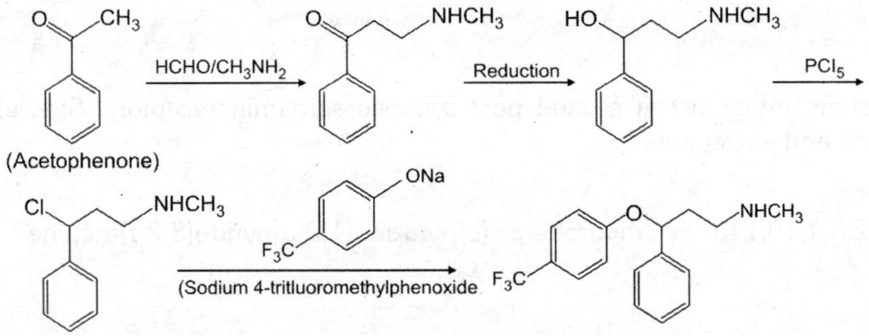

(Acetophenone)

(Sodium 4-trifluoromethylphenoxide)

It is a selective serotonin (27) reuptake inhibitor.

Fluvoxamine

(E)-5-Methoxy-1-[4-trifluoromethyl)phenyl]-1-pentanone O-(2-aminoethyl)oxime

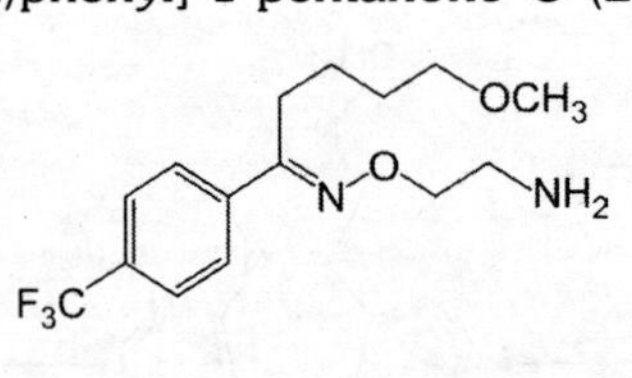

Synthesis

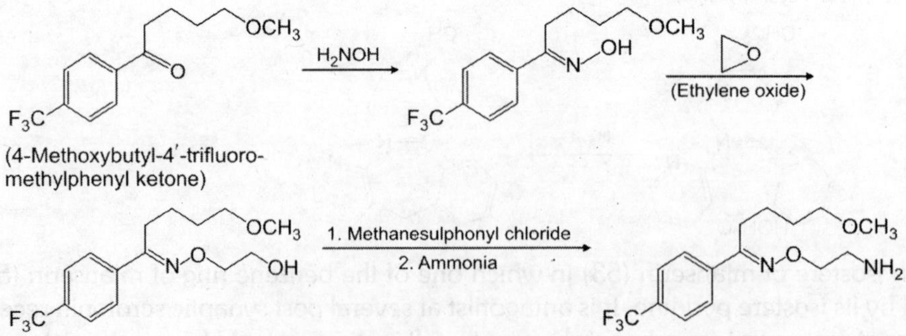

(4-Methoxybutyl-4′-trifluoro-
methylphenyl ketone)

1. Methanesulphonyl chloride
2. Ammonia

Same activity as fluoxetine (55). The E-isomer of the oxime is active.

Paroxetine

(–)-*trans*-4(*p*-Fluorophenyl)-3[[3,4-(methylenedioxy)phenoxy]methyl]piperidine

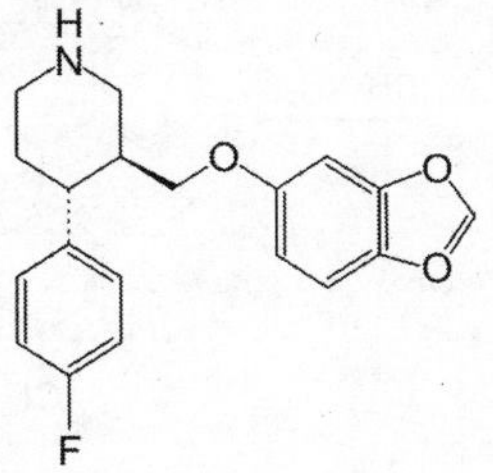

Synthesis

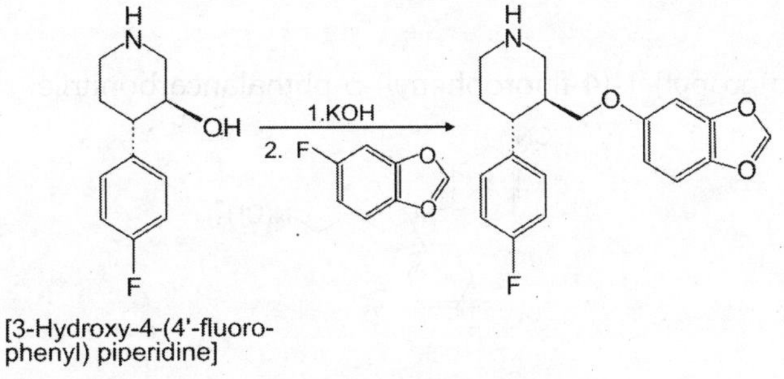

[3-Hydroxy-4-(4'-fluoro-phenyl) piperidine]

Same activity as fluoxetine (55). The *trans*-isomer is active.

Sertraline

(1*S*,4*S*)-4-(3, 4-Dichlorophenyl)-1,2,3,4-tetrahydro-*N*-methyl-1-naphthalenamine

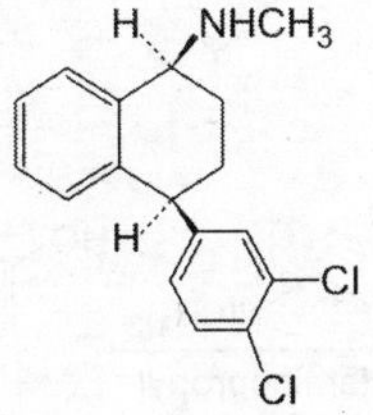

Synthesis

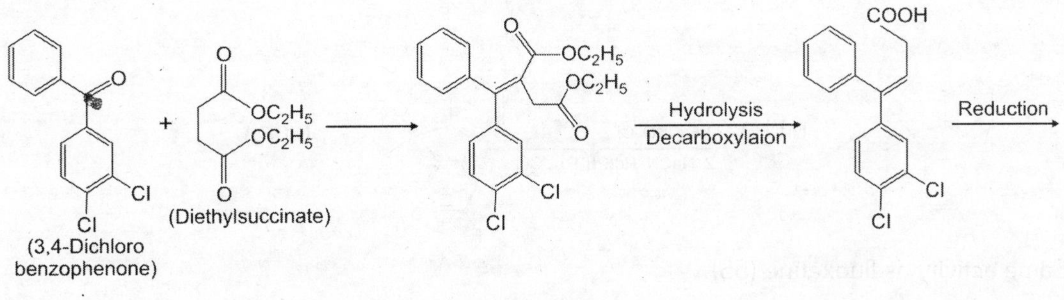

(3,4-Dichloro benzophenone)

(Diethylsuccinate)

Hydrolysis
Decarboxylaion

Reduction

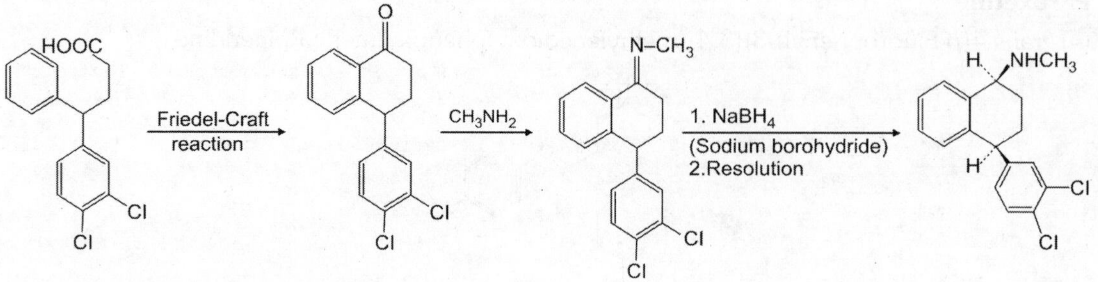

Same activity as fluoxetine (55).

Citalopram

1-[3-(Dimethylamino)propyl]-1-(4-fluorophenyl)-5-phthalancarbonitrile

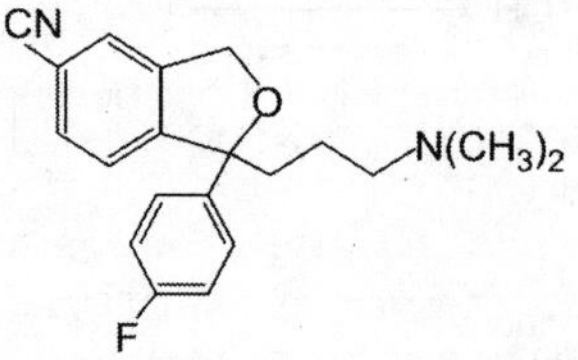

Synthesis

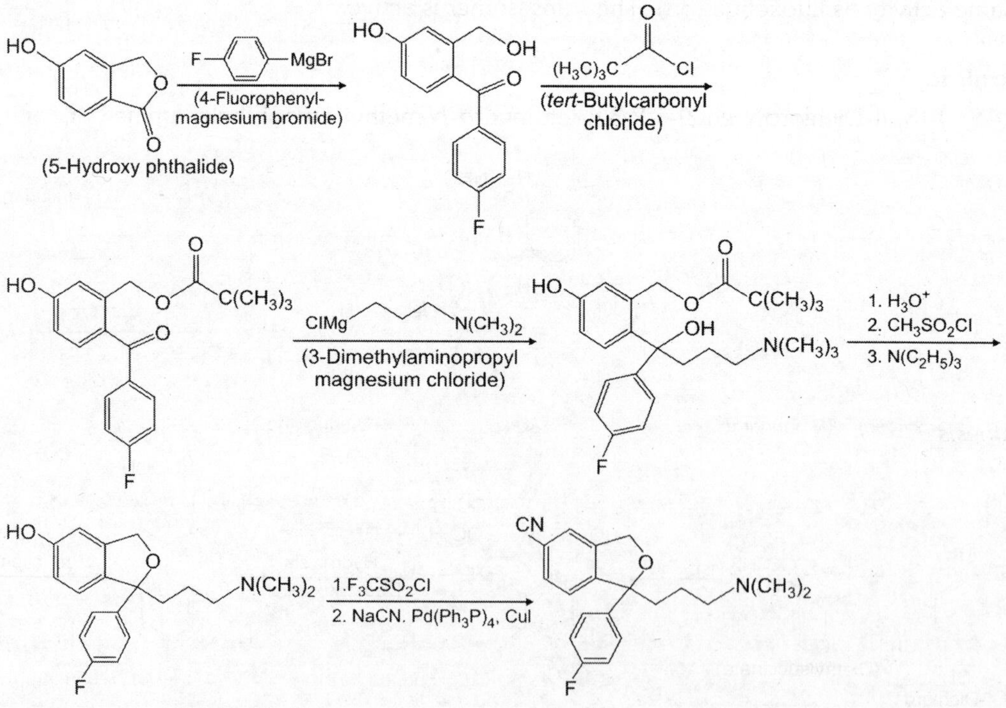

Same activity as fluoxetine (55).

ANTIDEPRESSANTS: MISCELLANEOUS COMPOUNDS

Reboxetine

(±)-(2R)-2-[(αR)-α-(o-Ethoxyphenoxy)benzyl]morpholine

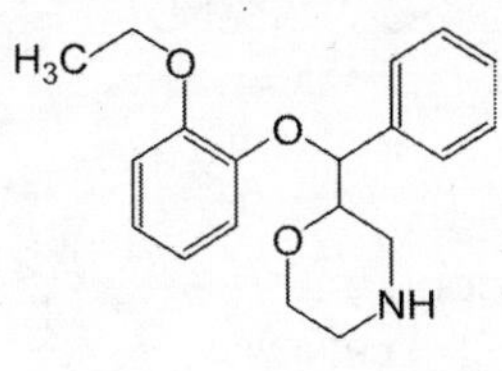

Synthesis

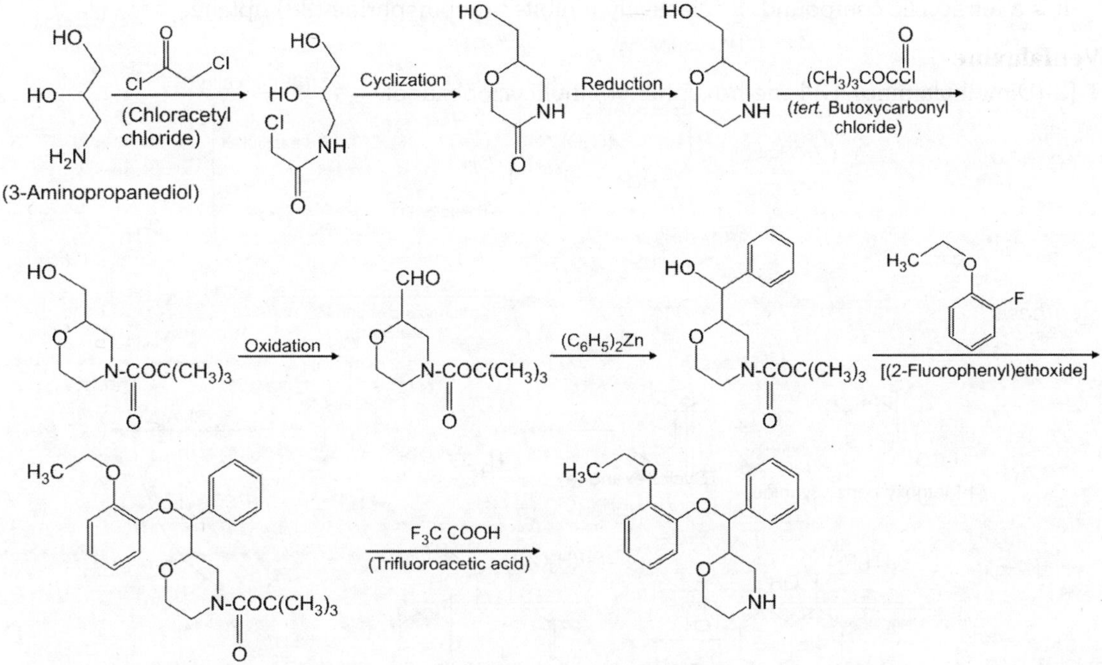

It selectively inhibits the reuptake of norepinephrine (28).

Maprotiline

N-Methyl-9, 10-ethanoanthracene-9(10H)-propanamine

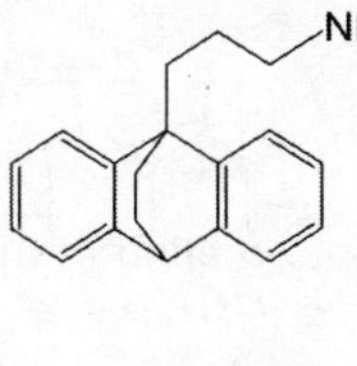

Synthesis

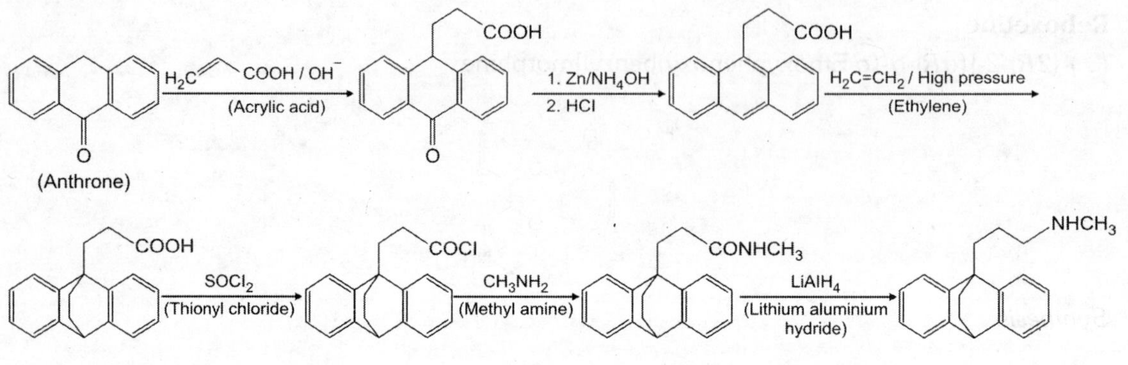

It is a tetracyclic compound. It selectively inhibits norepinephrine (28) uptake.

Venlafaxine

1-[2-(Dimethylamino)-1-(4-methoxyphenyl)ethyl]cyclohexanol

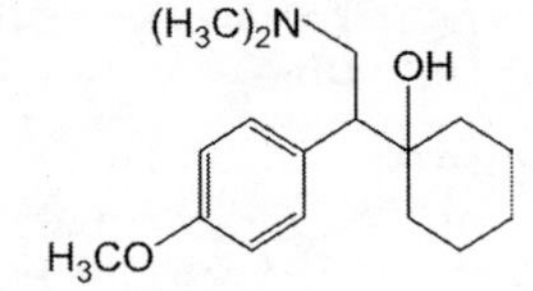

Synthesis

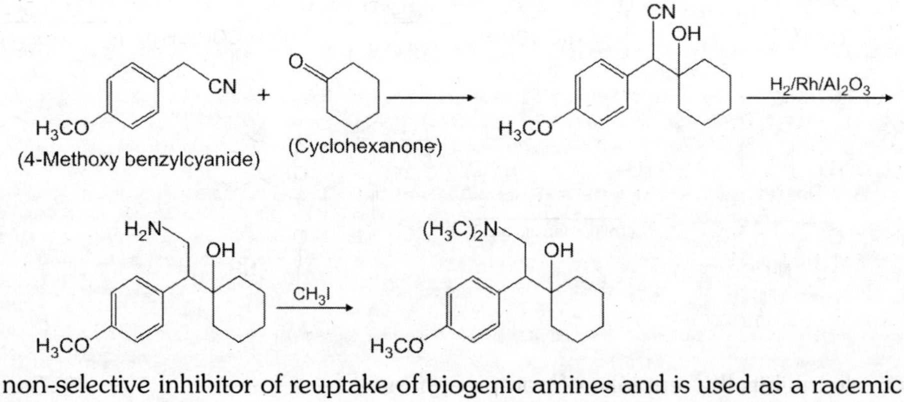

It is a non-selective inhibitor of reuptake of biogenic amines and is used as a racemic mixture.

Duloxetine

(+)-(S)-N-Methyl-γ-(1-naphthyloxy)-2-thiophenepropylamine

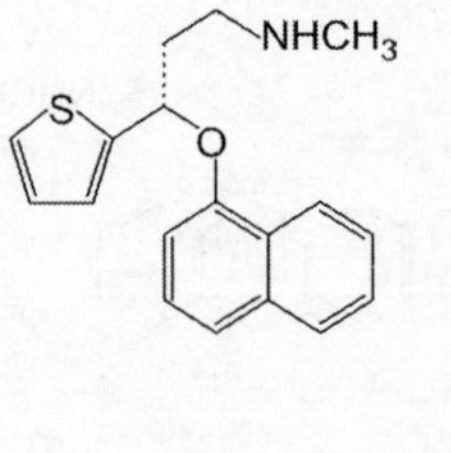

Synthesis

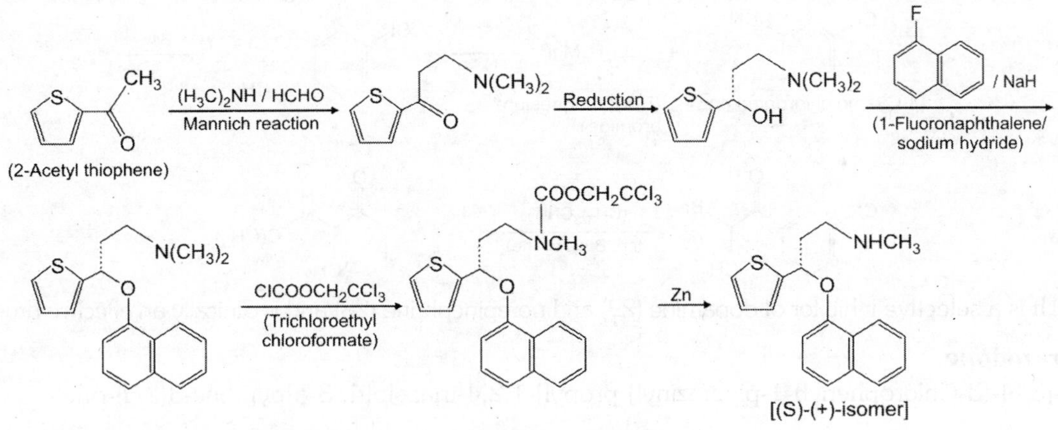
CH3
S
O
(2-Acetyl thiophene)
(H3C)2NH / HCHO
Mannich reaction
N(CH3)2
Reduction
OH
F
/ NaH
(1-Fluoronaphthalene/
sodium hydride)
ClCOOCH2CCl3
(Trichloroethyl
chloroformate)
COOCH2CCl3
NCH3
Zn
NHCH3
[(S)-(+)-isomer]

It is a nonselective inhibitor of various biogenic amines.

Nomifensine

1,2,3,4,-Tetrahydro-2-methyl-4-phenyl-8-isoquinolinamine

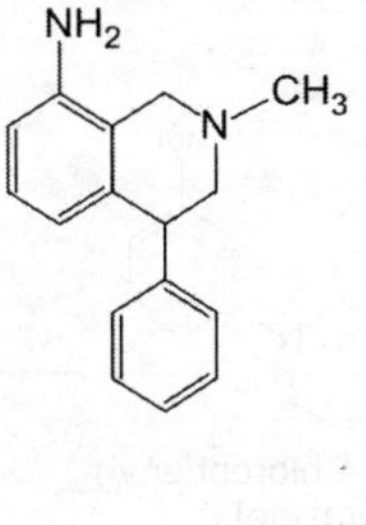
NH2
N
CH3

Synthesis

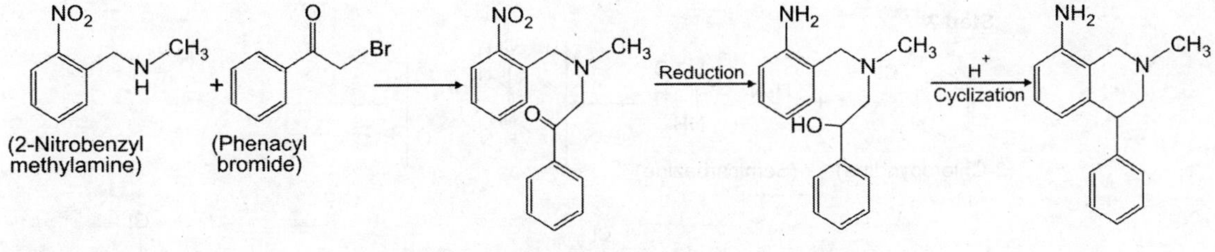
NO2
CH3
N
H
+
O
Br
(2-Nitrobenzyl
methylamine)
(Phenacyl
bromide)
Reduction
NH2
HO
H+
Cyclization

It is selective inhibitor of dopamine (29) and norepinephrine (28).

Bupropion

(±)-2-(*tert.*-Butylamino)-3´-chloropropiophenone

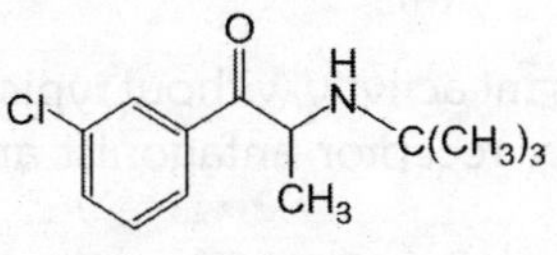
O
Cl
H
N
C(CH3)3
CH3

Synthesis

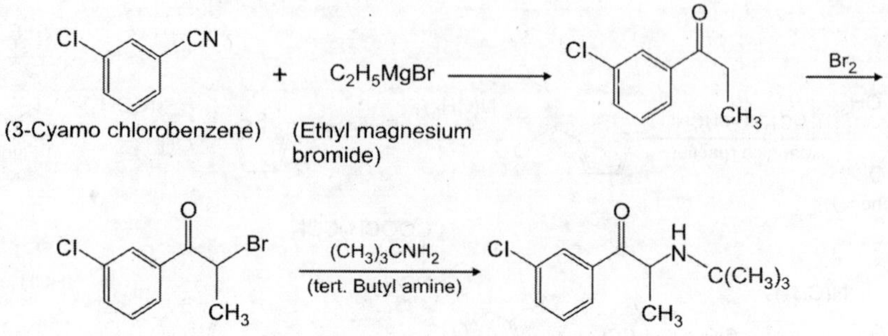
(3-Cyamo chlorobenzene)
(Ethyl magnesium bromide)
(tert. Butyl amine)

It is a selective inhibitor of dopamine (29) and norepinephrine (28) and is clinically an effective drug.

Trazodone

2-[3-[4-(3-Chlorophenyl)-1-piperazinyl] propyl]-1,2,4-triazolo[4, 3-a]pyridine-3(2*H*)-one

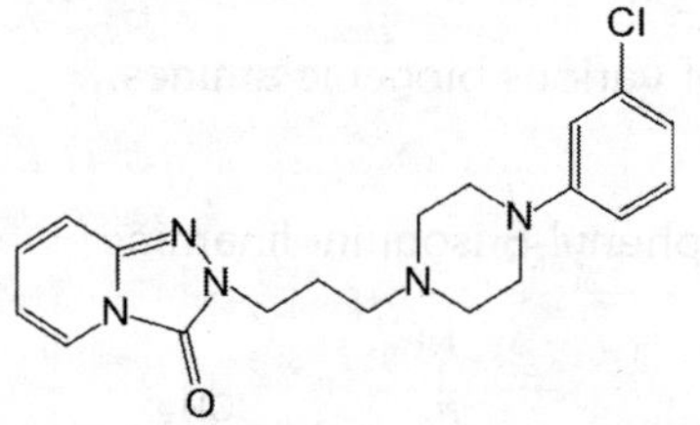

Synthesis

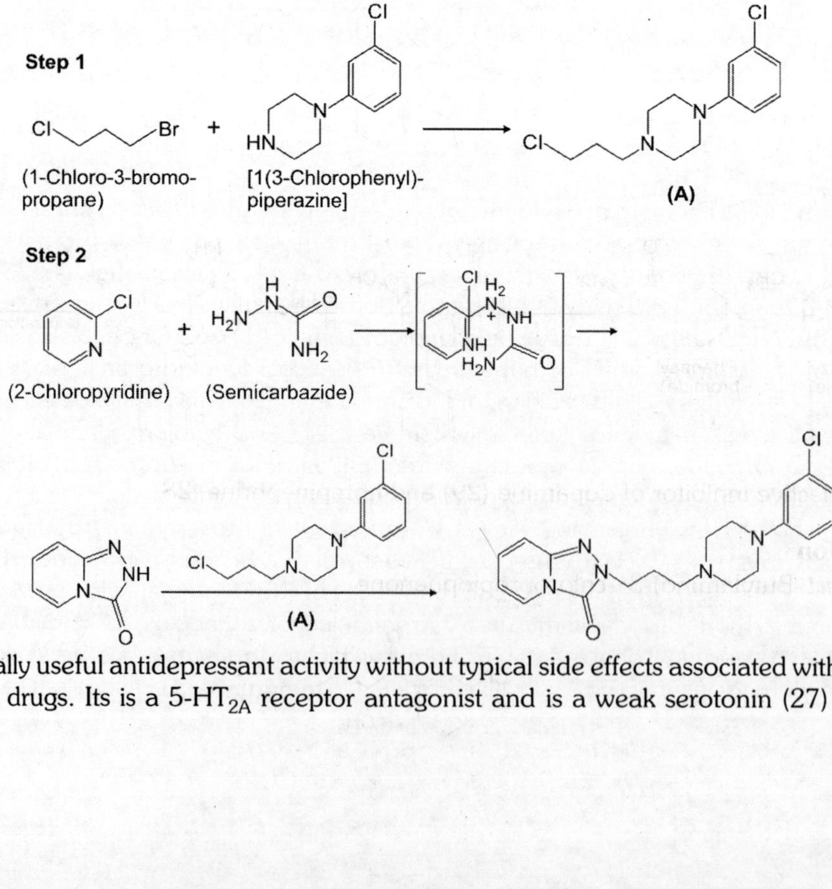
Step 1
(1-Chloro-3-bromo-propane)
[1(3-Chlorophenyl)-piperazine]
(A)
Step 2
(2-Chloropyridine)
(Semicarbazide)
(A)

It has clinically useful antidepressant activity without typical side effects associated with classical antidepressant drugs. Its is a 5-HT_{2A} receptor antagonist and is a weak serotonin (27) reuptake inhibitor.

Section III
Drug Therapy of Inflammation

ANTIHISTAMINICS AND
ANTIULCER AGENTS

HISTAMINE, 4(5)-(2-AMINOETHYL)-IMIDAZOLE (1), occurs in most of the body organs and body fluids. The two methylene carbons through which the amino group is attached to imidazole ring are designated as α and β. It exists in two tautomeric forms (1a) and (1b). In aqueous solutions, the equilibrium is towards left favouring (1a) by 4:1. Histamine (1) has two pK_a values of 9.40 (due to aliphatic primary amino group) and 5.80 (due to N). At physiological pH, it exists as equilibrium mixture of monocation (2) (96%) and dication (3) (3%). Conformational analysis studies have shown that histamine (1) exists in *trans* (4) and *gauche* (5) conformations, which are important for interaction with the receptors.

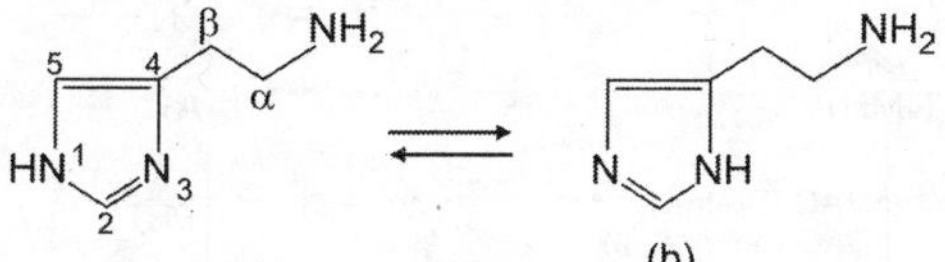

(a)   (b)

(1)

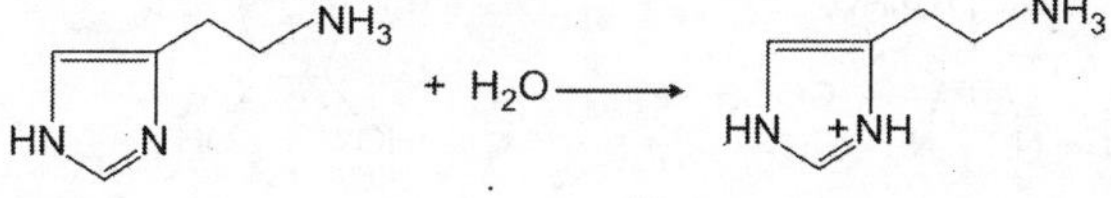

(2)   (3)

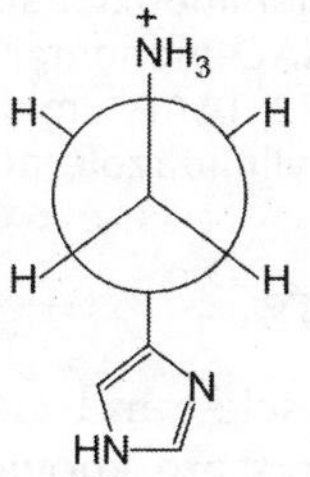

(4) 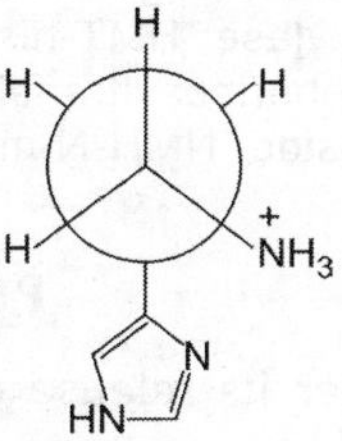   (5)

BIOSYNTHESIS, STORAGE, AND RELEASE OF HISTAMINE

Histamine (1) is formed from amino acid *S*-histidine (6) by the action of histidine decarboxylase or aromatic amino acid decarboxylase. In tissues, mast cells which store the histamine, are the site for histamine synthesis. In blood, it is basophil. Histamine (1) is released from mast cells by exocytosis during inflammatory or allergic reactions. The stimuli include interaction of antigen with IgE antibodies. Morphine and d-tubocurarine also release histamine (1). Agents which increase cAMP formation, such as β-adrenoreceptor agonists, inhibit histamine (1) release.

Histamine (1) is rapidly metabolized in liver to inactive metabolites which include *N*-methylhistamine (NMH), *N*-methyl imidazole acetic acid (NMIAA), imidazole acetic acid (IAA), and imidazole acetic acid riboside (IAAR) (Fig. 11.1).

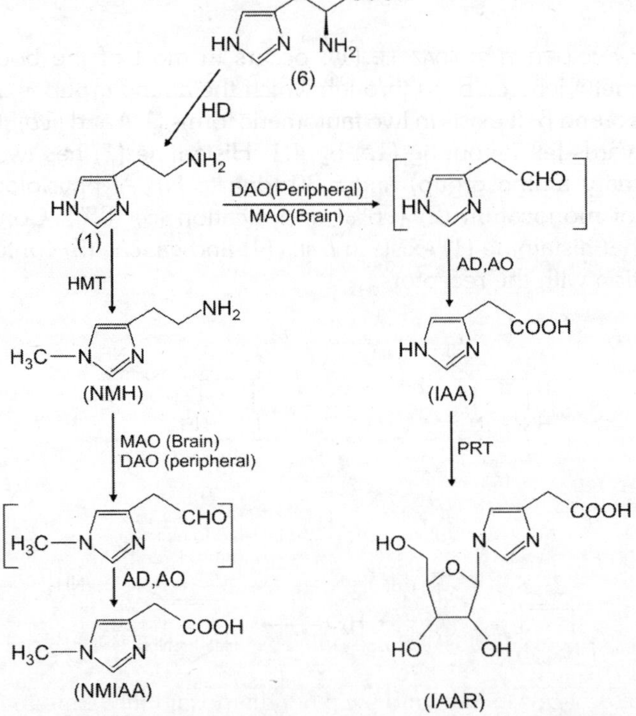

Fig. 11.1: Biosynthesis and metabolism of histamine (1).
(AD-aldehyde dehydrogenase; AO-aldehyde oxidase; DAO-diamineoxidase; HD-L-histidine decarboxylase; HMT-histamine N-methyltransferase; MAO-monoamineoxidase; PRT-phosphoribosyltransferase; IAA-imidazole acetic acid; IAAR- imidazole acetic acid riboside; NMH-N-methylhistamine; NMIAA-N-methylimidazole acetic acid.)

PHARMACOLOGICAL EFFECTS

Histamine (1) after its release exerts effects on smooth muscles and glands by interacting with receptors. At present three types of histamine (1) receptors are known and these include H_1-, H_2-and H_3-receptors. Interaction with H_1-receptors results in bronchoconstriction, contraction of gut, vasodilation, and increased vascular permeability. Cardiac stimulation and stimulation of gastric secretion is mediated through H_2-receptors. The significance of H_3-receptors is not known. Histamine (1) is also involved in vomiting through its action on CNS.

H_1- and H_2-receptors belong to G-protein coupled receptors. H_1-receptors are coupled to phospholipase C. Activation of H_1-receptors results in formation of inositol-1, 4, 5-triphosphate (IP_3) and diacylglycerol (DAG). IP_3 release causes rapid release of Ca^{++} from endoplasmic reticulum. Diacylglycerol activates protein kinase C and Ca^{++} activates Ca^{++}/calmodulin dependent protein kinases and phospholipase A_2 in the target tissues to generate the response.

H_2-receptors are linked to adenylyl cyclase which results in activation of c-AMP-dependent protein kinase in the target cell.

H_3-receptors which are found at presynaptic site inhibit release of a variety of neurotransmitters.

The pathophysiological role of histamine (1) as mediator of allergic reactions is treated with histamine release inhibitors, H_1-antagonists, and compounds possessing both these activities. The other pathophysiological condition of increased gastric secretion leading to peptic ulcers is overcome by use of H_2-antagonists and proton pump inhibitors.

HISTAMINE RELEASE INHIBITORS

Khellin (7), a natural product, has bronchodilating activity. This led to discovery of cromolyn (8) and nedocromil (9), the benzopyran analogs, and lodoxamide (10), and pemirolast (11) prossessing similar activity. All of these compounds act by inhibiting the release of histamine (1) through inhibition of mast cell degranulation, however, they have no effect on released histamine (1). They are mainly used in asthamatic conditions and in the eye for prevention of itching and conjunctivitis.

(7)   (8)   (9)

(10)   (11)

H_1-RECEPTOR ANTAGONISTS

H_1-antagonists inhibit the responses of smooth muscle to histamine (1). They also inhibit bronchospasm induced by histamine (1) in guinea pig but not in humans. Clinically, H_1-antagonists are used for allergic reactions such as rhinitis, urticaria, drug hypersensitivities. H_1-antagonists are also used against motion sickness and other causes of nausea and vomiting.

At present two types of H_1-antagonists are available, the classical or first generation H_1-antagonists and the second generation or non-sedating antihistaminics. Most of the structure activity relationship studies have been carried out on the first generation or classical antihistaminics. The structural requirements of this class of antihistaminics can be represented by (12), where Ar and Ar' are aromatic or hetero-aromatic rings, one of which may be separated from X by a methylene group. The two aromatic rings should not be co-planar. X may be O,C, or N, n is usually 2. The basic function, NRR' in which the nitrogen is carrying two alkyl groups could also be a nitrogen heterocycle. For optimum activity, the distance between the centre of aromatic rings and the nitrogen should be 5Å to 6 Å. This distance is achieved when the compound exists in *trans*-conformation. Antihistaminics with rigid structure have similar distance between aromatic rings and basic nitrogen.

$$\begin{array}{c} Ar \\ Ar' \end{array} X\text{-}(CH_2)_n\text{-}N \begin{array}{c} R \\ R' \end{array}$$

(12)

The classical antihistaminics have been classified on the basis of nature of connecting atom (X), variation in diaryl groups, and nature of basic nitrogen and these include:

1. Aminoalkyl ethers.
2. Ethylenediamines.
3. Piperazines.
4. Propylamines.
5. Tricyclic H_1-receptor antagonists.

Aminoalkyl Ethers

The general formula of this class of drugs is (13), where Ar is a benzene ring, Het, a hetrocyclic ring such as 2-pyridyl, R can be H or CH_3, R' and R" are small alkyl groups such as methyl. However, there are some aminoalkyl ethers, which differ from this general structure. The various compounds belonging to this class include diphenhydramine (14), chlorodiphenhydramine (15), bromodiphenhydramine (16), carbinoxamine (17), doxylamine (18), and setastine (19). The compounds which differ from general structure (13) include clemastine (20) and diphenylpyraline (21).

$$\begin{array}{c} R \\ Ar\text{---}C\text{-}O\text{-}(CH_2)_2\text{-}N \\ Het \end{array} \begin{array}{c} R' \\ R'' \end{array}$$

(13)

X

$N(CH_3)_2$

(14), X = H
(15), X = Cl
(16), X =Br

Introduction of substitution in one of the rings such as chloro, bromo, results in compounds which have better therapeutic effect. Thus, chlorodiphenhydramine (15) and bromodiphen-hydramine (16) are superior to diphenhydramine (14). Similarly, substitution of a heterocyclic ring for one of the aromatic rings as in carbinoxamine (17) and doxylamine (18) results in enhancement

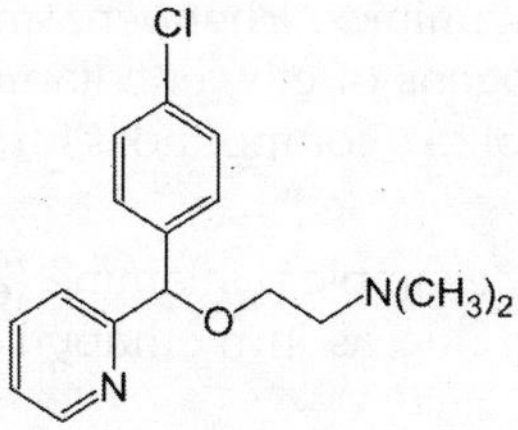

(17)

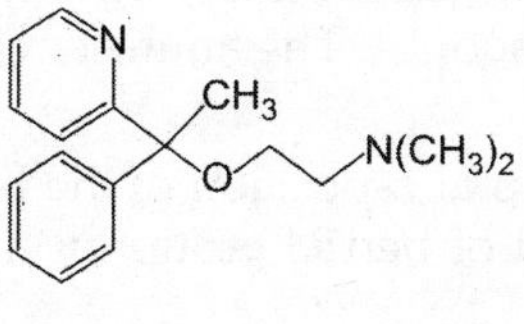

(18)

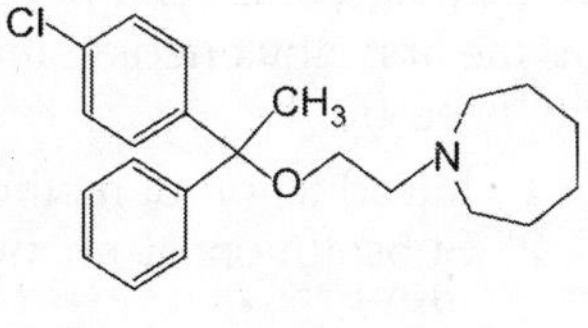

(19)

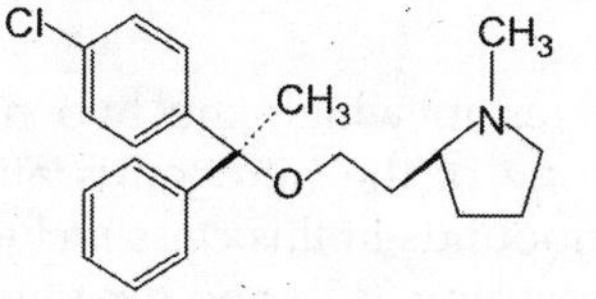

(20)

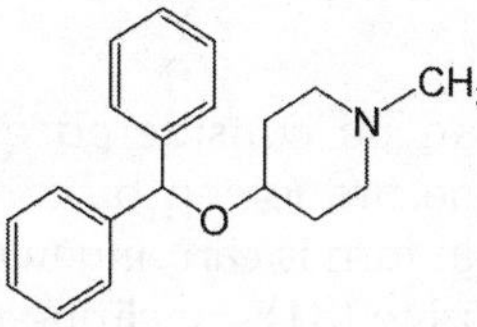

(21)

of antihistaminic activity. Substitution of hydrogen at benzylic carbon by methyl results in asymmetry as in case of doxylamine (18) and clemastine (20). Out of the two enantiomers, the S-enantiomer is more active. These drugs possess significant anticholinergic activity which may enhance the H_1-blocking action on exocrine secretions. These drugs also produce drowsiness, which is probably because they can pass the blood-brain barrier and bind to H_1-receptors in brain.

Ethylenediamines

This class of H_1-antagonists, excepting antazoline (22) have the general formula (23), the $X–(CH_2)_2–N$ of (12) being substituted by ethylenediamine residue. In antazoline (22), the second nitrogen forms part of the imidazole ring. The various compounds belonging to this class include antazoline (22), phenbenzamine (24), tripelennamine (25), pyrilamine (26), thonzylamine (27), and methapyrilene (28).

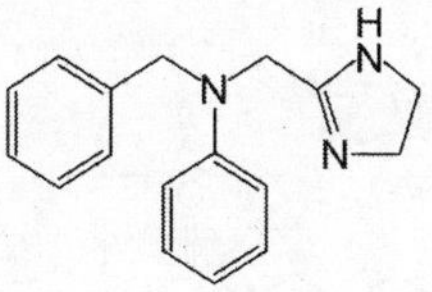

(22)

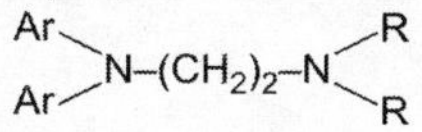

(23)

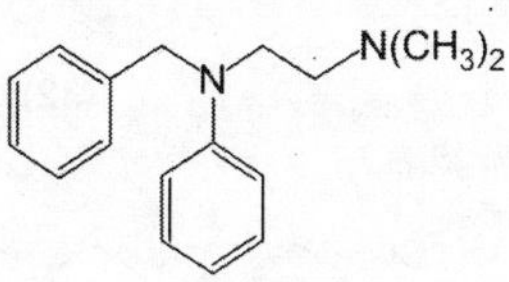

(24)

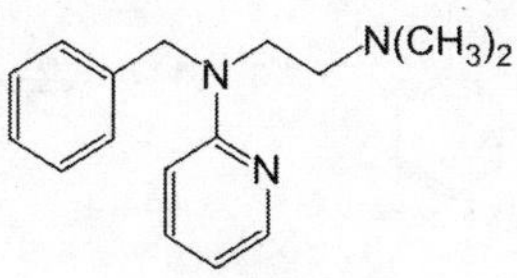

(25)

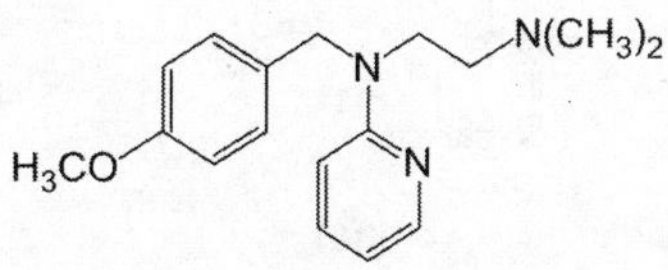

(26)

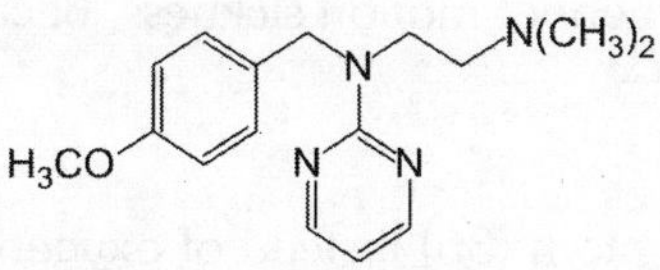

(27)

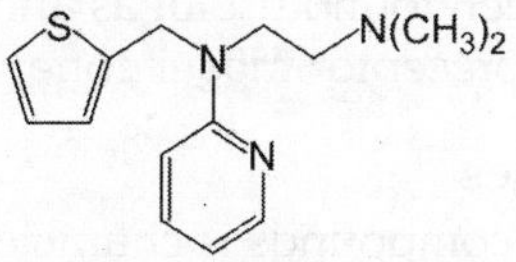

(28)

Ethylenediamine class of H_1-antagonists are highly effective antihistaminics. Phenbenzamine (24), which contains a phenyl and a benzyl moiety on one of the nitrogens of ethylenediamine, was the first ethylenediamine H_1-antagonist. The antihistaminic activity of this compound is further enhanced by:

1. Introduction of methoxyl group at *p*-position of the benzyl group, example pyrilamine (26).
2. Substitution of phenyl moiety of benzyl group by a heterocyclic ring as in methapyrilene (28).

Most of these compounds display CNS depressant activity as well as gastrointestinal side effects.

Piperazines

Piperazines can be considered ethylenediamine derivatives in which the two nitrogens of ethylenediamine are joined by a ethylene chain. Further, one of the nitrogen is attached to a carbon which in turn is carrying two aryl moieties (29). Compounds in this class include cyclizine (30), chlorcyclizine (31), meclizine (32), buclizine (33), hydroxyzine (34), and oxatomide (35).

(29)

(30), X=H
(31), X=Cl

(32)

(33)

(34)

(35)

Piperazines have slow onset and longer duration of action. The compounds belonging to this class have been found useful as antiemetic and in the treatment of motion sickness, because they act on chemoreceptor trigger zone.

Propylamines

This class of compounds is characterized by having carbon atom (36) instead of oxygen (ethers), or nitrogen (ethylenediamines and piperazines). The carbon may be sp^3 or sp^2 hybridized or may be a part of a ring. Compounds belonging to this series of antihistaminics include pheniramine (37), chlorpheniramine (38), brompheniramine (39), pyrrobutamine (40), triprolidine (41), dimethindene (42), and phenindamine (43).

(37), X = H
(38), X = Cl
(39), X = Br

(36)

(40)

(41)

(42)

(43)

Pheniramines which are chiral, have been resolved and the antihistaminic activity is almost exclusively found in the *S*-isomer.

Compounds with unsaturation, include pyrrobutamine (40), triprolidine (41), dimethindene (42), and phenindamine (43). Among the open chain unsaturated compounds, the *E*-isomers prossess much higher antihistaminc activity than the corresponding *Z*-isomers. From the studies on unsaturated propylamines, it has been suggested that a distance of 5-6Å between the tertiary aliphatic amine and one of the aromatic nucleus is necessary for binding to H_1-receptors.

Propylamines are the most active H_1-antagonists. These agents produce less sedation and anticholinergic effects than other H_1-antagonists.

Tricyclic H_1-Receptor Antagonists

These include phenothiazines and dibenzocycloheptenes. The phenothiazines which show H_1- antagonistic activity include promethazine (44), trimeprazine (45), methdilazine (46), and pyrathiazine (47). In addition to antihistaminic activity, phenothiazines also show antipsychotic activity. However, antihistaminic phenothiazines do not have substitution in aromatic rings and the side chain carrying the basic nitrogen is branched.

(44)

(45)

(46)   (47)

Phenothiazines with asymmetric carbon in the chain have been resolved and both enantiomers have been found to possess similar antihistaminic activity.

In addition to antihistaminic activity, phenothiazines, also possess antiemetic, anticholinergic, and sedative actions.

The dibenzocycloheptanes and benzocycloheptapyridines include cyproheptadine (48) and azatadine (49). Both of these compounds show potent antihistaminic activity.

(48)   (49)

Second Generation H₁-Receptor Antagonists

This class of H$_1$-antagonists comprises of diverse class of compounds having no similarity in chemical structure. However, all of these are selective H$_1$-antagonists and do not possess sedative effects associated with other H$_1$-antagonists. This is because they are not able to cross the blood-brain barrier. These compounds are contraindicated with antibiotics like erythromycin and clarithromycin. These antibiotics inhibit their metabolism resulting in higher blood levels which may cause arrhythmia.

Some of the compounds belonging to this class of H$_1$-antihistaminics include terfenadine (50), fexofenadine (51), astemizole (52), loratidine (53), desloratidine (54), cetirizine (55), acrivastine (56), ebastine (57), carebastine (58), and mizolastine (59).

(50), R = CH$_3$
(51), R = COOH

(52)

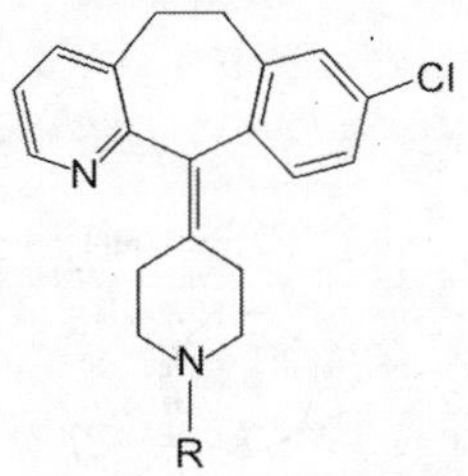

(53), R = COOC$_2$H$_5$

(54), R = H

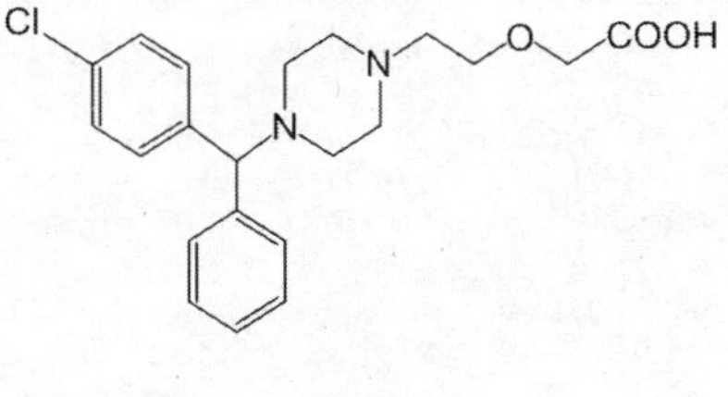

(55)

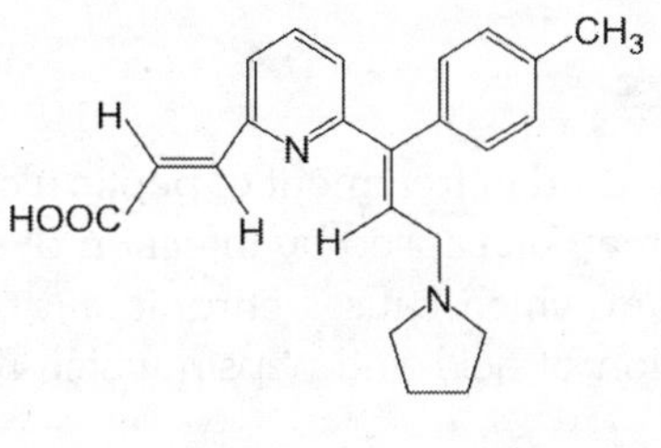

(56)

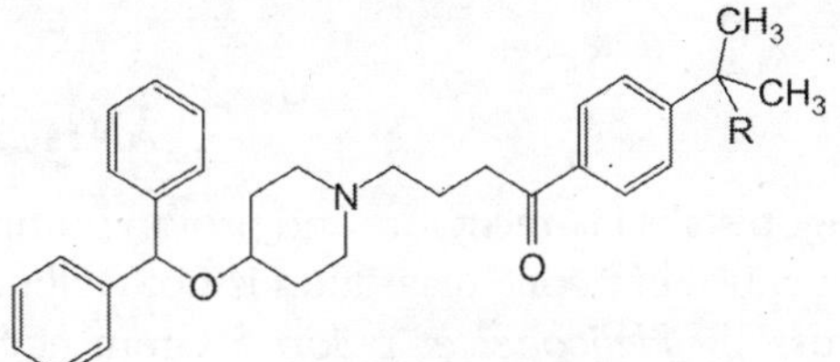

(57), R = CH$_3$

(58), R = COOH

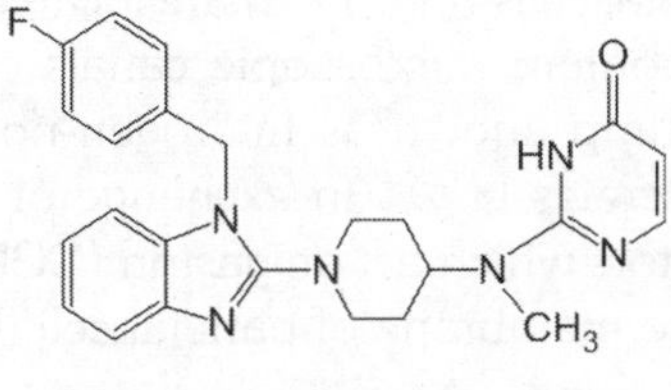

(59)

HISTAMINE RELEASE INHIBITORS WITH H$_1$-RECEPTOR ANTAGONISTIC ACTIVITY

In recent times antihistaminic agents have been developed which prossess dual action. They not only stabilize the mast cells and thus prevent the release of histamine but also act as H$_1$-antagonists. These type of antihistaminics are used topically to relieve itching in eye, congestion in conjuctiva, and erythema. Some of these include, olopatadine (60), levocabastine (61), emedastine (62), azelastine (63), ketotifen (64), and epinastine (65).

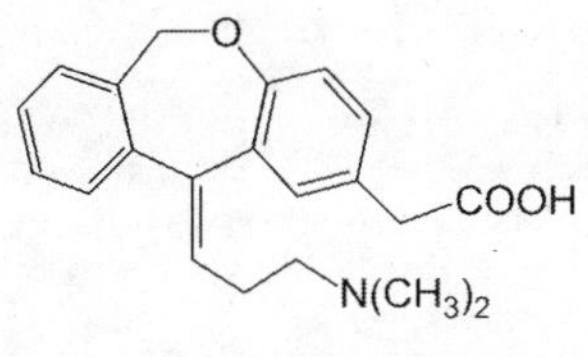

(60)

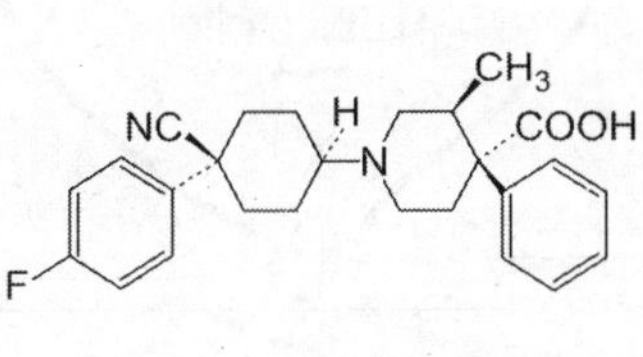

(61)

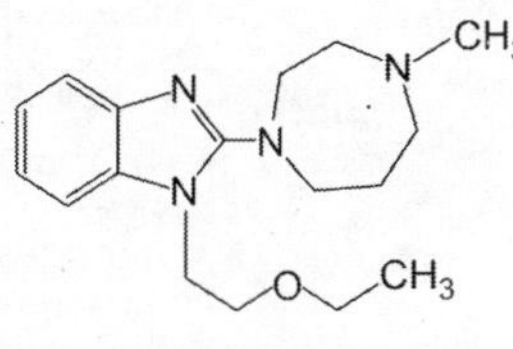

(62)

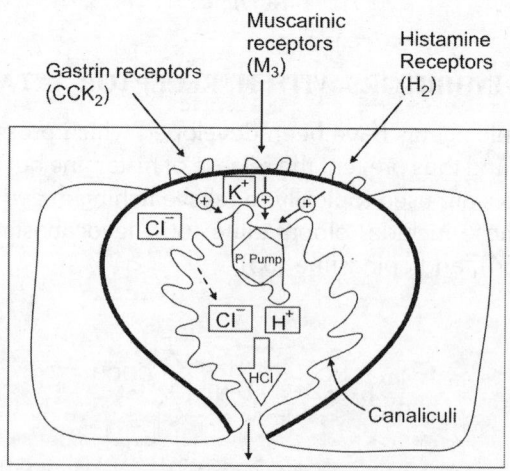

(63)   (64)   (65)

ANTIULCER AGENTS

Antagonists of H_2-receptors and proton pump inhibitors are used in treatment of peptic ulcers. The exact cause of peptic ulceration is not well understood. It may be caused by infection of stomach mucosa by *Helicobacter pylori* a Gram-negative bacterium which causes chronic gastritis. The other factors involved can be increased secretion and action of acid and pepsin which results in mucosal damage and ultimately in ulceration.

Mechanism of Gastric Acid Secretion

The acid secreting cells called parietal cells (Fig. 11.2) are located in lower part of the stomach. The apical area of the parietal cells contain microscopic canals called canaliculi. The wall of this canaliculus contain the proton pump known as hydrogen-potassium adnosine triphosphatase (H_3O^+-K^+-ATPase) system that secretes H_3O^+ in exchange of K^+. Secretion of acid by parietal cells is regulated by various mediators which act on gastrin (CCK_2), muscarinic-M_3, and histamine H_2-receptors located on the surface membrane of parietal cell (Fig. 11.3).

Gastrin receptors
(CCK_2)

Muscarinic
receptors
(M_3)

Histamine
Receptors
(H_2)

Fig. 11.2: Parietal cell

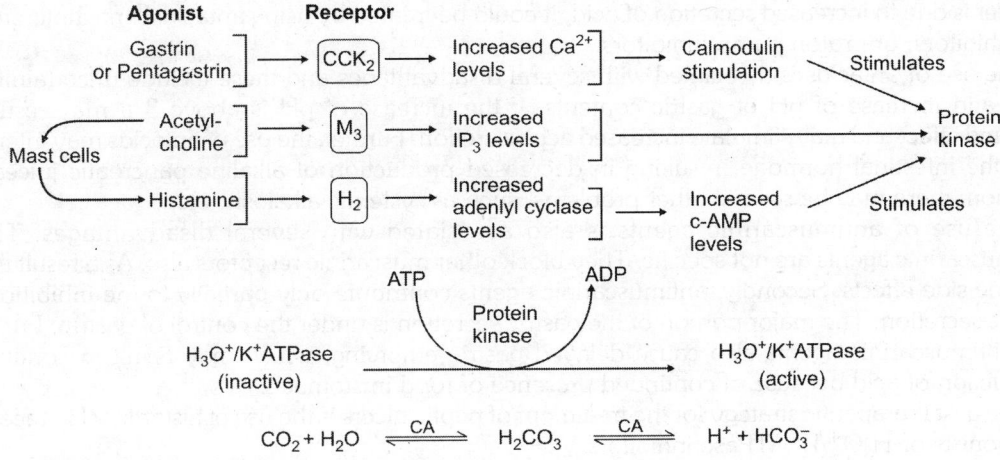

Fig. 11.3: Physiological control of hydrochloric acid secretion.
(CA-carbonic anhydrase; IP_3-Inositol triphosphate.)

Gastrin receptors are stimulated by gastrin and pentagastrin, secreted by G cells located in pyloric region of stomach. The stimulation of gastrin receptors alters the permeability of cell membrane for Ca^{2+}. The Ca^{2+} stimulates the enzyme calmodulin which leads to the activation of protein kinase which in turn activates the protein pump.

Stimulation of muscarinic M_3-receptors leads to increased inositol triphosphate (IP_3) in parietal cells. The (IP_3) in presence of Ca^{2+} activates protein kinase which in turn activates proton pump. Acetylcholine also triggers degranulation of mast cells leading to histamine release.

Stimulation of H_2-receptors by histamine leads to increased levels of adenlyl cyclase which in turn results in increased c-AMP levels. The c-AMP activates the protein kinase.

The activated protein kinase then activates the inactive proton pump H_3O^+/K^+ ATPase by phosphorylating it which enabels it to carry H^+ ions.

In the parietal cells, carbon dioxide combines with water in presence of carbonic anhydrase to form carbonic acid, which splits into H^+ and bicarbonate ions. The HCO_3^- ions are transported out of parietal cells in exchange of chloride ions. The H^+ gets attached to proton pump, which carries these across the cell membrane to release them in exchange of potassium ions. The proton pump then goes back across the membrane and releases potassium ion and gets inactivated.

The H^+ combine with the Cl^- which are already present in canal to form HCl. The acid formed in canalicular space is transported through the canals into the orifice of parietal cells which opens into gastric glands which lead into the lumen of the stomach. The hydrochloric acid so formed along with the pepsin constitutes the gastric juice.

As indicated above, excess secretion of gastric juice results in peptic ulcers. Ulcers can also be caused by *H. pylori*, NSAIDs and malignancy.

Prostaglandins, the synthesis of which is inhibited by NSAIDs, inhibit histamine-stimulated adenlyl cyclase activity in parietal cell. They also stimulate the secretion of mucous and bicarbonate, thus, contributing to cytoprotective effects of endogenous prostaglandins.

When the ulceration is due to *H. pylori* appropriate antimicrobial agents are used. If the cause of ulcer is due to increased secretion of acid, it could be treated by using antacids, anticholinergics, H_2-inhibitors, or proton pump inhibitors.

The use of antacids is associated with several disadvantages and these include uncertainity of dose and increase of pH of gastric contents. If the increase of pH is above 3 it may result in rebound effect and may stimulate increased acid secretion. Further, the use of antacids may interfere with the intestinal hormone, resulting in decreased production of alkaline pancreatic juices. In addition, there may be several other problems, such as systemic alkalosis, etc.

The use of antimuscarinic agents is also associated with several disadvantages. Thus, antimuscarinic agents are not specific. They block other muscarinic receptors also. As a result there may be side effects. Secondly, antimuscarinic agents contribute only partially to the inhibition of gastric secretion. The major portion of the gastric secretion is under the control of gastrin. Further, the antimuscarinic agents also cause delayed gastric emptying, which may result in continued production of acid because of continued presence of food in stomach.

The best therapeutic strategy for the treatment of peptic ulcers is the use of histamine H_2-receptor antagonists or H_3O^+/K^+ATPase inhibitors.

H_2-Receptor Antagonists

The H_2-antagonists have been found effective in management of peptic ulcers. This is attributed to inhibition of gastric secretion by histamine as well as gastrin. They also reduce to a large extent the acid secretion due to acetylcholine. The decreased acid secretion results in reduction in pepsin secretion and consequently the decreased secretion of gastric juice. The decreased secretion of gastric juice in stomach results in healing of ulcers. With the stoppage of treatment, relapses have been reported.

The various H_2-antagonists used in clinical practice include, burimamide (66), metiamide (67), cimetidine (68), famotidine (69), nizatidine (70), and ranitidine (71).

(66)

(67), X = S
(68), X = NCN

(69)

(70)

(71)

Proton Pump Inhibitors

As indicated earlier, the final step in the production of hydrochloric acid is the extrusion of protons. This is catalyzed by H^+/K^+-ATPase, which is responsible for the exchange of proton with K^+.

Inhibition of this pump can lead to inhibition of hydrochloric acid formation. In 1972, Swedish workers reported the discovery of proton pump inhibitory properties of pyridylmethyl-sulfinylbenzimidazoles (72). The pyridylmethylsulfinylbenzimidazoles (72) in acidic pH are converted to highly reactive intermediate (73) which reacts with thiol group of $H^+/K^+/ATPase$ to yield (74) and inhibit them it. Further, benzimidazoles have antimicrobial activity against *H. pylori* and therefore, are effective antiulcer agents. Some of the proton pump inhibitors are omeprazole (75), lansoprazole (76), rabeprazole (77), and pantoprazole (78).

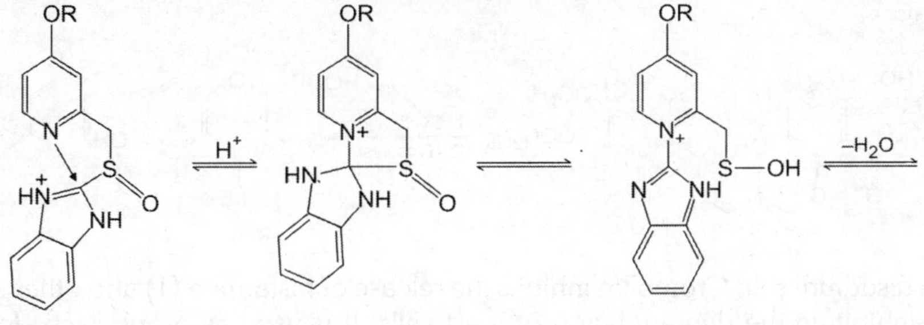

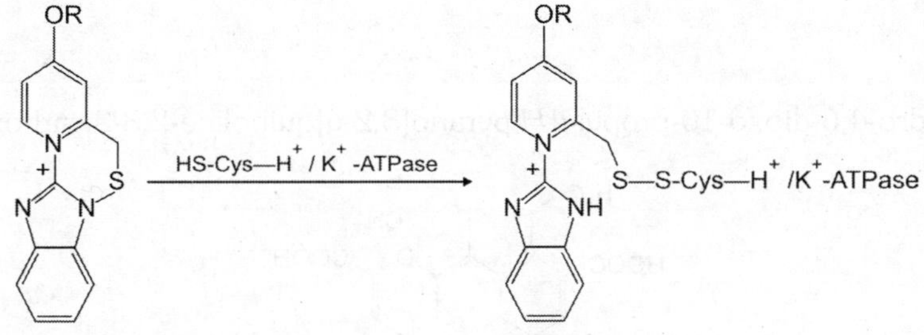

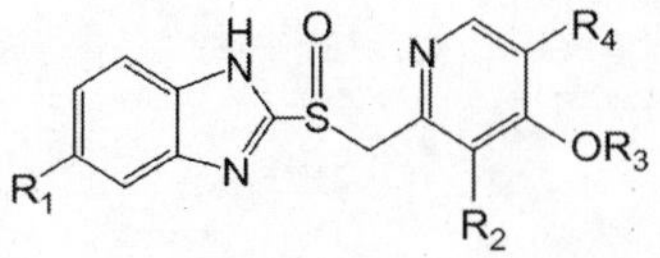

(75), $R_1 = OCH_3$, $R_2 = R_3 = R_4 = CH_3$

(76), $R_1 = R_4 = H$, $R_2 = CH_3$, $R_3 = CH_2CF_3$

(77), $R_1 = R_4 = H$, $R_2 = CH_3$, $R_3 = (CH_2)_3OCH_3$

(78), $R_1 = OCHF_2$, $R_2 = OCH_3$, $R_3 = CH_3$, $R_4 = H$

INDIVIDUAL COMPOUNDS

ANTIHISTAMINICS : HISTAMINE RELEASE INHIBITORS
Cromolyn
1,3-Bis(2-carboxy-chromon-5-yloxy)-2-hydroxypropane

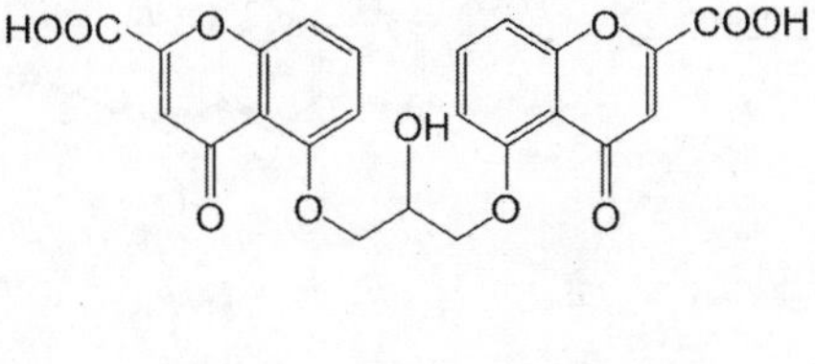

Synthesis

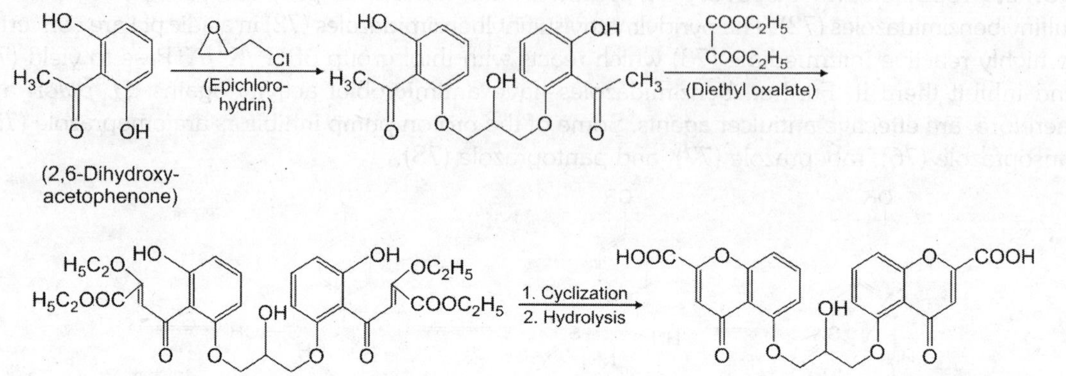

(2,6-Dihydroxy-
acetophenone)

It is used as disodium salt. Cromolyn inhibits the release of histamine (1) and other inflammatory mediators by inhibiting the degranulation of mast cells. It is used as prophylactic for asthamatic attacks.

Nedocromil

9-Ethyl-6,9-dihydro-4,6-dioxo-10-propyl-4*H*-pyrano[3,2-g]quinoline-2,8-dicarboxylic acid

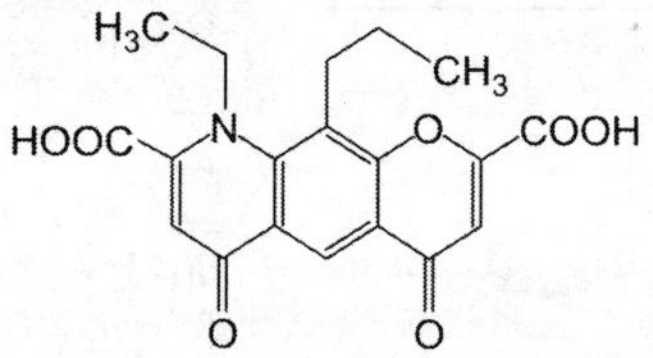

Synthesis

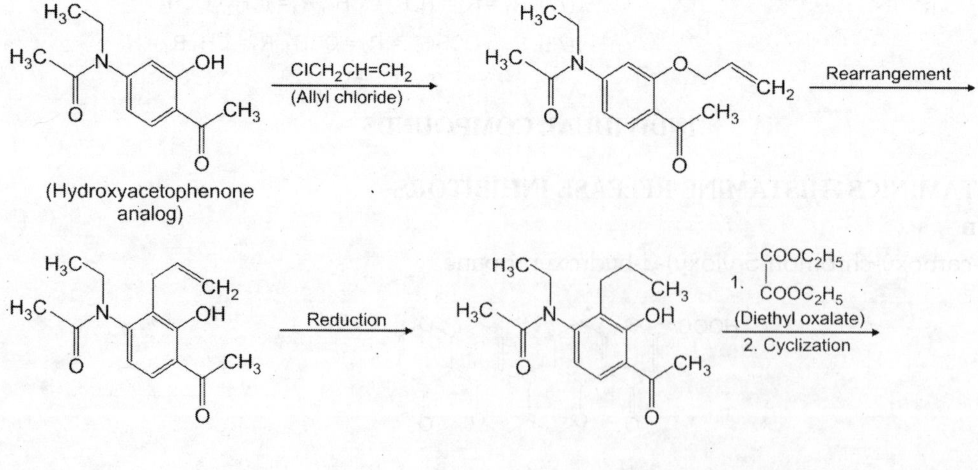

(Hydroxyacetophenone
analog)

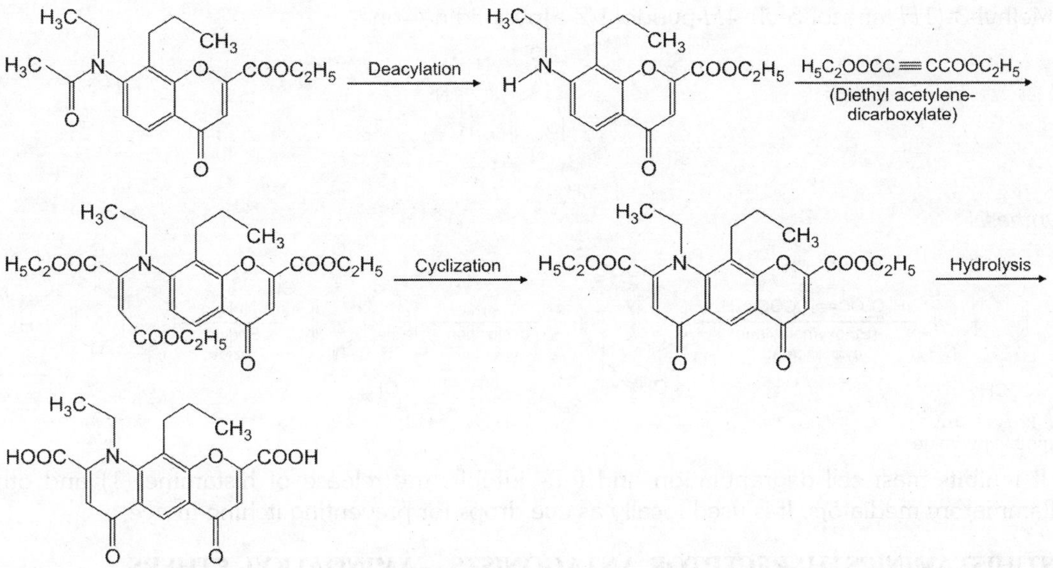

It is used as disodium salt. It shows broader pharmacological action than cromolyn (8). The mechanism of action is similar to cromolyn (8).

Lodoxamide

N, N-(2-Chloro-5-cyano-*m*-phenylene)dioxamic acid

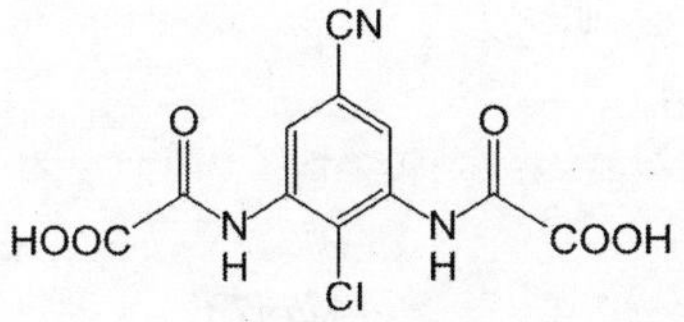

Synthesis

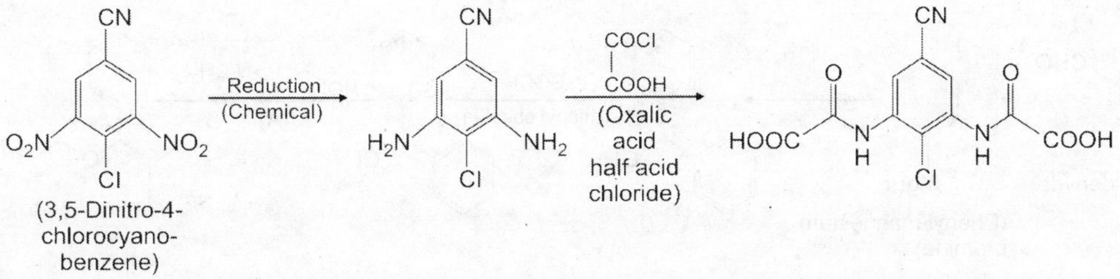

It inhibits the release of histamine (1) through inhibition of mast cells degranulation. It is used topically in eye to prevent conjunctivitis and itching.

Pemirolast

9-Methyl-3-(1*H*-tetrazol-5-yl)-4*H*-pyrido[1,2-a]pyrimidin-4-one

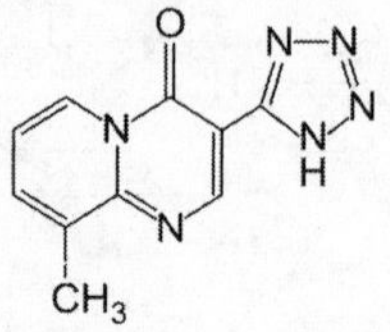

Synthesis

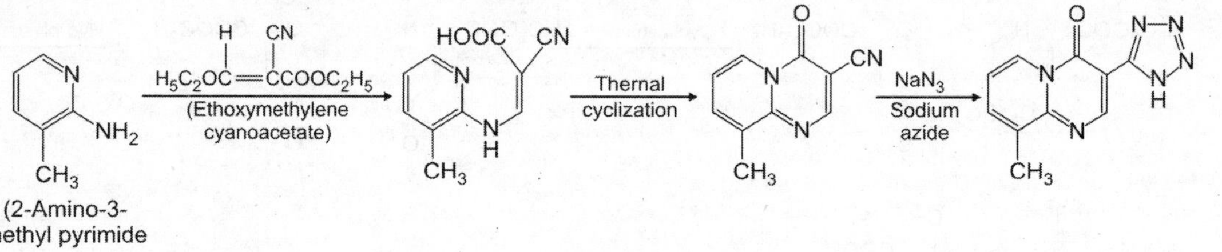

It inhibits mast cell degranulation and thus inhibits the release of histamine (1) and other inflammatory mediators. It is used locally as eye drops for preventing itching in eye.

ANTIHISTAMINICS : H₁-RECEPTOR ANTAGONISTS—AMINOALKYL ETHERS

Diphenhydramine

2-Diphenylmethoxy-*N,N*-dimethylethanamine

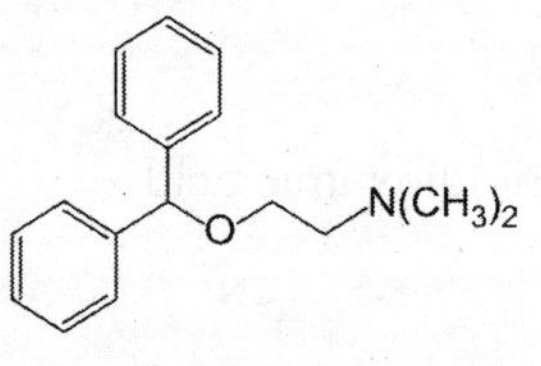

Synthesis

Step 1

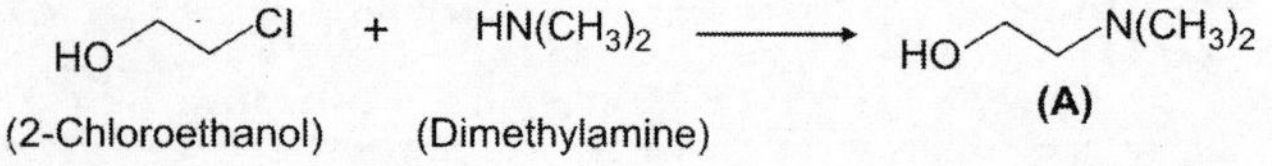

(2-Chloroethanol)   (Dimethylamine)

Step 2

(Benzaldehyde)   MgBr
(Phenyl magnesium bromide)

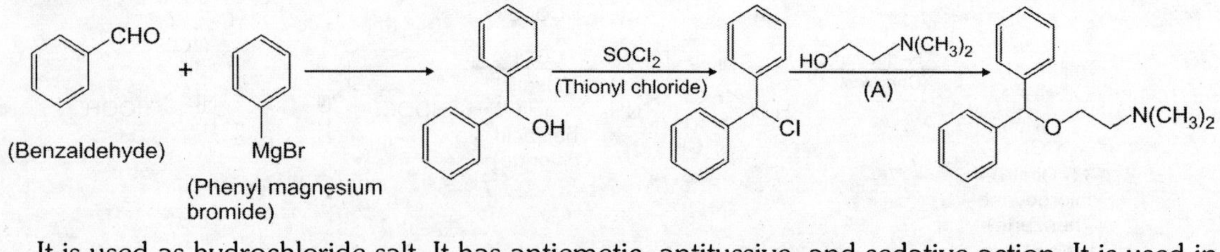

It is used as hydrochloride salt. It has antiemetic, antitussive, and sedative action. It is used in various allergic condition. Concurrent use of alcoholic beverages and other CNS depressants are contraindicated.

Another salt of diphenhydramine known as dimenhydrinate (79), is a salt of 8-chlorotheophylline and diphenhydramine. It is used in nausea of motion sickness and pregnancy.

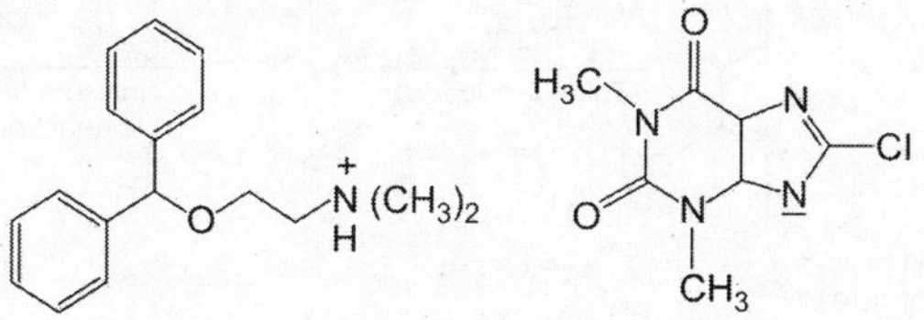

(79)

Chlorodiphenhydramine

2-[(4-Chlorophenyl)phenylmethoxy]-N,N-dimethylethanamine

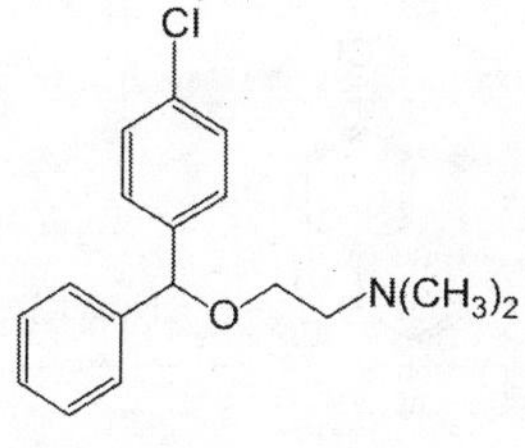

Synthesis

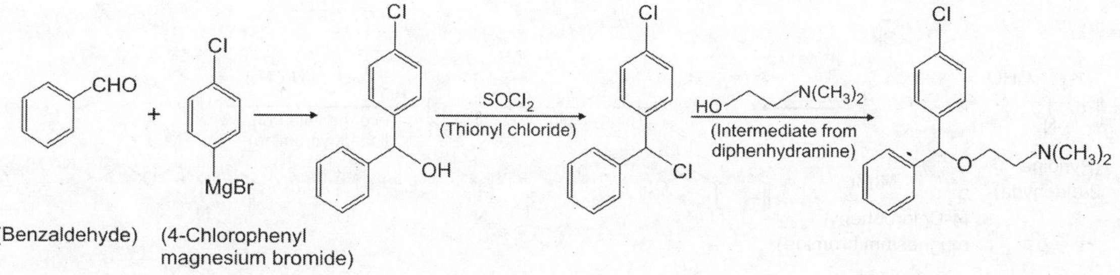

(Benzaldehyde) (4-Chlorophenyl magnesium bromide)

It is also used as hydrochloride salt.

Bromodiphenhydramine

2-[(4-Bromophenyl)phenylmethoxy]-N,N-dimethyletanamine

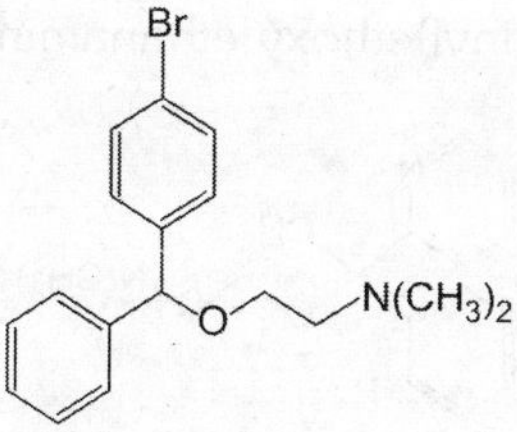

Synthesis

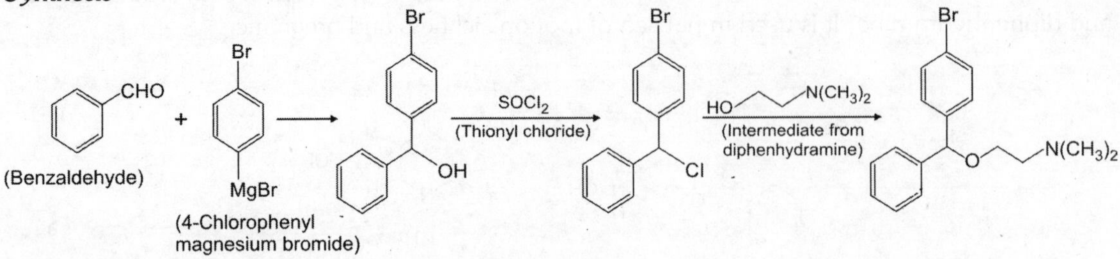

It is used as a hydrochloride salt. Bromodiphenhydramine is more lipid soluble and is more effective.

Carbinoxamine

2-[(4-Chlorophenyl)-2-pyridinylmethoxy]-*N*,*N*-dimethylethanamine

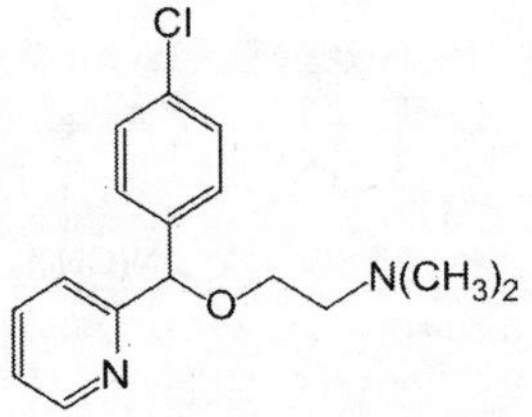

Synthesis

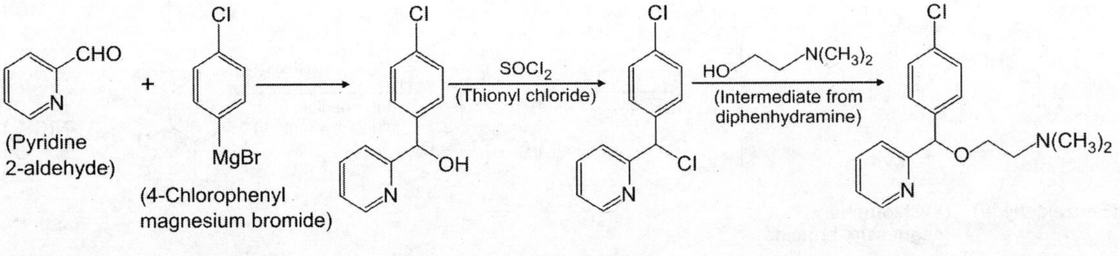

Carbinoxamine is used as a maleate salt. It contains an asymmetric carbon atom. The *levo*-isomer which has *S*-configuration is more active than *dextro*-isomer. In clinical practice, however, the racemic form is used. It is a potent antihistaminic.

Doxylamine

N,*N*-Dimethyl-2-[1-phenyl-1-(2-pyridinyl)ethoxy]ethanamine

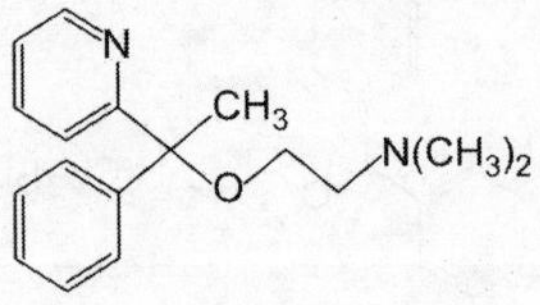

Synthesis

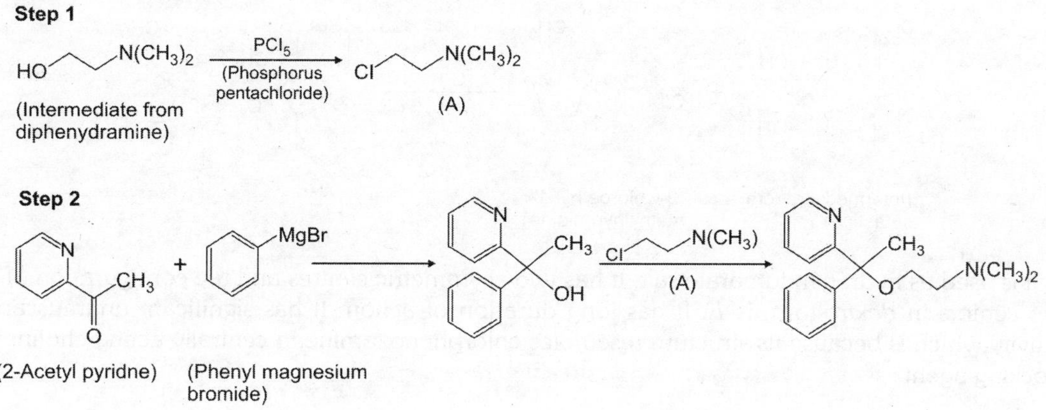

Step 1

(Intermediate from
diphenydramine)

(A)

Step 2

(2-Acetyl pyridne) (Phenyl magnesium
bromide)

It is used as succinate salt. Its potency is comparable to that of diphenhydramine (14). It is also a good hypnotic agent.

Setastine

1-[2-[1-(4-Chlorophenyl)-1-phenylethoxy]ethyl]hexahydro-1*H*-azepine

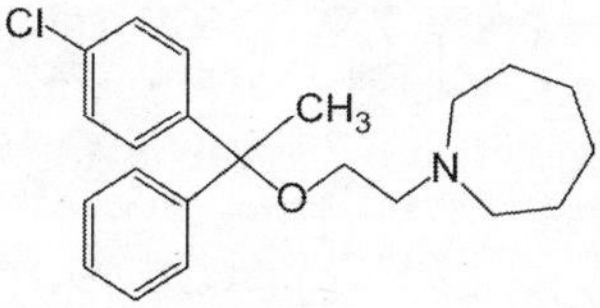

Synthesis

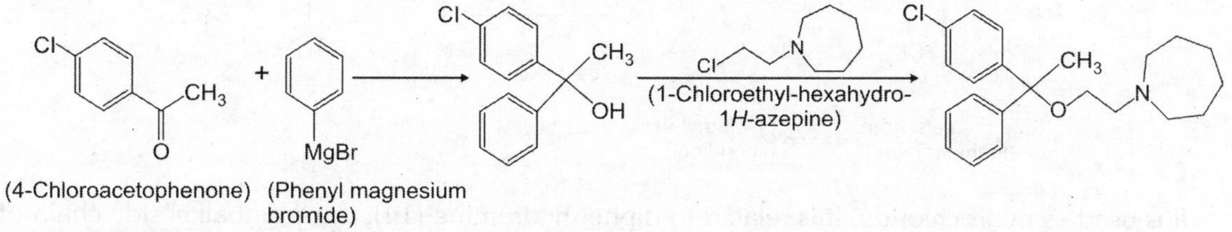

(4-Chloroacetophenone) (Phenyl magnesium
bromide)

(1-Chloroethyl-hexahydro-
1*H*-azepine)

It is claimed to be non-sedating antihistaminic.

Clemastine

(+)-2-[2-[(*p*-Chloro-α-methyl-α-phenylbenzyl)oxy]ethyl]-1-methylpyrrolidine

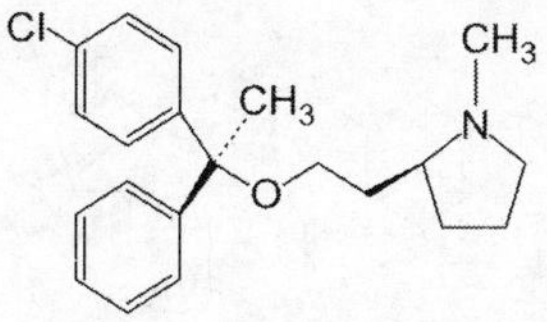

Synthesis

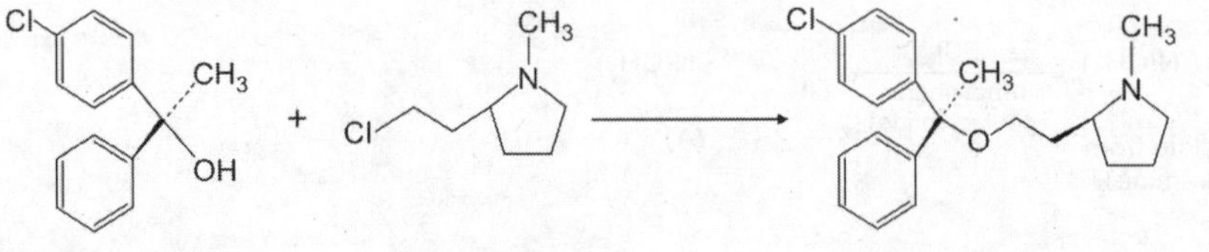

| (Intermediate from setastine) | (2-Chloroethyl-1-methylpyrrolidine) | |

It is used as hydrogen fumarate salt. It has two asymmetric centres and the configuration of the two centers in *dextro*-form is *R*. It has long duration of action. It has significant antimuscarinic activity which is because its structure resembles chlorphenoxamine, a centrally acting cholinergic blocking agent.

Diphenylpyraline
4-(Diphenylmethoxy)-1-methylpiperidine

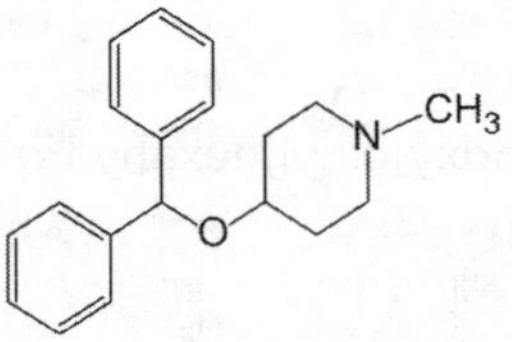

Synthesis

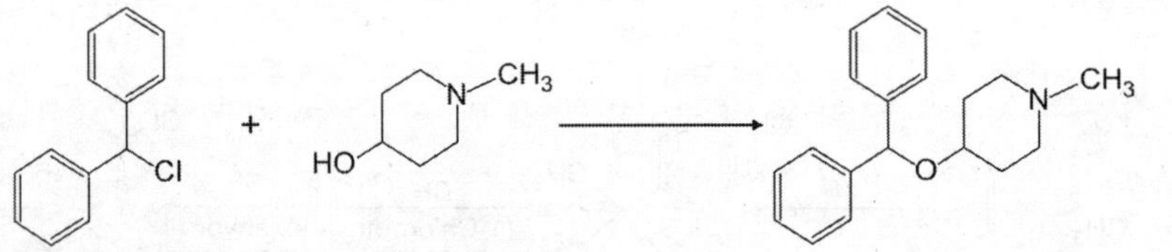

| (Intermediate from diphenhydramine) | (1-Methyl-4-piperidinol) | |

It is used as hydrochloride. It is related to diphenhydramine (14), the aminoalkyl side chain of which is incorporated in piperidine ring of diphenylpyraline. It is a potent antihistaminic.

ANTIHISTAMINICS: H$_1$-RECEPTOR ANTAGONISTS—ETHYLENEDIAMINES

Antazoline
2-[(*N*-Benzylanilino)methyl]-2-imidazoline

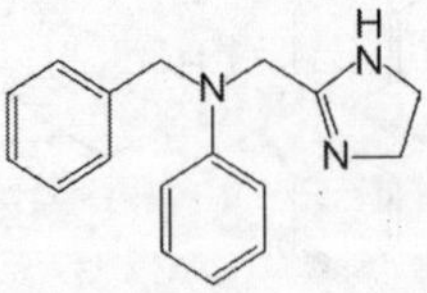

Synthesis

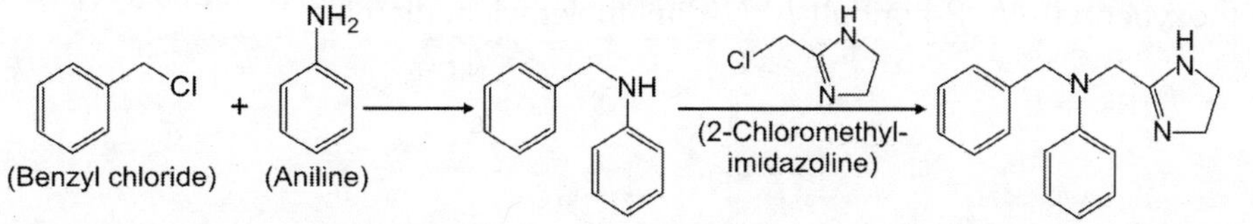

It is used as a dihydrogenphosphate salt. It is less active and is used topically for the eye.

Phenbenzamine
N-Benzyl-*N*-phenyl-*N*',*N*'-dimethylethylenediamine

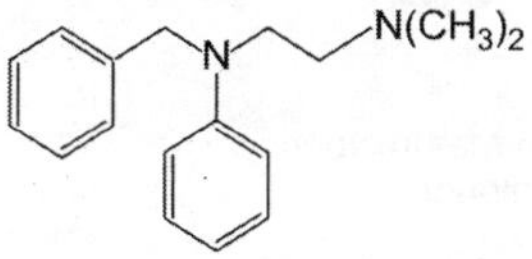

Synthesis

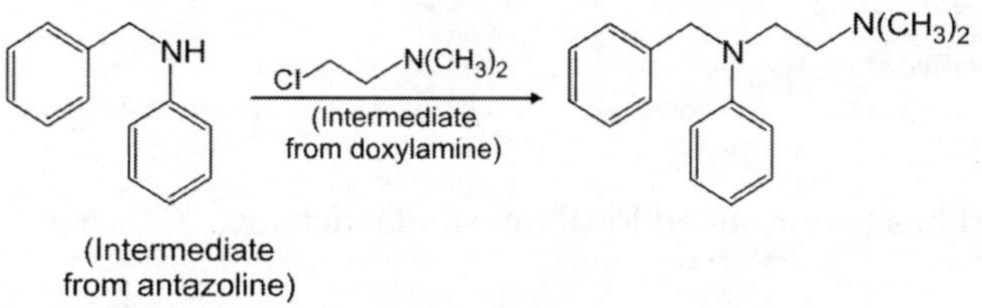

It was the first H_1-antagonist used in clinical practice. It is less active than other compounds of this series.

Tripelennamine
N-Benzyl-*N*-(2-pyridyl)-*N*',*N*'-dimethylethylenediamine

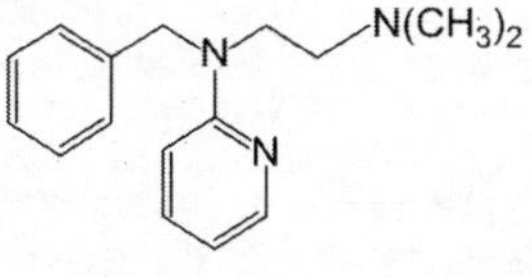

Synthesis

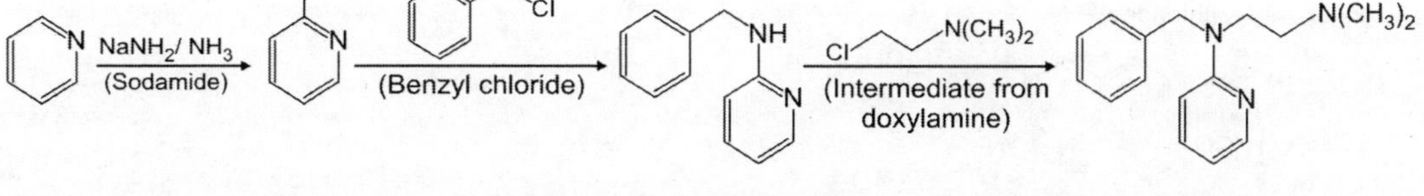

It is used as hydrochloride and citrate salt. It is as effective as diphenhydramine (14) and has fewer side effects. Use of alcohol is contraindicated.

Pyrilamine

N-(p-Methoxybenzyl)-N-(-2-pyridyl)-N',N'-dimethylethylenediamine

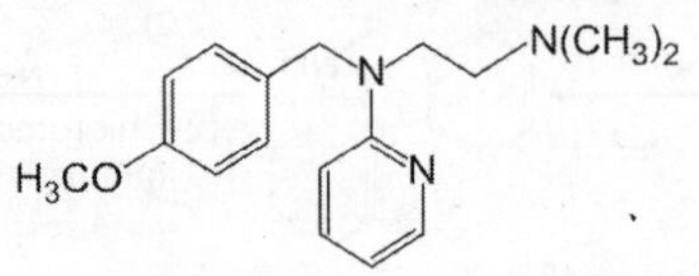

Synthesis

(2-Aminopyridine, intermediate from tripelenamine)

(p-Methoxybenzyl chloride)

(Intermediate from doxylamine)

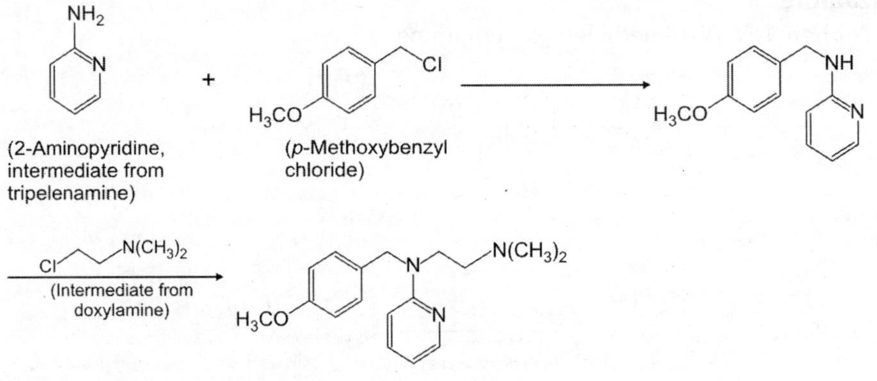

It is less potent and has pronounced local anesthetic activity.

Thonzylamine

N-(p-Methoxybenzyl)-N-(2-pyrimidinyl)-N',N'-dimethylethylenediamine

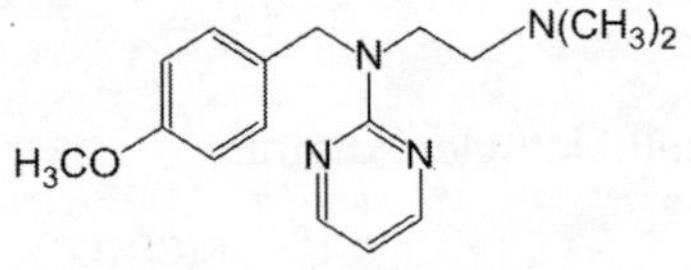

Synthesis

(p-Methoxybenzyl chloride)

(2-Aminopyrimidine)

(Intermediate from doxylamine)

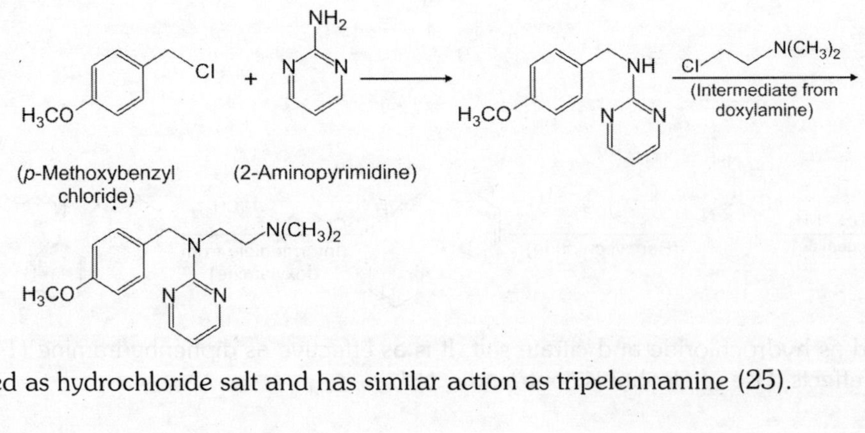

It is used as hydrochloride salt and has similar action as tripelennamine (25).

Methapyrilene

N-(2-Pyridinyl)-*N*-(2-thienylmethyl)-*N'*,*N'*-dimethylethylenediamine

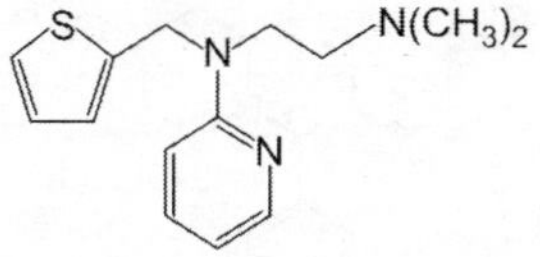

S
N
N(CH3)2
N

Synthesis

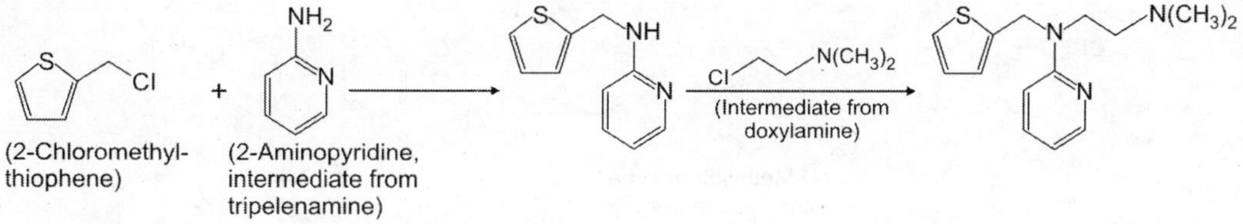

S
Cl
+
NH2
N
(2-Chloromethyl-
thiophene)
(2-Aminopyridine,
intermediate from
tripelenamine)
NH
Cl
N(CH3)2
(Intermediate from
doxylamine)
N(CH3)2

It has similar activity as tripelennamine (25).

ANTIHISTAMINICS : H_1-RECEPTOR ANTAGONISTS—PIPERAZINES

Cyclizine

1-Diphenylmethyl-4-methylpiperazine

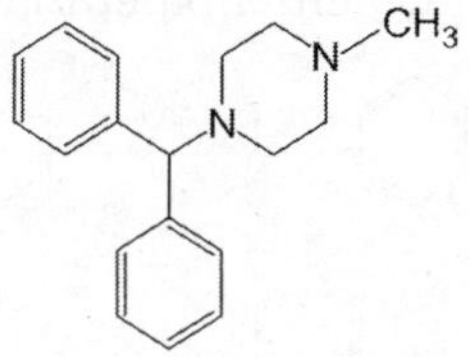

CH3
N
N

Synthesis

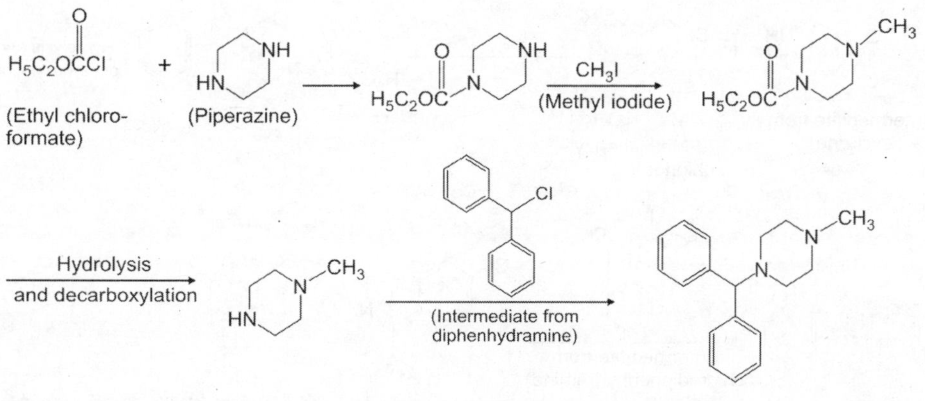

H5C2OCCl
(Ethyl chloro-
formate)
+
NH
HN
(Piperazine)
H5C2OC
CH3I
(Methyl iodide)
CH3
Hydrolysis
and decarboxylation
HN
Cl
(Intermediate from
diphenhydramine)

It is used as hydrochloride and lactate salt. Since the lactate salt is more water soluble, it is used for intramuscular administration. It is primarily used for motion sickness.

Chlorcyclizine

1-(p-Chloro-α-phenylbenzyl)-4-methylpiperazine

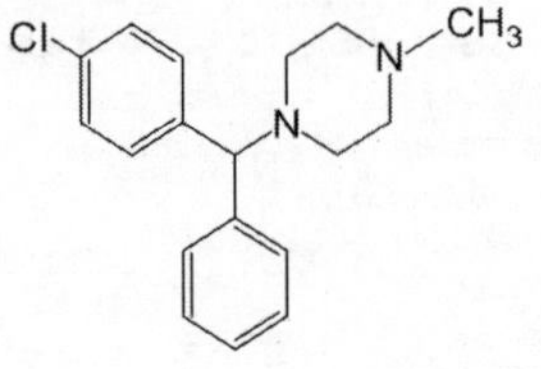

Synthesis

(Intermediate from chlorodiphenhydramine)

(N-Methylpiperazine intermediate from cyclizine)

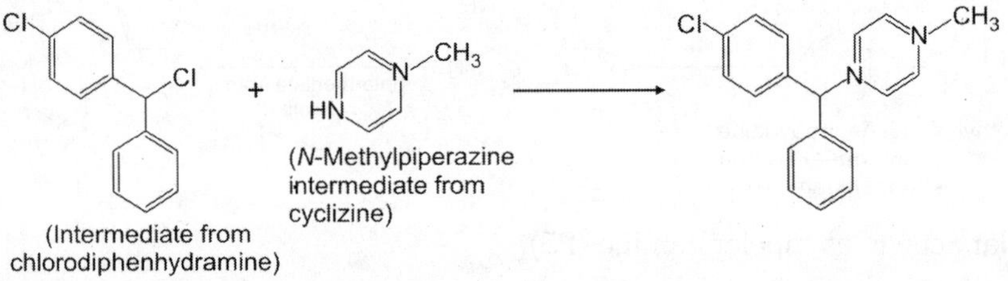

It is more active and less toxic than diphenhydramine (14) and is indicated in number of allergic conditions, such as urticaria, hay fever, sinusitis, and in asthma. It is used as hydrochloride salt.

Meclizine

1-(p-Chloro-α-phenylbenzyl)-4-(m-methylbenzyl)piperazine

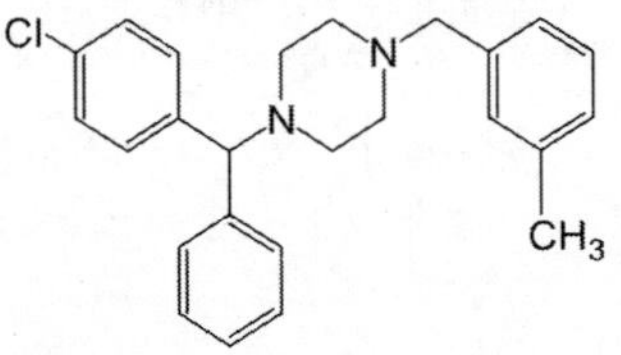

Synthesis

(Intermediate from cyclizine)

(3-Methylbenzyl chloride)

Hydrolysis and decarboxylation

(Intermediate from chlorodiphenhydramine)

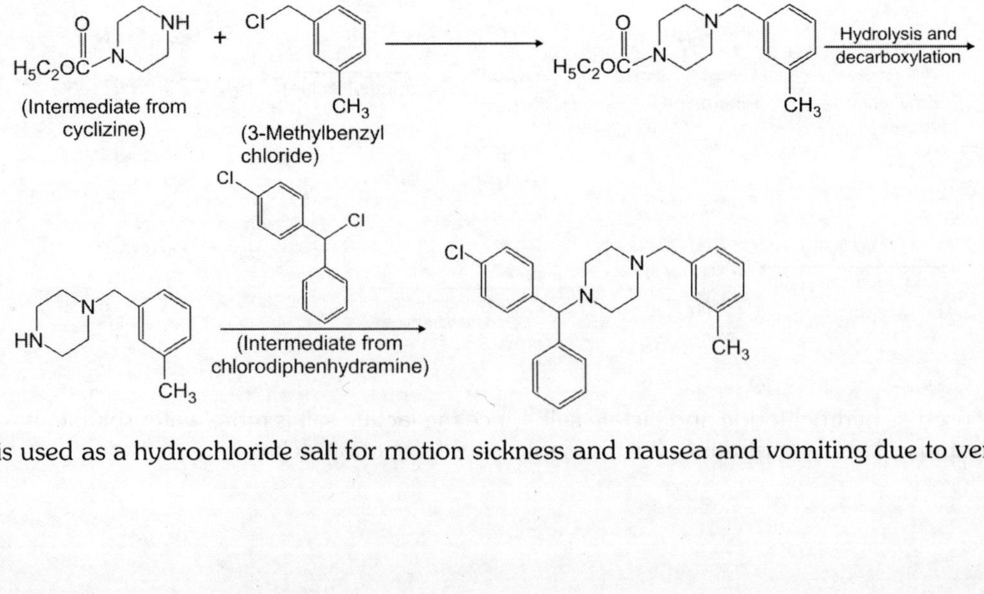

It is used as a hydrochloride salt for motion sickness and nausea and vomiting due to vertigo.

Buclizine

1-(*p*-Chloro-α-phenylbenzyl)-4-(*p-tert*-butylbenzyl)piperazine.

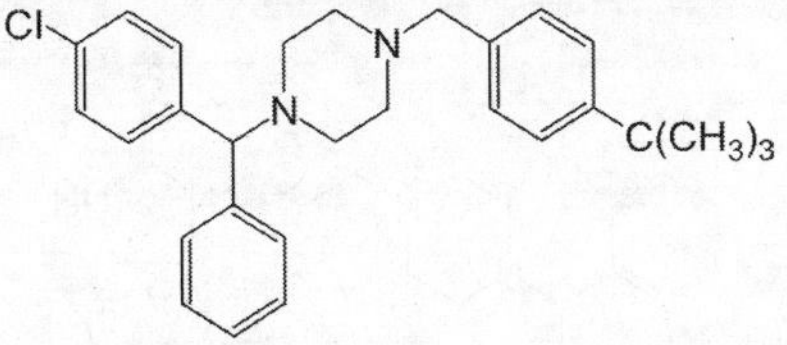

Synthesis

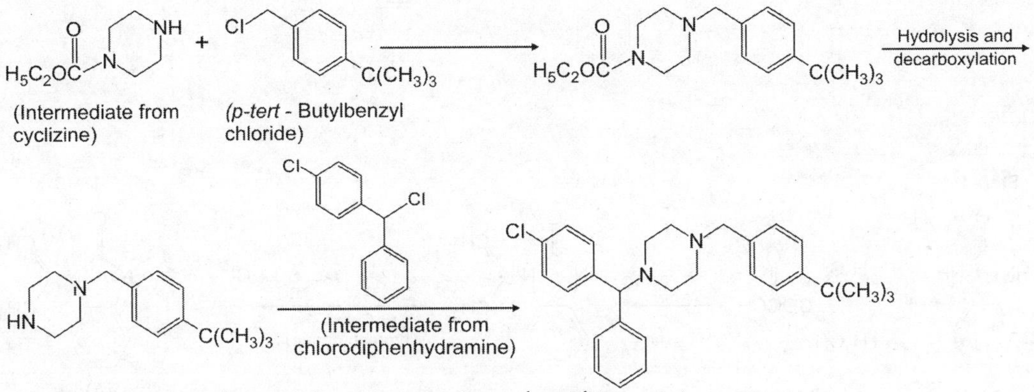

Its hydrochloride salt is used as antiemetic and antihistaminic.

Hydroxyzine

1-(*p*-Chloro-α-phenylbenzyl)-4-(2-hydroxyethoxyethyl)piperazine

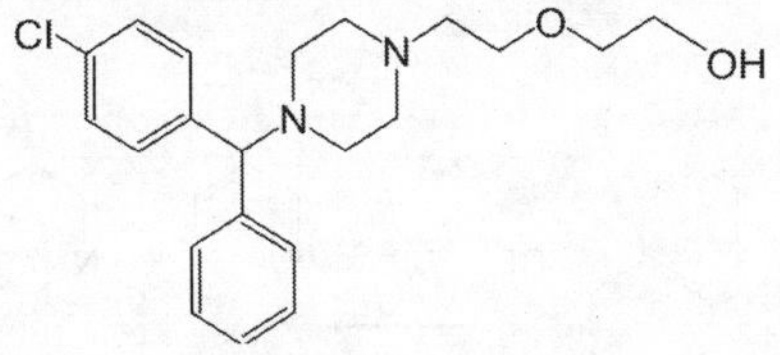

Synthesis

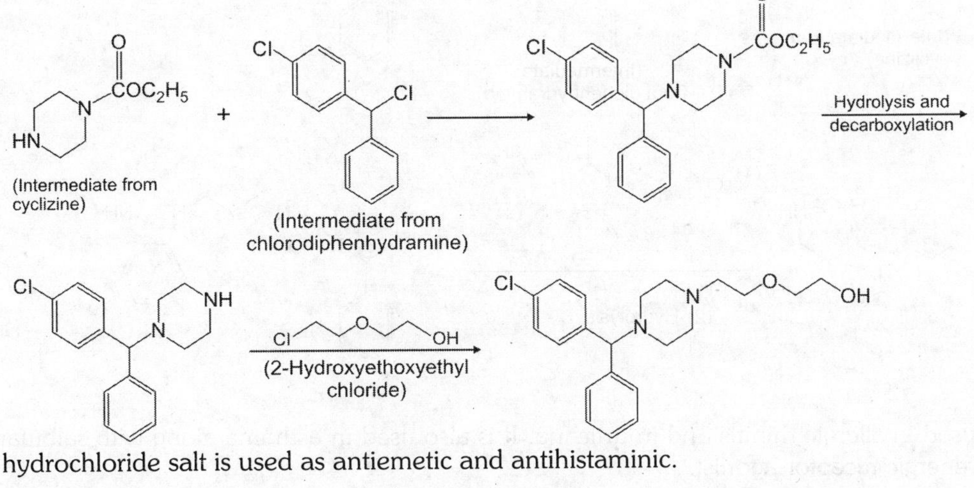

Its hydrochloride salt is used as antiemetic and antihistaminic.

Oxatomide

1-[3-[4-(Diphenylmethyl)-1-piperazinyl]propyl]-2-benzimidazolinone

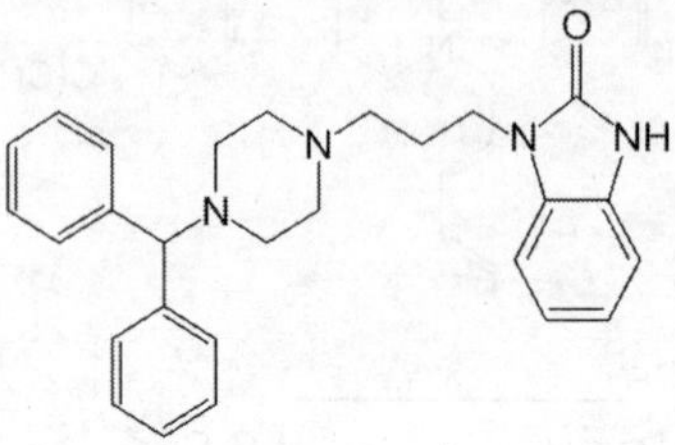

Synthesis

Step 1

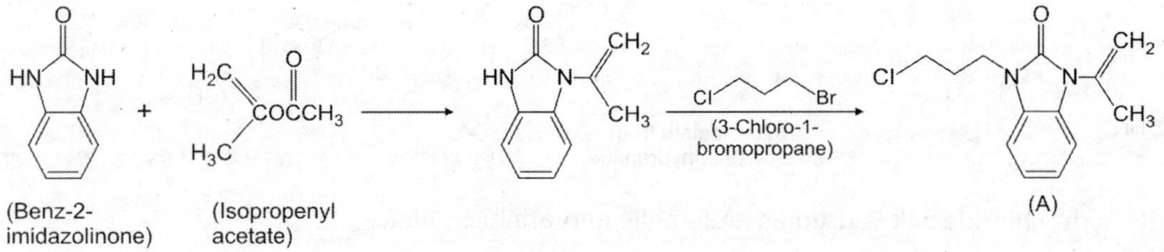

(Benz-2-
imidazolinone)

(Isopropenyl
acetate)

(3-Chloro-1-
bromopropane)

(A)

Step 2

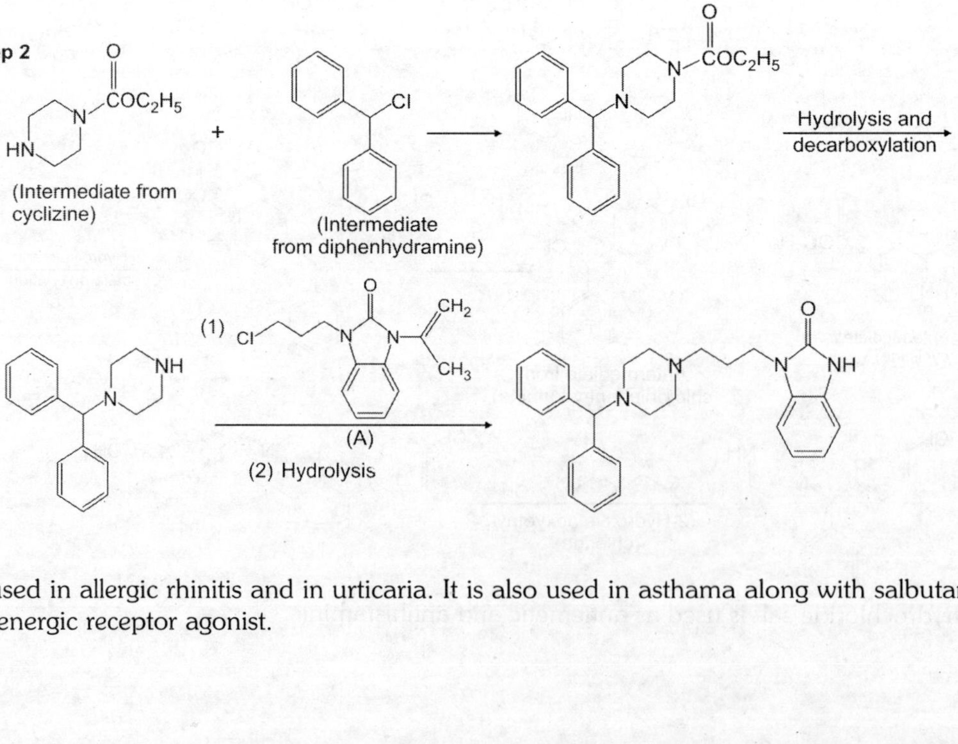

(Intermediate from
cyclizine)

(Intermediate
from diphenhydramine)

Hydrolysis and
decarboxylation

(1)

(A)

(2) Hydrolysis

It is used in allergic rhinitis and in urticaria. It is also used in asthama along with salbutamol, a β_2-adrenergic receptor agonist.

ANTIHISTAMINTICS: H_1-RECEPTOR ANTAGONISTS—PROPYLAMINES

Pheniramine

3-Phenyl-3-(2-pyridyl)-*N,N*-dimethylpropylamine

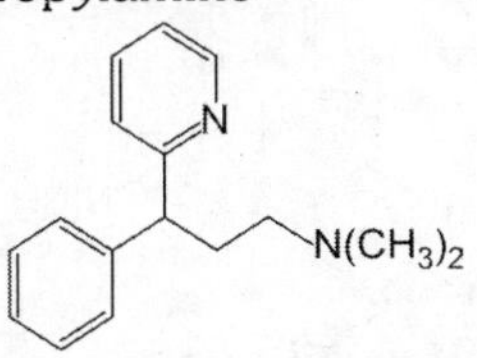
N
N(CH3)2

Synthesis

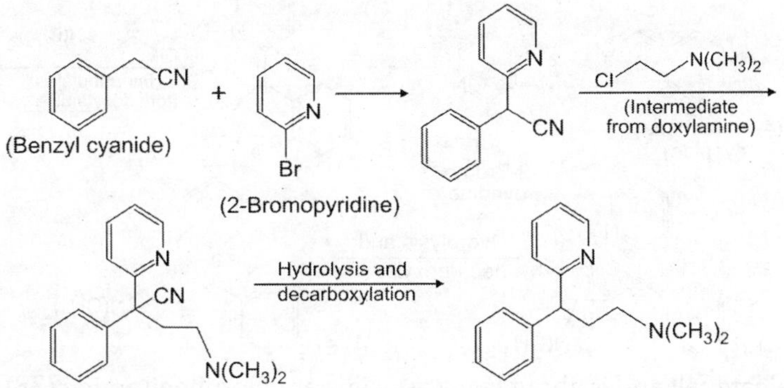
CN
(Benzyl cyanide)
+
N
Br
(2-Bromopyridine)
CN
Cl
N(CH3)2
(Intermediate
from doxylamine)
Hydrolysis and
decarboxylation
N(CH3)2

It is used as a maleate salt.

Chlorpheniramine

3-(*p*-Chlorophenyl)-3-(2-pyridyl)-*N, N*-dimethylpropylamine.

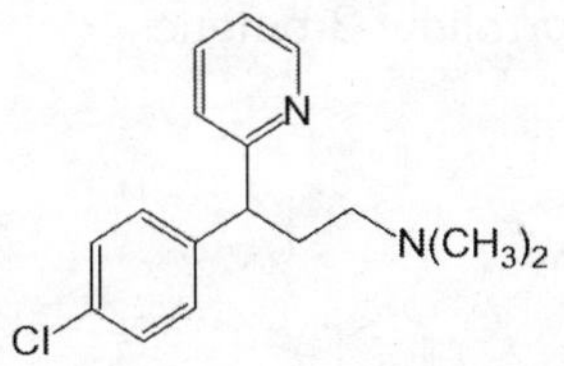
N
N(CH3)2
Cl

Synthesis

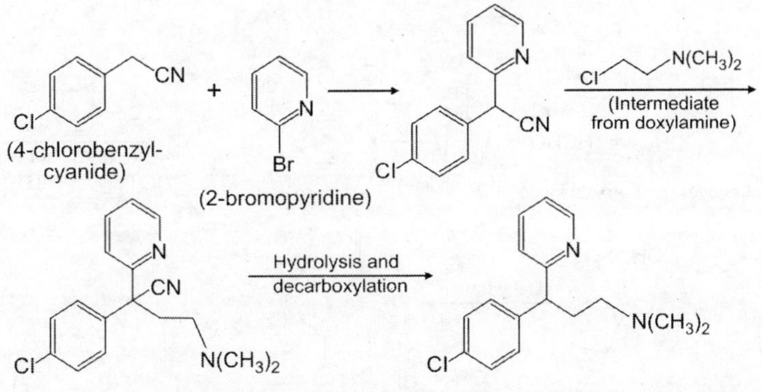
CN
Cl
(4-chlorobenzyl-
cyanide)
+
N
Br
(2-bromopyridine)
CN
Cl
N(CH3)2
(Intermediate
from doxylamine)
Hydrolysis and
decarboxylation
N(CH3)2

Although it is used as racemic mixture, most of the activity resides in dextro-isomer. It is about 10-times more active than pheniramine (37). Its maleate salt is used as antihistaminic.

Brompheniramine

3-(p-Bromophenyl)-3-(2-pyridyl)-N,N-dimethylpropylamine

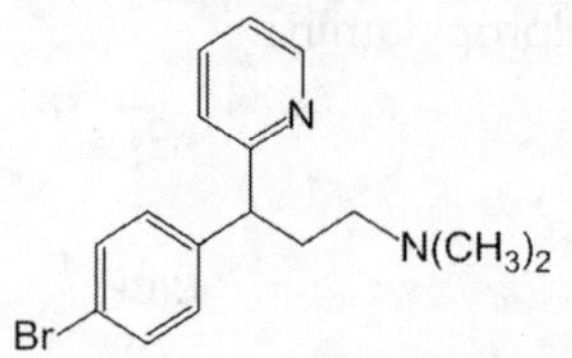

Synthesis

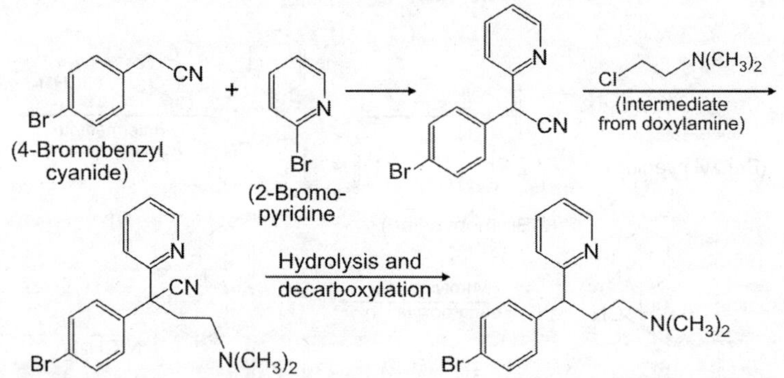

It is used as maleate salt and is about twice as active as chlorpheniramine (38) as H_1-antagonist. Dextro-form possesses maximum activity.

Pyrrobutamine

(E)-1-p-Chlorophenyl-2-phenyl-4-pyrrolidyl-2-butene

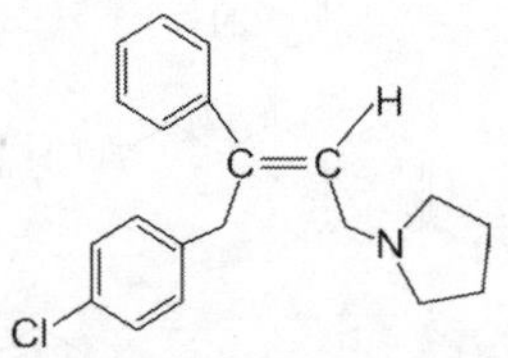

Synthesis

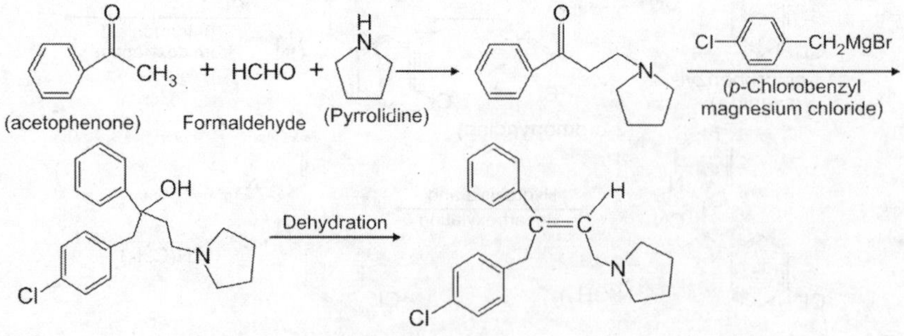

It is used as phosphate and hydrochloride salt.

Triprolidine

(*E*)-2-[3-(Pyrrolidin-1-yl)-1-*p*-tolylprop-1-enyl]pyridine

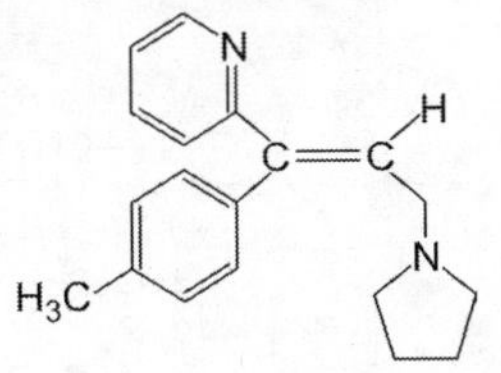

Synthesis

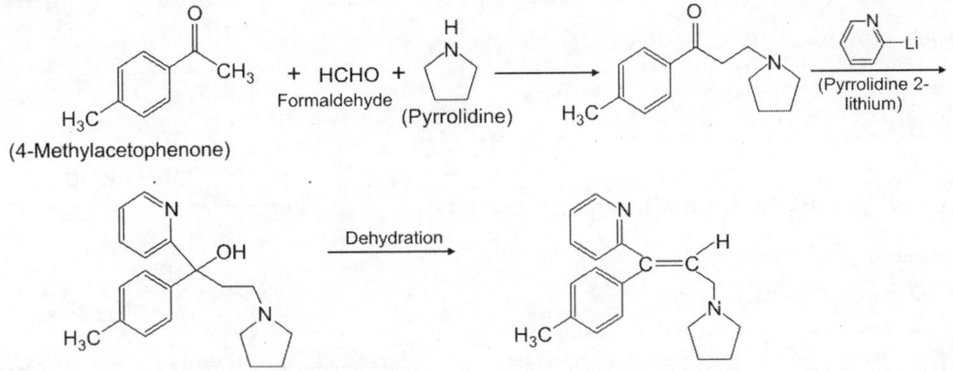

It is used as a tartrate salt. The activity is mainly in *E*-isomer. The potency is of the same order as that of chlorpheniramine (38).

Dimethindene

(±)-*N,N*-Dimethyl-3-[1-(2-pyridinyl)ethyl]-1-*H*-indene-2-ethanamine

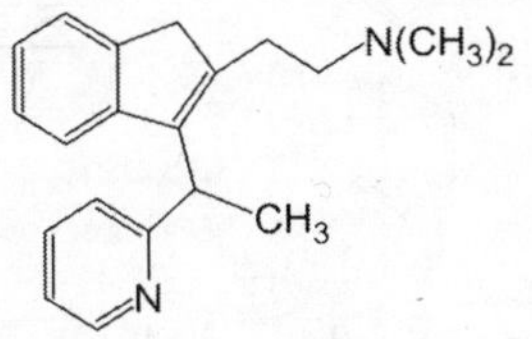

Synthesis

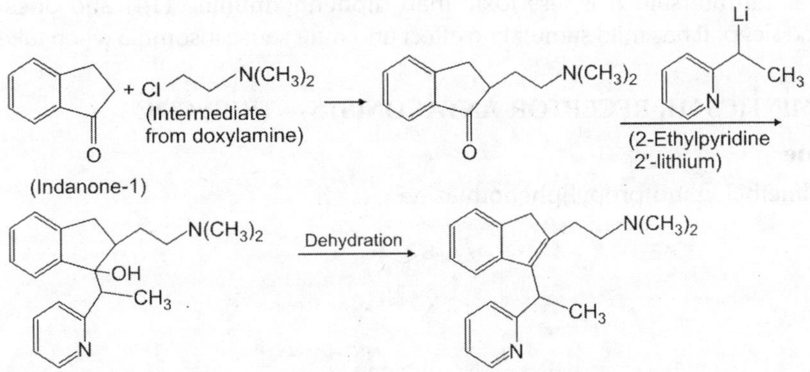

It is used as maleate salt. The antihistaminic activity lies mainly in levo-isomer. It is a potent antihistaminic. The side effects are sedation and drowsiness.

Phenindamine

2,3,4,9-Tetrahydro-2-methyl-9-phenyl-1H-indeno[2, 1-c]pyridine

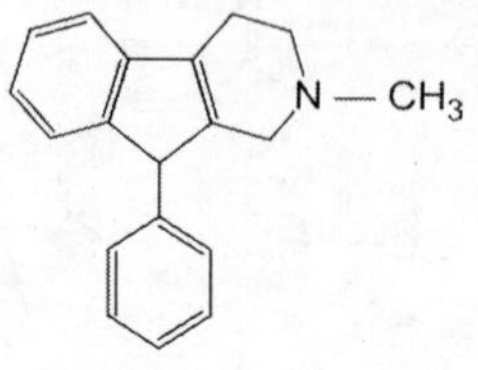

Synthesis

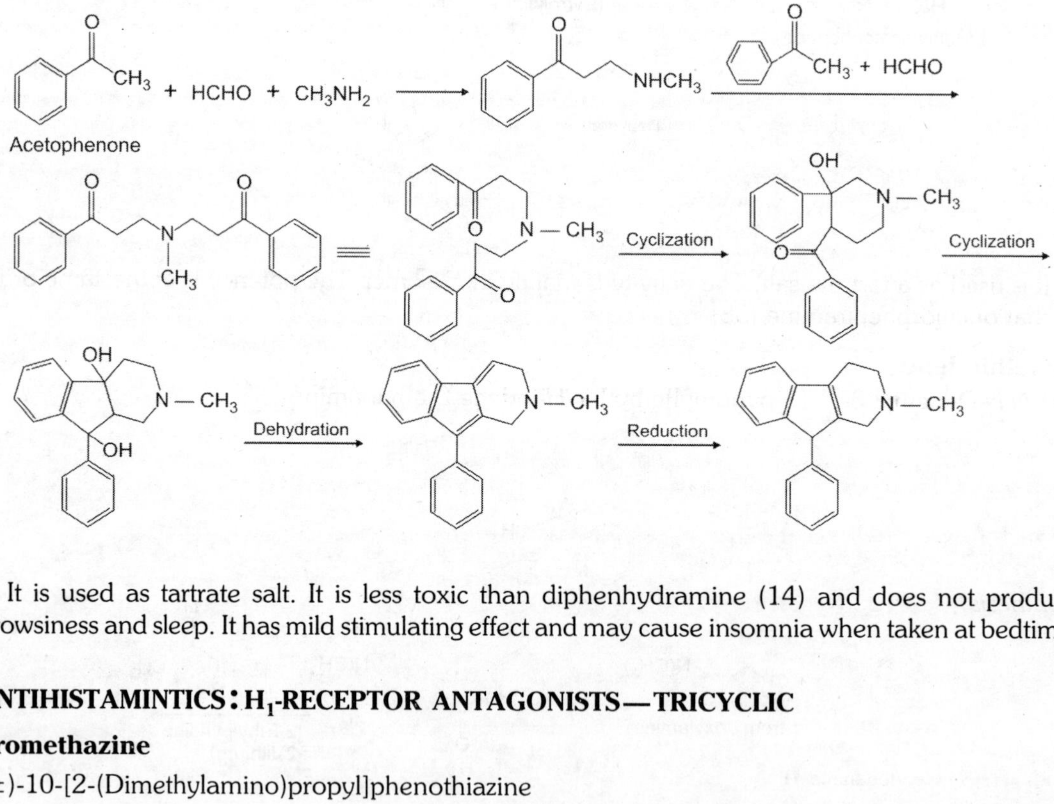

It is used as tartrate salt. It is less toxic than diphenhydramine (14) and does not produce drowsiness and sleep. It has mild stimulating effect and may cause insomnia when taken at bedtime.

ANTIHISTAMINTICS : H$_1$-RECEPTOR ANTAGONISTS—TRICYCLIC

Promethazine

(±)-10-[2-(Dimethylamino)propyl]phenothiazine

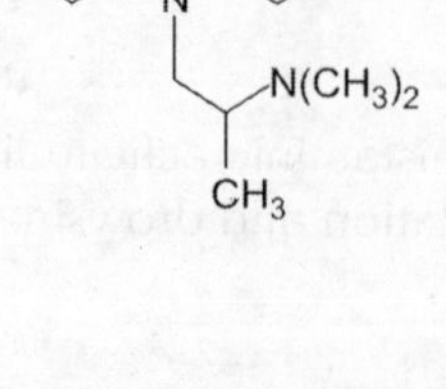

Synthesis

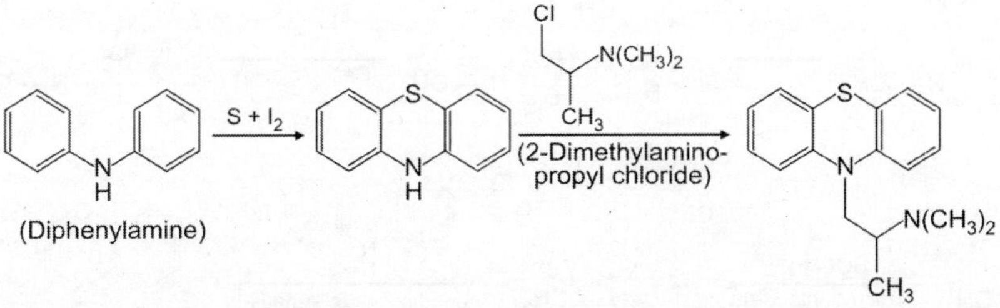

(Diphenylamine) → (2-Dimethylamino-propyl chloride)

It is used as hydrochloride and theocolate (8-chlorotheophylline) salt. It has prolonged duration of action and pronounced sedative effect. It possesses antiemetic and tranquillizing action also and potentiates the action of analgesics and sedatives.

Trimeprazine
($\pm$)-10[3-(Dimethylamino)-2-methylpropyl]phenothiazine

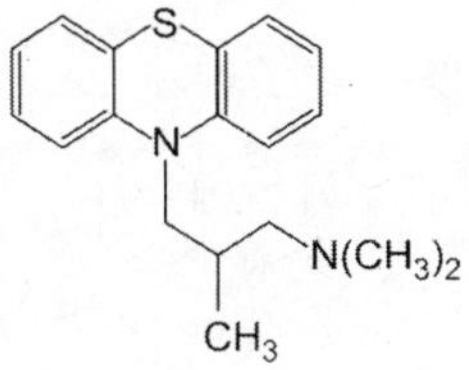

Synthesis

(Phenothiazine, intermediate from promethazine)

(3-Dimethylamino-2-methylpropyl chloride)

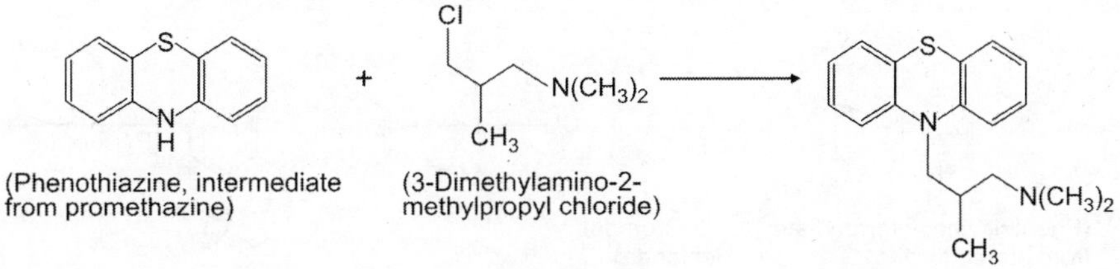

It is used as tartrate salt and is about 5 times as active as promethazine (44).

Methdilazine
10-[(1-Methyl-3-pyrrolidinyl)methyl]phenothiazine

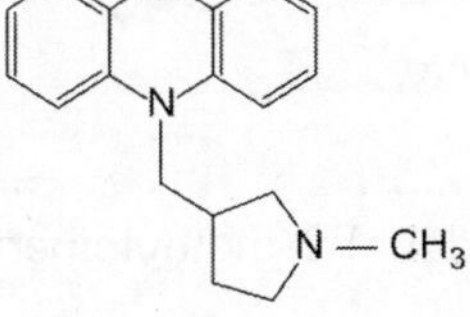

Synthesis

(1-Methyl-pyrrolidin-2-one)

(Ethyl oxalate half ester)

Reduction (Catalytic)

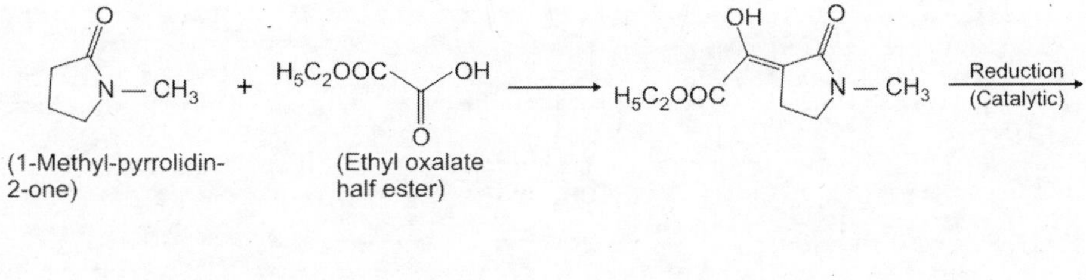

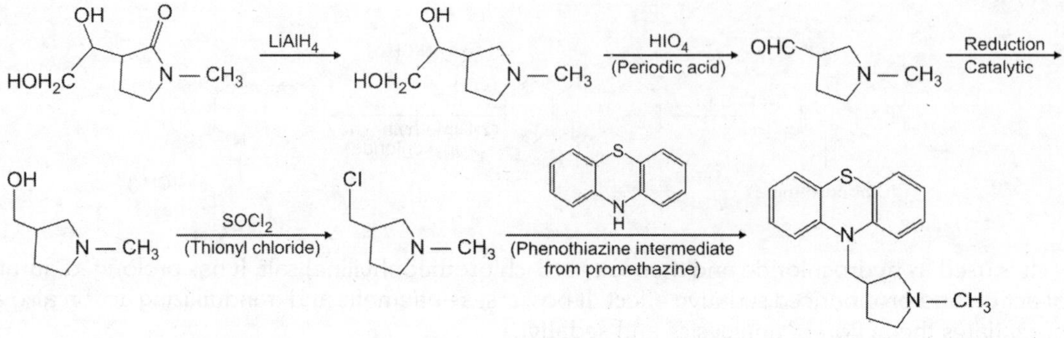

It is used as base as well as its hydrochloride salt. Base is used as a chewable tablet and salt is used orally.

Pyrathiazine
10-[2-(1-Pyrrolidinyl)ethyl]phenothiazine

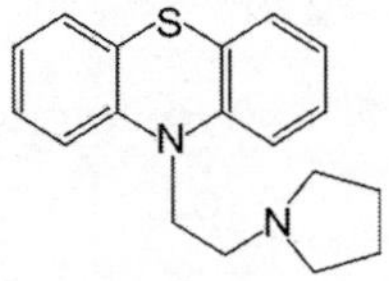

Synthesis

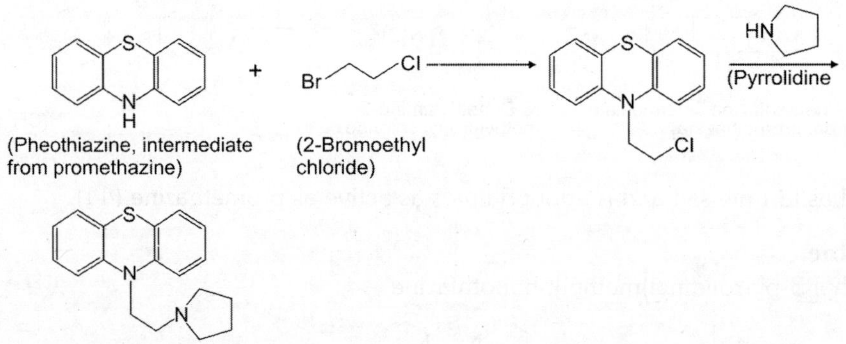

(Pheothiazine, intermediate from promethazine)

(2-Bromoethyl chloride)

(Pyrrolidine

It has moderate antihistaminic activity.

Cyproheptadine
4-(5*H*-Dibenzo[a, d]cyclohepten-5-ylidene)-1-methylpiperidine

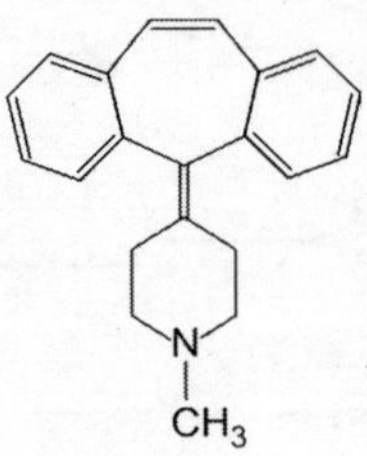

Synthesis

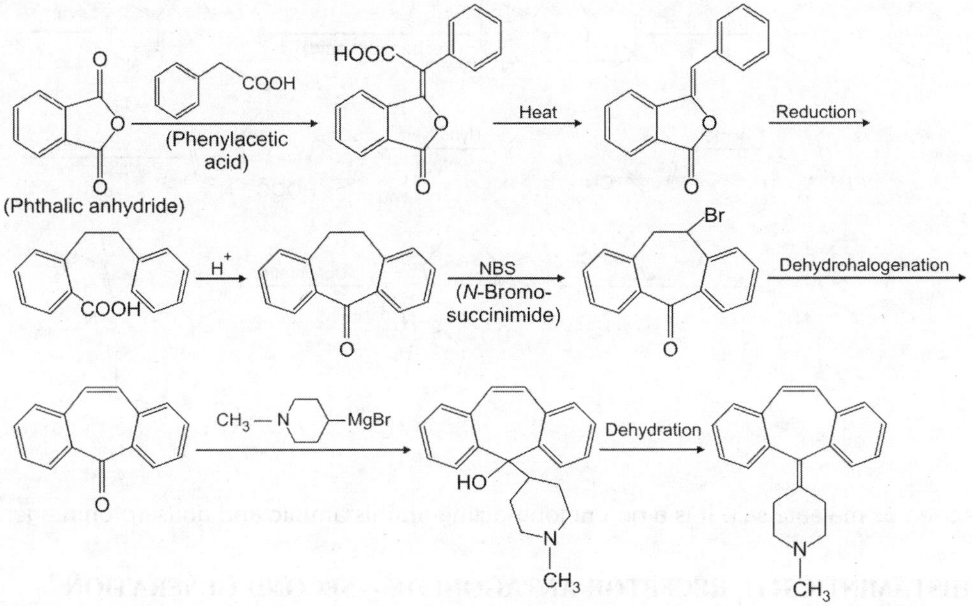

It is used as hydrochloride. It has both antihistaminic and antiserotonin activity. The antihistaminic activity is comparable to chlorpheniramine (38).

Azatidine

6,11-Dihydro-11-(1-methyl-4-piperidylidene)-5*H*-benzo[5, 6]cyclohepta [1, 2-b] pyridine

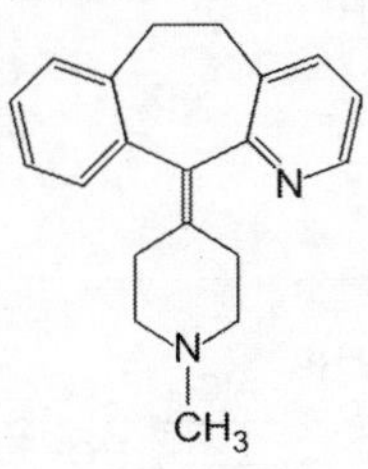

Synthesis

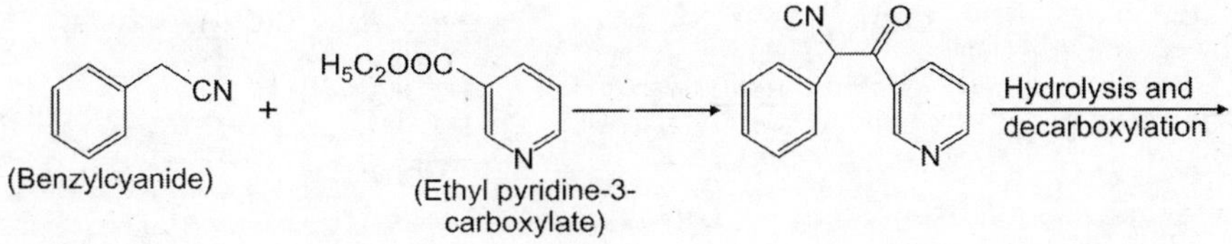

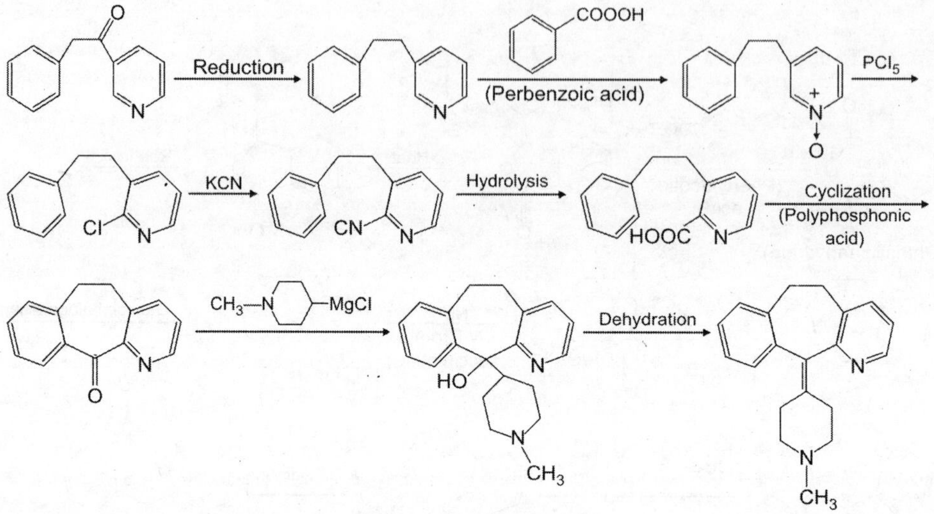

It is used as maleate salt. It is a potent long-acting antihistaminic and antiserotonin agent.

ANTIHISTAMINTICS : H₁-RECEPTOR ANTAGONISTS—SECOND GENERATION

Terfenadine
1-(*p-tert*-Butylphenyl)-4-[4'-(α-hydroxydiphenylmethyl)-1-piperidyl]-butanol

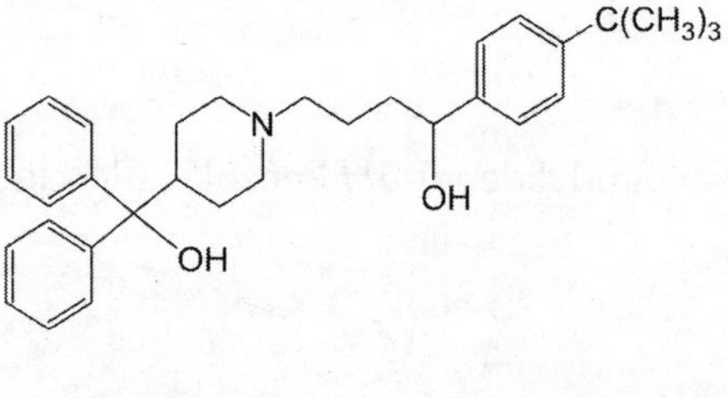

Synthesis

Step 1

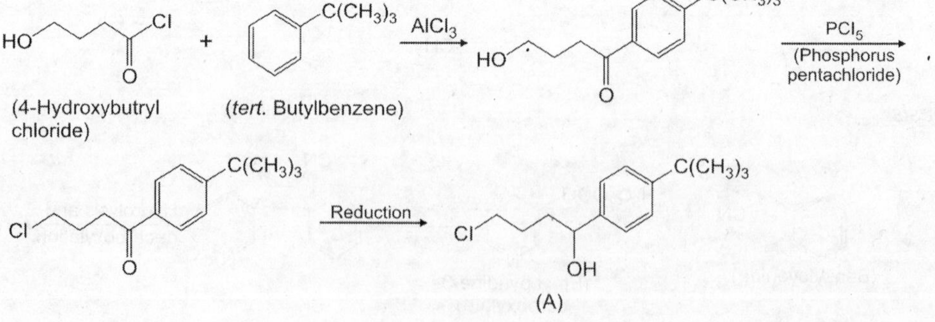

(A)

Step 2

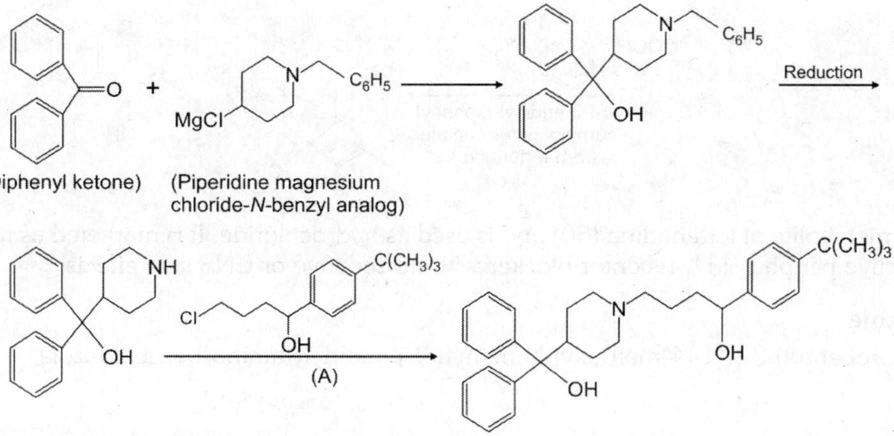

(Diphenyl ketone)   (Piperidine magnesium
                     chloride-*N*-benzyl analog)

It is a long-acting non-sedative H$_1$-antagonist.

Fexofenadine

(±)-4-[1-Hydroxy-4[4-(hydroxydiphenylmethyl)-1-piperidinyl]butyl-α, α-dimethyl benzeneacetic acid

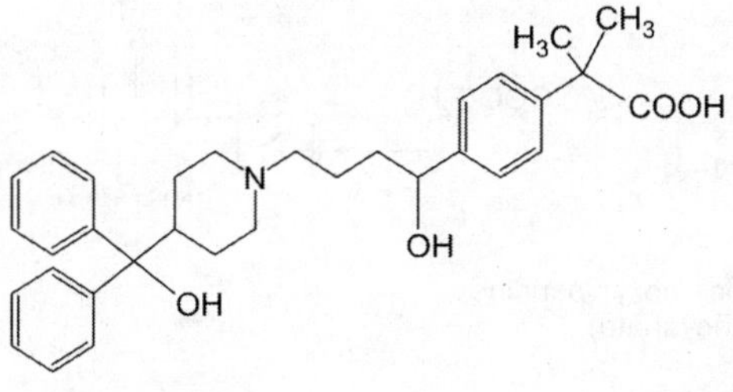

Synthesis

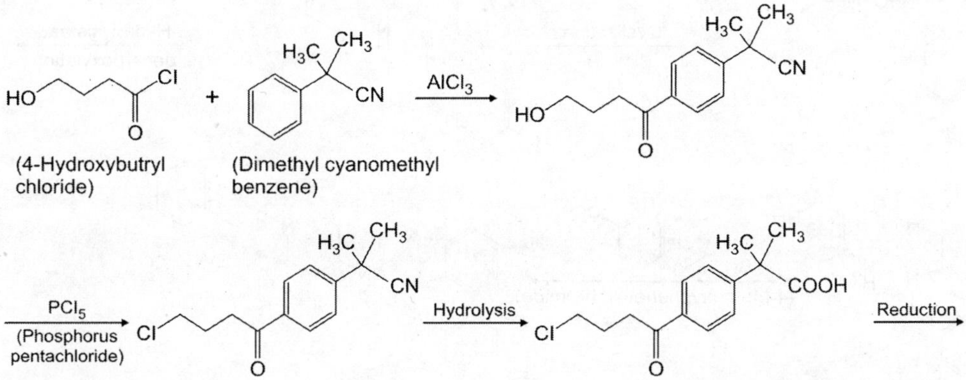

(4-Hydroxybutryl   (Dimethyl cyanomethyl
chloride)   benzene)

PCl$_5$
(Phosphorus
pentachloride)

Hydrolysis

Reduction

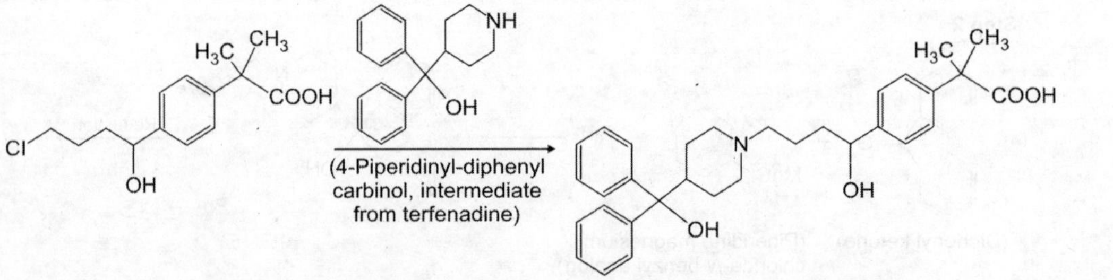

It is a metabolite of terfenadine (50) and is used as hydrochloride. It is marketed as racemate. It is a selective peripheral H_1-receptor blocker with no sedative or CNS side effects.

Astemizole

1-(4-Fluorobenzyl)-2-[[(1-(4-methoxyphenethyl)-4-piperidyl] amino]benzimidazole

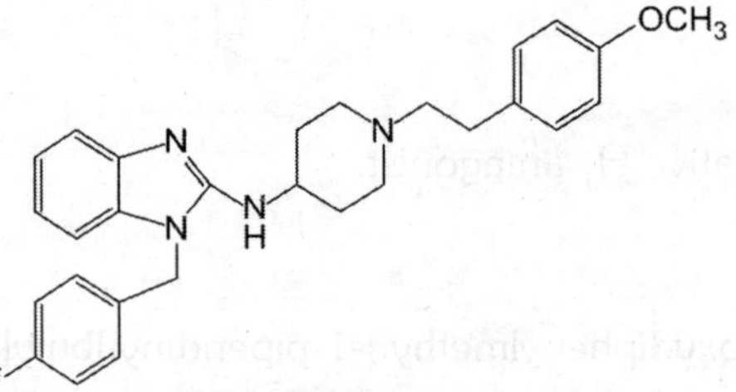

Synthesis

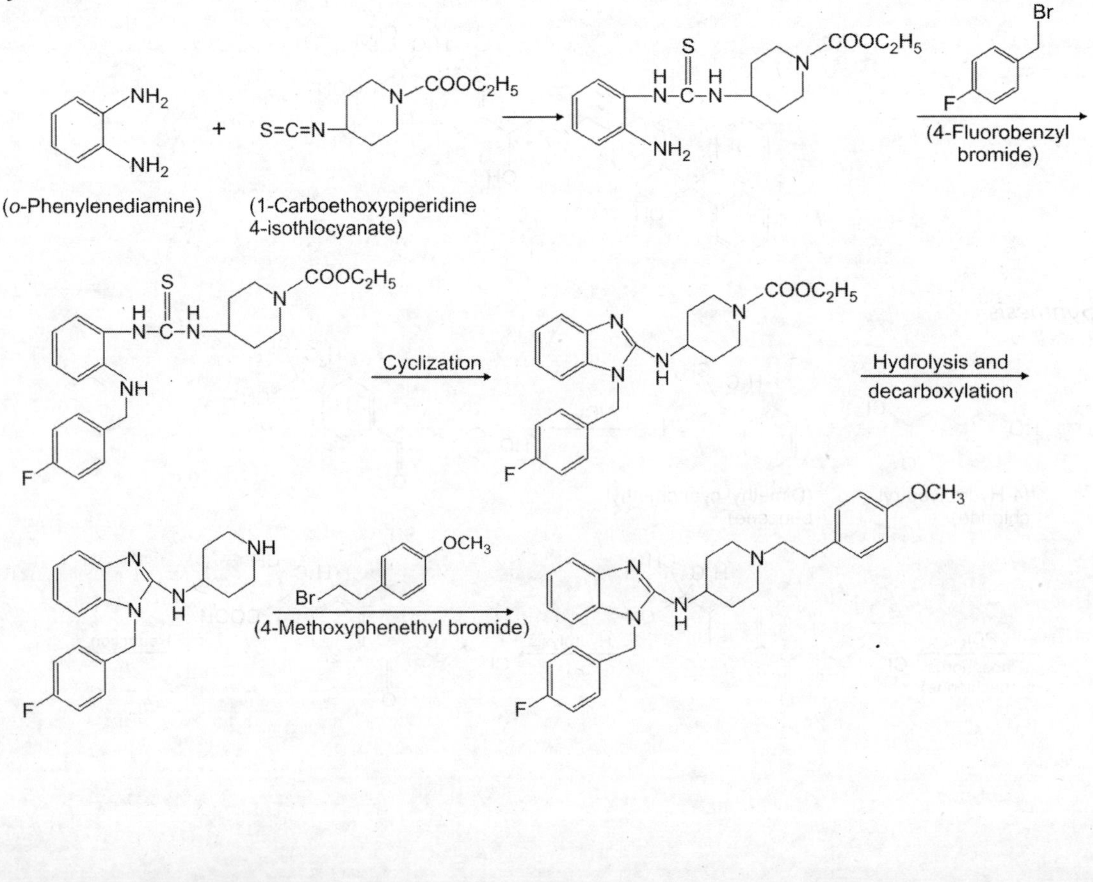

It is a potent selective H_1-antagonist without sedative effect. It has no muscarinic, serotogenic, adrenergic, or H_2-antagonistic activity.

Loratadine

4-(8-Chloro-5,6-dihydro-11H-benzo[5,6]cyclohepta[1, 2 b]pyridin-11-ylidene)-1-piperidinecarboxylic acid ethyl ester.

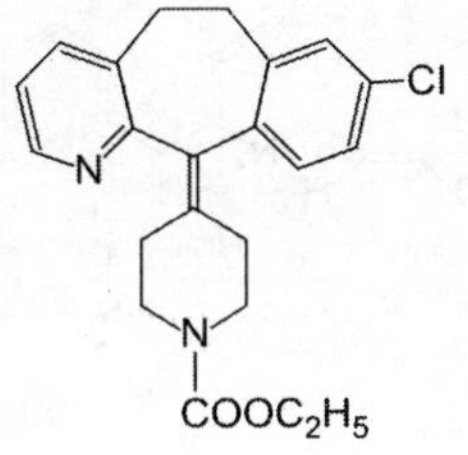

Synthesis

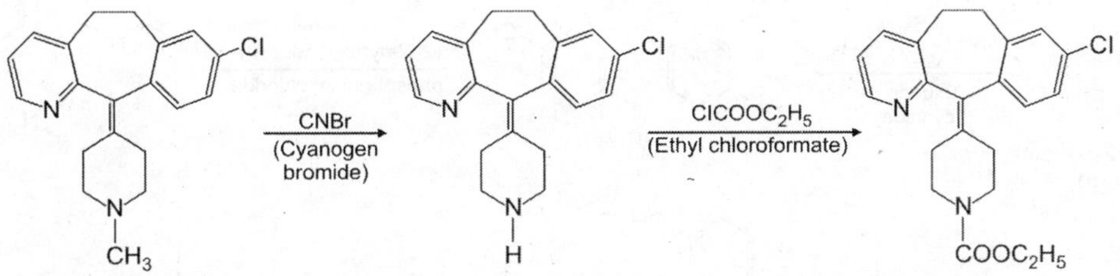

(8-Chloroazatadine)

The structure of loratadine is similar to azatidine (49) excepting that it contains a chloro group in benzene nucleus and there is carboxyethyl group on piperidine nitrogen instead of methyl group. It has less CNS effects because it cannot pass blood-brain barrier. It is metabolized to desloratidine (54) which is also active H_1-antagonist.

Cetirizine

[2-[4-[(4-Chlorophenyl)phenylmethyl]-1-piperazinyl]ethoxy]acetic acid

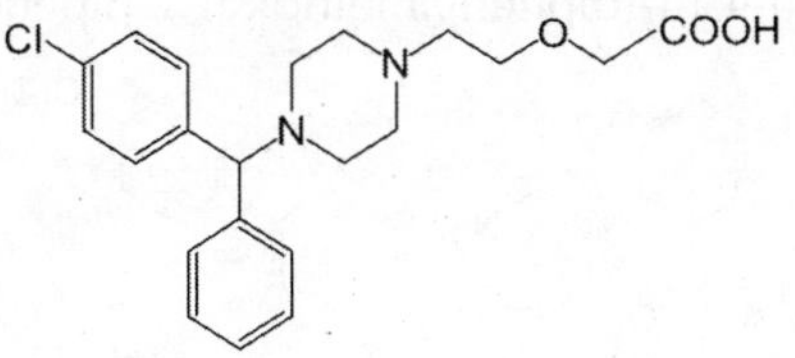

Synthesis

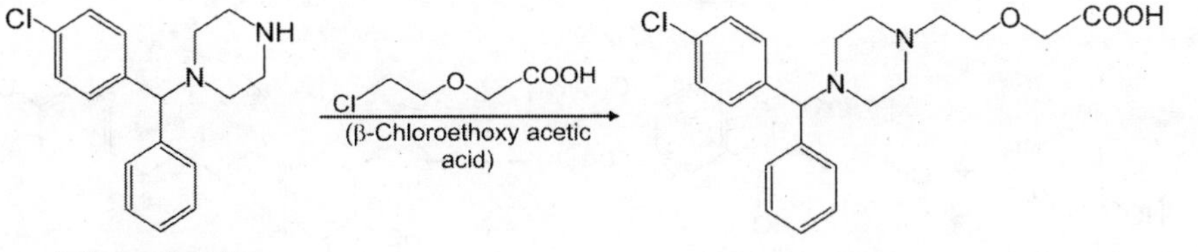

(Intermediate from hydroxyzine)

It is the carboxylic acid metabolite of hydroxyzine (34). Because of the carboxylic acid group it cannot pass the blood-brain barrier. It is highly selective H_1-antagonist without any central effects. It has rapid onset of action and longer duration of action.

Acrivastine

(E, E)-3-[6-[1-(4-methylphenyl)-3-(1-pyrrolidinyl)-1-propenyl]-2-pyridinyl]-2-propenoic acid

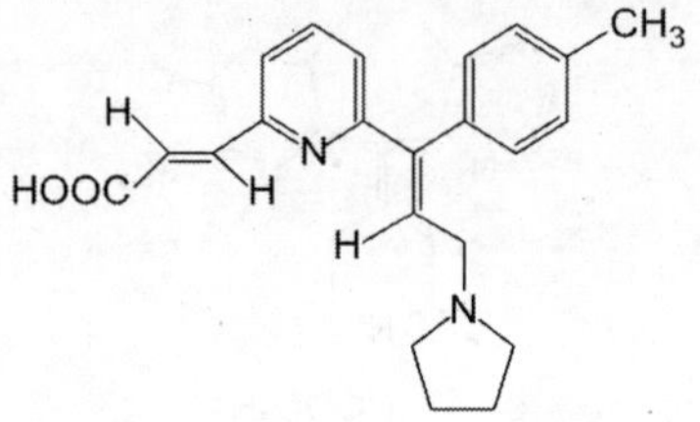

Synthesis

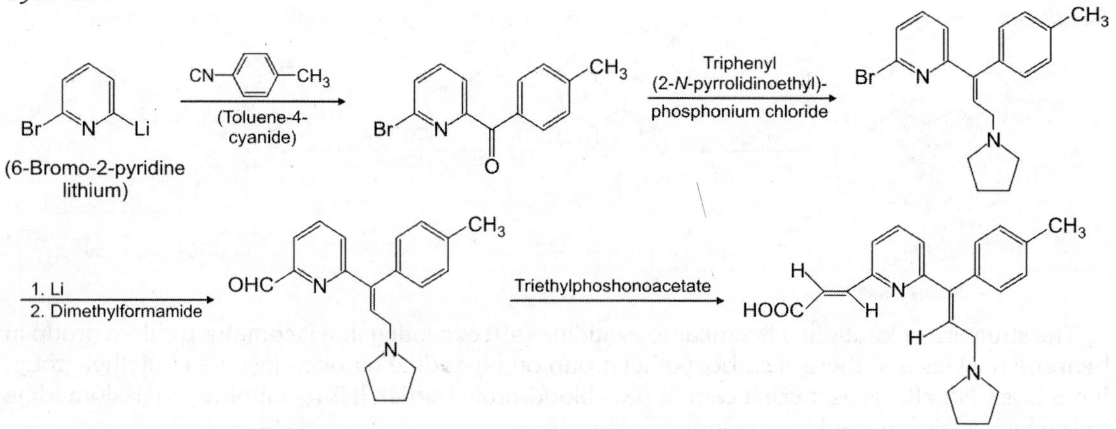

It is an analog of triprolidine (41). It has similar activity as triprolidine (41) but does not possess anticholinergic activity at the concentration used clinically.

Ebastine

1-[4-(1,1-Dimethylethyl)phenyl]-4-[4-(diphenylmethoxy)-1-piperidinyl]-1-butanone

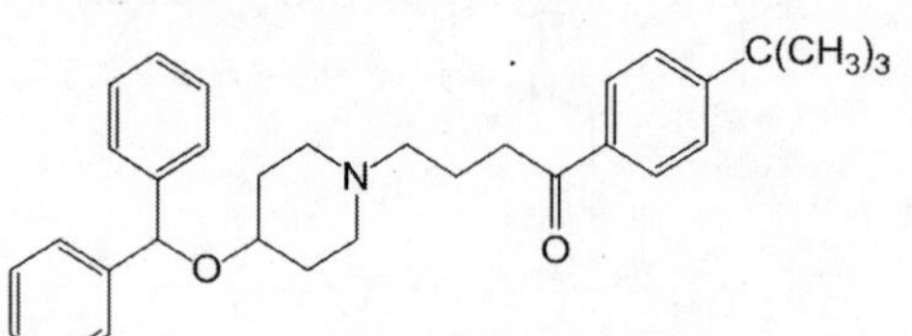

Synthesis

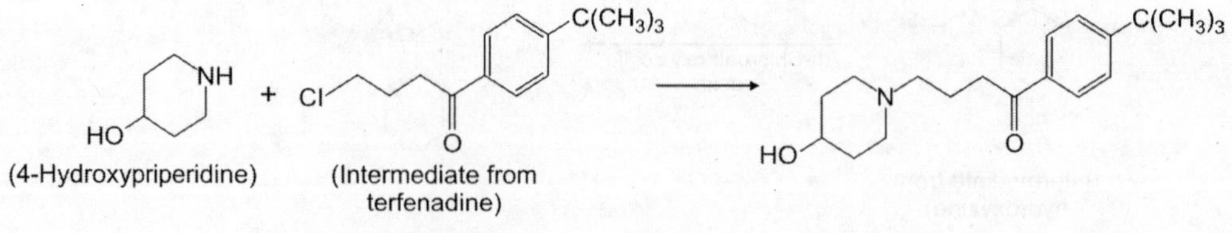

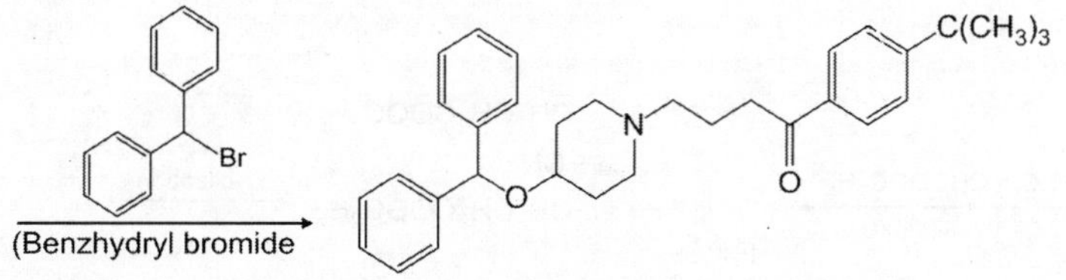

(Benzhydryl bromide)

It is similar to terfenadine (50) and is potent drug without sedation and anticholinergic activity. Carebastine (58), its carboxy metabolite is the active metabolite.

ANTIHISTAMINTICS : HISTAMINE RELEASE INHIBITORS WITH H$_1$-RECEPTOR ANTAGONISTIC ACTIVITY

Olopatadine

(11Z)-11-[3-Dimethylamino)propylidene[-6,11-dihydrodibenz[b,e]oxepin-2-acetic acid

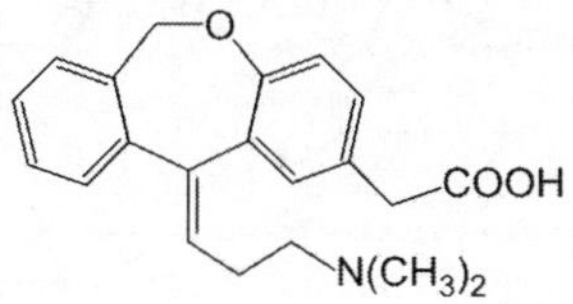

Synthesis

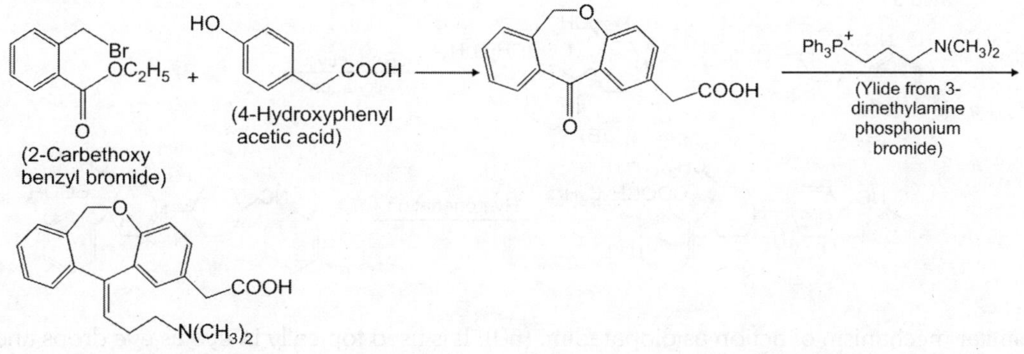

It inhibits the release of histamine (1) from mast cells as well as inhibits H$_1$-receptors. It is used topically for the relief of itching in the eye. It is related to tricyclic H$_1$-antagonists.

Levocabastine

(-)-*trans*-1-[*cis*-4-Cyano-4-(*p*-fluorophenyl)cyclohexyl]-3-methyl-4-phenylisonipecotic acid

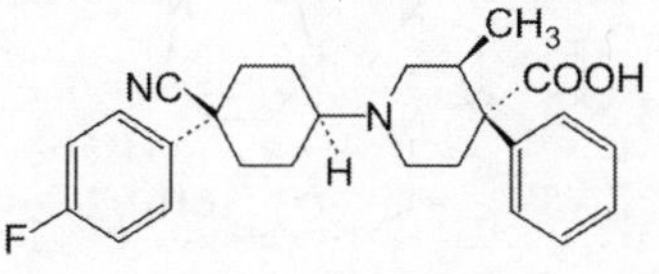

Synthesis

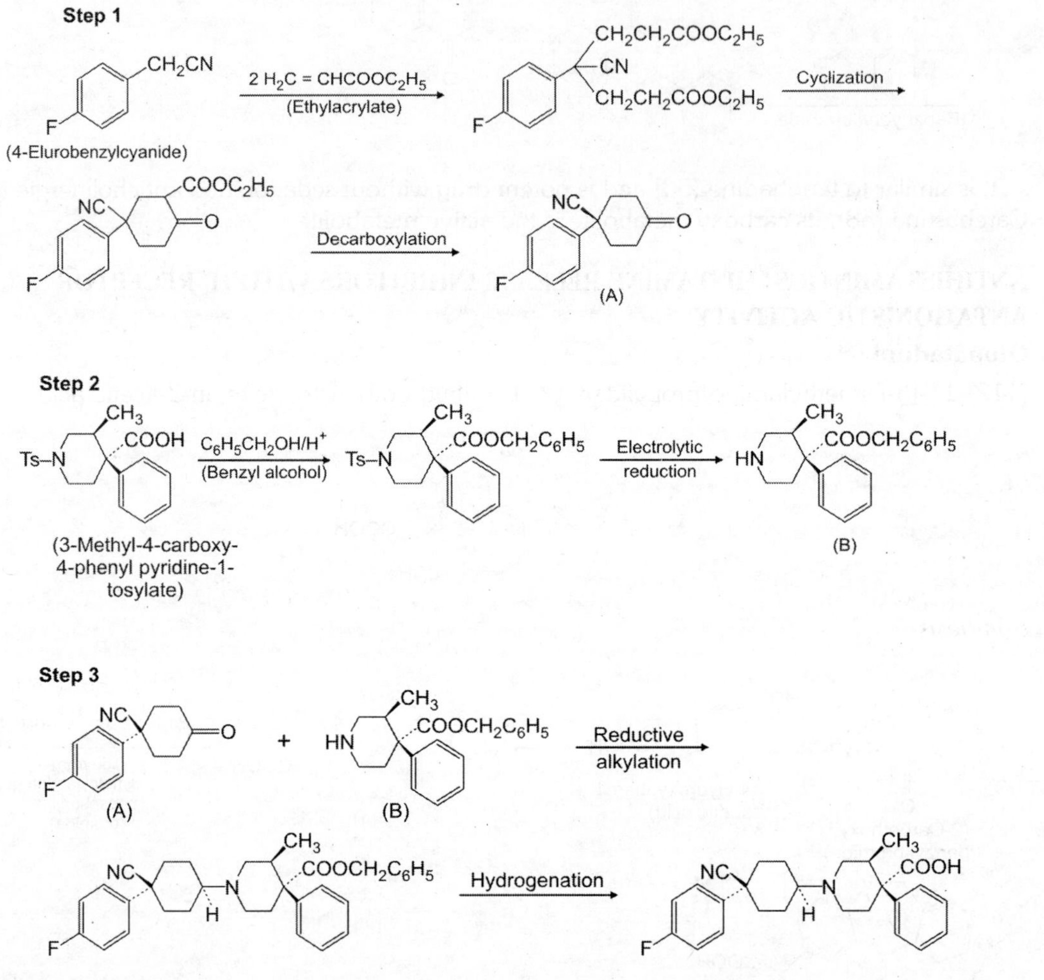

Step 1

(4-Elurobenzylcyanide)

2 H$_2$C = CHCOOC$_2$H$_5$
(Ethylacrylate)

Cyclization

Decarboxylation

(A)

Step 2

(3-Methyl-4-carboxy-
4-phenyl pyridine-1-
tosylate)

C$_6$H$_5$CH$_2$OH/H$^+$
(Benzyl alcohol)

Electrolytic
reduction

(B)

Step 3

(A)   +   (B)

Reductive
alkylation

Hydrogenation

Similar mechanism of action as olopatadine (60). It is used topically in eye as eye drops and as nasal spray.

Emedastine

1-(2-Ethoxyethyl)-2-(hexahydro-4-methyl-1*H*-1,4-diazepin-1-yl)-1*H*-benzimidaole

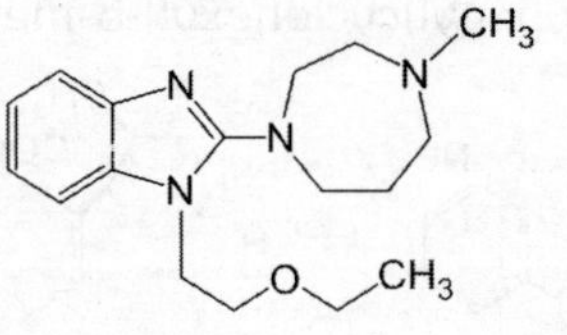

Synthesis

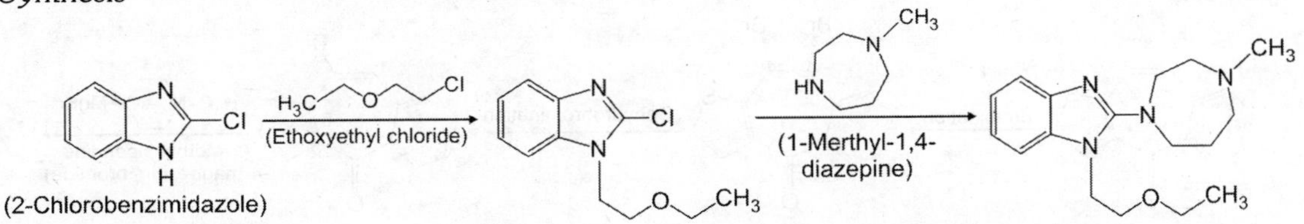

It is structurally related to astemizole (52) which is a second generation antihistaminic. It has similar action and use as levocabastine (61).

Azelastine
4-(*p*-Chlorobenzyl)-2-(hexahydro-1-methyl-1*H*-azepin-4-yl)-1(2*H*)-phthalazinone

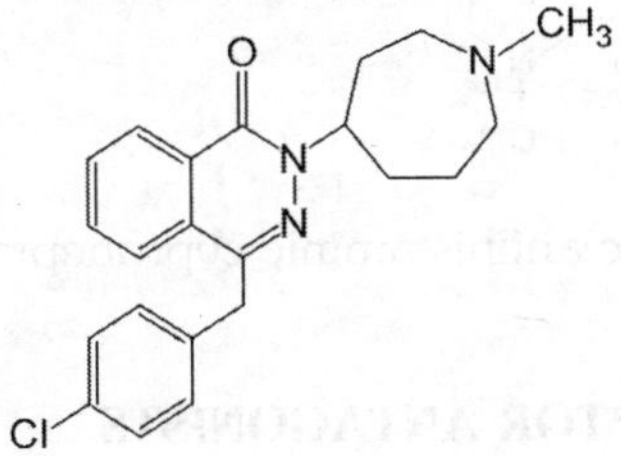

Synthesis

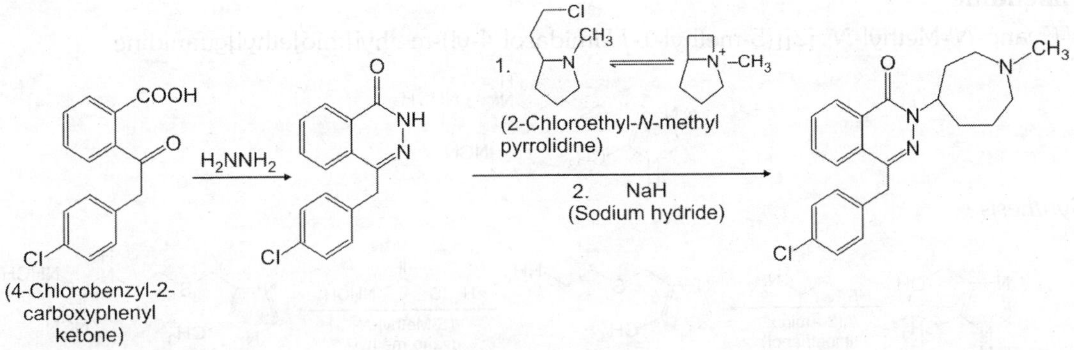

Same action and use as emedastine (62).

Ketotifen
4,9-Dihydro-4-(1-methyl-4-piperidinylidene)-10*H*-benzo[4, 5]cyclohepta[1, 2-b]thiophen-10-one

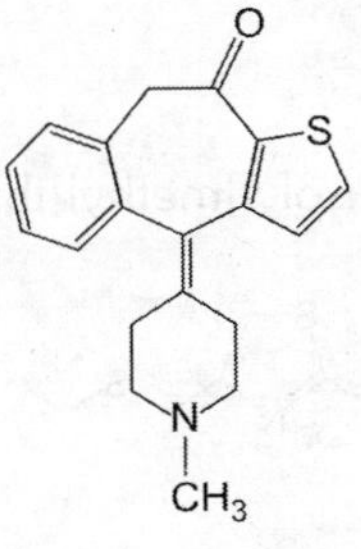

Synthesis

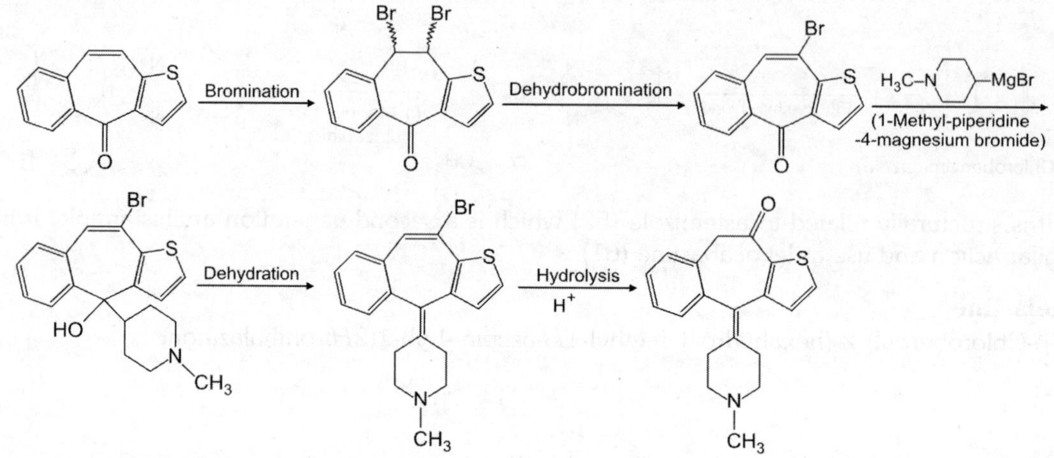

It is structurally similar to tricyclic antihistaminic cyproheptadine (48). It has similar action and use as emedastine (62).

ANTIULCER AGENTS : H$_2$-RECEPTOR ANTAGONISTS

Cimetidine

N-Cyano-*N'*-Methyl-*N"*-[2[[(5-methyl-1-*H*-imidazol-4-yl)-methyl]thio]ethyl]guanidine

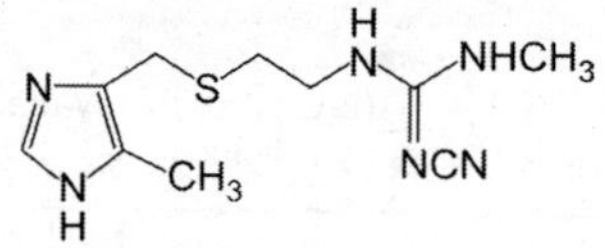

Synthesis

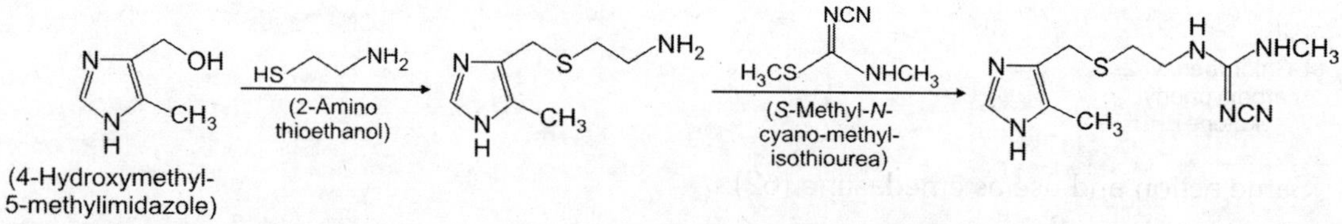

(4-Hydroxymethyl-5-methylimidazole)

Cimetidine is used orally for duodenal ulcers, hypersecretory condition, and benign gastric ulcer. Antacids interfere with the cimetidine absorption and they are administered at least an hour before or after the administration of cimetidine.

Famotidine

3-[[[2-[(Aminoiminomethyl)amino]4-thiazolyl]methyl]thio]-*N*-(aminosulfonyl) propanimidamide

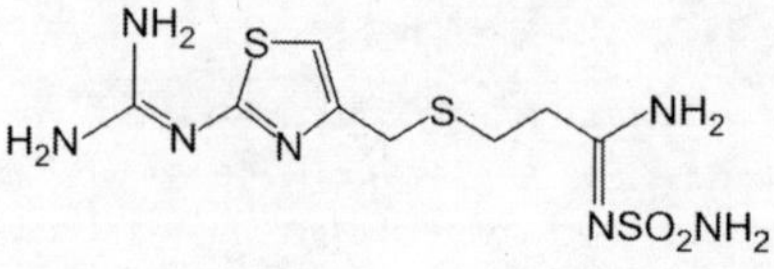

Synthesis

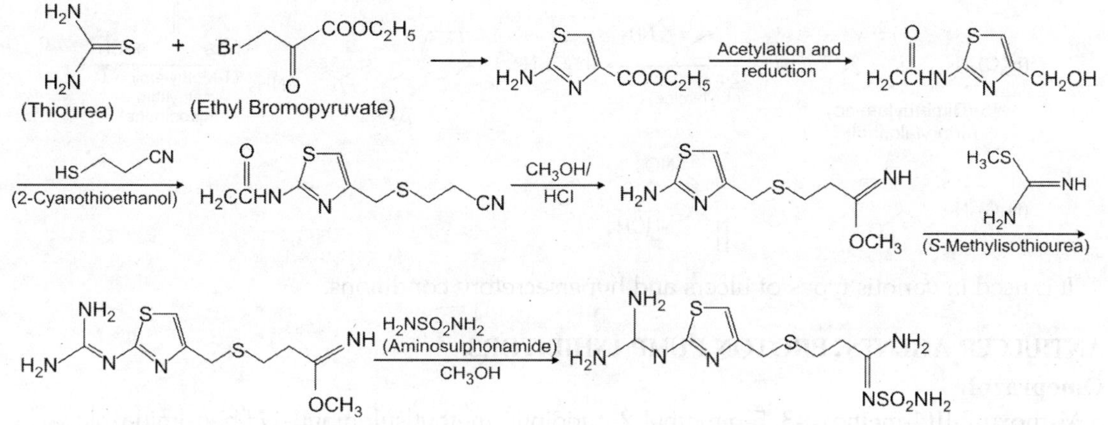

Famotidine is a competitive inhibitor of H_2-receptors and inhibits basal and nocturnal gastric secretion. It is used in duodenal ulcers, basal gastric ulcers, and hypersecretory conditions.

Nizatidine

N-[2-[[[2-[(Dimethylamino)methyl]-4-thiazolyl]-methyl]thio]ethyl]-*N*′methyl-2-nitro-1,1-ethene-diamine

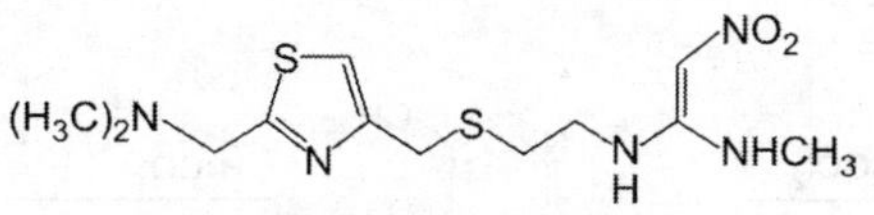

Synthesis

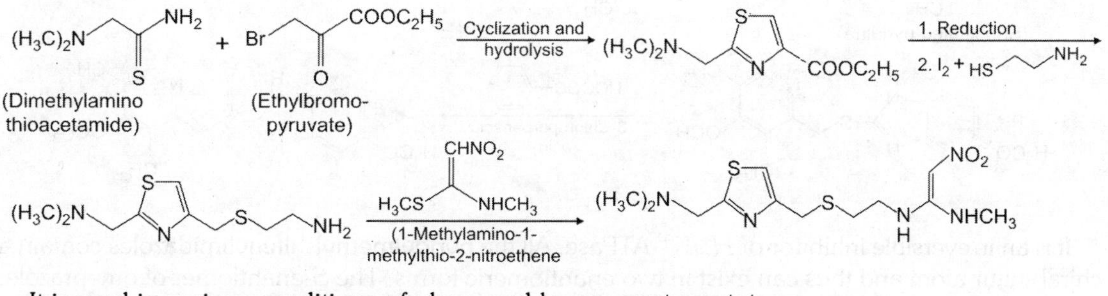

It is used in various conditions of ulcers and hypersecretory state.

Rantidine

N-[2-[[[5-[(Dimethylamino)methyl]2-furanyl]methyl]thio]ethyl]-*N*′-methyl-2-nitro-1,1-ethenediamine

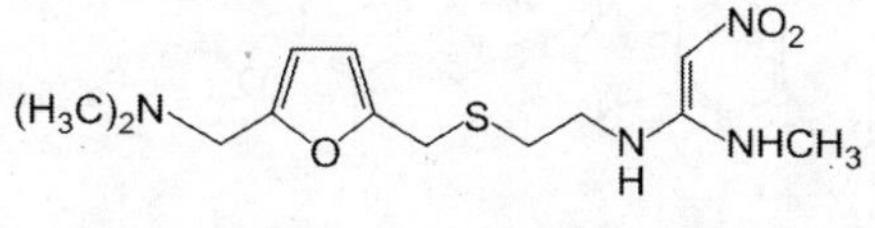

Synthesis

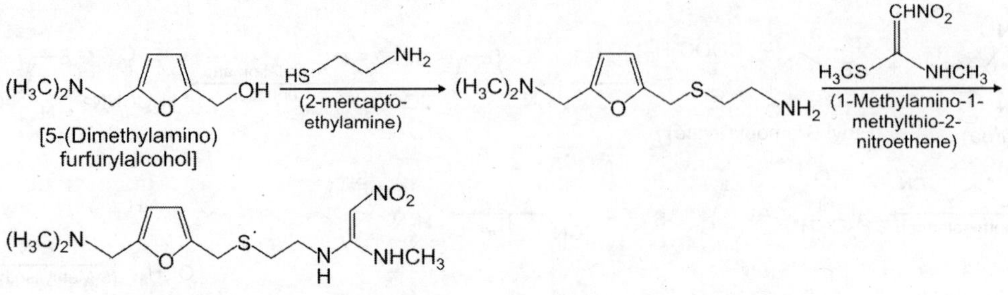

It is used in various types of ulcers and hypersecretory conditions.

ANTIULCER AGENTS : PROTON PUMP INHIBITORS

Omeprazole

5-Methoxy-2-[[(4-methoxy-3, 5-dimethyl-2-pyridinyl)-methyl]sulphinyl]-1*H*-benzimidazole

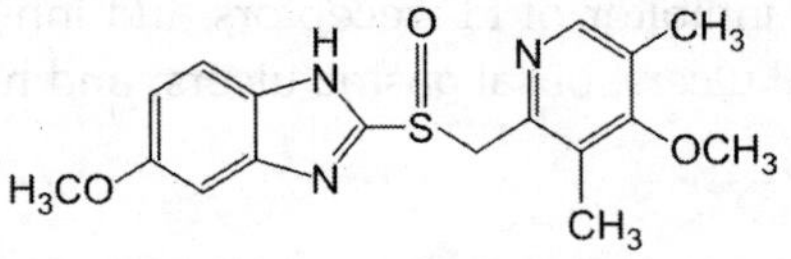

Synthesis

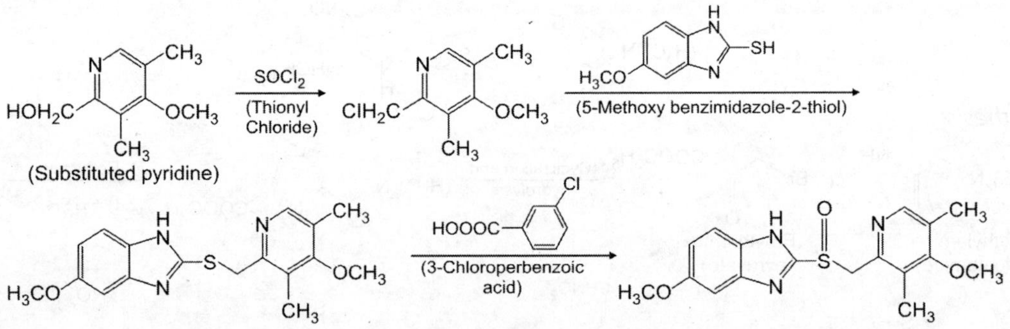

It is an irreversible inhibitor of H^+/K^+-ATPase. All the pyridylmethylsulfenylimidazoles contain a chiral sulfur atom and thus can exist in two enantiomeric forms. The *S*-enantiomer of omeprazole, commonly known as esomeprazole, is slightly more active than its *R*-enantiomer.

Lansoprazole

2-[[[3-Methyl-4-(2,2,2-trifluoroethoxy)-2-pyridinyl]methyl]sulphinyl]-1*H*-benzimidazole

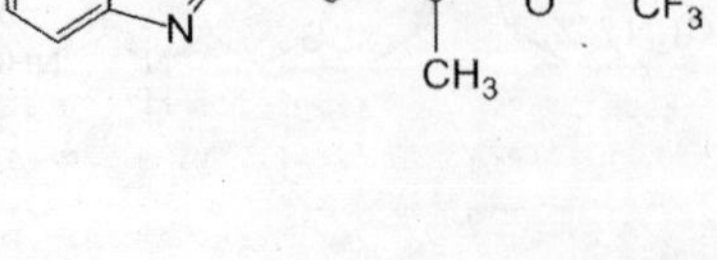

Synthesis

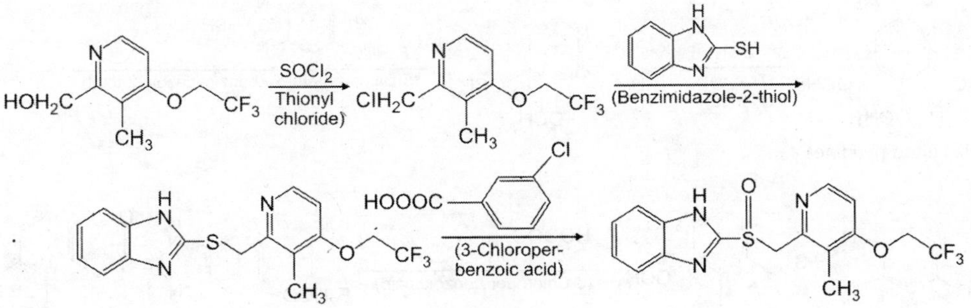

It is an inhibitor of H^+/K^+-ATPase.

Rabeprazole

2-[[[4-(3-Methoxypropoxy)-3-methyl-2-pyridinyl]methyl]sulphinyl]-1-*H*-benzimidazole

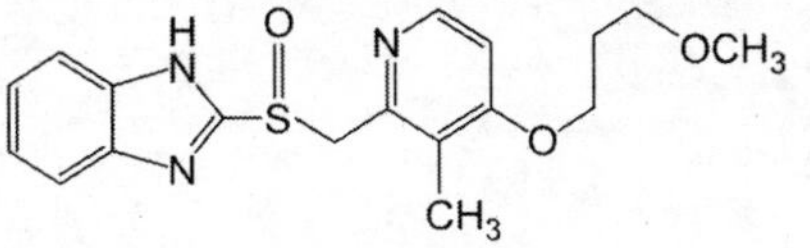

Synthesis

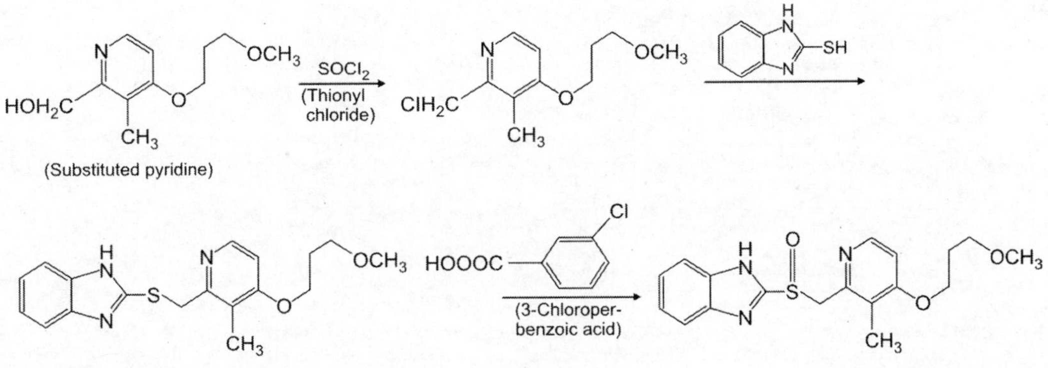

It is an inhibitor of H^+/K^+-ATPase.

Pantoprazole

5-(Difluoromethoxy)-2-[[(3,4-dimethoxy-2-pyridinyl)methyl]-sulphinyl]-1*H*-benzimidazole

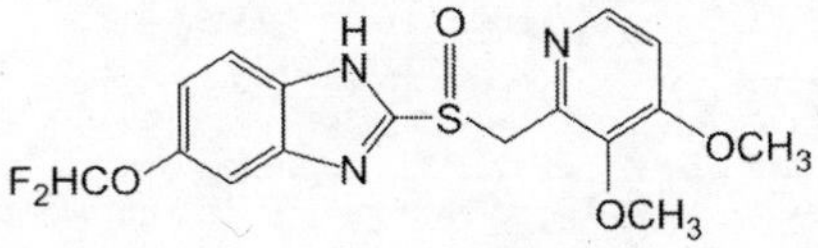

Synthesis

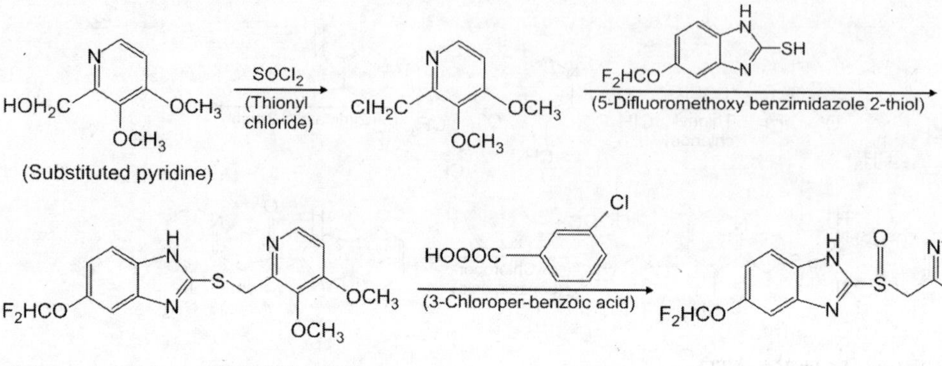

HOH₂C—(Substituted pyridine with N, OCH₃, OCH₃) →[SOCl₂ (Thionyl chloride)]→ ClH₂C—(pyridine with N, OCH₃, OCH₃) →[F₂HCO-benzimidazole-2-thiol (5-Difluoromethoxy benzimidazole 2-thiol)]→

F₂HCO—(benzimidazole)—S—CH₂—(pyridine, OCH₃, OCH₃) →[HOOOC—(3-Chloro)—benzene (3-Chloroper-benzoic acid)]→ F₂HCO—(benzimidazole)—S(=O)—CH₂—(pyridine, OCH₃, OCH₃)

It is an inhibitor of H⁺/K⁺-ATPase.

CHAPTER 12

ANALGESICS, ANTIPYRETICS, AND NONSTEROIDAL ANTI-INFLAMMATORY DRUGS

CERTAIN non-opioid non-steroidal structures possess analgesic and antiinflammatory activities. They constitute non-steroidal antiinflammatory drugs.

Antipyretics are drugs which have a specific effect on body temperature, this is due to their action on heat regulating centre in hypothalamus. They do not lower the normal body temperature and differ in this respect from hypothermic agents like chlorpromazine. The fall in temperature occurs at varying intervals after the injection of an antipyretics except in refractory cases where it begins within 2 to 3 hr.

The use of antipyretics is now restricted to cases where the temperature rise is so high as to constitute a danger in itself, to viral or other infections not amenable to chemotherapy, and to patients with febrile reactions secondary to Hodgkin's disease, heat stroke, and CNS involvement, etc. They are also used to relieve the neuralgic pain, headache, and general discomfort.

Many of these drugs are also used in rheumatoid diseases as anti-inflammatory agents. The rheumatoid diseases include rheumatoid arthritis, rheumatic fever, osteoarthritis, ankylosing spondylitis, etc. In arthritis, there can be limitation of joint function and destruction of bone, cartilage, and other articular structures.

The cause and mechanisms involved in different inflammatory diseases is not well understood. However, substances such as histamine (1), eicosanoids, platelet activating factor (2), bradykinin (3), and cytokines have been implicated as the mediators of inflammation.

$$H_3CCO-CH \begin{array}{c} O \\ \| \end{array} \quad H_2C-O-(CH_2)_nCH_3$$

(1)

(2), n = 15 or 17

Arg—Pro—Pro—Gly—Phe—Ser—Pro—Phe—Arg

(3)

As discussed earler, in 'Antihistaminics and Antiulcer Drugs', histamine (1) is synthesized by the body from histidine by the action of histidine decarboxylase. It is stored in mast cells and is released from these cells during inflammatory or allergic reactions. The action of histamine (1) are produced by binding to H_1-, H_2-, or H_3-receptors. The effects mediated through H_1-receptors include

335

contraction of smooth muscles other than blood vessels, vasodilation, and increased vascular permeabiliy. The effects mediated through H_2-receptors include stimulation of gastric secretion and cardiac stimulation. H_3-receptors which occur at presynaptic sites are involved in inhibition of the release of different neurotransmitter.

Eicosanoids include prostaglandins, thromboxanes, and leukotrienes. The eicosanoids are derived from arachidonic acid which is released by phospholipase A_2 from phospholipids.

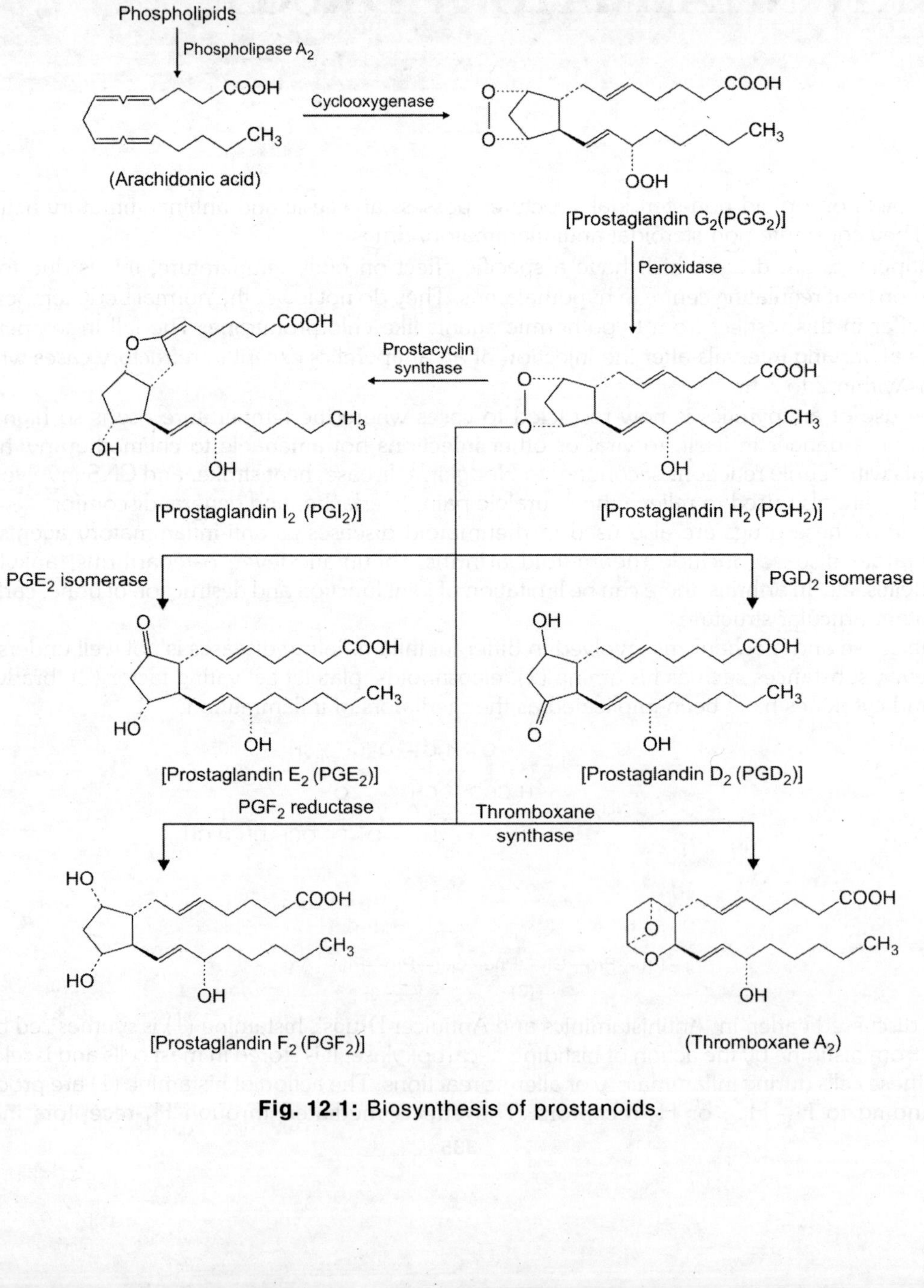

Fig. 12.1: Biosynthesis of prostanoids.

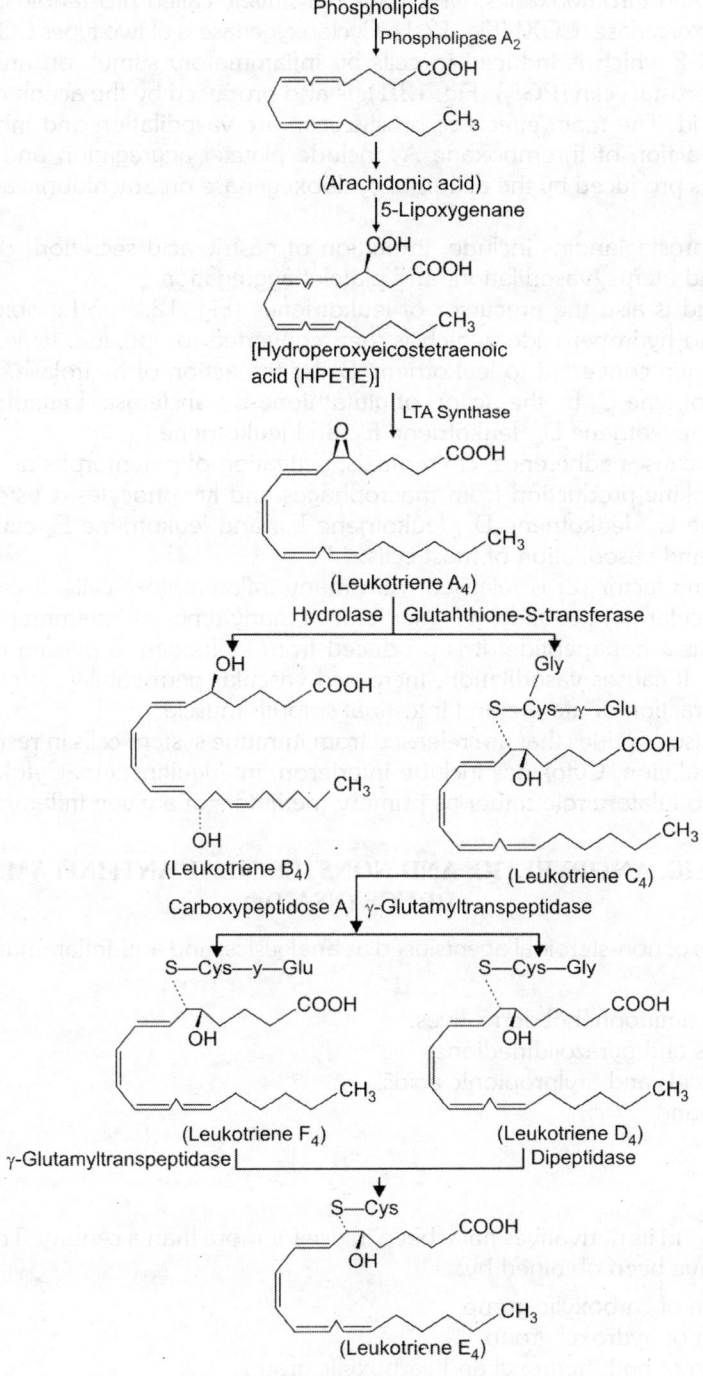

Fig. 12.2: Biosynthesis of leukotrienes.

Prostaglandins and thromboxanes, which are collectively called prostanoids, are produced by the action of cyclooxygenase (COX) (Fig. 12.1). Cyclooxygenase is of two types COX-1, a constitutive enzyme and COX-2 which is induced in cells by inflammatory stimuli on arachidonic acid. In addition to these, prostacyclin (PGI_2) (Fig. 12.1), is also produced by the action of cyclooxygenase on arachidonic acid. The main effects of prostacyclin are vasodilation and inhibition of platelet aggregation. The action of thromboxane A_2 include platelet aggregation and vasoconstriction. The prostaglandins produced by the action of cyclooxygenase on arachidonic acid include PGE_2, PGF_2, PGD_2.

The effects of prostaglandins include, inhibition of gastric acid secretion, contraction of GIT smooth muscle and uterus, vasodilation, and platelet aggregation.

Arachidonic acid is also the precursor of leukotrienes (Fig. 12.2). 5-Lipooxygenase converts arachidonic acid to hydroperoxide, which is then converted to epoxide, leukotriene A_4 by LTA synthase. This is then converted to leukotriene B_4 by the action of hydrolase. Leukotriene A_4 is converted to leukotriene C_4 by the action of glutathione-S-transferase. Leukotriene C_4 in turn is then converted to leukotriene D_4, leukotriene E_4, and leukotriene F_4.

Leukotriene B_4 causes adherence, chemotaxis, activation of polymorphs and monocytes, and stimulation of cytokine production from macrophages and lymphocytes. Cysteinyl leukotrienes, namely leukotriene C_4, leukotriene D_4, leukotriene E_4, and leukotriene F_4 cause contraction of bronchial muscle and vasodilation of mast cells.

Platelet activating factor (2) is released from many inflammatory cells. It causes vasodilation and increased vascular permeability. It is mediator in many types of inflammations.

Bradykinin (3) is a nonapeptide, it is produced from kininogen, a plasma α-globulin, by the enzyme kallikrein. It causes vasodilation, increased vascular permeability, stimulates pain nerve endings, and contraction of uterine and intestinal smooth muscle.

Cytokines are also peptides that are released from immune system cells in response to antigenic or mutagenic stimulation. Cytokines include interferon, interleukins, etc. Cytokines probably act primarily in the modulatory role rather as primary mediators of a given inflammatory response.

ANALGESIC, ANTIPYRETIC, AND NONSTEROIDAL ANTI-INFLAMMATORY DRUGS (NSAIDs)

The various classes of non-steroidal agents used as analgesics, and anti-inflammatory drugs include,

- (a) salicylates,
- (b) aniline and aminophenol derivatives,
- (c) pyrazolones and pyrazolidinediones
- (d) arylacetic acids and arylpropionic acids,
- (e) fenamates, and
- (f) oxicams.

Salicylate

Salicylic acid (4a) and its derivatives have been in use for more than a century. The various analogs of salicylic acid have been obtained by:

- (a) Modification of carboxylic group.
- (b) Substitution of hydroxyl group.
- (c) Modification of both hydroxyl and carboxylic groups.
- (d) Introduction of another substituent in the phenyl nucleus.

(a), R=H
(b), R=Na

(4)

The most common method of using salicylic acid (4a) is as its sodium salt (4b). Sodium salicylate (4b), because of its disagreeable taste and irritating properties, is not used now. Phenyl salicylate (5) or salol was the first ester of salicylic acid introduced in medicine. Its hydrolysis to phenol and salicylic acid (4a) is very slow in intestine. Methyl salicylate (6), which is present in oil of wintergreen, is used topically in neuralgia.

(5)   (6)   (7)

Among amides, salicylamide (7) has been claimed to be more potent than aspirin [acetylsalicylic acid, (8)] with fewer side effects.

One of the most important and widely used analog is aspirin (8). It is used as antipyretic, analgesic, anti-inflammatory, and antiplatelet drug. A serious drawback of aspirin (8) is that it causes gastrointestinal disturbances, which may be serious and can lead to bleeding. To overcome this, salts of aspirin (8) with calcium (9) and aluminium (10) have been used. The carboxylic group of aspirin (8) has been esterified with N-acetyl-p-aminophenol yielding benorylate (11). On hydrolysis in vivo, it yields paracetamol [acetaminophen, (12)] and aspirin (8).

(8)   (9)   (10)

(11)   (12)   (13)

Salsalate (13) in which the carboxylic group of salicylic acid (4a) is esterified with hydroxyl group of another salicylic acid (4a) molecule is claimed to cause less gastric distress. This is because it is insoluble in stomach and is absorbed in small intestines.

Metabolism of salicylic acid (4a) results in 2, 5-dihydroxybenzoic acid [gentisic acid (14)], and 2, 3, 5-trihydroxybenzoic acid (15). Various derivatives of these acids have been made and tested for their antipyretic, analgesic, and anti-inflammatory activities. Sodium gentisate (16) was found to be as effective as aspirin (8), but it produces side effects.

Diflunisal (17) which is salicylic acid substituted at position 5 by 2, 4-difluorophenyl group, has been found to be more active than aspirin (8).

(14), R = H
(16), R = Na

(15)

(17)

Aniline and Aminophenol Derivatives

Acetanilide (18) is an antipyretic, but is toxic. Its toxicity is due to its metabolite p-aminophenol (19). Various analogs of p-aminophenol were prepared in the hope that its toxicity will be lessened. Phenacetin (20) was one of these. However, it was found to cause methemoglobinemia and hemolytic anemia. Paracetamol (12), another analog, is one of the most widely used analgesic. Propacetamol (21) is a prodrug of paracetamol (12) and is used for pain and fever.

(18)   (19)   (20)   (21)

Pyrazolones and Pyrazolidinediones

This group comprises of analogs of 5-pyrazolone (22) and 3, 5-pyrazolidinediones (23). Among 5-pyrazolones (22), phenazone [antipyrine, (24)], aminopyrine (25), and analgin (26) have been the most successful.

(22)   (23)   (24)   (25)   (26)

A number of mixtures of active 5-pyrazolones with hypnotics in the molar ratios of 1:1 or 1:2 have been used as analgesic, antipyretics, and antirheumatics. Some of these are aminopyrine (25) and diethylbarbituric acid combination and aminopyrine (25), and isopropylphenyl barbituric acid.

Phenylbutazone (27), a pyrazolidinedione (23), is the most successful antiarthritic drug. It improves the symptoms of gout and various types of arthritis. Oxyphenbutazone (28) is the metabolite of phenylbutazone (27) and shows similar action.

Sulphinpyrazone (29), another pyrazolidinedione analog, has a phenylsulphinylethyl moiety at position 4. It is mainly used as uricosuric agent.

(27)   (28)   (29)

Azapropazone (30) is a benzotriazine derivative which has activity similar to phenylbutazone (27). It is also a potent uricosuric agent and is used in gout.

(30)

Arylacetic Acid and Arylpropionic Acids

Among the arylacetic acid derivatives, diclofenac (31), fenclofenac (32), amfenac (33), and sulindac (34) are some of the analogs used in clinical practice. Diclofenac (31) is used as sodium salt. It possesses analgesic, antipyretic, and anti-inflammatory activities. Sulindac (34) is a prodrug which is metabolized to sulphide, the active form.

(31)   (32)   (33)

Analogs containing a heterocyclic moiety with acetic acid include indomethacin (35), tolmetin (36), zomepirac (37), and etodolac (38). Indomethacin (35) is one of the potent anti-inflammatory drugs. It also possesses antipyretic and analgesic activity. The anti-inflammatory activity of tolmetin (36) is intermediate between phenylbutazone (27) and indomethacin (35). It inhibits polymorph migration and decreases capillary permeability.

(34)

(35)

(36)

(37)

(38)

Zomepirac (37) which is a structural variation of tolmetin (36) is used as an analgesic. Etodolac (38) is 50 times more active than aspirin (8) and 5 times more active than sulindac (34) but less potent than indomethacin (35). It produces less gastrointestinal bleeding than other non-steroidal anti-inflammatory drugs.

The α-aryl propionic acid derivatives include ibuprofen (39), flurbiprofen (40), ketoprofen (41), fenoprofen (42), loxoprofen (43), and naproxen (44). All of these compounds contain an asymmetric carbon atom and the activity is generally found in (S)-isomer.

(39)

(40)

(41)

(42)

(43)

(44)

Ibuprofen (39) is the most widely used anti-inflammatory analgesic. It is marketed as a racemic mixture although the activity is present in S (+)-isomer. It is more potent than aspirin (8) but less than indomethacin (35). Flurbiprofen (40) possesses antipyretic, anti-inflammatory, and analgesic activity. It is used in rheumatoid arthritis and osteoarthritis.

Ketoprofen (41), which also possesses anti-inflammatory, analgesic, and antipyretic activities, is however, less potent than indomethacin (35).

Fenoprofen (42) is used as a calcium salt. It is less active than indomethacin (35) but more potent than aspirin (8). It also possesses analgesic and antipyretic activities.

Loxoprofen (43) is a newly introduced drug used as sodium salt.

Naproxen (44) is marketed as (S)(+) – enantiomer. It is more potent than aspirin (8), phenylbutazone (27), and ibuprofen (39) as anti-inflammatory agent. It also possesses antipyretic activity.

Among the analogs containing propionic acid moiety with a heteroaromatic ring are carprofen (45), pranoprofen (46), benoxaprofen (47), flunoxaprofen (48), oxaprozin (49), and suprofen (50). Ketorolac (51) represents a cyclized hetroarylpropionic acid analog. All of these possess anti-inflammatory and analgesic activities.

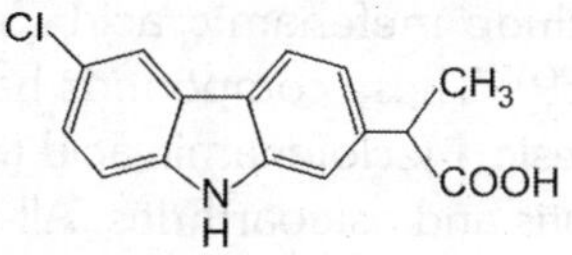

(45)

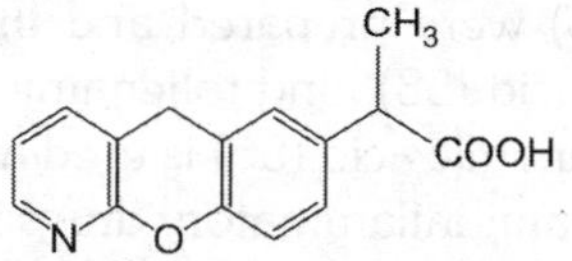

(46)

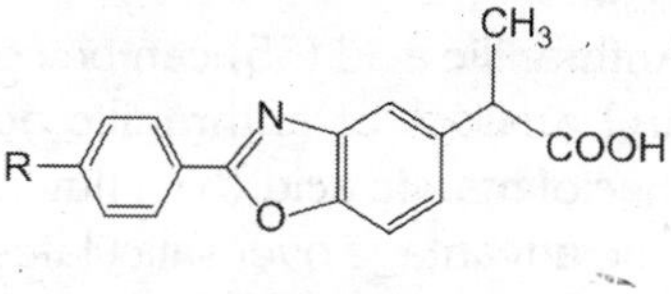

(47), R = Cl
(48), R = F

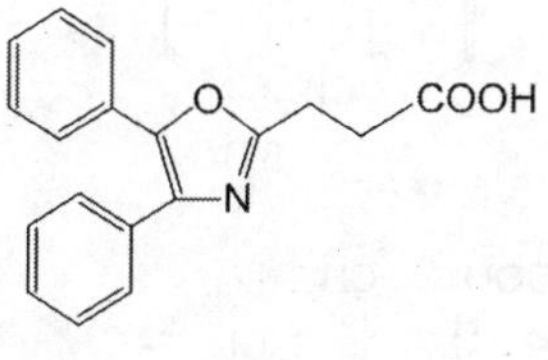

(49)

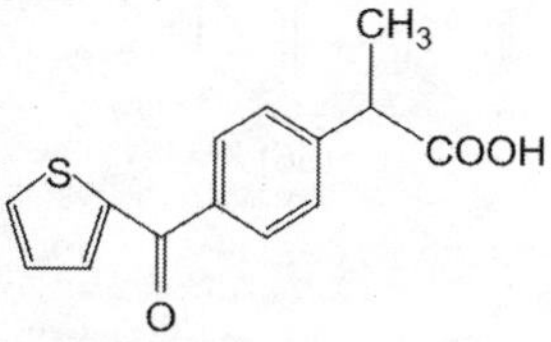

(50)

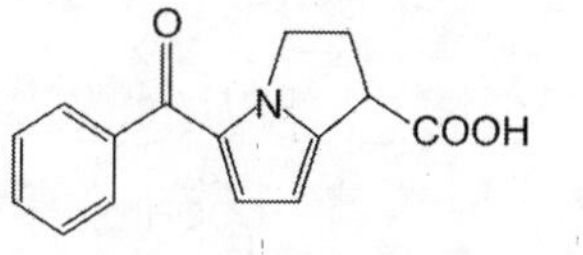

(51)

Fenbufen (52) which contains carbonyl propionic acid moiety attached to biphenyl possesses less GI side effects.

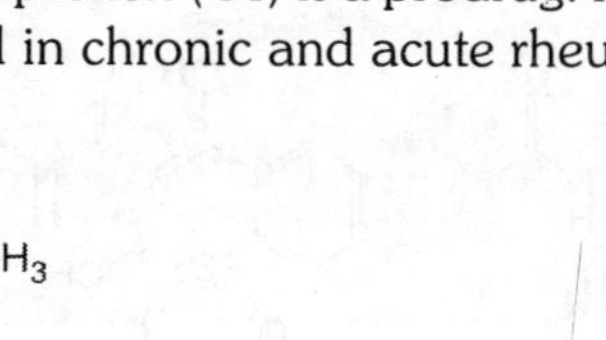

(52)

Nabumetone (53), a variant of naproxen (44) is a prodrug. Its active metabolite is 6-methoxy-2-naphthylacetic acid (53a). It is used in chronic and acute rheumatoid arthritis.

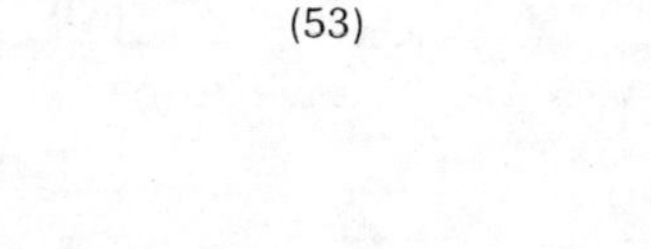

(53)

(53a)

An amide analog of ketoprofen (41), piketoprofen (54), is indicated in painful musculoskeletal disorders.

(54)

Fenamates

Anthranilic acid (55) can be considered as an isostere of salicylic acid (4a). Based on this, various aryl analogs of anthranilic acid (55) were prepared and these include mefenamic acid (56), meclofenamic acid (57), flufenamic acid (58), and tolfenamic acid (59). These compounds have little advantage over salicylates. Mefenamic acid (56) is used as analgesic. Meclofenamic acid (57) and flufenamic acid (58) are used as anti-inflammatory drugs in arthritis and osteoarthritis. All the fenamates cause diarrhea.

(55)   (56)   (57)

(58)   (59)

Oxicams

4-Hydroxy-1, 2-benzothiazine carboxamide (60), usually known as "oxicam" possess anti-inflammatory activity. Piroxicam (61) and meloxicam (62) are the compounds belonging to this class. Isosteric replacement of benzene ring of piroxicam (61) with thiophene ring results in tenoxicam (63). Piroxicam (61) possesses analgesic, antipyretic, and anti-inflammatory activity. It has a long half-life. Meloxicam (62) and tenoxicam (63) which possess analgesic and anti-inflammatory activity are used in osteoarthritis.

(60)   (61)   (62)   (63)

Structure-Activity Relationship Studies

All of the non-specific cyclooxygenase inhibitors contain an acidic group represented by enolic group (pyrazole, pyrazolidinediones, and oxicams), a carboxylic group (arylacetic acid, aryl- and heteroaryl-propionic acid, and fenamates). The activity of nabumetone (53), which is non-acidic drug, is attributed to its conversion to its acid metabolite (53a). The acidic group is located about one carbon away from an aromatic or a heteroaromatic ring (acetic acid and α-propionic acid analogs). Any increase in the cabon atoms between carboxylic group and the aromatic ring usually results in decrease in activity. In case of α-propionic acid analogs, which contain an asymmetric centre, the activity is generally associated with (S)-isomer.

Mechanism of Action

The non-steroidal anti-inflammatory agents act by inhibiting the enzyme cyclooxygenase (Fig. 12.1) used in the first step for conversion of arachidonic acid to prostaglandins. Cyclooxygenase is of two types, cyclooxygenase-1 (COX-1) and cyclooxygenase-2 (COX-2). COX-1 is constitutive enzyme expressed in most tissues including blood platelets. It is also involved in stimulating bicarbonate secretion and mucus which results in producing an overall reduction in acidity in GI tract. COX-2 is induced in inflammatory cells when they are activated.

Most of the non-steroidal anti-inflammatory drugs described are non-selective inhibitors of cyclooxygenases. Aspirin (8), sulindac (34), indomethacin (35), and piroxicam (61) are more selective for COX-1. Those which are equipotent for both enzymes are diclofenac (31), flurbiprofen (40), naproxen (44), and nabumetone (53). Compounds such as paracetamol (12) and ibuprofen (39) are more selective inhibitors of COX-2.

Some of the side effects, such as gastrointestinal bleeding and disturbances, are because of inhibition of COX-1.

The antipyretic, analgesic and anti-inflammatory effects of these agents are due to inhibiton of prostaglandin sysnthesis. The E-type prostaglandin production during inflammatory processes disturb the "Thermostat" located in hypothalamus. As a results, there is increase in body temperature. The non-steroidal antiinflammatory drugs, by virtue of inhibition of prostaglandin synthesis, prevent this disturbance in heat regulating centre and thus the thermostat is reset.

The analgesic action of non-steroidal anti-inflammatory agents during inflammation is also due to inhibition of prostaglandin synthesis. Similarly, the inflammatory processes which are also associated with the synthesis and release of prostaglandin, are also inhibited. The other action of non-steroidal anti-inflammatory drugs is oxygen radical scavanging effect. The oxygen radical, produced by neutrophils and macrophages, is necessary for the production of prostaglandin, and is implicated in the inflammatory processes (Fig. 12.1). Scavanging of oxygen radical as well as inhibition of COX-1 and COX-2 contribute to the anti-inflammatory action of these agents.

CYCLOOXYGENASE-2 (COX-2) INHIBITORS

Some of the selective COX-2 inhibitors include nimesulide (64), lumiracoxib (65), etoricoxib (66), rofecoxib (67), celecoxib (68), valdecoxib (69), and parecoxib (70). These compounds are claimed to possess activity comparable to non-selective cyclooxygenase inhibitors. However, they do not possess the toxic effects of non-selective cyclooxygenase inhibitors on gastrointestinal tract which is due to inhibition of COX-1.

(64)   (65)   (66)   (67)

(68)   (69)   (70)

DISEASE MODIFYING ANTIRHEUMATOID DRUGS (DMARDs)

The various classes of drugs discussed earlier do not stop the progress of rheumatic disease, but help in suppressing pain and inflammation. Drugs which retard the progress of disease are known as "disease modifying antirheumatoid drugs" or DMARDS. These drugs include gold compounds, penicillamine, 4-aminoquinolines, and immunomodulators.

The organic gold compounds used in rheumatoid diseases include sodium aurothiomalate (71), aurothioglucose (72), and auranofin (73). The exact mechanism by which gold compounds act is not yet fully understood. However, they inhibit lysosomal enzymes, the release of which promotes inflammatory process. They also decrease the production of toxic O_2 metabolites from phagocytes.

Penicillamine (74), a product of hydrolysis of penicillin, is thought to decrease interleukin-1 (cytokine) generation. Penicillamine (74) can chelate metals and is used in Wilson's disease in which there is copper accumulation in kidney, liver, and brain.

(71)   (72)   (73)   (74)

Among 4-aminoquinolines which are used as antimalarials, hydroxychloroquine (75), has found use in rheumatoid diseases. The exact mechanisms of hydroxychloroquine (75) is not known but it is thought to inhibit the release of lysosomal enzymes and reduce generation of interleukin-1 (cytokins). It also inhibits phospholipase A_2 and therefore reduces the formation of eicosanoids.

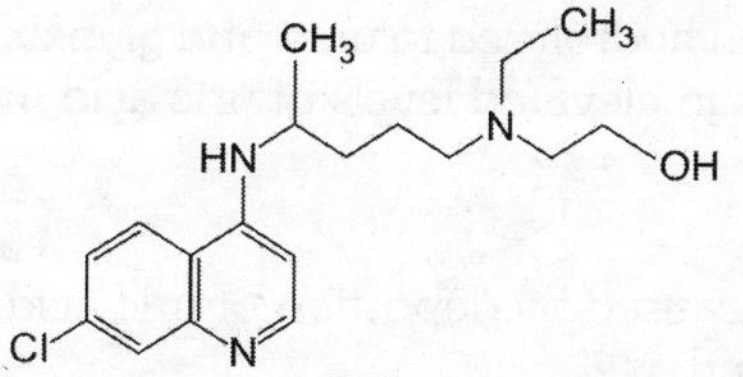

(75)

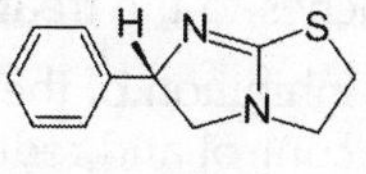

(76)

In rheumatic disease, a defect in immune system is involved. Both immunostimulants as well as immunosuppressant show beneficial action in these diseases. Levamisole (76), an anthelmintic with immunostimulatory effect has shown significant antirheumatic activity. Antineoplastic agents such as methotrexate (77), leflunomide (78), etc. which are immunosuppressants, have also shown beneficial action.

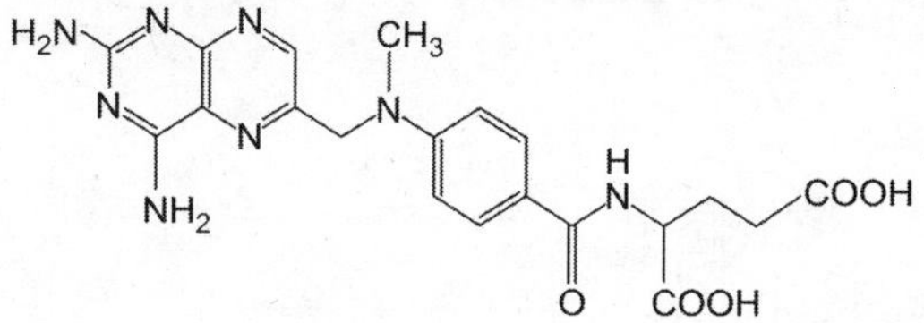

(77)

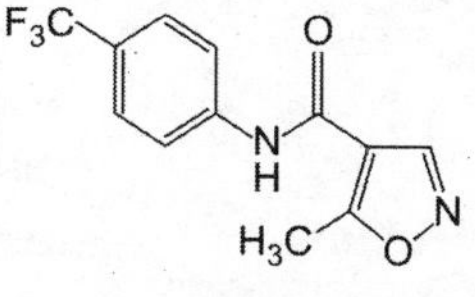

(78)

DRUGS USED IN GOUT

Gout is a metabolic disease characterized by high levels of uric acid in plasma and urine. It can be of two types acute and chronic. In acute gouty arthritis, there is accumulation of monosodium urate within the joints. In chronic form of disease, there appears erosive joint deformity. Uric acid is an excretory product of purine metabolism formed from guanine or adenine via xanthine (Fig. 12.3).

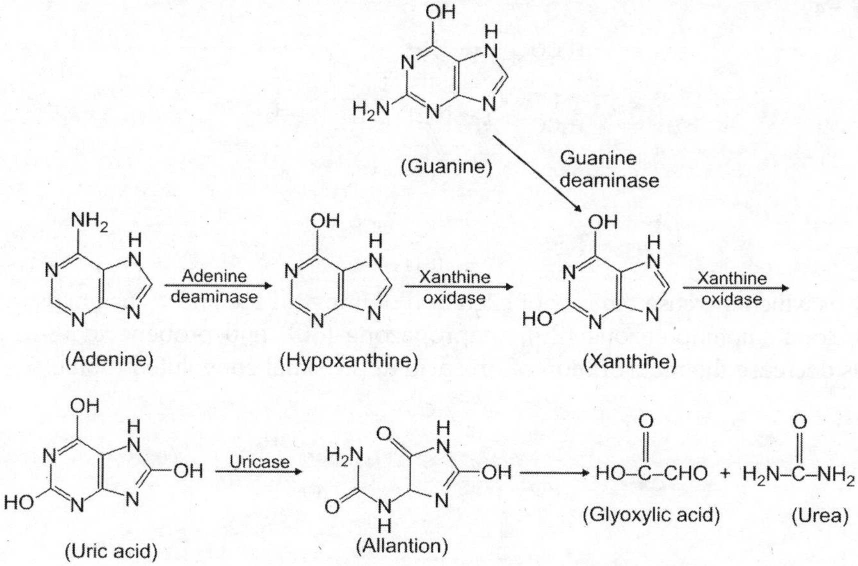

Fig. 12.3: Biosynthesis and metabolism of uric acid.

Uric acid is converted to allantoin by uricase which is then hydrolyzed to urea and glyoxylic acid. Overproduction or decreased excretion of uric acid results in elevated levels of uric acid in blood.
   The approaches to the treatment of gout has been:

   (a) through inhibition of the synthesis of uric acid,
   (b) through control and reduction of the inflammation caused by depostion of uric acid,
   (c) through increasing the rate of uric acid excretion, and
   (d) by non-steroidal anti-inflammatory analgesics.

Allopurinol (79) is an antimetabolite of hypoxanthine and it inhibits the enzyme xanthine oxidase. Xanthine oxidase converts allopurinol (79) to alloxanthine (80) which acts as an effective non-competitive inhibitor of xanthine oxidase. This way the concentration of a highly water insoluble uric acid is reduced and at the same time the concentration of water soluble hypoxanthine and xanthine is increased. It is a drug of choice in long-term treatment of gout but is ineffective in acute attacks.

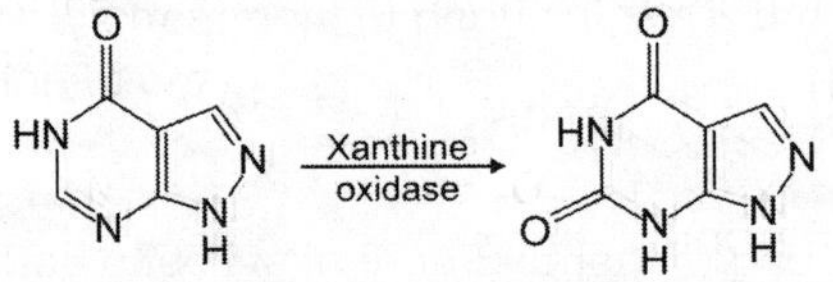

(79)   (80)

Colchicine (81) is an alkaloid obtained from *Colchicum autumnale*. It dramatically relieves the pain and inflammation of gouty arthritis in 12-24 hr. It is effective in this disorder because of its anti-inflammatory properties. Recent studies have shown that monosodium urate activates the lipooxygenase pathway leading to the formation of leukotriene B_4 (Fig. 12.2). Colchicine (81) appears to inhibit the leukocyte migration and phagocytosis and also inhibits the formation of leukotriene B_4.

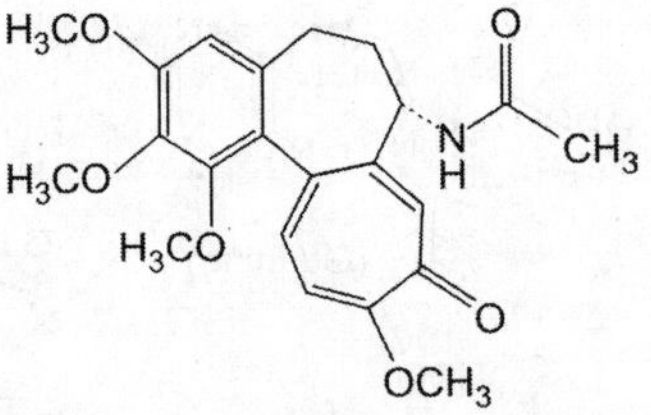

(81)

Substances which increase the rate of excretion of uric acid are known as uricosuric agents. To this class belong sulphinpyrazone (29), azapropazone (30), and probenecid (82). All of these compounds decrease the reabsorption of uric acid at proximal convoluted tubule.

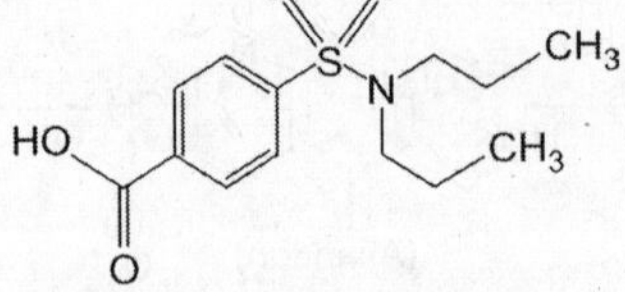

(82)

INDIVIDUAL COMPOUNDS

ANALGESICS, ANTIPYRETICS AND NONSTEROIDAL ANTIINFLAMMATORY DRUGS (NSAIDS)

NSAIDS : SALICYLATES

Sodium Salicylate

2-Hydroxybenzoic acid sodium salt

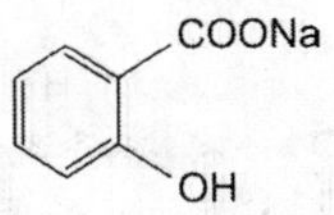

It is prepared by treating salicylic acid (4a) with sodium bicarbonate in aqueous medium. Sodium salicylate is a salt of choice for administration of salicylates. It has anti-inflammatory analgesic activity.

Salicylamide

2-Hydroxybenzamide

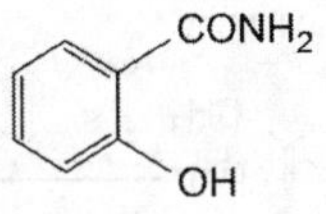

Synthesis

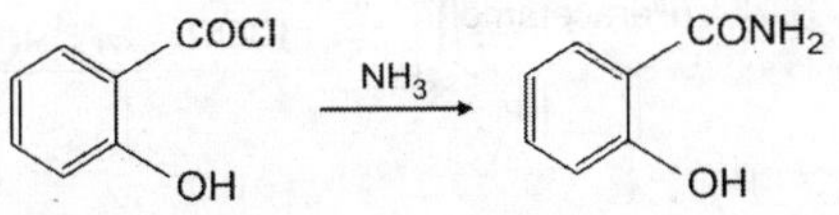

(Salicylic acid chloride)

It does not cause gastric irritation and is used in patients who are allergic to aspirin (8). It causes sedation and drowsiness which is because it enters CNS rapidly as compared to other salicylates. It possesses analgesic and antipyretic effect but not the anti-inflammatory action.

Aspirin

Acetylsalicylic acid

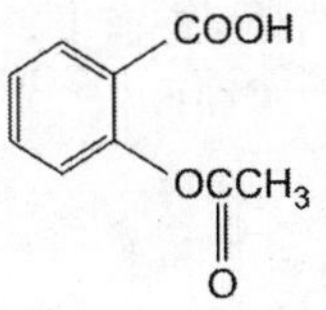

Synthesis

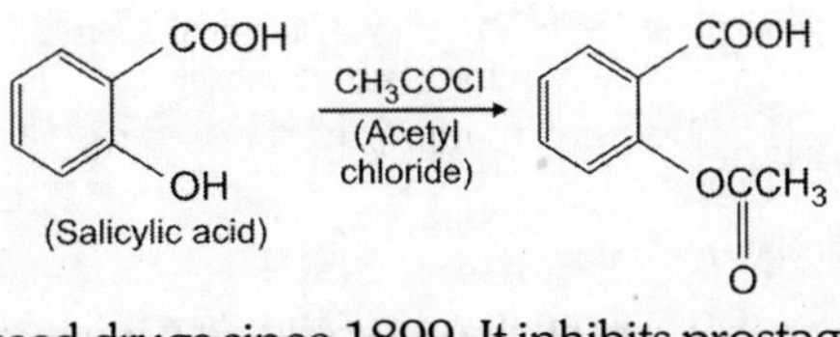

(Salicylic acid)

It is one of the most widely used drugs since 1899. It inhibits prostaglandin synthesis by irreversibly blocking the enzyme cyclooxygenase (Fig. 12.1). It inhibits granulocyte adherence to damaged vasculature, stabilizes the lysosomes and inhibits migration of leukocytes and macrophages to the site of inflammation. It also has analgesic and antipyretic effect. The normal body temperature is slightly affected.

Aloxiprin

It is a polymeric condensation product of aluminium oxide and aspirin (8). It is hydrolyzed in GI tract. It possesses analgesic, antipyretic, and anti-inflammatory activities.

Benorylate

2-Acetoxy-4´-(acetamino)phenylbenzoate

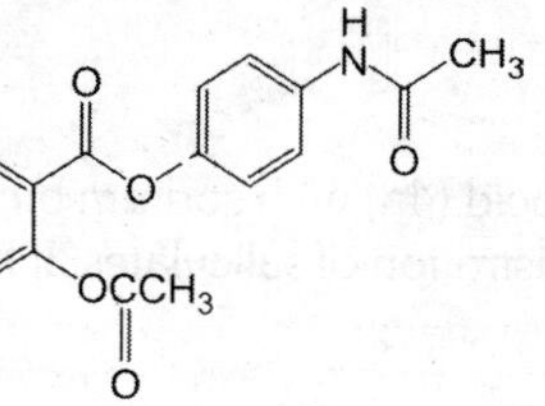

Synthesis

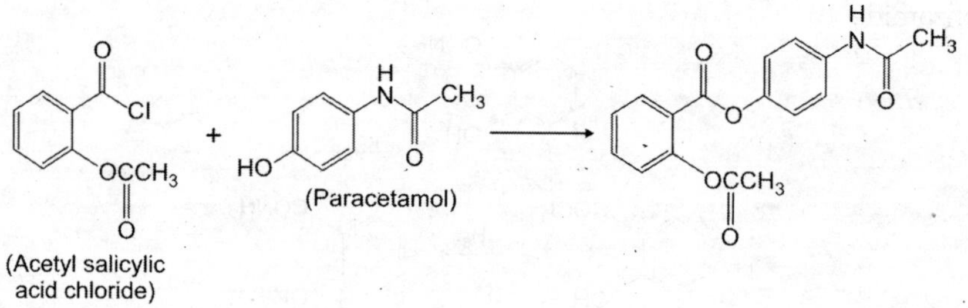

(Acetyl salicylic acid chloride)

(Paracetamol)

After absorption, benorylate is hydrolyzed to aspirin (8) and paracetamol (12). It is used as anti-inflammatory, antipyretic, and analgesic.

Salsalate

o-(2-Hydroxybenzoyl)salicylic acid

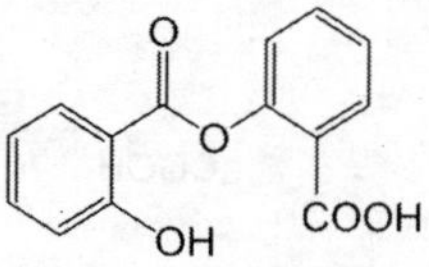

Synthesis

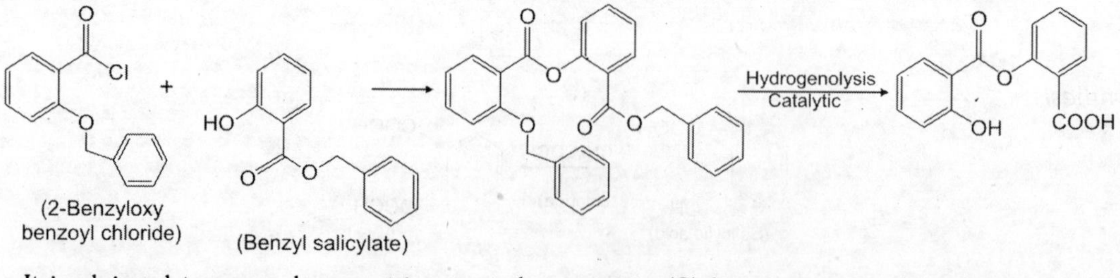

(2-Benzyloxy benzoyl chloride)

(Benzyl salicylate)

It is claimed to cause less gastric upset than aspirin (8) because it is relatively insoluble in stomach and is absorbed from small intestine. However, it is as effective as aspirin (8).

Diflunisal

5-(2, 4- Difluorophenyl)salicylic acid

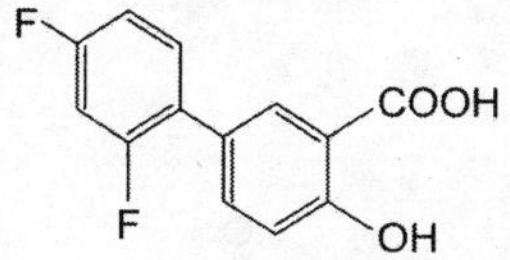

Synthesis

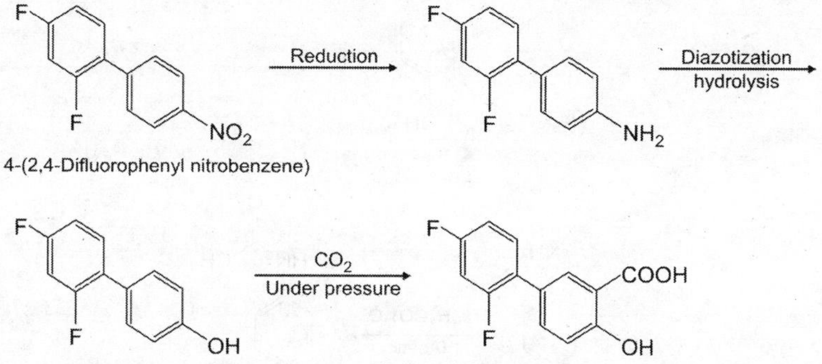

4-(2,4-Difluorophenyl nitrobenzene)

Diflunisal has analgesic and anti-inflammatory effects like aspirin (8) but no antipyretic effects. It is a potent competitive and reversible inhibitor of cyclooxygenase. It does not produce gastric or intestinal bleeding.

NSAIDS : ANILINES AND AMINOPHENOLS

Phenacetin

p-Ethoxyacetanilide

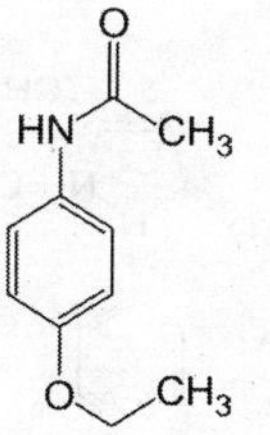

Synthesis

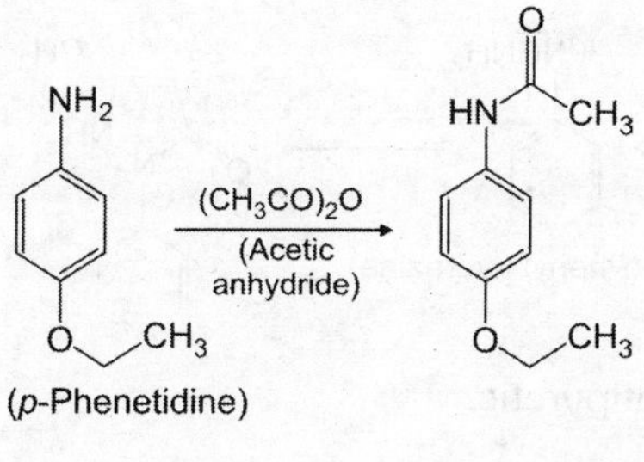

(*p*-Phenetidine)

It was once widely used analgesic and antipyretic. It causes damage to kidneys and has been shown to be carcinogenic to rats. It has been replaced in combination formulations by paracetamol (12).

Paracetamol

4-Hydroxyacetanilide

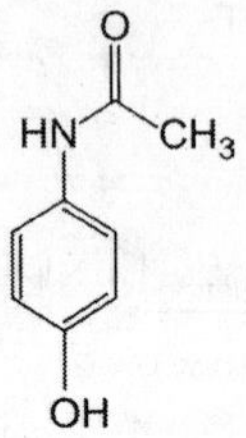

Synthesis

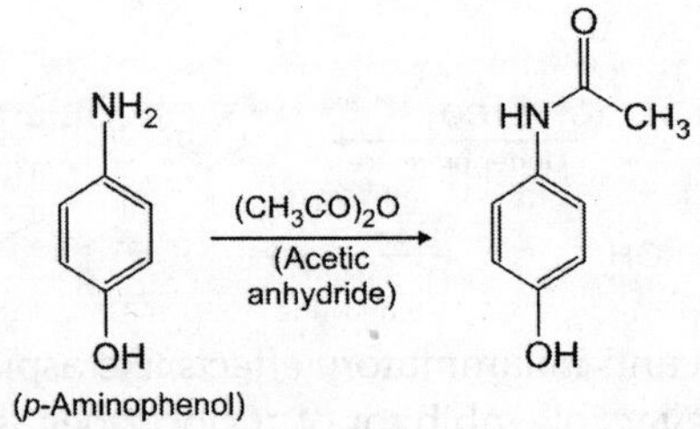

(*p*-Aminophenol)

It has analgesic and antipyretic activity comparable to acetanilide (18). It possesses same toxic effects as acetanilide (18) but they occur less frequently.

NSAIDS : PYRAZOLONES AND PYRAZOLIDINEDIONES

Phenazone

2, 3-Dimethyl-1-phenyl-3-pyrazolin-5-one

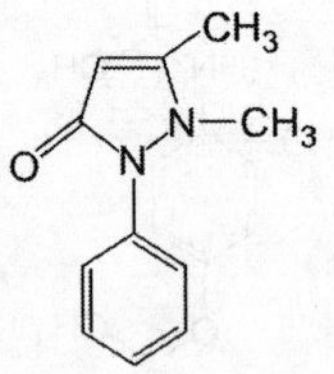

Synthesis

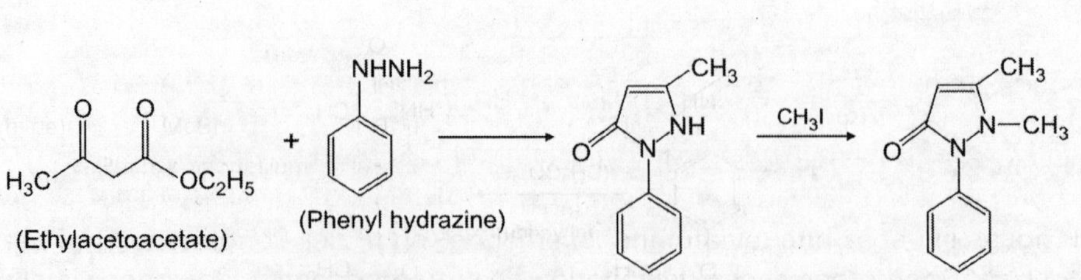

(Ethylacetoacetate)   (Phenyl hydrazine)

It is used as analgesic and antipyretic.

Analgin

1-Phenyl-2,3-dimethyl-5-pyrazolone-4-methylaminomethanesulfonate sodium.

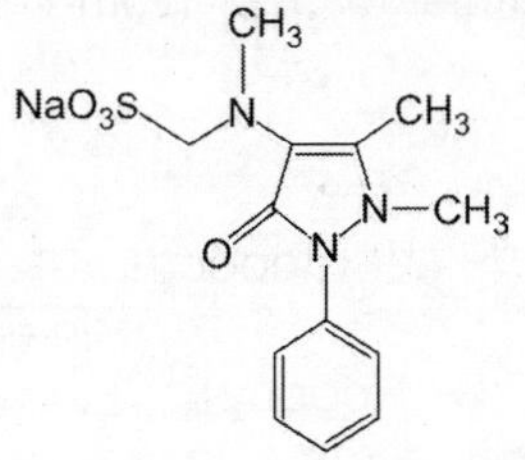

Synthesis

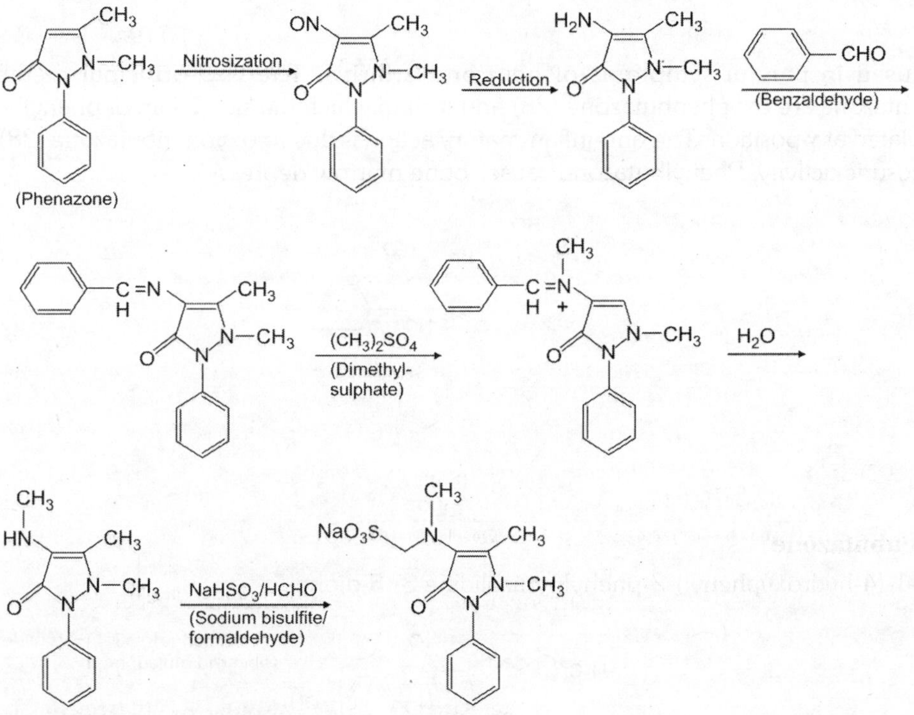

(Phenazone)

It is used as analgesic and antipyretic.

Phenylbutazone

4-Butyl-1,2-diphenyl-3,5-pyrazolidinedione

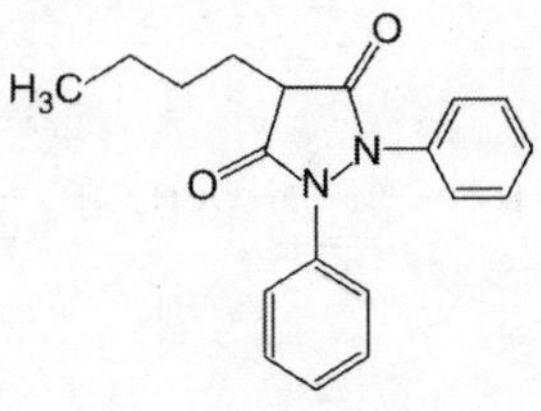

Synthesis

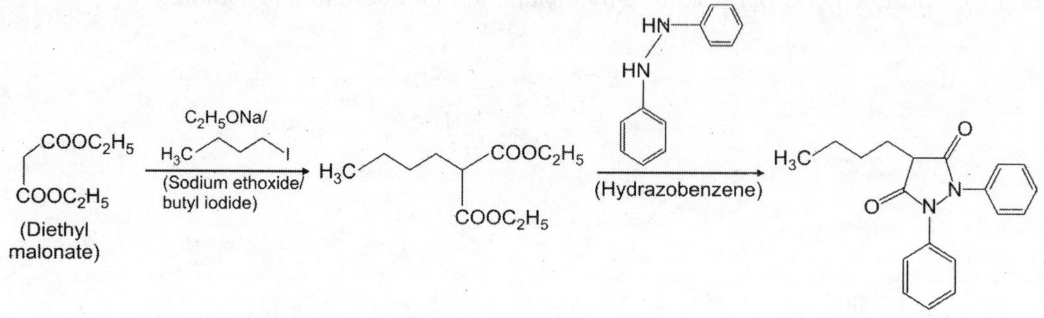

It is used in painful symptoms of gout and arthritis. The two principal metabolites of phenylbutazone are oxyphenbutazone (28) and (83) in which the side chain of phenylbutazone is hydroxylated at γ-position. The anti-inflammatory action is due to oxyphenbutazone (28) and (83) has uricosuric activity. Phenylbutazone causes bone marrow depression.

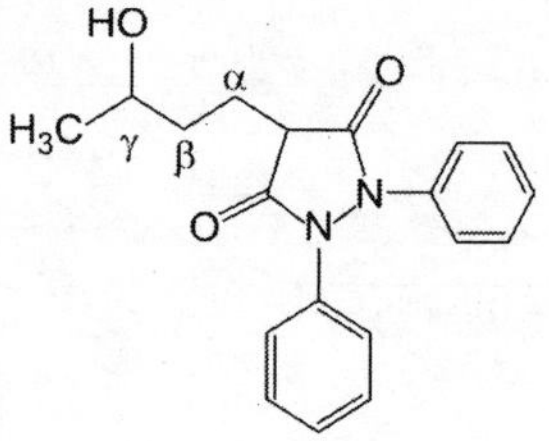

(83)

Oxyphenbutazone

4-Butyl-1-(4-hydroxyphenyl)-2-phenylpyrazolidine-3, 5-dione.

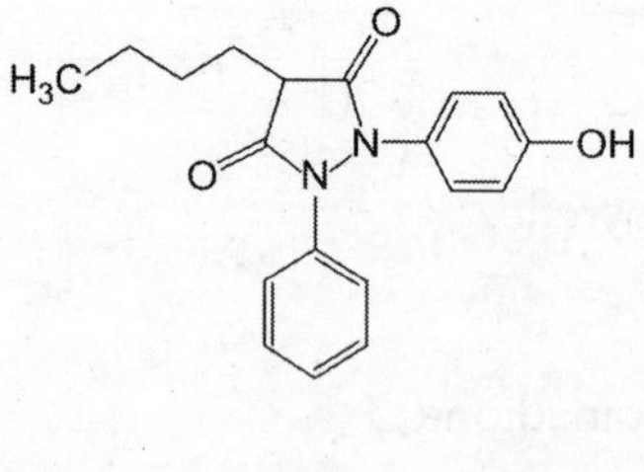

Syntehsis

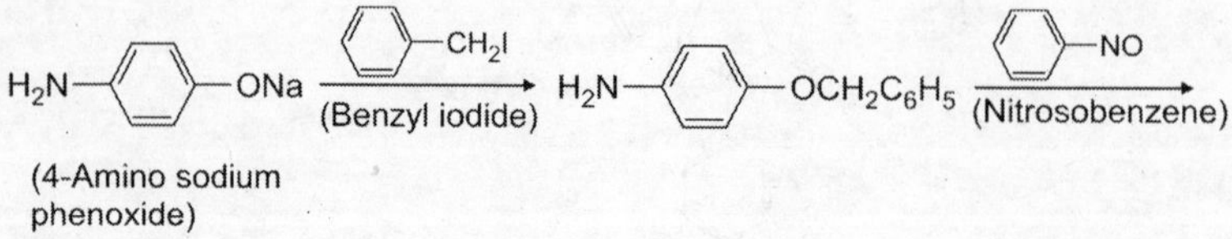

The drug is a metabolite of phenylbutazone (27) and has same effectiveness, indication, and side effects. It causes less gastric irritation. It is used as anti-inflammatory analgesic.

NSAIDS: ARYLACETIC ACIDS AND ARYLPROPIONIC ACIDS

Diclofenac Sodium

Sodium 2-[(2′,6′-dichlorophenyl)amino]phenylacetate

Synthesis

[N-(2'6'-Dichlorophenyl)aniline]

Diclofenac possesses structural segments of both anthranilic acid as well as arylacetic acid. It shows anti-inflammatory, analgesic, and antipyretic properties. It inhibits cyclooxygenase and lipooxygenase which results in reduced production of leukotrienes and release of arachidonic acid. It is used in the treatment of rheumatoid arthritis, osteoarthritis, and ankylosing spondylitis.

Fenclofenac

2-(2',4'-Dichlorophenoxy)phenylacetic acid

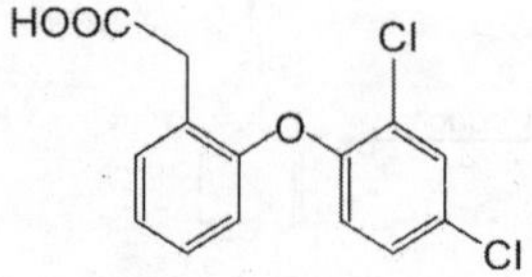

Synthesis

(2-Chloroacetophenone)   (Sodium 2,4-dichloro-
                            phenoxide)

Willgerodt reaction

$$\left(S + \quad O\overset{\frown}{\underset{\smile}{\quad}}NH \right)$$

Saponitication

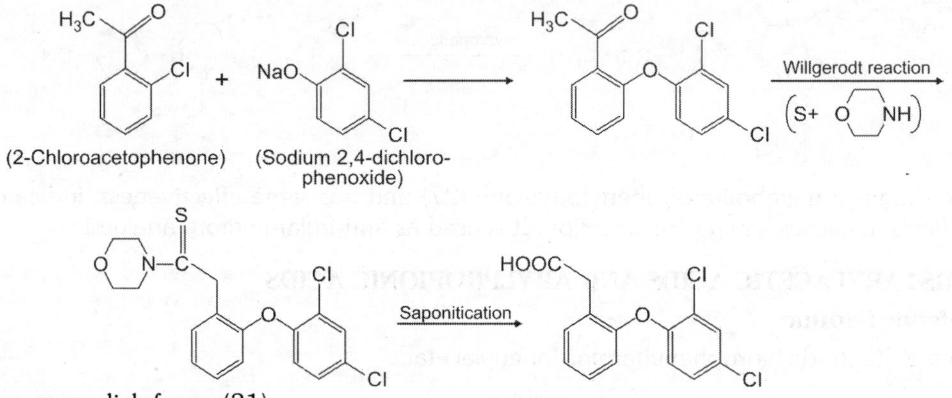

Same use as diclofenac (31).

Amfenac

2-Amino-3-benzoylphenylacetic acid

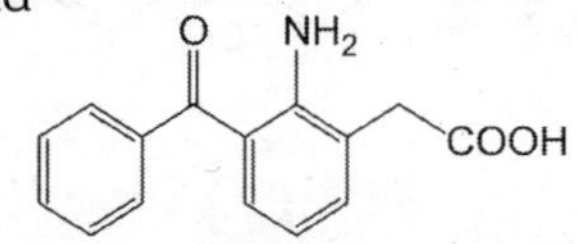

Synthesis

(1-Aminoindolin-
2-one)

(Phenylacetone)

HCl
C₂H₅OH

O₃
C₂H₅OH

HCl
Hydrolysis

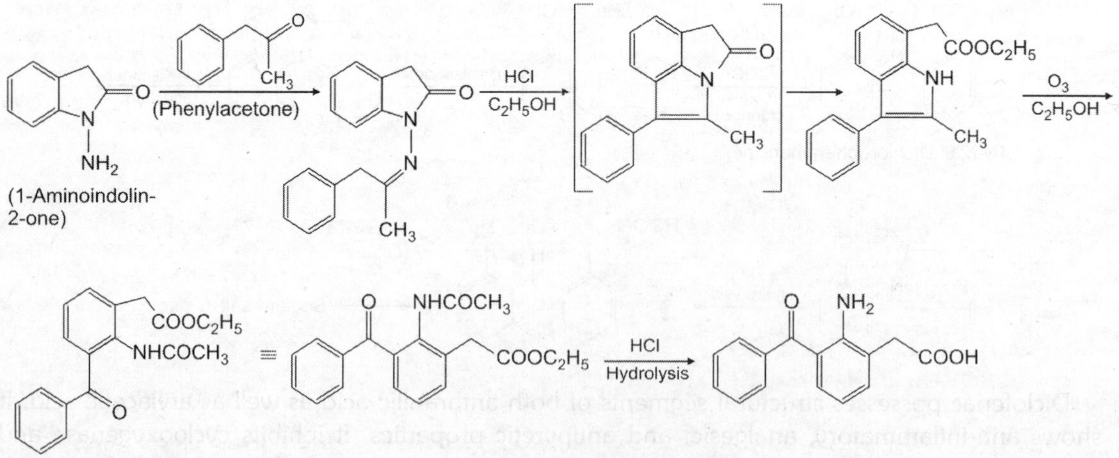

It is an anti-inflammatory agent. Its action is through inhibition of cyclooxygenase and is used after tooth extraction.

Sulindac

(Z)-5-Fluro-2-methyl-1-[4-(methylsulphinyl)benzylidene]indene-3-acetic acid.

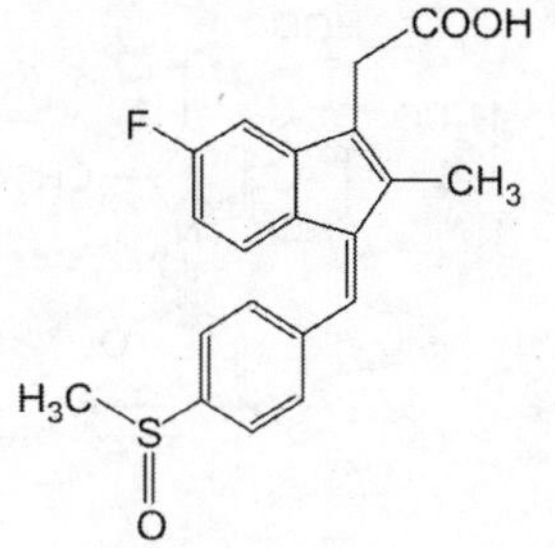

Synthesis

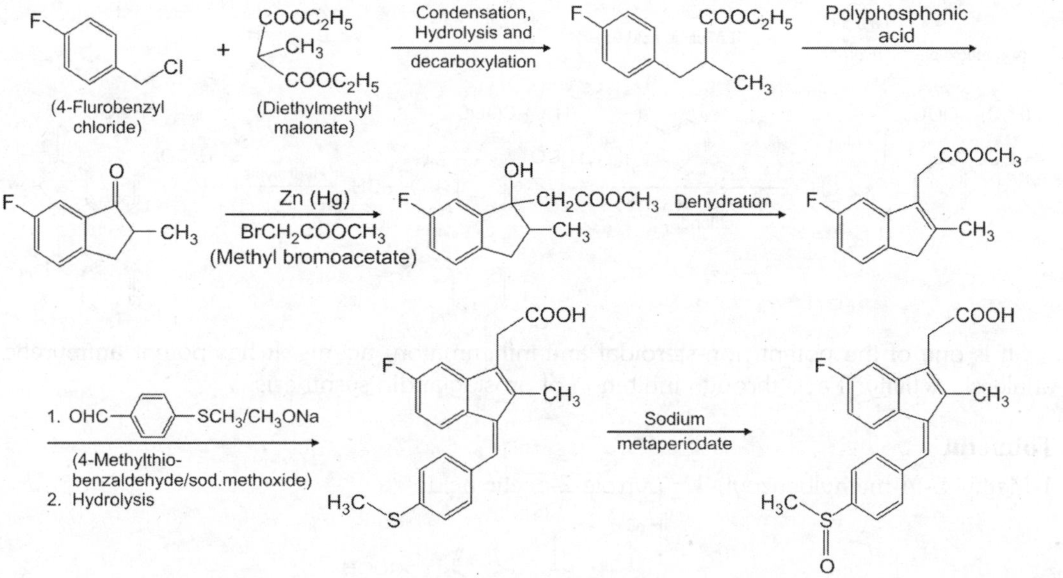

(4-Flurobenzyl chloride) + (Diethylmethyl malonate) → Condensation, Hydrolysis and decarboxylation → Polyphosphonic acid →

Zn (Hg) / BrCH$_2$COOCH$_3$ (Methyl bromoacetate) → Dehydration →

1. OHC——SCH$_3$/CH$_3$ONa (4-Methylthio-benzaldehyde/sod.methoxide)
2. Hydrolysis → Sodium metaperiodate →

Sulindac is a prodrug and is converted to active sulfide metabolite (84) which inhibits cyclooxygenase in joints. It produces much less GI disturbances. It is used as anti-inflammatory, antipyretic analgesic.

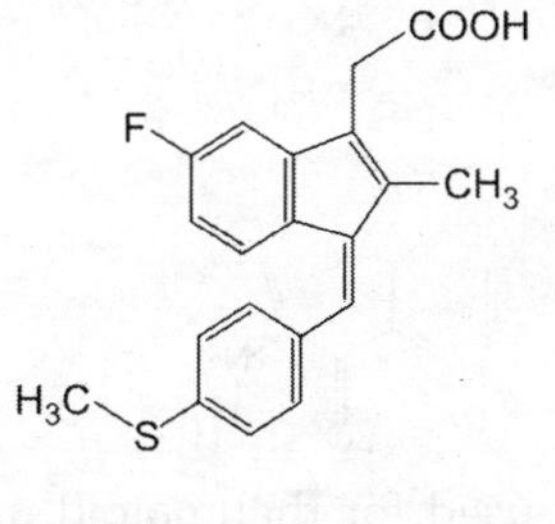

(84)

Indomethacin

1-(4-Chlorobenzoyl)-5-methoxy-2-methyl-1*H*-indole-3-acetic acid.

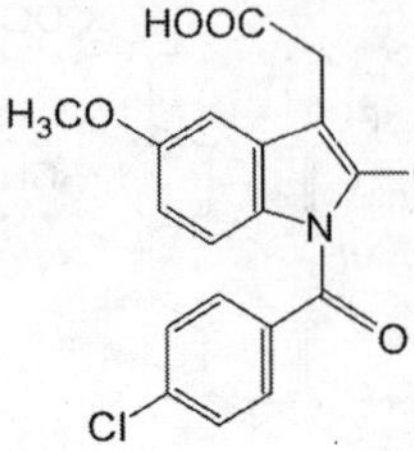

Synthesis

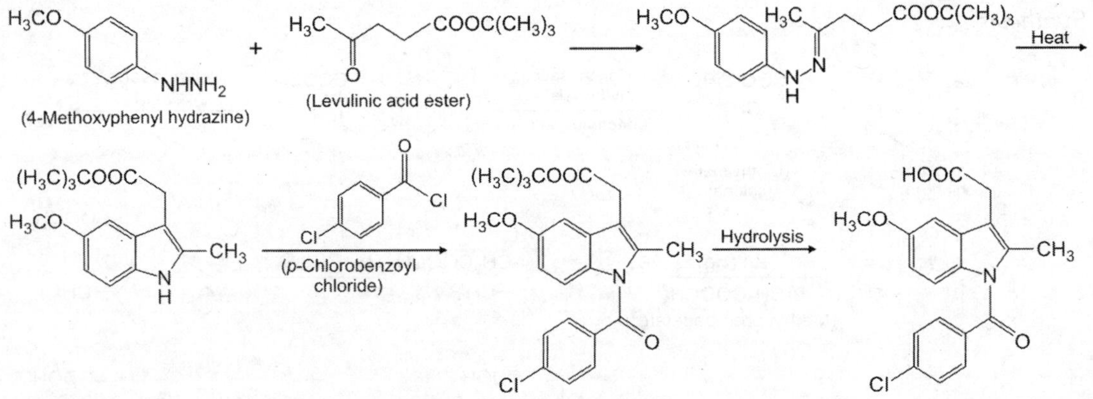

It is one of the potent non-steroidal anti-inflammatory agents. It has potent antipyretic and analgesic activity. It acts through inhibition of prostaglandin sysnthesis.

Tolmetin

1-Methyl-5-(4-methylbenzoyl)-1*H*-pyrrole-2-acetic acid

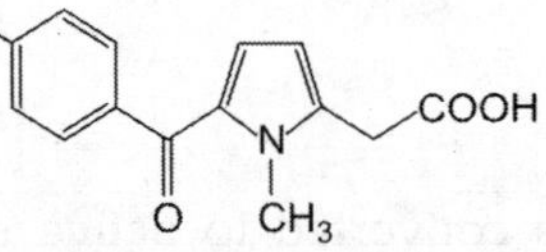

Synthesis

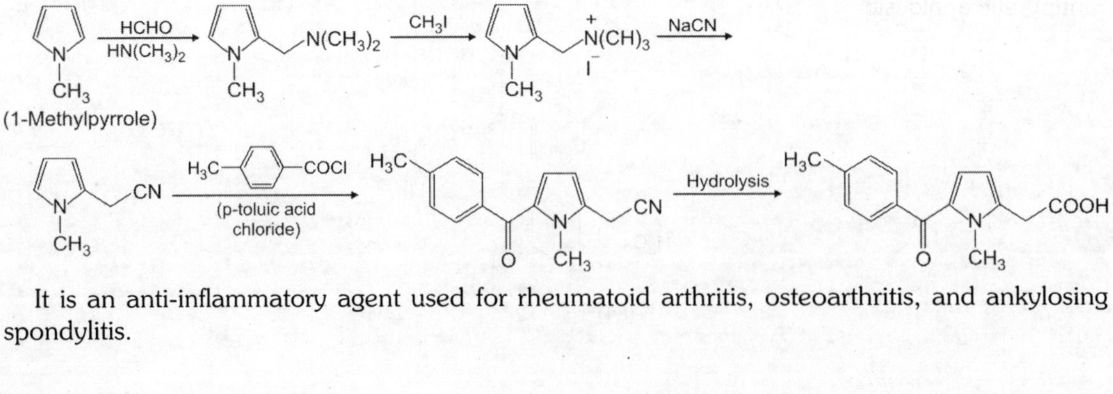

It is an anti-inflammatory agent used for rheumatoid arthritis, osteoarthritis, and ankylosing spondylitis.

Zomepirac

5-(4-Chlorobenzoyl)-1, 4-dimethyl-1*H*-pyrrole-2-acetic acid.

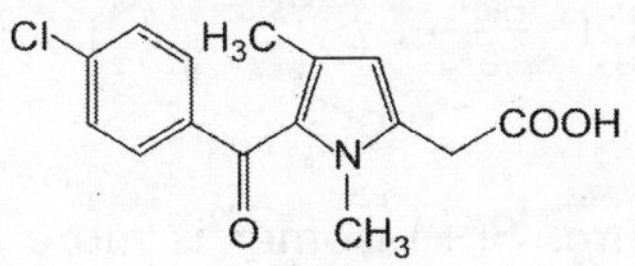

Synthesis

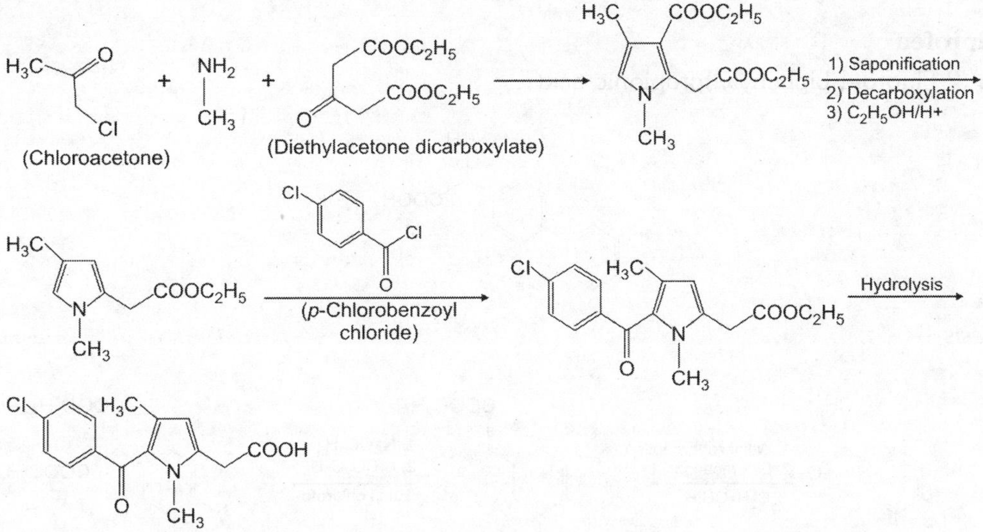

Zomepirac is mainly used as an analgesic, particularly in case of arthritis, and musculoskeletal injuries.

Ibuprofen

(*RS*)-2-(4-Isobutylphenyl)propionic acid

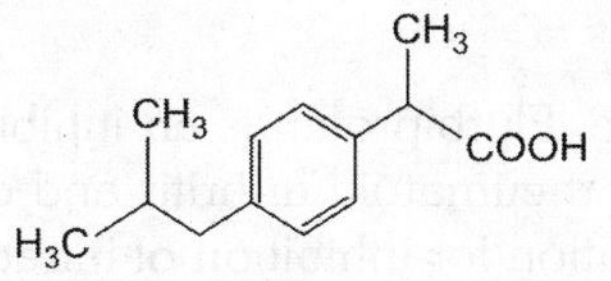

Synthesis

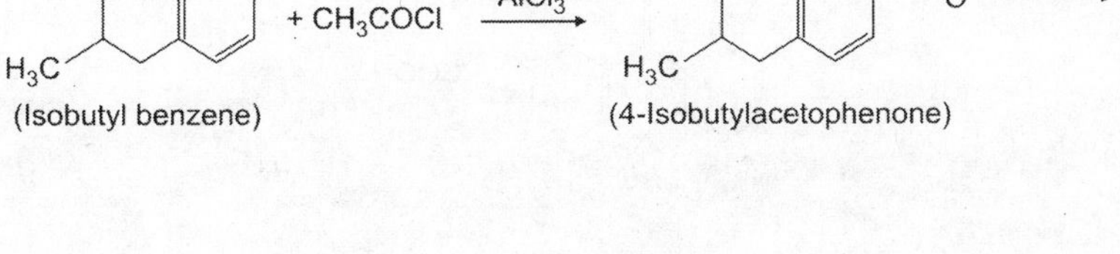

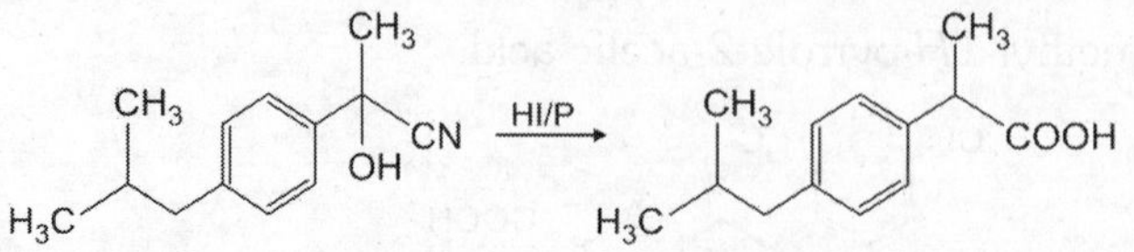

It is marketed as racemic mixture. $S(+)$-isomer is more active. It appears comparable to aspirin (8) in rheumatoid arthritis with lower incidence of side effects. It is indicated in rheumatoid arthritis and osteoarthritis and also in reduction of pain and fever.

Flurbiprofen

(RS)-2-(2-Fluoro-4-biphenylyl)propionic acid

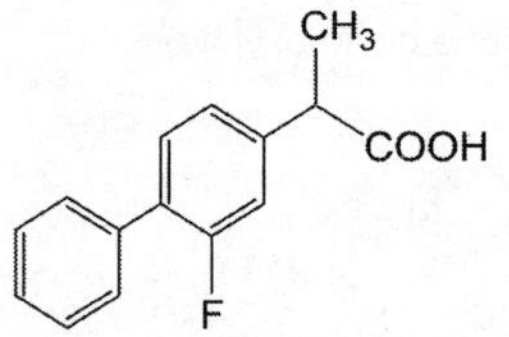

Synthesis

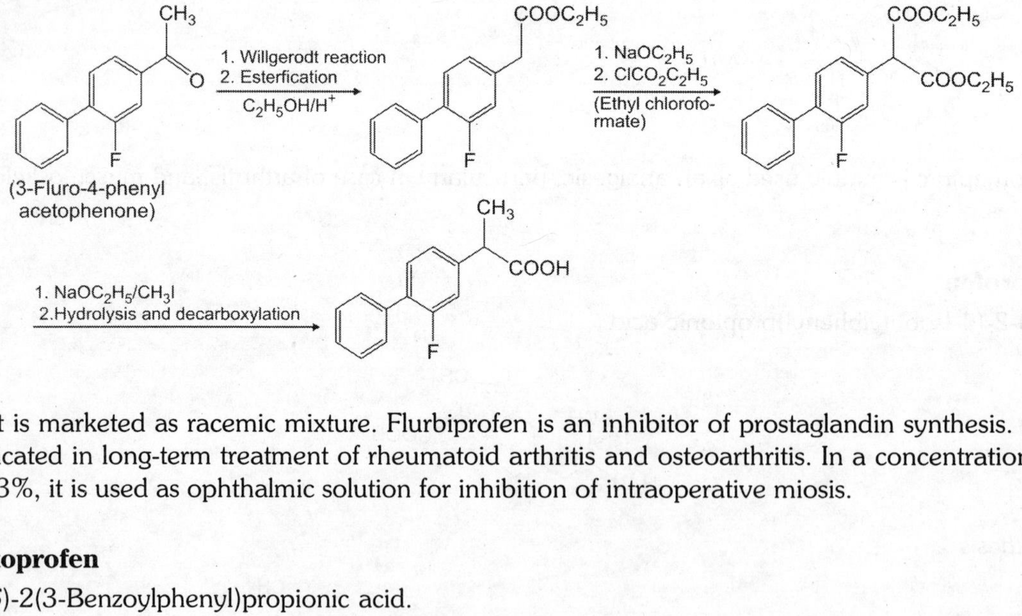

(3-Fluro-4-phenyl acetophenone)

It is marketed as racemic mixture. Flurbiprofen is an inhibitor of prostaglandin synthesis. It is indicated in long-term treatment of rheumatoid arthritis and osteoarthritis. In a concentration of 0.03%, it is used as ophthalmic solution for inhibition of intraoperative miosis.

Ketoprofen

(RS)-2(3-Benzoylphenyl)propionic acid.

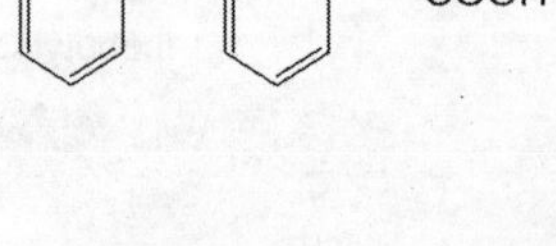

Synthesis

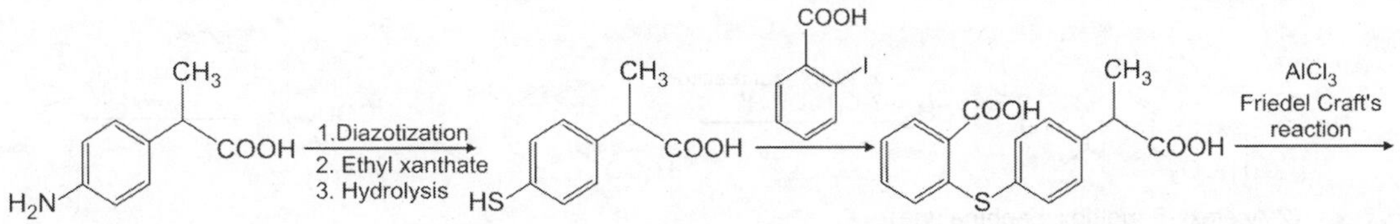

[2-(4-Aminophenyl propionic acid)]

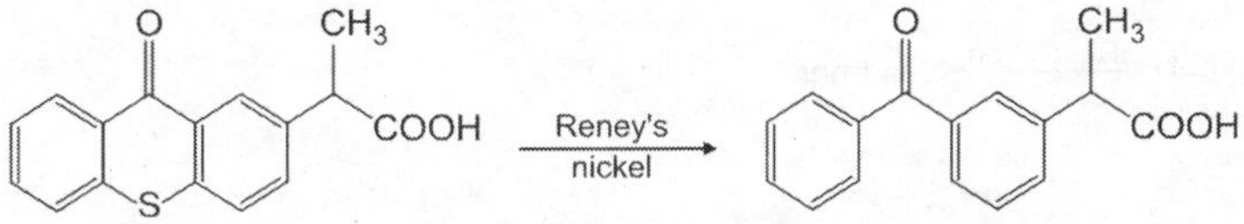

It is marketed as racemic mixture. In addition to inhibition of prostaglandin synthesis, it also inhibits the synthesis of leukotrienes and leukocyte migration into the inflamed tissues. It possesses anti-inflammatory, analgesic, and antipyretic properties.

Fenoprofen calcium

Calcium (*RS*)-2-(3-phenoxyphenyl)propionate dihydrate

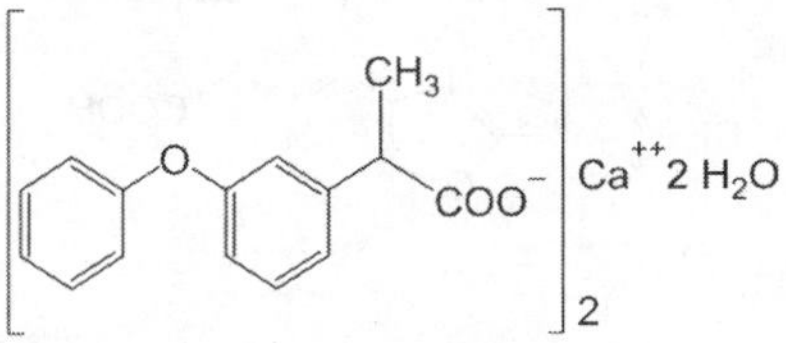

Synthesis

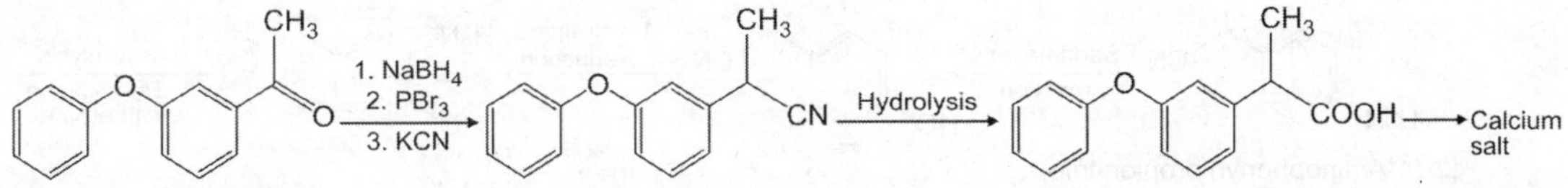

(3-Phenoxyacetophenone)

It is marketed as racemic mixture although *S*(+)-isomer is more active. Like other non-steroidal anti-inflammatory agents, it inhibits prostaglandin synsthesis. It is used in rheumatoid arthritis and osteoarthritis.

Naproxen

(*S*)-2-(6-Methoxy-2-naphthyl)propionic acid

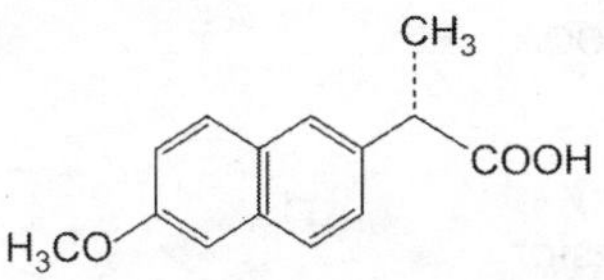

Synthesis

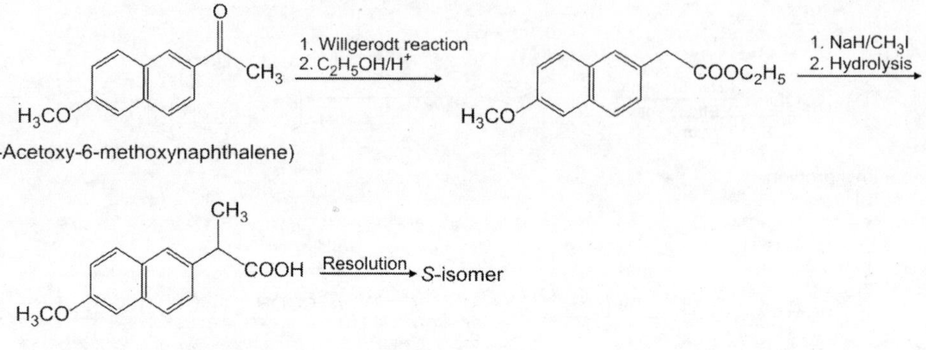

(2-Acetoxy-6-methoxynaphthalene)

It is the only arylpropionic acid analog which is marketed as *S*(+)-enantiomer. It is a powerful prostaglandin inhibitor. Naproxen is recommended for use in rheumatoid and gouty arthritis. It shows good analgesic activity. Side effects include drowsiness and nausea.

Benoxaprofen

2-(4-Chlrophenyl)-α-methyl-5-benzoxazolacetic acid

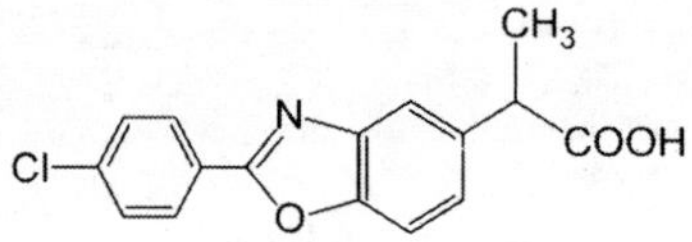

Synthesis

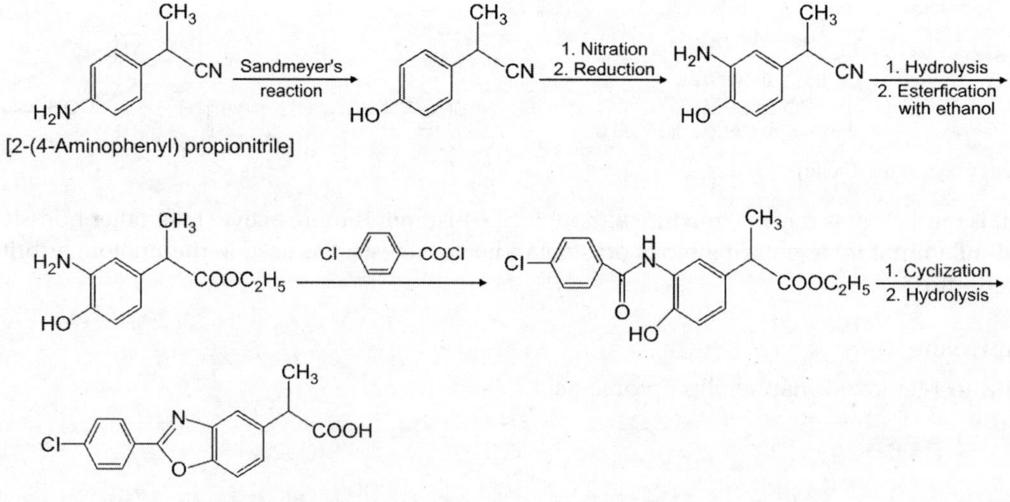

[2-(4-Aminophenyl) propionitrile]

It is an anti-inflammatory analgesic.

Oxaprozin

4,5-Diphenyl-2-oxazolepropionic acid

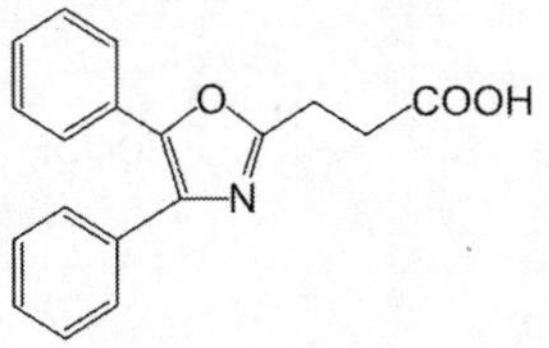

Synthesis

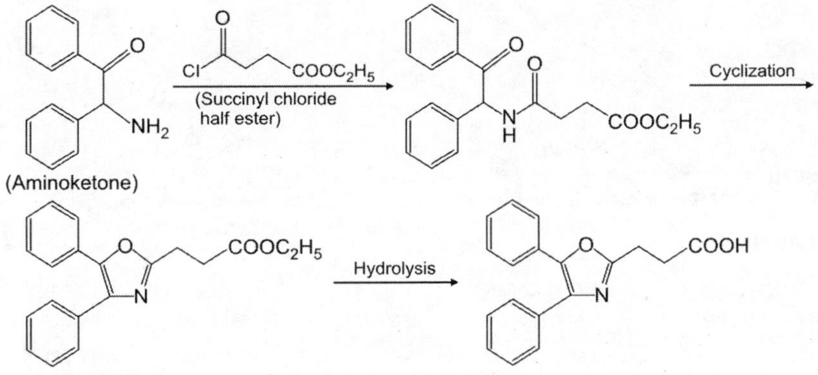

It is used for long-term treatment of osteoarthritis and rheumatoid arthritis.

Suprofen

α-Methyl-4-(2-thienylcarbonyl)benzeneacetic acid.

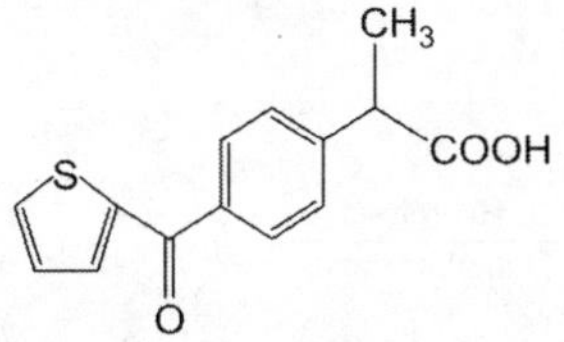

Synthesis

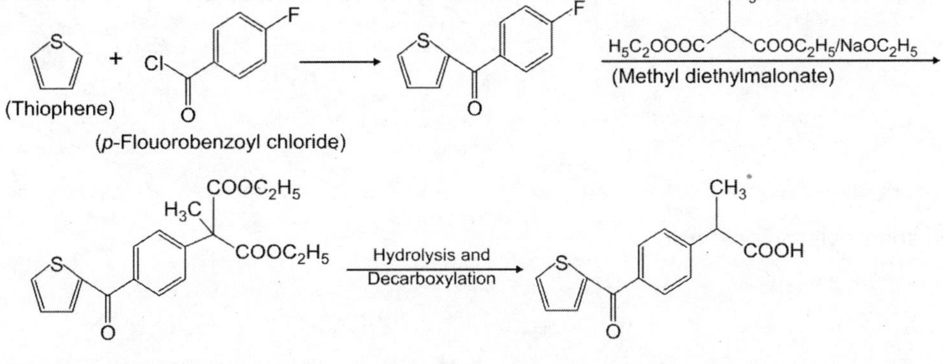

It is used as 1% ophthalmic solution for preventing surgically induced miosis during cataract extraction. It acts through inhibition of prostaglandin synthesis. It is anti-inflammatory analgesic.

Ketorolac

(*RS*)-5-Benzoyl-2, 3-dihydro-1*H*-pyrrolizine-1-carboxylic acid

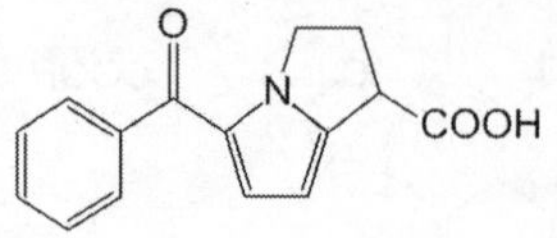

Synthesis

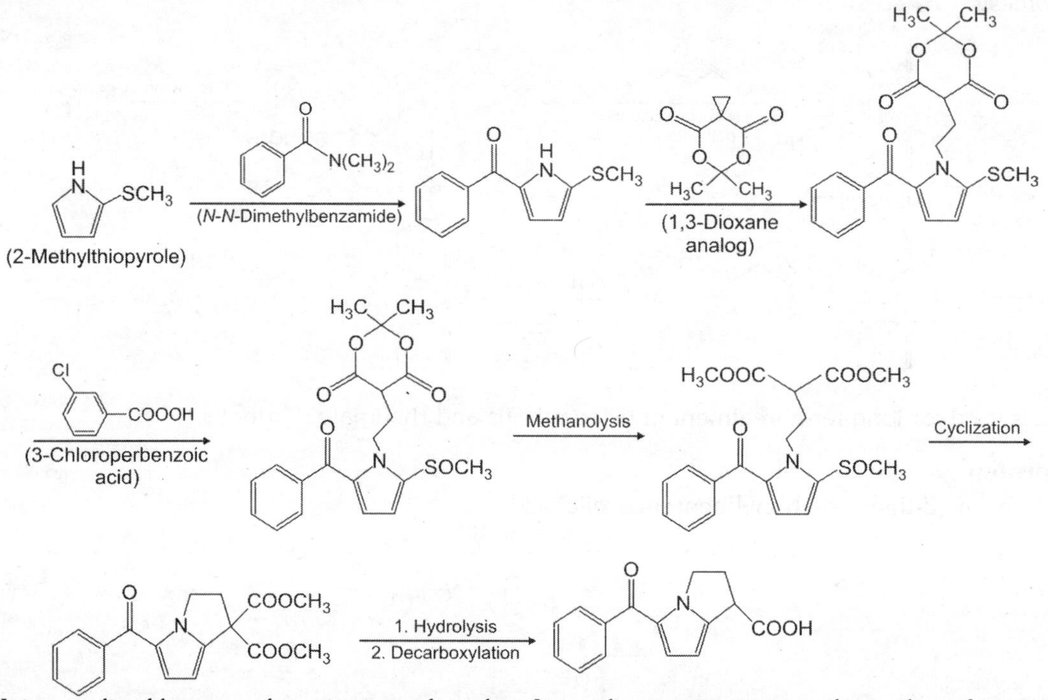

It is a cyclized heteroarylpropionic acid analog. Its analgesic activity is similar to that of centrally acting analgesic and acts by inhibiting prostaglandin synthesis. It is used as a tromethamine (85) salt.

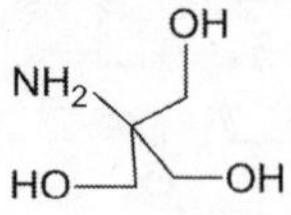

(85)

Fenbufen

β-*p*-Phenylbenzoylpropionic acid.

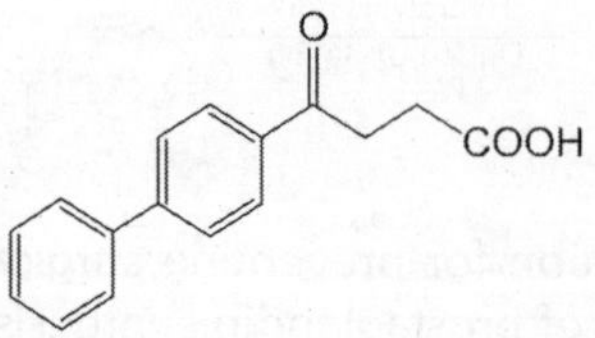

Synthesis

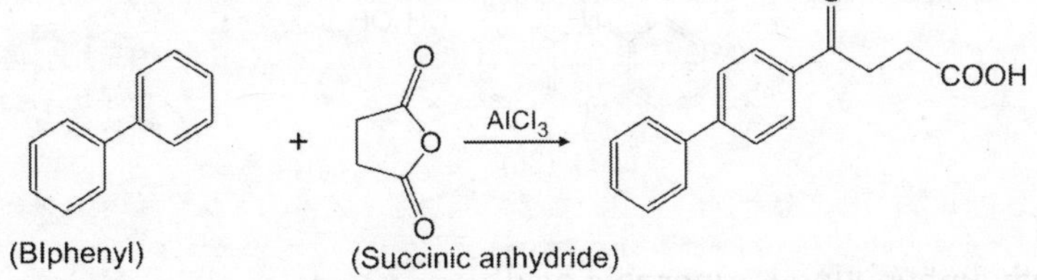

(Biphenyl) + (Succinic anhydride) $\xrightarrow{AlCl_3}$

It is an anti-inflammatory drug with less gastric irritation. Its metabolite biphenyl acetic acid is also active.

NSAIDS : FENAMATES

Mefenamic Acid

N-(2, 3-Xylyl)anthranilic acid

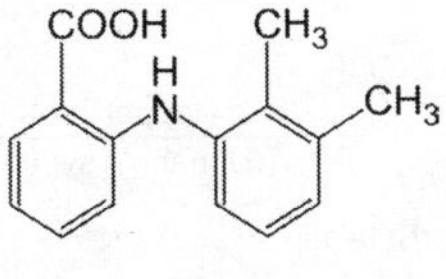

Synthesis

(2-Chlorobenzoic acid) + (2,3-Dimethyl-aniline) $\xrightarrow[\text{(Ulmann's synthesis)}]{\text{Copper-bronze}}$

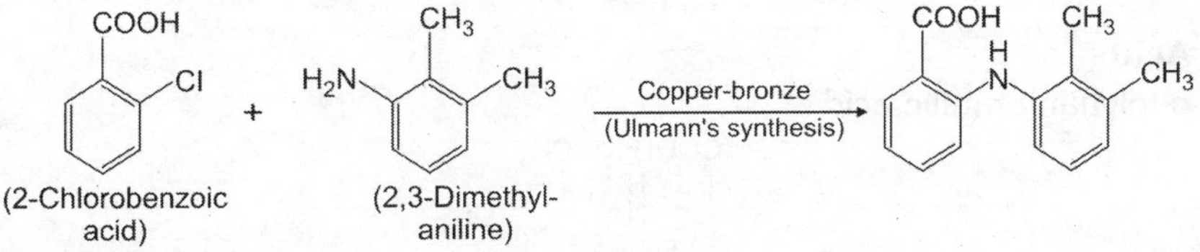

Mefenamic acid is used as anti-inflammatory analgesic.

Meclofenamic Acid

N-(2, 6-Dichloro-*m*-tolyl)anthranilic acid

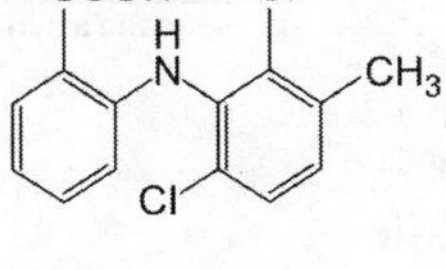

Synthesis

(2-Iodobenzoic acid) + (2,6-Dichloro-3-methylaniline) $\xrightarrow[\text{(Ulmann's synthesis)}]{\text{Copper-bronze}}$

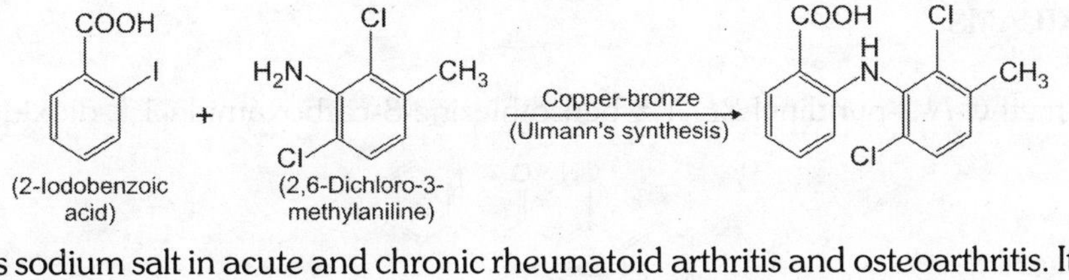

It is used as sodium salt in acute and chronic rheumatoid arthritis and osteoarthritis. Its metabolite, the hydroxymethyl analog (86) obtained by oxidation of methyl group possesses anti-inflammatory activity.

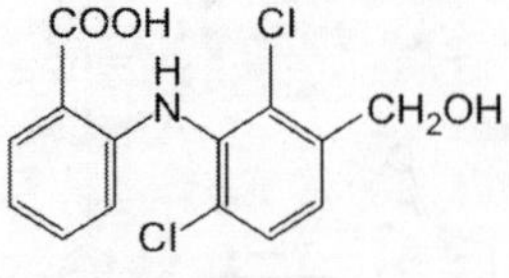

(86)

Flufenamic Acid

2-[[3-(Trifluoromethyl)phenyl]amino]benzoic acid

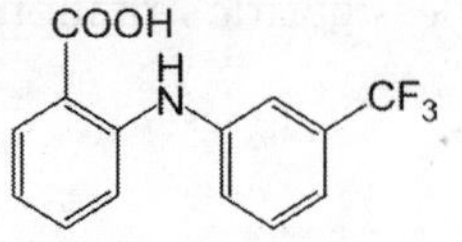

Synthesis

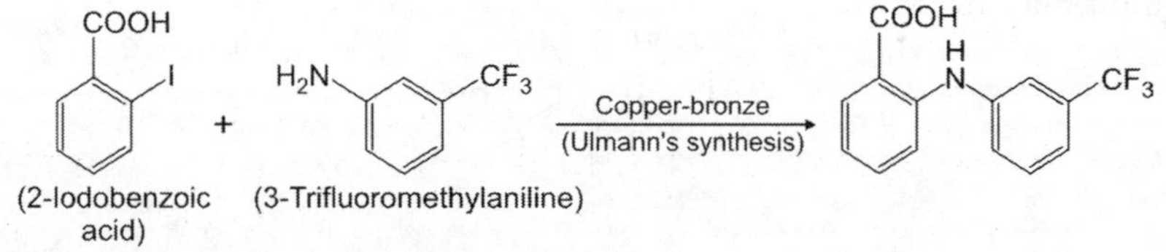

(2-Iodobenzoic acid) + (3-Trifluoromethylaniline) → [Copper-bronze (Ulmann's synthesis)]

It is used as anti-inflammatory analgesic.

Tolfenamic Acid

N-(3-Chloro-o-tolyl)anthranilic acid

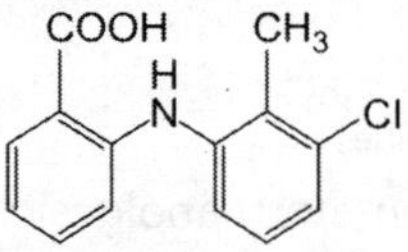

Synthesis

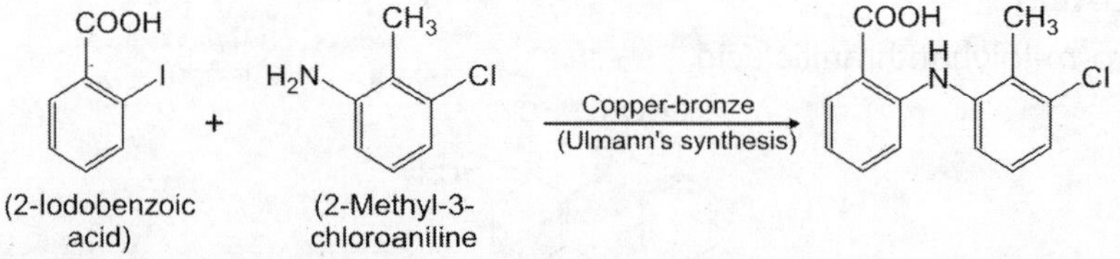

(2-Iodobenzoic acid) + (2-Methyl-3-chloroaniline) → [Copper-bronze (Ulmann's synthesis)]

It is used as anti-inflammatory analgesic.

NSAIDS—OXICAMS
Piroxicam

4-Hydroxy-2-methyl-N-2-pyridinyl-2H-1,2-benzothiazine-3-carboxamide-1,1-dioxide

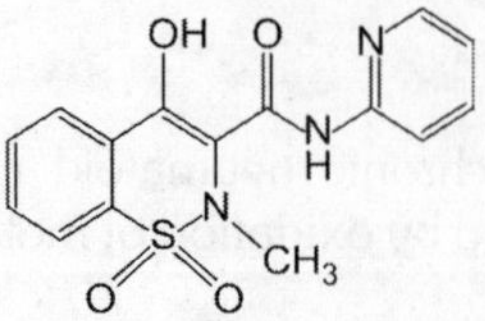

Synthesis

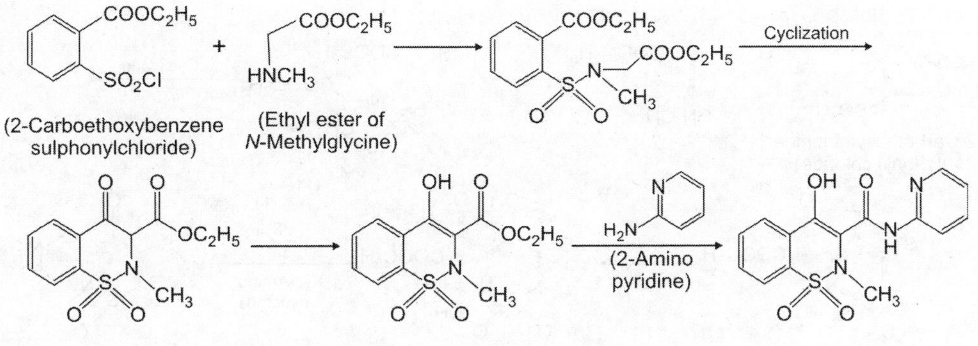

(2-Carboethoxybenzene sulphonylchloride)

(Ethyl ester of N-Methylglycine)

Cyclization

(2-Amino pyridine)

It is an anti-inflammatory drug with a long plasma half-life.

Meloxicam

4-Hydroxy-2-methyl-N-(5-methyl-2-thioazolyl)-2H-1, 2-benzothiazine-3-carboxamide 1, 1-dioxide

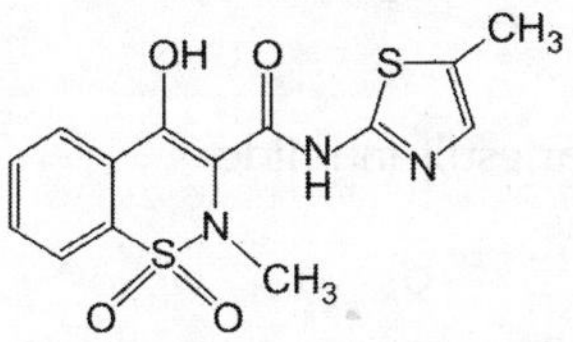

Synthesis

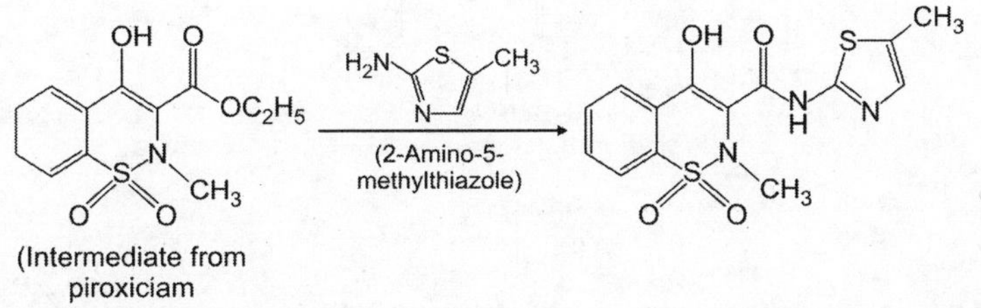

(Intermediate from piroxiciam

(2-Amino-5-methylthiazole)

Meloxicam has some selective COX-2 inhibiting activity. But not as other COX-2 specific inhibitors. It is used in treatment of osteoarthritis.

Tenoxicam

4-Hydroxyl-2-methyl-N-2-pyridinyl-2H-thieno [2,3-e]-1,2-thiazine-3-carboxamide 1, 1-dioxide

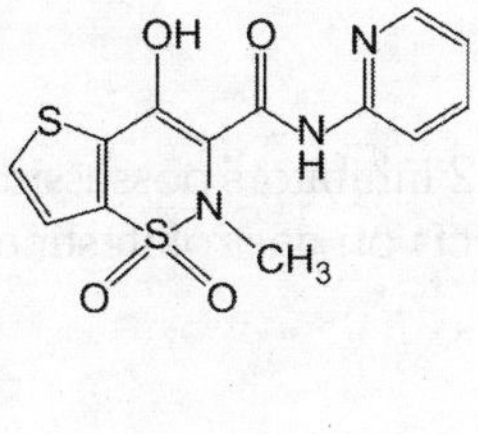

Synthesis

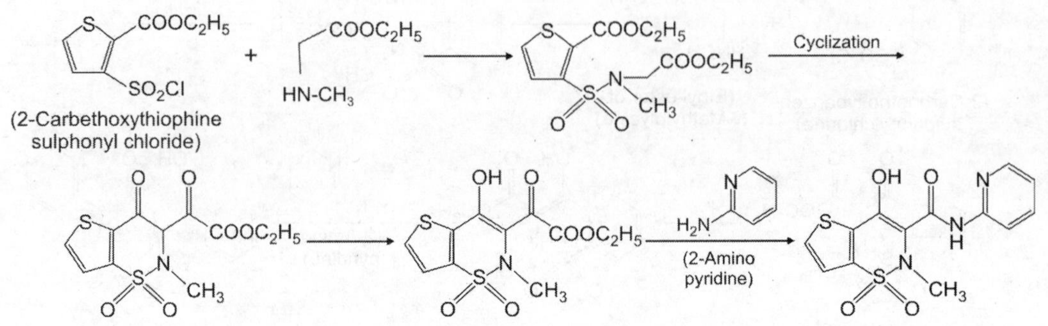

(2-Carbethoxythiophine sulphonyl chloride)

(2-Amino pyridine)

The benzene ring of piroxicam (61) when replaced by thiophene ring results in tenoxicam. It is used as antininflammatory analgesic.

NSAIDS : CYCLOOXYGENASE -2 (COX-2) INHIBITORS

Nimesulide

N-(4-Nitro-2-phenoxyphenyl)methanesulfonamide

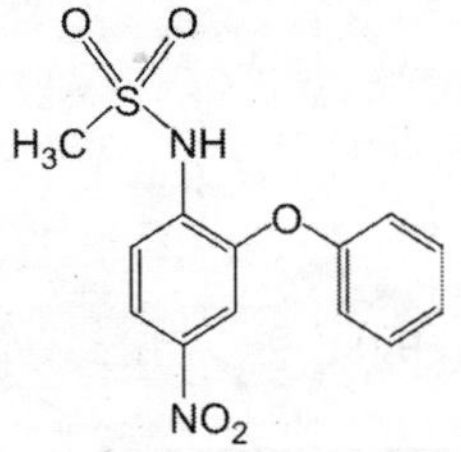

Synthesis

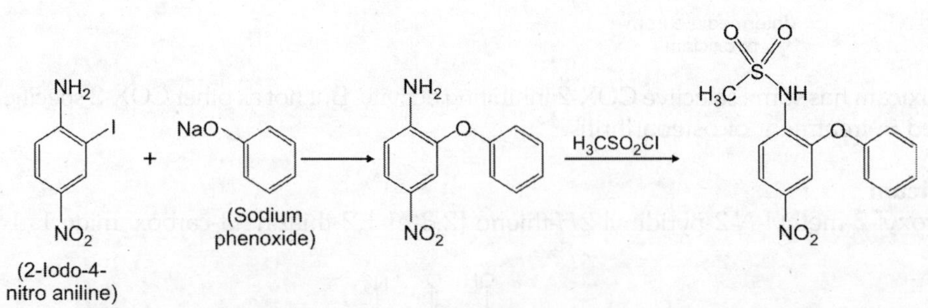

(2-Iodo-4-nitro aniline)

(Sodium phenoxide)

It belongs to 'sulide' group of COX-2 inhibitors possessing high degree of selectivity for inhibition of COX-2 and is therefore free of effects on gastrointestinal tract.

Lumiracoxib

2-(2'-Chloro-6'-fluoroanilino)-5-methylphenylacetic acid

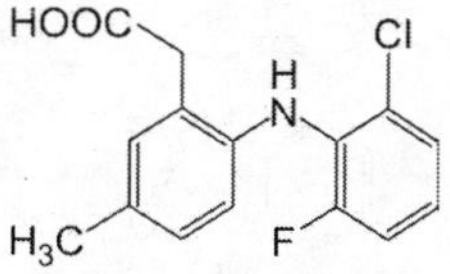

Synthesis

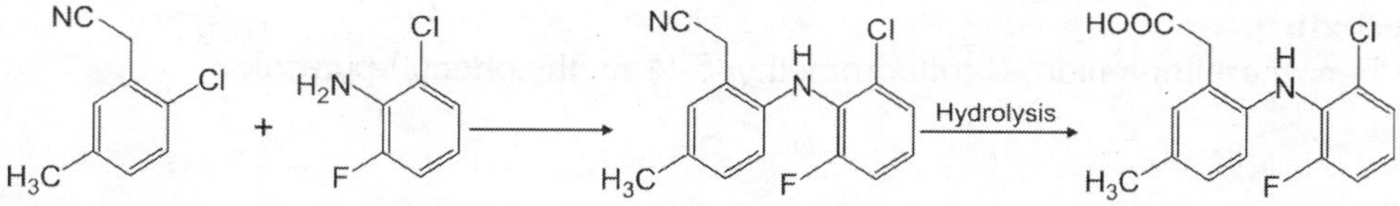

(2-Chloro-5- methyl benzylcyanide)   (2-Chloro-6-pluroaniline)

Lumiracoxib is effective in treatment of osteoarthiritis, rheumatoid arthiritis, and the acute pain associated with these inflammatory diseases.

Rofecoxib

4-(4-Methylsufonylphenyl)-3-phenyl-5*H*-2-furanone

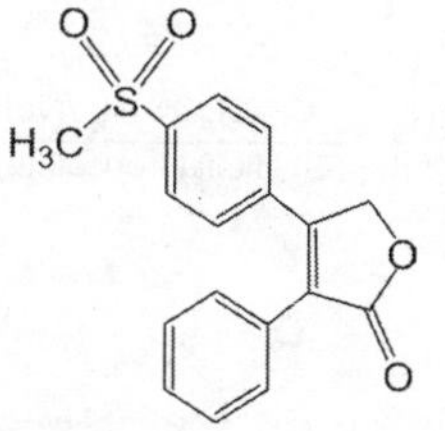

Synthesis

Step 1

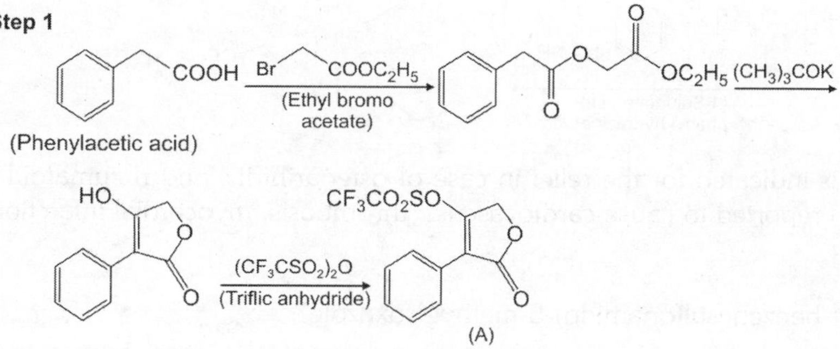

(Phenylacetic acid)   (Ethyl bromo acetate)

Step 2

(4-Bromo Thioanisole)   (B)

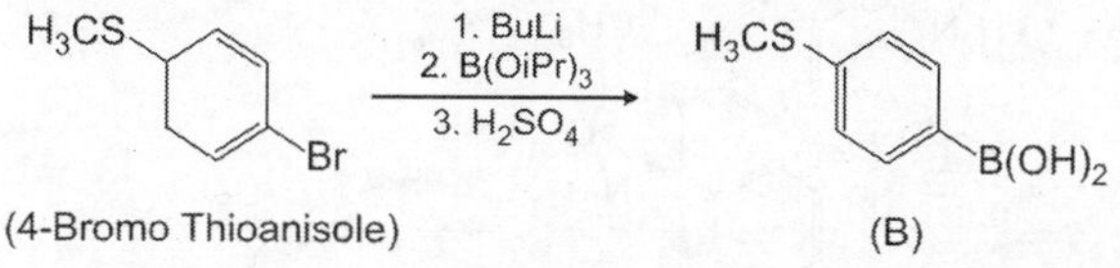

Step 3

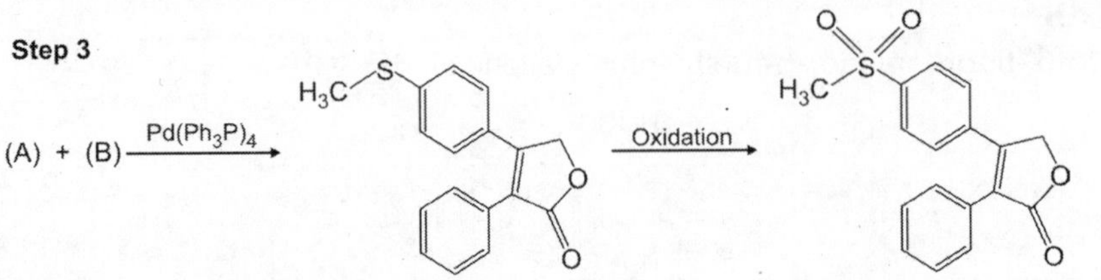

$$(A) + (B) \xrightarrow{Pd(Ph_3P)_4}$$

Oxidation →

Rofecoxib is indicated in ostoarthiritis

Celecoxib

1-(4-Benzenesulfonamido)-3-trifluoromethyl-5-(4-methylphenyl)-pyrazole

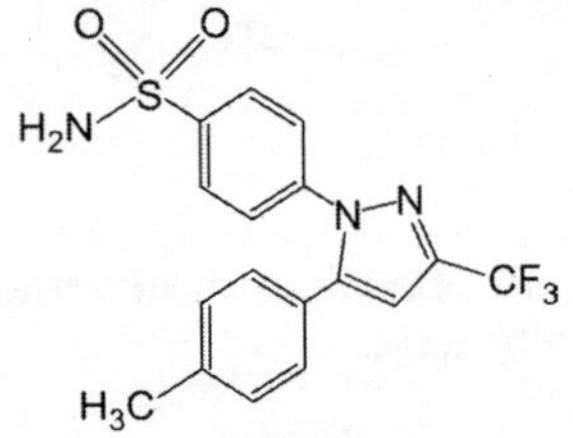

Synthesis

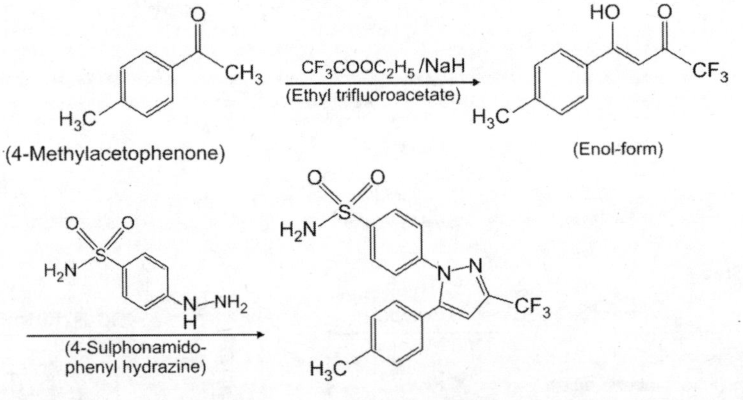

(4-Methylacetophenone) $\xrightarrow[\text{(Ethyl trifluoroacetate)}]{CF_3COOC_2H_5 \text{ /NaH}}$ (Enol-form)

(4-Sulphonamido-phenyl hydrazine)

Celecoxib is indicated for the relief in case of osteoarthiritis and rheumatoid arthiritis. Celec-oxib has been reported to cause cardiovascular thrombosis, myocardial infarction, and stroke.

Valdecoxib

3-Phenyl-4-(4-benzenesulfonamido)-5-methyl-isoxazole

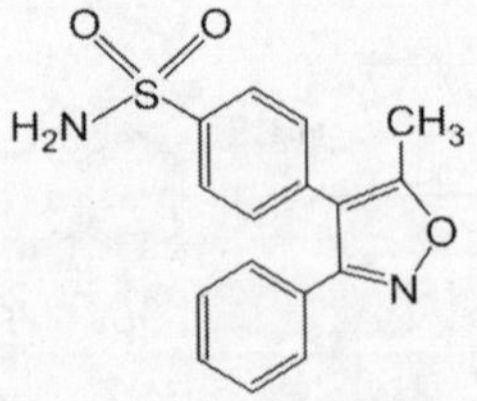

Synthesis

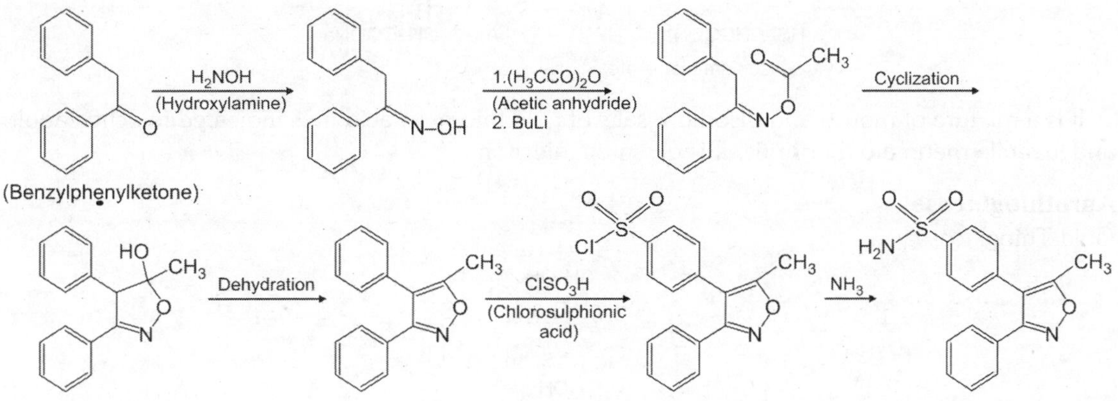

It is indicated in osteoarthiritis and rheumatoid arthiritis. However it has been withdrawn because of sefety concerns.

Parecoxib

3-Phenyl-4-(4-*N*-propionoxybenzenesulfonamido)-5-methyl-isoxazole

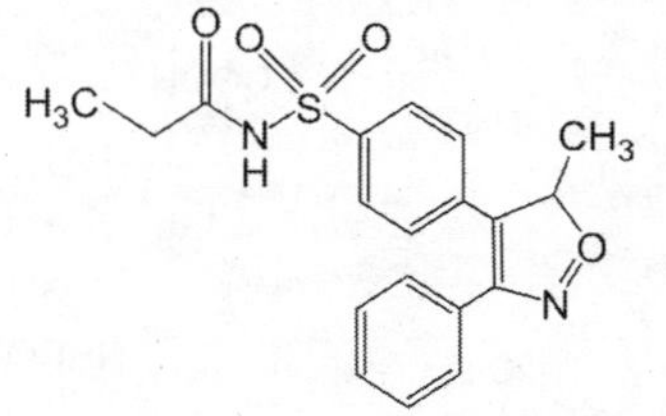

Synthesis

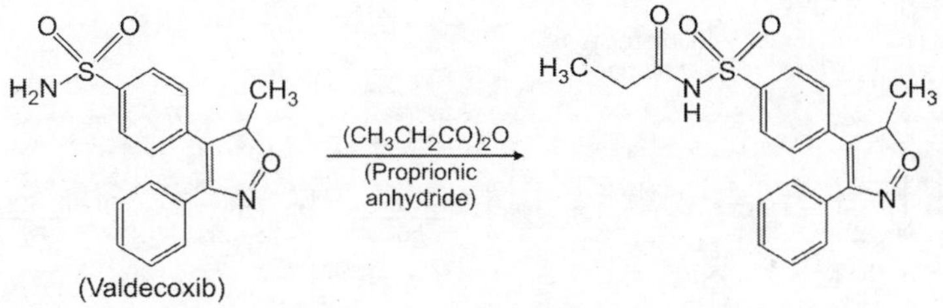

It is a prodrug of valdecoxib (69) and undergoes rapid hydrolysis to its.

DISEASE MODIFYING ANTIRHEUMATIC DRUGS (DMARDs)
Sodium Aurothiomalate

Gold sodium thiomalate

$$CH_2COONa$$
$$|$$
$$Au-S-CH-COONa$$

Synthesis

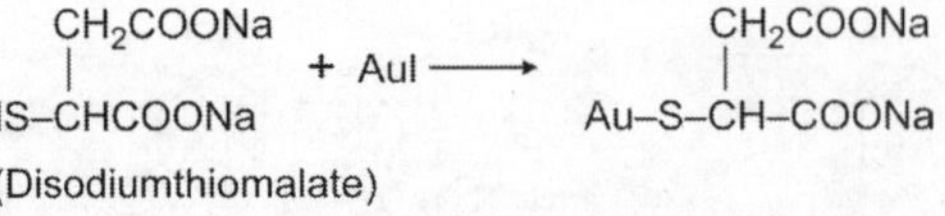

$$CH_2COONa \quad CH_2COONa$$
$$| \qquad + AuI \longrightarrow \qquad |$$
$$HS-CHCOONa \qquad Au-S-CH-COONa$$

(Disodiumthiomalate)

It is a mixture of mono- and disodium salts of gold thiomalic acid. It is indicated in active adult and juvenile rheumatoid arthritis. It is given by injection.

Aurothioglucose
Gold Thioglucose

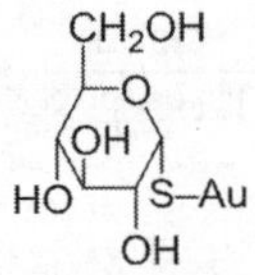

CH₂OH structure (thioglucose with S–Au)

It is prepared by adding a solution of aurous bromide to an aqueous solution of thioglucose saturated with sulphur dioxide. It is also administered by parentral routes. It is indicated for the adjunctive treatment of adult and juvenile rheumatoid arthritis.

Penicillamine
3, 3-Dimethyl-D-cysteine

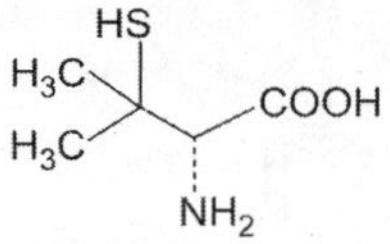

Penicillamine structure

Synthesis

Reaction scheme: DL-Valine + Chloracetyl chloride → intermediate → (CH₃CO)₂O (Acetic anhydride) → Azlactone → H₂S → thiazoline → H₂O boil → intermediate → HCl/boil Pyridine → Racemic mixture → HCOOH → Brucine salt → Resolve → D-form

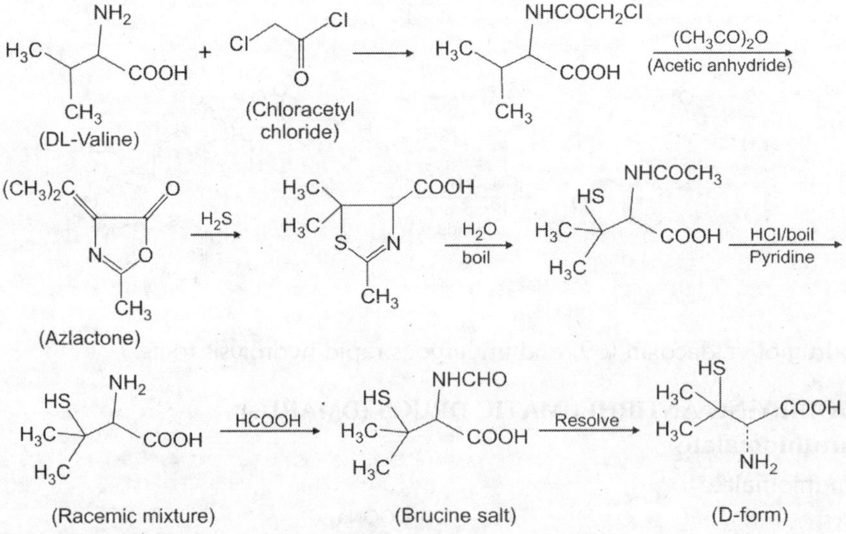

It is used to treat severe rheumatoid arthritis.

Hydroxychloroquine

See "ANTIPROTOZOAL DRUGS I: CHEMOTHERAPY OF MALARIA"

Hydroxychloroquine is used for the treatment of rheumatoid arthritis, lupus erythematosus, and malaria.

Methotrexate

See ANTICANCER AGENTS

It is used in rheumatoid arthiritis in patients who do not respond to NSAIDS.

Leflunomide

5-Methyl-*N*-[4-(trifluoromethyl)phenyl]-4-isoxazolecarboxamide

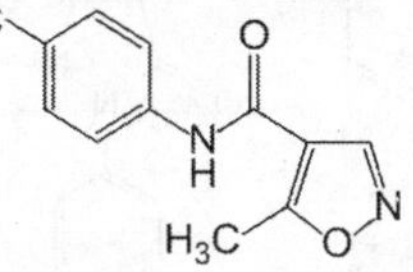

Synthesis

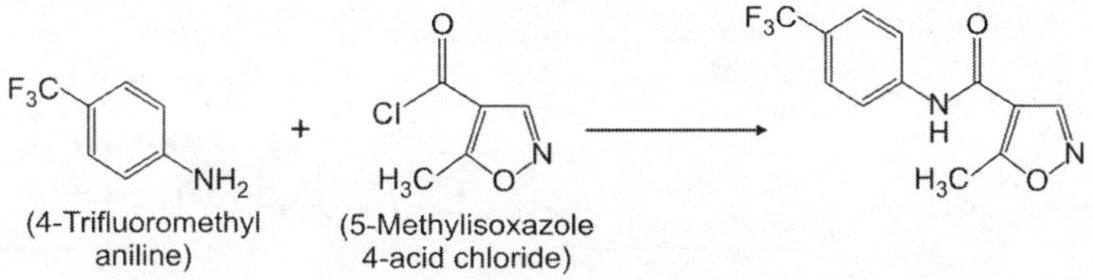

(4-Trifluoromethyl
aniline)

(5-Methylisoxazole
4-acid chloride)

It is an immunosuppressant used in rheumatoid arthiritis. It is indicated in patients where the NSAIDS fail. It is a prodrug and is converted to teriflunomide (87) the active form.

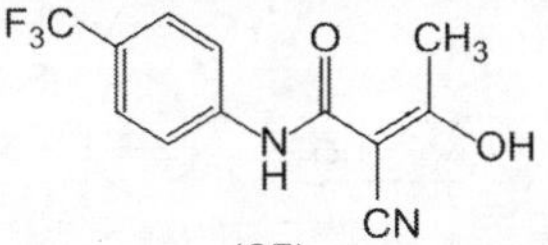

(87)

DRUGS USED IN GOUT

Allopurinol

1,5-Dihydro-4*H*-pyrazolo[3,4-d]pyrimidine-4-one

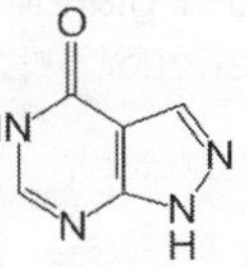

Synthesis

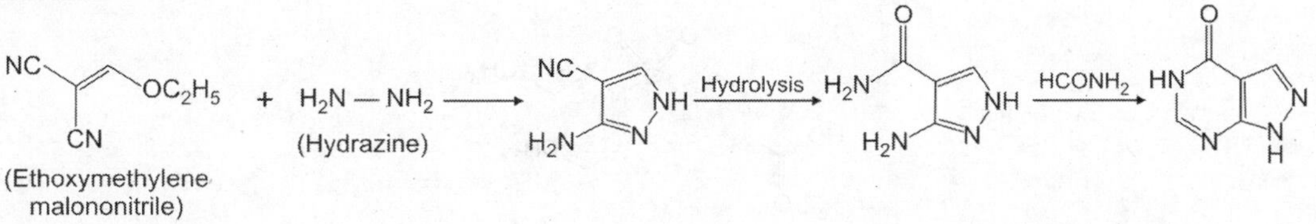

(Ethoxymethylene
malononitrile)

(Hydrazine)

It is an isomer of hypoxanthine. It has higher affinity for xanthine oxidase than xanthine and is converted to alloxanthine (80) which acts as a non-competitive inhibitor of xanthine oxidase. Thus, the synthesis of uric acid, a highly water insoluble substance, is inhibited and at the same time there is increase in concentration of water soluble hypoxanthine and xanthine which are excreted through urine.

Sulphinpyrazone

1,2-Diphenyl-4-[2-(phenylsulphinyl)ethyl]pyrazolidine-3, 5-dione

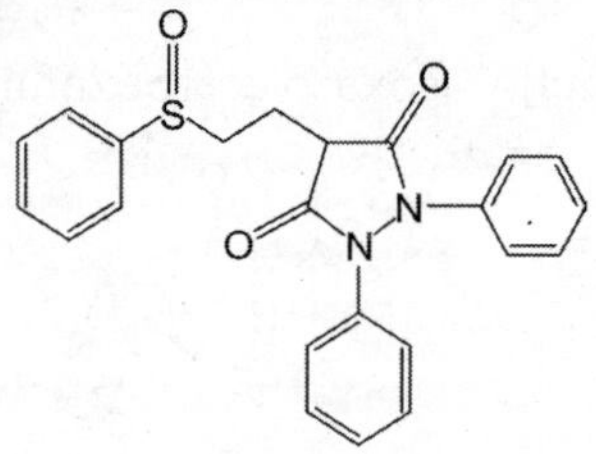

Synthesis

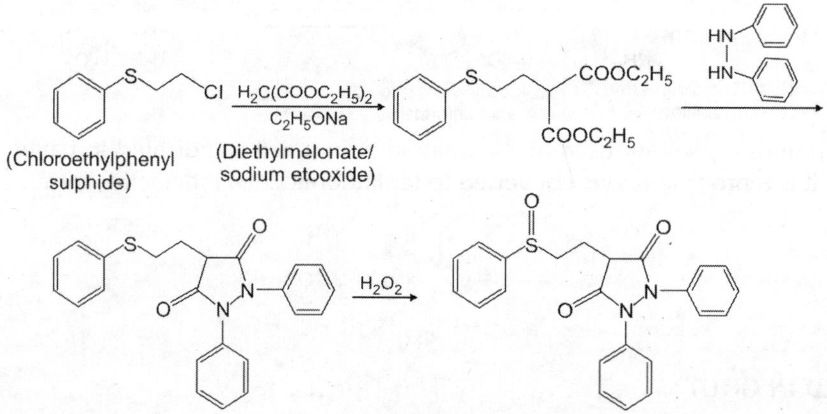

(Chloroethylphenyl sulphide)

(Diethylmelonate/ sodium etooxide)

It decreases plasma uric acid by decreasing its reabsorption. It produces stonger uricosuric effect than probenecid (82). It also inhibits human platelet prostaglandin synthesis at cyclooxygenase level but has no analgesic and antipyretic effects.

Probenecid

4-[(Dipropylamino)sulphonyl]benzoic acid

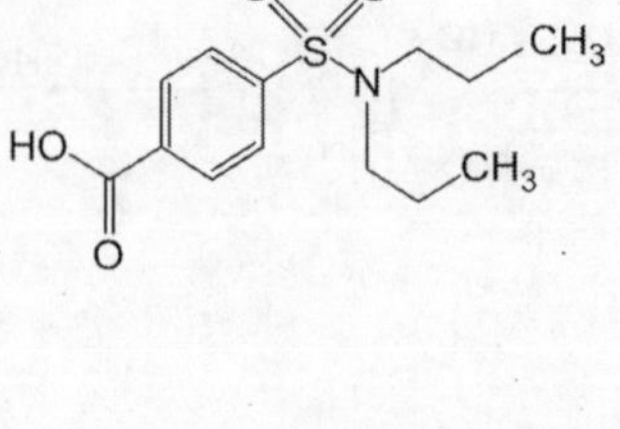

Synthesis

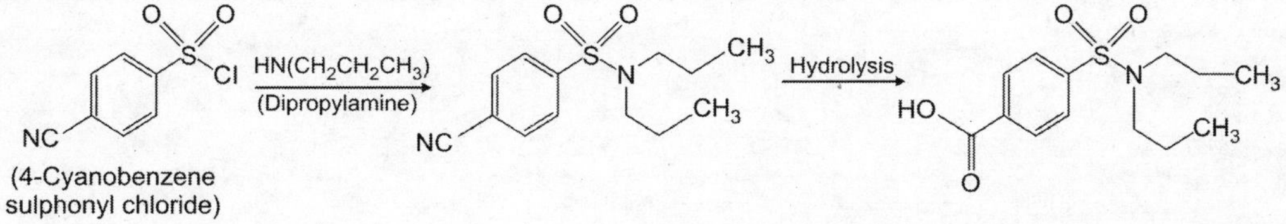

(4-Cyanobenzene
sulphonyl chloride)

It is a uricosuric agent and is used in acute gout. It reduces uric acid level by decreasing its reabsorption.

Section IV
Renal and Cardiovascular Drugs

CHAPTER
13

DIURETICS

DIURETICS are substances that increase the excretion of urine by kidneys. Kidney is one of the paired glandular organ which lie on the posterior abdominal wall, one on each side of the vertebral column behind the peritonium and below the diaphragm. The increased excrertion of urine results in decrease in body fluids, especially the extracellular fluids.

The function of kidney is regulation of volume and compostion of body fluids which it accomplishes by elimination of variable amounts of Na^+, K^+, H^+, Cl^-, HPO_4^{2-}, and SO_4^{2-}, excrection of waste products such as urea, uric acid, creatinine, etc. and the maintenance of acid-base balance. The intracellular fluid is in osmotic equilibrium with extracellular fluid. Thus, any change in extracellular fluid results in change in composition of intracellular fluid.

The functional unit of kidney is nephron (Fig. 13.1) and there are approximately one million nephrons in each kidney. The nephron consists of a tubule closed on one end and the other end opening into a collecting tubule. The closed end which is cup-shaped is known as Bowman's capsule. It almost completely encloses a network of arterial capillaries, called glomerulus. The renal tubule after the Bowman's or glomerular capsule consists of 3 parts, namely, proximal convoluted tubule, the loop of Henle or medullary loop, and the distal convoluted tubule, leading into a collecting tubule.

After the blood is delivered to each glomerulus, many of its components, excepting the substances with molecular weight of 67,000 and above, are filtered into Bowman's capsule. In this way, serum, albumin and globulins are retained. As the filtrate passes down the renal tubule, reabsorption process takes place at straight portion and proximal convoluted tubule. This reabsorption is of 65–70 % of sodium, chloride, water and calcium ions, 80–90% of bicarbonate and phosphate ions, 100% of glucose, amino acids, and low molecular weight proteins.

As the fluid moves down, the descending limb of loop of Henle, it becomes more concentrated. After passing through ascending limb of loop of Henle, it becomes dilute, because half of the sodium and chloride ions are reabsobed. Distal convoluted tubule is the third major site where the sodium ions reabsorption takes place through cation exchange which is under the control of aldosterone. The fourth and the final site where the sodium ions reabsorption takes place is cortical collecting tubule. Sodium ions from renal tubular fluid is exchanged for potassium ions and to a lesser extent with hydrogen ions from blood. The amount of sodium ions reabsorbed at this site depends on:

(a) Plasma and renal level of mineralocorticoids like aldosterone. The higher its level, the greater reabsorption of sodium ions and greater the excretion of potassium and hydrogen ions.

(*b*) The flow rate of fluid in tubule and percentage of filtered load of sodium ions at the exchange sites. The greater the flow rate and the load of sodium, the greater the amount of exchange.

(*c*) Acid-base status of individual. Acidosis favours exchange of sodium ions, with hydrogen ions whereas alkalosis favours exchange of sodium ions with potassium.

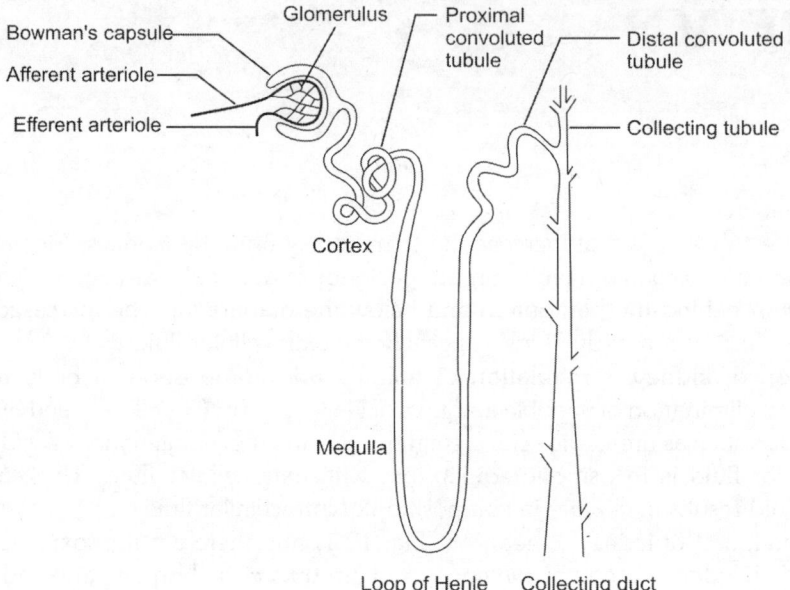

Fig. 13.1: Nephron.

The kidney is able to respond to changes in glomerular filtration rate. An increase in glomerular filtration rate results in increased excretion of water and sodium chloride. This results in release of renin which in turn leads to the formation of angiotensin II. Angiotensin II formation results in renal vasoconstriction which decreases glomerular filtration rate. Another mechanism by which urine formation is controlled is through the production of vasopressin or antidiuretic hormone released from posterior pituitary. Vasopressin increases the reabsorption of water in the distal convoluted tubule.

The disturbances in kidney function arise from glomerular filtration rate or in the capacity of tubular reabsorption. This results in abnormal increase in volume of extracellular fluid that produces a condition known as edema. The main diseases associated with edema are congestive heart failure, premenstrual tension, edema of pregnancy, renal edema, and cirrhosis with ascites.

One of the application of diuretics is in hypertension. Mild hypertension is controlled with diuretics. Moderate to severe cases of hypertension are treated with diuretics in combination with other drugs.

There are four sites of diuretic action in renal tubule and these include, proximal sites, one medullary and the other cortical. The third site is thick ascending limb of Henle and the fourth site the distal convoluted tubule.

The various classes of diuretics are:

1. Water and osmotic agents.
2. Acidifying salts.
3. Organomercurials.
4. Phenoxyacetic acids.
5. Purines and related heterocyclic.
6. Sulphonamides which include,

   (a) carbonic anhydrase inhibitors, and
   (b) thiazides and hydrothizides.

7. Aldosterone antagonists and inhibitors.

WATER AND OSMOTIC AGENTS

When large amount of water is taken, it increases the blood volume which inhibits antidiuretic hormone resulting in diuresis. The electrolyte concentration is, however, not affected and there is no net loss of water from tissues because it is retained in proportion to concentration of electrolyte present.

Osmotic diuresis occurs naturally in diabetes. With the increase in blood concentration of glucose, the tubular maximum is exceeded. So excretion of glucose necessitates excretion of an osmotically equivalent volume of water. This is how osmotic diuretics act.

Substances used as osmotic diuretics include substances which have limited tubular reabsorption. When they are administered in high concentration, it results in passing of large quantity of water from body into the tubule and this results in diuresis. Examples of osmotic diuretics include urea, (H_2NCONH_2), polyhydroxy compounds such as mannitol (1), sorbitol (2), isosorbide (3), and glycerol (4).

(1)   (2)   (3)   (4)

Mannitol (1) is one of the most commonly used substances as osmotic diuretic. It is administered intravenously in a concentration of 5-50%. Isosorbide (3) is used mainly in glaucoma. The site of action of osmotic diuretics is proximal tubule, loop of Henle, and collecting tubule.

ACIDIFYING SALTS

Acidifying salts such as ammonium chloride and ammonium nitrate have a weak diuretic effect. Their administration results in excess of anions such as Cl^- and NO_3^-. The ammonium ion is metabolized to urea. Increased anions result in increased Na^+ output. The Na^+ reabsorption leads to increase in H^+ output and consequent acidification of urine. The same mechanism is involved when calcium nitrate [$Ca(NO_3)_2$] or calcium chloride ($CaCl_2$) is administered. Ca^{++} are removed by deposition in bone or excreted as phosphates. The kidney rapidly develops a compensating mechanism to neutralise the acid formed. This compensatory mechanism involves increased formation of ammonia, resulting in acidifying salts losing their effectiveness as diuretics. Other disadvantages of acidifying salts include, gastric irritation, anorexia, nausea, and vomiting.

ORGANOMERCURIALS

Organomercurials were the only effective diuretics earlier. However with the advent of newer and safer diuretics, they have been largely replaced. The use of organomercurials started with merbaphen (5), a drug originally used for syphilis. Since it was highly toxic, search for newer organomercurials started. This resulted in the synthesis of mersalyl (6) which was less toxic.

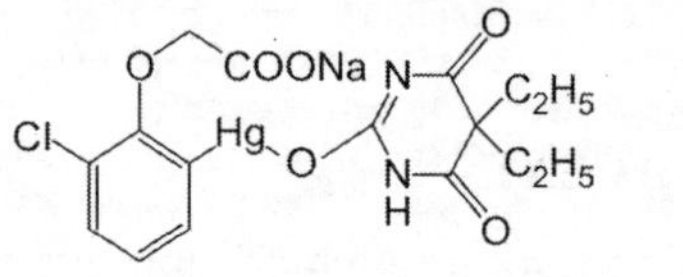

(5) 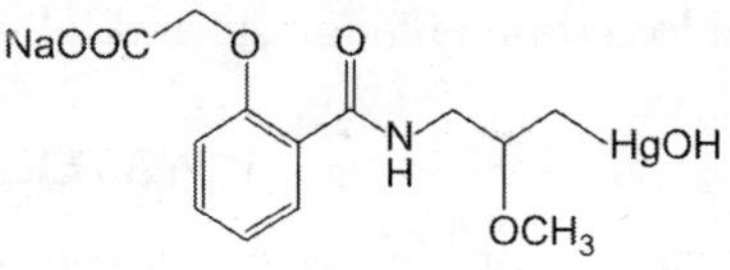   (6)

All of the organomercurials used as diuretics contain an alkoxymercuripropyl group (7) attached to an amide derivatives of an acid, where R could be aliphatic, alicyclic, aromatic, or heterocyclic. R´ could be — H, CH_3, — C_2H_5, or — CH_2CH_2 OCH_3, X could be — OH, — Cl. — Br, — O_2CCH_3, — SCH_2COONa, — $SCH_2(CHOH)_4CH_2OH$, or theophylline.

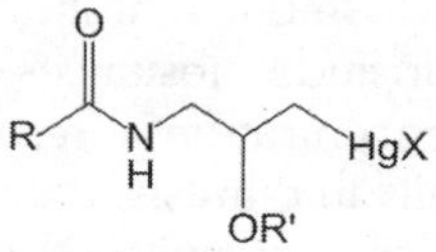

(7)

Organomercurials act at proximal convoluted tubule site. Their action is believed to be due to Hg^{++} which is released from the organomercurials. The Hg^{++} combines with sulfhydryl groups (Fig. 13.2) of renal enzymes which are necessary for reabsorption. This results in increased loss of sodium chloride and water. The blocking of enzyme by the mercuric ions is established by the observation that with the administration of dimercaprol (8) the diuretic activity of mercurial diuretics is not observed. This is because Hg^{++} reacts with thiol groups of dimercaprol (8) rather than of enzyme.

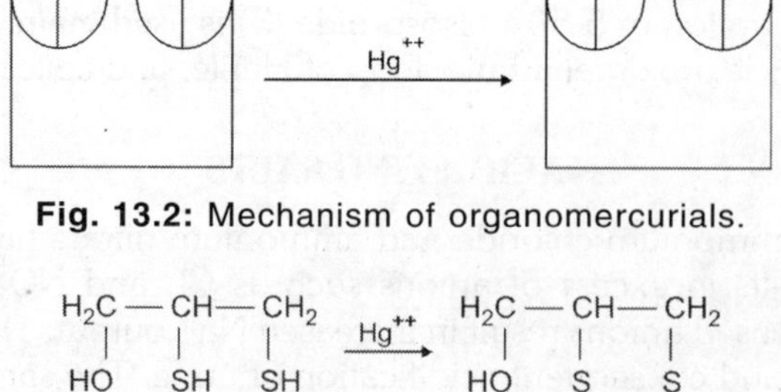

Fig. 13.2: Mechanism of organomercurials.

(8)   (9)

Some of the advantages of organomercurials include:

1. With the exception of potassium sparing diuretics and aldosterone antagonists, the organomercurials produce less potassium loss than most of other diuretics.
2. They do not significantly alter the excretion of K^+, NH_4^+, HCO_3^-, or PO_4^- and therefore, do not produce marked disturbances in electrolyte balance of the body fluid.
3. They do not affect the carbohydrate metabolism and therefore do not affect the blood sugar levels.
4. The uric acid elimination also remains unaffected and therefore they do not produce uricacidemia.

One of the disadvantages of organomercurials is that they are not well absorbed from GI tract. However, they produce a rapid and reliable onset of action when given parenterally. Some of the toxic reactions include local irritation, necrosis, and when used orally for prolonged period their use may result in mercurialism.

PHENOXYACETIC ACIDS

Working on the hypothesis that organomercurials acted by blocking of sulfhydryl enzyme, which is necessary for sodium reabsorption, α, β-unsaturated ketones (10), which also could reversibly react with sulfhydryl groups, were investigated for their diuretic activity. Derivatives of phenoxyacetic acids (11) containing α, β-unsaturated carbonyl group were investigated and found to possess high diuretic activity. The purpose for using free carboxylic acid was that it will increase the excretion by the kidney.

(10)

Structure-Activity Relationships Studies (11)

R = R' = R" = H or lower alkyl
X = Y = H, lower alkyl or Cl

(11)

1. For maximum action, at least one position on aromatic ring should be substituted with halogen or methyl. Disubstitution increases the activity, but more substitution results in loss of activity.
2. For maximum activity, the β-position of the unsaturated ketone should be unsubstituted.
3. Reduction of double bond diminishes the activity.
4. The oxyacetic acid residue should be *para*- to the α, β-unsaturated ketone moiety.

These studies on the α, β-unsaturated ketones have resulted in the synthesis of one of the most powerful diuretics, ethacrynic acid (12). It inhibits $Na^+/K^+/2Cl^-$ co-transporter in the thick ascending loop of Henle. This inhibition is thought to be due to adduct formed between $= CH_2$ of ethacrynic acid (12) and the cysteine. The inhibition results in increased excretion of sodium, potassium, calcium, and chloride ions which results in diuresis. The side effects of ethacrynic acid (12) include excessive loss of fluid, hypokalemia and metabolic alkalosis due to hydrogen ion excretion.

(12)

PURINES AND RELATED HETEROCYCLICS

Purines

Caffeine (13), theophylline (14) and theobromine (15) are the three xanthines which possess diuretic activity. They have been used for centuries by the humans in form of tea and coffee. Among the three, theophylline (14) is about 3 times as active as caffeine (13) and theobromine (15) occupying the intermediate position. In addition to their diuretic activity, they also are CNS stimulants. Clinically, they are not used as diuretics. Theophylline (14) and theobromine (15) have been used in combination with other substances. The most widely used combination is aminophylline (16) which is a combination of ethylenediamine with theophylline (14). It is used as cardiac stimulant, coronary dilator, and antiasthmatic agent.

(13)   (14)   (15)

(16)

Xanthines act both by decreasing tubular electrolyte reabsorption and by increasing glomerular filtration rate through increased blood flow which is because of improved cardiac output. They also increase excretion of sodium and chloride ions. They are not used nowadays.

Pteridines

The observation that xanthopterin (17) was capable of affecting kidney led to investigation of pteridines as diuretics. One of the compounds, 2, 4-diamino-6, 7-dimethylpterdine (18) showed good diuretic activity. Further studies led to the discovery of a potent diuretic triamterene (19). Triamterene (19) is one of the K$^+$ sparing diuretic. It inhibits sodium and water reabsorption by blocking the sodium channels in distal convoluted tubule.

(17)   (18)   (19)

Structure-Activity Relationship Studies

1. Replacement of one of the primary amino group with a lower alkylamino group did not affect the activity,
2. phenyl group seemed to be essential for activity. Its replacement by other groups such as tolyl or p-hydroxy phenyl led to less active or inactive compounds. Similarly, replacement by smaller alkyl groups also showed lower activity.

Triamterene (19) acts on distal convoluted tubule, inhibiting sodium reabsorption through blockade of sodium channel, thus making less sodium available for transport across the membrane. One of the serious side effect is hyperkalemia.

Pyrazines

Pyrazines of the type (20) can be considered as open chain analogs of pteridine structure. Such compounds were found to produce diuretic activity. Maximum activity was found in amiloride (21), which is N-amidino-3, 5-diamino-6-chloropyrazine-2-carboxamide. Like triamterene (19), it is also a potassium sparing diuretic and acts in the same manner by making less sodium available for reabsorption through blockade of sodium channels in distal collecting tubule.

(20)   (21)

SULPHONAMIDES

Carbonic Anhydrase Inhibitors

The systemic acidosis caused by sulphanilamide (22) has been attributed to inhibition of the enzyme carbonic anhydrase. Carbonic anhydrase catalyzes the reversible hydration of carbon dioxide leading to the formation of carbonic acid which decomposes to H$^+$ and HCO$_3^-$ (Eq. 1). The H$^+$ are exchanged with Na$^+$ in renal tubule or they may combine with HCO$_3^-$ to form H$_2$CO$_3$ which forms CO$_2$ and H$_2$O. Inhibition of carbonic anhydrase reduces the concentration of H$^+$ in renal tubules and leads to increased excretion of Na$^+$ and HCO$_3^-$, thereby, producing diuresis. There is also significant loss of K$^+$. The urine which is normally acidic becomes alkaline and systemic acidosis occurs. During acidosis, the carbonic anhydrase inhibitors are not effective till the acid-base balance is restored. Sulphonamides act by competing with carbonic acid for the receptor surface on the enzyme. (Fig. 13.3)

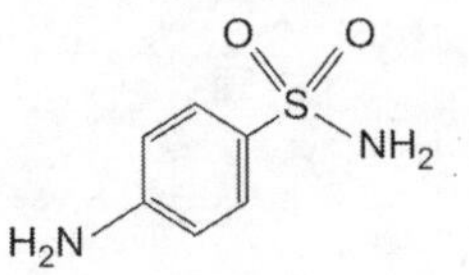

(22)

$$CO_2 + H_2O \xrightleftharpoons[\text{Carbonic anhydride}]{} H_2CO_3 \xrightleftharpoons{} H^+ + HCO_3^- \cdots\cdots (Eq\text{-}1)$$

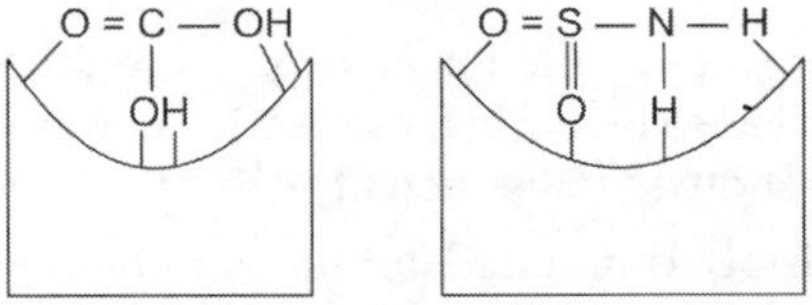

Fig. 13.3: Active site of carbonic anhydrase.

Aliphatic sulphonamides are less active as compared to heterocyclic sulphonamides. Of the various heterocyclic systems, 1,3,4-thiadiazoles were the most effective. One of the compounds in this series was acetazolamide (23), it was the most active compounds. Other compounds in the series include methazolamide (24) and ethoxzolamide (25). Among the aromatic sulphonamides, dichlorphenamide (26) was found to be an effective carbonic anhydrase inhibitor. Carbonic anhydrase inhibitors are also used in ophthalmology for reducing the intraocular pressure in glaucoma.

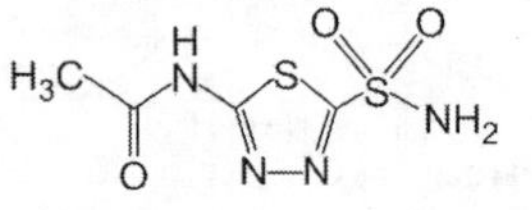

(23)

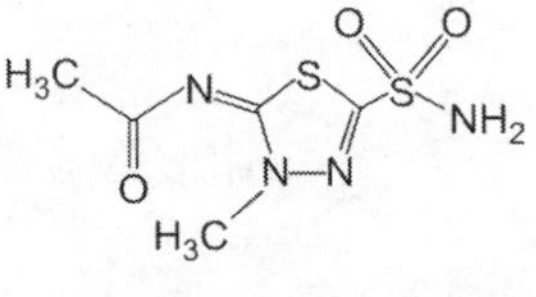

(24)

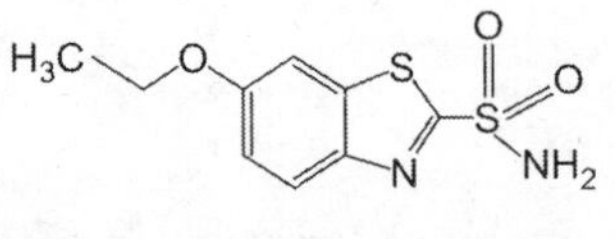

(25)

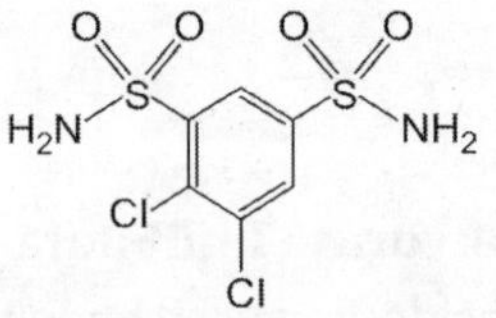

(26)

5-Sulphamoylanthranilic acid in which the amino group is substituted showed very high degree of diuretic activity. The most potent compound in this series was furosemide (27) containing furfuryl ring on amino nitrogen. Furosemide (27) is an orally effective loop diuretic. It acts on the thick segments of the ascending loop of Henle inhibiting $Na^+/K^+/2Cl^-$ carrier in the luminal membrane. This results in inhibition of reabsorption of $Na^+/K^+/Cl^-$ and their increased excretion.

Other sulphonamides which act in similar fashion as furosemide (27) include bumetanide (28), piretanide (29), torsemide (30), azosemide (31), and tripamide (32).

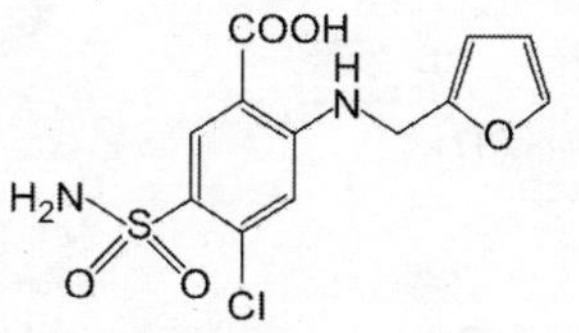

(27) 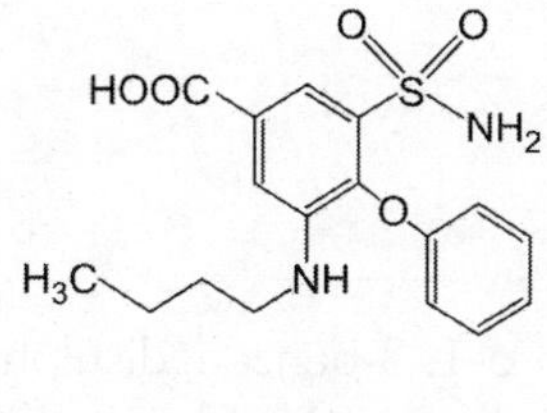   (28) 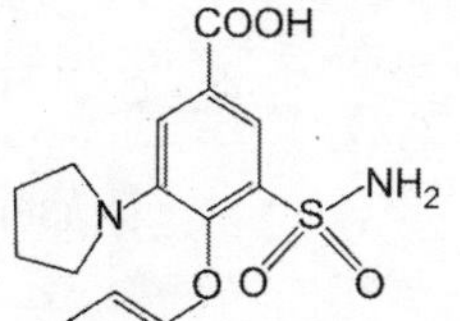   (29)

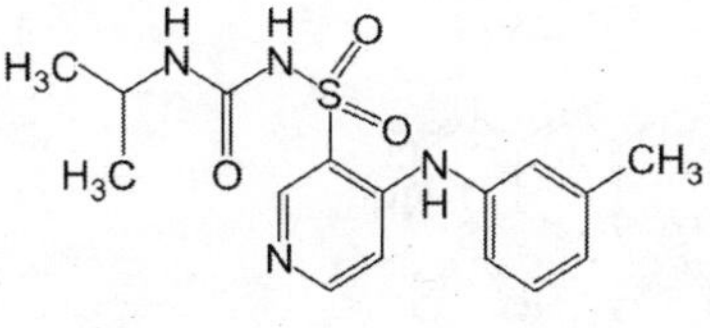

(30) 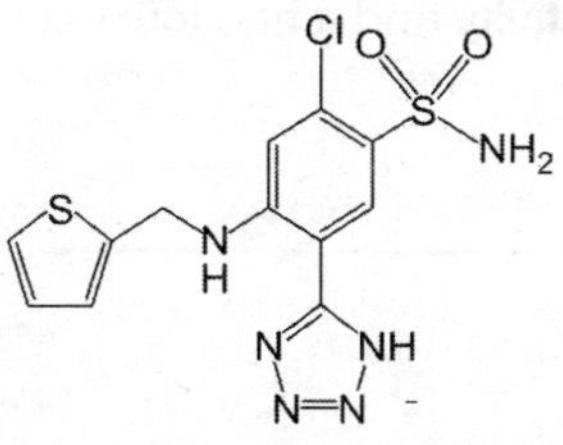   (31) 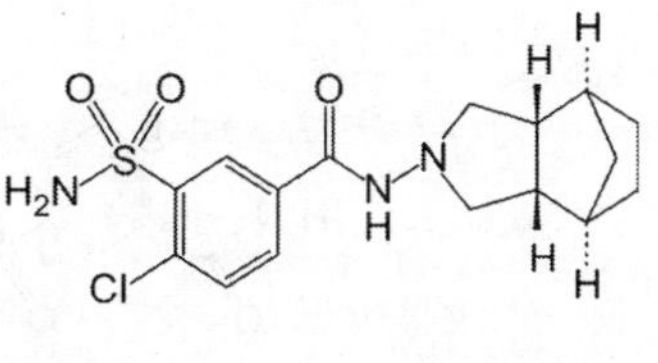   (32)

Benzophenones with a sulphonamide moiety have been found to possess diuretic activity. Optimum activity was observed in chlorthalidone (33) which is a tautomeric form of *ortho*-substituted benzophenone. Chlorthalidone (33) acts on distal convoluted tubule. It decreases reabsorption of Na$^+$ and Cl$^-$ by binding to the chloride site of Na$^+$/Cl$^-$ co-transport system and inhibiting it.

The other sulphonamides in this category include xipamide (34), indapamide (35), the quinazolin-4-one analogs, metolazone (36), and quinethazone (37). They act in same manner as chlorthalidone (33) by binding to Na$^+$/Cl$^-$ co-transport system and inhibiting the reabsorption of Na$^+$ and Cl$^-$ in distal convoluted tubule.

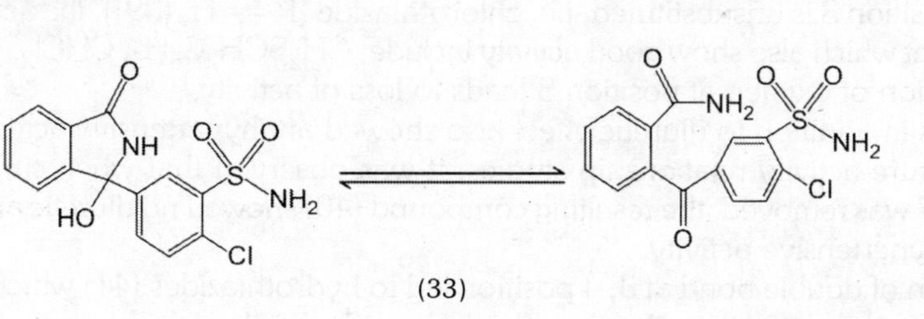

(33)

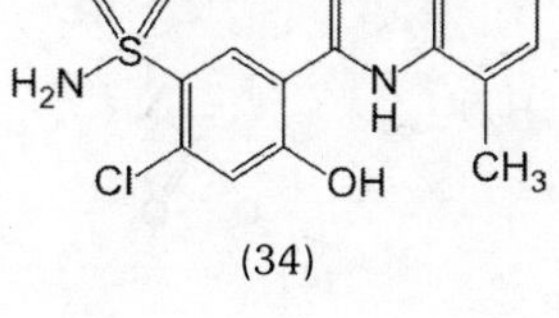

(34) 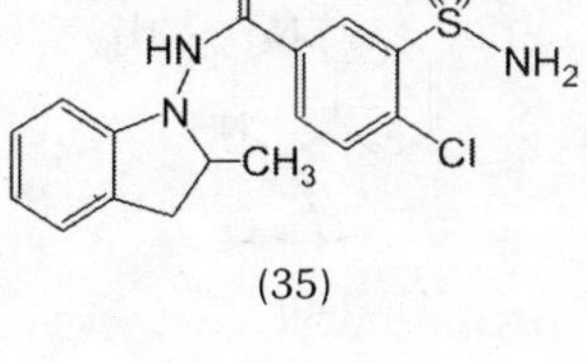   (35)

(36)

(37)

Thiazides and Hydrothiazides

While working on 4-acylamino-6-chloro-1, 3-benzenedisulphonamides (38), it was observed that when it was heated, it underwent cyclization readily to give (39). These compounds were designated as thiazides, and the parent compound where R = H (39) is known as chlorothiazide. When tested, it was found that it showed diuretic activity and it had low toxicity with favourable excretion pattern.

(38)   (39)

Structure-Activity Relationship Studies in Thiazides

1. Of the various substitutents at position 6, chlorine and bromine has the most favourable effect on activity.
2. The best position for the sulphamido group is 7, i.e. *meta* to sulphamido moiety which forms part of thiadiazine ring.
3. Sulphamido moiety at position 7 is essential for activity, its methyl or acyl derivatives lead to campounds which are either inactive or weakly active.
4. When position 3 is unsubstituted, i.e. chlorothiazide [R = H, (39)], the activity is high. Other substituent which also show good activity include, $CH_2SCH_2C_6H_5$, $CHCl_2$, cyclopentylmethyl. Introduction of oxygen at position 3 leads to loss of activity,
5. Thiazides in addition to diuretic effect also showed antihypertensive activity. While carrying out structure-activity relationship studies, it was observed that when sulphamido group at position 7 was removed, the resulting compound (40) showed no diuretic activity but retained the antihypertensive activity.
6. Reduction of double bond at 3, 4 position led to hydrothiazides (41) which were found to be 10 times more active than the parent compounds. Further, the reduction product had also weak carbonic anhydrase inhibiting activity.

(40)   (41)

Structure-Activity Relationship Studies in Hydrothiazide

1. Substituents at position 3 which had the most favourable effect on diuretic activity were, alkyl,cycloalkyl, haloalkyl and aralkyl groups.
2. Unlike thiazides, substitution at position 3 by an alkyl group resulted in better diuretic activity. The activity was maximum when the alkyl group was ethyl.
3. As regards the substitution in benzene nucleus, it followed the same pattern as in thiazides.

Some of the thiazides (39) used clinically include, chlorothiazide (39a) and benzthiazide (39b). The clinically useful hydrothiazides (41), include hydrochlorothiazide (41a), hydroflumethiazide (41b), trichlormethiazide (41c), cyclopenthiazide (41d), bendroflumethiazide (41e), methyclothiazide (41f), and polythiazide (41g).

(**a**), R = R$_1$ = H; R$_2$ = Cl
(**b**), R = R$_1$ = H; R$_2$ = CF$_3$
(**c**), R = H; R$_1$ = CHCl$_2$; R$_2$ = Cl

(**d**), R = H; R$_1$ = H$_2$C— ; R$_2$ = Cl

(**e**), R = H; R$_1$ = H$_2$C— ; R$_2$ = CF$_3$

(39)
(**a**), R = H
(**b**), R = H$_2$C

(41)

(**f**), R = CH$_3$; R$_1$ = CH$_2$Cl ; R$_2$ = Cl

(**g**), R = CH$_3$; R$_1$ = H$_2$C—S— CF$_3$; R$_2$ = Cl

Thiazides and hydrothiazides act on distal convoluted tubule by inhibiting Na$^+$/Cl$^-$ co-transport system, thus inhibiting the reabsorption of Na$^+$ and Cl$^-$. They also increase significantly the potassium loss which is because of high flow rate of filtrate produced by these agents.

ALDOSTERONE ANTAGONISTS AND INHIBITORS

Mineralocorticoids secreted by adrenal cortex are responsible for maintaining the water and mineral balance in the body. Aldosterone (42) is the most powerful mineralocorticoid and is responsible for reabsorption of Na$^+$ in distal convoluted tubule. It stimulates Na$^+$/H$^+$ exchanger by binding to aldosterone receptors in the membrane. Further, in the cells after binding to its receptors a specific protein is synthesized which activates the sodium channels. It is also believed to increase the number of basolateral sodium pumps.

The action of aldosterone (42) can be counteracted either by blocking its action on distal convoluted tubule or by inhibiting its synthesis. Either of these would result in diuresis through increased excretion of Na$^+$.

(42)

Aldosterone Antagonists

While working on aldosterone (42) antagonists, it was observed that steroidal spirolactones were specific aldosterone antagonists. The first of these compounds was 3-(3-oxo-17β-hydroxy-4-androsten-17α-yl) propionic acid lactone (43).

(43)   (44)

For maximum activity:

1. The 5-membered spirolactone ring at C-17 and the 3-keto-Δ^4-function in ring A was necessary.
2. The isomer with an inverted configuration at C-17 was inactive.
3. 19-Nor analogs of (43) were more active when given parenterally but not orally.
4. Activity could be increased by introduction of acetylthio group at position 7.

These studies resulted in the synthesis of spironolactone (44). Structure-activity relationships have shown that inversion of acetylthio group at position 7 leads to loss of activity. Other modifications including introduction of various groups such as alkyl, keto, hydroxyl at different positions, did not have any beneficial effect.

Mechanism of Action

Spironolactone (44) is metabolized to canrenone (45) and then to canrenoate (46). Canrenone (45) is the active form of spironolactone (44). It competes with aldosterone (42) for binding to intracellular aldosterone-receptors, thereby, inhibiting the action of aldosterone (42). This results in excretion of sodium and decrease in potassium excretion. Spironolactone (44) is effective only when sodium retention is due to excessive amounts of aldosterone (42). It is ineffective in patients with cirrhosis.

Use of spironolactone (44) with thiazides results in increased diuresis than when spironolactone (44) is used alone. Further, since thiazides increase and spironolactone (44) decreases the K$^+$ excretion, the administration of such a combination results in favourable electrolyte excretion pattern.

Eplerenone (47) is a new aldosterone-receptor antagonist. Its action and mechanism is similar to that of spironolactone (44).

(44) $\longrightarrow$

(45)   (46)   (47)

Aldosterone Inhibitors

Amphenone B (48) has been found to inhibit the enzymes responsible for 11β-, 17α-, and 21-hydroxylation. This results in inhibition of aldosterone (42) biosynthesis. Amphenone B (48) has also been found to inhibit the secretion of aldosterone (42). All these effects result in diuresis. However, it is not effective in adrenolactomized animals. Structure-activity relationships studies have shown that modification and shifting of amino group to other positions results in loss of activity. Similarly, increase in size of the methyl group to ethyl group also results in loss of activity.

(48)

Studies on desoxybenzoins (49) resulted in the synthesis of metyrapone (50). Metyrapone (50) inhibits 11β-hydroxylation resulting in inhibition of biosynthesis of hydrocortisone, corticosterone, and aldosterone (42). Lower blood levels of hydrocortisone result in stimulation of ACTH by the anterior pituitary. The net result is increase in secretion of 11-desoxyhydrocortisone and 11-desoxycorticosterone in large quantities. 11-Desoxycorticosterone is a potent salt retaining hormone. Thus, administration of metyrapone (50) elicits a compensatory mechanism which negates its diuretic effect. The diuretic effect can, however, be restored by preventing the secretion of 11-desoxycorticods. This can be achieved by suppressing ACTH release through administration of prednisone and dexamethasone. Metyrapone (50) is not used as a diuretic. It has found use as a diagnostic agent.

R = H, R' = NH₂
R = NH₂, R' = H
R = R' = NH₂

(49)

(50)

HIGH CEILING DIURETICS

High ceiling diuretics include ethacrynic acid (12), the sulphonamides furosemide (27), bumetanide (28), piretanide (29), torsemide (30), azosemide (31), and tripamide (32). Muzolimine (51), a pyrazolin-5-one analog is another of the high ceiling diuretics. These diuretics produce peak diuresis which is much greater than other diuretics. They inhibit $Na^+/K^+/2Cl^-$ carrier in the thick ascending loop of Henle.

(51)

POTASSIUM SPARING DIURETICS

Triamterene (19), amiloride (21), spironolactone (44), and eplerenone (47), constitute the potassium sparing diuretics. While triamterene (19) and amiloride (21) inhibit sodium channel in distal convoluted tubule, spironolactone (44), and eplerenone (47) act by inhibiting the action of aldosterone by binding to the aldosterone receptor.

INDIVIDUAL COMPOUNDS

PHENOXYACETIC ACIDS
Ethacrynic Acid
[2, 3-Dichloro-4-(2-ethylacryloyl)phenoxy]acetic acid

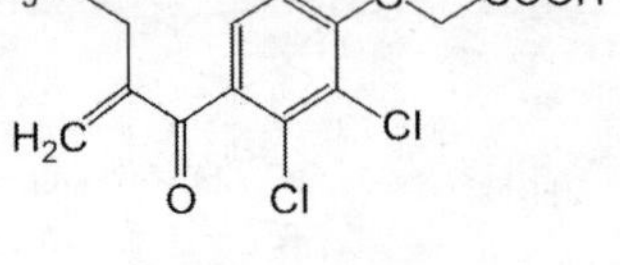

Synthesis

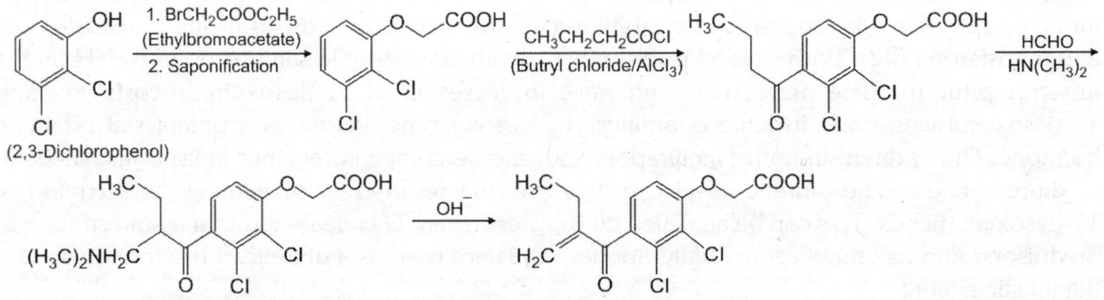

It is a high-ceiling diuretic. It acts on thick ascending limb of loop of Henie inhibiting $Na^+/K^+/2Cl^-$ carrier, thus preventing the reabsorption of Na^+, K^+, and Cl^- ions.

PURINES AND RELATED HETEROCYCLICS – PURINES
Caffeine, Theophylline, and Theobromine
See CENTRAL NERVOUS SYSTEM STIMULANTS

PURINES AND RELATED HETEROCYCLICS : PTERIDINES
Triamterene
2,4,7-Triamino-6-phenylpteridine

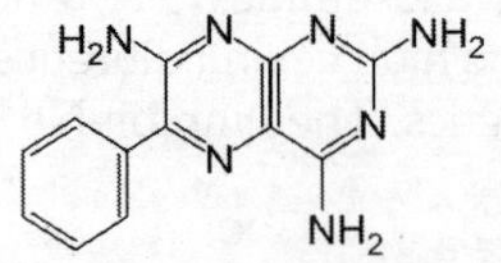

Synthesis

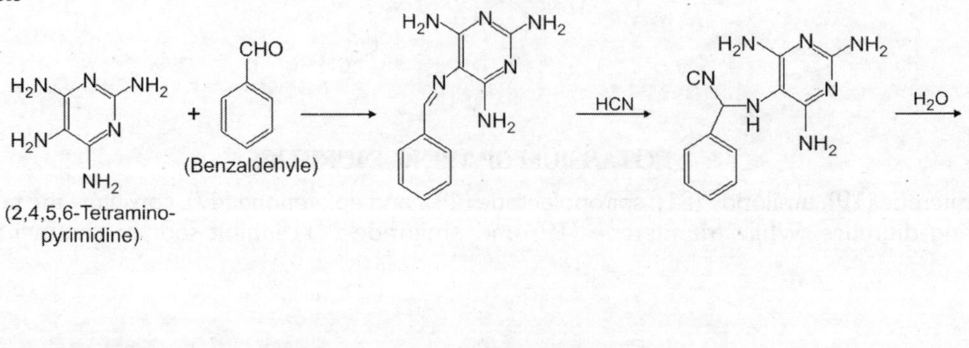

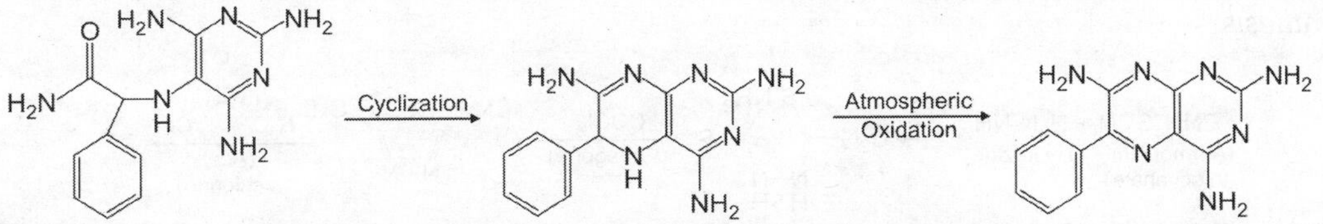

Triamterene is a potassium sparing diuretic which inhibits Na$^+$ channel thus preventing Na$^+$ reabsorption in distal convoluted tubule it is contraindicated in presence of renal diseases.

PURINES AND RELATED HETEROCYCLICS : PYRAZINES
Amiloride
N-Amidino-3,5-diamino-6-chloropyrazine-2-carboxamide

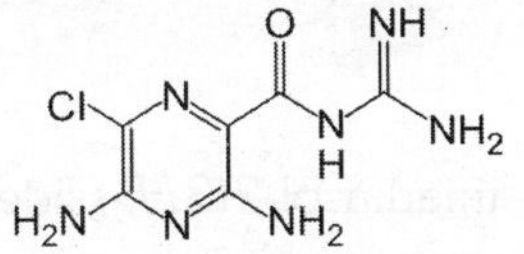

Synthesis

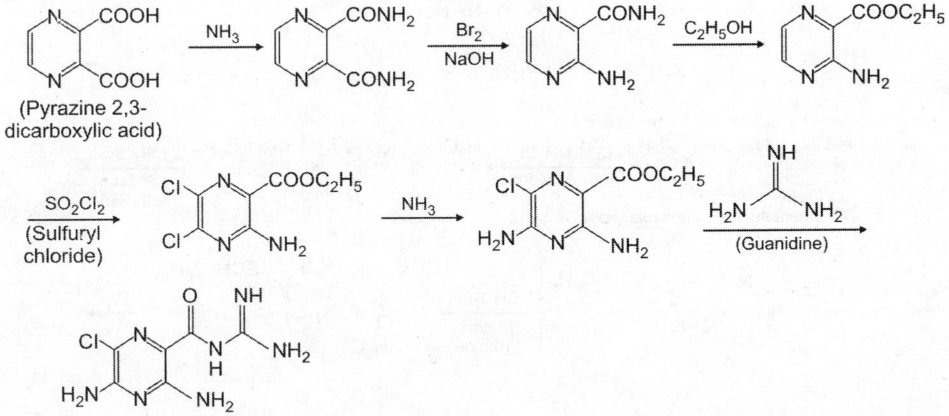

Amiloride is a long lasting K$^+$ sparing diuretic that potentiates the effect of thiazides. Like triamterene (19), it acts on distal convoluted tubule inhibiting sodium channel thereby inhibiting sodium reabsorption and consequent diuresis.

SULPHONAMIDES : CARBONIC ANHYDRASE INHIBITORS
Acetazolamide
2-Acetylamino-1,3,4-thiazdiazole-5-sulphonamide

Synthesis

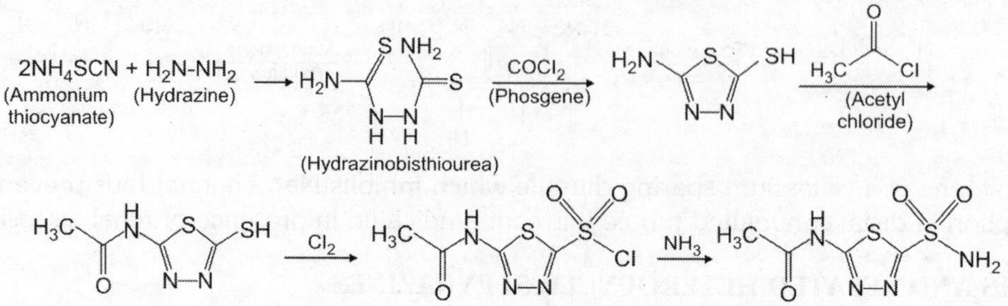

It inhibits carbonic anhydrase, an enzyme responsible for reversible hydration of carbon dioxide and thereby decreasing reabsorption of sodium bicarbonate. It causes systemic acidosis which may necessitate the interruption of the therapy. It is also used in glaucoma.

Methazolamide

N-[5-(Aminosufonyl)-3-methyl-1,3,4-thiadiazol-2(3*H*)-ylidene]acetamide

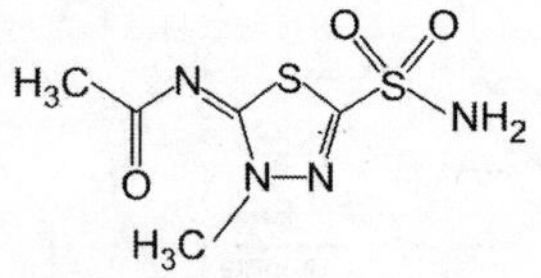

Synthesis

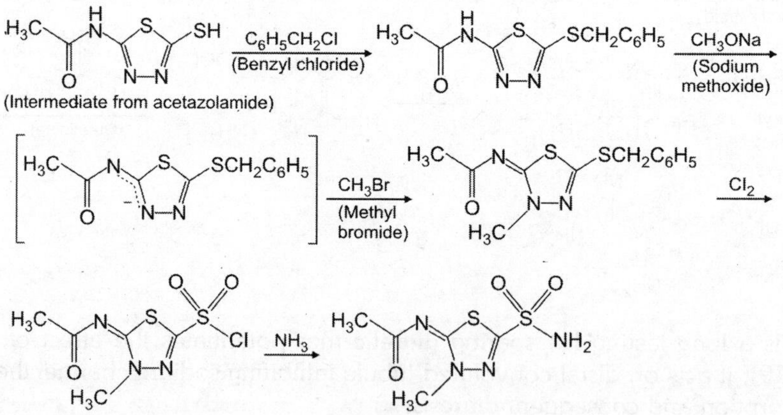

Similar activity and mechanism as acetazolamide (23).

Ethoxzolamide

6-Ethoxy-2-benzothiazolsulphonamide

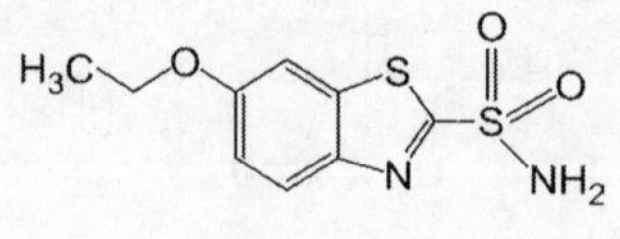

Synthesis

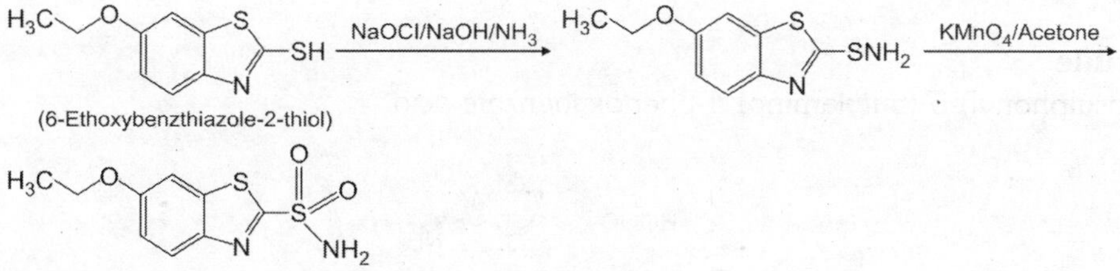

(6-Ethoxybenzthiazole-2-thiol)

Similar activity and mechanism as acetazolamide (23).

Dichlorphenamide

4,5-Dichloro-1,3-benzenedisulphonamide

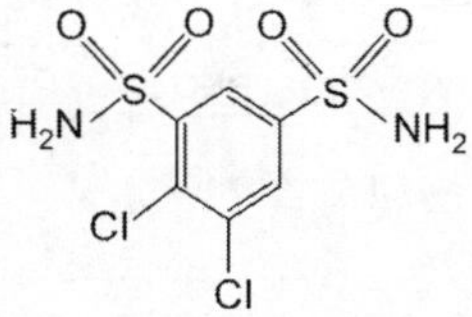

Synthesis

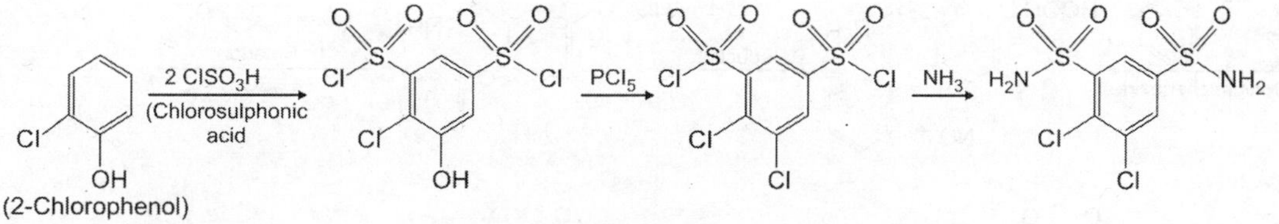

(2-Chlorophenol)

Like acetazolamide (23), it is an inhibitor of carbonic anhydrase.

Furosemide

4-Chloro-*N*-furfuryl-5-sulphamoylanthranilic acid

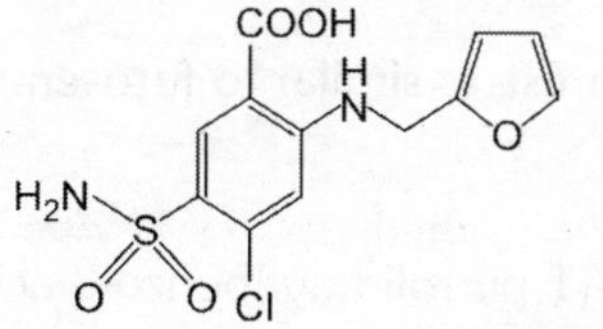

Synthesis

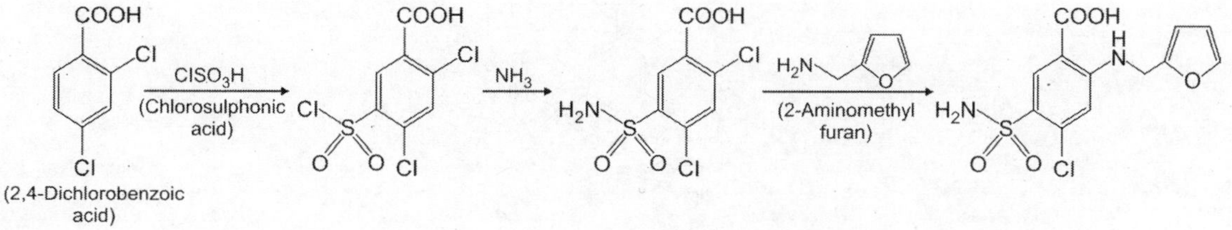

(2,4-Dichlorobenzoic acid)

Furosemide is also classified as high-ceiling loop diuretic. It increases excrection of Na^+, K^+ and Cl^- by the same mechanism as ethacrynic acid (12).

Bumetanide

3-(Aminosulphonyl)-5-(butylamino)-4-phenoxybenzoic acid.

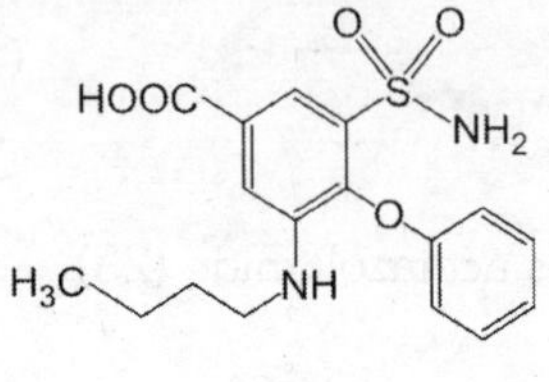

Synthesis

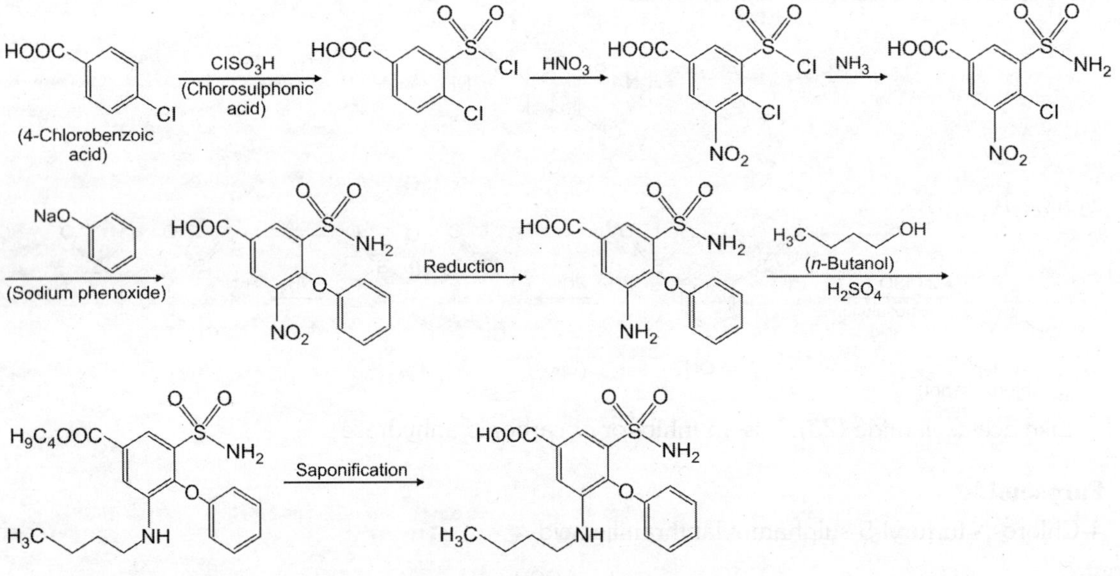

Its action and mechanism of diuresis is similar to furosemide (27).

Piretanide

3-(Aminosulphonyl)-4-phenoxy-5-(1-pyrrolidinyl)benzoic acid

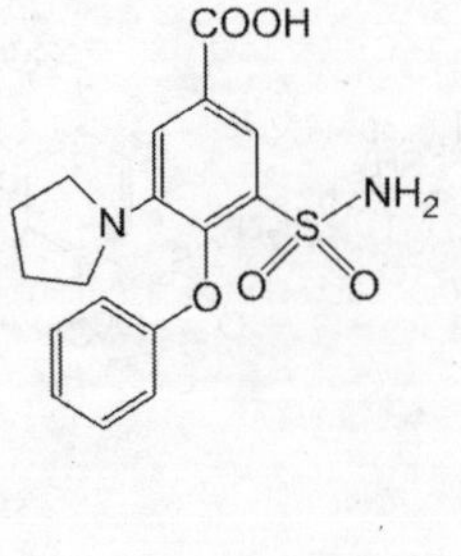

Synthesis

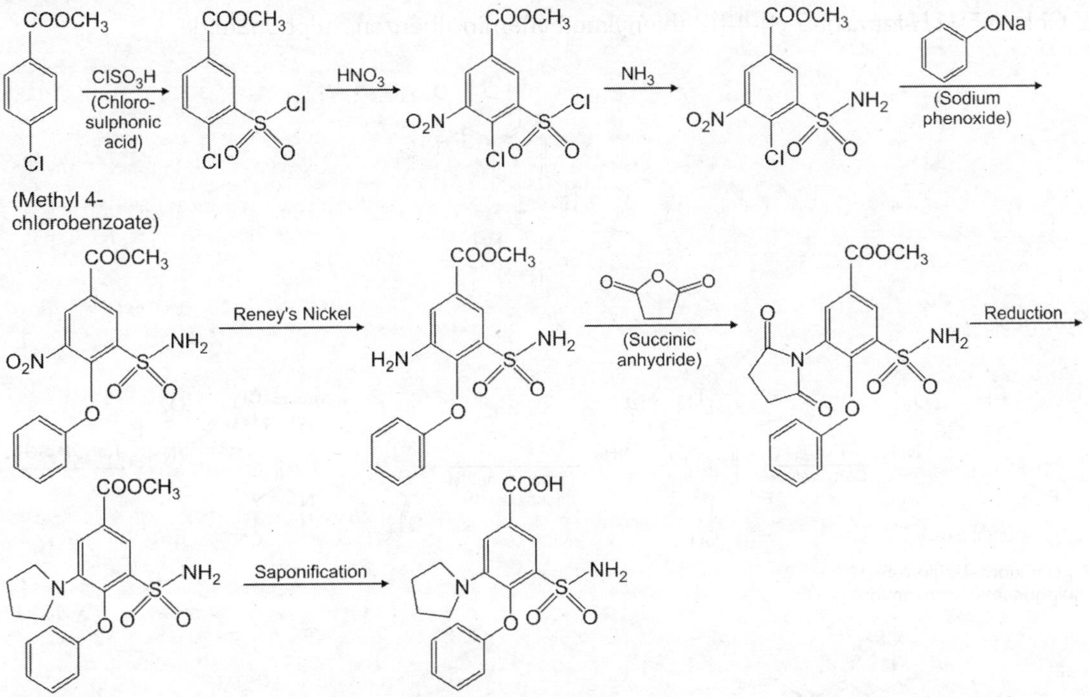

(Methyl 4-
chlorobenzoate)

It is also a high ceiling loop diuretic like furosemide (27) and bumetamide (28) and acts in similar fashion.

Torsemide

3-Isopropylcarbamylsuphonamido-4-(3'-methylphenyl) aminopyridine

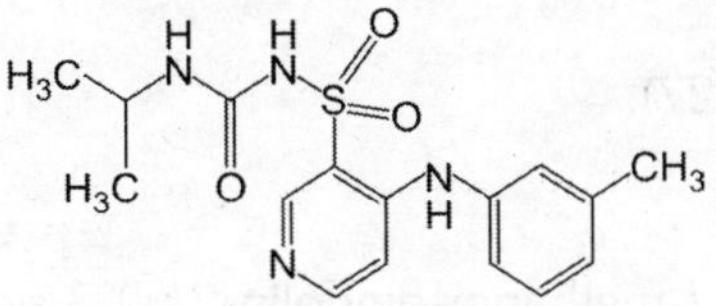

Synthesis

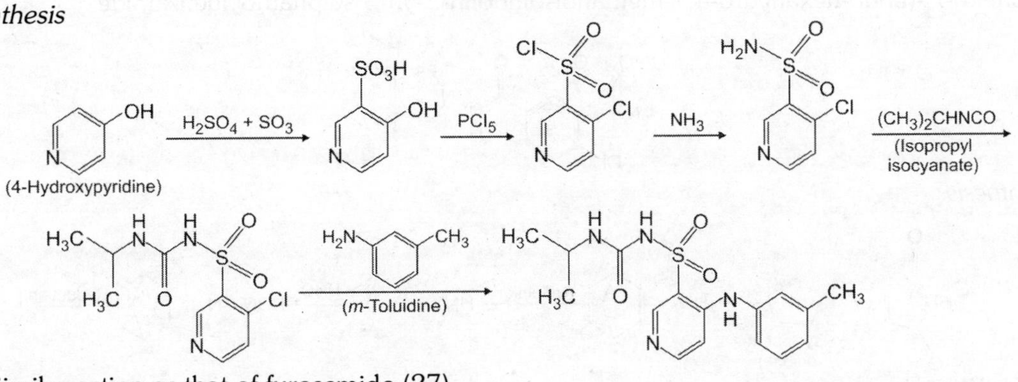

(4-Hydroxypyridine)

Similar action as that of furosemide (27).

Azosemide

2-Chloro-5-(1*H*-tetrazol-5-yl)-4-[(2-thienylmethyl)amino]benzenesulphonamide

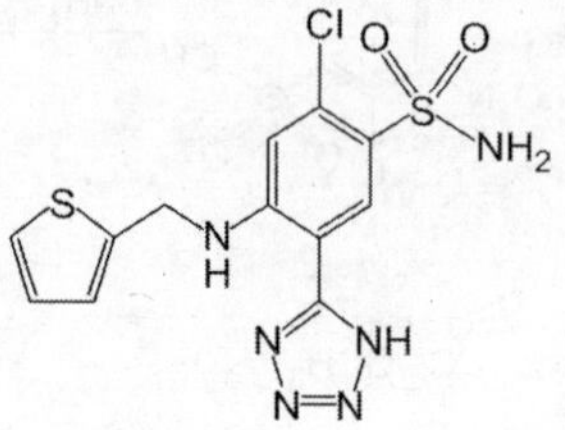

Synthesis

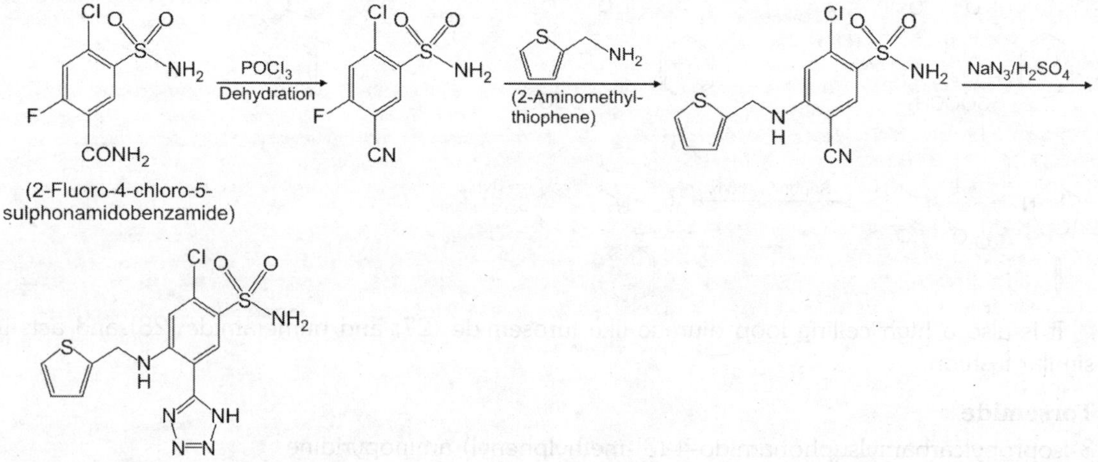

(2-Fluoro-4-chloro-5-sulphonamidobenzamide)

(2-Aminomethyl-thiophene)

Same activity as furosemide (27).

Tripamide

4-Chloro-*N*-(*endo*-hexahydro-4,7-methanoisoindolin-2-yl)-3-sulphamoylbenzamide

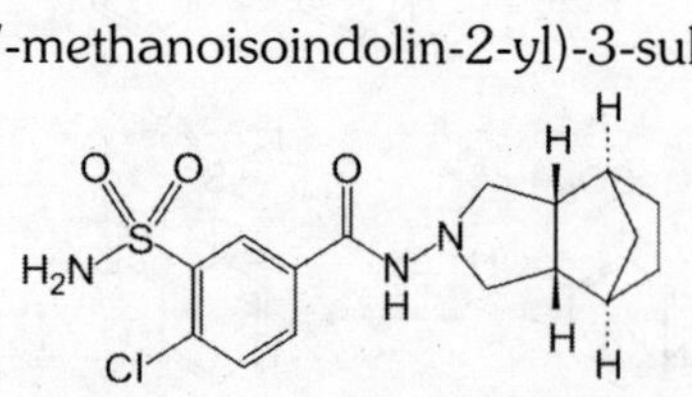

Synthesis

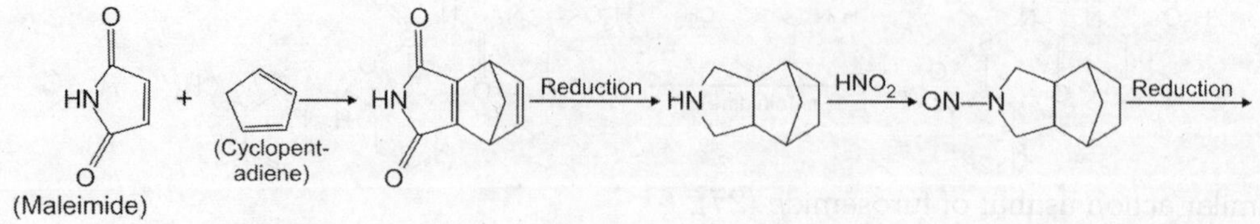

(Maleimide)

(Cyclopent-adiene)

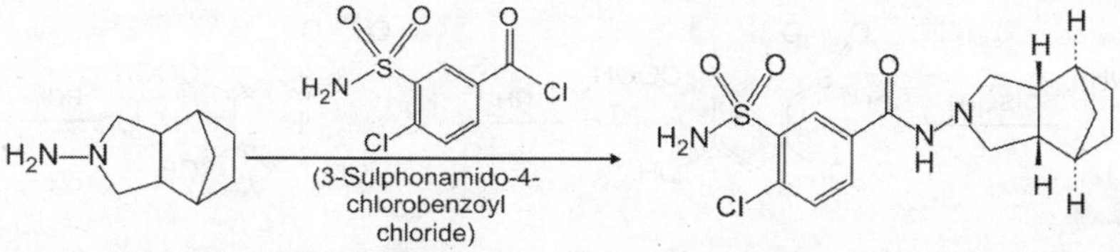

Same activity as furosemide (27).

Chlorthalidone

2-Chloro-5-(3-hydroxy-1-oxoisoindolin-3yl)benzenesulphonamide

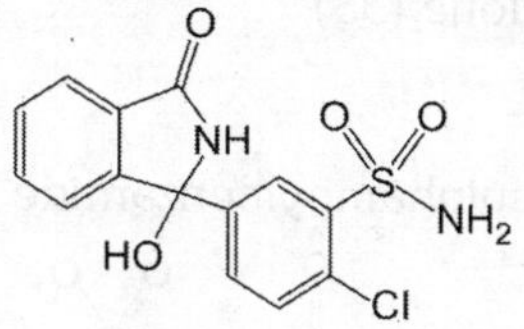

Synthesis

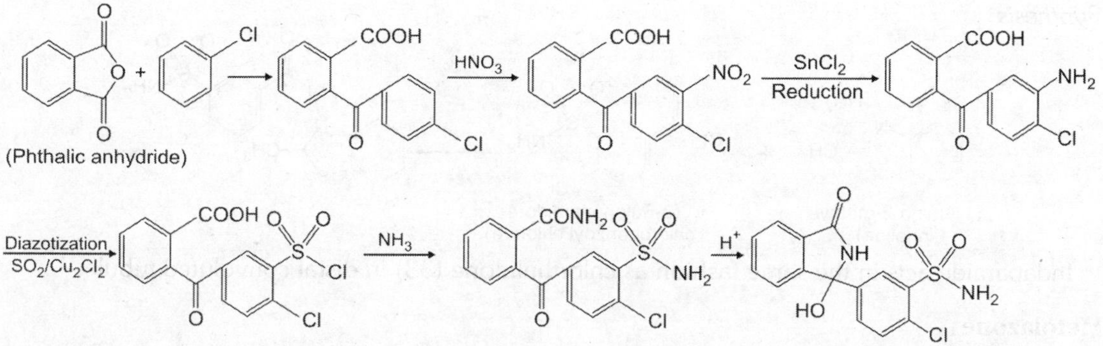

(Phthalic anhydride)

It is a potent, long acting diuretic, and antihypertensive agent. It acts on distal convoluted tubule.

Xipamide

4-Chloro-5-sulphamoyl-2', 6'-salicyloxylidide

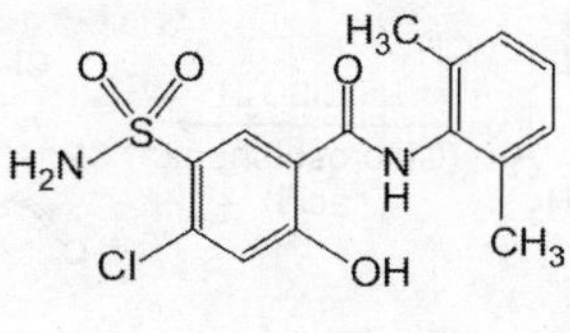

Synthesis

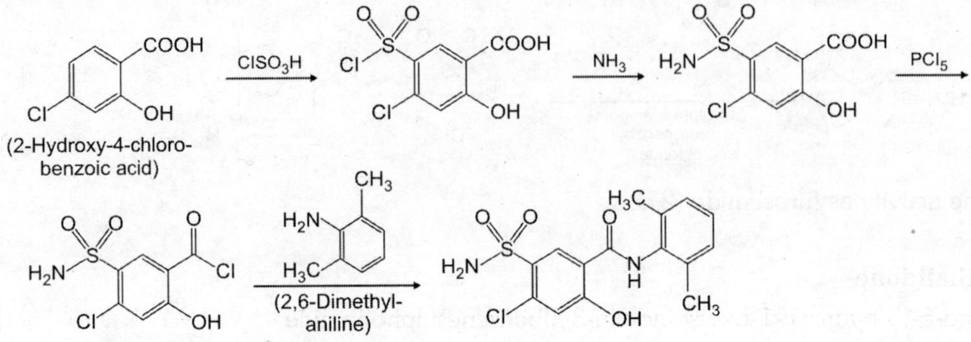

It has a similar aciton as chlorthalidone (33).

Indapamide

4-Chloro-*N*-(2-methyl-1-indolinyl)-3-sulphamoylbenzamide

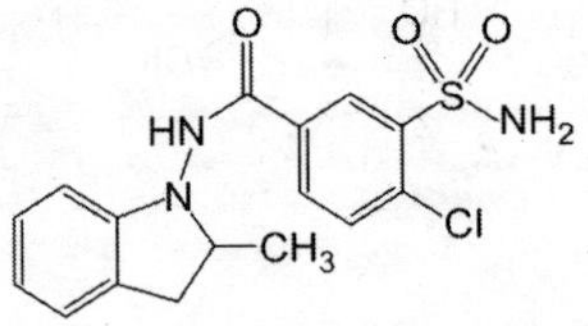

Synthesis

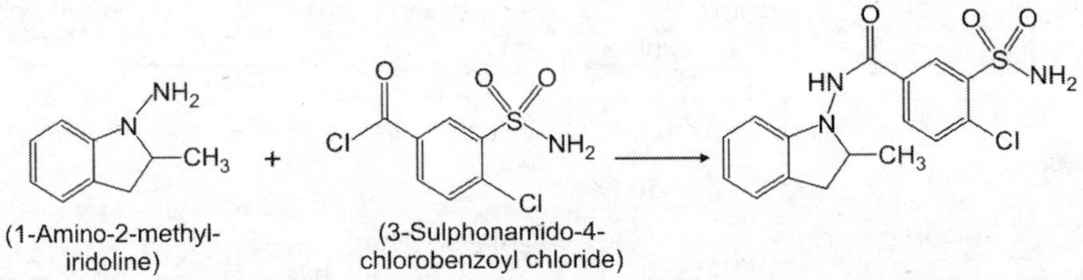

Indapamide acts in the same fashion as chlorthalidone (33) in distal convoluted tubule.

Metolazone

7-Chloro-1,2,3,4-tetrahydro-2-methyl-3-(2-methylphenyl)-4-oxo-6-quinazolinesulphonamide

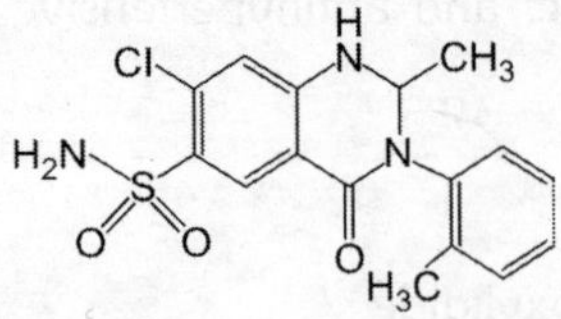

Synthesis

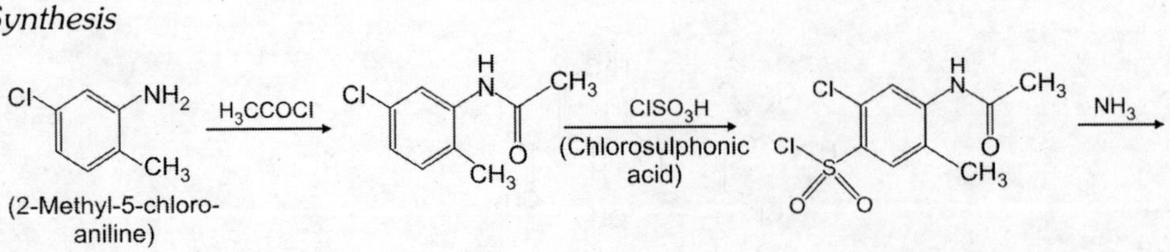

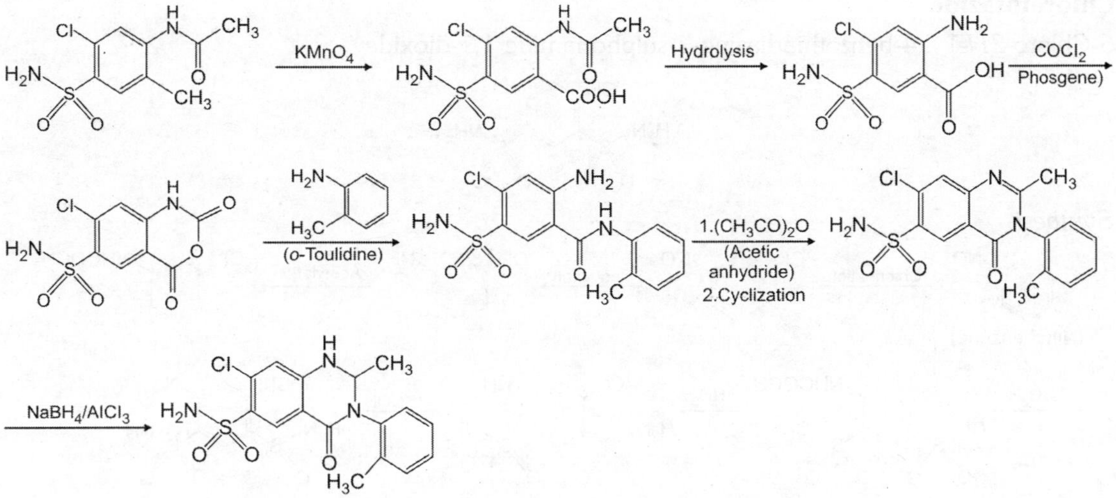

Metolazone acts in the same fashion as chlorthalidone (33) inhibiting the Na$^+$ reabsorption in distal convoluted tubule.

Quinethazone

7-Chloro-2-ethyl-1,2,3,4-tetrahydro-4-oxo-6-quinazolinesulphonamide

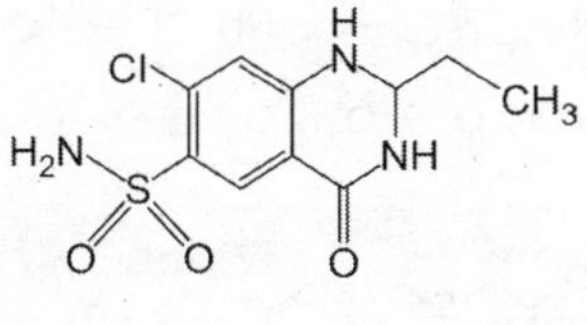

Synthesis

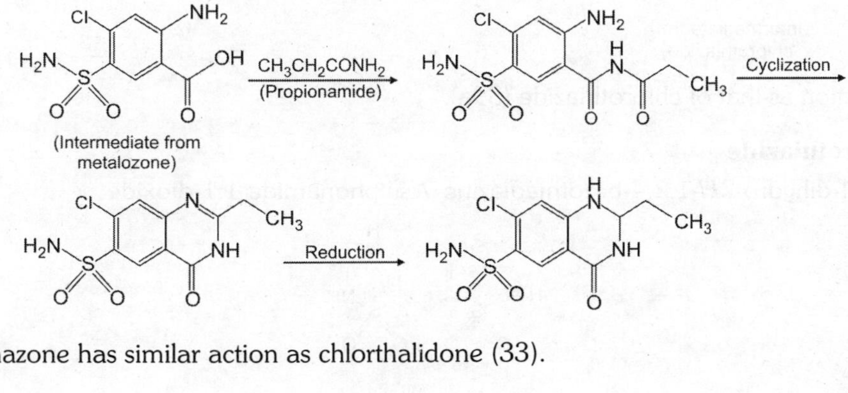

(Intermediate from metalozone)

Quinethazone has similar action as chlorthalidone (33).

SULPHONAMIDES : THIAZIDES AND HYDROTHIAZIDES

Chlorothiazide

6-Chloro-2H-1,2,4-benzothiadiazine-7-sulphonamide 1,1-dioxide

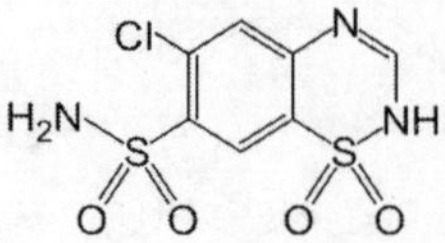

Synthesis

(Nitrobenzene)

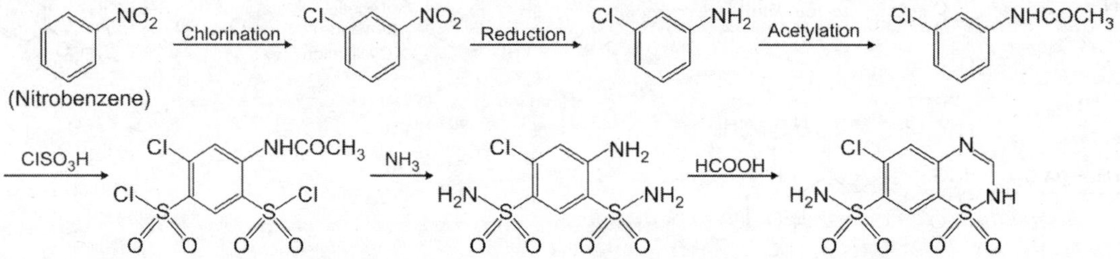

It is a potent diuretic and is used in all types of edema. It causes significant loss of K^+. It acts on distal convoluted tubule inhibiting Na^+/Cl^- co-transport system which results in inhibition of reabsorption of Na^+ and Cl^-. The high K^+ loss is because of high flow rate of filtrate.

Benzthiazide

6-Chloro-3-[[(phenylmethyl)thio]methyl]-2H-1,2,4-benzothiadiazine-7-sulphonamide 1, 1-dioxide

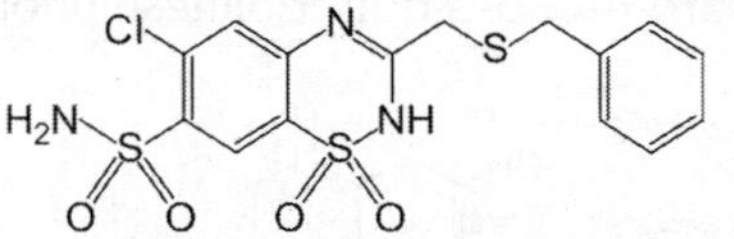

Synthesis

(Intermediate from
chlorothiazide)

(Benzyl mercaptoacetic
acid)

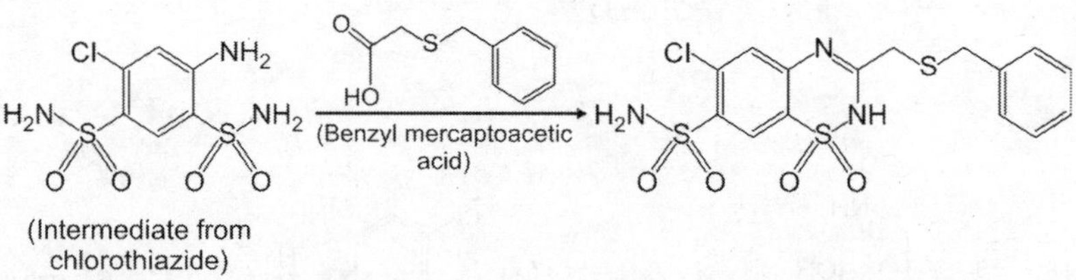

Similar action as that of chlorothiazide (39a).

Hydrochlorothiazide

6-Chloro-3,4-dihydro-2H-1,2,4-bezothiadiazine-7-sulphonamide 1,1-dioxide

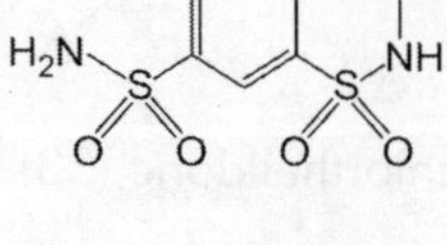

Synthesis

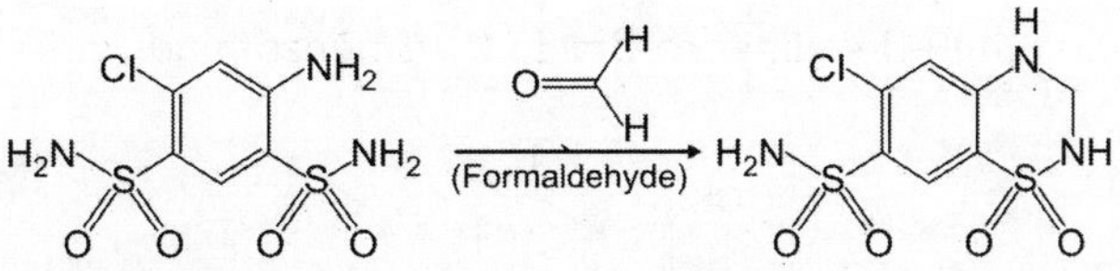

(Intermediate from
chlorothiazide)

It is more potent than chlorothiazide (39a). Mechanism of action is same as that of chlorothiazide (39a).

Hydroflumethiazide

3,4-Dihydro-6-(trifluoromethyl)-2H-1,2,4-benzothiadiazine-7-sulphonamide 1,1, dioxide

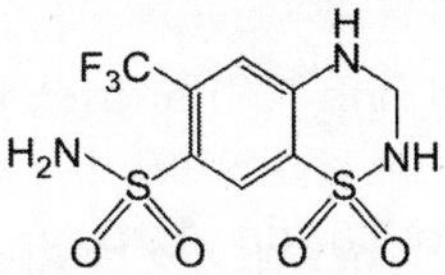

Synthesis

(Trifluoromethylbenzene)

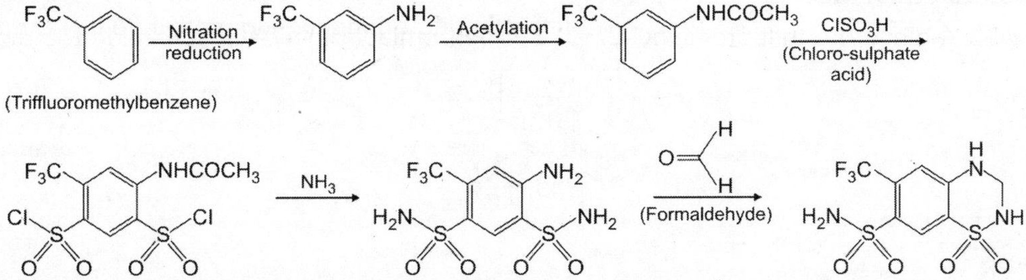

The activity, the excretion pattern, and the mechanism of action are similar to that of hydrochlorothiazide (41a).

Trichlormethiazide

6-Chloro-3-(dichloromethyl)-3, 4-dihydro-2H-1, 2, 4-benzothiadiazine-7-sulphonamide 1, 1-dioxide

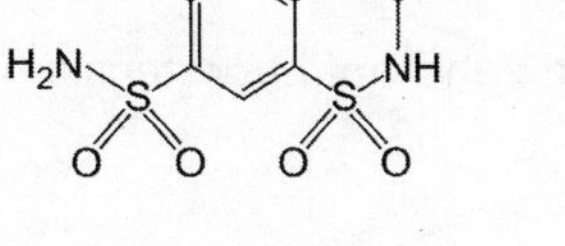

Synthesis

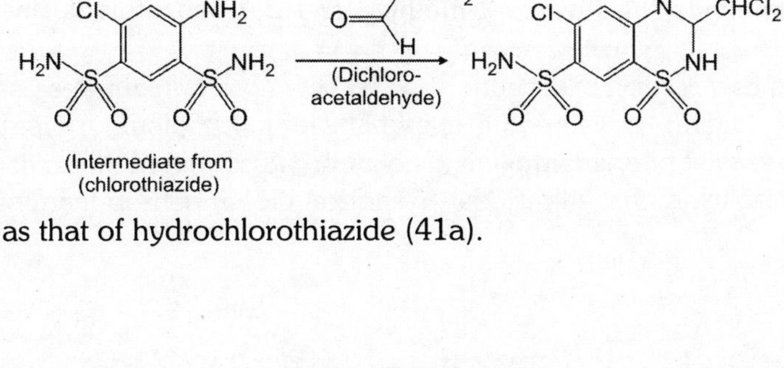

(Intermediate from
(chlorothiazide)

Similar activity as that of hydrochlorothiazide (41a).

Cyclopenthiazide

6-Chloro-3-(cyclopentylmethyl)-3-4-dihydro-2H-1, 2, 4-benzothiadiazine-7-sulphonamide 1, 1-dioxide

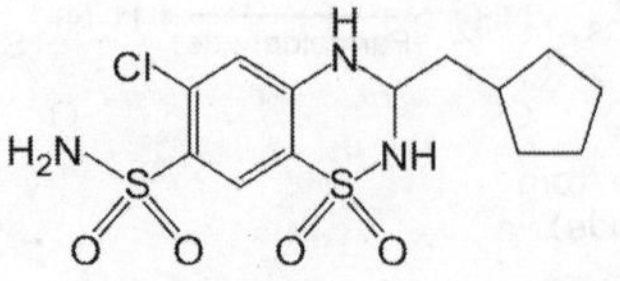

Synthesis

(Intermediate from chlorothiazide)

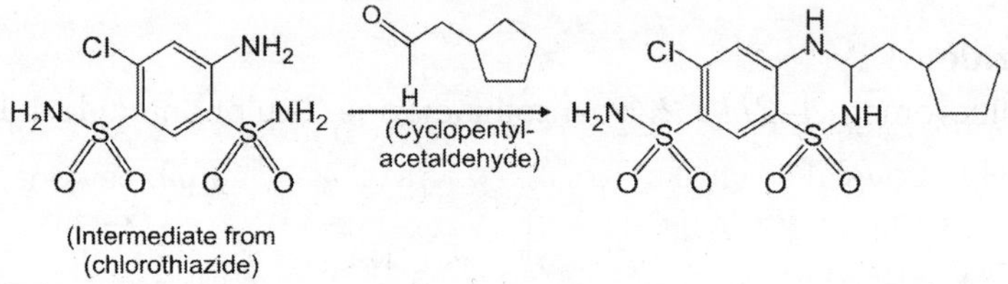

Similar activity as that of hydrochlorothiazide (41a).

Bendroflumethiazide

3-Benzyl-3, 4-dihydro-6-trifluoromethyl-2H-1, 2, 4-benzothiadiazine-7-sulphonamide 1, 1-dioxide.

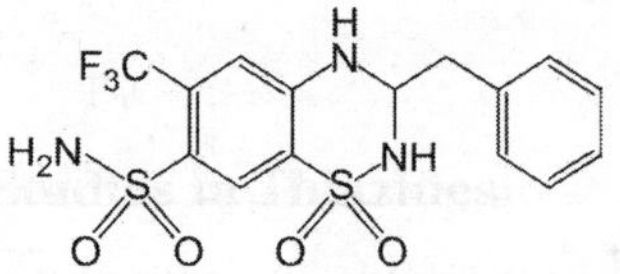

Synthesis

(Intermediate from hydroflumethiazide)

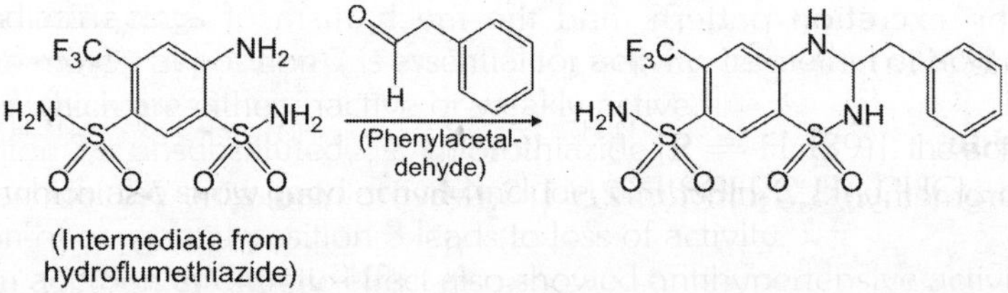

It is one of the most potent diuretic and antihypertensive agent mechanism of action same as chlorothiazide (39a).

Methyclothiazide

6-Chloro-3-(chloromethyl)-3,4-dihydro-2-methyl-2H-1,2,4-benzothiadiazine-7-sulphonamide 1, 1-dioxide

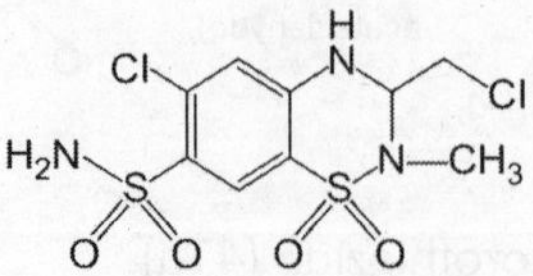

Synthesis

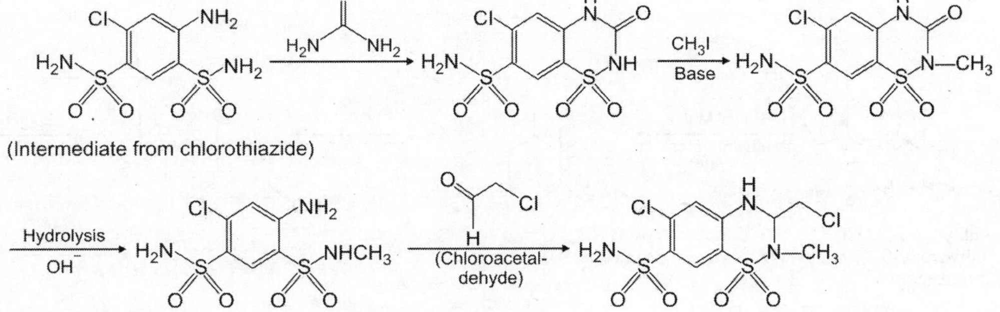

(Intermediate from chlorothiazide)

(Chloroacetal-dehyde)

Similar action as that of hydrochlorothiazide (41a).

Polythiazide

6-Chloro-3, 4-dihydro-2-methyl-3-[[(2, 2, 2-trifluoroethyl) thio]methyl]-2*H*-1, 2, 4-benzothiadiazine-7-sulphonamide 1, 1-dioxide

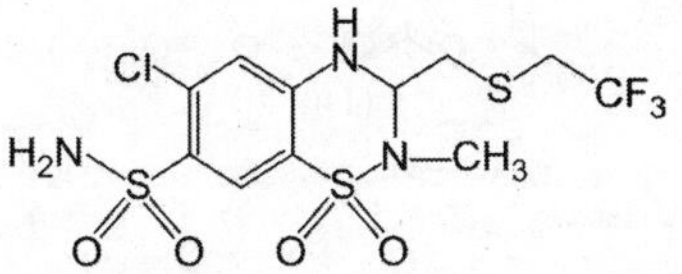

Synthesis

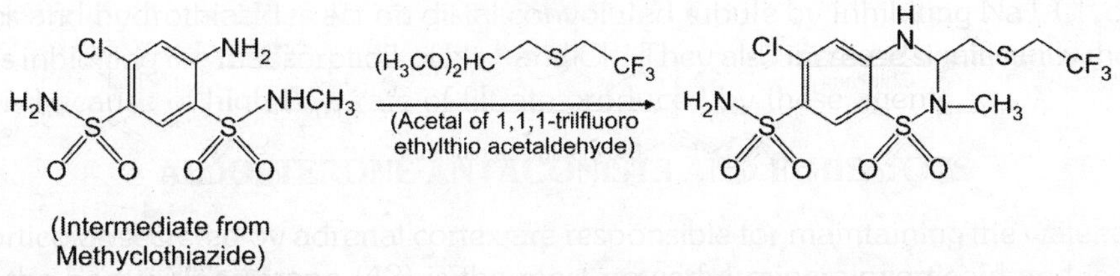

(Intermediate from Methyclothiazide)

(Acetal of 1,1,1-triflouro ethylthio acetaldehyde)

It has a lesser effect on K^+ excretion as compared to other thiazides and hydrothiazides. and possesses longer duration of action.

ALDOSTERONE ANTAGONISTS

Spironolactone

7α-(Acetylthio)-17β-hydroxy-3-oxopregn-4-ene-21-carboxylic acid, γ-lactone

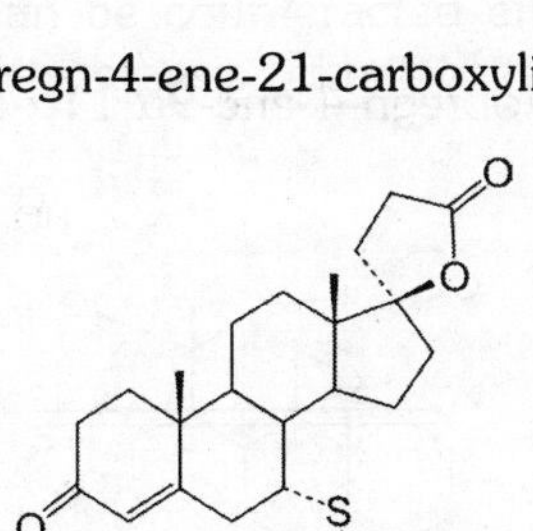

Synthesis

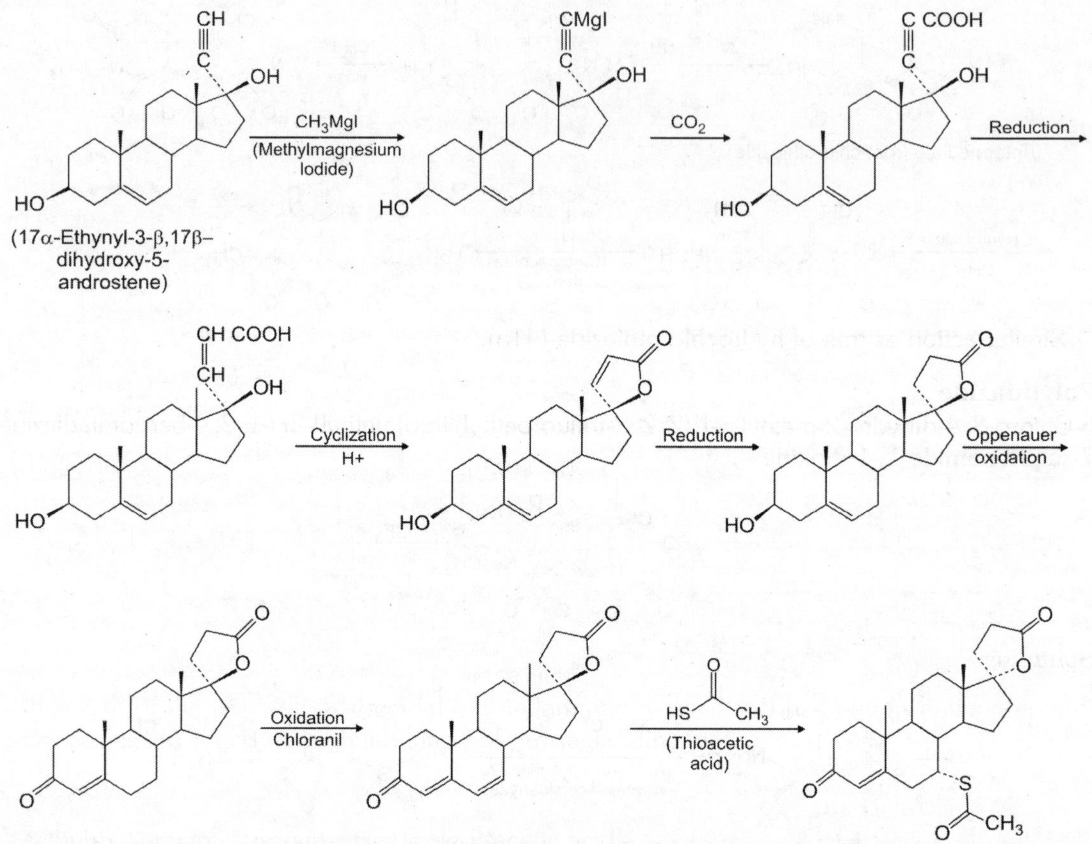

(17α-Ethynyl-3-β,17β–
dihydroxy-5-
androstene)

It is a potassium sparing diuretic. It competes with aldosterone (42) for binding to intracellular aldosterone receptors. This results in inhibition of Na^+ retention property of aldosterone (42) and decrease in K^+ excretion. It is effective when sodium retention is due to excessive-aldosterone and is effective in patients with cirrhosis.

Eplerenone

7α-Carbomethoxy-17β-hydroxy-3-oxopregn-4-ene-9α,11α-epoxide-21-carboxylic acid, γ-lactone

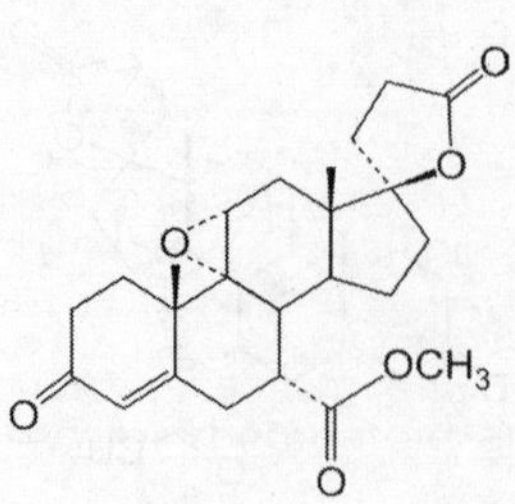

Synthesis

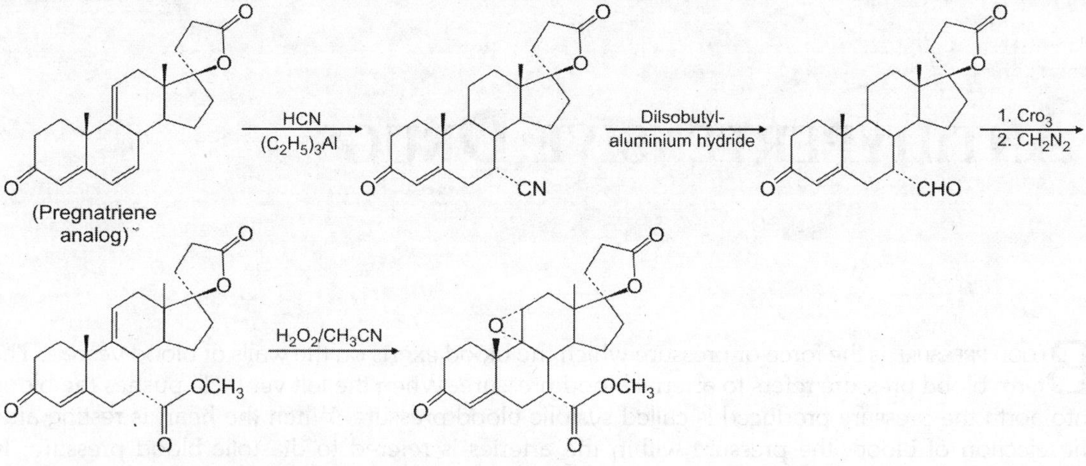

(Pregnatriene analog)

HCN / $(C_2H_5)_3Al$

Diisobutyl-aluminium hydride

1. Cro$_3$ 2. CH_2N_2

CHO

OCH$_3$

H_2O_2/CH_3CN

OCH$_3$

It has similar activity as spironolactone (44).

HIGH CEILING DIURETICS

PYRAZOLINES
Muzolimine

3-Amino-1-(3,4-dichloro-α-methylbenzyl)-2-pyrazolin-5-one

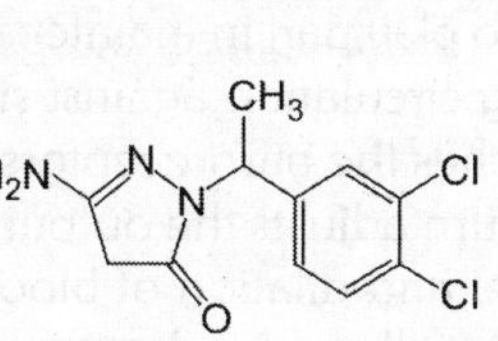

Synthesis

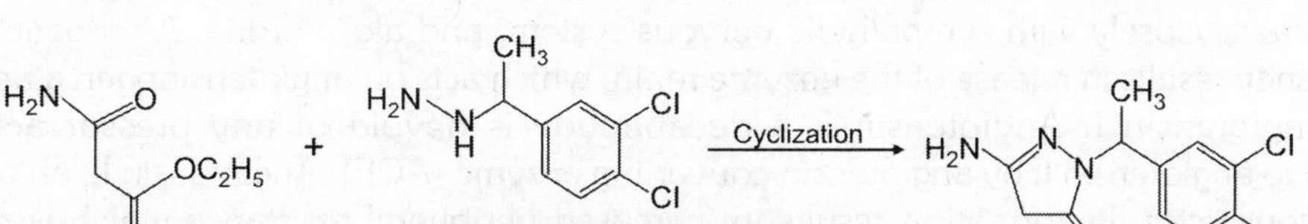

(Malonylester halfamide)

+

(Substituted phenylhydrazine analog)

Cyclization

It is a high ceiling diuretic.

CHAPTER 14

ANTIHYPERTENSIVE DRUGS

BLOOD PRESSURE is the force or pressure which the blood exerts on the walls of blood vessels. The term blood pressure refers to arterial blood pressure. When the left ventricle pushes the blood into aorta the pressure produced is called systolic blood pressure. When the heart is resting after the ejection of blood, the pressure within the arteries is refered to diastolic blood pressure. In adults, systolic blood pressure is usually 120 mm Hg and the diastolic 80 mm Hg. However, it varies according to age. According to WHO, hypertension is a state in which systolic blood pressure is 150 mm Hg and above and the diastolic 95 mm Hg or more.

Hypertension has been divided into two major divisions according to etiology. Primary or essential hypertension in which the cause of increase in blood pressure is not known and secondary hypertension in which the cause is known. Thus, secondary hypertension may originate from pathological states in CNS, tumor of medulla, renal, and endocrine glands.

Blood pressure is the function of cardiac output and the peripheral vascular resistance. The peripheral vascular resistance is exerted at arterioles, post-capillary venules, and heart. In addition to these, baroreceptors and kidney also play part in maintenance of the blood pressure. Baroreceptor reflexes are responsible for protecting circulation against stress. When one stands up from a lying position a rise in blood pressure stretches the baroreceptors increasing their input to cardiovasuclar centre. The cardiovascular centre in turn adjusts the output to the heart and blood vessels, through decrease in stroke volume, heart rate, and dilation of blood vessels. The net result is fall in blood pressure. Conversely, the tendency to fall in blood pressure is prevented by increased heart rate and peripheral resistance.

Kidney contributes to the maintenance of blood pressure by regulating the volume of intravascular fluid. The humoral system, which operates through kidney, involves renin-angiotensin system, which interacts closely with sympathetic nervous system, and aldosterone. A reduction in blood flow to kidney results in release of the enzyme renin, which acts on angiotensinogen a polypeptide, to give angiotensin I. Angiotensin I, a decapeptide is devoid of any pressor activity. It is converted to angiotensin II by angiotensin converting enzyme (ACE). Angiotensin II, an octapeptide is a vasoconstrictor. Its formation results in increased peripheral resistance which is responsible for increased blood pressure. Angiotensin II is converted to angiotensin III, a heptapeptide, which stimulates the aldosterone secretion. Aldosterone secretion results in retention of sodium and water. This in turn increases the cardiac output resulting in increased blood pressure (Fig. 14.1).

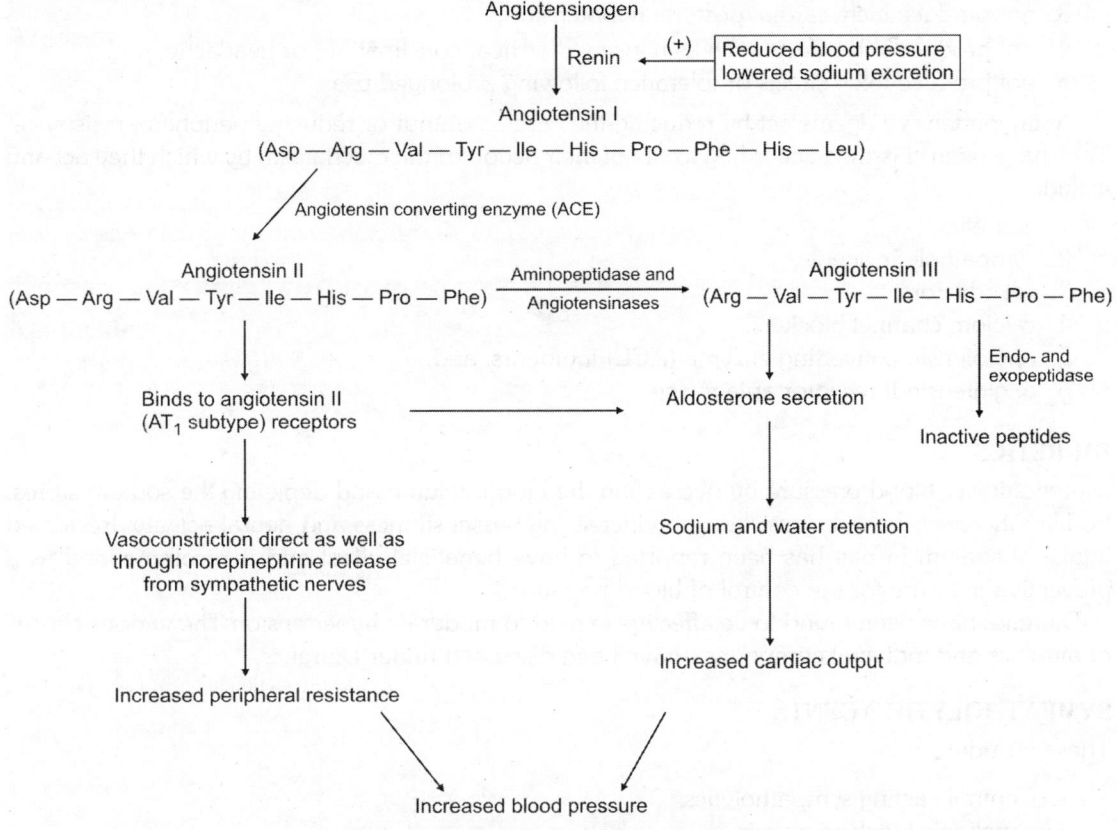

Fig. 14.1: Renin–Angiotensin system.

The antidiuretic hormone, vasopressin, is produced by hypothalamus. Release of hormone is controlled by osmoreceptors. An increase in osmolality stimulates vasopressin release. It facilitates reabsorption of water in distal tubule and thus is involved in control of blood pressure.

The increased blood pressure by renin-angiotensin system is counteracted by release of vasodilators such as "Kinins". Kallikrein acts on kininogen converting it into bradykinin, which is responsible for the release of prostaglandin E_2 (PGE_2) and prostacyclin which have a vasodilatory effect.

Atrial natriuretic peptide, ANP, is released by atria and antagonises the action of various vasoconstrictor agents thus lowering the blood pressure. However, its exact role is not known, apparently it affects Na^+ excretion.

Hypertension if left untreated can lead to various cardiac, cerebrovascular and renal complication, which may result in shortening of life.

ANTIHYPERTENSIVE DRUGS

An ideal antihypertensive drug should:

1. Lower the blood pressure gradually and equally in all body positions,
2. produce lower capillary resistance without lowering the cardiac output,

3. not produce tachycardia, postural hypotension,
4. not produce side effects such as nausea, diarrhea, constipation, or headache, and
5. not produce toxic effects or tolerance following prolonged use.

Antihypertensive agents act by reducing the cardiac output or reducing peripheral resistance. They have been classified according to site of their action or the mechanism by which they act and include:

1. Diuretics,
2. sympatholytic agents,
3. vasodilators,
4. calcium channel blockers,
5. angiotensin converting enzyme (ACE) inhibitors, and
6. angiotensin II receptor antagonists.

DIURETICS

Diuretics lower blood pressure by decreasing the blood volume and depleting the sodium stores. Sodium increases vascular resistance by increasing vessel stiffness and neural activity. Restricted intake of sodium in diet has been reported to have beneficial effect and is recommended as a preventive measure for the control of blood pressure.

Diuretics have been found to be effective in mild to moderate hypertension. The various classes of diuretics and indiviual compounds have been discussed under Diuretics.

SYMPATHOLYTIC AGENTS

These include:

1. Centrally acting sympatholytics,
2. ganglionic blocking agents,
3. drugs affecting noradrenergic neurons, and
4. adrenergic receptor blockers.

Centrally Acting Sympatholytics

Centrally acting sympatholytics agents include metyrosine (1) methyldopa (2), clonidine (3), guanabenz (4), and guanfacine (5).

(1)   (2)   (3)

(4)   (5)

Metyrosine (1) is a competitive inhibitor of tyrosine hydroxylase, an enzyme responsible for conversion of tyrosine (6) to dopa (7) in the biosynthesis of norepinephrine (8). Inhibiton of tyrosine hydroxylase results in blockade of biosynthesis of norepinephrine (8) (See Adernergic drugs). Metyrosine (1) is useful in controlling the blood pressure in pheochromocytoma but not for tretment of essential hypertension.

(6)   (7)   (8)

Methyldopa (2) is an analog of dopa (7). After being transported to CNS by an amino acid transport mechanism, it is converted to α-methylnorepinephrine (10) via α-methyldopamine (9).

α-Methylnorepinephrine (10) is an α_2-adrenergic receptor agonist. Binding of α-methylnor-epinephrine (10) to α_2-adrenegic receptors leads to decrease in peripheral resistance which results in hypotensive effect. Reduction in plasma renin activity has also been reported to contribute to the antihypertensive action of methyldopa (2). Methyldopa (2) is unstable in alkaline medium. For parentral formulations, hydrochloride of its ethyl ester, methyldopate (11) is used.

(9)   (10)

(11)

Clonidine (3), guanabenz (4) and guanfacine (5), the α_2-adrenergic agonists, act by stimulating the α_2-adrenergic receptors and imidazoline I_1-receptors in CNS. This results in inhibition of sympathetic output and consequent decrease in peripheral resistance. The overall effect is decrease in blood pressure.

Recently, centrally acting antihypertensives which are selective for imidazoline I_1 receptors have been developed. These include moxonidine (12) and rilmenidine (13). These agents are free from side effects such as sedation, bradycardia, and mental depression.

(12)   (13)

Ganglionic Blocking Agents

Ganglionic blocking agents block the transmission of impulses in sympathetic and parasympathetic autonomic ganglia.

The hypotensive effect of ganglionic blocking agents is due to reduction of norepinephrine (8) release from the postganglionic sympathetic nerve endings. They also reduce the cardiac output by reducing venous return which is due to venous dilation. Ganglionic blocking agents are no more used because of their toxicity, development of resistance, and erratic absorption from GI tract. One drug worth mention is trimethaphan camsylate (14). It produces extremely transient hypotension and is used to produce controlled transient hypotension. Mecamylamine (15) is another drug used earlier.

(14)   (15)

Drugs Affecting Noradrenergic Neurons

The drugs of this class include guanethidine (16), guanadrel (17), bethanidine (18), and reserpine (19). Guanethidine (16), guanadrel (17) and bethanidine (18) act by affecting the norepinephrine (8) release, while as reserpine (19) affects the norepinephrine (8) storage site.

(16)   (17)

(18)   (19)

Guanethidine (16) is transported across the sympathetic nerve membrane by the same mechanism that transports norepinephrine (8). Once it enters neurone it gets concentrated in norepinephrine (8) storage sites where it replaces the norepinephrine (8). This results in gradual depletion of norepinephrine (8) in its storage sites. It also inhibits norepinephrine (8) release from nerve endings when sympathetic nerves are stimulated. Since neuronal uptake is necessary for the hypotensive action of guanthidine (16), drugs which affect this uptake, block its action. Examples of these are cocaine, tricyclic antidepressants, phenothiazines, etc.

The hypotensive action of guanethidine (16) is associated with sodium and water retention. Administration of a diuretic, therefore, becomes necessary to avoid the tolerance to the drug.

Guanadrel (17) and bethanidine (18), which also contain a guanidine moiety, act in the same fashion as guanethidine (16).

Reserpine (19), an alkaloid obtained from *Rauwolfia* species, acts by affecting norepinephrine (8) storage. It inhibits ATP-driven monoamine transporter responsible for the transport of norepinephrine (8), dopamine, and serotonin in both central and peripheral neurons. Norepinephrine (8) instead accumulates in cytoplasm where it is degraded by monoamine oxidases. This results in decreased concentration of norepinephrine (8) and sympathetic transmission is thus blocked.

Adrenergic Receptor Blockers

These can be further classified as:

1. *α_1-Adrenergic receptor blockers,*
2. *β-adrenergtic receptor blockers,*
3. *mixed α- and β-adrenergic receptor blockers.*

α_1-Adrenergic Receptor Blockers

Some of the drugs which selectively block α_1-adrenergic receptors include prazosin (20), terazosin (21), and doxazosin (22). The antihypertensive action of these is because of peripheral vasodilation caused by blockade of post-synaptic α_1-adrenergic receptor in smooth muscle and bladder. The blockade of α_1-receptors in bladder results in diuresis which contributes to antihypertensive action.

β-Adrenergic Receptor Blockers

The selective β_1-adrenoreceptor blockers used as antihypertensive agents include acebutolol (23), atenolol (24), betaxolol (25), bisoprolol (26), esmolol (27), and metoprolol (28). Some of the non-selective β-adrenoreceptor blockers include propranolol (29), carteolol (30), nadolol (31), penbutolol (32), pindolol (33), and timolol (34). β-Adrenergic blockers antagonise catecholamine competitively at β_1- and β_2-receptors in heart and blood vessels. They reduce the contractility of myocardium, decrease heart rate, and inhibit renin release. After sometime, the cardiac output returns to normal and the blood pressure remains low because of decreased peripheral vascular resistance. The inhibition of the renin release, which is mediated through blockade of β_2-receptor is also contributing to reduction of blood pressure.

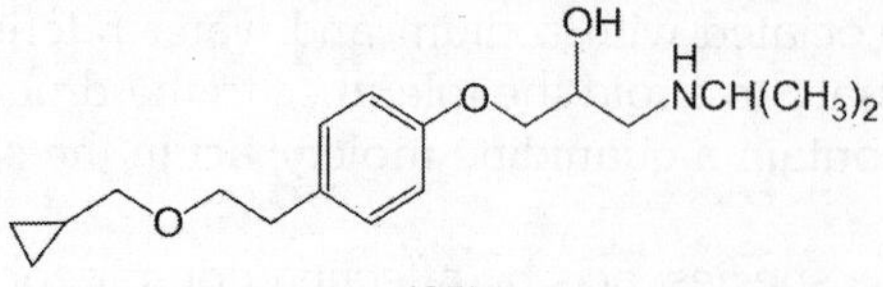

(25)

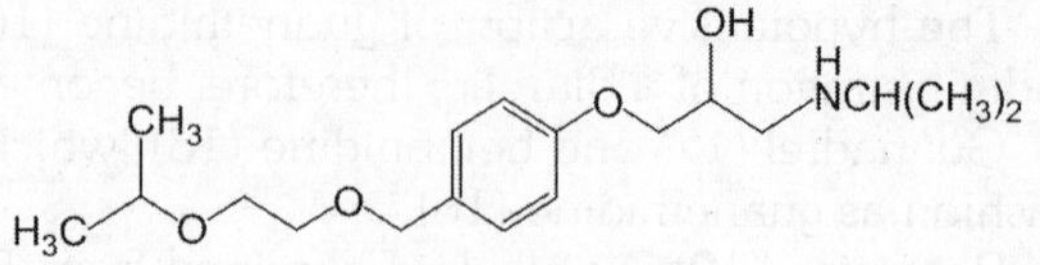

(26)

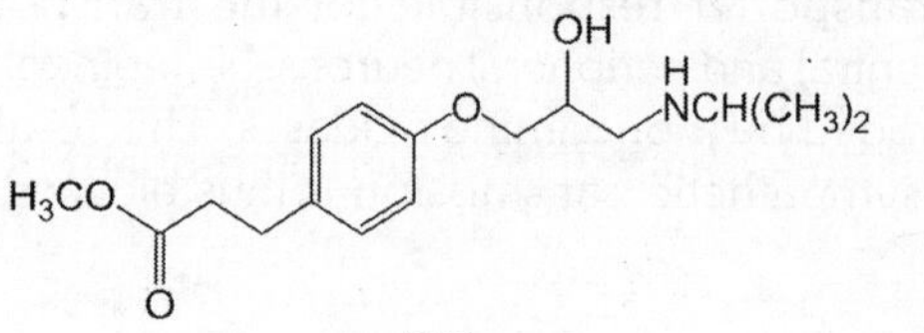

(27)

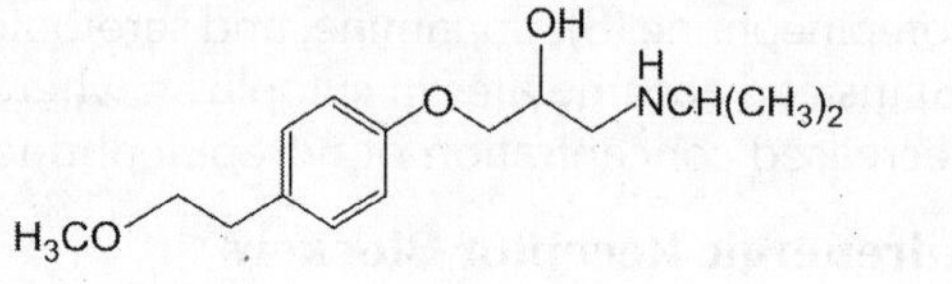

(28)

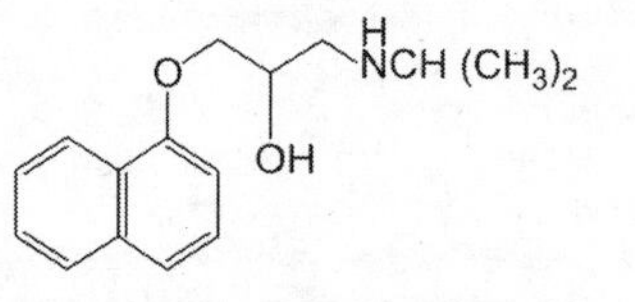

(29)

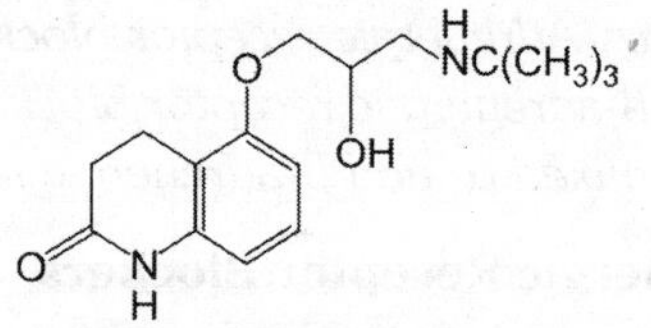

(30)

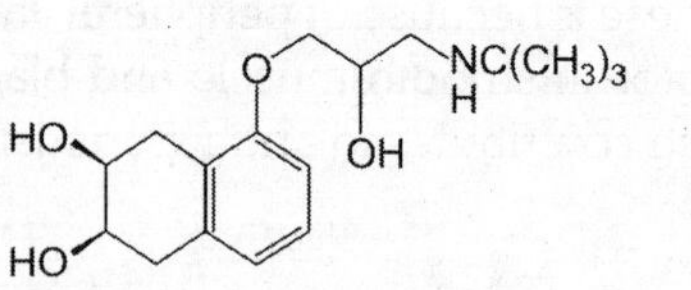

(31)

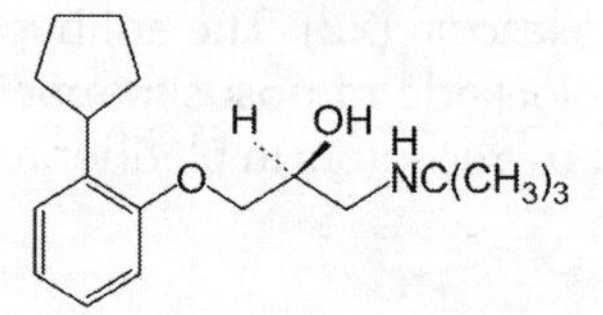

(32)

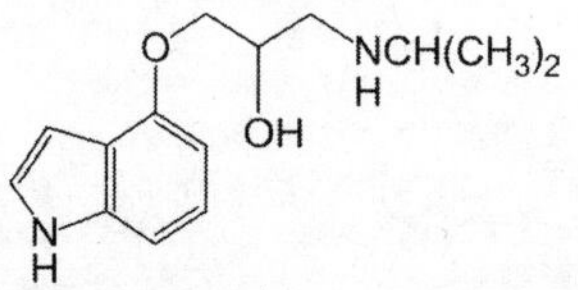

(33)

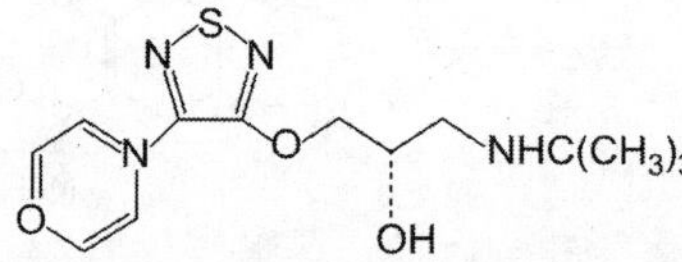

(34)

Mixed α- and β-Adrenergic Receptor Blockers

The two drugs available in this category include labetalol (35) and carvedilol (36). Both of these compounds are used as racemates. The mechanism of their action is through blockade of both α- and β-adrenoreceptors. The blockade of both receptors gives these agents advantage over other classes of antihypertensives. α_1-Blockade results in lowering of peripheral vascular resistance, without affecting cardiac output. This prevents bradycardia, β-blockade helps to prevent reflex tachycardia which is usually observed in many of the vasodilators.

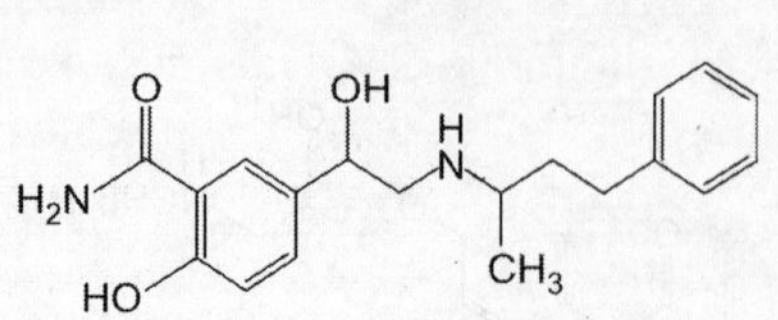

(35)

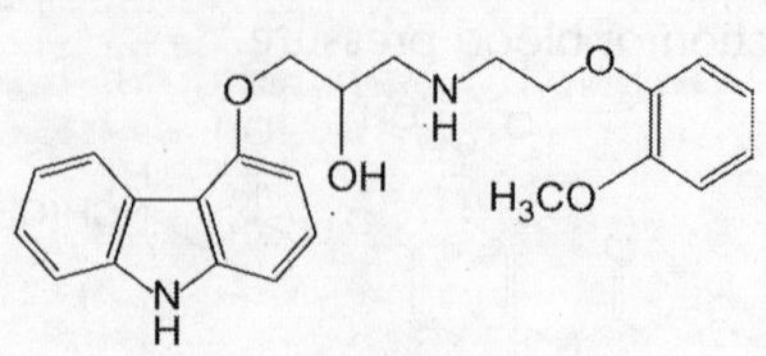

(36)

VASODILATORS

Vasodilators act by relaxing smooth muscles of arterioles and veins and thereby reducing the vascular resistance. The net result is decreased arterial blood pressure. The reflex response to this, which counteract the hypotensive effect, include increased cardiac heart rate, and output and an increased plasma renin activity. All these reflex responses are mediated through baroreceptors, sympathetic nervous system, renin-angiotensin system, and aldosterone.

Vasodilators are usually used in combination with sympatholytics and diuretics. Sympatholytics block the effects on heart and plasma-renin levels. Diuretics prevent the fluid retention and plasma volume expansion. Some of the drugs used as vasodilators include hydralazine (37), minoxidil (38), diazoxide (39), and sodium nitroprusside (40).

(37)

(38)

(39)

(40)

Hydralazine (37) is a phthalazine analog. It relaxes smooth muscles by opening the ATP-modulated potassium channels. This causes efflux of potassium resulting in hyperpolarization of vascular smooth muscle cells resulting in inhibitory action on membrane excitation and subsequent vasodilation. The effect is greater on arterioles than on veins. As discussed earlier, administration of vasodilators elicits compensatory responses which counteracts the hypotensive effect. To overcome this, they are usually given along with other antihypertensive agents including diuretics.

Minoxidil (38) and diazoxide (39) cause vasodilation in the same manner as hydralazine (37). They are also administered along with sympatholytics and diuretics to counteract the compensatory responses. Both of these are arterial vasodilators.

Sodium nitroprusside (40) is metabolized to nitric oxide, which activates guanylate cyclase. This results in vasodilation of arteries as well as veins. Sodium nitroprusside (40) is usually given in emergency. The serious toxic effect of sodium nitroprusside (40) are accumulation of cyanide, metabolic acidosis, arrhythmias, and excessive hypotension, all these may lead to death.

CALCIUM CHANNEL BLOCKERS

In addition to antiarrhythmic and antianginal activity, calcium channel blockers also dilate peripheral arterioles and reduce blood pressure. Because of this property, they have found use as antihypertensive agents. These substances act by blocking the calcium channel and thus the influx of calcium into the smooth muscle. Some of these include amlodipine (41), felodipine (42), isradipine (43), nicardipine (44), nifedipine (45), nimodipine (46), bepridil (47), dilitiazem (48), verapamil (49), and ziconotide (50).

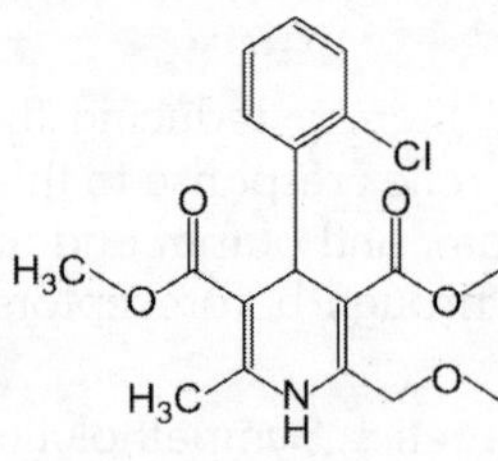

(41)

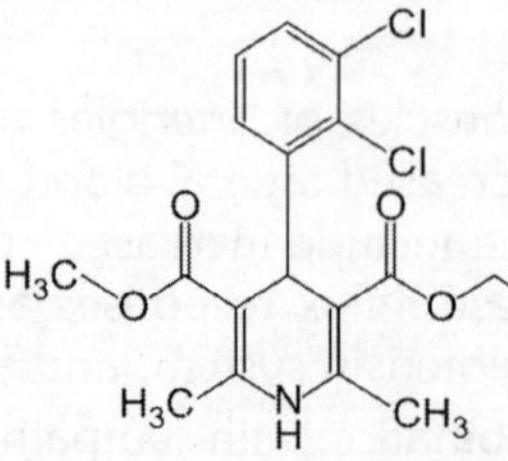

(42)

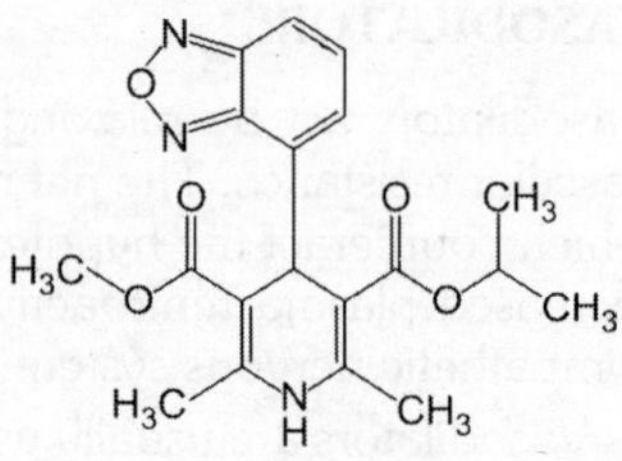

(43)

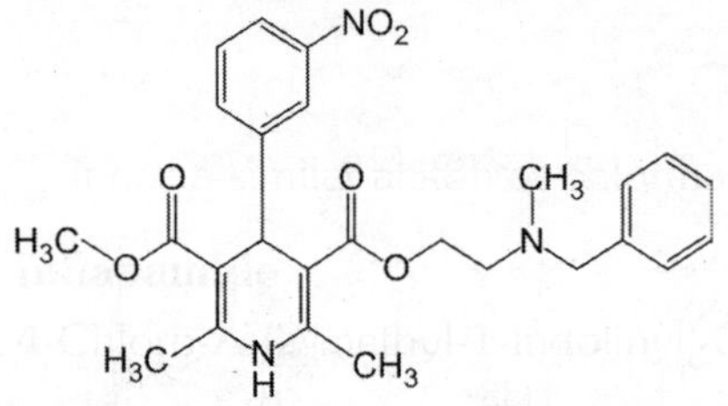

(44)

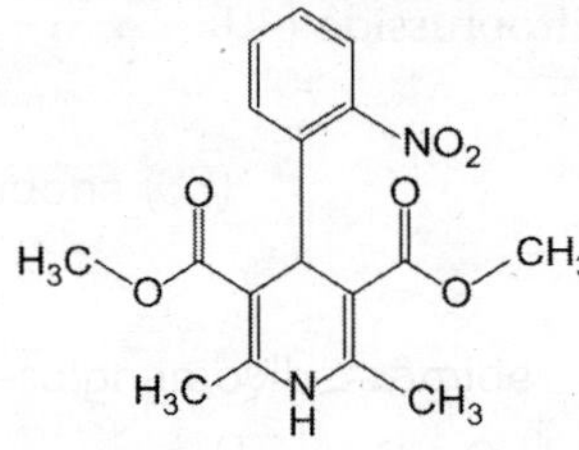

(45)

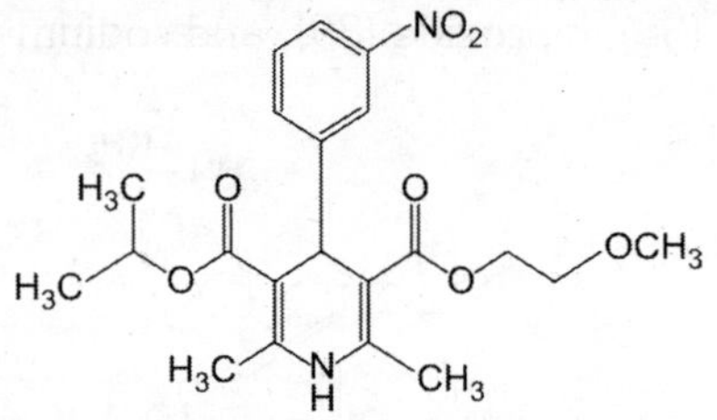

(46)

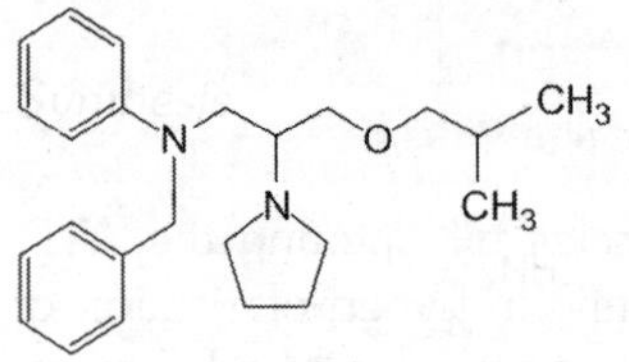

(47)

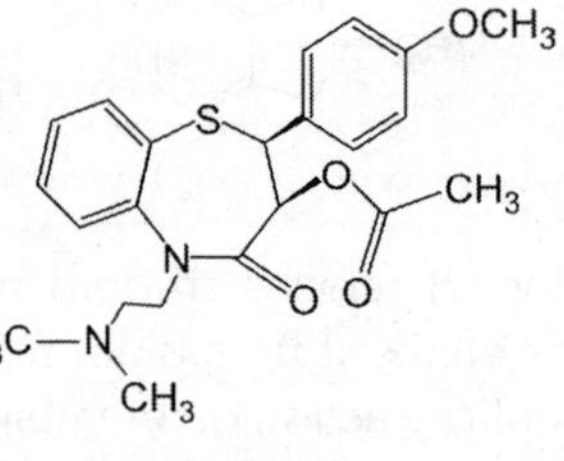

(48)

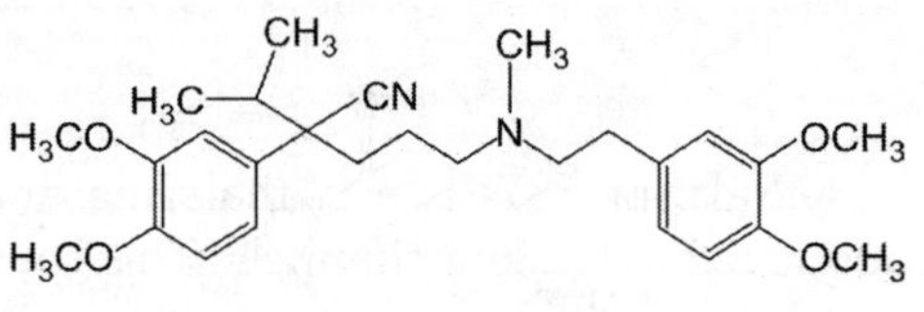

(49)

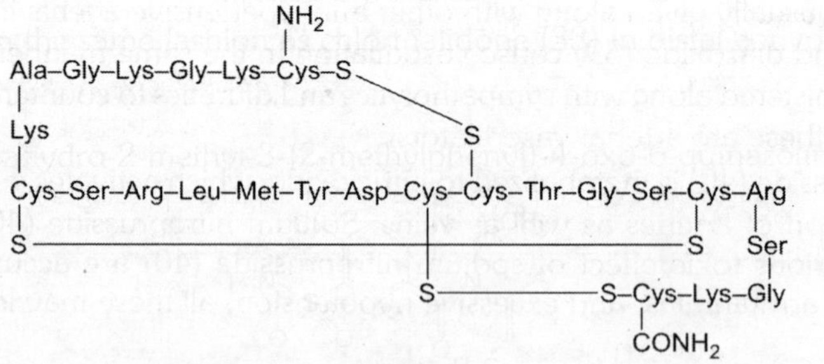

(50)

ANGIOTENSIN CONVERTING ENZYME INHIBITORS

These include:

(a) α-Amino-γ-phenyl butyric acid analogs such as benazepril (51), enalapril (52), lisinopril (53), moexipril (54), quinapril (55), ramipril (56), spirapril (57), and trandolapril (58), (*b*) α-aminopentanoic acid analogs such as perindopril (59),

(*c*) thiols, captopril (60), and

(*c*) phosphonates, fosinopril (61).

Angiotensin converting enzyme inhibitors inhibit the conversion of angiotensin I to angiotensin II, which results in decreased peripheral resistance. They also increase bradykinin levels which results in vasodilation as well as increase in prostaglandin synthesis, this also contributes to vasodilation.

Benazepril (51), enalapril (52), moexipril (54), quinapril (55), ramipril (56), spirapril (57), trandolapril (58), perindopril (59), and the phosphonate analog, fosinopril (61) are the prodrugs. They get activated by esterases and are converted to dicarboxylic acids, benazeprilat (62), enalaprilat (63), moexiprilat (64), quinaprilat (65), ramiprilat (66), spiraprilat (67), trandolaprilat (68), perindoprilat (69), and fosinoprilat (70), respectively.

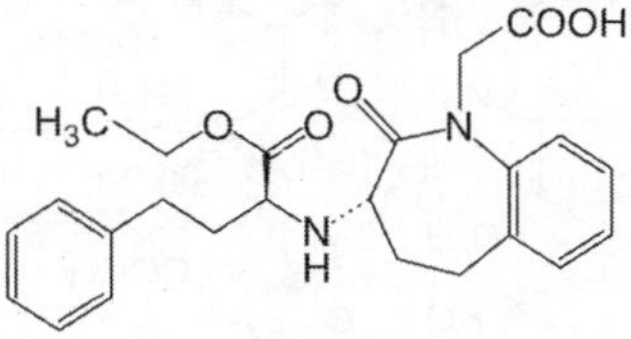

(51)

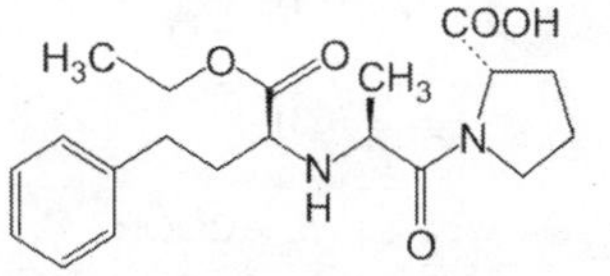

(52)

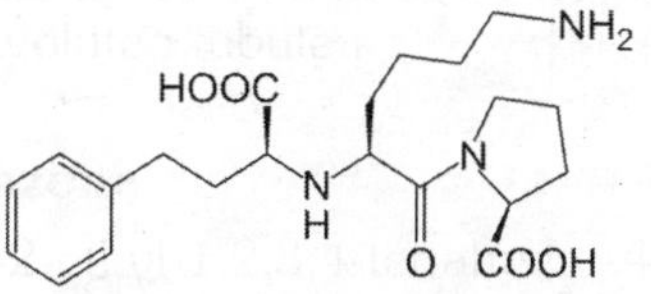

(53)

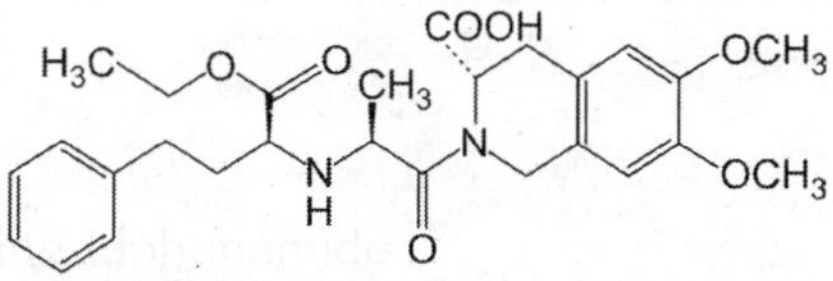

(54)

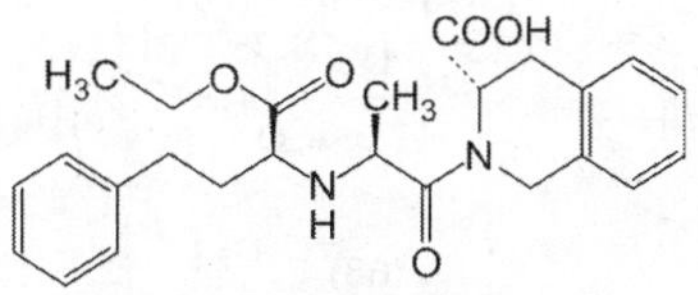

(55)

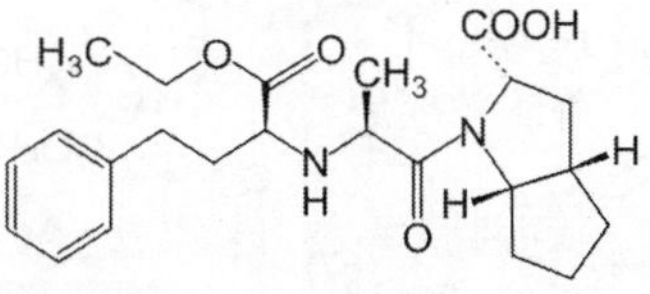

(56)

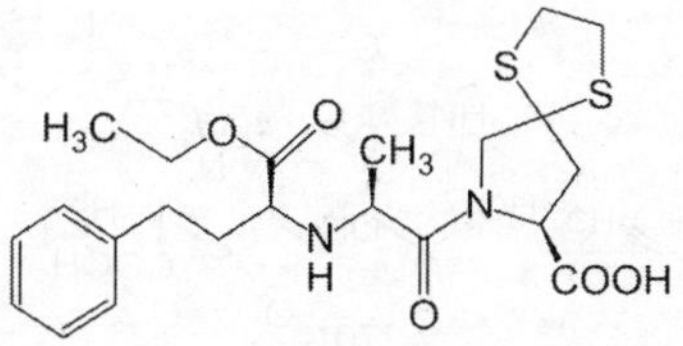

(57)

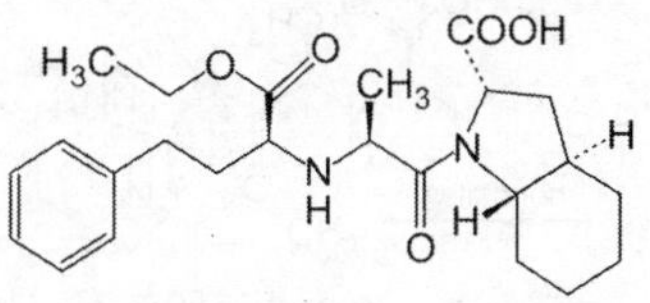

(58)

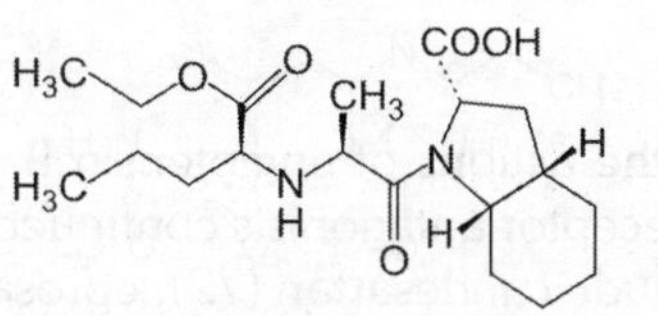

(59)

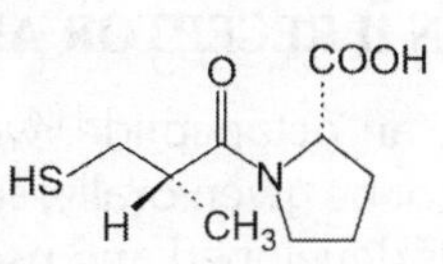

(60)

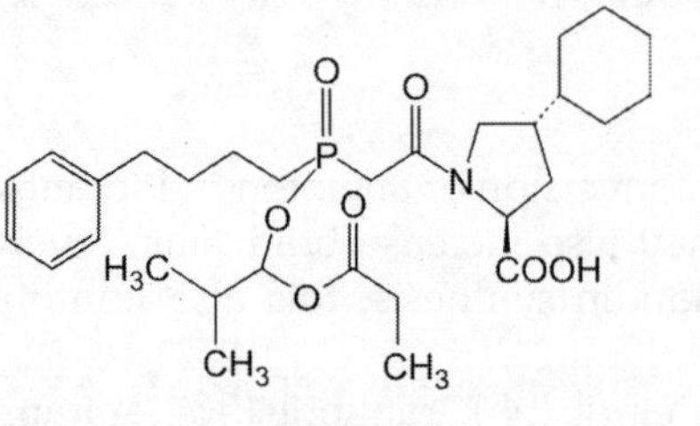

(61)

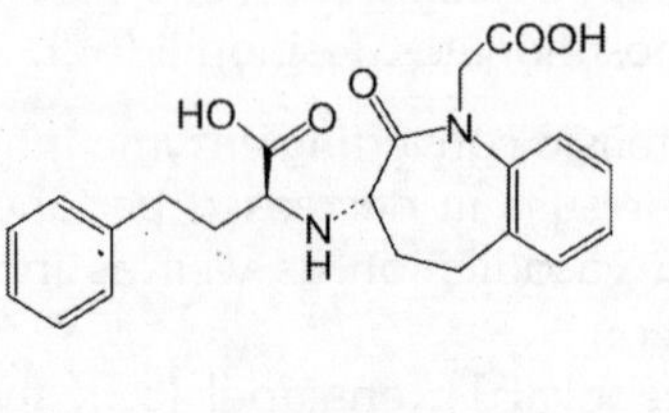

(62)

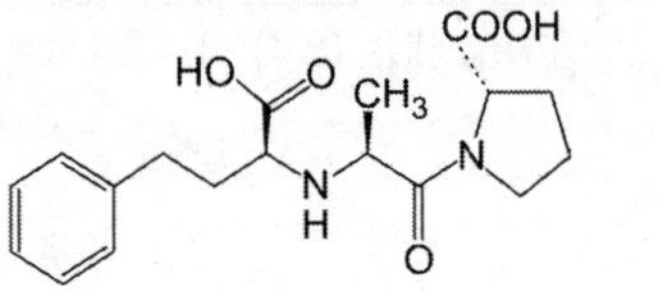

(63)

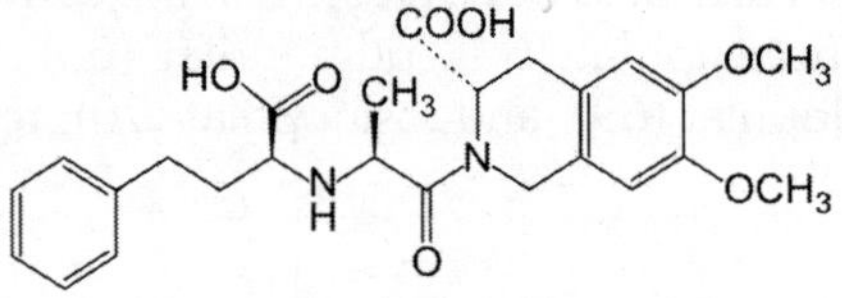

(64)

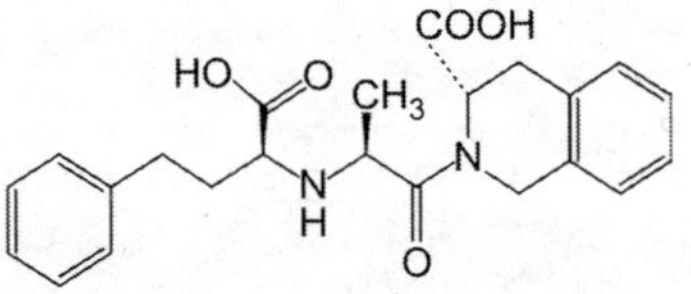

(65)

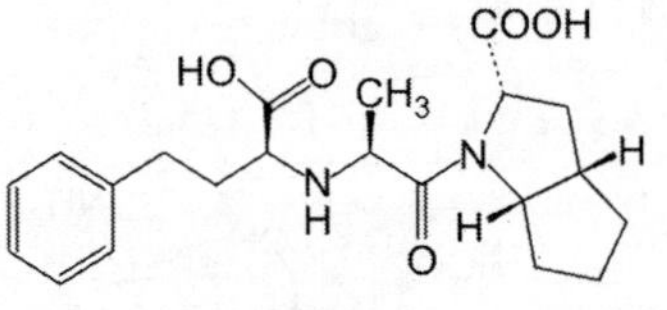

(66)

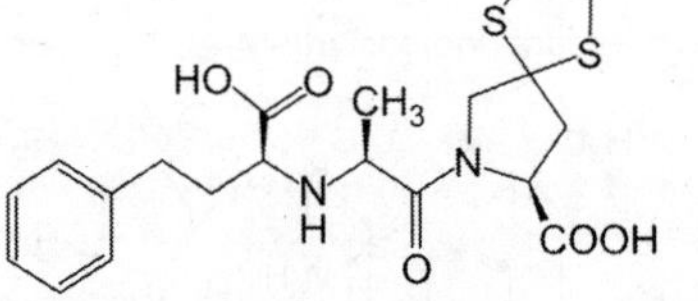

(67)

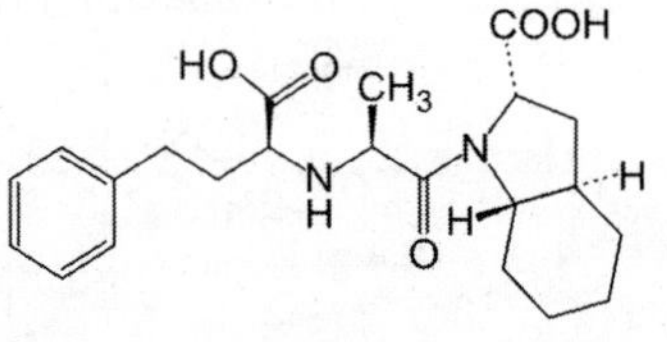

(68)

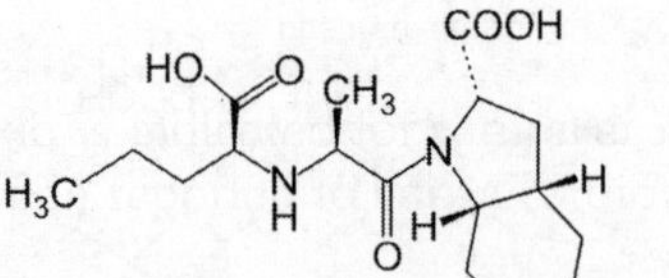

(69)

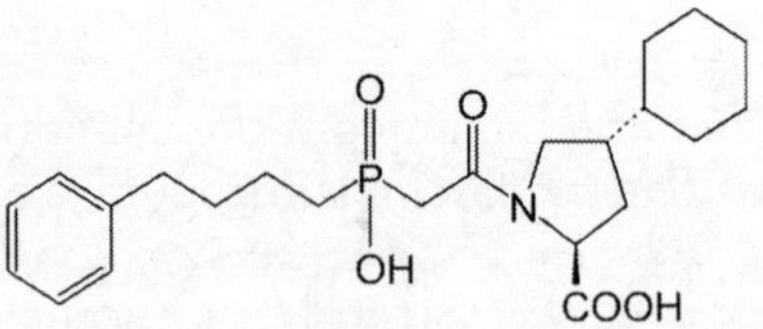

(70)

ANGIOTENSIN II RECEPTOR ANTAGONISTS

Saralasin (71), an octapeptide, was found to antagonize the actions of angiotensin II. However, since it could not be given orally, search for angiotensin II receptor antagonists continued. Some of the compounds developed and used in clinical practice include candesartan (72), eprosartan (73), irbesartan (74), losartan (75), olmesartan (76), telmisartan (77), and valsartan (78). Two subtypes of angiotensin II receptors are known. These include Type I or AT_1 and Type 2 or AT_2. All the angiotensin II receptor blockers are more selective for AT_1 subtype receptor of angiotensin II receptors and act by competitive antagonism, preventing and reversing the effects of angiotensin II.

The role of AT_2 subtype receptors of angiotensin II receptors is not known.

Sar — Arg — Val — Tyr — Val — His — Pro — Ala

(71)

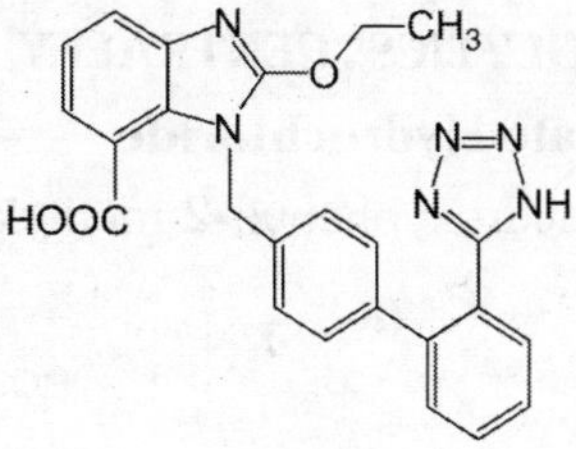

(72)

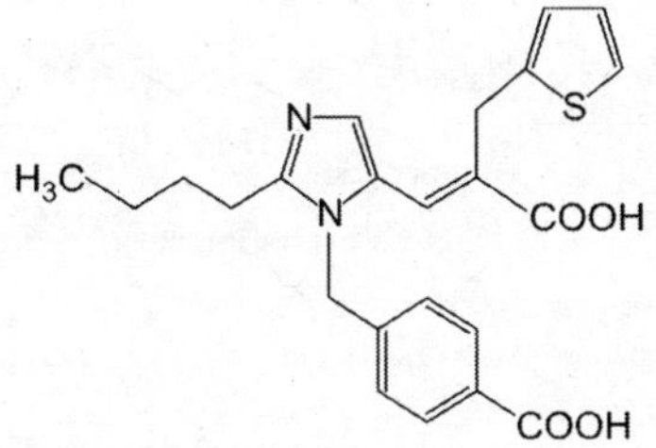

(73)

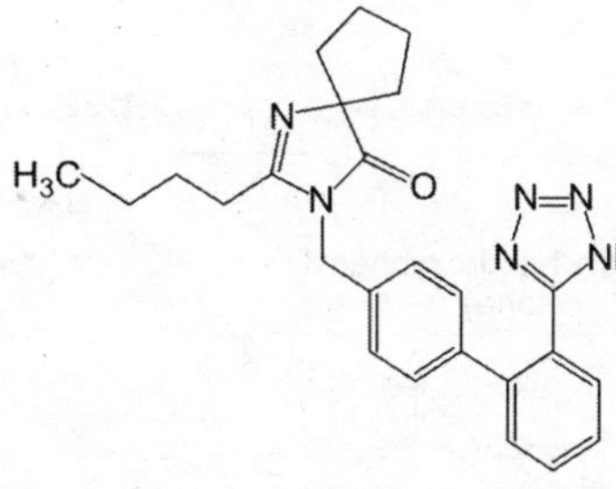

(74)

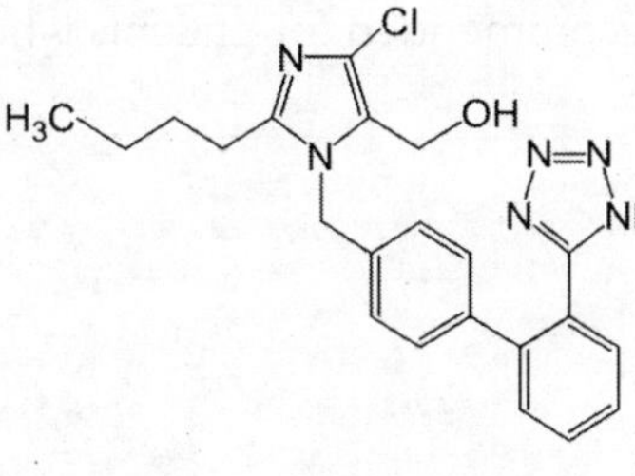

(75)

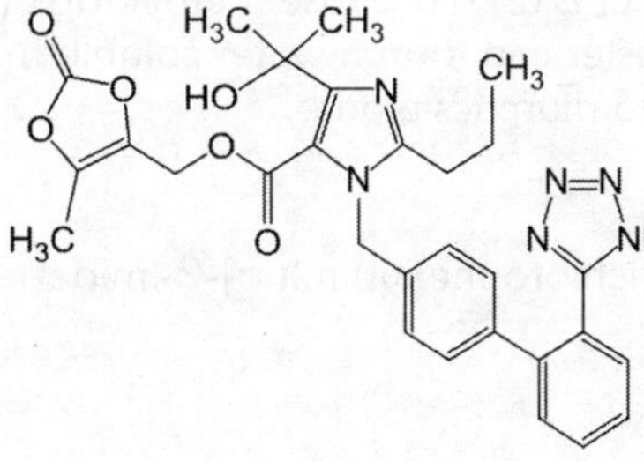

(76)

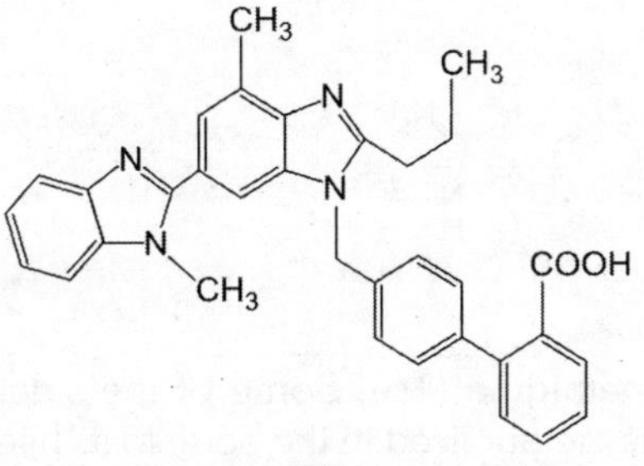

(77)

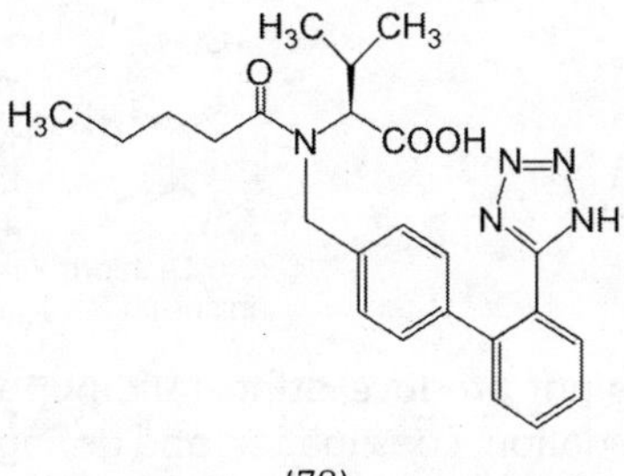

(78)

INDIVIDUAL COMPOUNDS

DURETICS

See DIURETICS

SYMPATHOLYTICS : CENTRALLY ACTING

Methyldopate Hydrochloride

L-3-(3,4-Dihydroxyphenyl)-2-methylalanine ethyl ester hydrochloride

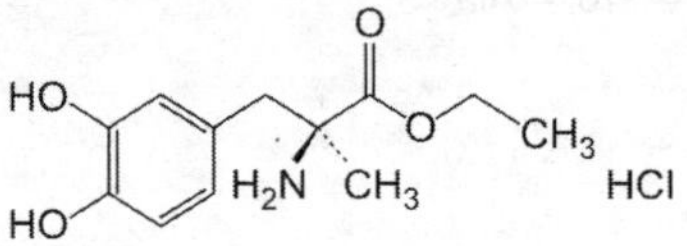

Synthesis

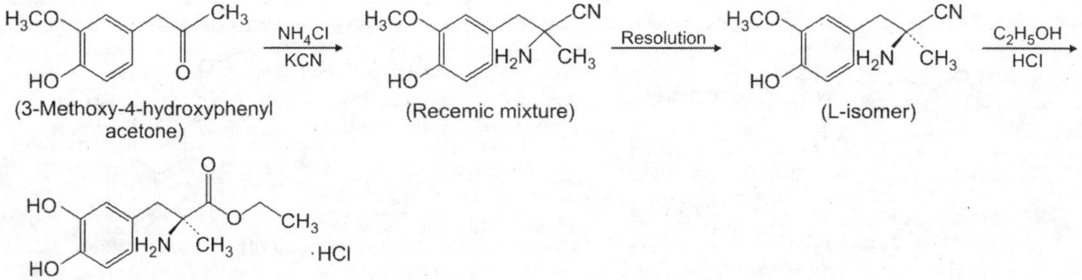

(3-Methoxy-4-hydroxyphenyl acetone)   (Recemic mixture)   (L-isomer)

The ester is used because methyldopa (2) is a zwitterion and is not soluble enough for parenteral use, the ester can form a water soluble hydrochloride. It is recommended for patients who do not respond to diuretics alone.

Clonidine

2-[(2,6-Dichlorophenyl)imino]-2-imidazoline

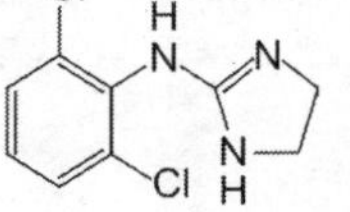

Synthesis

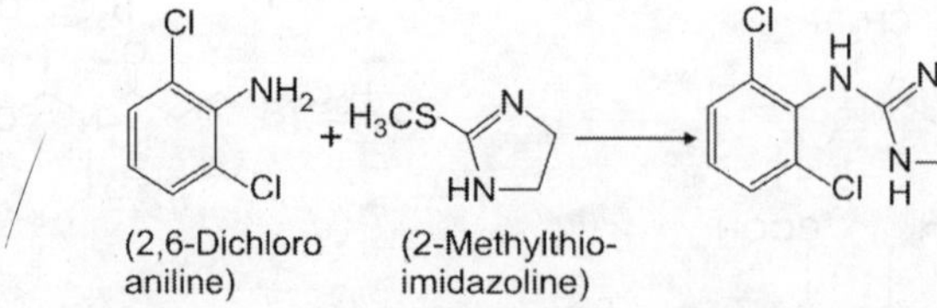

(2,6-Dichloro aniline)   (2-Methylthio-imidazoline)

It does not produce orthostatic hypotension like guanethidine (16). Some of the side effects include sedation, constipation and drying of the mouth. It is metabolized in the body to its hydroxide which is then converted to glucuronide and sulphate.

Guanabenz

2-[(2,6-Dichlorophenyl)methylene]hydrazinecarboximidamide

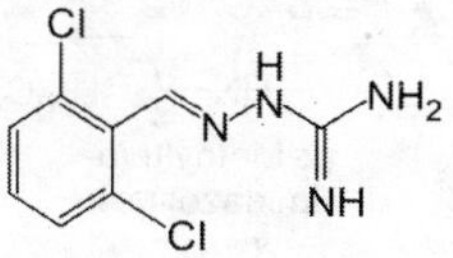

Synthesis

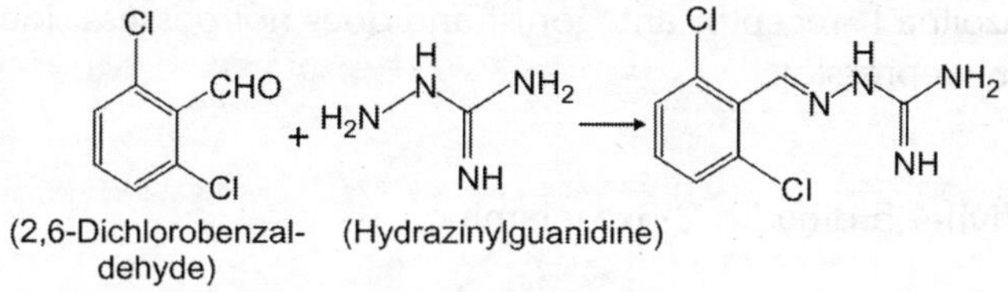

(2,6-Dichlorobenzal-   (Hydrazinylguanidine)
dehyde)

Like clonidine (3) it also does not produce orthostatic hypotension. It is also converted to its hydroxy derivative and then to glucuronide and sulfate.

Guanfacine

N-(Aminoiminomethyl)-2,6-dichlorobenzeneacetamide

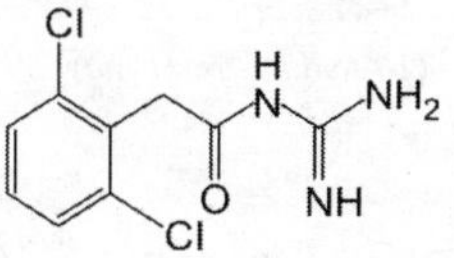

Synthesis

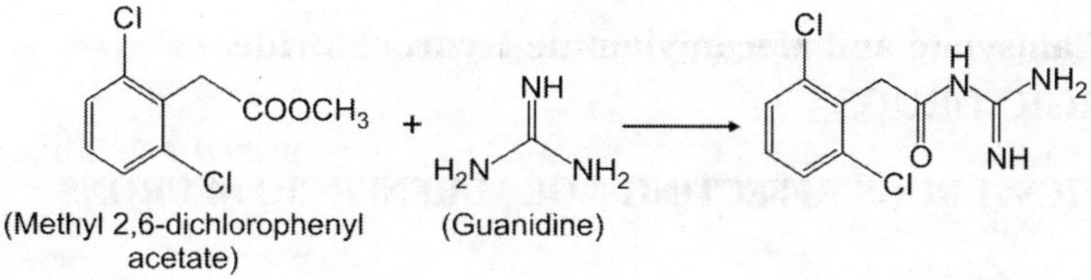

(Methyl 2,6-dichlorophenyl   (Guanidine)
acetate)

The drug has a longer duration of action and has fewer CNS side effects as compared to other related drugs.

Moxonidine

4-Chloro-6-methoxy-2-methyl-5-(2-imidazolin-2-yl)aminopyrimidine

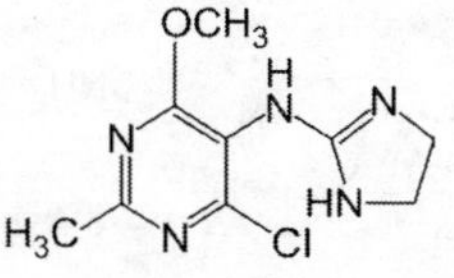

Synthesis

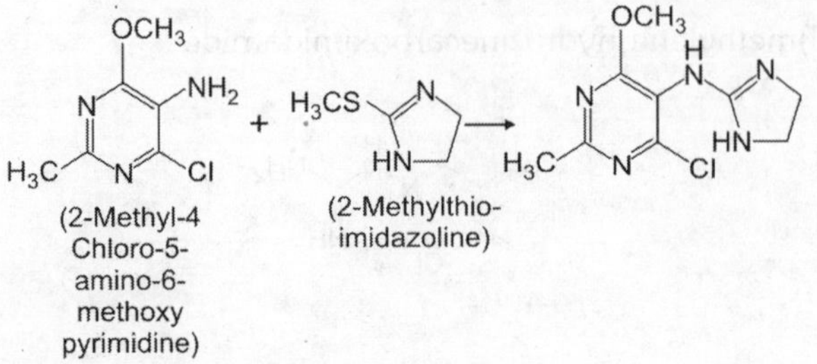

It is selective imidazoline I_1-receptor antagonist and does not possess side effects like sedation, bradycardia, or mental depression.

Rilmenidine

N-(Dicyclopropylmethyl)-4,5-dihydro-2-oxazolamine

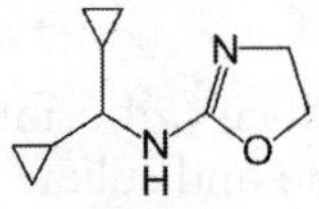

Synthesis

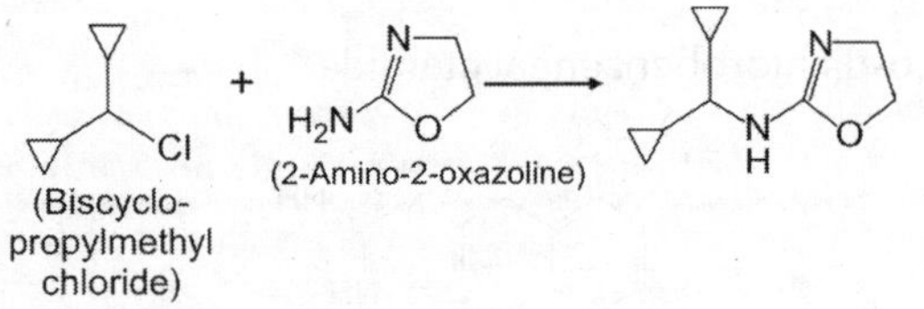

Same activity and mechanism as moxonidine (12).

SYMPATHOLYTICS : GANGLIONIC BLOCKING AGENTS

Trimethaphan Camsylate and Mecamylamine Hydrochloride

See CHOLINERGIC DRUGS

SYMPATHOLYTICS : DRUGS AFFECTING NORADRENERGIC NEURONS

Guanethidine

1-[2-(Perhydroazocin-1-yl)ethyl] guanidine

Synthesis

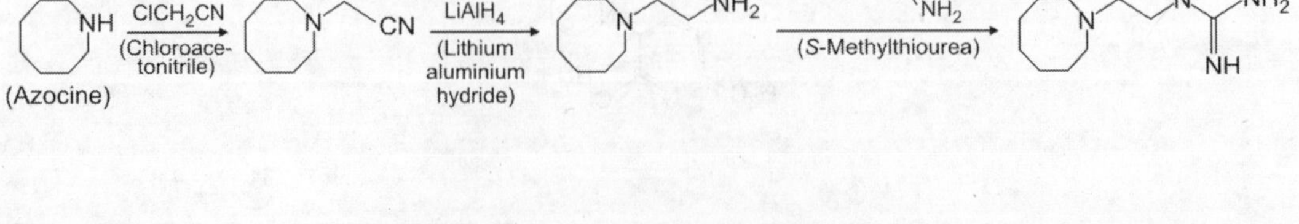

It produces a gradual fall in blood pressure and has a much longer half-life (several days). Since it is highly polar, therefore, it cannot pass the blood-brain barrier.

It is metabolized by microsomal enzymes to 2-(6-carboxy hexylamino) ethyl guanide (79) and guanethidine N-oxide (80), both of these have weak or no antihypertensive effects.

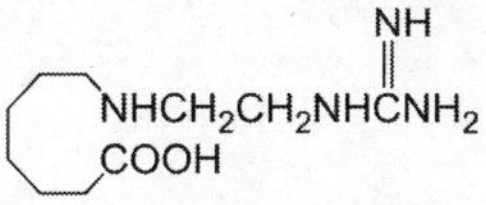

(79) 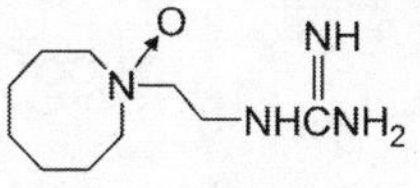   (80)

Guanadrel

(1,4-Dioxaspiro[4.5]dec-2-ylmethyl)guanidine

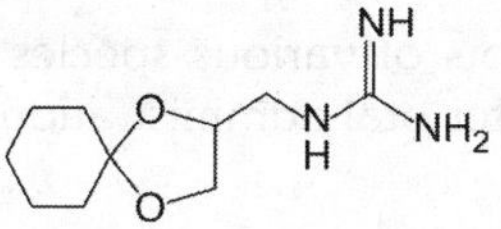

Synthesis

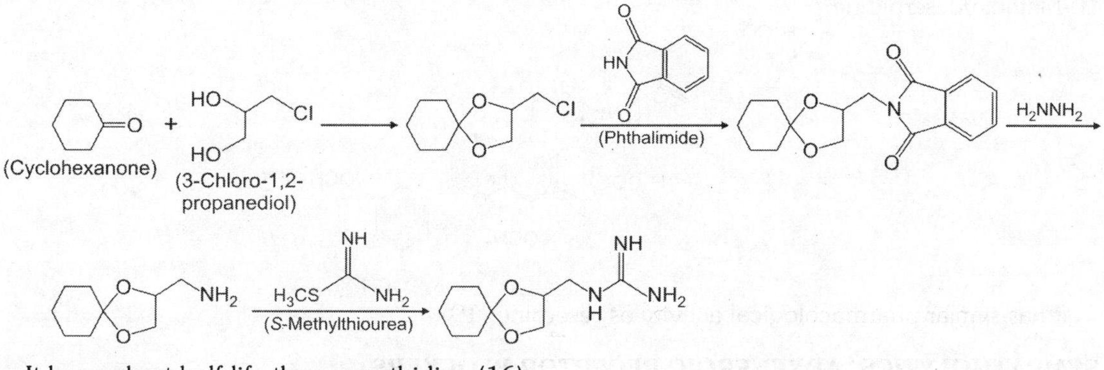

It has a short half-life than gunethidine (16).

Bethanidine

1-Benzyl-2,3-dimethylguanidine

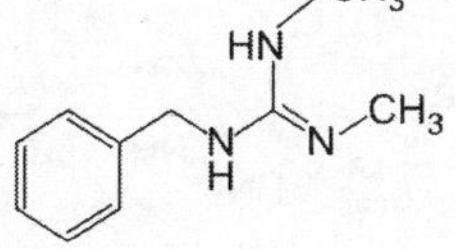

Synthesis

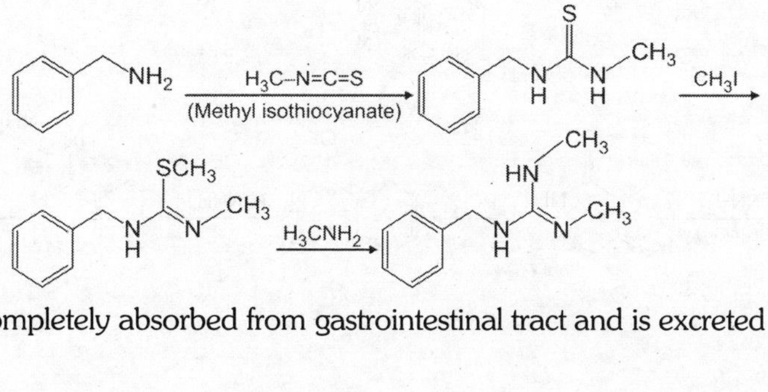

It is rapidly but completely absorbed from gastrointestinal tract and is excreted unchanged in urine.

Reserpine

11,17α-Dimethoxy-18β-[(3,4,5-trimethoxybenzoyl)oxy]-3β, 20α-yohimbane-16β-carboxylic acid methyl ester

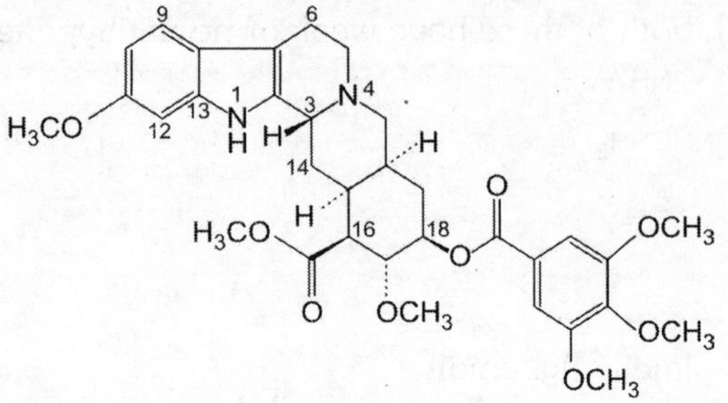

It is an alkaloid obtained from roots of various species of *Rauwolfia* belonging to the family *Apocynacea*. It is readily absorbed after oral administration.

Methoserpidine

10-Methoxydeserpidine

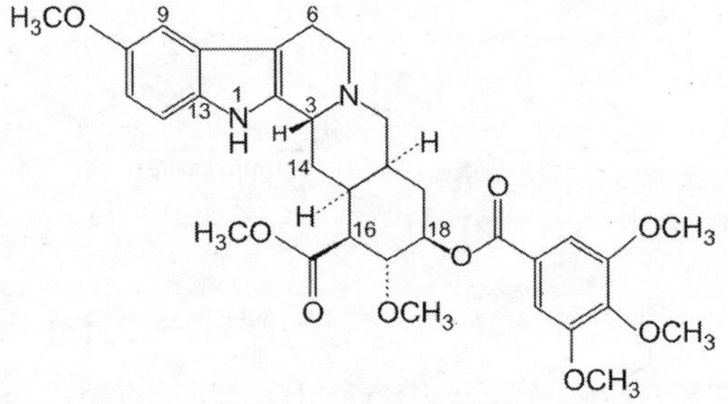

It has similar pharmacological activity as reserpine (19).

SYMPATHOLYTICS : ADRENERGIC RECEPTOR BLOCKERS

See ADRENERGIC DRUGS

VASODILATORS

Hydralazine Hydrochloride

Phthalazin-1-ylhydrazine hydrochloride

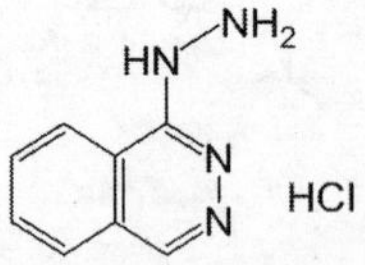

Synthesis

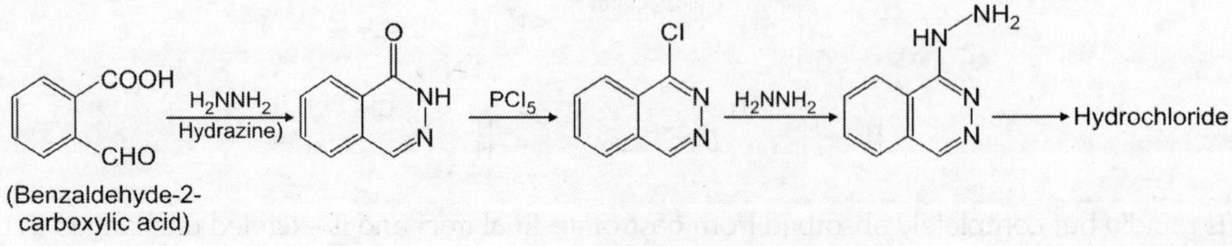

It is useful in the treatment of moderate to severe hypertension and is often used with β-blockers and diuretic.

Minoxidil

2,4-Diamino-6-piperidinopyrimidine 3-oxide

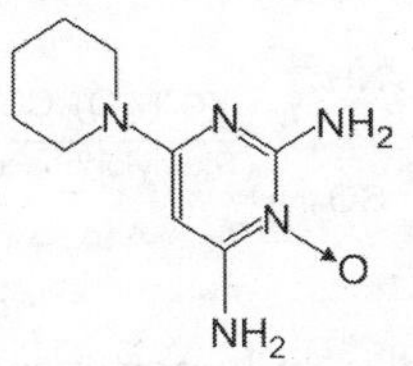

Synthesis

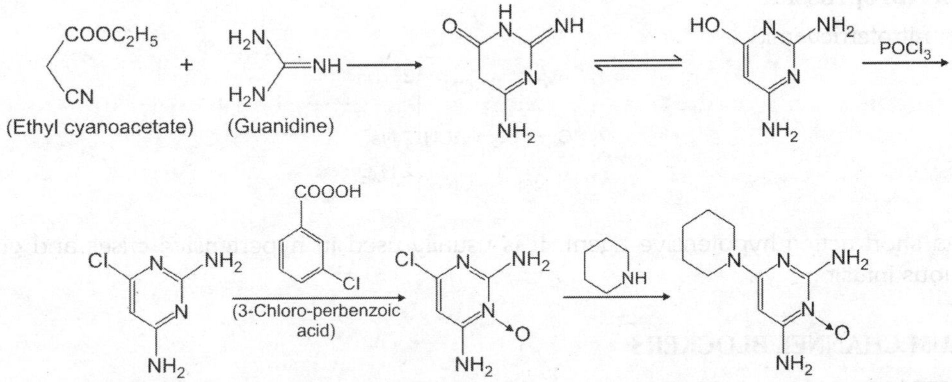

As such minoxidil is inactive. It is converted to its active form, minoxidil N-O-sulphate (81) in liver by sulphotransferase. It is used for severe hypertension along with diuretics to overcome the sodium and water retention. Minoxidil is also used for hair growth in alopecia androgenitica. The hair growing effect may be due to increase in cutaneous blood flow.

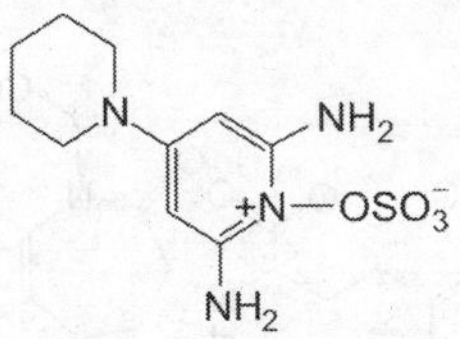

(81)

Diazoxide Sodium

Sodium 7-chloro-3-methyl-2H-1,2,4-benzothiadiazine 1, 1-dioxide

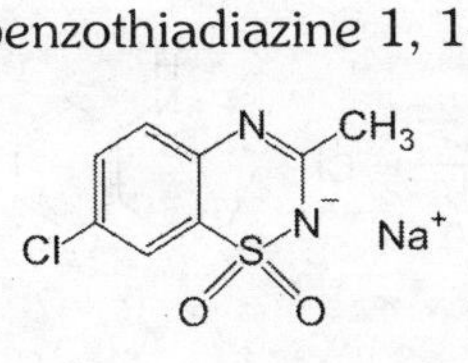

Synthesis

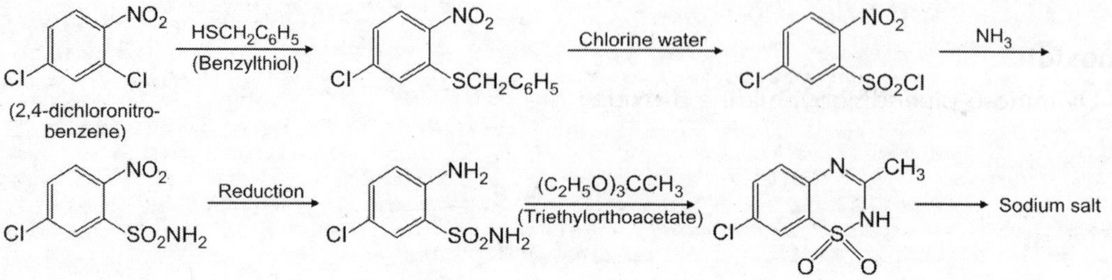

It is absorbed readily when given orally. In hypertensive emergencies, it is given parenterally.

Sodium Nitroprusside

Sodium nitroferricyamide

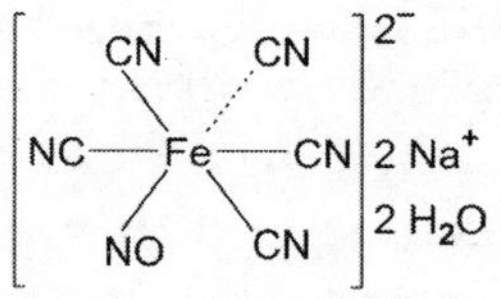

It is a short acting hypotensive agent. It is usually used in hypertensive crises and given by continuous infusion.

CALCIUM CHANNEL BLOCKERS

See ANTIANGINAL, ANTIARRHYTHMIC, AND CARIDOTONIC DRUGS

ANGIOTENSIN CONVERTING ENZYME INHIBITORS

Benazepril

(3S)-(1-Carboxymethyl)-[[(1S)-1-(ethoxycarbonyl)-3-phenylpropyl]amino]2,3,4,5-tetrahydro-1H-[1]benzazepine-2-one

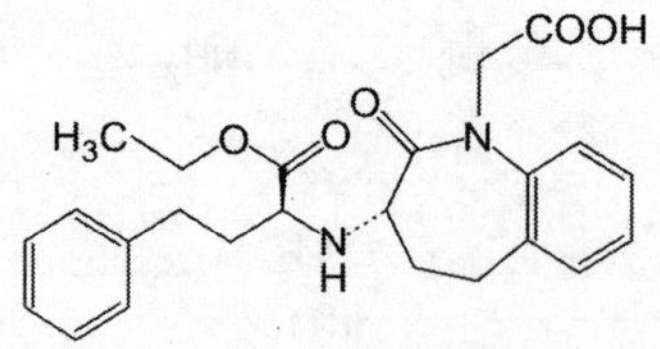

Synthesis

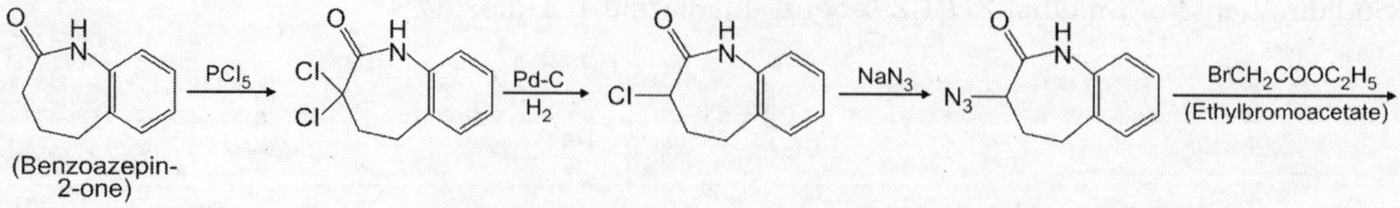

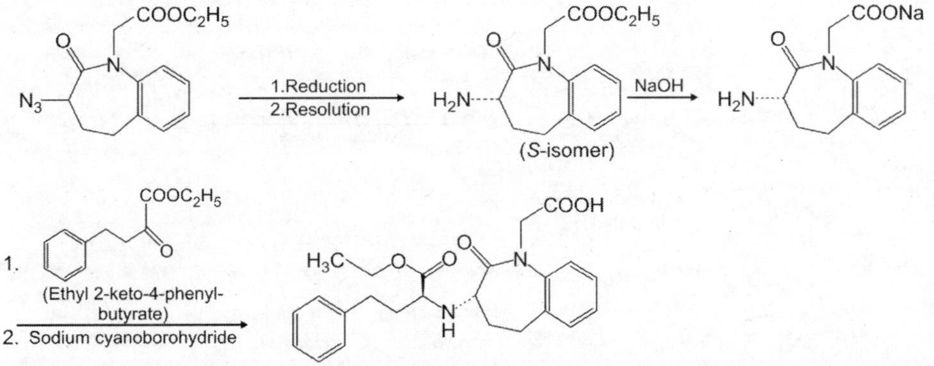

Its antihypertensive action is because of inhibition of angiotensin converting enzyme, the enzyme responsible for converting angiotensin I into angiotensin II which is responsible for vasoconstriction resulting in hypertension. It is hydrolyzed by esterases to benazeprilat (62), the active form.

Enalapril

1-[N[(S)-1-Carboxy-3-phenylpropyl]-L-alanyl]-L-proline 1′-ethylester

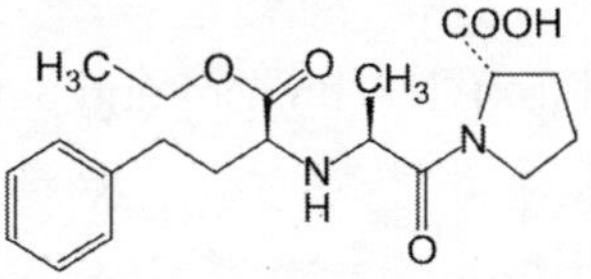

Synthesis

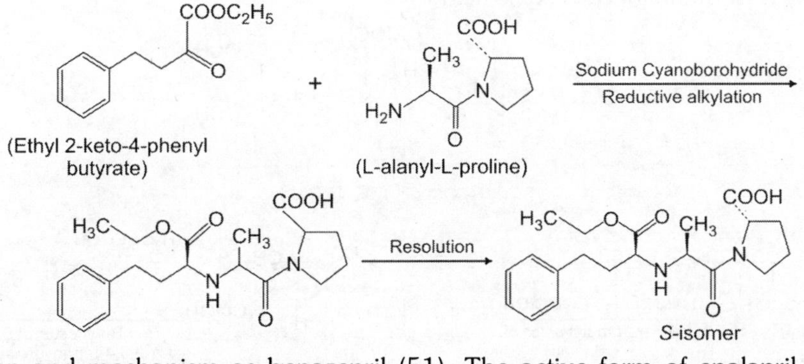

Same action and mechanism as benazepril (51). The active form of enalapril is the diacid enalaprilat (63).

Lisinopril

(S)-1-[N²-(1-Carboxy-3-phenylpropyl)-L-lysyl]-L-proline

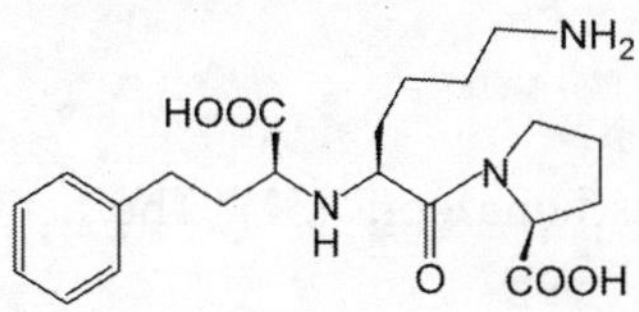

Synthesis

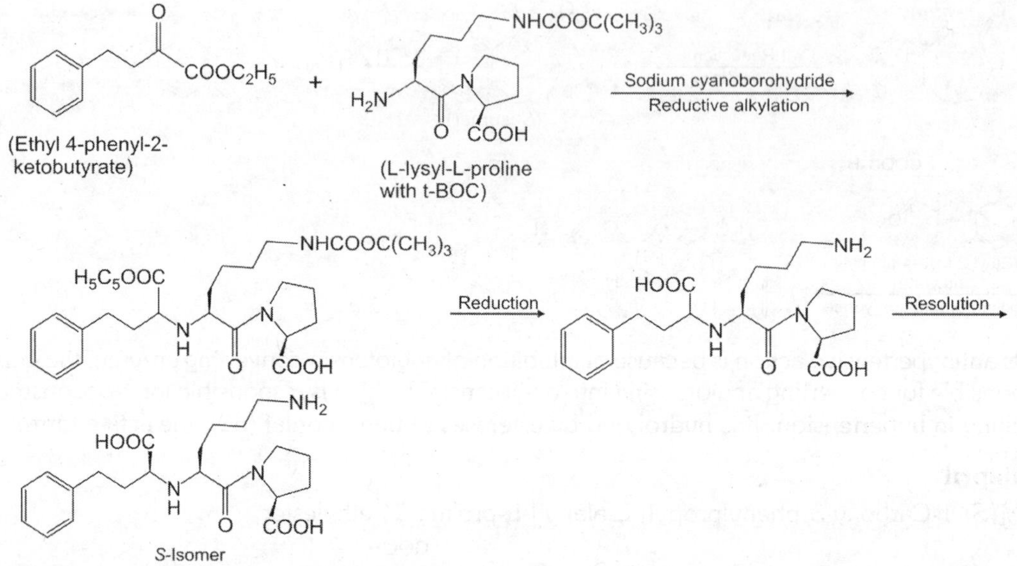
NHCOOC(CH3)3
COOC2H5
H2N
COOH
Sodium cyanoborohydride
Reductive alkylation
(Ethyl 4-phenyl-2-ketobutyrate)
(L-lysyl-L-proline with t-BOC)
H5C5OOC
NHCOOC(CH3)3
Reduction
HOOC
NH2
Resolution
S-Isomer

It is the lysine analog of enalapril (52). Mechanism and action is same as benazepril (51).

Moexipril

(3*S*)-2[(2*S*)-2-[[(1*S*)-1-(Ethoxycarbonyl)-3-phenylpropyl]amino]-1-oxopropyl]-1,2,3,4-tetrahydro-6,7-dimethoxy-3-isoquinolinecarboxylic acid

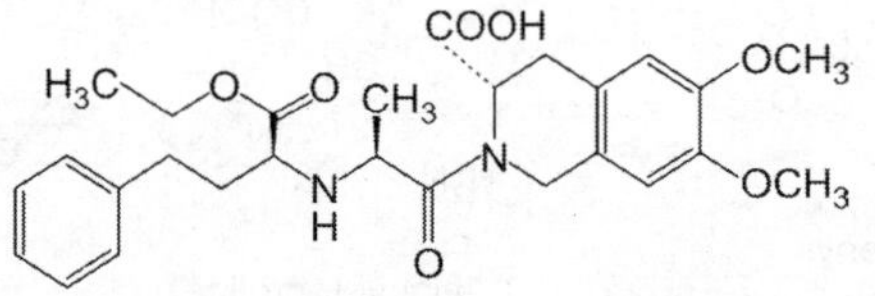
COOH
H3C
CH3
OCH3
OCH3

Synthesis

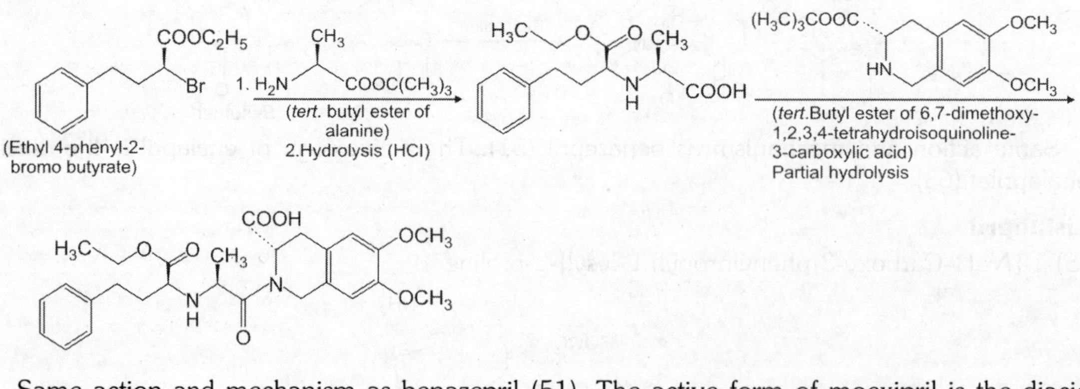
COOC2H5
Br
CH3
1. H2N
COOC(CH3)3
(tert. butyl ester of alanine)
2.Hydrolysis (HCl)
(Ethyl 4-phenyl-2-bromo butyrate)
H3C
CH3
COOH
(H3C)3COOC
HN
OCH3
OCH3
(tert.Butyl ester of 6,7-dimethoxy-1,2,3,4-tetrahydroisoquinoline-3-carboxylic acid)
Partial hydrolysis

Same action and mechanism as benazepril (51). The active form of moexipril is the diacid moexiprilat (64).

Quinapril

(*S*)-2-[(*S*)-*N*-[(*S*)-1-Carboxy-3-phenylpropyl] alanyl]-1, 2, 3, 4-tetrahydro-3-isoquinoline-carboxylic acid 1-ethylester

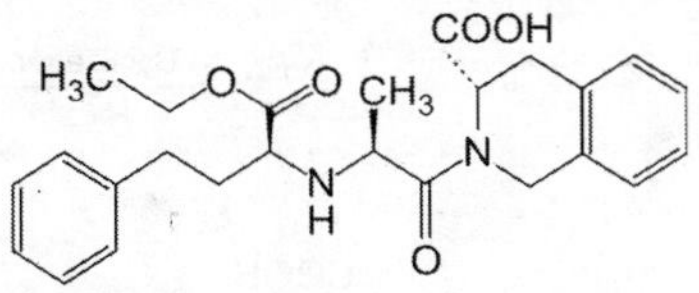
COOH
H3C
O
O
CH3
N
N
H
O

Synthesis

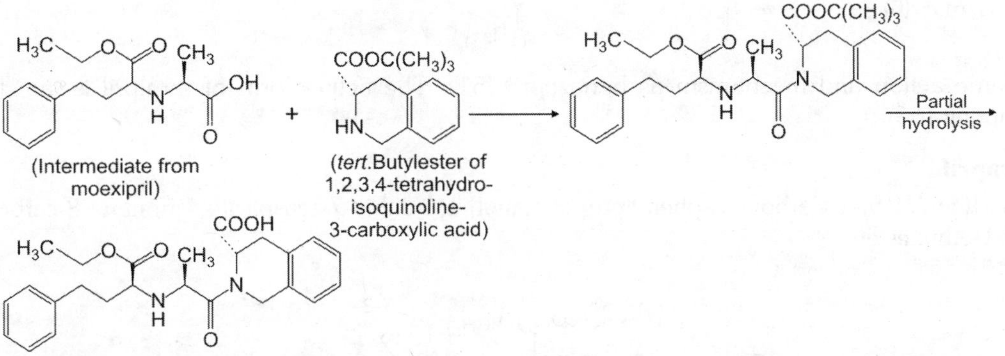
(Intermediate from moexipril)
(tert.Butylester of 1,2,3,4-tetrahydro-isoquinoline-3-carboxylic acid)
COOC(CH3)3
Partial hydrolysis
COOH

Same action and mechanism as benazepril (51). The active form of quinapril is the diacid quinaprilat (65).

Ramipril

(2*S*,3a*S*,6a*S*)-1-[(*S*)-*N*-[(*S*)-1-Carboxy-3-phenylpropyl] alanyl]octahydrocyclopenta[b]pyrrole-2-carboxylic acid 1-ethyl ester

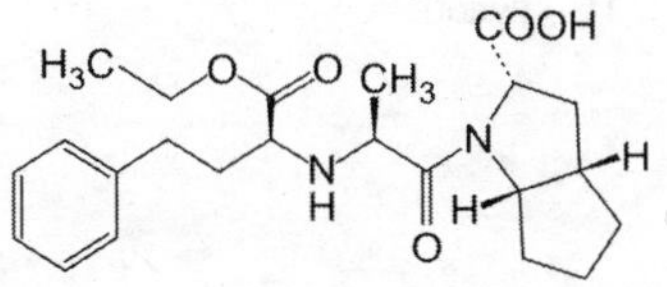
COOH
H3C
O
O
CH3
N
N
H
H
H
O

Synthesis

Step 1

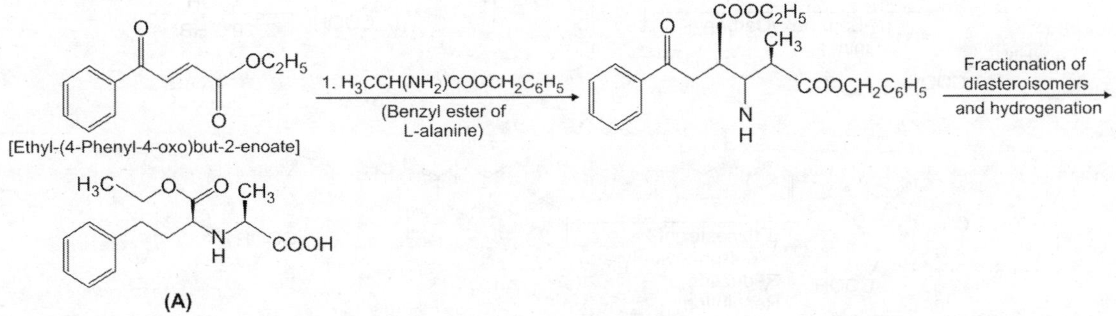
OC2H5
[Ethyl-(4-Phenyl-4-oxo)but-2-enoate]
1. H3CCH(NH2)COOCH2C6H5
(Benzyl ester of L-alanine)
COOC2H5
CH3
COOCH2C6H5
Fractionation of diasteroisomers and hydrogenation
COOH
(A)

Step 2

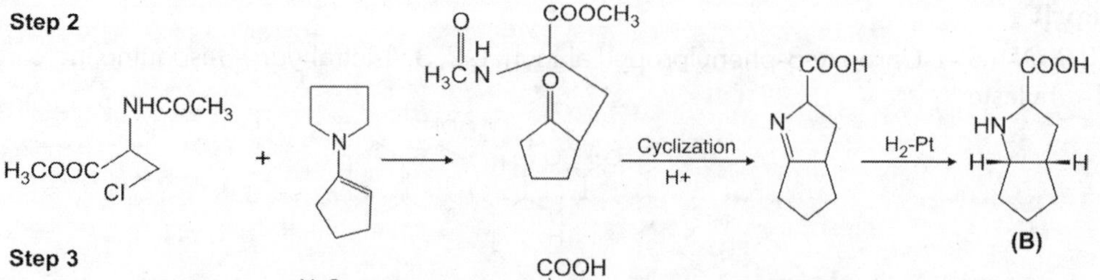

Step 3

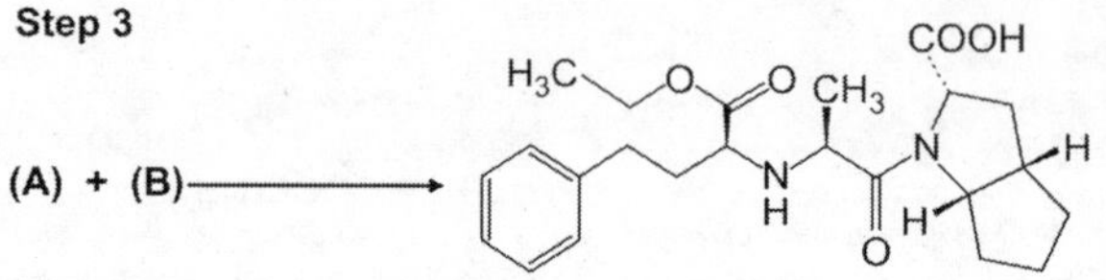

(A) + (B) ⟶

Same action and mechanism as benazepril (51). The active form of ramipril is the diacid ramiprilat (66).

Spirapril

[8S)-7[(S)-N-[(S)-1-Carboxy-3-phenylpropyl]alanyl]-1,4-dithia-7-azaspiro[4,4]nonane-8-carboxylic acid 1-ethyl ester

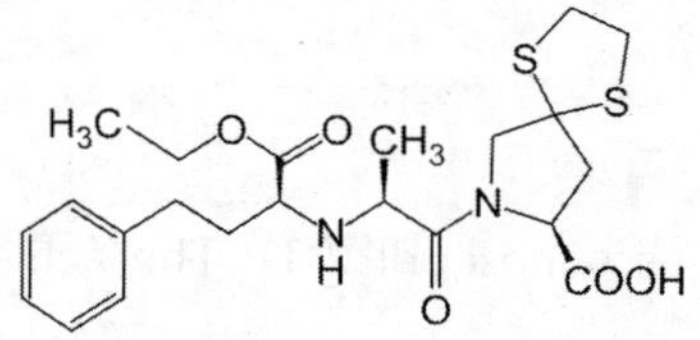

Synthesis

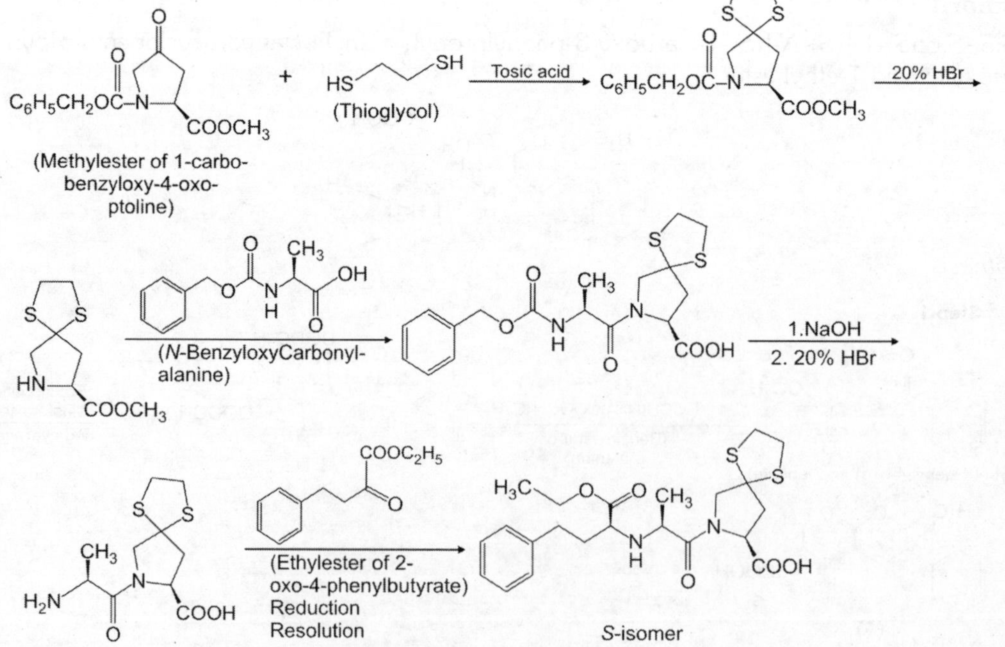

(Methylester of 1-carbo-
benzyloxy-4-oxo-
ptoline)

(Thioglycol)

(N-BenzyloxyCarbonyl-
alanine)

1.NaOH
2. 20% HBr

(Ethylester of 2-
oxo-4-phenylbutyrate)
Reduction
Resolution

S-isomer

Same action and mechanism as benazepril (51). The active form of spirapril is the diacid spiraprilat (67).

Perindopril

(2S,3aS,7aS)-1-[(S)-N-[(S)-1-Carboxybutyl]alanyl]hexahydro-2-indolinecarboxylic acid 1-ethyl ester

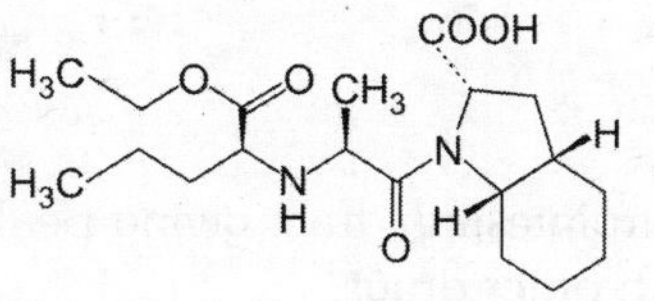

Synthesis

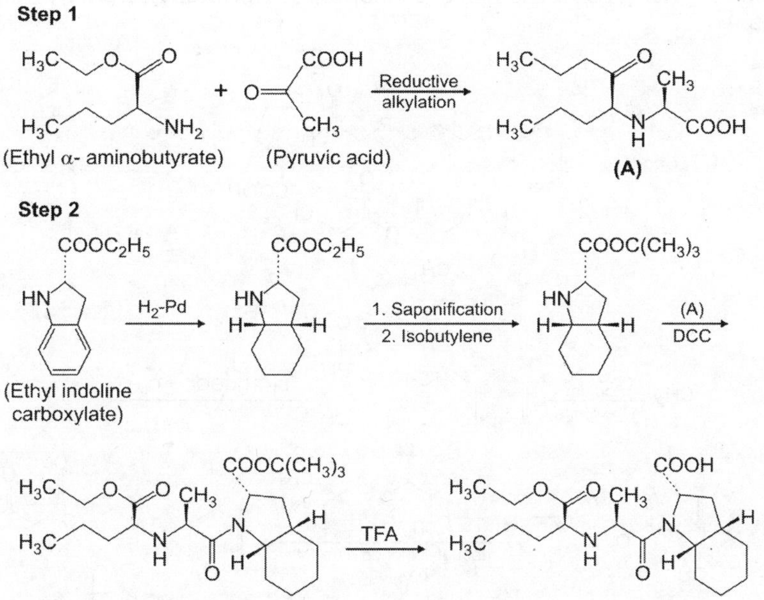

Step 1

(Ethyl α- aminobutyrate) (Pyruvic acid) (A)

Step 2

(Ethyl indoline carboxylate)

Same action and mechanism as benazepril (51). The active form of perindopril is the diacid perindoprilat (69).

Captopril

1-[(2S)-3-Mercapto-2-methyl-1-oxopropyl]-L-proline

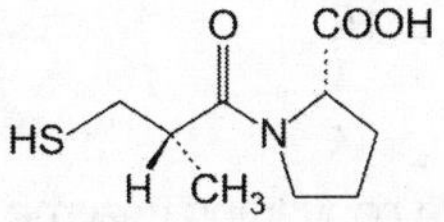

Synthesis

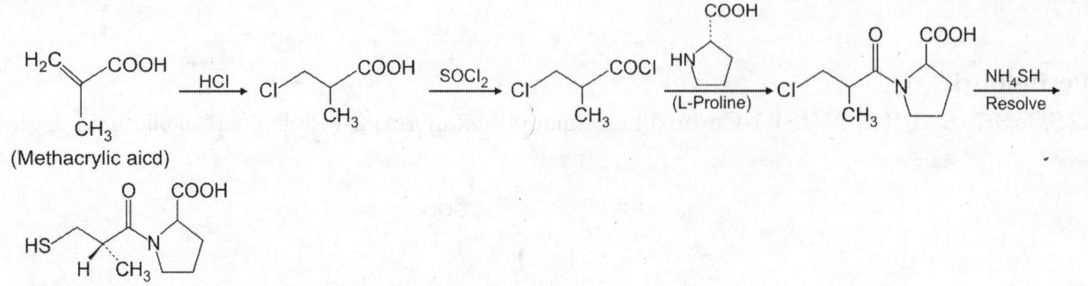

(Methacrylic aicd)   (L-Proline)

It is rapidly absorbed from gastrointestinal tract giving peak plasma concentrations within an hour. It is used in combination with other drugs.

Fosinopril

(4S)-4-Cyclohexyl-1-[[(R)-[(1S)-2-methyl-1-(1-oxopropoxy)propoxy](4-phenylbutyl) phosphinyl]-acetyl]-L-proline

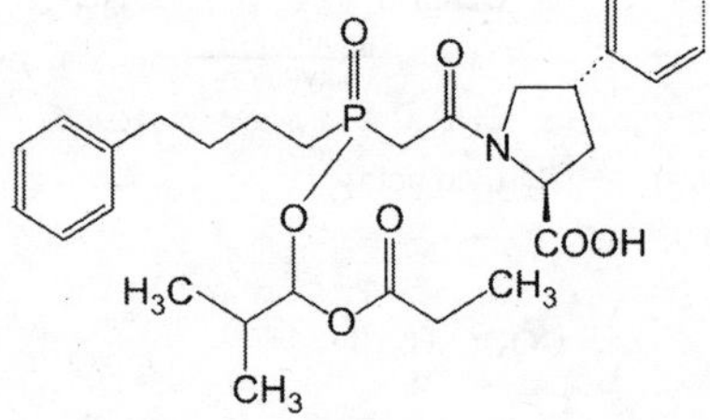

Synthesis

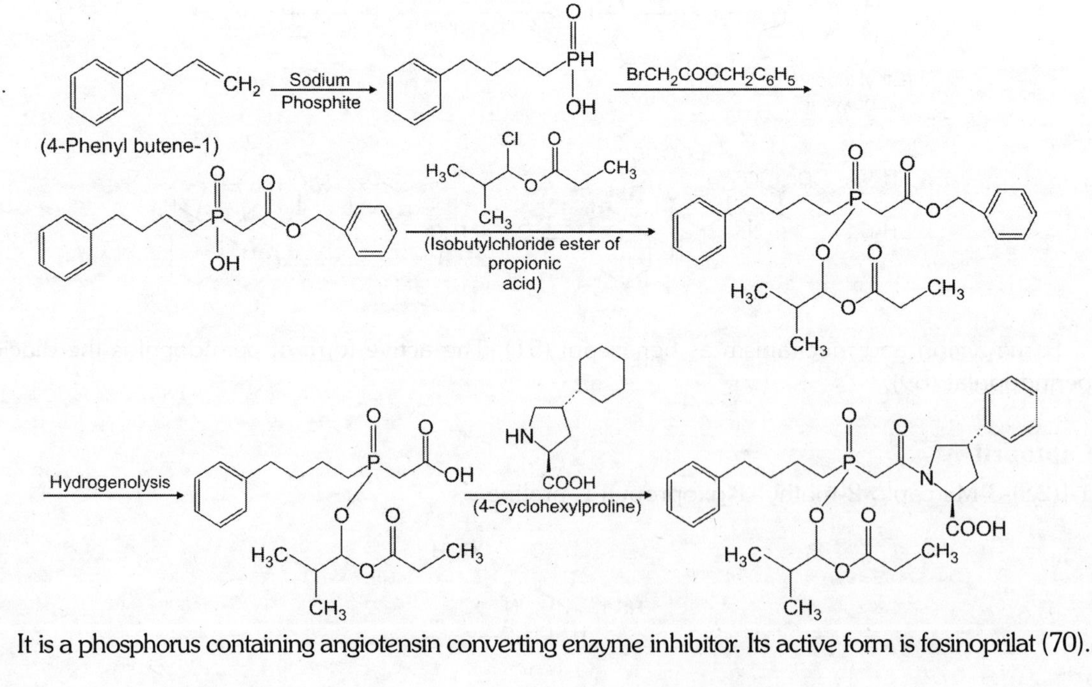

(4-Phenyl butene-1)

(Isobutylchloride ester of propionic acid)

(4-Cyclohexylproline)

It is a phosphorus containing angiotensin converting enzyme inhibitor. Its active form is fosinoprilat (70).

ANGIOTENSIN II RECEPTOR ANTAGONISTS
Candesartan

2-Ethoxy-1-[[2'-(1*H*-tetrazol-5-yl)(1,1'-biphenyl]-4-yl]methyl]-1*H*-benzimdazole-7-carboxylic acid

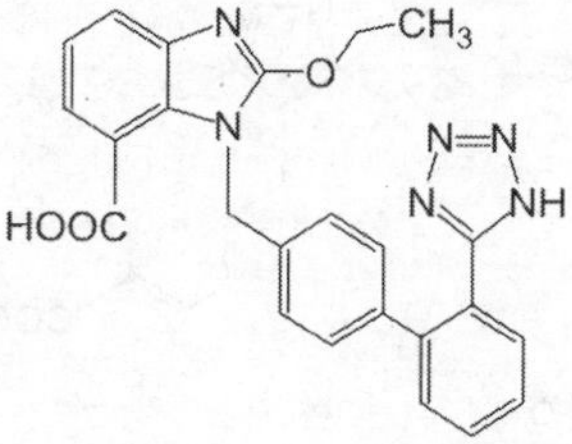

Synthesis

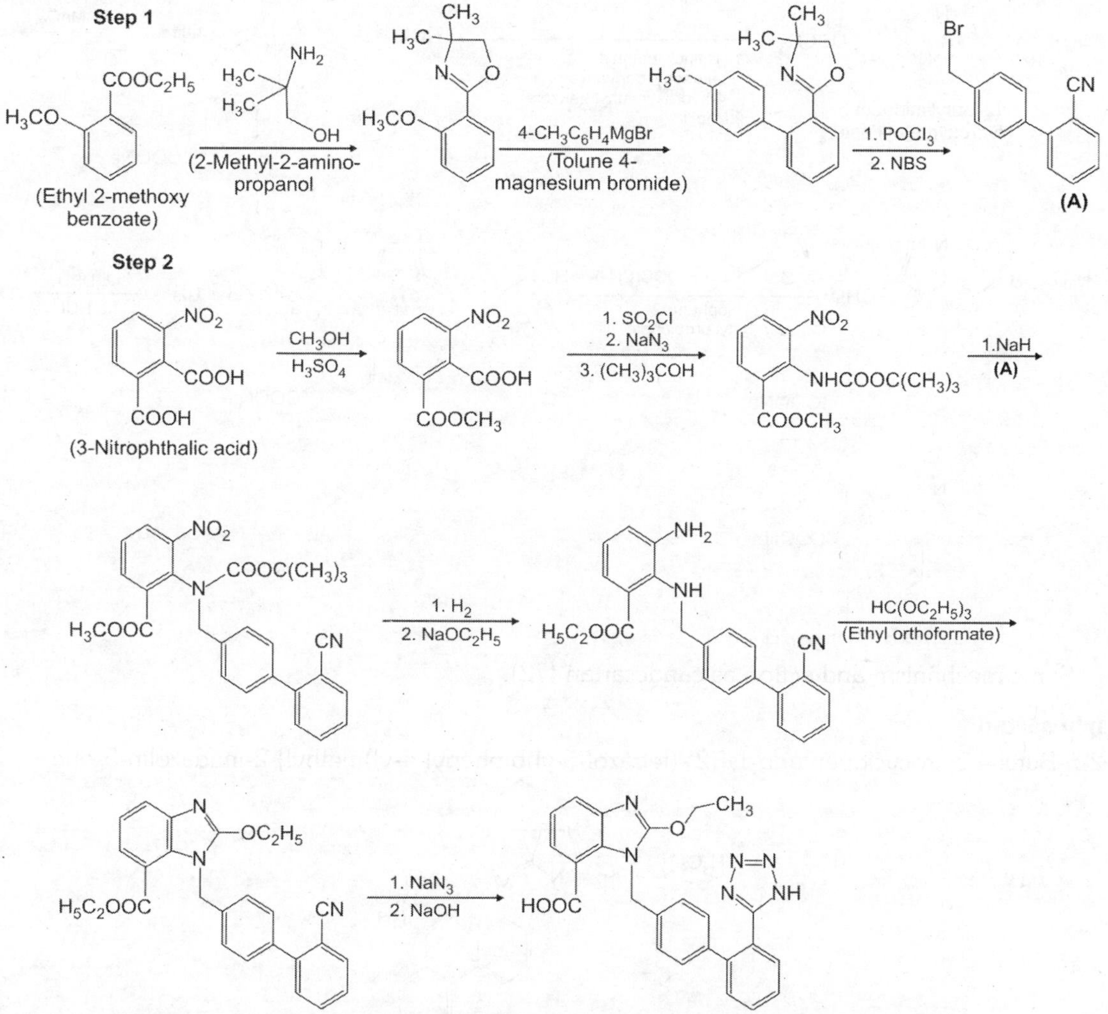

Step 1

Step 2

It is a competitive blocker of angiotensin II receptor blocking AT_1 subtype receptor.

Eprosartan

(*E*)-3-[2-Butyl-1-[(4-carboxyphenyl)-methyl]-imidazol-5-yl]-2-(2-thienylmethyl)-2-propenoic acid

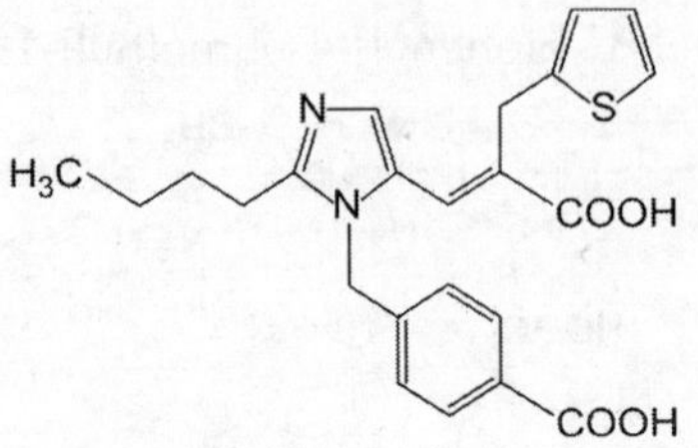

Synthesis

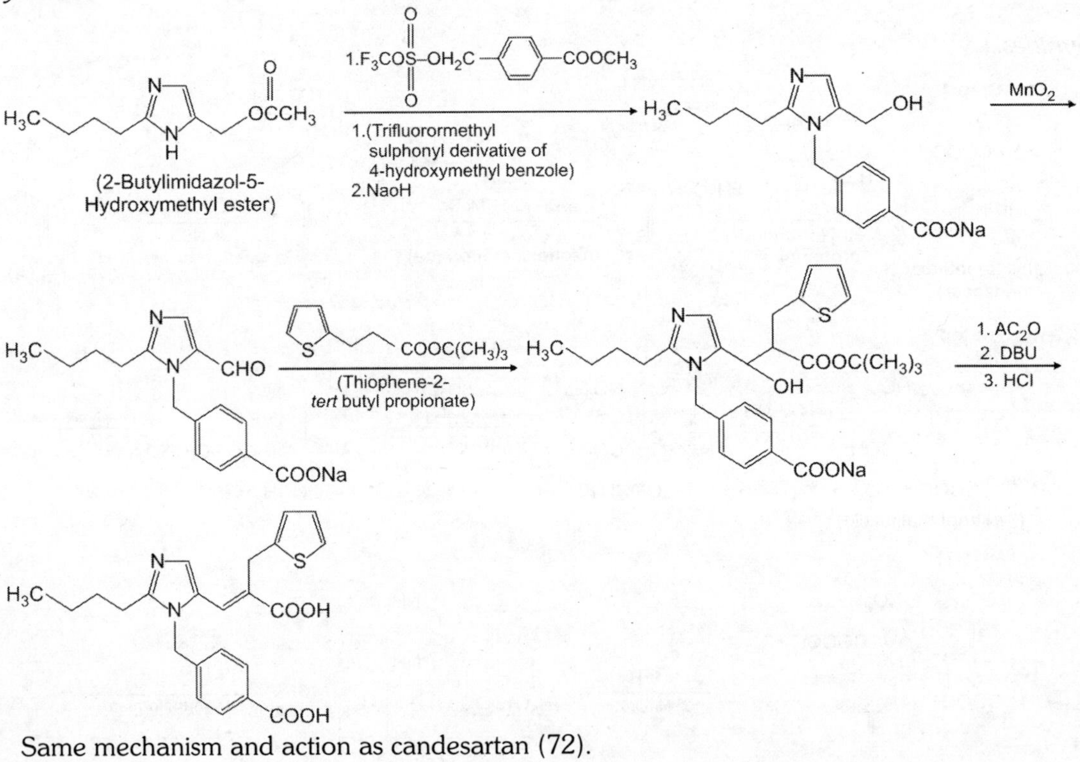

(2-Butylimidazol-5-
Hydroxymethyl ester)

1.(Trifluorormethyl
  sulphonyl derivative of
  4-hydroxymethyl benzole)
2.NaoH

(Thiophene-2-
tert butyl propionate)

1. AC₂O
2. DBU
3. HCl

Same mechanism and action as candesartan (72).

Irbesartan

2-*n*-Butyl-4-spirocyclopentane-1-[(2'-(tetrazol-5-yl)biphenyl-4-yl)methyl]-2-imidazolin-5-one

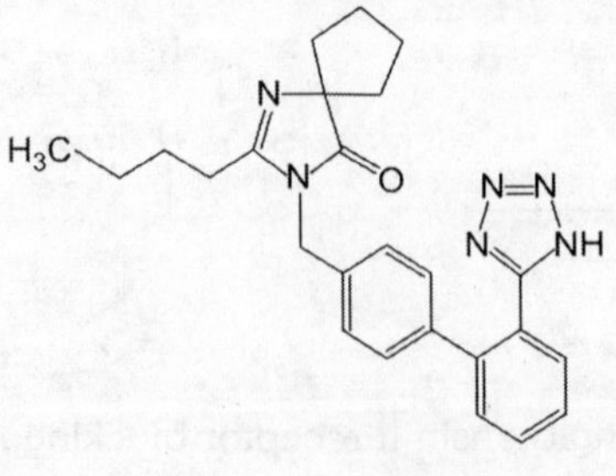

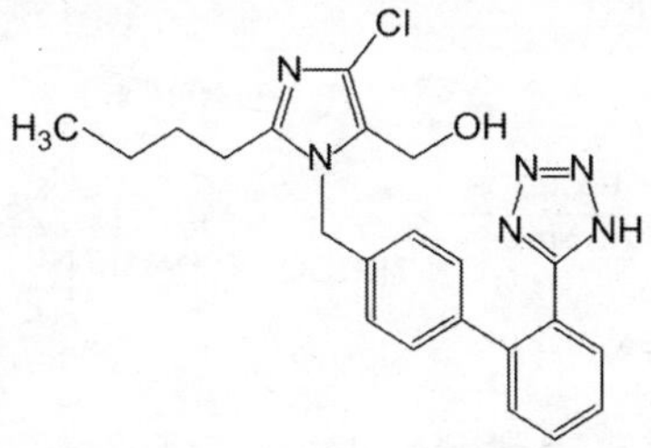

Synthesis

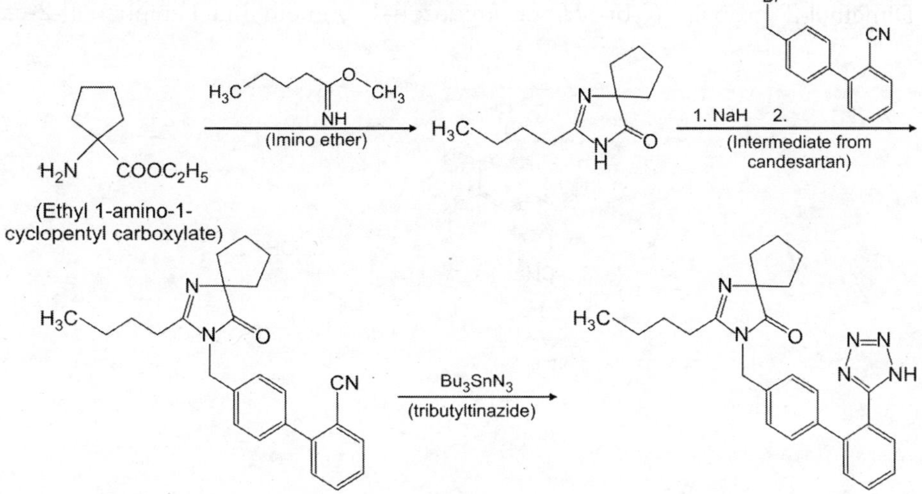

Same mechanism and action as candesartan (72).

Losartan

2-*n*-Butyl-4-chloro-1-[[2'(1*H*-tetrazol-5-yl)[1,1'-biphenyl]-4-yl]methyl]-1-*H*-imidazol-5-methanol

Synthesis

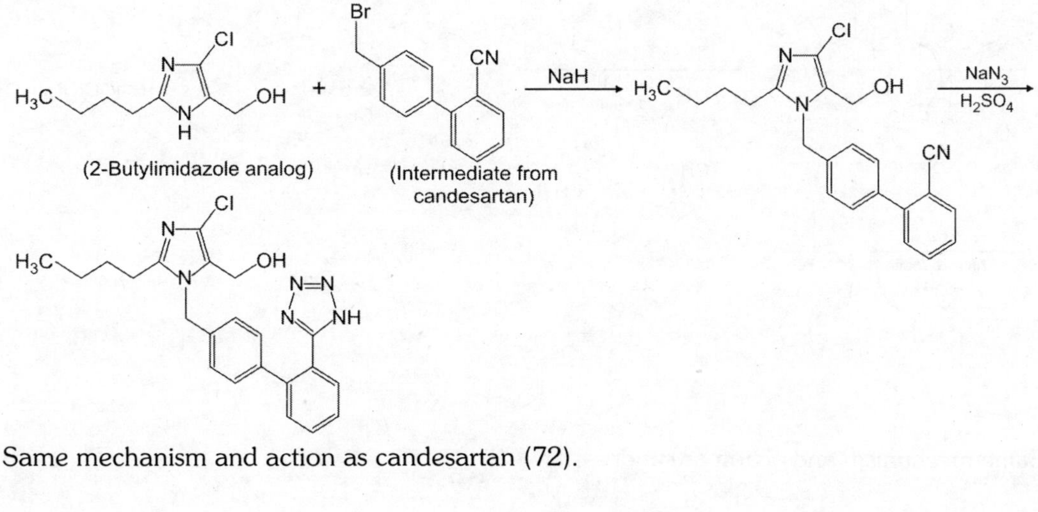

(2-Butylimidazole analog)　　(Intermediate from candesartan)

Same mechanism and action as candesartan (72).

Telmisartan

4'-[(1,4'-Dimethyl-2'-propyl[2,6'-bi-1H-benzimidazol]-1'-yl)methyl][1,1'-biphenyl]-2-carboxylic acid

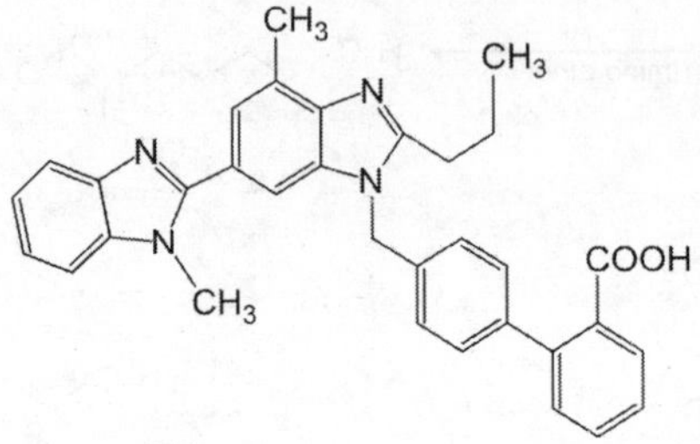

Synthesis

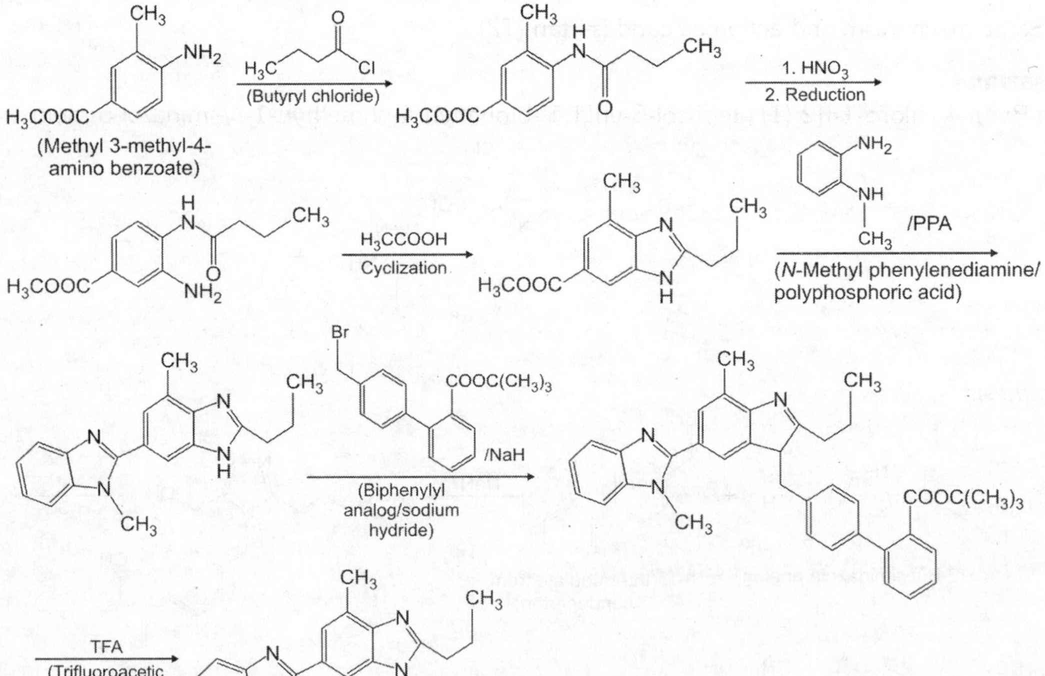

Same mechanism and action as candesartan (72).

Valsartan

(S)-N-(1-Carboxy-2-methylprop-1-yl)-N-pentanoyl-N-[2'-(1H-tetrazol-5-yl)-biphenyl-4-ylmethyl]amine

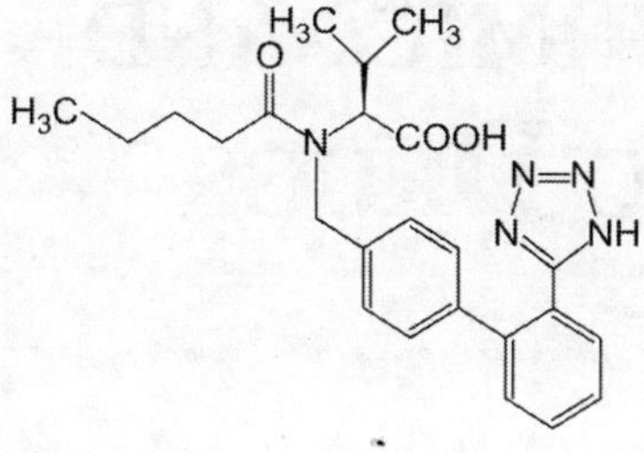

Synthesis

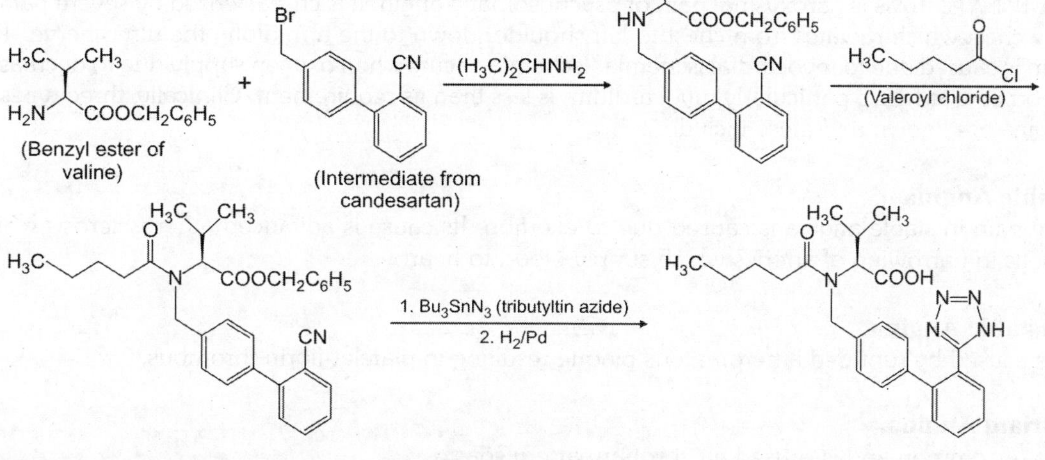

Same mechanism and action as candesartan (72).

CHAPTER 15

ANTIANGINAL, ANTIARRHYTHMIC, AND CARDIOTONIC DRUGS

ANTIANGINAL DRUGS

ANGINA PECTORIS is paroxysmal pain of psychosomatic origin. It is characterized by severe pain in chest which radiates from chest to left shoulder down to the arm along the ulnar nerve. The pain is caused due to myocardial ischemia. Ischemia occurs when oxygen supply due to decreased blood flow to heart, particularly myocardium, is less than its requirement. Clinically, three types of angina are known and these include:

Stable Angina
The pain in stable angina is caused due to exertion. Its cause is advanced atherosclerosis which results in narrowing of arteries which supply blood to heart.

Unstable Angina
It is caused by ruptured atheromatous plaque resulting in platelet-fibrin thrombus.

Variant Angina
It is uncommon and is caused by coronary artery spasm.

The treatment for anginal attacks is directed towards the increased blood flow through the use of vasodilators such as organic nitrates, decreased heart rate and contraction through the use of calcium antagonists, β-adrenoreceptor blockers, together with the treatment for atheromatous deposits, and antiplatelet drugs such as aspirin.

The drugs used for angina include:

1. Organic nitrites and nitrates,
2. calcium channel blockers,
3. β-adrenergic receptor blocking agents, and
4. modulators of myocardial metabolism.

Organic Nitrites and Nitrates
These include esters of nitrous acid and nitric acid with alcohols. Some of these are amyl nitrite (1), nitrogycerin (2), erythrityl tetranitrate (3), pentaerythritol tetranitrate (4), tenitramine (5), propatyl nitrate (6), and isosorbide dinitrate (7).

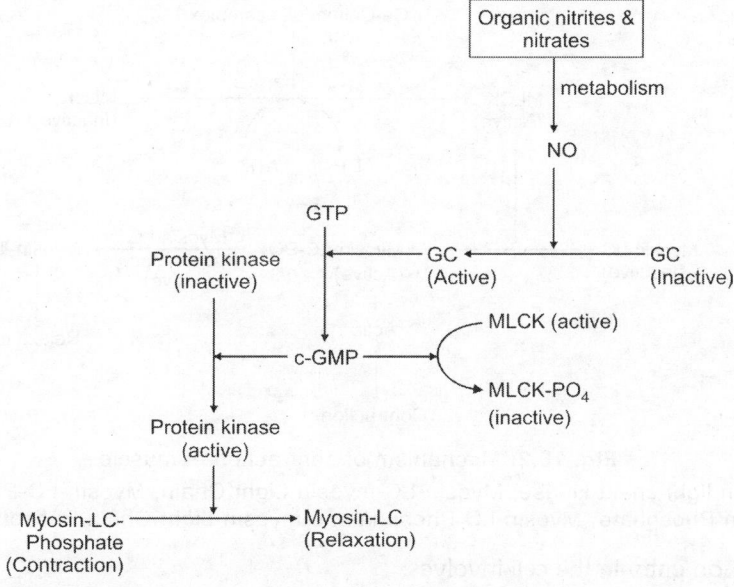

For longer duration of action and higher activity, higher lipophilicity seems to be essential.

The tissue sulphydryl containing enzymes act on organic nitrites and nitrates and give nitric oxide (NO). In smooth muscles, NO activates gaunylate cyclase (GC). The activated GC converts gaunosine triphosphate (GTP) to cyclic gaunosine monophosphate (c-GMP) which phosphorylates myosin light chain kinase (MLCK). Phosphorylation of MLCK results in its inactivation and consequent smooth muscle relaxation, c-GMP also activates protein kinase that leads ultimately to dephosphorylation of myosin light chain (Myosin-LC) and sequestration of intracellular Ca^{2+} (Fig. 15.1).

Fig. 15.1: Events leading to smooth muscle relaxation following administration of organic nitrites and nitrates. (NO-nitric oxide; GC-gaunylate cyclase; GTP-gaunosine triphosphate; c-GMP-cyclic gaunosine monophosphate; MLCK-myosin light chain kinase; MLCK-Po4-myosin light chain kinase phosphate; Myosin-LC-myosin light chain; Myosin-LC-phosphate-myosin light chain phosphate.)

Molsidomine (8), a syndone, produces vascular smooth muscle relaxation by generating nitric oxide, like organic nitrites and nitrates, after it is converted to linsodimine (9), the active form, by esterases. The linsodimine (9) is than converted to nitroso metabolite SIN-1A (10). Nitric oxide is generated from SIN-1A (10) after reaction with molecular oxygen.

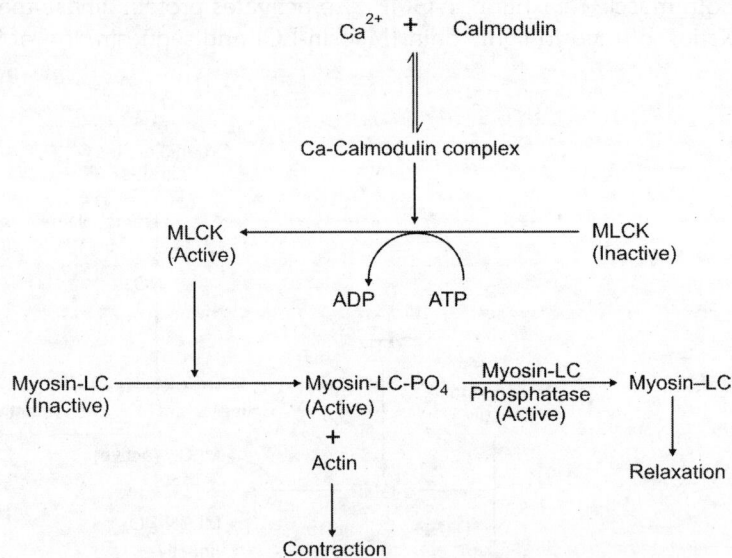

Calcium Channel Blockers

Calcium ion is involved in many processes of short-time duration which include excitation contraction and secretion. The mechanism of contraction by calcium ion involves complexation of calcium ion with calmodulin. This complex activates myosin light chain kinase (MLCK), which in turn phosphorylates myosin. The myosin phosphate then combines with actin which results in contraction of muscle (Fig. 15.2).

Fig. 15.2: Mechanism of contraction of muscle.
(MLCK-myosin light chain kinase; Myosin-LC-myosin Light Chain; Myosin-LC-PO$_4$-myosin Light Chain Phosphate; Myosin-LC Phosphatase-myosin Light Chain Phosphatase.)

The calcium ion entry in the cell involves:

(a) Voltage gated calcium channels,
(b) ligand gated calcium channels,
(c) Na$^+$-Ca^{2+} exchange, and
(d) store-operated calcium channels.

They are located in different parts. Four types of voltage gated Ca^{2+} channel have been identified and include L-type, located in cardiac and smooth muscle and responsible for contraction of these muscles. N-type of ion channel, which are found in neurons and responsible for transmitter release. T-type of channel found in pacemaker cells and P-type are located in Purkinje cells, their functions are not known yet.

Ligand gated Ca^{2+} channels are activated by excitatory neurotransmitters. They are relatively non-selective and conduct other ions including Ca^{2+}.

Store operated Ca^{2+} channels occur in plasma membrane and operate when endoplasmic retriculum Ca^{2+} stores are depleted.

The mechanism of excitation-contraction coupling in cardiac muscle involves opening of L-type of channel and entry of Ca^{2+}. These Ca^{2+} act on ryanodine receptors to release Ca^{2+} from sarcoplasmic reticulum. The released Ca^{2+} combine with troponin to give troponin-Ca^{2+} complex which results in contraction of heart muscle.

The calcium channel blockers act on L-channel, which is made up of 5 different subunits α_1, α_2, β, γ, and δ. The subunit form the central pore of the calcium ion channel. It is to these units that calcium channel blockers bind and then inactivate the channel and do not allow the channel to open. Examples of these blockers are amlodipine (11), felodipine (12), isradipine (13), nicardipine (14), nifedipine (15), nimodipine (16), bepridil (17), dilitiazem (18), and verapamil (19).

(11)

(12)

(13)

(14)

(15)

(16)

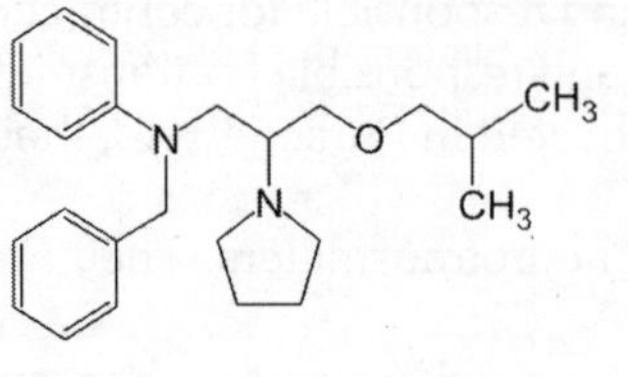

(17)

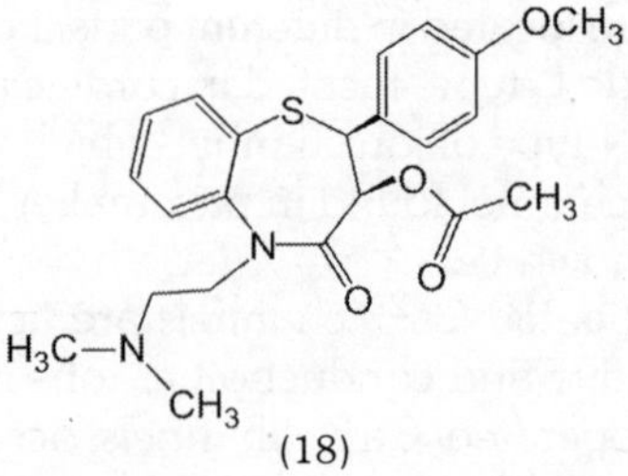

(18)

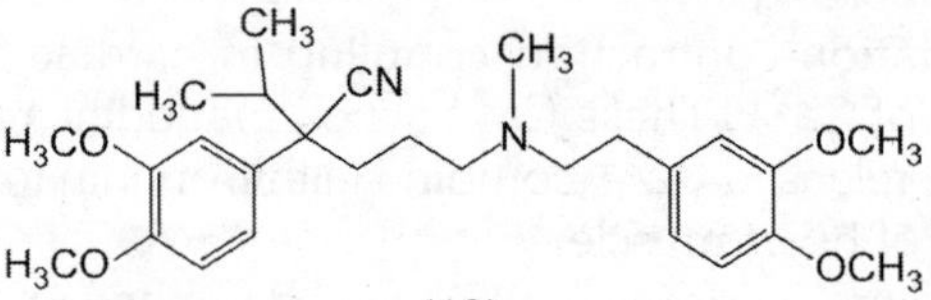

(19)

β-Adrenergic Receptor Blocking Agents

These agents are used in exertion-induced angina. Some of these blockers used in angina include atenolol (20), metoprolol (21), propranolol (22), and timolol (23). They are used either alone or in combination with other classes of antianginal drugs such as calcium channel blockers.

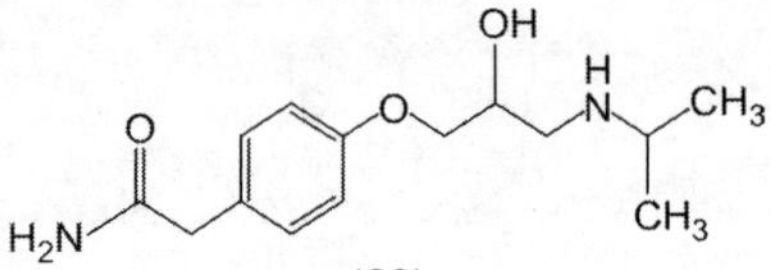

(20)

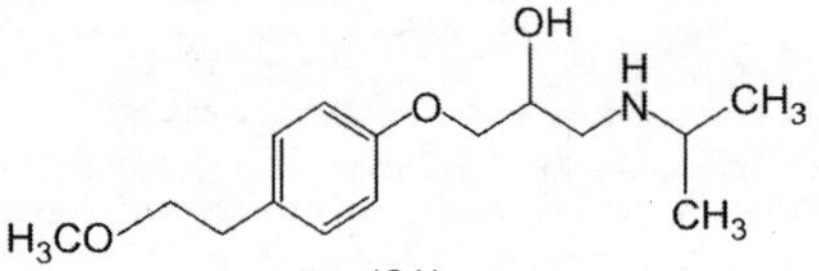

(21)

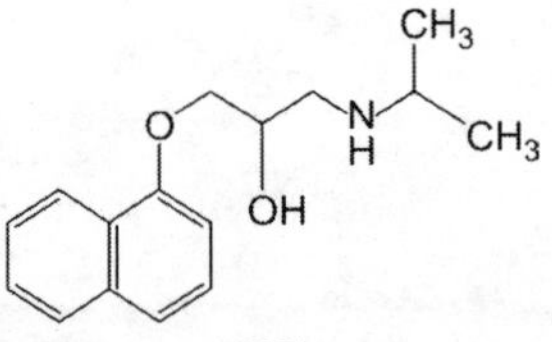

(22)

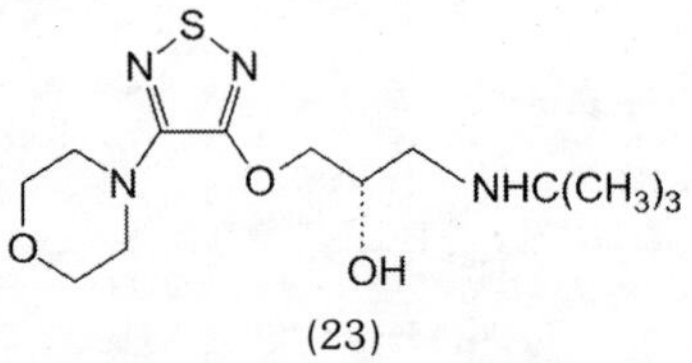

(23)

Modulators of Myocardial Metabolism

Ranolazine (24) in combination with calcium channel blockers, β-blockers, or nitrates has been found effective in patients with chronic stable angina. The exact mechanism of ranolazine (24) is not known. It seems to inhibit the free fatty acid oxidation and increase the glucose oxidation thus generating more ATP per molecule of oxygen. It also inhibits late Na^+ current which reduces the energy required for myocardial repolarization.

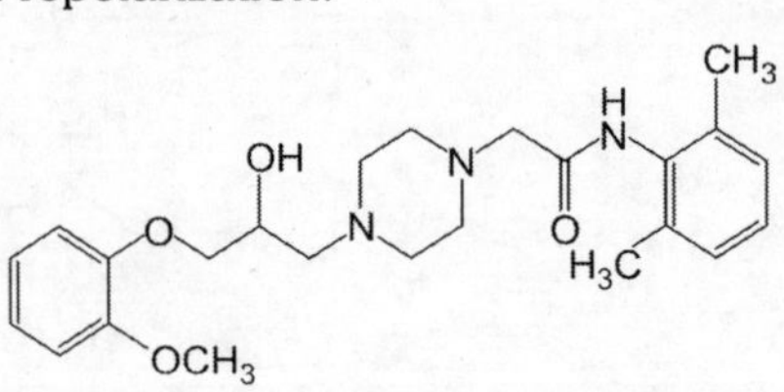

(24)

ANTIARRHYTHMIC DRUGS

The normal cardiac contraction is initiated by the electrical impulse which originates in the sinoatrial (SA) node or pacemaker cells. The electrical impulse spreads rapidly through atria and then enters atrioventricular node. The impulse then propagates over the His-Purkinje system and spreads all over the ventricle. Contraction of ventricular muscle is synchronous and hemodynamically effective. When the initiation and propagation of cardiac impulse deviates from above, arrhythmias result. It is manifested in abnormality in rate, in the site from where the impulse originates, or in conduction of the impulse. Some of the causes responsible for arrhythmias include:

1. Malfunctioning of pacemaker cells.
2. Blockade of impulse transmission through atreoventricular node.
3. Diseases like atherosclerosis or hyperthyroidism or myocardial ischemia.
4. The electrical signals may originate from cells other than pacemaker cells and then compete with the normal impulses. Such arrhythmias are known as ectopic.
5. An electrical impulse may not die out after firing but continues to circulate and re-excite the resting heart cells, resulting in re-entrant rhythms. This phenomenon which is called reentry, is found in coronary atherosclerosis.

Antiarrhythmic drugs have been classified on the basis of their electrophysiological effect and include class I to class IV drugs.

Class I Drugs
These have been further classified into:

Class Ia drugs and include quinidine (25), procainamide (26), and disopyramide (27).

Class Ib drugs include lignocaine (28), phenytoin (29), tocainide (30), and mexiletine (31).

Class Ic drugs include flecainide (32), encainide (33), propafenone (34), and moricizine (35).

(25)   (26)   (27)

(28)   (29)   (30)   (31)

(32)

(33)

(34)

(35)

Class I drugs act on nerve and myocardial membrane to slow conduction by inhibiting phase O of action potential. This they do by blocking the sodium channels. These drugs reduce the maximum rate of depolarization. They also increase the threshold of the excitability, decrease conduction velocity, and decrease polarization in pacemaker cells. They increase the effective refractory period and decrease conduction velocity. Increase of the refractory periods tends to abolish re-entry arrhythmia.

Class II Drugs

Class II antiarrhythmic drugs include β-adrenergic blocking agents such as propranolol (22). They block the role of sympathetic nervous system in genesis of certain cardiac arrhythmias such as ventricular arrhythmias. Similarly sympathetic activity is also responsible for AV conduction and β-blockers increase the refractory period of AV node.

Class III Drugs

The drugs belonging to this class act by prolonging the cardiac action potential. This they do by blocking some of the potassium channels involved in cardiac repolarization. Prolongation of action potential increases the refractory period. The drugs in this category include amiodarone (36), bretylium tosylate (37), dofetilide (38), ibutilide (39), sotalol (40), and azimilide (41).

(36)

(37)

(38)

(39)

(40)

(41)

Class IV Drugs

These include calcium channel blockers. They act on L-type of calcium channels. They slow conduction of sinoatrial and atrioventricular nodes. These effects block the conduction of premature impulses of AV node and thus are effective in preventing supraventricular arrhythmias. The drugs include diltiazem (18) and verapamil (19).

CARDIOTONIC DRUGS

These include:

1. Cardiac glycosides.
2. Phosphodiesterase inhibitors.
3. Drugs that increase calcium ion sensitivity to myocardium contractile proteins.
4. Adenylyl cyclase stimulants.
5. β-Adrenergic receptor stimulants.

Cardiac Glycosides

Cardiac glycosides are a class of steroidal glycosides which when injected have the ability to exert a powerful and specific action on cardiac muscles. When used in small amounts they exert a beneficial stimulation of diseased heart, but in excessive doses cause death in systole. They are used in congestive heart failure and associated edema.

Cardiac glycosides are found in plants and animals. In plants, they occur in almost every part, i.e seeds, leaves, stems, root, or bark. The cardiac glycoside bearing plants belong to the families *Apocynaceae, Scrophulariaceae, Liliaceae, Moraceae,* and *Ranunculaceae.* Some of the important sources of cardiac glycosides include, digitalis, squill, and strophanthus. Cardiac glycosides are made up of sugar component and aglycone portion which is steroidal. Some of the sugars found in cardiac glycoside include D-glucose (42), L-rhamnose (43), D-digitoxose (44), D-fucose (45), L-talomethylose (46), D-antiarose (47), D-allomethylose (48), D-thevetose (49), D-digitalose (50), L-acovenose (51), L-acofriose (52), D-cymarose (53), D-sarmentose (54), L-oleandrose (55), D-diginose (56), and D-boivinose (57).

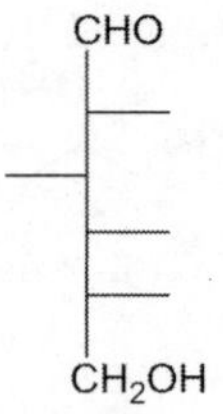

CHO   CHO   CHO   CHO   CHO   CHO

CH₂OH   CH₃   CH₃   CH₃   CH₃   CH₃

(42) 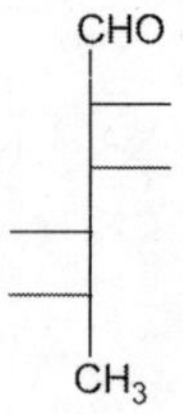   (43) 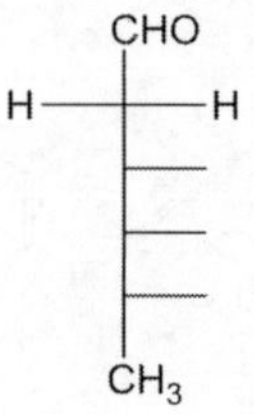   (44) 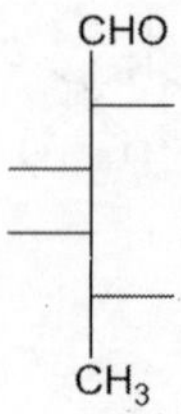   (45) 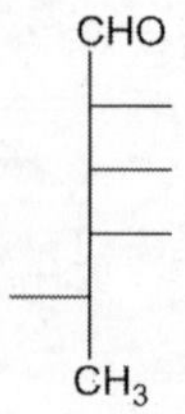   (46) 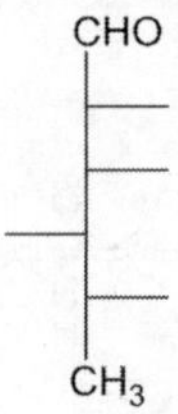   (47)

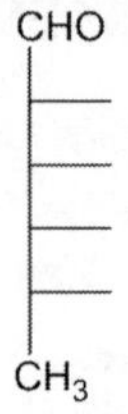

CHO   CHO   CHO   CHO   CHO   CHO

CH₃   CH₃   CH₃   CH₃   CH₃   CH₃

(48) 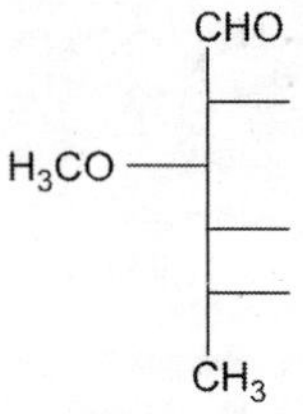   (49) 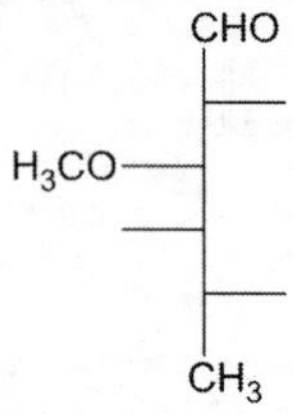   (50) 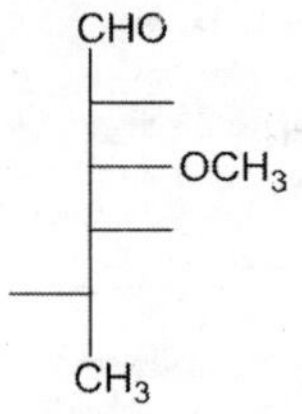   (51) 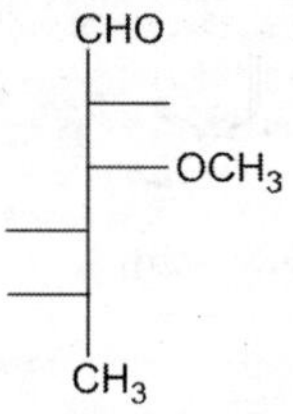   (52) 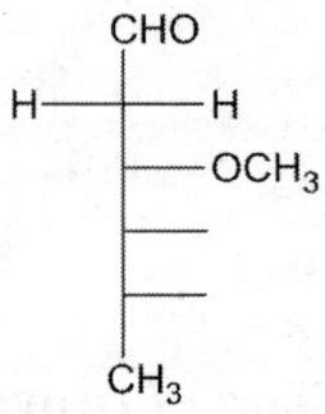   (53)

CHO   CHO   CHO   CHO

CH₃   CH₃   CH₃   CH₃

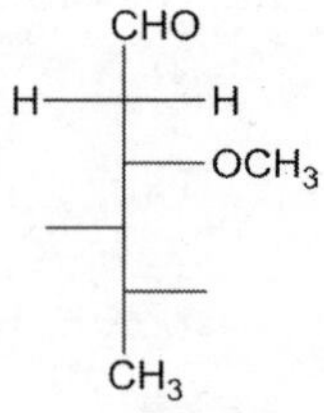

(54) 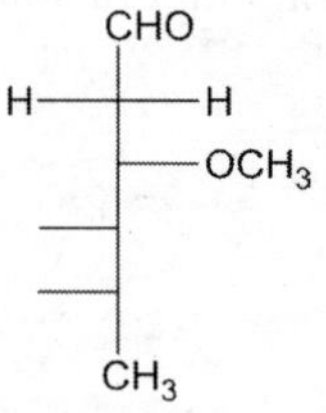   (55) 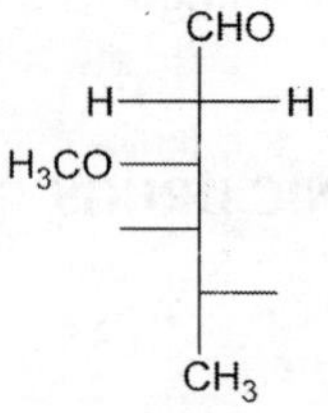   (56) 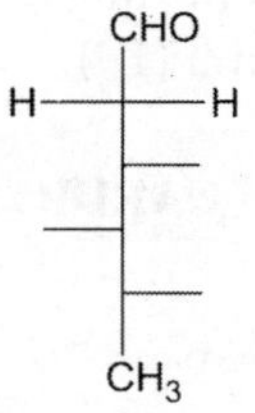   (57)

The aglycone part is of two types called cardenolide (58) and bufadienolide (59). A cardenolide (58) has a five-membered unsaturated lactone ring at position 17 and bufadienolide (59) a six-membered lactone ring with two double bonds. The rings A/B and C/D are *cis*-fused and rings B/C *trans*-fused. The other important features include a 3β-hydroxyl and or 14β-hydroxyl groups. In addition to these hydroxyl groups, there can be hydroxyl groups at other positions also. The 3β-hydroxyl group is involved in the glycosidal linkage.

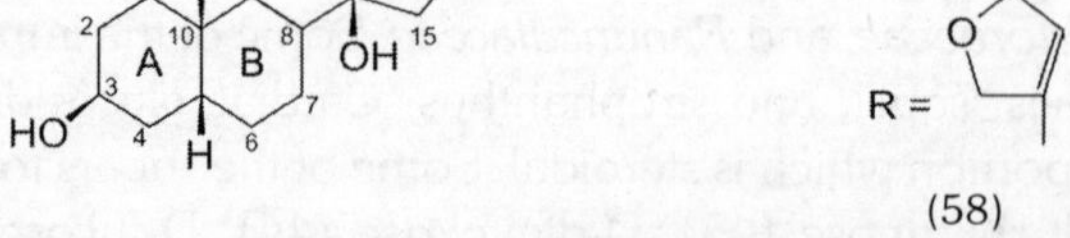

(58)

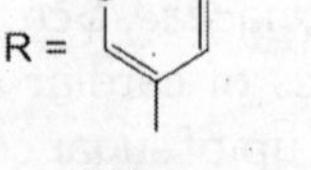

(59)

Cardenolides occur as plant glycosides and bufadienolide are found in both plants and animals. Some of the cardiac glycosides together with the structure of their aglycones and sugar moieties are given in Table 15.1.

Table 15.1: Cardiac glycosides and their aglycones

Glycoside	*Aglycone*

Source: Digitalis species

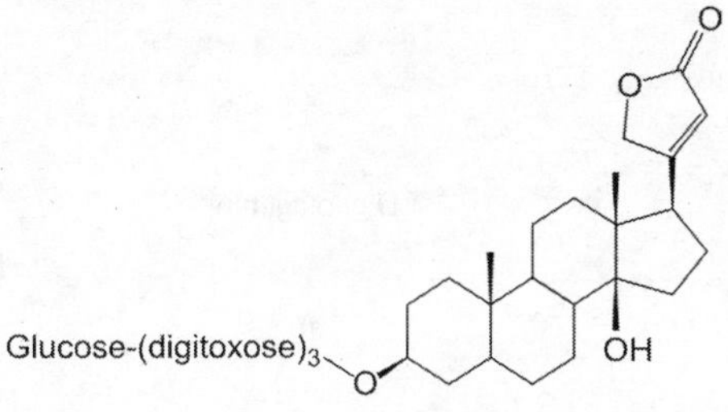

Glucose-(digitoxose)$_3$-O

(Purpurea glycoside A)

HO

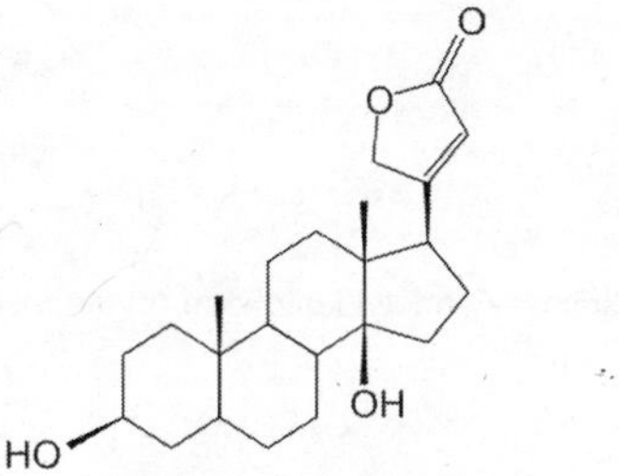

(Digitoxigenin)

(Digitoxose)$_3$-O

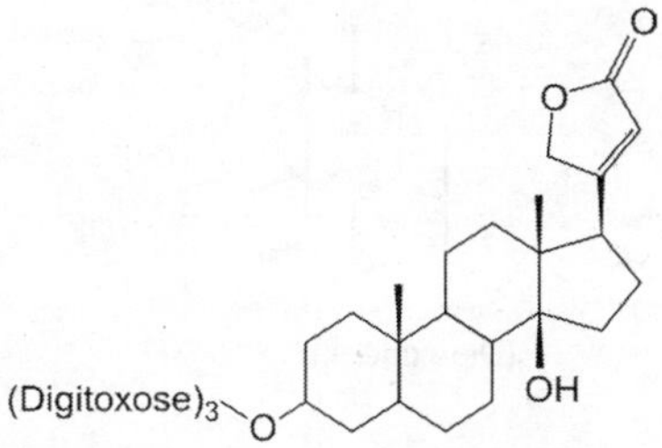

(Digitoxin)

Digitoxigenin

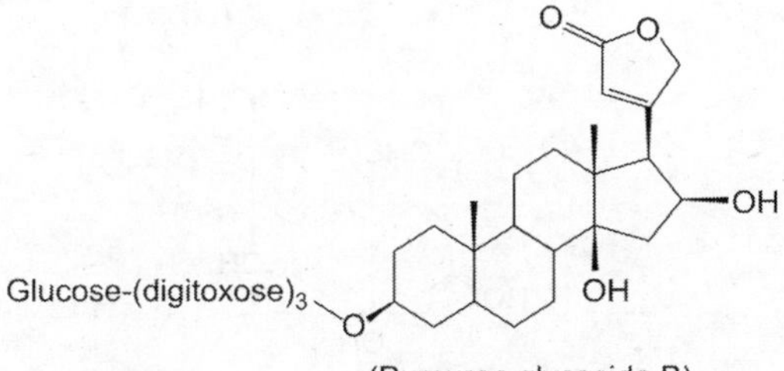

Glucose-(digitoxose)$_3$-O

(Purpurea glycoside B)

HO

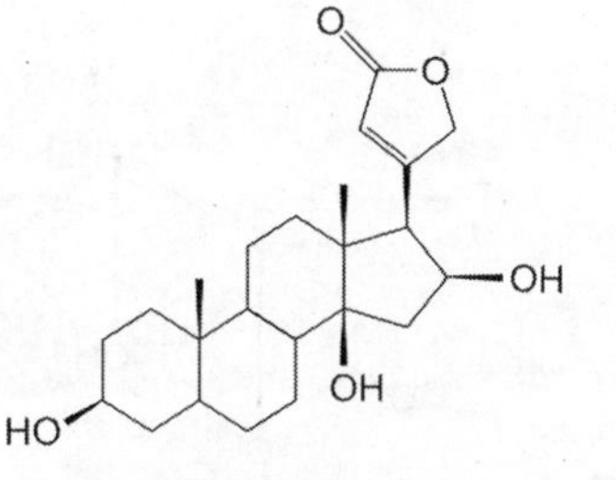

(Gitoxigenin)

(Digitoxose)$_3$-O

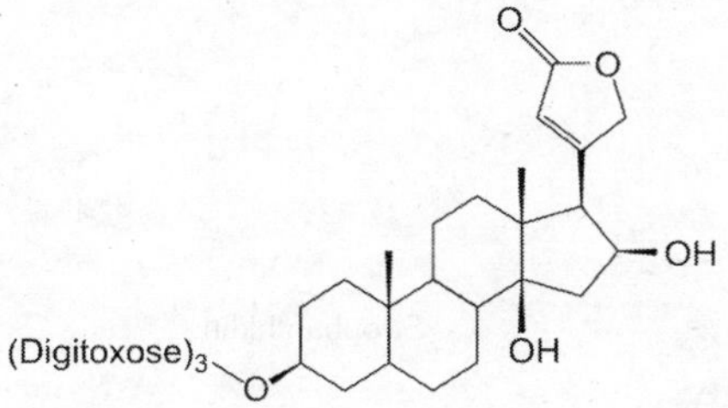

(Gitoxin)

Gitoxigenin

Contd.

Table 15.1: Cardiac glycosides and their aglycones (Contd.)

Glycoside	Aglycone

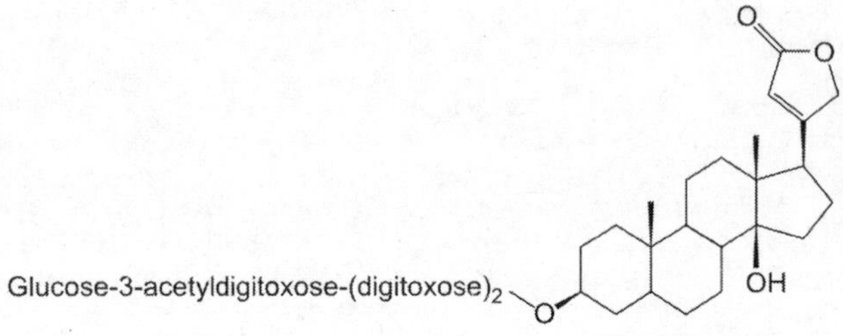

Glucose-3-acetyldigitoxose-(digitoxose)$_2$—O

(Lenatoside A)

Digitoxigenin

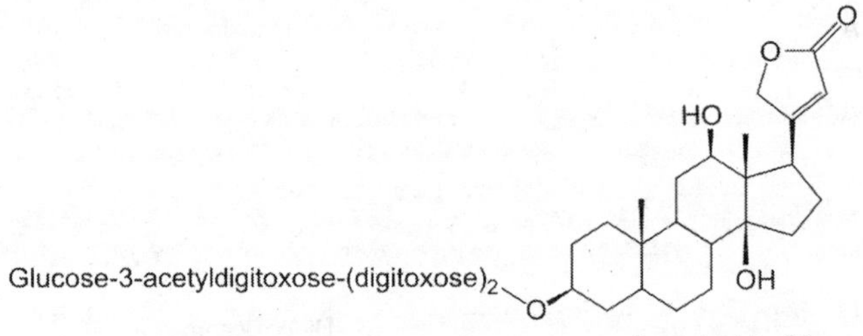

Glucose-3-acetyldigitoxose-(digitoxose)$_2$—O

(Lanatoside C)

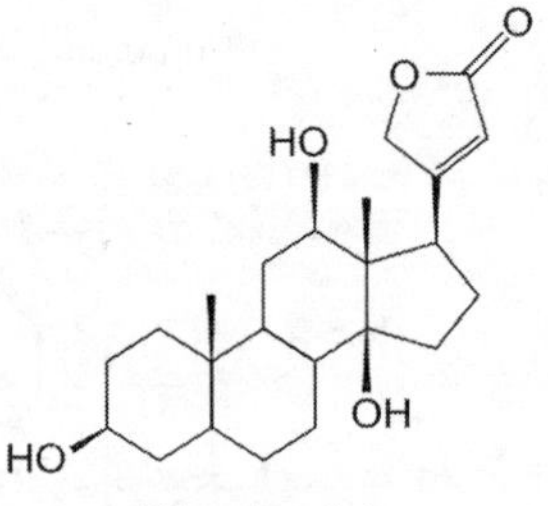

(Digoxigenin)

Source: Strophanthus species

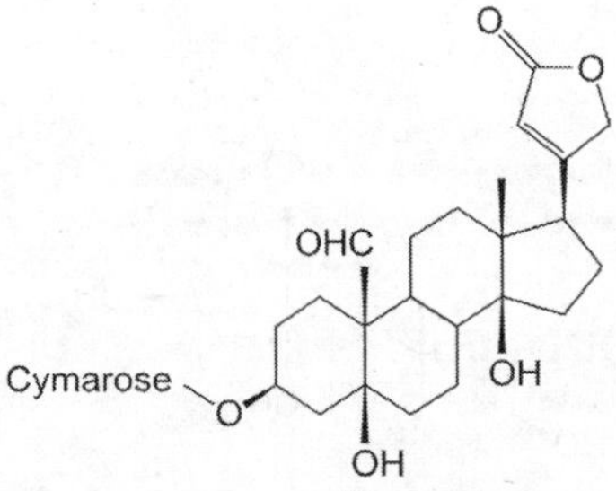

Cymarose—O

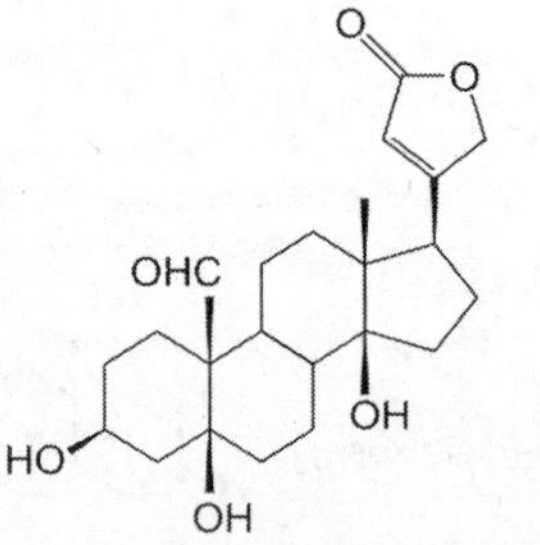

(Cymarin)

(Strophanthidin)

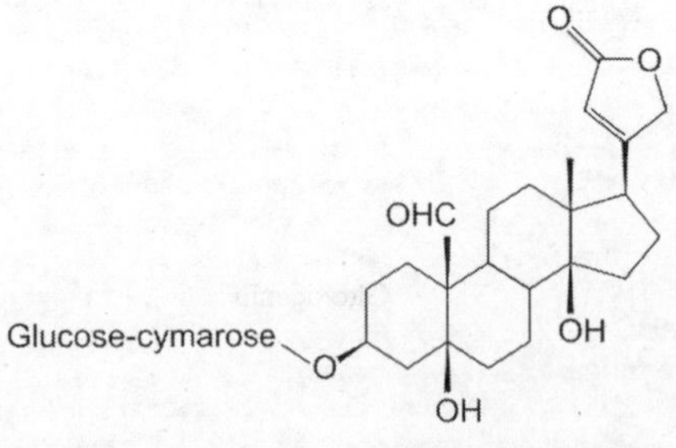

Glucose-cymarose—O

(K-Strophanthin-β)

Strophanthidin

Contd.

Table 15.1: Cardiac glycosides and their aglycones (Contd.)

Glycoside	*Aglycone*

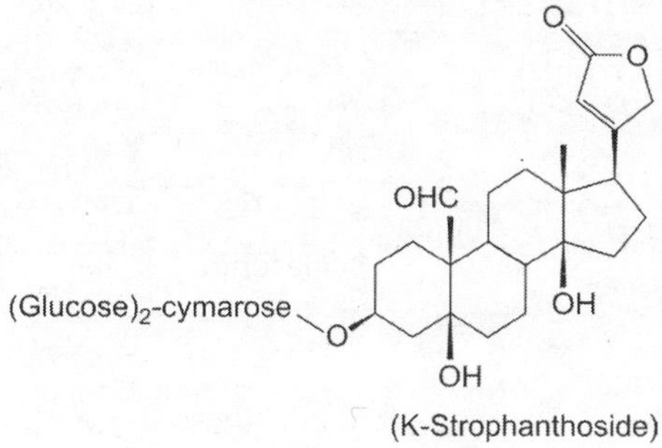

(Glucose)₂-cymarose—O

(K-Strophanthoside)

Strophanthidin

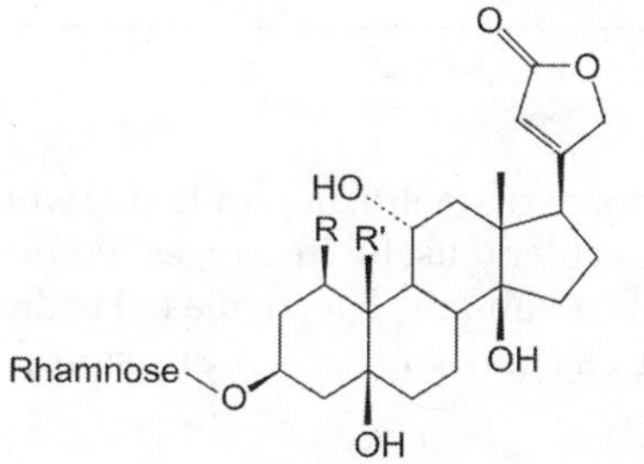

Rhamnose—O

R = OH
R' = CH₂OH

(Ouabain)

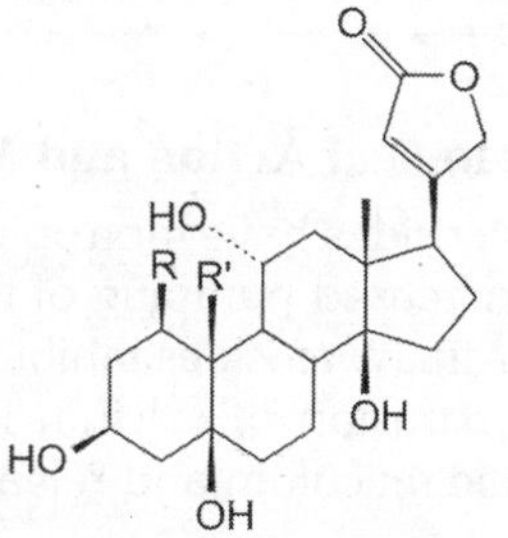

R = OH
R' = CH₂OH

(Ouabagenin)

Source: Squill species

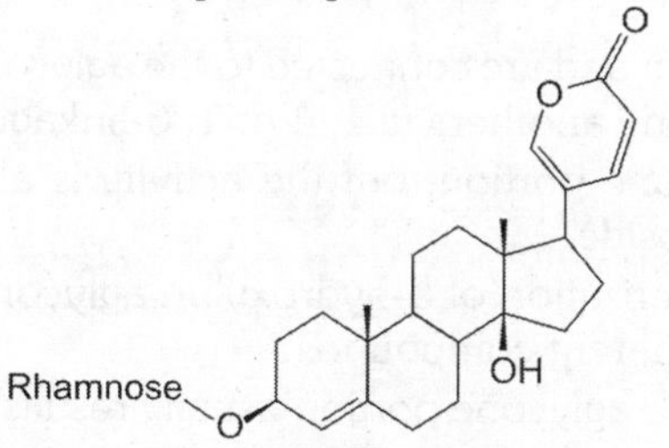

Rhamnose—O

(Proscillaridin A)

HO

(Scillarenin)

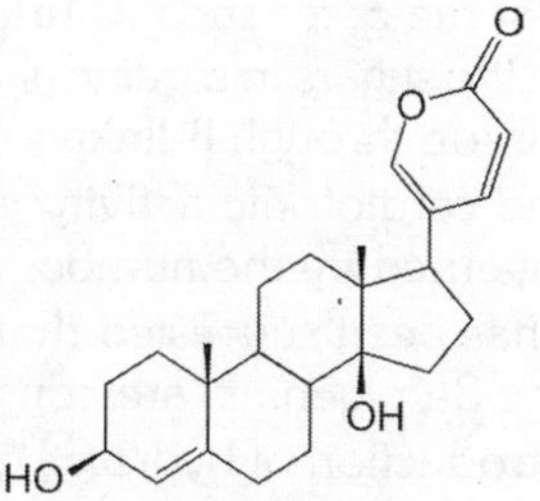

Glucose-rhamnose—O

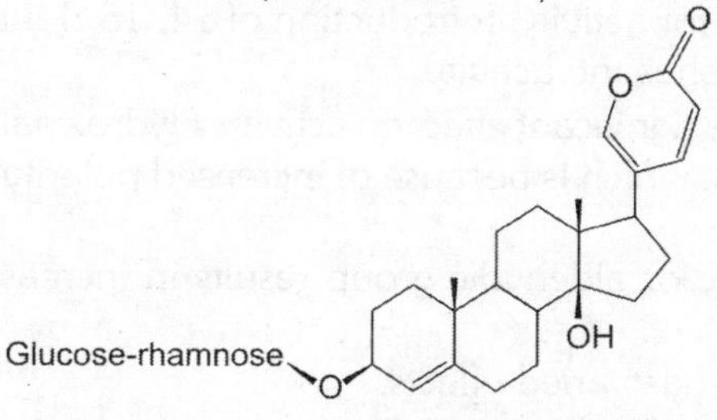

(Scillaren A)

scillarenin

Contd.

Table 15.1: Cardiac glycosides and their aglycones (Contd.)

Glycoside	Aglycone

(Glucose)$_2$- rhamnose

(Glucoscillaren A)

Scillarenin

Pharmacological Action and Mechanism of Action

Cardiac glycosides have inotropic action, i.e. they increase the force of contraction of heart, which results in increased pumping of the blood. These drugs are particularly useful in congestive heart failure. Cardiac glycosides inhibit Na^+/K^+ pump by binding to its α-subunit. The increased sodium ions slow extrusion of calcium ions. This results in increased calcium ions which are stored in sarcoplasmic reticulum and released by each action potential.

Structure-Activity Relationship Studies

1. The steroidal aglycone in cardiac glycosides has *trans* B/C ring fusion and *cis* C/D ring fusion. The A/B ring fusion which in most of the cases is *cis*, has also been found to be *trans* in some cases such as urarigenin and cartoxigenin.
2. All the sugars in cardiac glycosides occur in pyranose form and are connected to the aglycone portion through β-linkage. The sugars are attached to one another via 1, 4 or 1, 6-linkages.
3. The cardiotonic activity is essentially present in aglycone portion, but the activity is also governed by the number and kind of sugar in the glycoside.
4. It has been suggested that the sugar prevents the epimerization of 3-hydroxyl in aglycone. The 3-epigenins are considerably less active than the parent compounds.
5. Introduction of hydroxyl groups at other positions on the aglycone portion usually results in varied effects.
6. The C-14 β-hydroxyl group seems to be essential for activity. Introduction of 14, 15-double bond by dehydration of 14-hydroxyl group abolishes the activity.
7. Additional hydroxyl groups at 5, 11, 12, or 16 have significant effect on activity. Hydroxylated cardiac glycosides have shorter duration of action, which is because of increased polarity of hydroxylated analogs.
8. Conversion of methyl group at C-19 to alcoholic or aldehydic group results in increased cardiac activity.
9. Introduction of double bond at different position has varied effects.
10. The β-oriented lactone ring is essential for activity. Reduction of double bonds of lactone ring results in loss of activity.

Phosphodiesterase Inhibitors

Phosphodiesterase degrades c-AMP. Inhibition of phosphodiesterase, therefore, results in increased concentration of c-AMP. The increased c-AMP levels results in increased activity of c-AMP dependent protein kinases responsible for increased Ca^{2+} influx through calcium ion channel and increased release and faster reaccumulation by the sarcoplasmic reticulum. Thus, with the increased c-AMP levels more Ca^{2+} become available for cardiac contraction. Amrinone (60) and milrinone (61), the bipyridines are selective inhibitors of phosphodiesterase. These drugs are used for only short-term treatment because they increase mortality in patients with heart failure.

(60)   (61)

Drugs that Increase Calcium Ion Sensitivity of Myocardial Contractile Proteins

Sulmazole (62) and pimobendan (63) increase the sensitivity of myocardial contractile proteins towards Ca^{2+}.

(62)   (63)

Adenylyl Cyclase Stimulant

Forskolin (64), the diterpene has been found to stimulate adenylyl cyclase. This results in increased c-AMP levels in myocardium, which in turn results in activation of protein kinases and increased intracellular Ca^{2+}, necessary for contraction of cardiac muscle. It has also direct effect on voltage dependent potassium ion channel.

(64)   (65)

β-Adrenergic Receptor Stimulants

Increased levels of adenylyl cyclase can also result by stimulation of β-adrenergic receptors. Stimulation of these receptors results in increased levels of adenylyl cyclase which ultimately results in increased intracellular Ca^{2+} required for cardiac muscles. Dobutamine (65) is a potent β_1-agonist. It is active only by intravenous route because of its rapid first pass metabolism.

INDIVIDUAL COMPOUNDS

ANTIANGINAL DRUGS: ORGANIC NITRITES AND NITRATES

Amyl Nitrite

3-Methylbutylnitrite

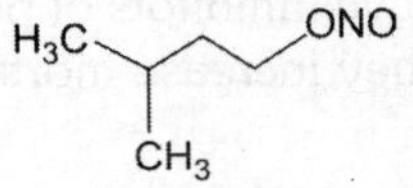

Synthesis

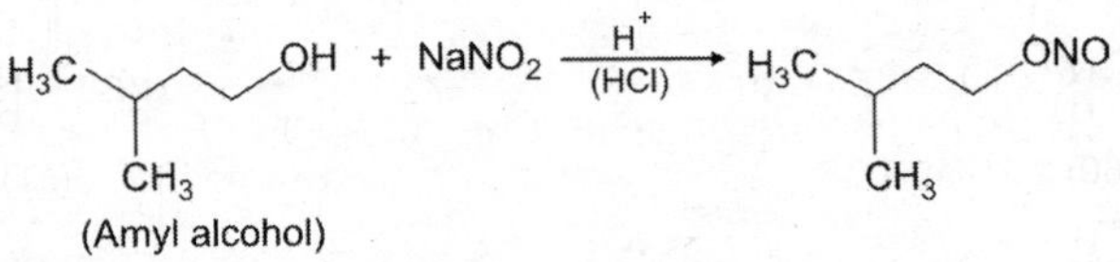

(Amyl alcohol)

It consists chiefly of isoamyl nitrite but other isomers are also present. It is a yellowish liquid with ethereal odour and pungent taste.

Nitroglycerin

1,2,3-Propanetriol trinitrate

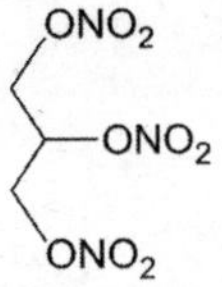

Synthesis

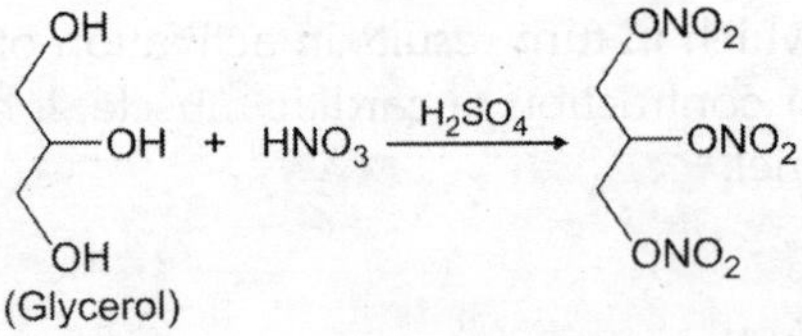

(Glycerol)

It is a colourless liquid, with a sweet burning taste. It is used extensively as an explosive in dynamite. Nitroglycerin tablets loose their potency during storage which is because of volatilization of nitroglycerin. This problem is overcome by incorporation of polyethylene glycol 400 or polyethylene glycol 4000 in the sublingual tablets.

Erythrityl Tetranitrate

(2*R*, 3*S*)-1,2,3,4-Butanetetroltetranitrate.

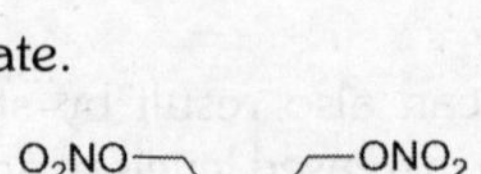

Synthesis

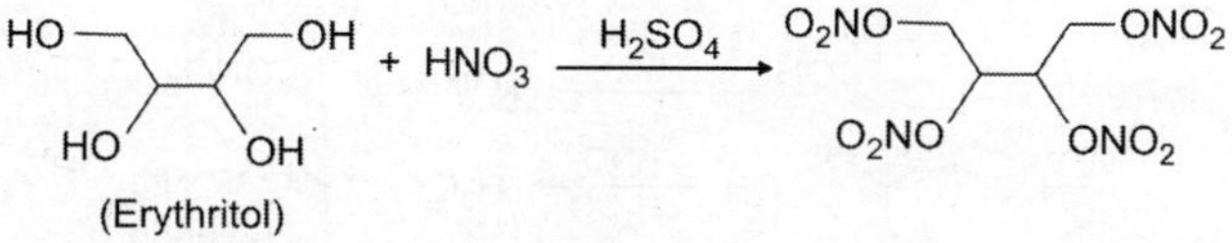

(Erythritol)

It is a solid, mp 61°, insoluble in water but soluble in organic solvents. It has delayed and longer action than nitroglycerin (2). *It is used in angina and in reduction of blood pressure.

Pentaerythritol Tetranitrate

2,2-Bis[(nitrooxy)methyl]-1, 3-propanediol dinitrate

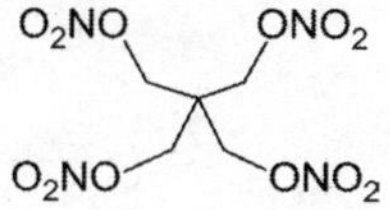

Synthesis

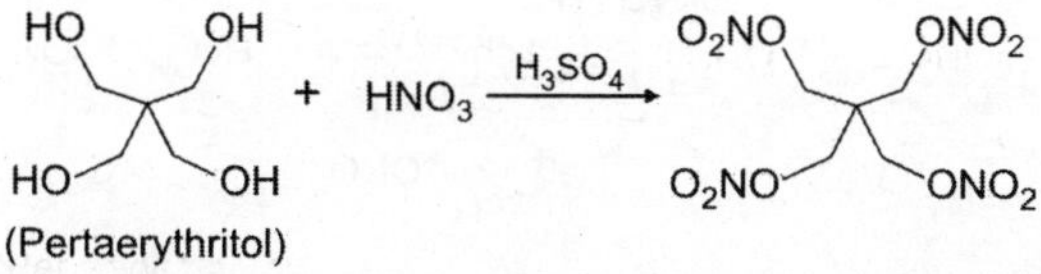

(Pertaerythritol)

It is a white crystalline substance, mp 140°. It is insoluble in water, slightly soluble in alcohol and highly soluble in acetone. It is highly explosive. For handling purposes, it is usually diluted with some inert material such as lactose.

It relaxes smooth muscles and is usually used as prophylactic inform of sustained release preparation.

Tenitramine

N,N,N,N-Tetra[(nitrooxy)ethyl]ethylenediamine

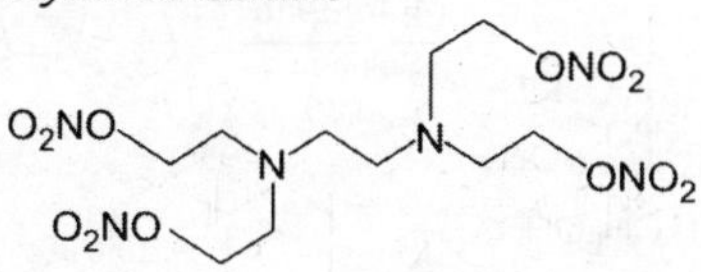

Synthesis

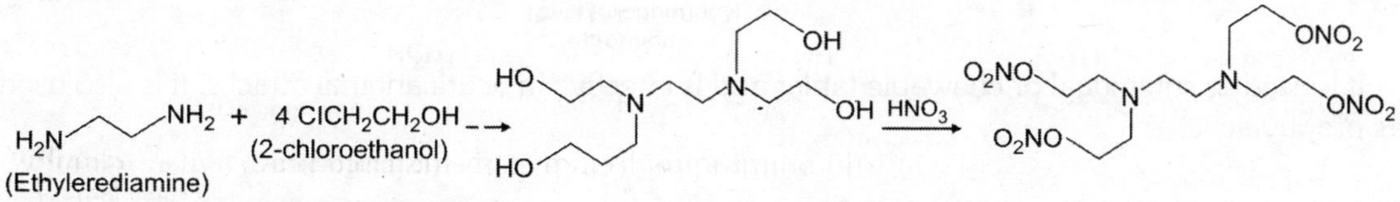

(Etheleredidiamine)

Used as vasodilator in angina

Propatyl Nitrate

2,2-Bis(hydroxymethyl)-1-butanol trinitrate

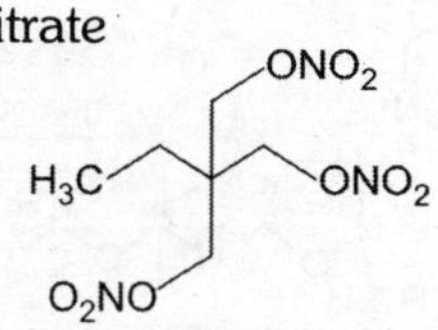

Synthesis

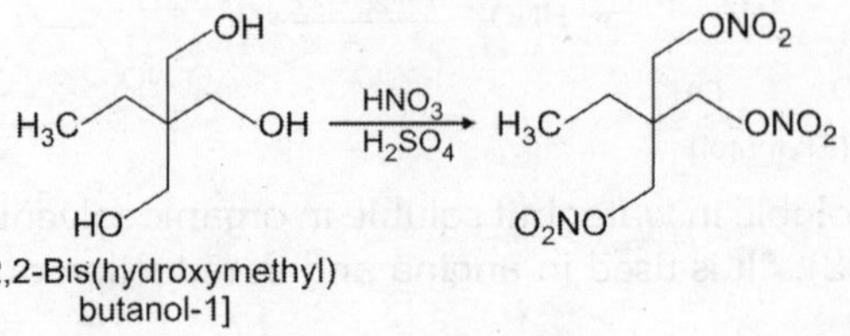

[2,2-Bis(hydroxymethyl)
butanol-1]

Used as vasodilator in angina.

Isosorbide Dinitrate

1,4:3,6-Dianhydro-D-glucitol dinitrate

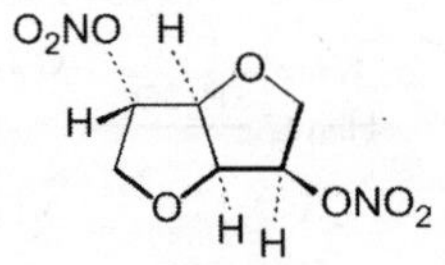

Synthesis

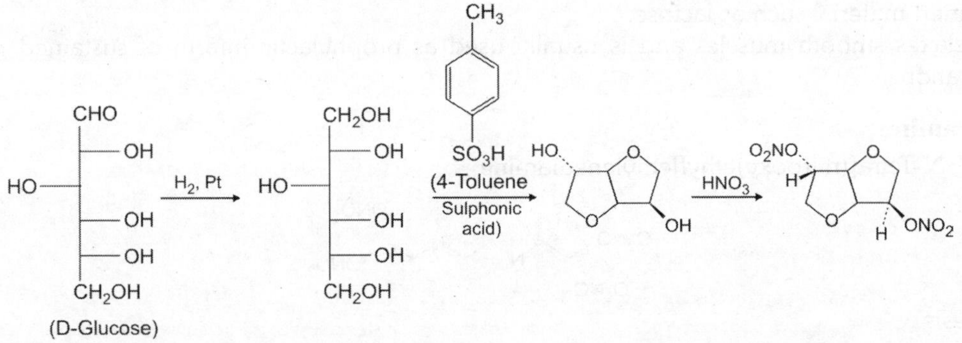

(D-Glucose)

It is used as sublingual or chewable tablet and is effective in acute anginal attacks. It is also used as prophylactic.

Molsidomine

N-(Ethoxycarbonyl)-3-(4-morpholinyl)syndone imine

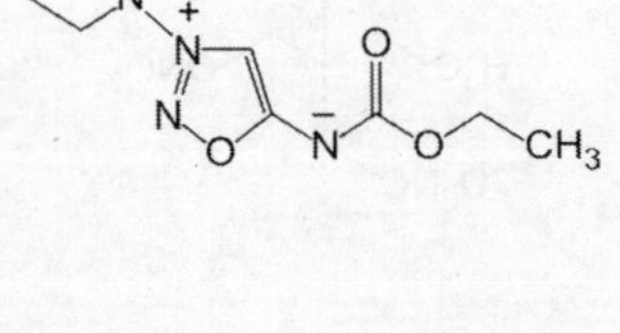

Synthesis

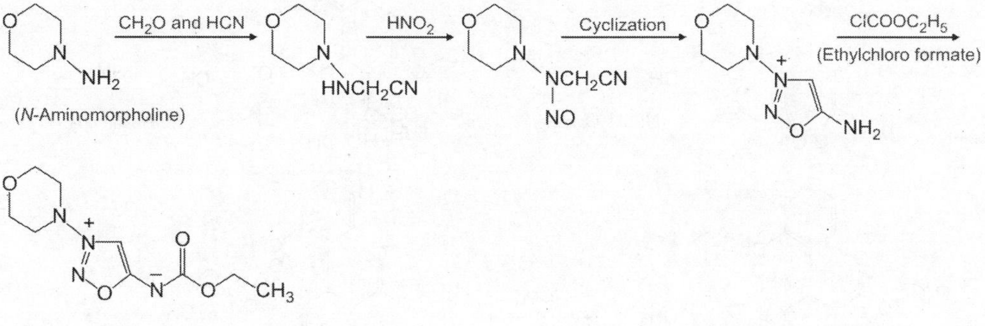

Molsidomine produces vascular smooth muscle relaxation by generating nitric oxide like nitrites and nitrates.

ANTIANGINAL DRUGS: CALCIUM CHANNEL BLOCKERS

Amlodipine

(±)-2-[(2-Aminoethoxy)methyl]-4-(2-chlorophenyl)-3-ethoxycarbonyl-5-methoxycarbonyl-6-methyl-1, 4-dihydropyridine

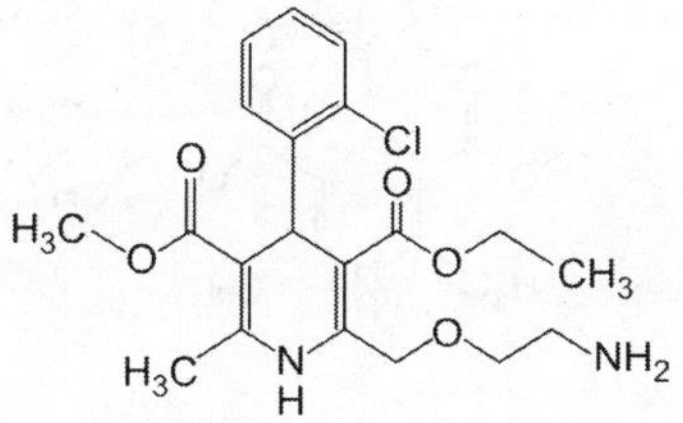

Synthesis

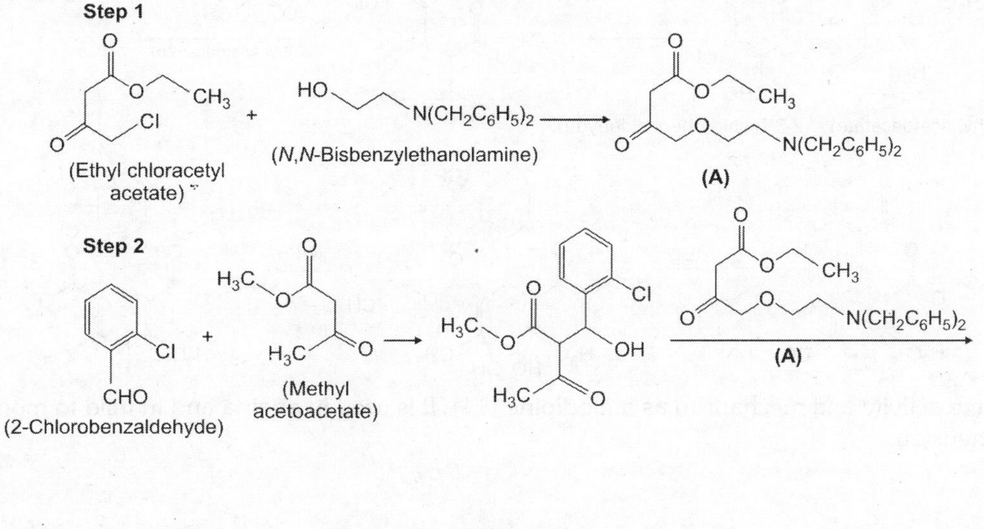

Step 1

(Ethyl chloracetyl acetate)

(*N,N*-Bisbenzylethanolamine)

(A)

Step 2

(2-Chlorobenzaldehyde)

(Methyl acetoacetate)

(A)

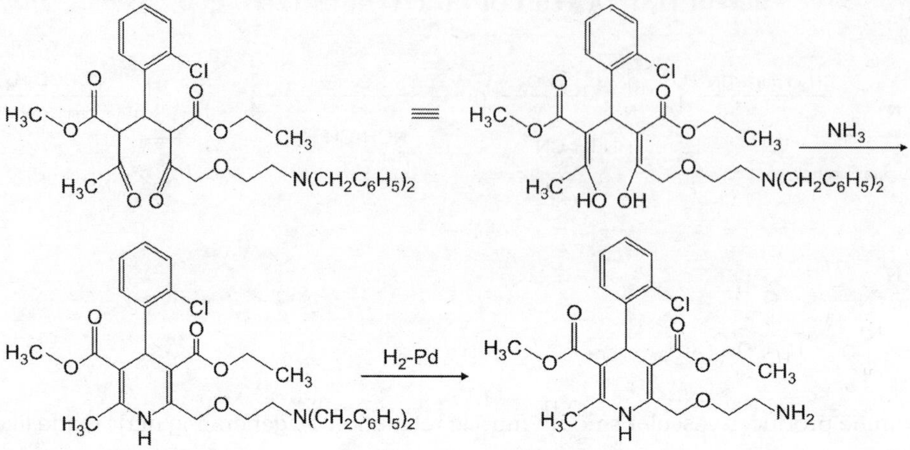
NH3
H2-Pd
N(CH2C6H5)2
NH2

It has a longer half-life. It is used in chronic stable angina and mild to moderate essential hypertension.

Felodipine

4-(2,3-Dichlorphenyl)-1,4-dihydro-2,6-dimethyl-3,5-pyridinedicarboxylic acid ethyl methyl ester

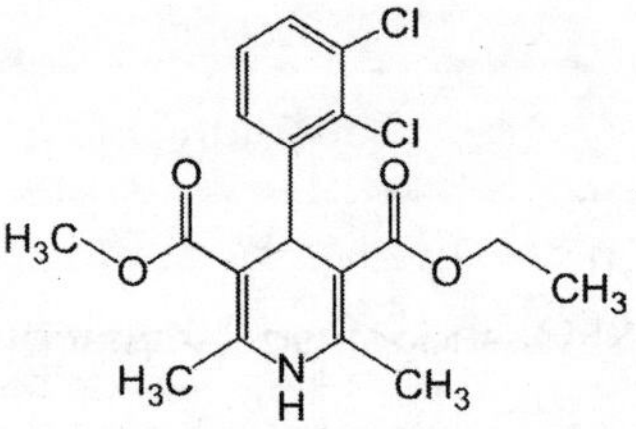

Synthesis

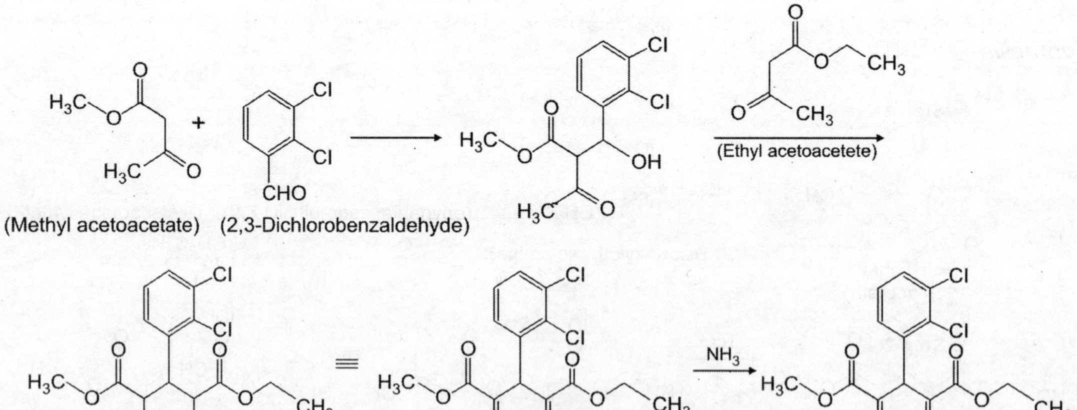
(Methyl acetoacetate)
(2,3-Dichlorobenzaldehyde)
(Ethyl acetoacetete)
NH3

Same activity and mechanism as amlodipine (11). It is used in angina and in mild to moderate hypertension.

Isradipine

Isopropyl 4-(2,1,3-benzoxadiazol-4-yl)1,4-dihydro-5-methoxycarbonyl-2,6-dimethyl-3-pyridinecarboxylate

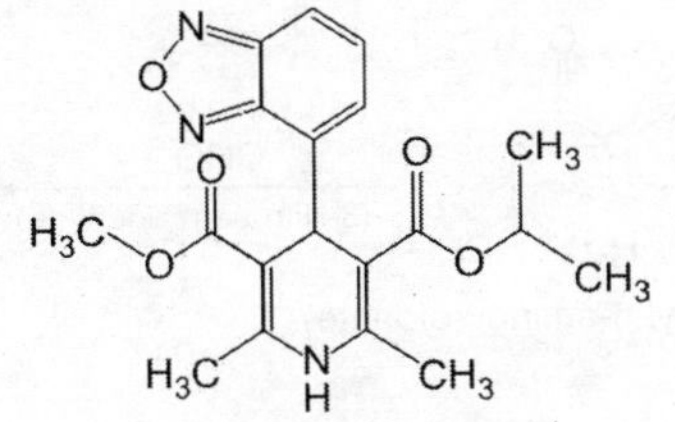

Synthesis

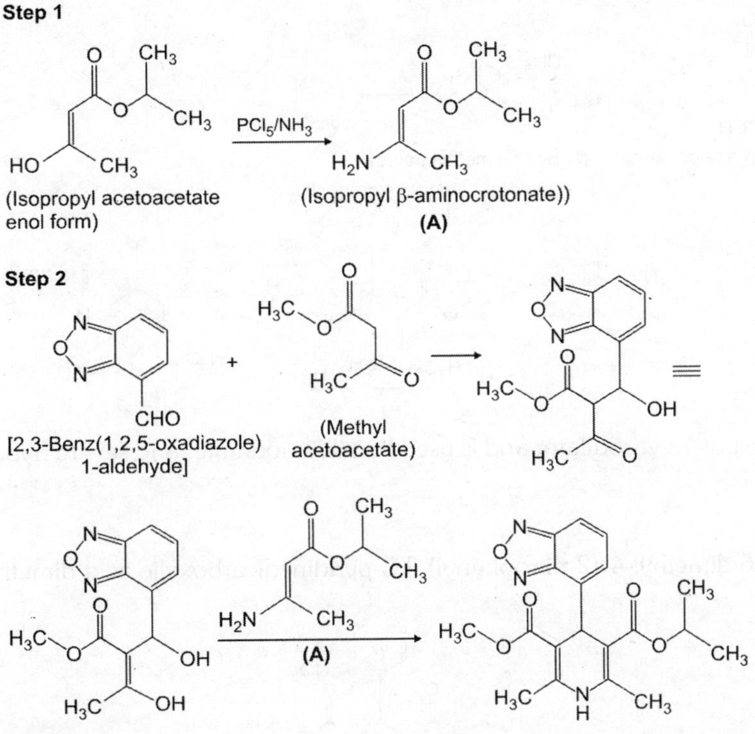

Step 1

(Isopropyl acetoacetate enol form)   (Isopropyl β-aminocrotonate))
(A)

Step 2

[2,3-Benz(1,2,5-oxadiazole) 1-aldehyde]   (Methyl acetoacetate)

Used for stable angina.

Nicardipine

1,4-Dihydro-2,6-dimethyl-4-(3-nitrophenyl)-3,5-pyridinedicarboxylic acid methyl 2-[methyl-(phenylmethyl) amino]ethyl ester.

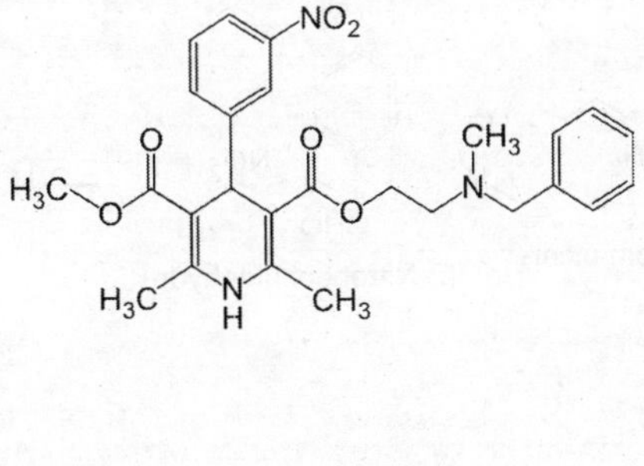

Synthesis

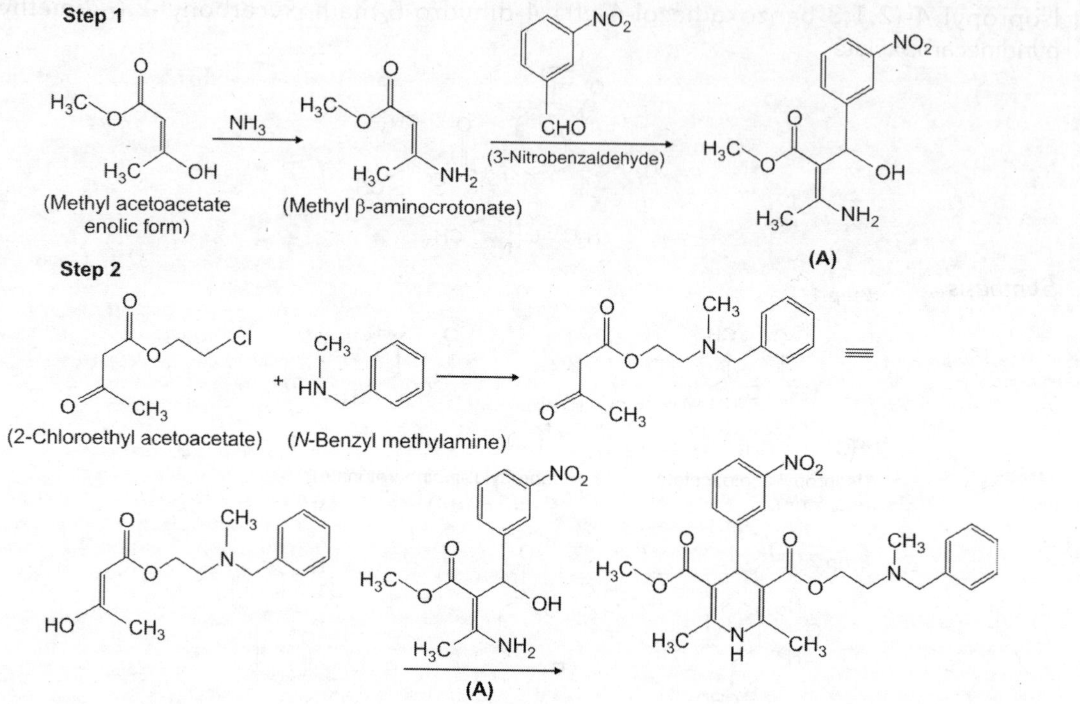

Step 1

(Methyl acetoacetate enolic form) → (Methyl β-aminocrotonate) → (A)

(3-Nitrobenzaldehyde)

Step 2

(2-Chloroethyl acetoacetate) + (N-Benzyl methylamine)

(A)

Nicardipine is potent vasodilator and is used in mild, moderate, and severe hypertension and in stable angina.

Nifedipine

1,4-Dihydro-2, 6-dimethyl-4-(2-nitrophenyl)-3,5-pyridinedicarboxylic acid dimethyl ester.

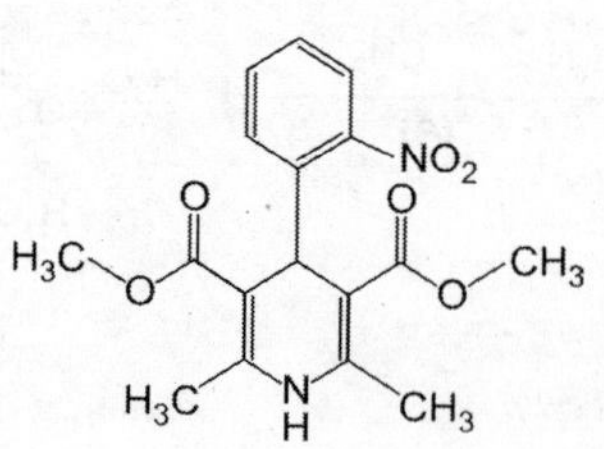

Synthesis

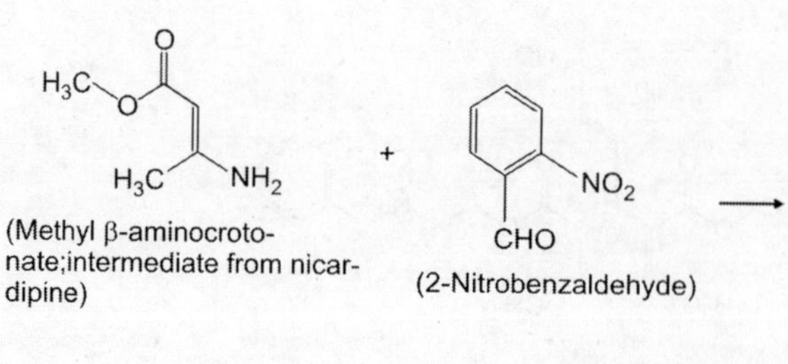

(Methyl β-aminocroto-nate;intermediate from nicar-dipine) + (2-Nitrobenzaldehyde)

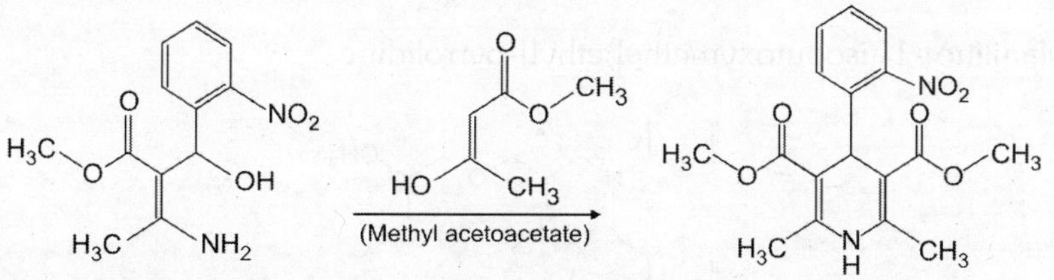

(Methyl acetoacetate)

It has a potent peripheral vasodilatory effect. It is used in angina as well as for treatment of hypertension.

Nimodipine

1, 4-Dihydro-2,6-dimethyl-4-(3-nitrophenyl)-3,5-pyridinedicarboxylic acid 2-methoxyethyl 1-methylethyl ester

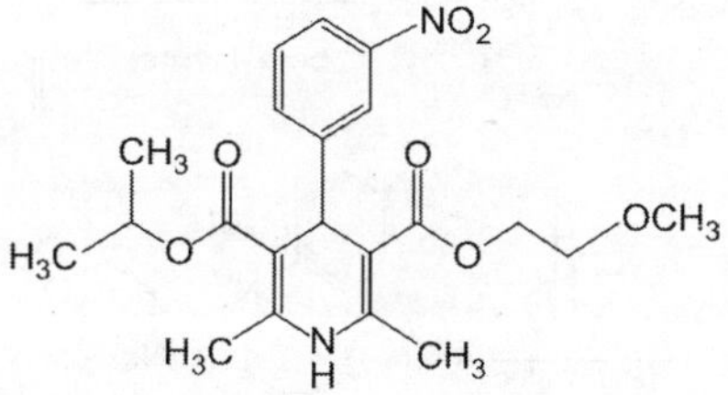

Synthesis

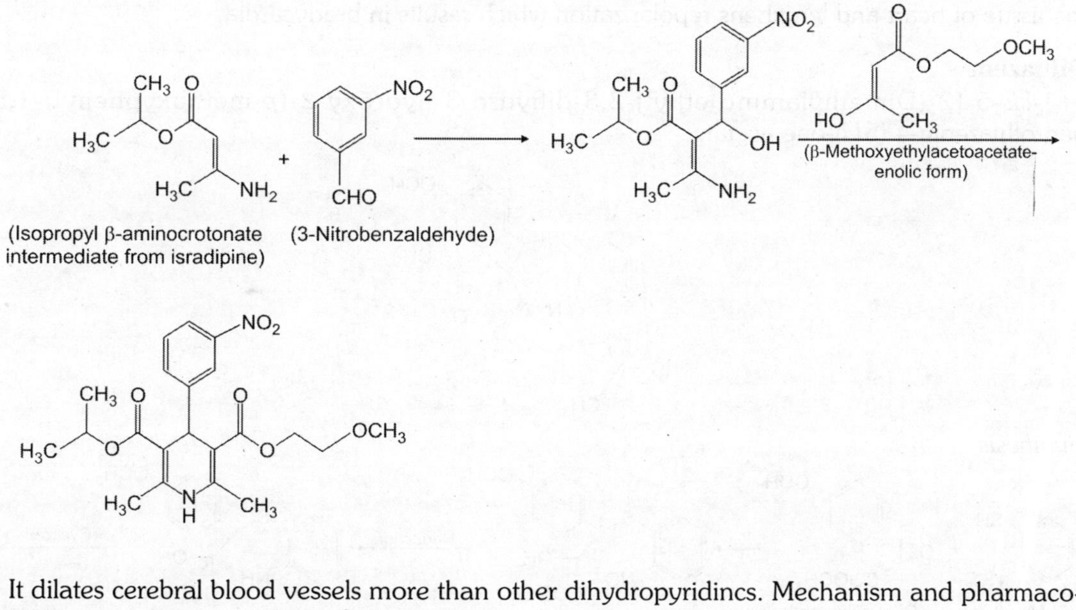

(Isopropyl β-aminocrotonate intermediate from isradipine)   (3-Nitrobenzaldehyde)

(β-Methoxyethylacetoacetate-enolic form)

It dilates cerebral blood vessels more than other dihydropyridincs. Mechanism and pharmacological action similar as that amlodipine (11).

Bepridil

1-[2-(N-benzylanilino)-1-(isobutoxymethyl)ethyl]-pyrrolidine

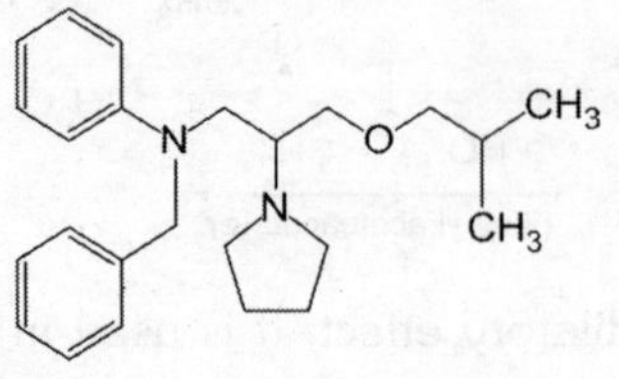

Synthesis

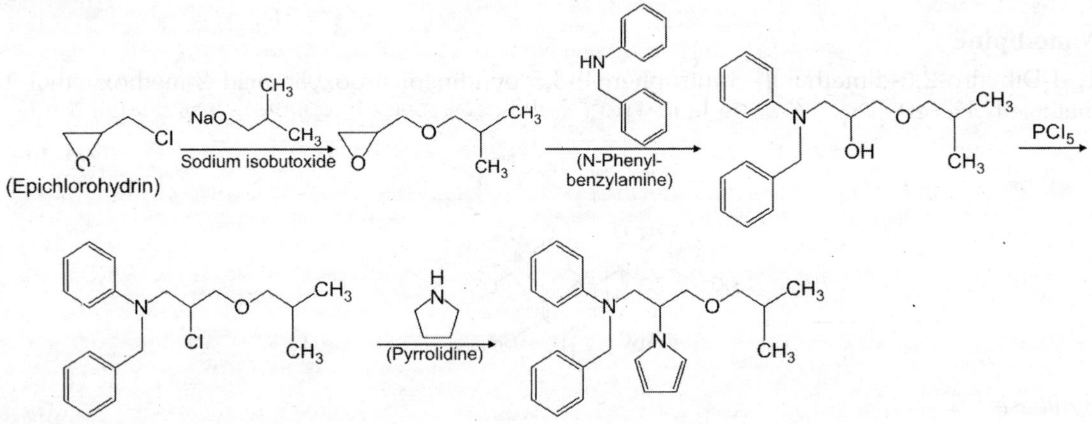

It is used as hydrochloride. In addition to calcium channel blocker, it also inhibits sodium flow in the tissue of heart and lengthens repolarization which results in bradycardia.

Diltiazem

(+)-cis-5-[2-(Dimethylamino)ethyl]-2,3-dihydro-3-hydroxy-2-(p-methoxyphenyl)-1,5-benzothiazepin-4 (5H)-one acetate

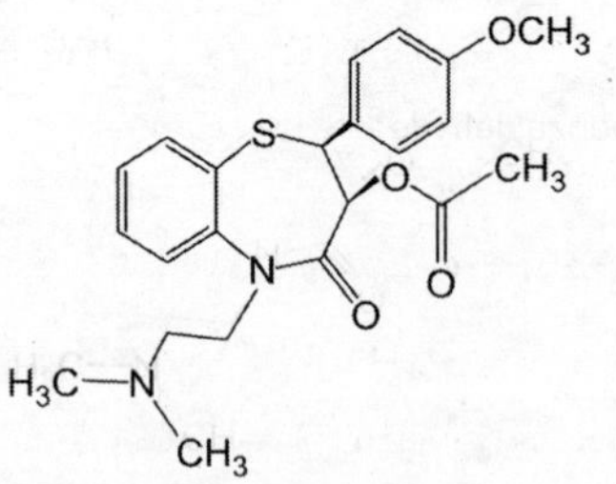

Synthesis

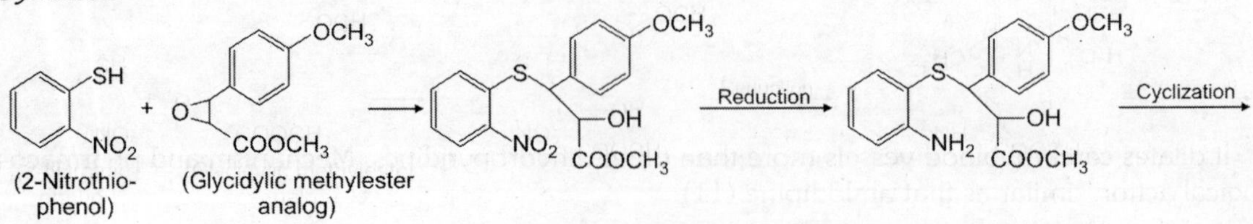

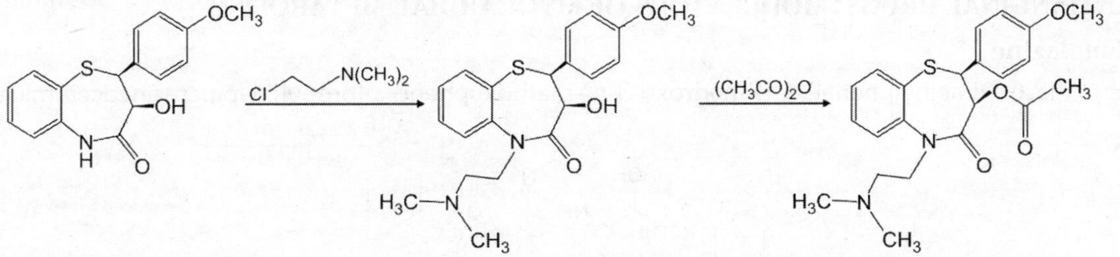

It is used as hydrochloride. The active metabolite of dilitiazem is deacetyldiltiazem (66).

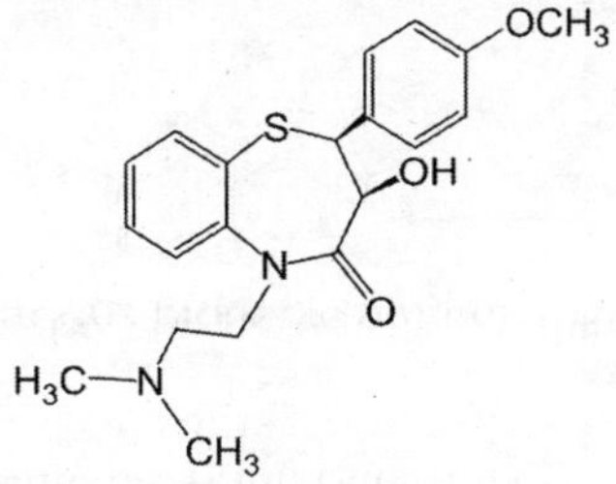

(66)

Verapamil

α-Isopropyl-α-[(*N*-methyl-*N*-homoveratryl)-γ-aminopropyl]-3, 4-dimethoxyphenylacetonitrile

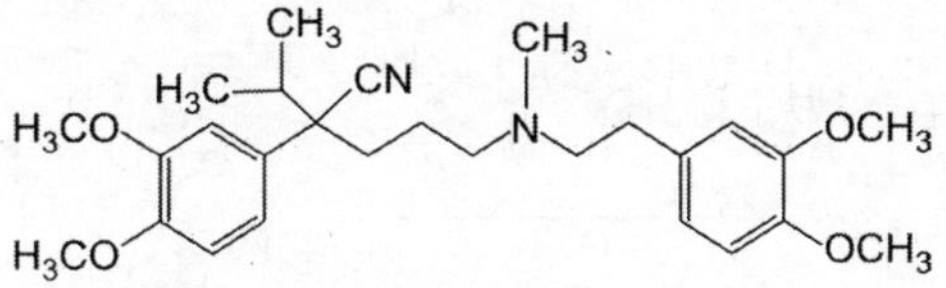

Synthesis

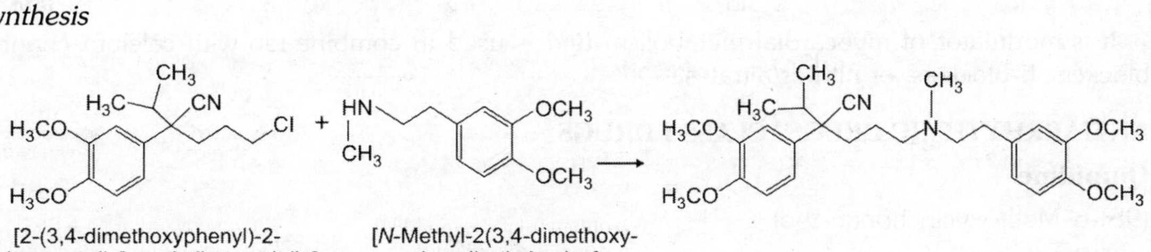

[2-(3,4-dimethoxyphenyl)-2-
(chloropropyl)-3-methylbutyronitrile]

[*N*-Methyl-2(3,4-dimethoxy-
phenyl) ethylamine]

It is absorbed rapidly after oral administration. It reduces systemic vascular resistance and mean blood pressure. Its major effect is on slow Ca^{2+} channel.

ANTIANGINAL DRUGS: β-ADRENERGIC RECEPTOR BLOCKING AGENTS

Atenolol, Metoprolol, Propranolol, and Timolol
See ADRENERGIC DRUGS

ANTIANGINAL DRUGS : MODULATORS OF MYOCARDIAL METABOLISM

Ranolazine

(±)-*N*-(2,6-Dimethylphenyl)-4-[2-hydroxy-3-(2-methoxyphenoxy)propyl]-1-piperazineacetamide

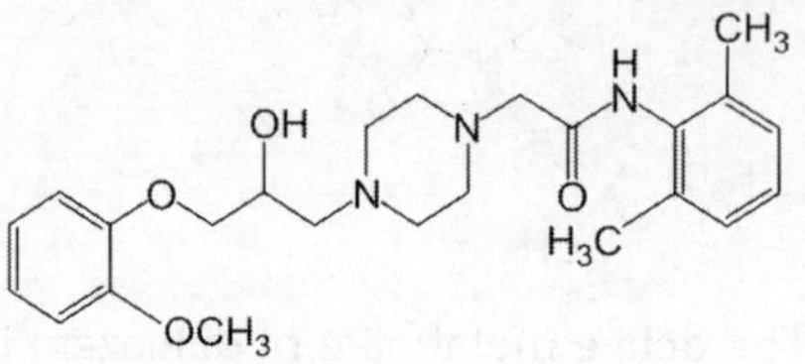

Synthesis

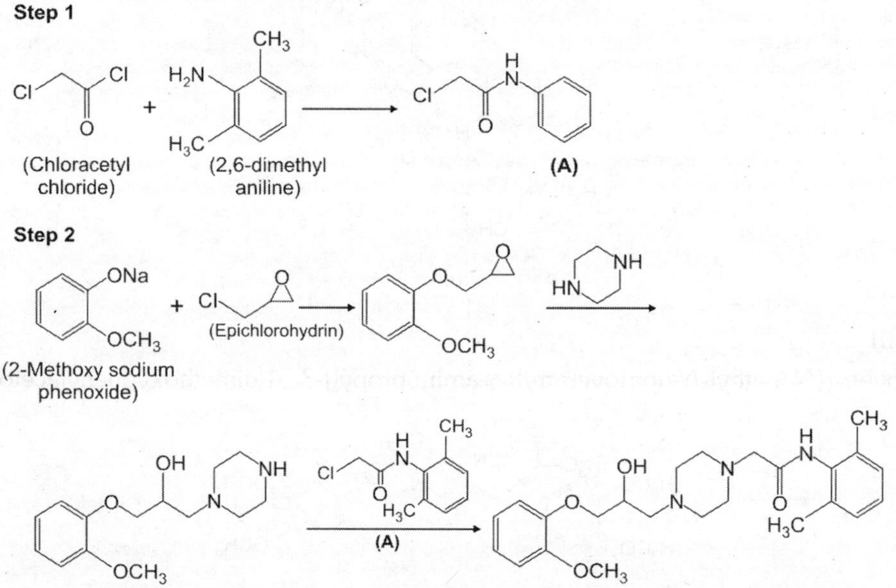

Step 1

(Chloracetyl chloride) + (2,6-dimethyl aniline) → **(A)**

Step 2

(2-Methoxy sodium phenoxide) + (Epichlorohydrin) →

It is modulator of myocardial metabolism and is used in combination with calcium channel blockers, β-blockers, or nitrites/nitrates.

ANTIARRHYTHMIC DRUGS : CLASS I DRUGS

Quinidine

(9S)-6'-Methoxycinchonan-9-ol

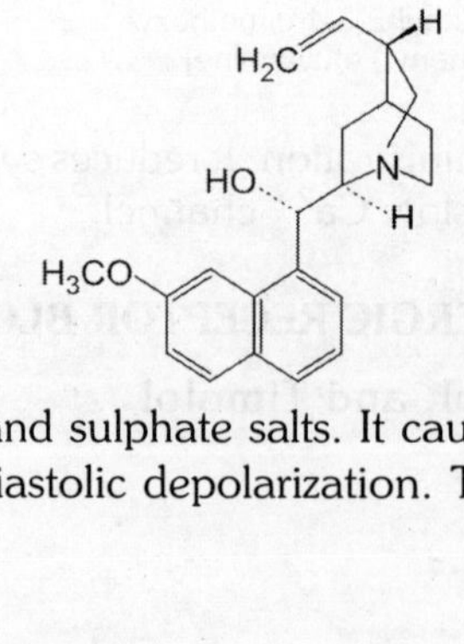

It is used as hydrogen sulphate and sulphate salts. It causes decreased sodium ion entry into myocardial cells causing phase 4 diastolic depolarization. The sodium channel block decreases

automaticity. It also decreases the conduction sufficiently to extinguish the propagating re-entrant wave front.

It is used orally and occasionally intramuscularly.

Procainamide

4-Amino-N-[2-(diethylamino)ethyl]benzamide

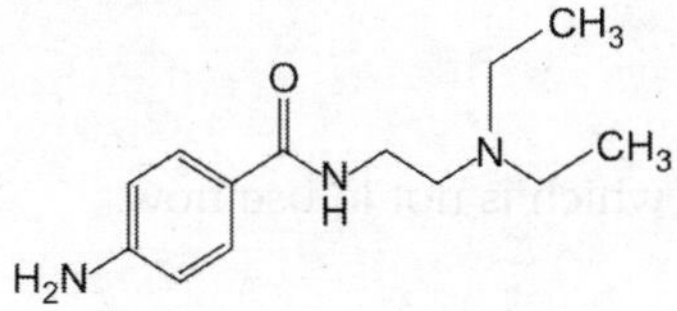

Synthesis

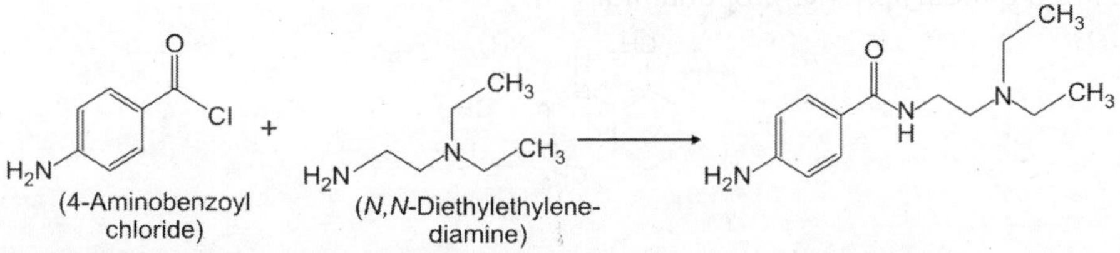

(4-Aminobenzoyl chloride)

(N,N-Diethylethylene-diamine)

It also belongs to class Ia antiarrhythmic drugs and is used as hydrochloride. It is a sodium channel blocker. It decreases conduction velocity and automaticity. It also increases the action potential duration and thereby refractory period.

Disopyramide

α-[2-(Diisopropylamino)ethyl]-α-phenyl-2-pyridineacetamide

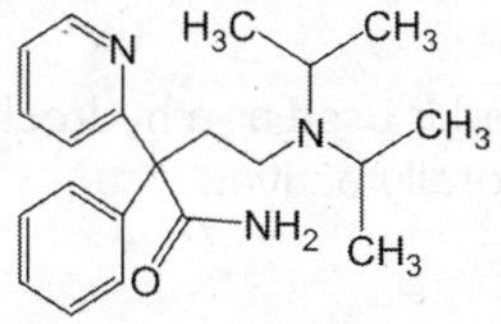

Synthesis

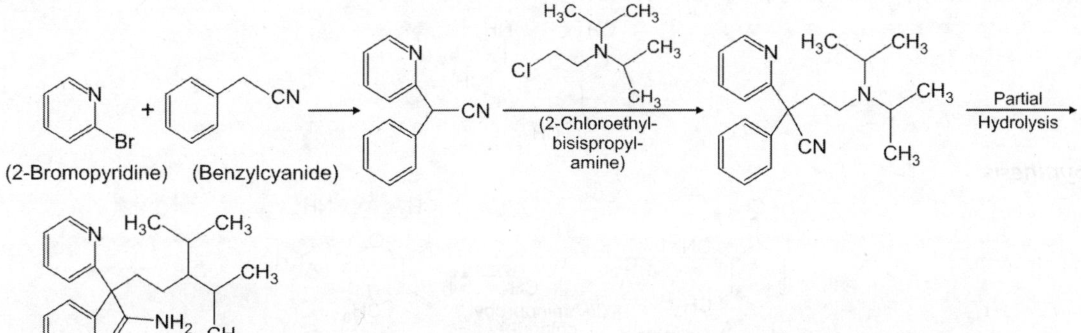

(2-Bromopyridine)   (Benzylcyanide)

(2-Chloroethyl-bisispropyl-amine)

Partial Hydrolysis

It belongs to class Ia antiarrhythmic drugs. It is used as phosphate clinically in the treatment of refractory, life-threatening ventricular tachyarrhythmias.

Lignocaine

See **LOCAL ANESTHETICS**

It is a class Ib antiarrhythmic agent and is used as hydrochloride. It is used intravenously for ventricular arrhythmias. It depresses sodium ion influx during diastole. It also alters membrane responsiveness in Pinkinje fibers.

Phenytoin

See **ANTIEPILEPTIC DRUGS**

It is a class Ib antiarrhythmic drug which is not in use now.

Tocainide

2-Amino-N-(2,6-dimethylphenyl)propanamide

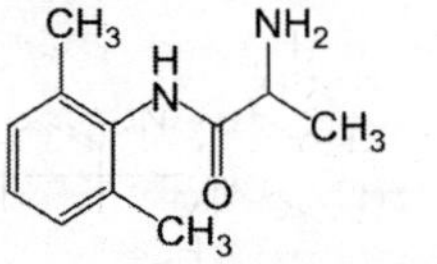

Synthesis

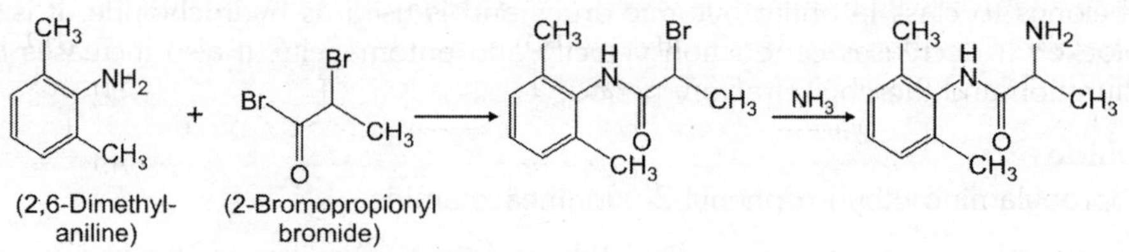

(2,6-Dimethyl-aniline)   (2-Bromopropionyl bromide)

It is a class Ib antiarrhythmic drug and is used as a hydrochloride. It is an analog of ligocaine (28) and has similar action. However, it is orally active.

Mexiletine

1-(2,6-Dimethylphenoxy)-2-propanamine

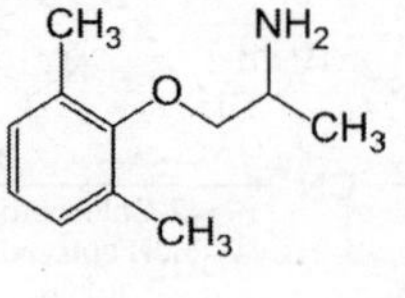

Synthesis

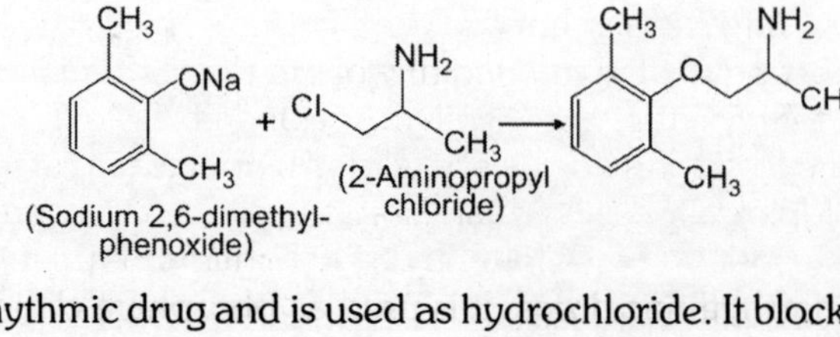

(Sodium 2,6-dimethyl-phenoxide)   (2-Aminopropyl chloride)

It is a class Ib antiarrhythmic drug and is used as hydrochloride. It blocks fast sodium ion channel. It increases the threshold of excitability of myocardial cells and is used as a long-term prophylactic orally.

Flecainide

N-(2-Piperidinylmethyl)-2,5-bis (2,2,2-trifluoroethoxy) benzamide

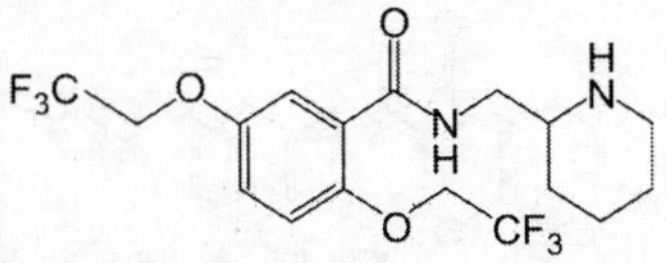

Synthesis

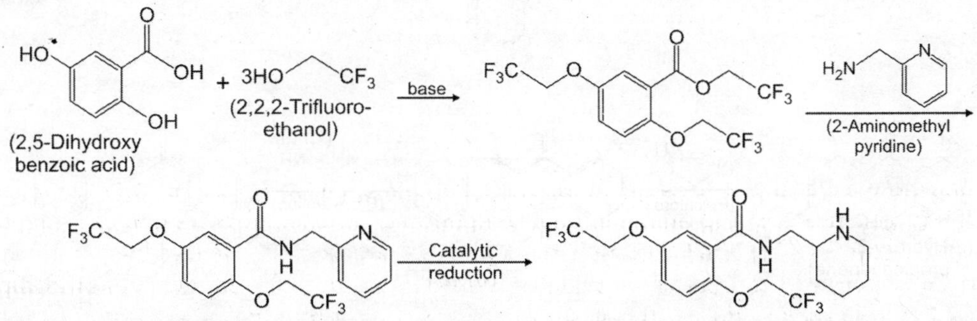

It is used as an acetate and belongs to class Ic of antiarrhythmic drugs. It suppresses ventricular ectopic beats and is used as prophylactic orally.

Encainide

(±)-4-Methoxy-*N*-[2-[2-(1-methyl-2-piperidinyl)ethyl]phenyl]benzamide

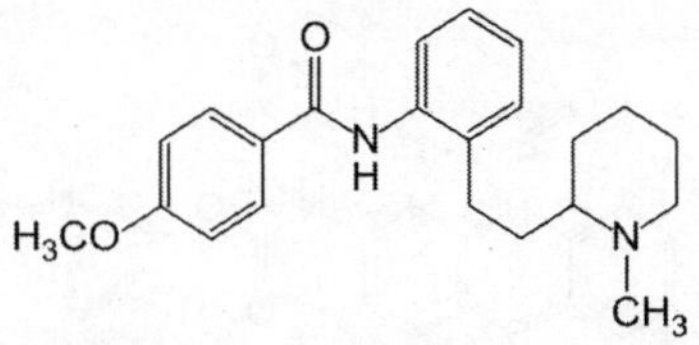

Synthesis

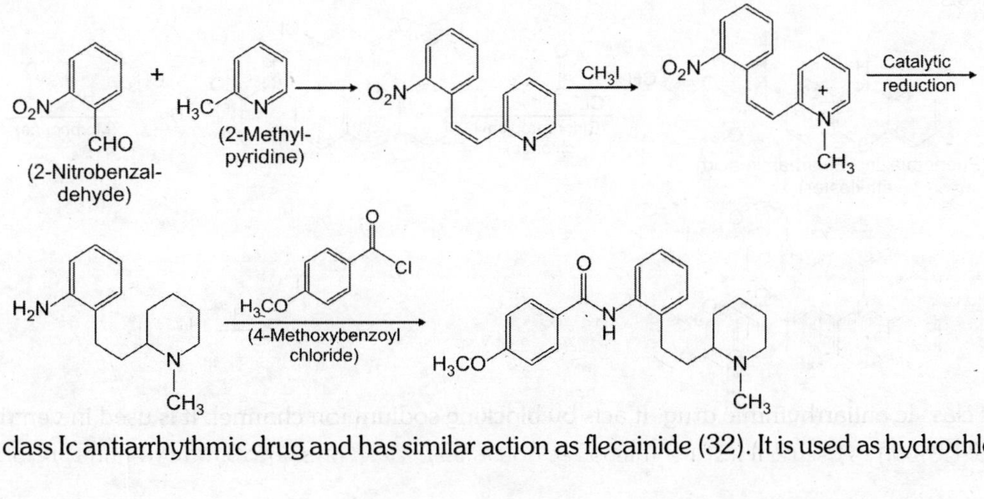

It is a class Ic antiarrhythmic drug and has similar action as flecainide (32). It is used as hydrochloride.

Propafenone

2'-(2-Hydroxy-3-(propylamino)propoxy]-3-phenylpropiophenone

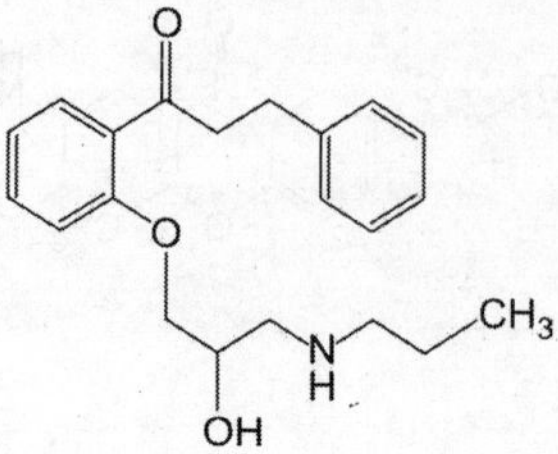

Synthesis

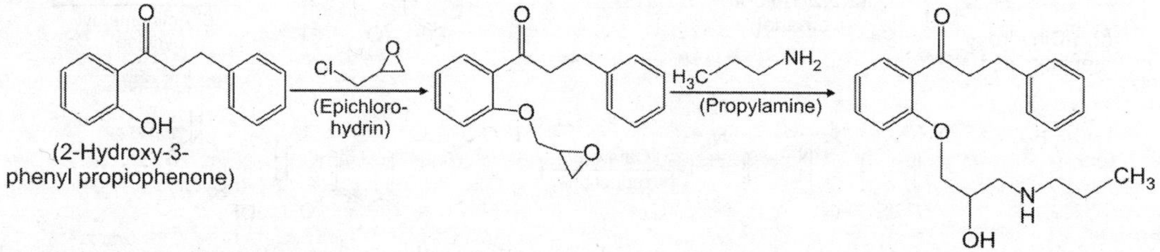

(2-Hydroxy-3-
phenyl propiophenone)

(Epichloro-
hydrin)

(Propylamine)

It is a class IC antiarrhythmic drug.

Moricizine

[10-[3-(4-Morpholinyl)-1-oxopropyl]-10 *H*-phenothiazin-2-yl] carbamic acid ethyl *ester*

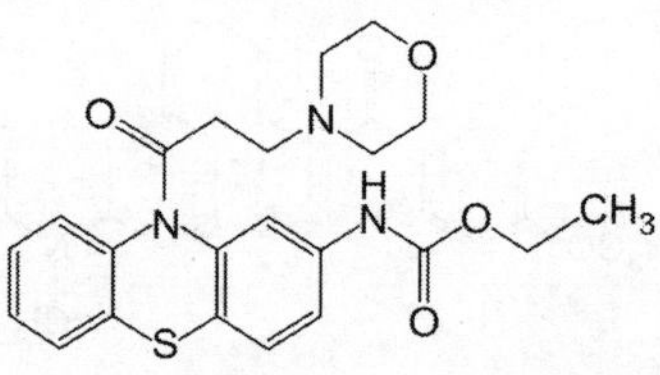

Synthesis

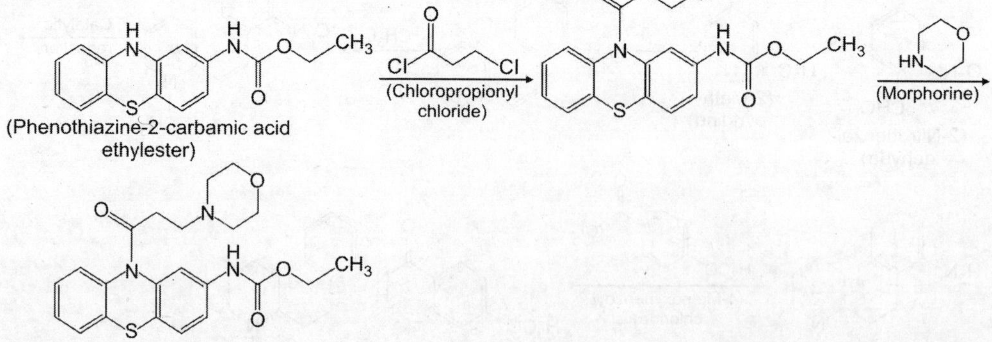

(Phenothiazine-2-carbamic acid
ethylester)

(Chloropropionyl
chloride)

(Morphorine)

It is class Ic antiarrhythmic drug. It acts by blocking sodium ion channel. It is used in ventricular arrhythmias.

ANTIARRHYTHMIC DRUGS : CLASS II DRUGS

Propranolol

See ADRENERGIC DRUGS

It is a class II antiarrhythmic drug. It is a β-adrenoreceptor blocker which may be conributing to its antiarrhythmic action.

ANTIARRHYTHMIC DRUGS : CLASS III DRUGS

Amiodarone

2-Butyl-3-benzofuranyl-4-[2-(diethylamino)-ethoxy]-3,5-diiodophenyl ketone

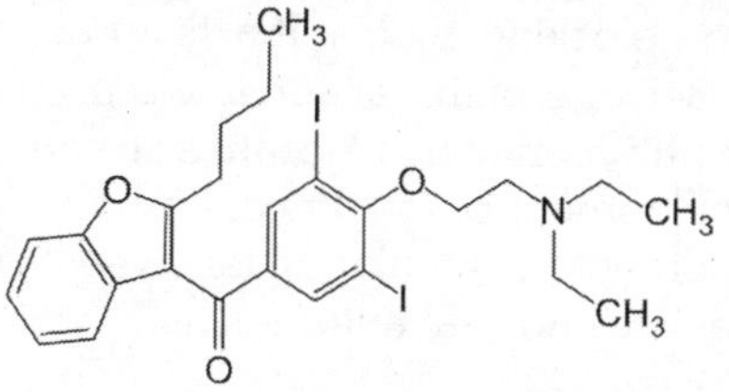

Synthesis

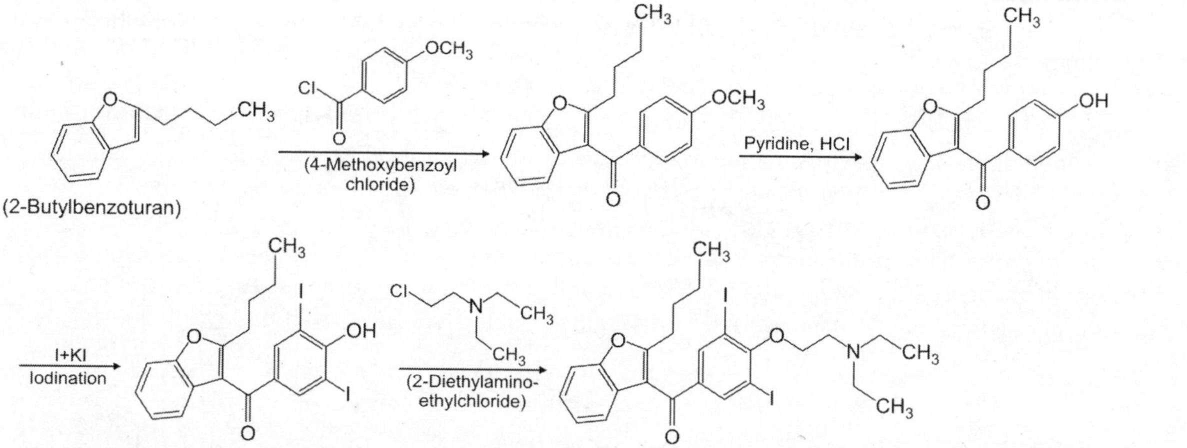

(2-Butylbenzoturan)
(4-Methoxybenzoyl chloride)
Pyridine, HCl

I+KI
Iodination
(2-Diethylamino-ethylchloride)

It is cardiac depressant drug useful in treatment of ventricular arrhythmia and is class III antiarrhythmic drug. It prolongs the action potential in all the cardiac tissues. Since it contains iodine, it has some effect on thyroid hormones.

Bretylium Tosylate

(*o*-Bromobenzyl)ethyldimethylammonium tosylate

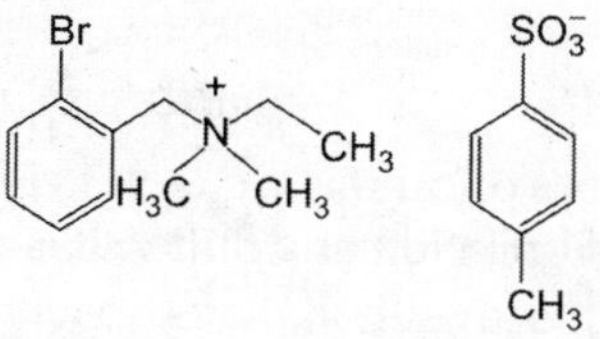

Synthesis

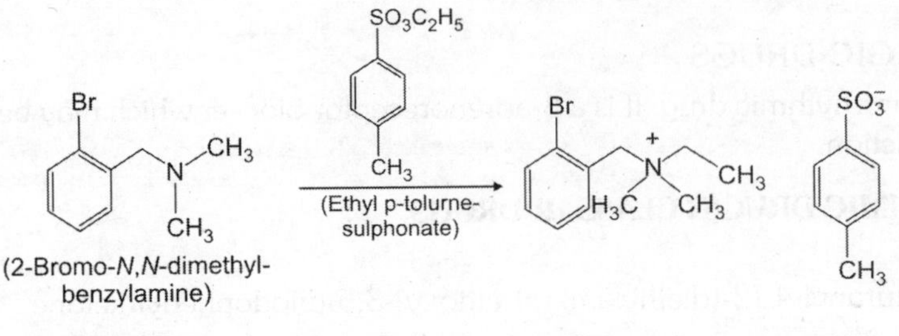

(2-Bromo-*N,N*-dimethyl-
benzylamine)

(Ethyl p-tolurne-
sulphonate)

Bretylium is adrenergic neuron blocking agents. It acts by accumulating in adrenergic neurons and displacing norepinephrine. Because of this action it was used as antihypertensive. However, it is not used nowadays as an antihypertensive because it causes postural hypotension, other disadvantages in its use are development of tolerance, and erratic oral absorption. It is a class III antiarrhythmic drugs. It acts by adrenergic stimulation followed by ganglionic blockade. It increases action potential duration and reduces normal automaticity.

Dofetilide

1-(4-Methanesulphonamidophenoxy)-2-[*N*-(4-methanesulphonamidophenethyl)-N-methylamino]-ethane

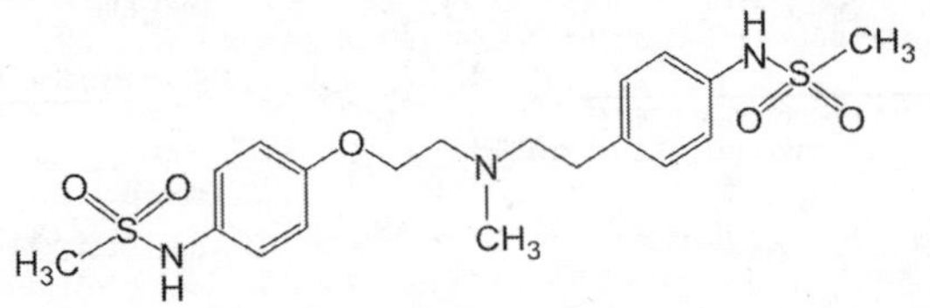

Synthesis

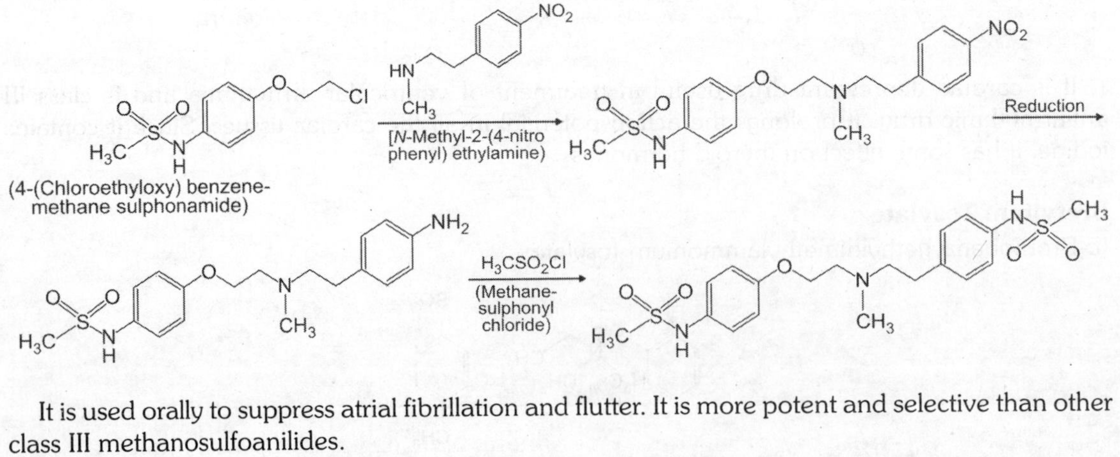

(4-(Chloroethyloxy) benzene-
methane sulphonamide)

[*N*-Methyl-2-(4-nitro
phenyl) ethylamine]

Reduction

(Methane-
sulphonyl
chloride)

It is used orally to suppress atrial fibrillation and flutter. It is more potent and selective than other class III methanosulfoanilides.

Ibutilide

N-[4-[4-Ethylheptylamino)-1-hydroxybutyl]phenyl]methanesulphonamide

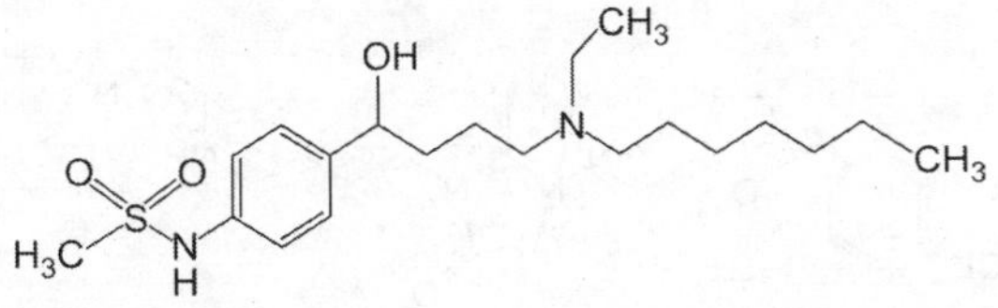

Synthesis

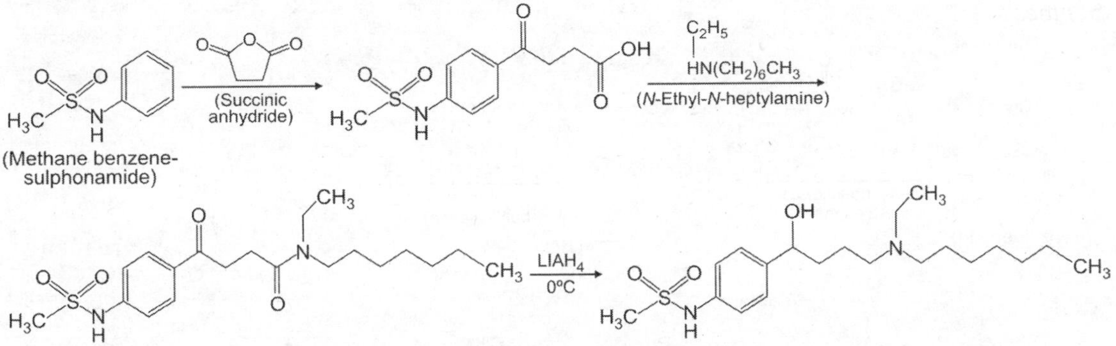

It has a similar activity as that of dofetilide (38) and is used as fumarate salt by intravenous infusion.

Sotalol

N-[4-[1-Hydroxy-2-[(1-methylethyl) amino]ethyl]phenyl]methanesulphonamide

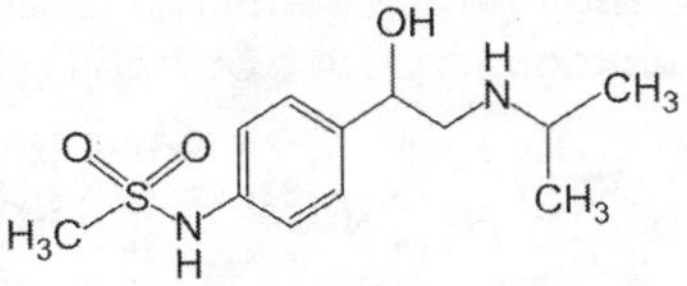

Synthesis

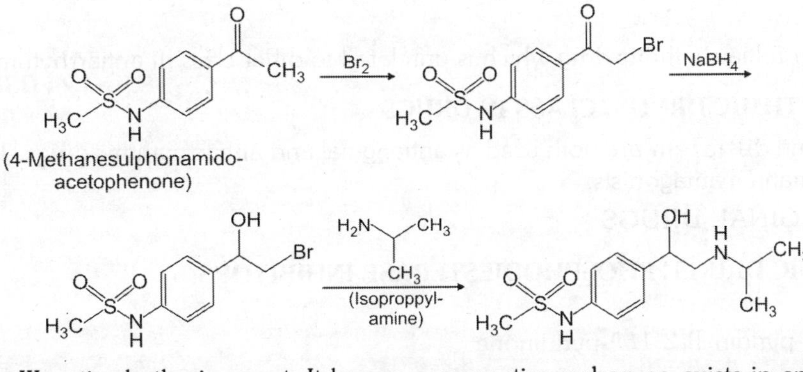

It is a class III antiarrhythmic agent. It has an asymmetirc carbon so exists in enantiomorphic forms. The (–) -isomer has β-blocking activity which is associated with class II antiarrhythmic drugs and potassium ion channel blocking activity—a property associated with class III antiarrhythmic drugs. The (+)-isomer has class III antiarrhythmic properties but the activity is much lower than the (–) -isomer. It is used to suppress ventricular ectopic beats and paroxysm supraventricular arrhythmias.

Azimilide

1-[[[5-(4-Chlorophenyl)-2-furanyl]methylene]amino]-3-[4-(4-methyl-1-piprazinyl)butyl]-2,4-imidazolidinedione

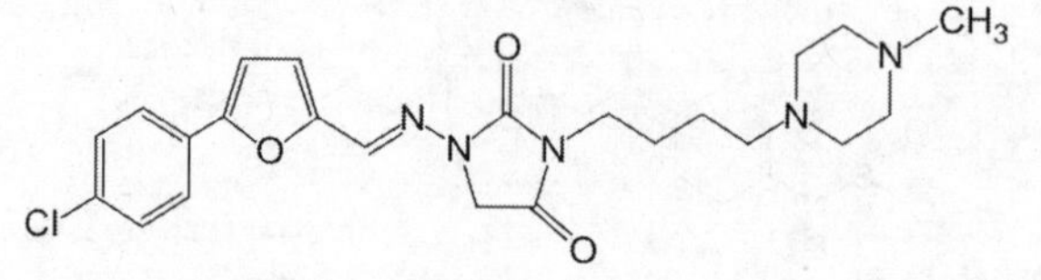

Synthesis

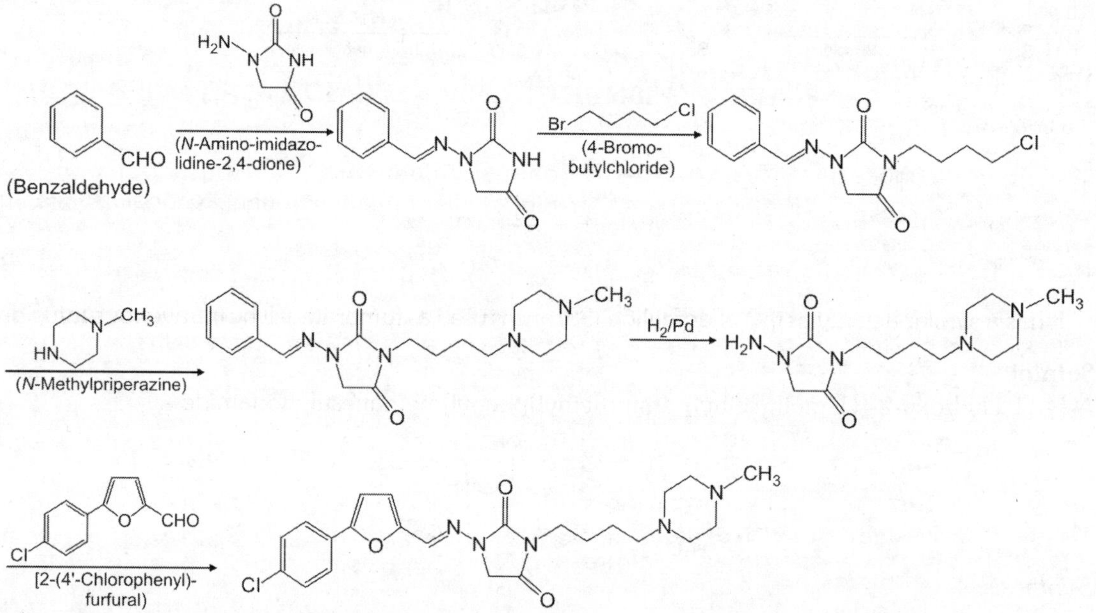

It is another antiarrhythmic drug which is unrelated to other class III antiarrhythmic agents.

ANTIARRHYTHMIC DRUGS: CLASS IV DRUGS

Verapamil and **diltiazem** are both used as antianginal and antiarrhythmic drugs. They both are calcium ion channel antagonists.

See **ANTIANGINAL DRUGS**

CARDIOTONIC DRUGS: PHOSPHODIESTERASE INHIBITORS

Amrinone

3-Amino-5-(4-pyridinyl)-2(1*H*)-pyridinone

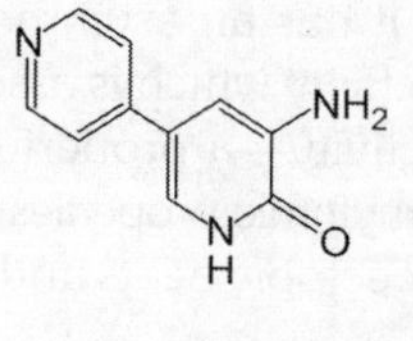

Synthesis

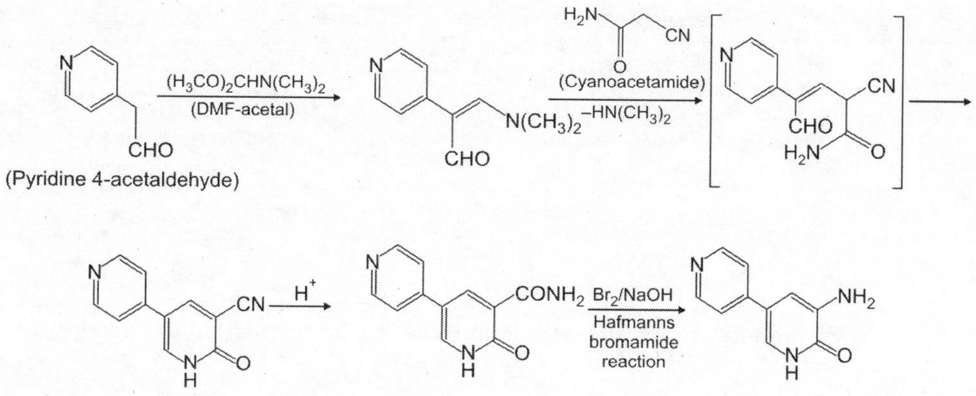

(Pyridine 4-acetaldehyde)

It inhibits phosphodiesterase, which results in increased levels of c-AMP. c-AMP activates protein kinases which increases calcium ion influx resulting in positive inotropic action. It is used only for short-term treatment of patients with heart failure.

Milrinone

1, 2-Dihydro-6-methyl-2-oxo-5-(4-pyridinyl)nicotinonitrile

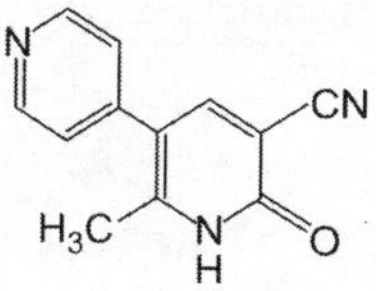

Synthesis

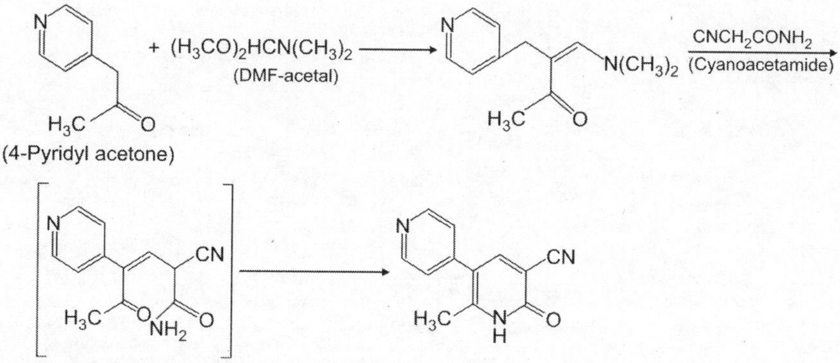

(4-Pyridyl acetone)

Activity similar to that of amrinone (60).

CARDIOTONIC DRUGS: β-ADRENERGIC RECEPTOR STIMULANTS
Dobutamine
See ADRENERGIC DRUGS

Section V
Drugs Acting on Blood

ANTICOAGULANTS, ANTIPLATELET, AND THROMBOLYTIC DRUGS

Hemostasis is the spontaneous arrest of bleeding from a damaged blood vessel. The responses which immediately follow hemostasis are vasoconstriction and then the platelets stick to the injured blood vessel and to each other resulting in primary hemostatic plug. This plug is reinforced by fibrin for long-term plugging. The fibrin formation results due to stimulation of plasma coagulation factors by platelets. As the wound heals, platelet aggregate, and fibrin clot are degraded.

Thrombosis is a pathological process in which platelet aggregate and fibrin clot are formed within the blood vessel in the absence of bleeding. Such a clot occlude the blood vessels.

Clots are formed in static blood in vitro and they consist of diffuse fibrin meshwork in which all the cells of the blood are trapped. Thrombus on the other hand is formed within the blood and is a pathological formation. It can be arterial or venous. Arterial thrombosis, which results in white thrombus (due to leukocytes and platelet in fibrin mesh) is associated with atherosclerosis. It results in ischemic necrosis. Thus, for example, myocardial infarction is due to thrombosis of coronary artery. Venous thrombosis, which results in red thrombus is similar to blood clot. It results in edema and inflammation of tissue which is drained by the vein. Thrombus can also travel to different parts of the body such as heart, lungs, and brain and can lead to ischemia and infarction.

Increased coagulability of blood is called thrombophilia and is associated with the use of certain contraceptives. Decreased coagulability results due to excessive use of anticoagulants or is hereditary as in case of hemophilia.

BLOOD COAGULATION

Blood coagulation is a process by which the fluid state of the blood is changed to a compact jelly-like mass. Number of factors are involved in coagulation (Table. 16.1). Coagulation involves activation of inactive precursors (zymogens) which are present in blood. The activation involves proteolysis and they are designated by the suffix "a". There are two pathways in coagulation, the intrinsic and the extrinsic pathway. Both these lead to the formation of factor Xa which converts prothrombin to thrombin. Thrombin converts fibrinogen to fibrin which is then converted to its insoluble form (polymer) by the factor XIII a (Fig. 16.1). Diseases associated with blood coagulation are either due to defect in coagulation or due to increased coagulation.

Table 16.1: Blood clotting factors

Factor	*Name*
I	Fibrinogen
I'	Fibrin monomer
I"	Fibrin polymer
II	Prothrombin
III	Tissue thromboplastin
IV	Ca^{2+}
V	Proaccelerin
VII	Proconvertin
VIII	Antihemophilic globulin (AHG)
IX	Christmas factor
X	Staurt-Power factor
XI	Plasma throboplastin antecedent (PTA)
XII	Hageman factor
XIII	Fibrin stabilizing factor
HMW-K	High molecular weight kininogen
Pre-K	Prekalikrein
Ka	Kallikrein
PL	Platelet phospholipid

Hemophilia A and hemophilia B, the hereditary diseases, caused by the deficiency of factors VIII and IX, respectively, are treated by giving fresh plasma or concentrated preparations of these factors.

Liver diseases, excessive treatment with oral anticoagulants and vitamin K deficiency, are treated by administering vitamin K. Vitamin K, a fat soluble vitamin, occurs in different forms and include vitamin K_1 [phylloquinone, (1)], vitamin $K_{2(30)}$ [menaquinone 6, (2)] and vitamin K_3 [(menadione, (3)].

O
R
CH3
O
CH3
CH3
CH3
CH3
(1) R = H2C
CH3
CH3
CH3
CH3
(2) R = CH2CH=C CH2 [CH2CH=C CH2]4CH2CH = C-CH3
(3) R = H

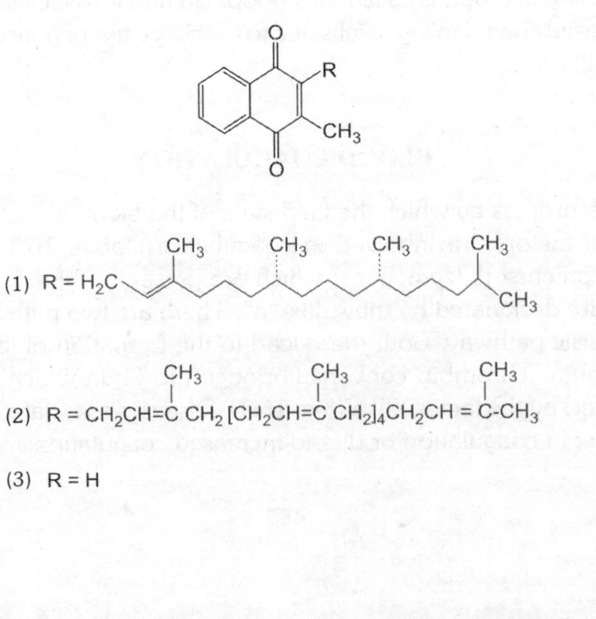

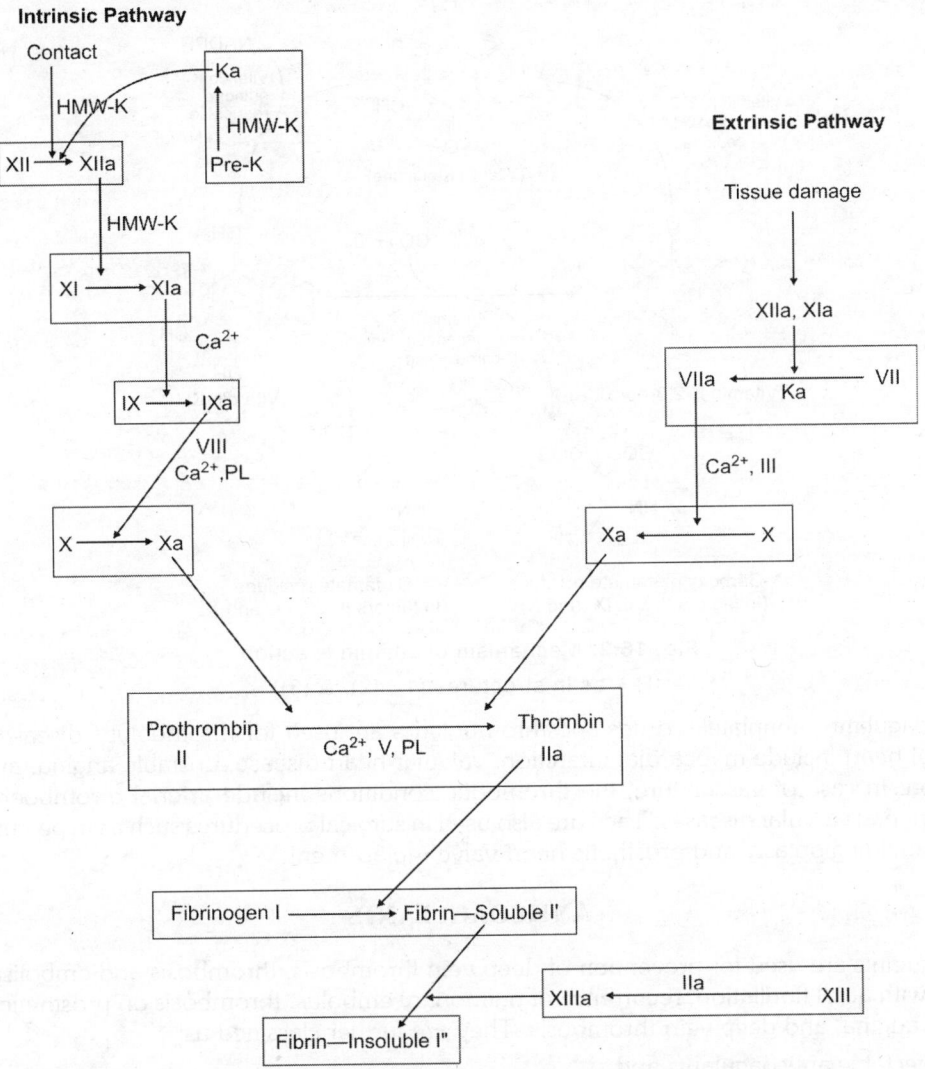

Fig. 16.1: Mechanism of blood coagulation.

Vitamin K is essential for the formation of clotting factors like II, VII, IX, and X. It is involved in the carboxylation of 10 or more glutamate residues to γ-carboxy glutamate. This carboxylation results in chelation of Ca^{2+} resulting in conformational changes in protein. These conformational changes in protein allow the four vitamin K-dependent clotting factors to bind to phospholipids of membrane during clotting process. Vitamin K-quinone is reduced by vitamin K-2,3-quinone reductase to hydroquinone vitamin KH_2 (Fig. 16.2). The reduced hydroquinone then in presence of vitamin K-dependent carboxylase and CO_2 and O_2 carboxylates the glutamic acid residues and itself is converted to vitamin K-2, 3-epoxide. The epoxide so formed, is converted to quinone by vitamin K-2, 3-epoxide reductase.

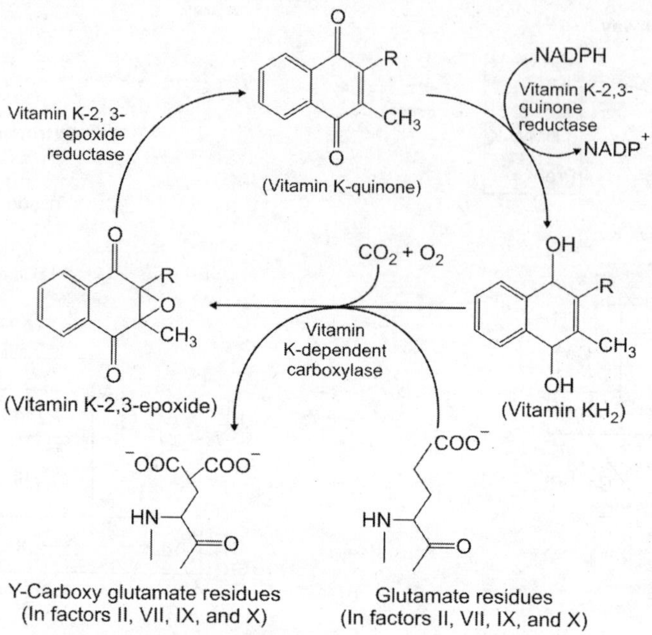

Fig. 16.2: Mechanism of vitamin K action.

[R = as in structures (1), (2), & (3)]

Anticoagulants, antiplatelet drugs and thrombolytics are used for thrombolytic diseases which in case of heart include myocardial infarction, valvular heart disease, unstable angina, and atrial fibrillation. In case of vasculature, the thrombotic conditions include arterial thromboembolism and peripheral vascular diseases. They are also used in surgical procedures such as in percutaneous transluminal angioplasty and prosthetic heart valve replacement.

ANTICOAGULANTS

Anticoagulants are used for prevention of deep vein thrombosis, thrombosis and embolisation in patients with atrial fibrillation, recurrence of pulmonary embolus, thrombosis on prosthetic valves, unstable angina, and deep vein thrombosis. They are further classified as:

1. Injectable anticoagulants and
2. oral anticoagulants.

Characteristics of an Ideal Anticoagulant

1. It should have high therapeutic index.
2. It should be equally effective whether administered orally or parenterally.
3. The drug should have a rapid onset and duration of action.
4. The effect on coagulation should terminate within reasonable period of time after the drug has been withdrawn.
5. Its effect should be rapidly reversed by a non-toxic antagonist.
6. It should not produce a toxic or cumulative effect.
7. Its therapeutic value must be clearly established.

INJECTABLE ANTICOAGULANTS

Injectable anticoagulants have been further classified as:

1. Heparin based anticoagulants,
2. direct thrombin inhibitors, and
3. selective Factor Xa inhibitors.

Heparin Based Anticoagulants

Heparin based anticoagulants include heparin and low molecular weight heparins. The unfractionated heparin (4) or high molecular weight heparin is mixture of straight chain and sulphated mucopolysaccharide (polymer of N-aetylglucosamine, D-glucuronic acid, or iduronic acid) with a molecular weight of 5-30 kDa (mean approx 15 kDa). It is found in secretory cells of mast cells. Heparin acts both in vitro and in vivo. It activates antithrombin III which is an inhibitor of thrombin and serine protease. Heparin also inhibits factor X.

$$R = H \text{ or } SO_3^-; \quad R' = SO_3^- \text{ or } COCH_3$$

(4)

Since heparin (4) is not absorbed from gut, it is administered subcutaneously. It is absorbed to the extent of 30% only. It binds to various protein receptors because of which there is decrease in bioavailability. Further, its non-specific binding results in heparin induced thrombocytopenia, a major drawback, caused by interaction of heparin to platelet factor 4.

It recent times fractionated heparins obtained by gel filtration chromatography or differential precipitation by ethanol, known as low molecular weight heparins, are also used as anticoagulants. These include dalteparin, enoxaparin, and tinzaparin. Their molecular weight varies from 4-6kDa. The low molecular weight heparins have better pharmacokinetic and pharmacodynamic profiles. Low molecular weight heparins have low protein binding affinity as well as lower interaction with platelet factor 4. As a result, there is lower incidence of heparin induced thrombocytopenia with the use of low molecular weight heparin. The mechanism of their action is similar to that of heparin.

Various approaches to increasing the absoption of heparin have been investigated and include the use of amine salt in enteric coated tablets, salts with organic lipophilic amines, oil-water emulsions, liposomes, and microsphere encapsulations.

Direct Thrombin Inhibitors

Thrombin plays an important role in coagulation which includes conversion of fibrinogen to fibrin, activation of factor XIII which is responsible for cross linking of fibrin polymers, and activation of platelets. Direct inhibition of thrombin, therefore, could be one of the methods to achieve anticoagulant effect. In recent times many direct thrombin inhibitors have been developed as a result of structure-based drug design and recombinant technology. These anticoagulants include lepirudin, desirudin, hirudin, bivalirudin, and argatroban.

Lepirudin and desirudin are proteins with 65 amino acids. Both of them inhibit thrombin irreversibly and are recombinant hirudin derivatives. Hirudin, a protein of 65 amino acids, was isolated from salivary glands of leech. Lepirudin is administered as an intravenous infusion and desirudin subcutaneously. They are used for treatment of heparin induced thrombocytopenia and thrombotic syndrome.

Bivalirudin has been used for unstable angina. It is a 20 amino acid peptide with reversible action. It is administered via intravenous bolus followed by continuous infusion. It has a rapid onset of action.

Argatroban (5) is used as prophylactic for the treatment of thrombosis in heparin induced thrombocytopenia. It is a reversible inhibitor of thrombin as well as clot bound thrombin.

(5)

Selective Factor Xa Inhibitors

Fondaparinux (6), a synthetic sulphated pentasaccharide, contains five essential sugars necessary for binding to antithrombin III. After binding to antithrombin III, it induces a conformational change in antithrombin III required for conjugation to factor Xa. It is a specific inhibitor of Xa with negligible antithrombin activity. It is used for treatment of deep vein thrombosis and is administered subcutaneously. It does not cause heparin induced thrombocytopenia.

(6)

ORAL ANTICOAGULANTS

Oral anticoagulants include:

1. Coumarins and
2. indanediones

Coumarins

The discovery of 3, 3′ methylene bis (4-hydroxycoumarin) or dicoumarol (7) as a causative agent for the death of cattle due to bleeding led to development of oral anticoagulants. At present number of oral anticoagulants are known and these include 4-hydroxycoumarin (8), warfarin (9), phenprocoumon (10), and acenocoumarol (11).

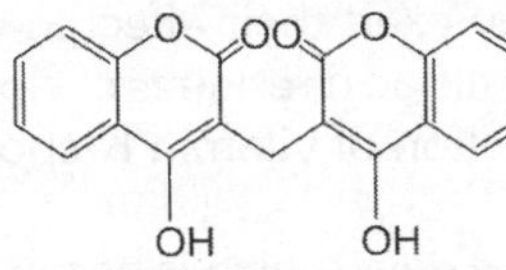

(7) 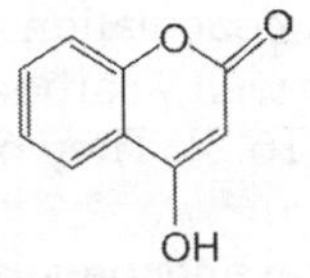   (8) 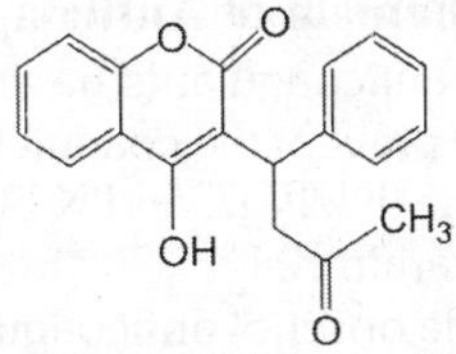   (9)

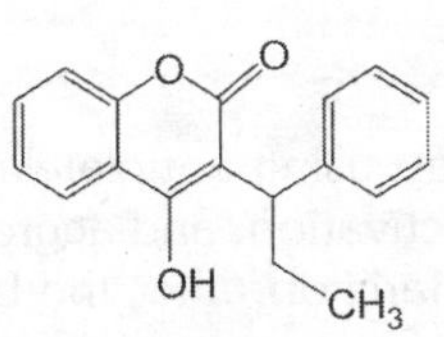

(10) 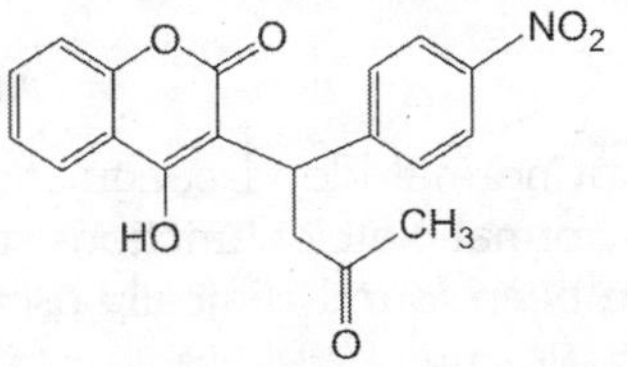   (11)

Structure-Activity Relationship Studies

Coumarin (12) shows only moderate anticoagulant activity. Substitution at position 3 by groups like hydroxyl or a benzamido group results in inactive compounds. However, when position 3 is substituted by methyl, ethyl, methoxy, or phenyl group, moderate activity appears. Substitution by hydroxyl group at position 4 results in significant anticoagulant activity. Substitution in the benzene nucleus at position 7 or 8 by a methoxy group results in powerful anticoagulants.

Structure-activity relationship studies on dicoumarol (7) have shown that for optimum activity a substituent on methylene bridge with 3 to 4 carbons and containing a carbonyl function at 2′ or 3′- position is necessary. Example of such compounds include ethyl biscoumacetate (13).

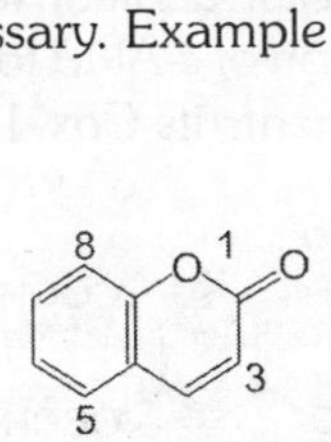

(12) 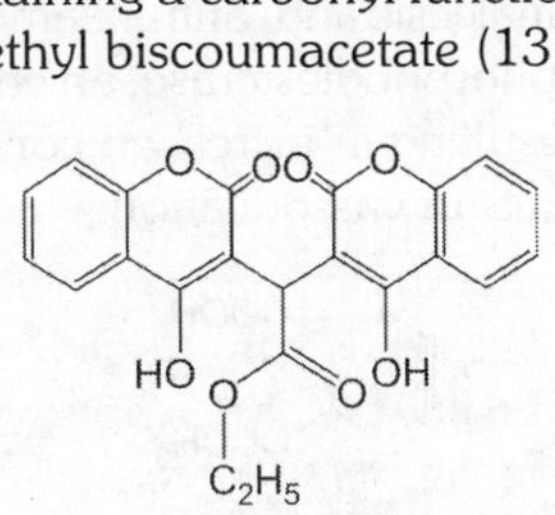   (13)

Indanedione

Indane-1, 3-dione (14) has certain structural resemblance to coumarin (12). Some of the compounds in this series include phenindione (15), clorindione (16), bromindione (17) anisindione (18) and diphenadione (19).

15, x = H
16, x = Cl
17, x = Br
18, x = OCH₃

(14)   (19)

Mechanism of Anticoagulants and Action of Oral Anticoagulants

Oral anticoagulants have no influence on coagulation in vitro, but they exert their effect in vivo. They prevent the coagulation by interfering with γ-carboxylation of glutamic acid residues of clotting factors II, VII, IX and X by vitamin K (Fig. 16.2). They prevent the reduction of vitamin K-epoxide to vitamin KH_2.

The onset of anticoagulant activity of oral anticoagulants takes several days which is because of time taken for the degradation of carboxylated factors.

ANTIPLATELET DRUGS

Inhibition of normal blood coagulation can also be achieved by using antiplatelet drugs which inhibit the normal platelet functions such as platelet adhesion, activation, and aggregation. These drugs have been found clinically useful in acute myocardial infarction, after the bypass surgery and in angioplasty.

Antiplatelet drugs include:

1. Cox-1 inhibitors,
2. phosphodiesterase inhibitors,
3. glycoprotein IIb/IIIa receptor antagonists, and
4. inhibitors of P2Y receptors.

Cox-1 Inhibitors

Some of these include aspirin (20), triflusal (21), sulphinpyrazone (22), and indobufen (23).

Aspirin (20) is a well known antiplatelet drug and acts through inhibition of Cox-1. It has antipyretic, analgesic and, anti-inflammatory activity also. Triflusal (21), in addition to Cox-1 inhibitor, also inhibits phosphodiesterase, an enzyme responsible for degradation of c-AMP to AMP in platelets and blood resulting in increased conc. of c-AMP. This effect auguments its Cox-1 inhibition effect and also results in vassodilation.

(20)   (21)

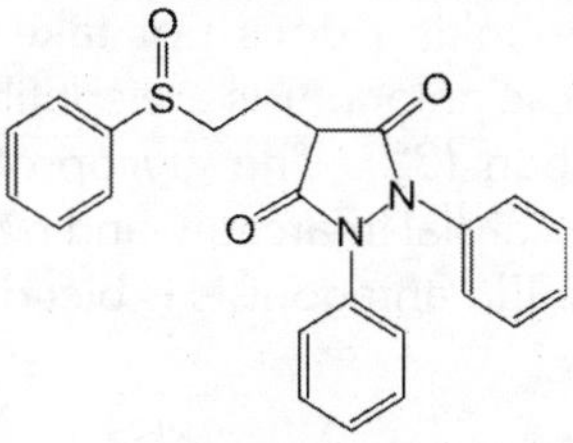

(22)

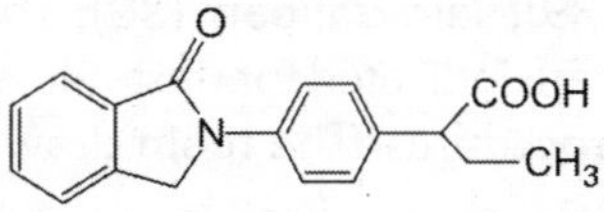

(23)

Sulphinpyrazone (22) is a structural analog of phenylbutazone (24). However, it does not have any significant anti-inflammatory effect. Both sulphinpyrazone (22) and its sulphide (25) metabolite possess Cox-1 inhibition activity.

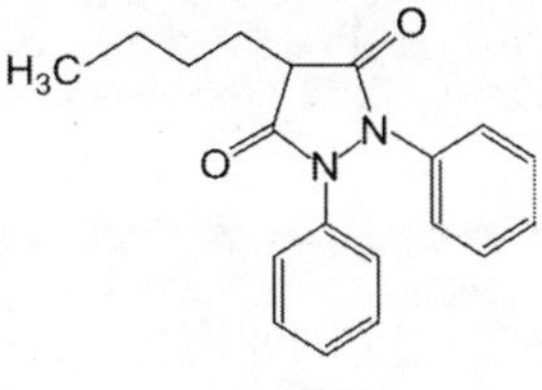

(24)

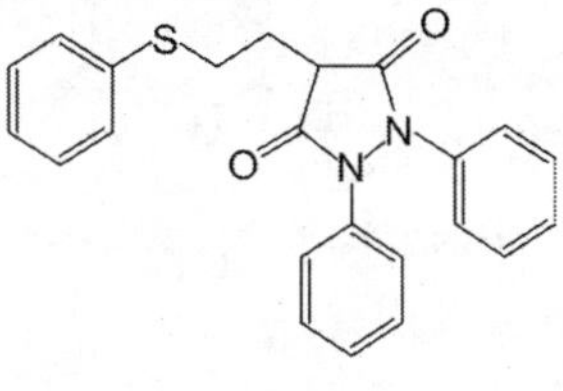

(25)

Indobufen (23) is a potent reversible inhibitor of Cox -1

Phosphodiesterase Inhibitors

As indicated above phosphodiestrase is an enzyme which converts c-AMP to AMP. Inhibition of this enzyme leads to higher concentrations of c-AMP in blood and platelets which results in inhibition of platelet aggregation and vasodilation. Some of these inhibitors include cilostazol (26) and dipyridamole (27). In addition to inhibition of phosphodiesterase they also block reuptake of adenosine and act at A_2-adenosine receptor to stimulate platelet adenylyl cyclase. Both of these effects result in increased blood and platelet levels of adenylyl cyclase.

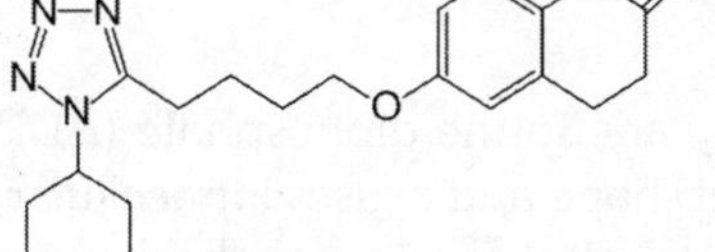

(26)

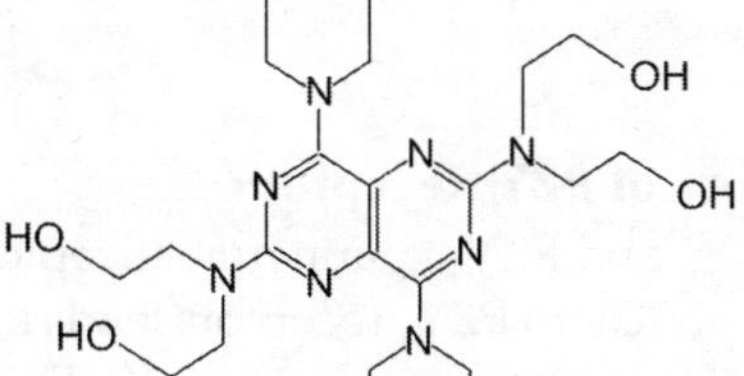

(27)

Gylcoprotein IIb/IIIa Receptor Antagonists

The final step of platelet aggregation is the expression of platelet membrane glycoprotein IIb/IIIa receptors. The normal substrate of these recptors is fibrinogen. One fibrinogen molecule acts to cross-link two platelets via binding of glycoprotein IIb/IIIa receptors. If the platelet surface receptors are occupied by another molecule then binding and crosslinking does not take place and consequently the aggregation does not take place. Some of these antagonists are eptifibatide (28), lamifiban (29), lefradafiban (30), roxifiban (31), and tirofiban (32). The glycoprotein IIb/IIIa antagonists are indicated for unstable angina, non-Q-wave myocardial infarction, and percutaneous coronary procedures. The main draw back of glycoprotein IIb/IIIa antagonists is bleeding.

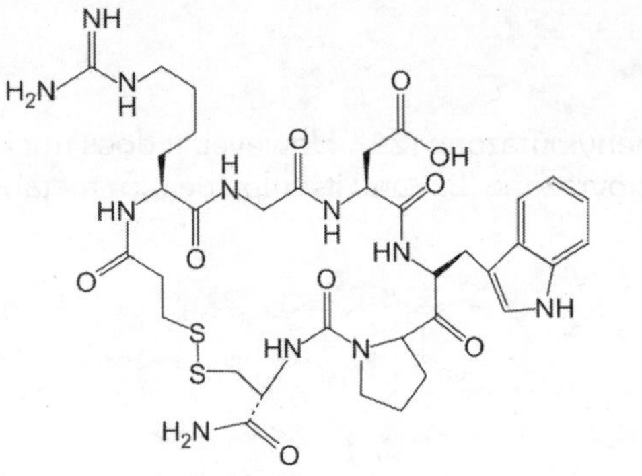

(28) 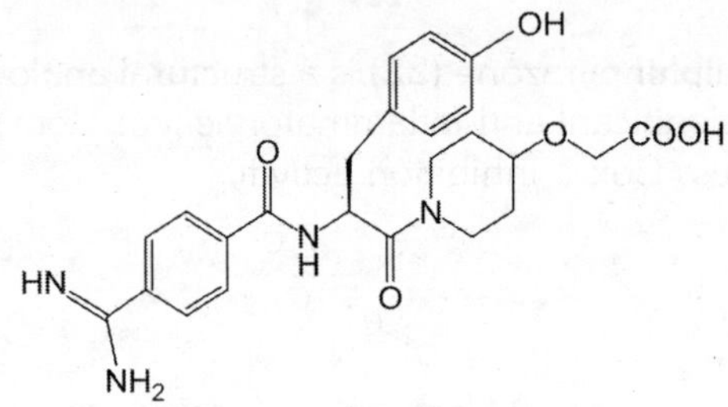　　　　　　　　　　　　(29)

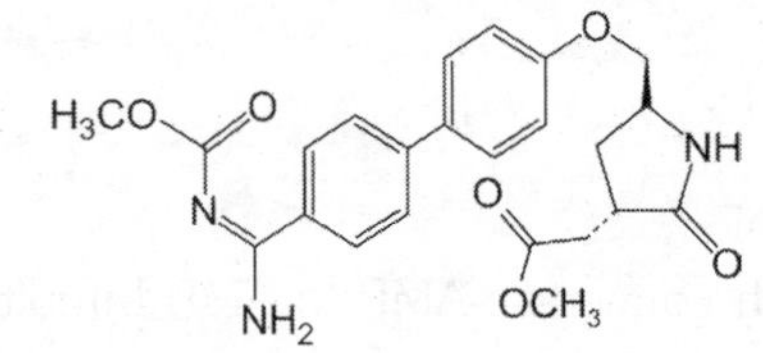

(30) 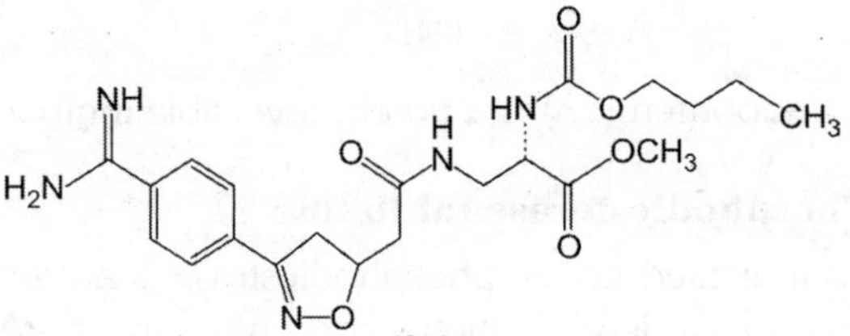　　　　　　　　　　　　(31)

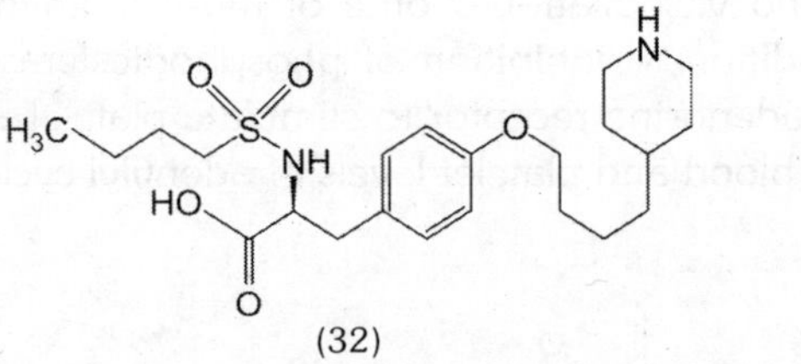

(32)

Inhibitors of P2Y Receptors

Both P2Y$_1$ and P2Y$_{12}$ purinergic receptors are activated by adenosine diphosphate (ADP). Initial binding of ADP to P2Y$_1$ receptors leads to change in platelet shape and causes intracellular calcium mobilization. Subsequent binding of ADP to P2Y$_{12}$ receptors results in sustained platelet aggregation by inhibiting adenylyl cyclase resulting in decrease in c-AMP levels. Ticlopidine (33) and clopidogrel (34) are the drugs which inhibit P2Y$_{12}$ receptors irreversibly.

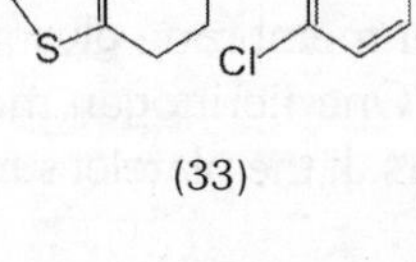

(33) 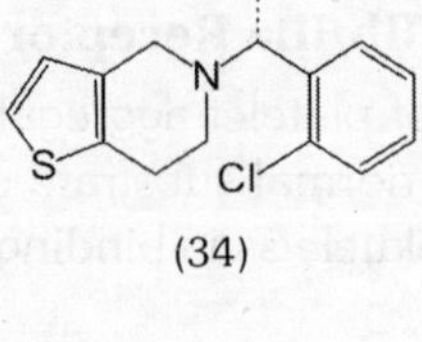　　　　　　　　　　　　(34)

THROMBOLYTIC DRUGS

Anticoagulants like unfractionated and low molecular weight heparins, direct thrombin inhibitors, selective Factor Xa inhibitors, and oral anticoagulants, prevent the formation, and propagation of thrombi. These agents are not, however, effective against preformed thrombi. This results in occluded or partially obstructed blood vessels. Thrombolytic agents dissolve the preformed clot by converting inactive zymogen plasminogen to the active protease plasmin. The plasmin than converts cross-linked fibrin polymer to fibrin degradation products. One of the disadvantage of thrombolytic agents is that it not only dissolves pathological thrombi but also the physiological thrombi formed in response to an injury. This may lead to bleeding.

Some of the thrombolytic agents include streptokinase, urokinase, alteplase, prourokinase, reteplase, and tenecteplase.

Stteptokinase is a first generation thrombolytic agent. It is a protein purified from cultures of β-hemolytic *Streptococci* bacteria. It is a protein with 414 amino acids and a molecular weight of 47kDa. Streptokinase acts by first complexing with plasminogen to form 1:1 activator complex. This complex then converts uncomplexed plasminogen to fibrinolytic enzyme plasmin. Streptokinase is non-specific in its action because it not only degrades fibrin but also catalyzes the breakdown of fibrinogen and factors V to VII. Further streptokinase may have antigenicity because it is foreign to the human body.

Urokinase which is found in urine degrades directly the fibrin and fibrinogen. It is isolated from human fetal kidney cells. Urokinase dos not possess antigenicity associated with streptokinase.

Alteplase is tissue plaminogen activator (tPA) that has high affinity for plasminogen bound to fibrin but low affinity for free plasminogen. It is unmodified human tpa and is produced commercially by recombinant technology.

Prourokinase, a urokinase-like tPA, is composed of 411 amino acids. It is a thrombolytic agent which does not interfere with hemostasis and nonimmunogenic. It is useful in the treatment of peripheral vascular occlusion.

Reteplase is a modified tPA in which first 172 amino acids that are present in alteplase have been removed. It contains 355 amino acids with a molecular weight of 39kDa.

Another genetically variant of tPA is tenecteplase. It is more resistant to plasminogen activator inhibitors. It is composed of 527 amino acids with 17 disulphide linkages.

INDIVIDUAL COMPOUNDS

ANTICOAGULANTS : INJECTABLE—HEPARIN BASED

Heparin
Heparinic acid

R = H or SO_3^-; R'= SO_3^- or $COCH_3$

Heparin is heterogenous mixture of variably sulphated polysaccharide chain composed of repeating units of N-actyl glucosamine and either iduronic or D-glucuronic acid. It is biosynthesized and stored in mast cells of tissues such as liver, lung, or gut. It is prepared from the lungs of oxen (heparin lung) or intestinal mucosa (heparin mucosa).

Heparin has the property of delaying the clotting of the blood. It acts by activating antithrombin III (AT III) a natural inhibitor that inactivates factor Xa and thrombin. It acts both in vivo and in vitro

Heparin is administered intravenously in two ways:

1. The intermittent dose method. In this, a dose of 50 mg is repeatedly given every 4 hours until a total of 250 mg/day has been given.
2. Continuous drip method. Slow infusion of heparin containing solution in the vein.

ANTICOAGULANTS : INJECTABLE—DIRECT THOMBIN INHIBITOS

Argatroban

(2R,4R)-1-[(2S)-5-[(Aminoiminomethyl)amino]-1-oxo-2-[[1,2,3,4-tetrahydro-3-methyl-8-quinoliny)sulphonyl]amino]pentyl]-4-methyl-2-piperidinecarboxylic acid

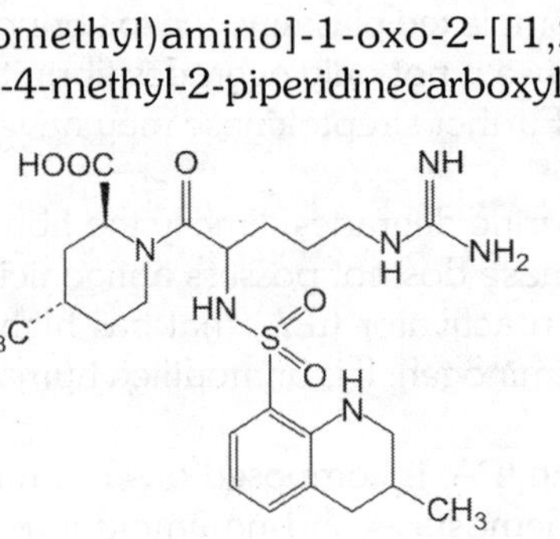

Synthesis

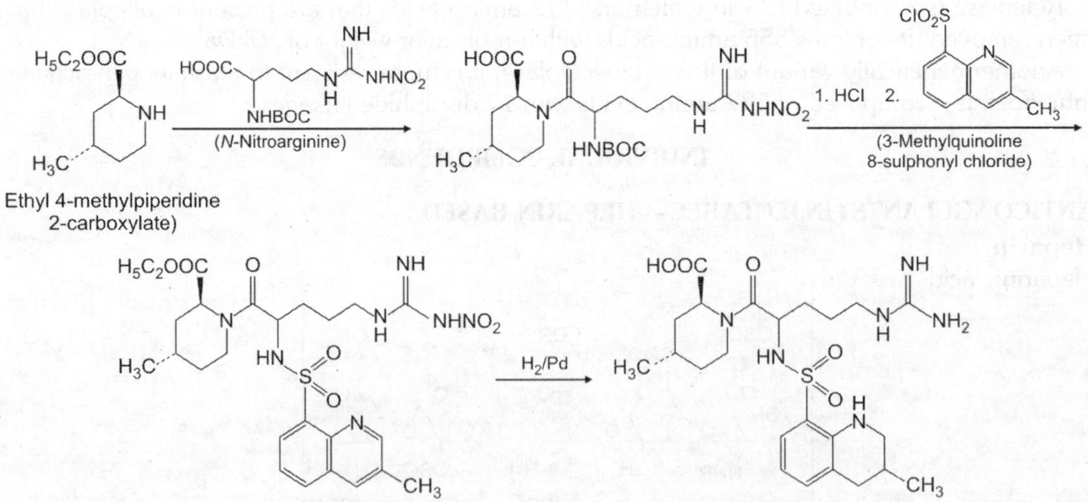

It is a direct inhibitor of thrombin.

ANTICOAGULANTS : INJECTABLE—SELECTIVE FACTOR Xa INHIBITORS
Fondaparinux

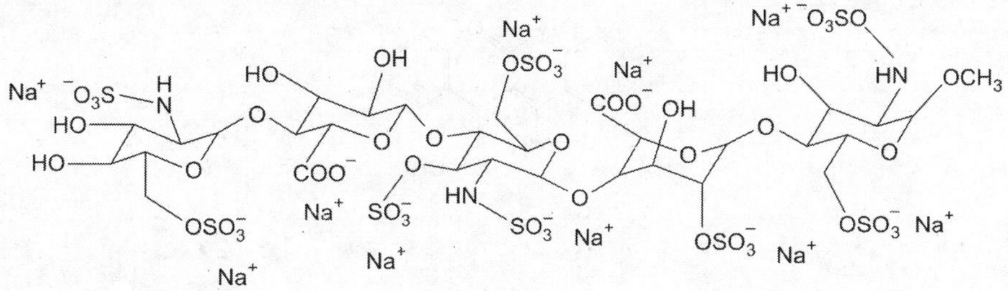

It is a synthetic sulphated pentasaccharide and is selective Factor Xa inhibitor

ANTICOAGULANTS : ORAL—COUMARINS
4-Hydroxycoumarin

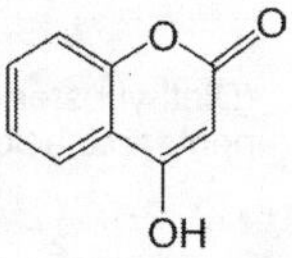

Synthesis

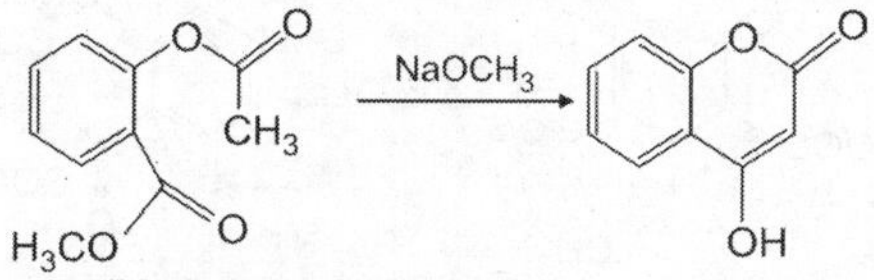

(Methylacetylsalicylate)

Warfarin Sodium
Sodium salt of 4-Hydroxy-3-(3-oxo-1-phenylbutyl)coumarin

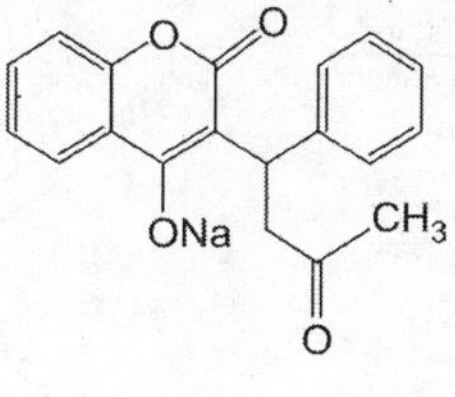

Synthesis

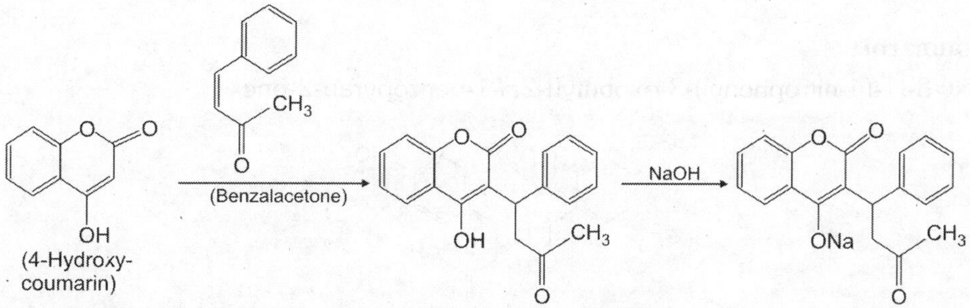

(4-Hydroxy-
coumarin)   (Benzalacetone)

It is a very good anticoagulant when used in proper dosage.

Phenprocoumon

4-Hydroxy-3-(1-phenylpropyl)-2-*H*-1-benzopyran-2-one

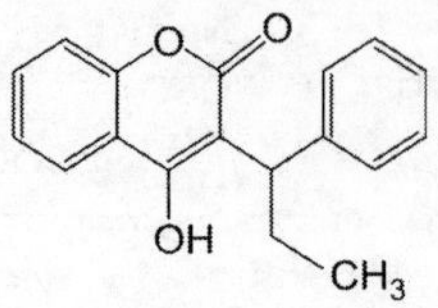
O
O
OH
CH3

Synthesis

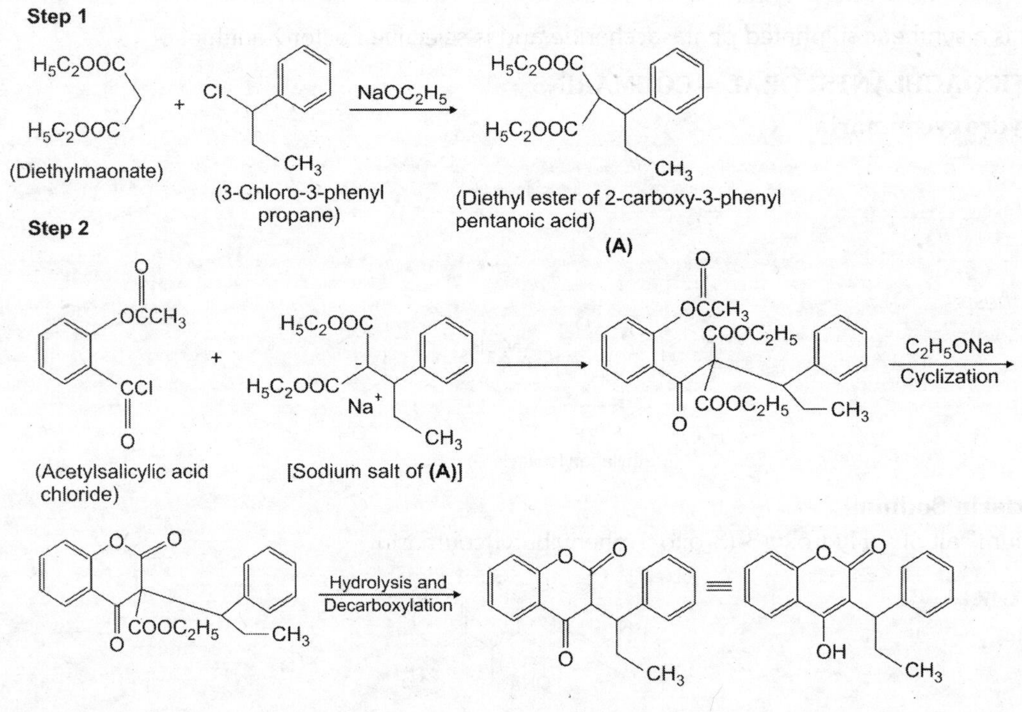
Step 1
H5C2OOC
H5C2OOC
(Diethylmaonate)
Cl
CH3
(3-Chloro-3-phenyl propane)
NaOC2H5
H5C2OOC
H5C2OOC
CH3
(Diethyl ester of 2-carboxy-3-phenyl pentanoic acid)
(A)
Step 2
OCCH3
CCl
(Acetylsalicylic acid chloride)
H5C2OOC
H5C2OOC
Na+
CH3
[Sodium salt of (A)]
OCCH3
COOC2H5
COOC2H5
CH3
C2H5ONa
Cyclization
COOC2H5
CH3
Hydrolysis and Decarboxylation
CH3
OH
CH3

Same activity as other coumarins.

Acenocoumarol

4-Hydroxy-3-[1-(4-nitrophenyl)-3-oxobutyl]-2*H*-1-benzopyran-2-one

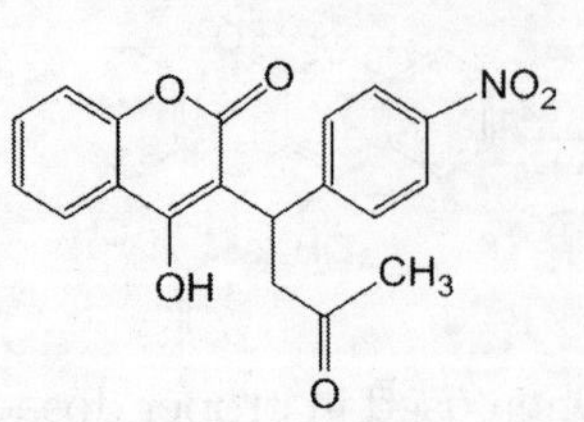
NO2
OH
CH3
O

Synthesis

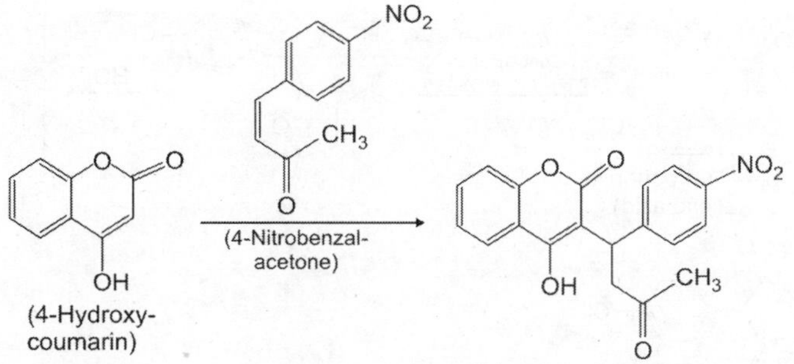

It is claimed to be the most active anticoagulant.

ANTICOAGULANTS : ORAL — INDANEDIONES

Phenindione

2-Phenylindane-1,3-dione

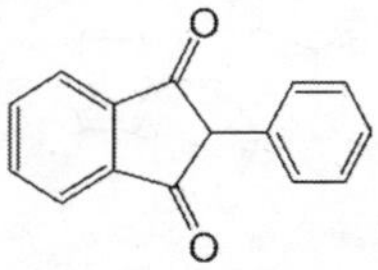

Synthesis

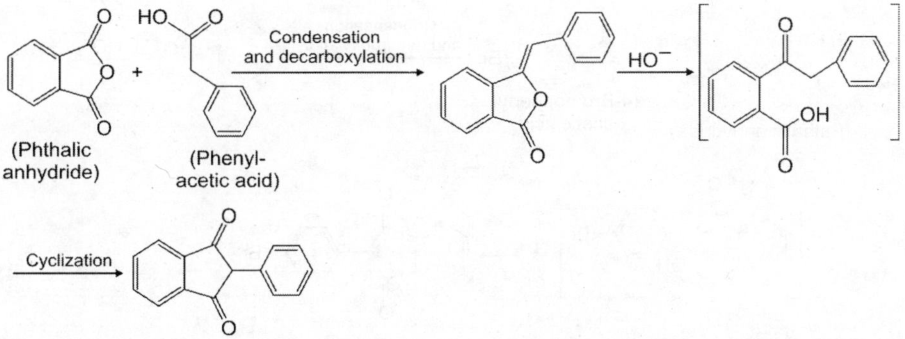

Phenindione is a prompt acting drug which is eliminated faster and is thus a safer drug.

Clorindione

2-(*p*-Chlorophenyl)indane-1,3-dione

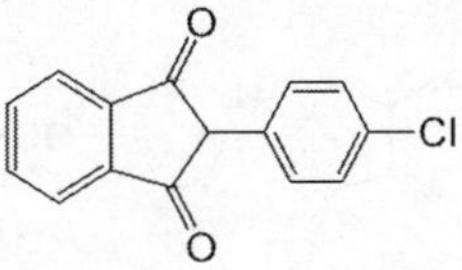

Synthesis

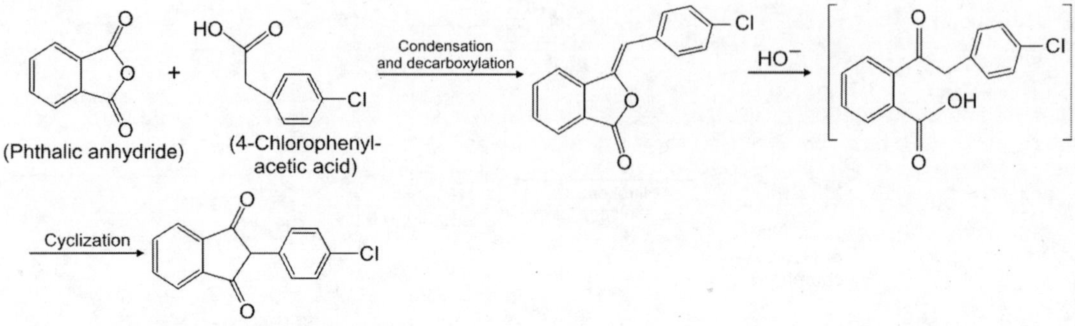

(Phthalic anhydride) + (4-Chlorophenyl-acetic acid) → Condensation and decarboxylation → HO⁻ →

Cyclization →

Similar in action to phenindione (15).

Bromindione

2-(*p*-Bromophenyl)indan-1,3-dione

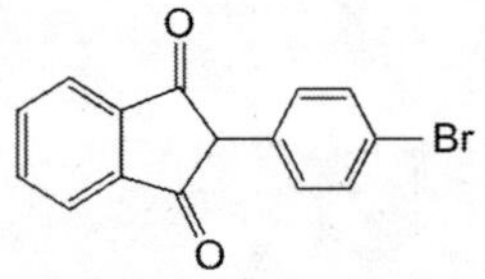

Synthesis

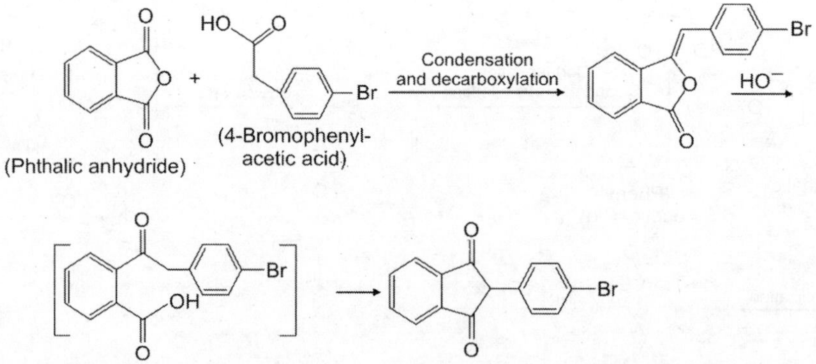

(Phthalic anhydride) + (4-Bromophenyl-acetic acid) → Condensation and decarboxylation → HO⁻ →

Similar action as clorindone (16).

Anisindione

2-(*p*-Methoxyphenyl)indan-1,3-dione

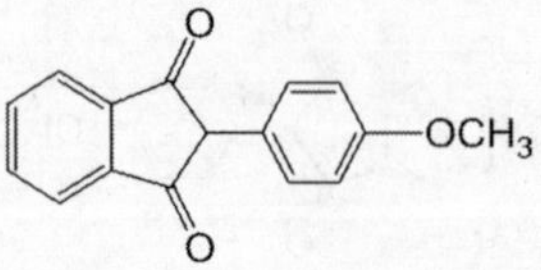

Synthesis

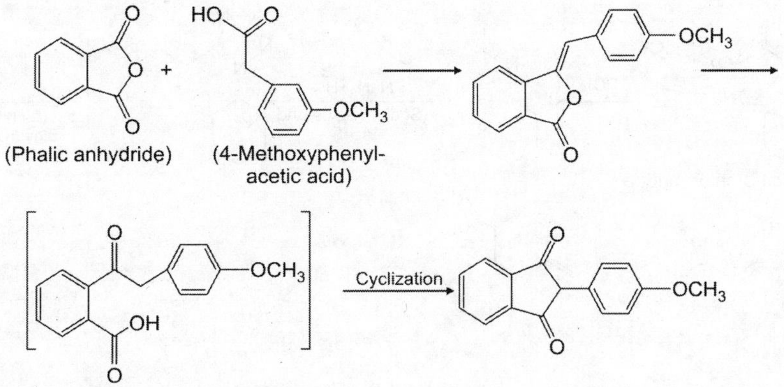
(Phalic anhydride)
(4-Methoxyphenyl-acetic acid)
OCH3
HO
OH
Cyclization

It is well absorbed after oral administration.

Diphenadione

2-(Diphenylacetyl)indan-1,3-dione

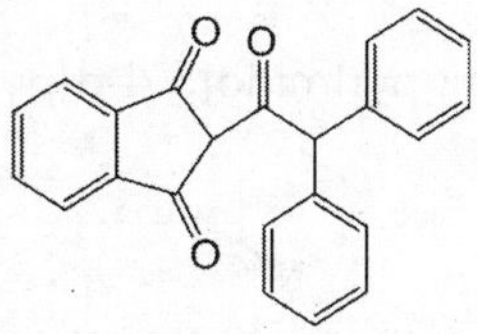

Synthesis

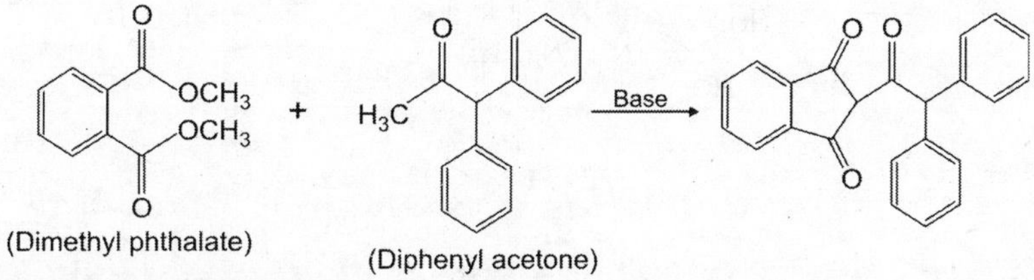
OCH3
H3C
Base
(Dimethyl phthalate)
(Diphenyl acetone)

Similar action as other indandiones.

ANTIPLATELET DRUGS: COX I INHBIBITORS

Aspirin and Sulphinpyrazone

See ANALGESICS, ANTIPYRETIC, AND NON-STEROIDAL ANTI-INFLAMMATORY DRUGS

ANTIPLATELET DRUGS: PHOSPHODIESTERASE INHIBITORS

Cilostazol

6-[4-(1-Cyclohexyl-1*H*-tetrazol-5-yl)butoxy]-3,4-dihydro-2(1*H*)quinolinone

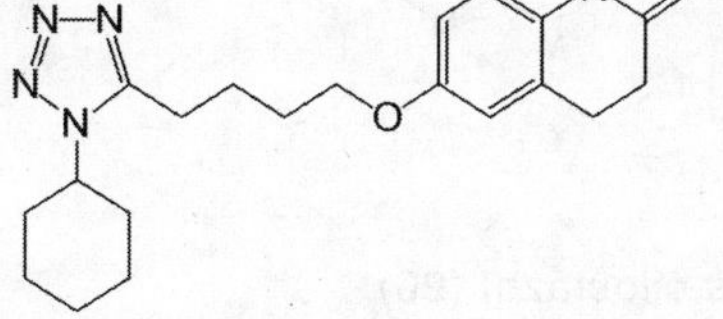

Synthesis

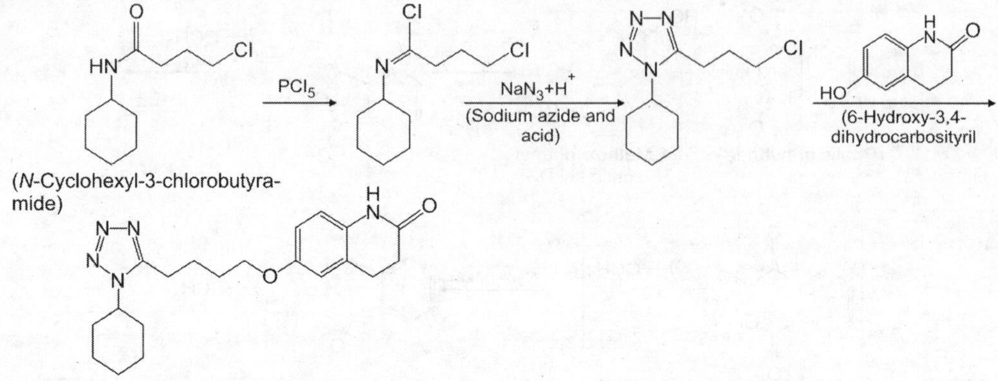

(*N*-Cyclohexyl-3-chlorobutyra-mide)

Cilostazol acts by inhibiting phosphodiesterase and blockade of adenosine reuptake and stimulation of A_2-adenosine receptor All this results in increase in c-AMP.

Dipyridamole

2,6-Bis(diethanolamino-4,8-dipiperidinopyrimido[5,4-d]pyrimidine

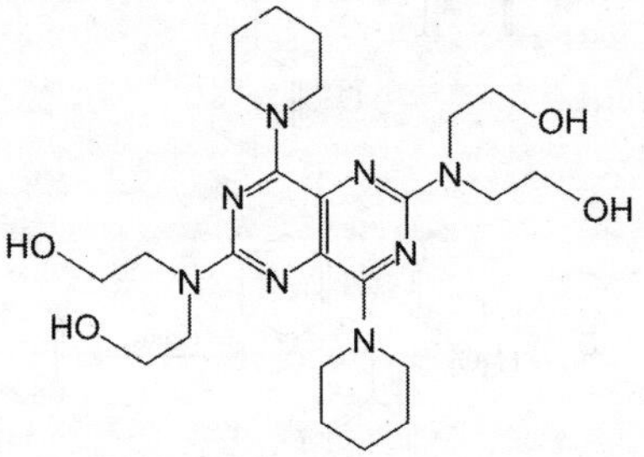

Synthesis

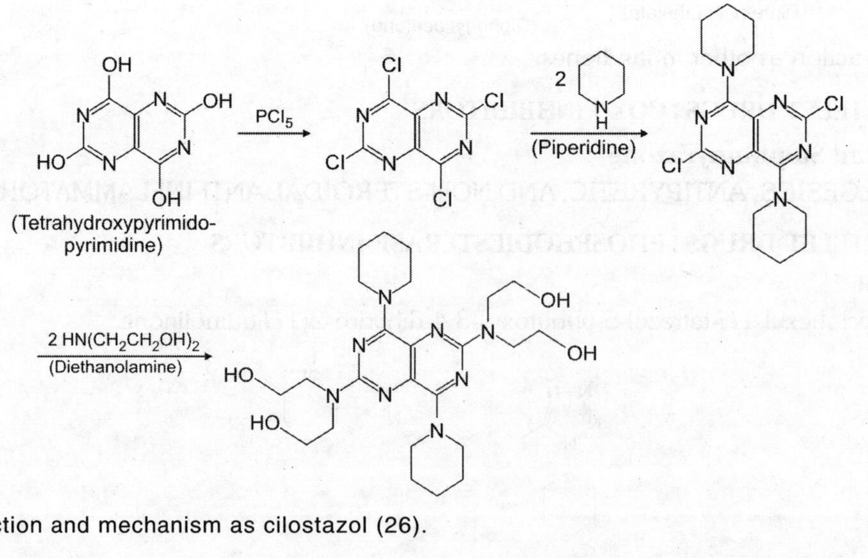

(Tetrahydroxypyrimido-pyrimidine)

Same action and mechanism as cilostazol (26).

ANTIPLATELET DRUGS : GLCOPROTEIN IIb/IIIa RECEPTOR ANTAGONISTS

Lamifiban

(S)-[[1-[2-[[4-(Aminoiminomethyl)benzoyl]amino]-3-(4-hydroxyphenyl)-1-oxopropyl]-4-piperidinyl]oxy]acetic acid

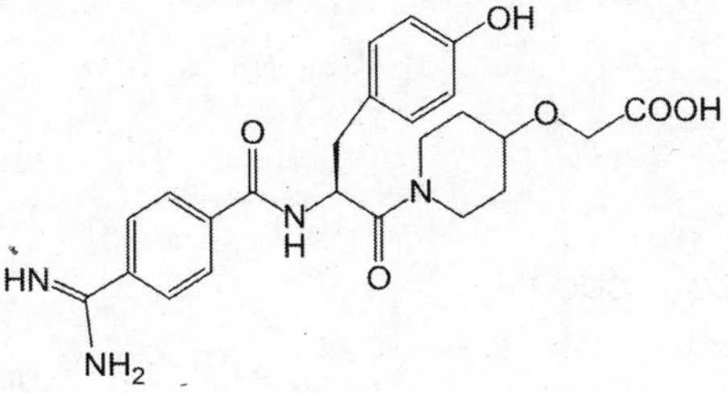

Synthesis

Step 1

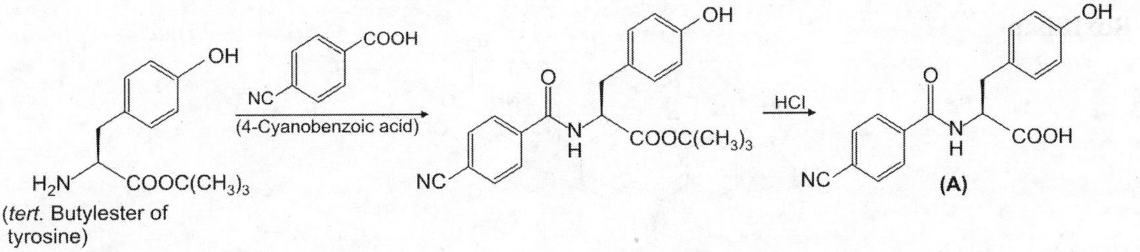

(tert. Butylester of tyrosine)

(4-Cyanobenzoic acid)

(A)

Step 2

(Sodium salt of *N-*benzyl piperidine 4-ol)

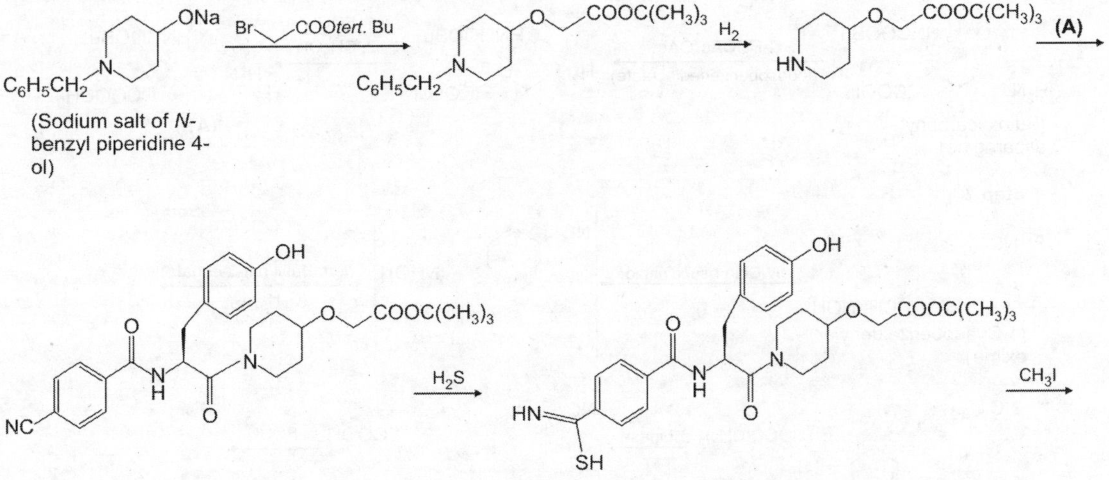

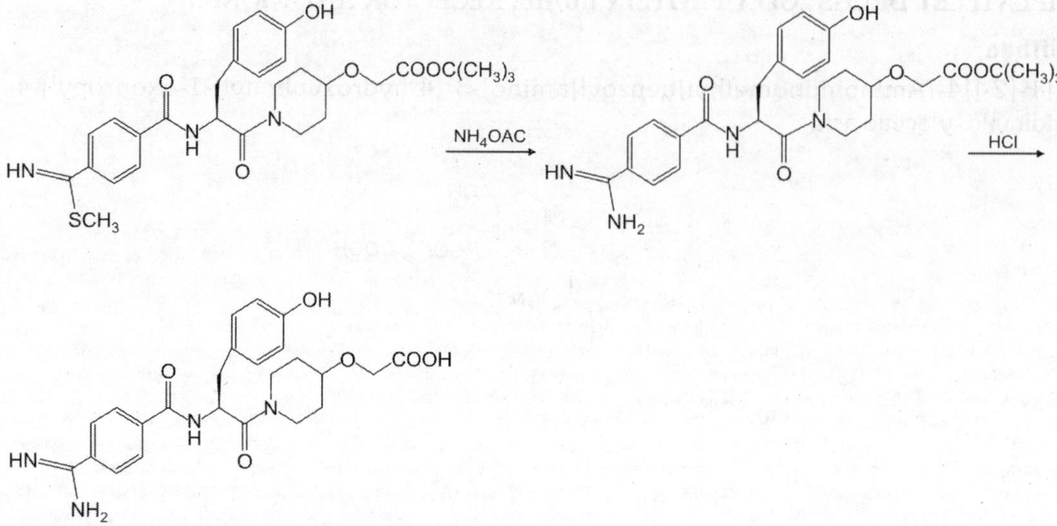

It is a glycoprotein IIb/IIIa receptor antagonist

Roxifiban

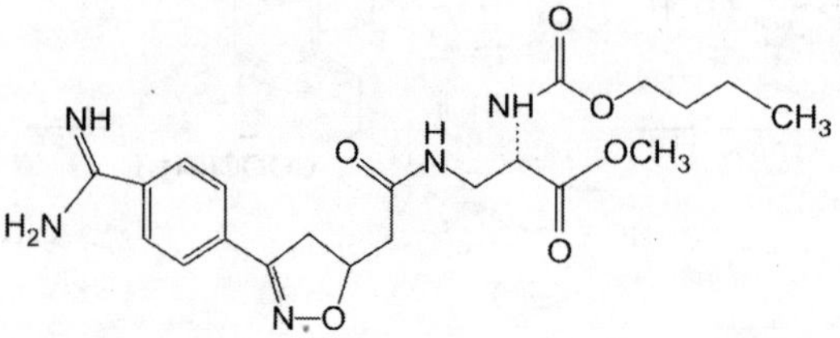

Synthesis

Step 1

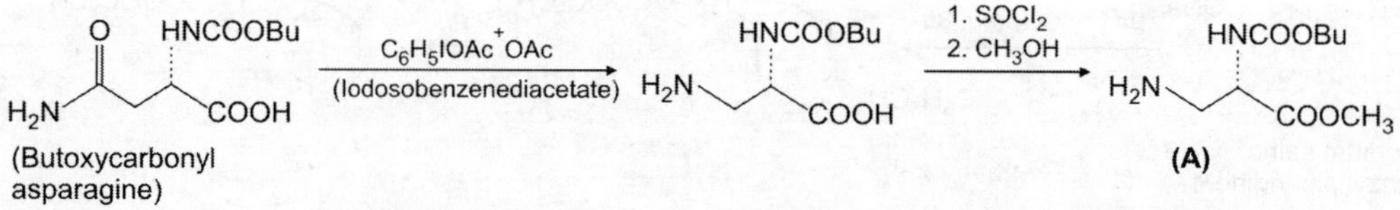

(Butoxycarbonyl asparagine)

C₆H₅IOAc⁺OAc (Iodosobenzenediacetate)

1. SOCl₂
2. CH₃OH

(A)

Step 2

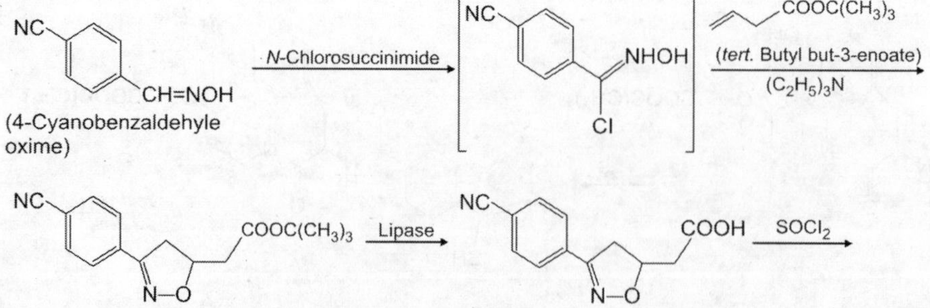

(4-Cyanobenzaldehyle oxime)

N-Chlorosuccinimide

COOC(CH₃)₃
(tert. Butyl but-3-enoate)
(C₂H₅)₃N

COOC(CH₃)₃   Lipase   COOH   SOCl₂

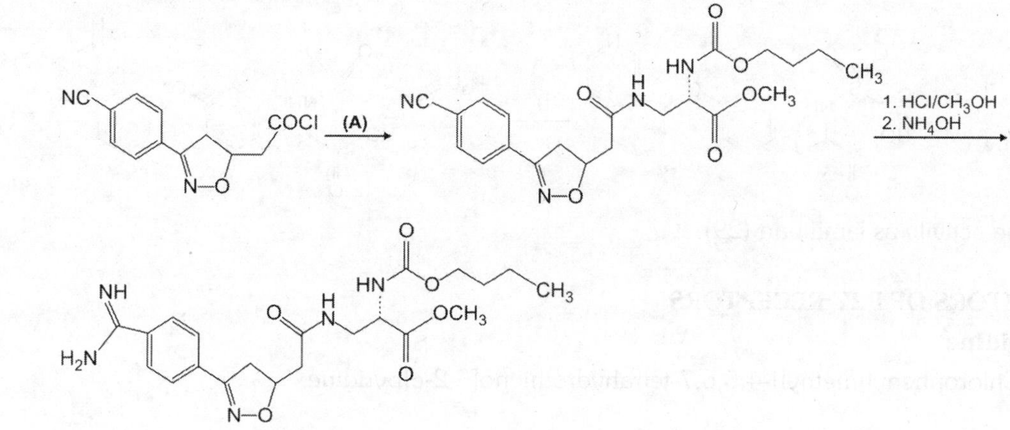

Same activity as lamifiban (29).

Tirofiban

N-(Butylsulphonyl)-*O*-[4-(4-piperidinyl)butyl]-L-tyrosine

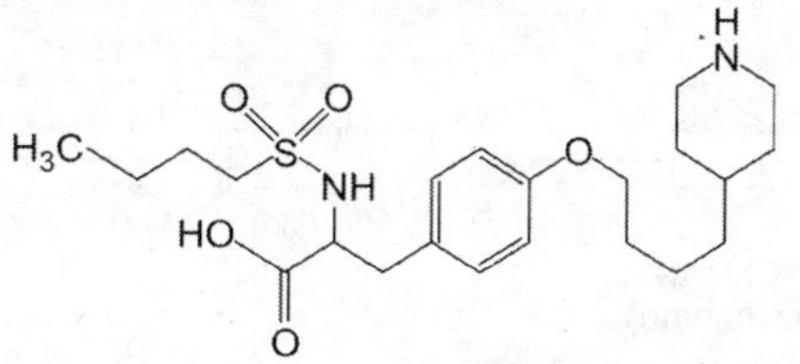

Synthesis

Step 1

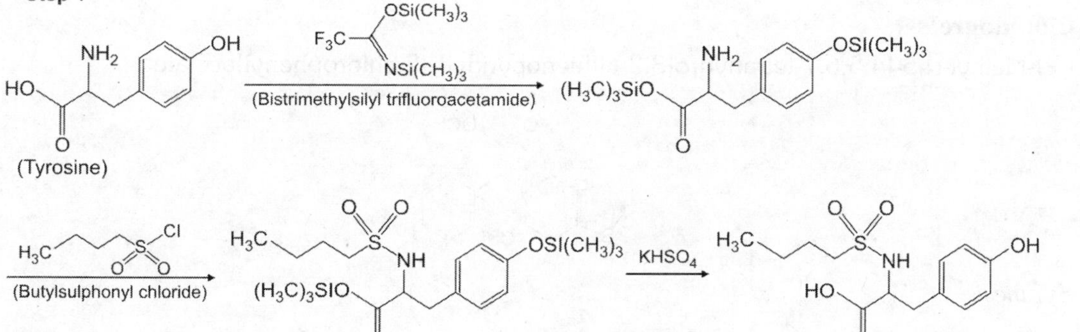

(Tyrosine)

(Bistrimethylsilyl trifluoroacetamide)

(Butylsulphonyl chloride)

(A)

Step 2

1. Butyl lithium
2. Br⟍⟍CL

(3-Bromopropyl chloride)

(4-Methylpyridine)

(A)

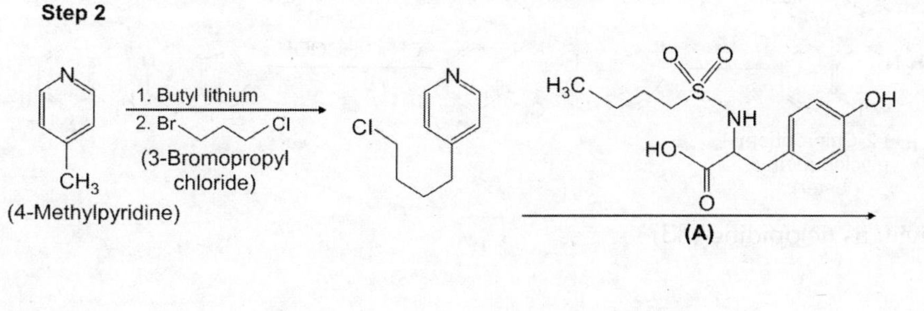

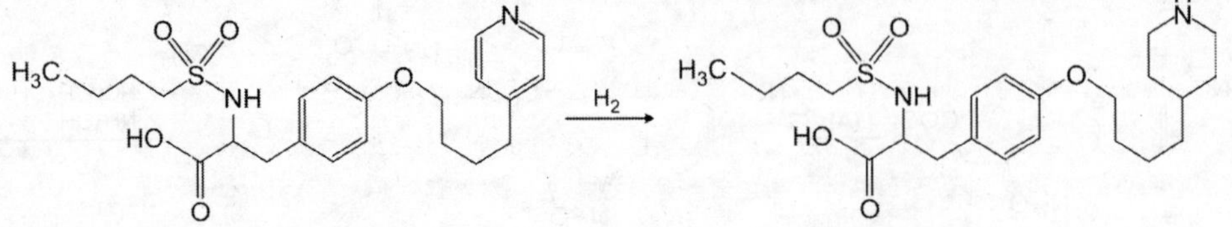

Same activity as lamifiban (29).

INHIBITORS OF P2Y RECEPTORS

Ticlopidine

5-[(2-Chlorophenyl)methyl]-4,5,6,7-tetrahydrothieno[3,2-c]pyridine

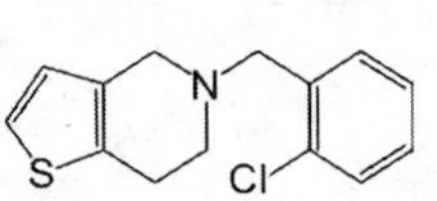

Synthesis

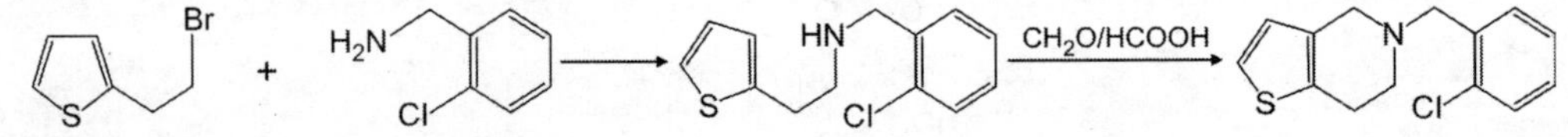

| [2-(2-Thienyl)-ethylbromide) | (2-Chloro-benzylamine) |

It is an inhibitor of $P2Y_{12}$ receptor.

Clopidogrel

(+)-Methyl-α-5-[4,5,6,7-tetrahydro[3,2-c]thienopyridyl]-(2-chlorophenyl)acetate

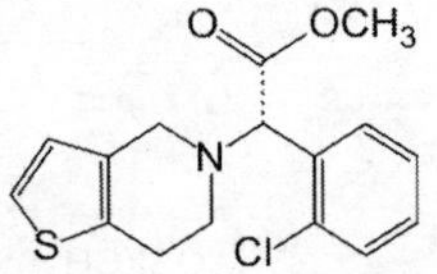

Synthesis

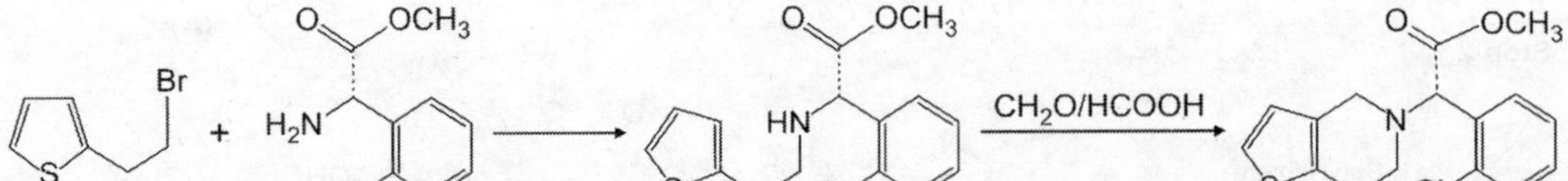

[2-(2-Thienyl)-ethylbromide]   [(+)-2-Chlorophenyl-glycine methyl ester]

It has similar activity as ticlopidine (33).

Section VI
Hormones and Antihormonal Drugs

STEROIDS AND STEROIDAL DRUGS

S TEROIDS are a class of compounds which are structurally related and distributed in nature, both in plant and animal kingdom. They possess wide variety of therapeutic activity and are the most widely and extensively used. The major therapeutic effects exhibited include hormonal (male and female sex hormones, and cortex hormones), female contraceptives, anti-inflammatory, cardiotonic, diuretic, vitamin, and antibiotic. The basic structure of steroid is 1, 2-cyclopentenophenanthrene (1) and all the steroids are derivatives of cyclopentanoperhydrophenanthrene (2). All the steroids, on selenium dehydrogenation at 360°, give Diel's hydrocarbon (3). The carbon system and designation of ring system is as shown in (4). The four rings are designated as A, B, C, and D. Out of these, rings A, B and C are six-membered and ring D a five-membered. The methyl groups at position 10 and 13 are called angular methyl groups and constitute C_{18} and C_{19}.

(1)

(2)

(3)

(4)

The stereochemical studies have shown that rings A/B can either be *cis*- or *trans*-fused, rings B/C are always *trans*-fused while rings C/D are in most cases *trans*-fused. The two angular methyl groups (C_{18} and C_{19}) project above the plane of the ring.

The convention of the nomenclature in the steroids is as follows:

1. Assuming the plane of the paper is the plane of the rings, the angular methyl groups project above this plane. All the configurations in the molecule are then referred with respect to angular methyl groups. Those groups or atoms which are on the same side as methyl groups are

referred to as β and are shown by a thick valence line. Those on the opposite side are referred to as α and are shown as broken line. Those atoms or groups whose configuration is not known are shown as wavy line and are designated by the Greek letter ξ (ky).

2. The naming of a compound is based on the parent hydrocarbon.
3. When all the ring fusions are *trans*, the series is known as allo-series. When A/B fusion is *cis* and B/C and C/D fusions *trans*, the series is called a normal series.
4. The parent hydrocarbons are:

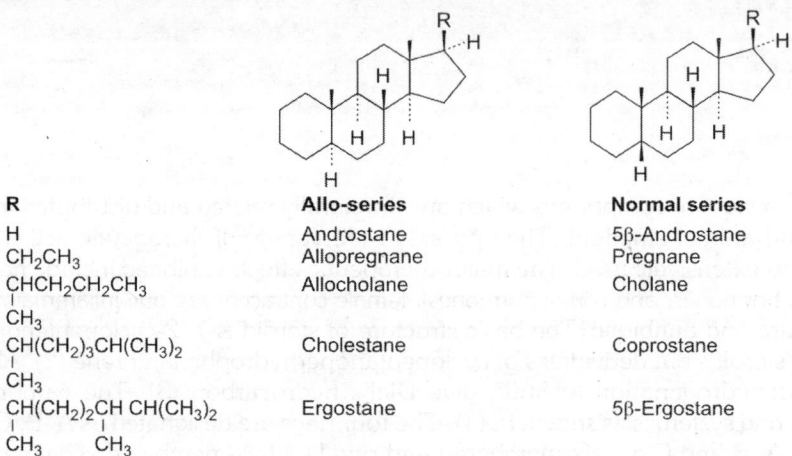

R	Allo-series	Normal series
H	Androstane	5β-Androstane
CH$_2$CH$_3$	Allopregnane	Pregnane
CHCH$_2$CH$_2$CH$_3$ | CH$_3$	Allocholane	Cholane
CH(CH$_2$)$_3$CH(CH$_3$)$_2$ | CH$_3$	Cholestane	Coprostane
CH(CH$_2$)$_2$CH CH(CH$_3$)$_2$ | | CH$_3$ CH$_3$	Ergostane	5β-Ergostane

5. When there is unsaturation at C$_5$, the compound is named as a derivative of androstane, pregnane, cholane, or cholestane.

Sterols are hydroxy derivatives. They can be classified on the basis of their source. Thus, those obtained from animals are known as zoosterols, e.g. cholesterol, coprostanol, and cholestanol. Those derived from plant kingdom are known as phytosterols, e.g. stigmasterol. Another class, known as mycosterols are derived from yeast and fungi, e.g. ergosterol. Sterols are usually found in oils and fats and occur as free or esters of fatty acids. They are isolated from unsaponifiable portion of oils or fats.

CHOLESTEROL

Cholesterol (5) is a sterol of higher animals, found free or as ester in all animal cells particularly in brain and spinal cord. The main sources of cholesterol (5) are fresh liver oils, brain, and spinal cord. Lanoline, the fat from wool, is a mixture of cholesteryl esters, mainly cholesteryl palmitate, stearate, and oleate.

Cholesterol (5) and other sterols give various colour reactions and include:

(*a*) **Salkowski reaction:** Addition of concentrated sulphuric acid to chloroformic solution of cholesterol (5) gives red colour in chloroform layer.

(*b*) **Liebermann-Burchard reaction:** When a chloroformic solution of cholesterol (5) is treated with concentrated sulphuric acid and acetic anhydride a greenish colour is developed.

A white precipitate of cholesterol (5) digitonide is obtained when an ethanolic solution of cholesterol (5) is treated with ethanolic solution of digitonin, a saponin. Cholesterol (5) digitonide is 1:1 complex of cholesterol-digitonin. The cholesterol (5) can be recovered from this complex by dissolving the complex in pyridine and adding ether. Cholesterol (5) remains in solution and digitonin is precipitated. Steroids having 3β-hydroxyl group form digitonide complex.

Cholesterol (5) plays an important role in biological system, it is used for incorporation in cell membrane, synthesis of other steroid hormones, and bile acids. It also is required for the absorption of fats from intestine. Cholesterol (5) has been implicated in atherosclerosis.

PHYTOSTEROLS AND MYCOSTEROLS

Stigmasterol (6) and ergosterol (7) belong to this category. Stigmasterol (6), a C_{29} sterol is obtained from soyabean oil. It has C_{10} side chain at C_{17} and double bonds at C_5 and C_{22} positions. Ergosterol which occurs in yeast is a C_{28} sterol with three double bonds at C_5, C_7 and C_{22}. Ergosterol is precursor of ergocalciferol.

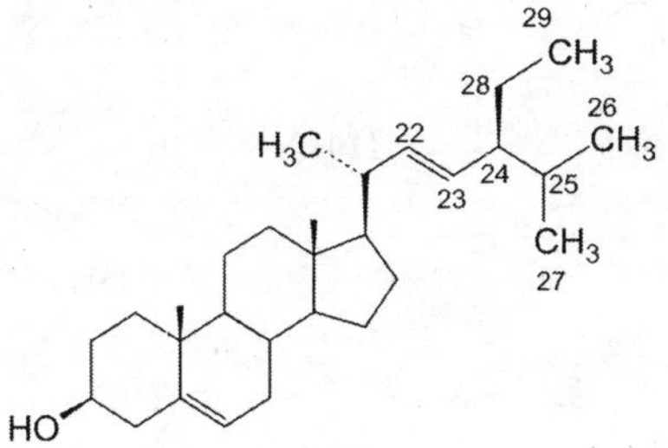

(6)

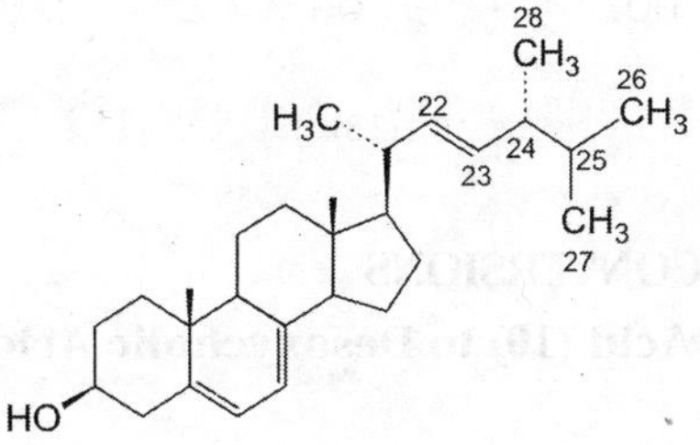

(7)

BILE ACIDS

Bile acids occur as sodium and potassium salts of conjugates of glycine (H_2NCH_2COOH) and taurine ($H_2NCH_2CH_2SO_3H$). They are secreted by liver and stored in gallbladder. They function as emulsifying agents in the intestine for fats and help their absorption.

Bile acids are hydroxy derivatives of either cholanic acid (8) or allocholanic acid (9). The hydroxyl

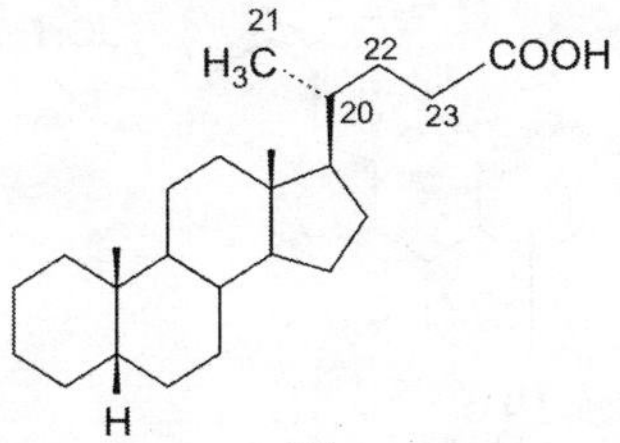

(8)

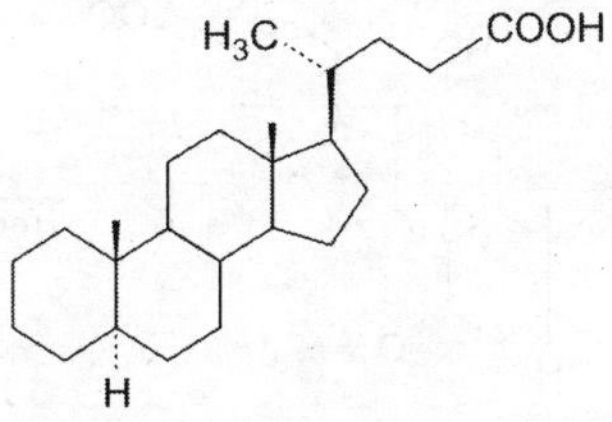

(9)

groups are found at position 3, 6, 7, 11, 12 or 23. The configuration of the hydroxyl groups in all the natural bile acids is α. Some of the important natural bile acids are cholic acid (10), desoxycholic acid (11), lithocholic acid (12), chenodesoxycholic acid (13), and hyodesoxycholic acid (14).

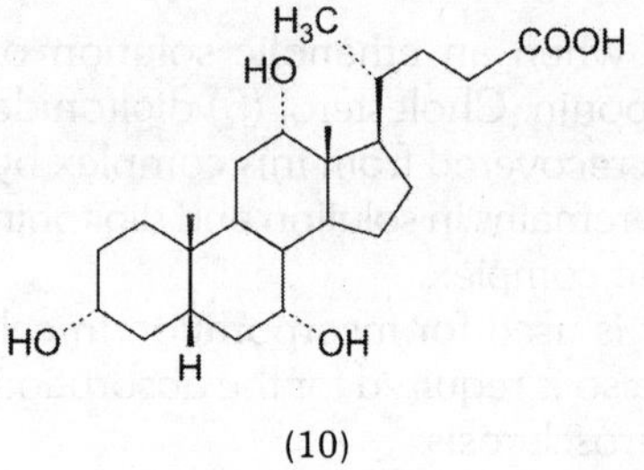

(10) 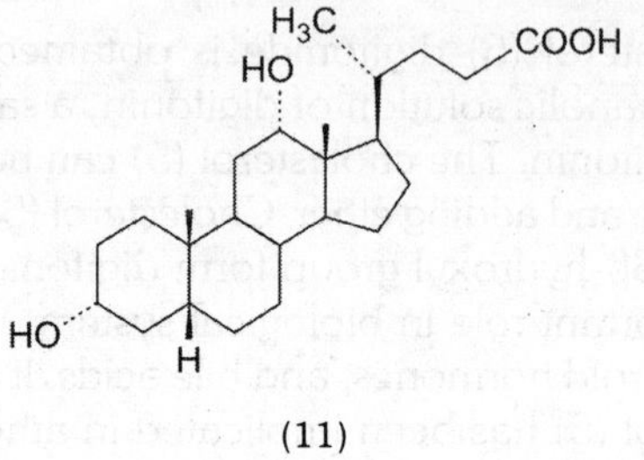   (11) 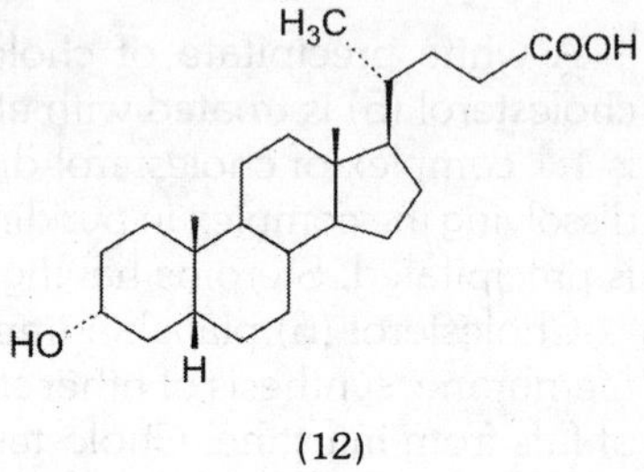   (12)

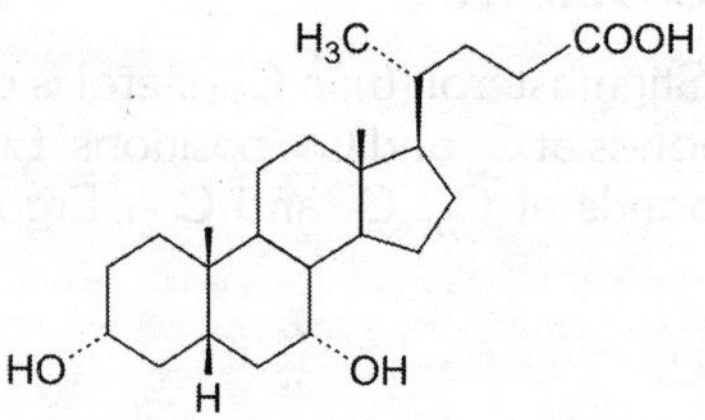

(13) 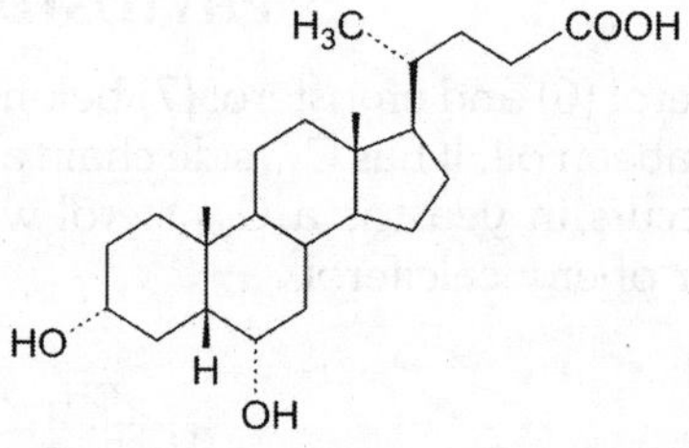   (14)

SOME CONVERSIONS
Cholic Acid (10) to Desoxycholic Acid (11)

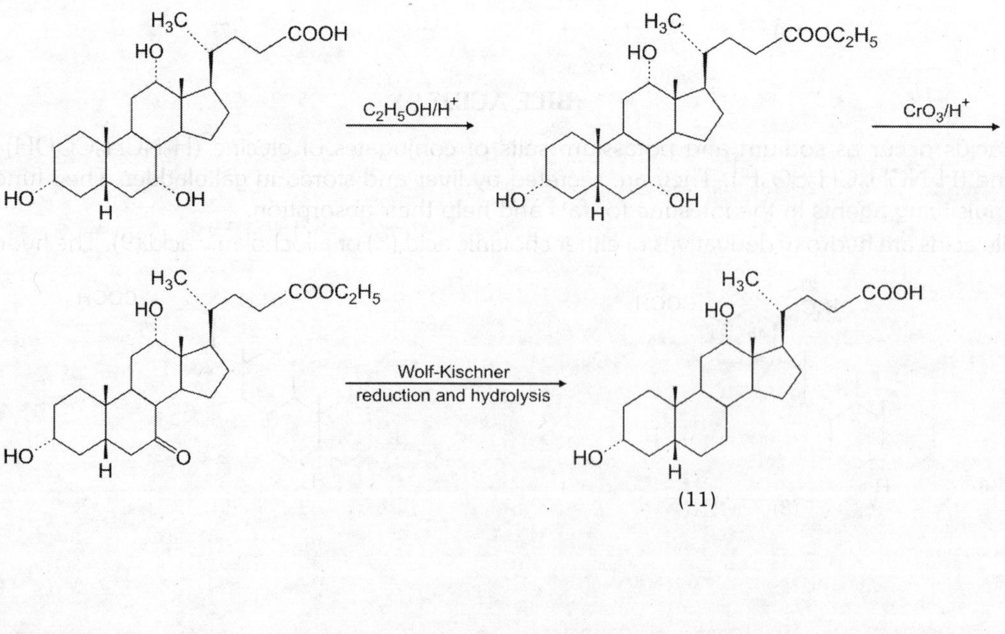

Cholic Acid (10) to Chenodesoxycholic Acid (13)

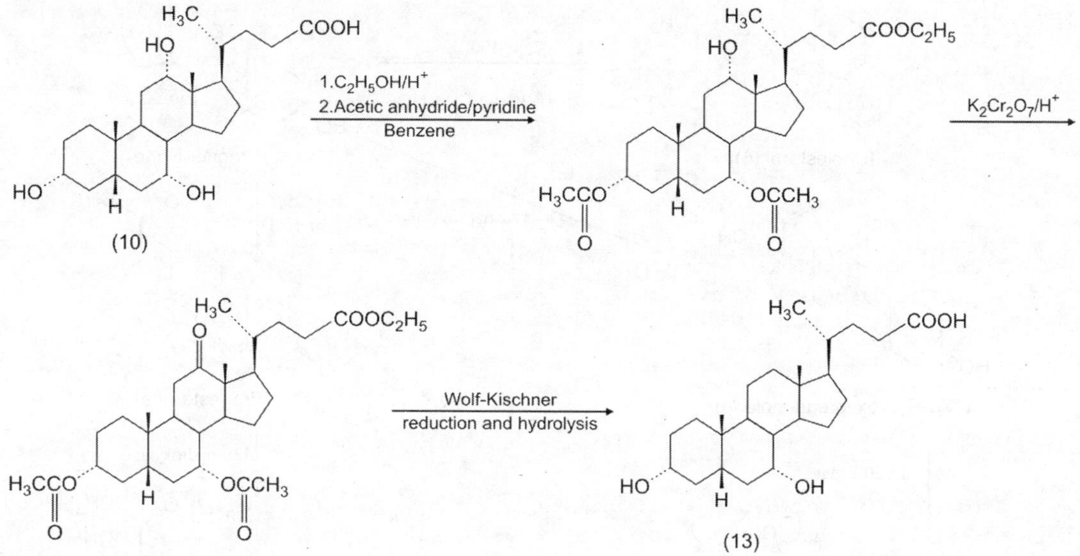

(10)

1.C_2H_5OH/H^+
2.Acetic anhydride/pyridine
Benzene

$K_2Cr_2O_7/H^+$

Wolf-Kischner
reduction and hydrolysis

(13)

SEX HORMONES

Sex hormones include:

(a) Androgens, the male sex hormones.

(b) Estrogens and progesterone the female sex hormones.

Although all of these are produced by both males and females but androgens are produced more by males and estrogens and progesterone more by females. The activity of these hormones seems to be controlled by hormones of anterior pituitary lobe. Because of this, the sex hormones are sometimes called secondary sex hormones and the hormones of anterior pituitary, the primary sex hormones. The biosynthetic precursor of sex hormones is cholesterol (5) (Fig. 17.1).

ANDROGENS

Androgens constitute the simplest class of steroidal hormones. They are non-benzenoid, do not have a side chain at C_{17} and have an oxygen function at C_3 and C_{17}. The principal androgen is testosterone (15), the other hormones are androsterone (16) and dehydroepiandrosterone (17).

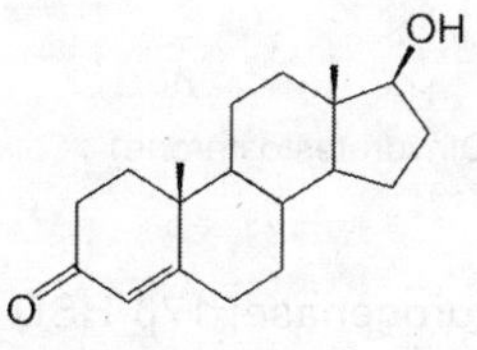

(15) 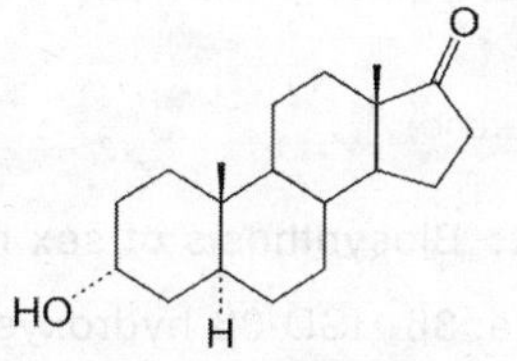   (16) 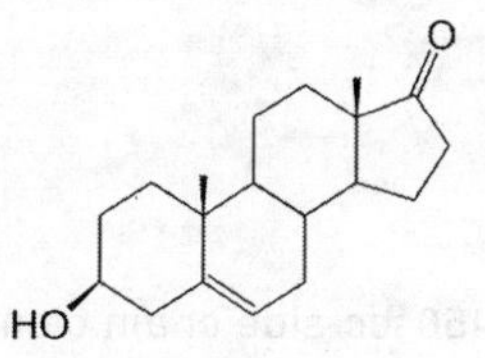   (17)

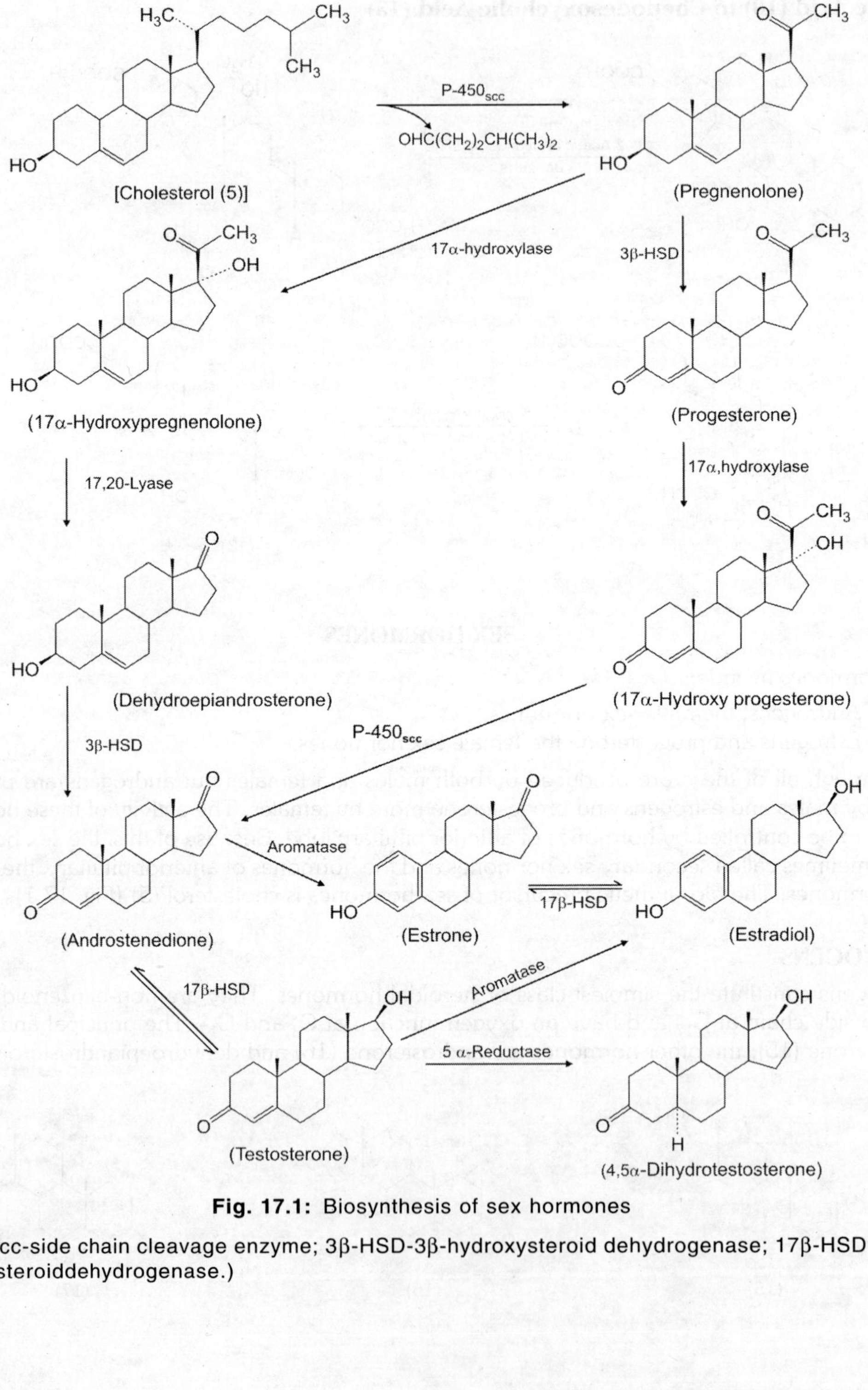

Fig. 17.1: Biosynthesis of sex hormones

(P. 450scc-side chain cleavage enzyme; 3β-HSD-3β-hydroxysteroid dehydrogenase; 17β-HSD - 17β-hydroxysteroiddehydrogenase.)

Androgens are responsible for the development of primary and secondary sex characteristics of various animals. In addition to this, androgens have anabolic or growth promoting activities. This anabolic effect is associated with increased blood supply to the tissues. They also increase the sebacious secretion which results in inhibition of scalp hair growth and stimulation of skin hair growth. Androgens also stimulate the growth of bone.

Testosterone (15) is not itself active, it is converted to its active metabolite (18), 17β-hydroxy-5α-androstan-3-one or 4,5α-dihydrotestosterone (18), by the action of 5α-reductase. Both testosterone (15) and 4,5α-dihydrotestosterone (18) modify gene transcription by binding with intracellular steroidal receptor which results in increased polymerase activity and increased synthesis of specific RNA and protein.

(18)

The testosterone preparations are mainly used for replacement therapy in testicular failure and as anabolic agents.

Testosterone Analogs and Anabolic Steroids

Testosterone (15) when given orally is rapidly absorbed and converted to inactive metabolite and only 1/6th of the dose administered is available in active form. Since metabolic inactivation involves oxidation of 17β-hydroxyl to 17-one, 17α-alkyl derivatives were prepared to overcome this. Further, efforts were made to separate the androgenic activity from the useful anabolic activity. However, complete separation of these activities has not been achieved.

17α-Methyltestosterone (19) is about half as active as testosterone (15) but it can be taken orally. Any further increase in the size of alkyl group at 17α-position reduces the activity. Thus, 17α-ethyltestosterone (20) has greatly reduced activity.

(19)

(20)

Fluoxymesterone (21), which is 9α-fluoro-11β-hydroxy analog of 17α-methyltestosterone (19) is about 5 to 10 times more active than testosterone (15). However, the separation of anabolic and androgenic activities have not been achieved in these analogs and the ratio is 1:1 in all these analogs including testosterone (15). One of the disadvantages of 17α-alkyl analogs is that they cause hepatic disorders, even jaundice. Analogs with longer duration of action have been prepared by esterifying the 17β-hydroxyl group and include, testosterone propionate (22), enanthate (23), and cypionate (24). They are used as intramuscular depot preparations.

Although complete separation of anabolic activity from androgenic activity has not been achieved but improved anabolic/androgenic ratio has been achieved. Removal of 19-methyl group results in nandrolone (25), which is orally active. Its esters decanoate (25a) and phenylpropionate (25b) are used as intramuscular depot preparations. Norethandrolone (26), which is 17α-ethyl analog, is orally active and possesses high anabolic and weak androgenic activity. Removal of keto function at position 3 of norethandrolone (26) results in ethylestrenol (27), which is more potent anabolic agent than norethandrolone (26).

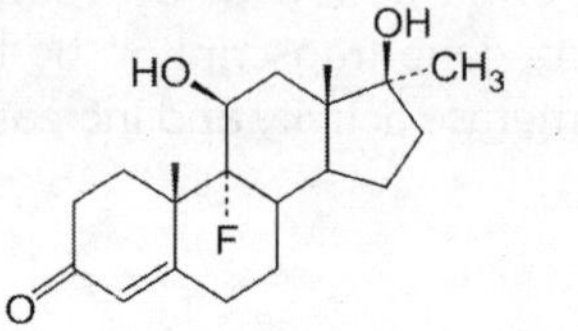

OH
HO
CH3
F
O

(21)

O
OC–R
O
(22), R=C2H5
(23), R=(CH2)5CH3
(24), R=CH2CH2

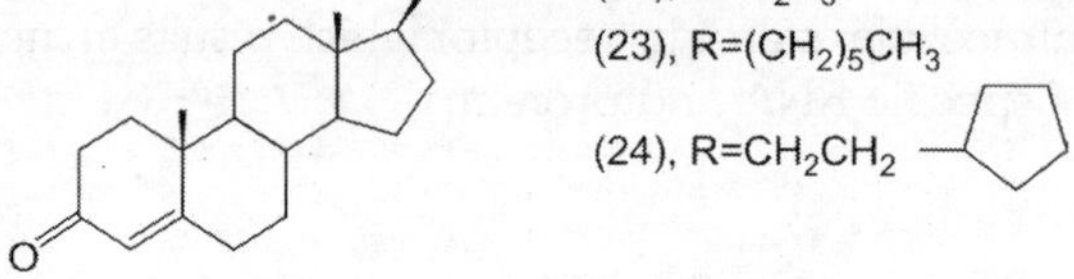

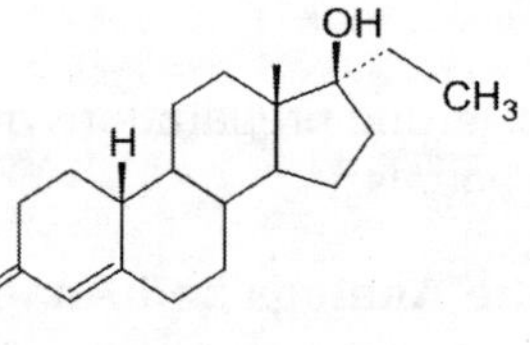

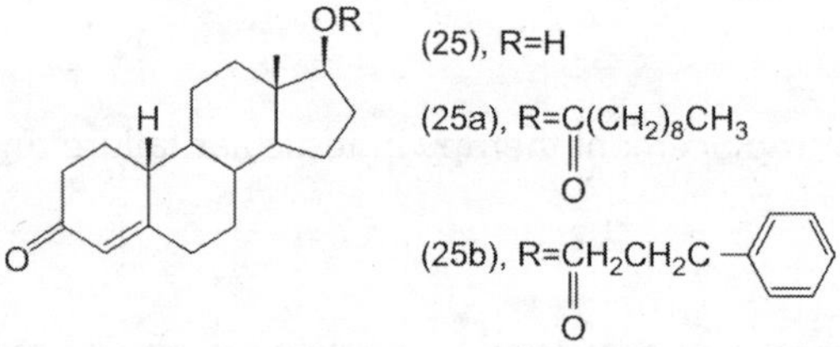

OR
H
O
(25), R=H
(25a), R=C(CH2)8CH3
O
(25b), R=CH2CH2C
O

OH
CH3
H
O

(26)

OH
CH3
H

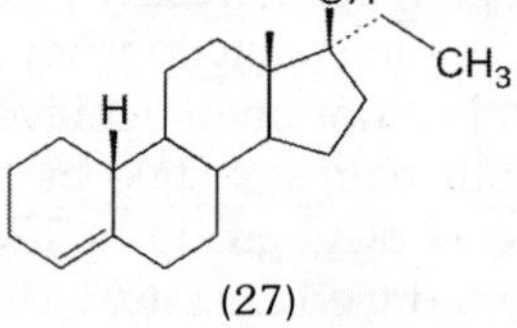

(27)

Introduction of an alkyl group at 1, 2, 7, or 18 position, as in case of methenolone acetate (28) or introduction of halogen in ring A, as in case of 4-chlorotestosterone acetate (29) also results in increase in the anabolic activity.

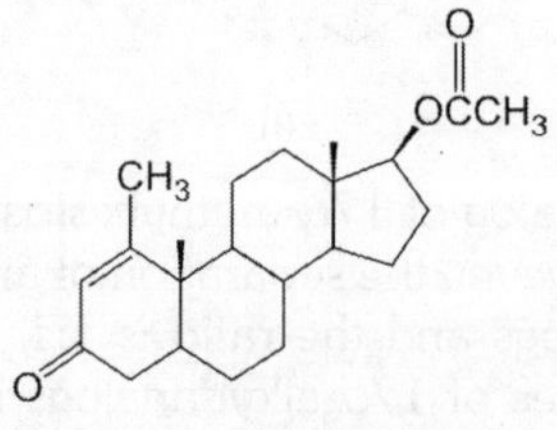

O
OCCH3
CH3
O

(28)

O
OCCH3
O
Cl

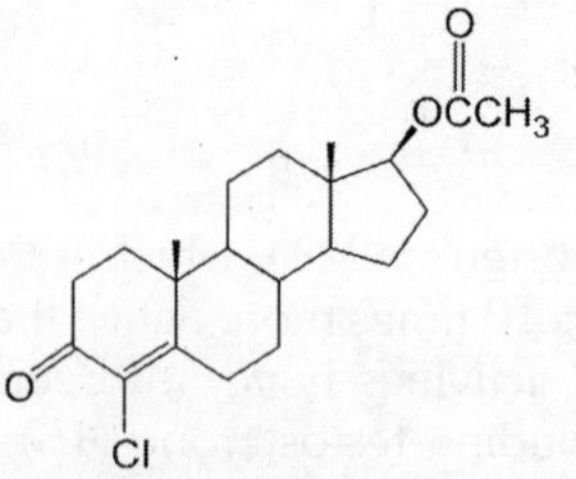

(29)

Introduction of oxygen in ring A as in oxandrolone (30) and heterocyclic steroid stanozolol (31), where pyrazole nucleus has been fused with ring A, also showed higher anabolic activity as compared to androgenic activity. (3:1). Oxymetholone (32), another anabolic steroid, is used to stimulate production of erythropoietin in the treatment of anemia due to bone marrow failure.

(30) (31) (32)

The D-homo-oxasteroid, testolactone (33) possesses some anabolic activity with weak androgenic activity. It is used in the treatment of breast cancer.

(33)

5α-Reductase Inhibitors and α₁-Adrenergic Receptor Antagonist

As indicated, 5α-reductase converts inactive testosterone (15) into active 4,5α-dihydrotestosterone (18). Two types of 5α-reductase are known and include type I and type II. Type I is found in liver and is involved in the metabolism of testosterone (15). Type II is located in prostate gland and testes. It is responsible for conversion of testosterone (15) to 4,5α-dihydrotestosterone (18). 4,5α-Dihydrotestosterone (18) is involved in pathogenesis of benign prostrate hyperplasia. In benign prostrate hyperplasia there is obstruction of urethra due to enlarged prostate. This results in gradual loss of bladder function and ultimately in incomplete emptying of bladder. The symptoms of benign prostate hyperplasia include poor urine stream and large residual urine volume. The enlarged prostate also results in increase in adrenergic tone. Severe benign prostate hyperplasia can result in problems such as retention and strain in bladder and this may lead to urinary tract infection, bladder, or kidney damage, and bladder stones.

Inhibition of 5α-reductase type II results in decreased concentration of 4,5α-dihydrotestosterone (18) in plasma and prostate which ultimately results in blockade of local action due to testosterone (15). The first of these inhibitors was the progestogen, medrogestone (34). The other inhibitors include finasteride (35) and dutasteride (36).

(34) (35) (36)

Finasteride (35) and dutasteride (36) are mechanism base inhibitors of type I and type II 5α-reductase. Further finasteride (35) is more selective for type II 5α-reductase than dutasteride (36).

The symptoms of benign prostatic hyperplasia can also be alleviated by use of α_1-adrenergic receptor antagonists. These antagonists relax the muscles of bladder and in prostate, thereby, reducing the pressure on urethra and increasing the flow of the urine. These antagonists include prazosin (37), terazosin (38), doxazosin (39), alfuzosin (40), and tamsulosin (41). They, however, do not cure benign prostatic hyperplasia but allevate the symptoms.

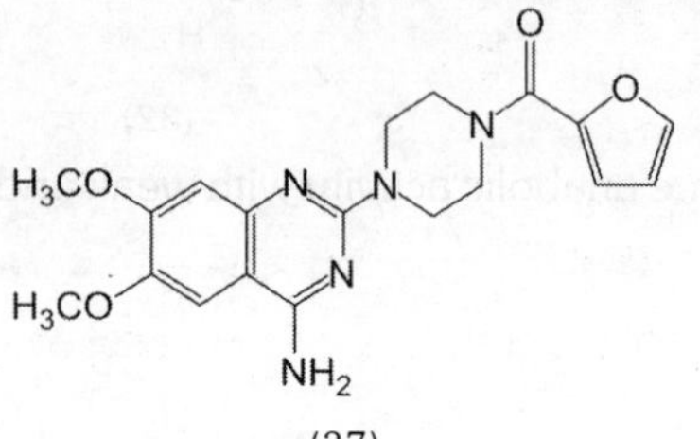

(37)

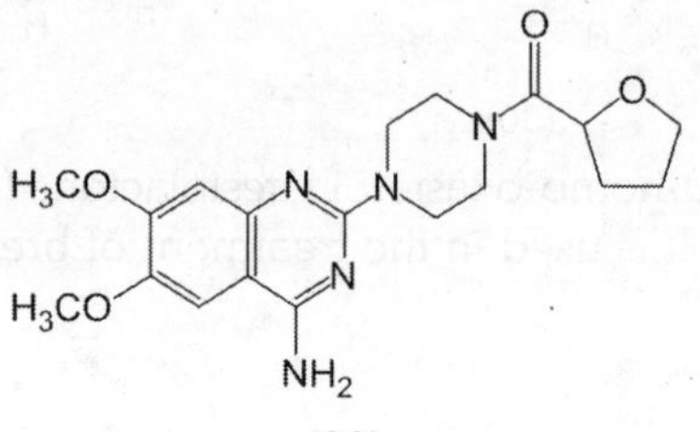

(38)

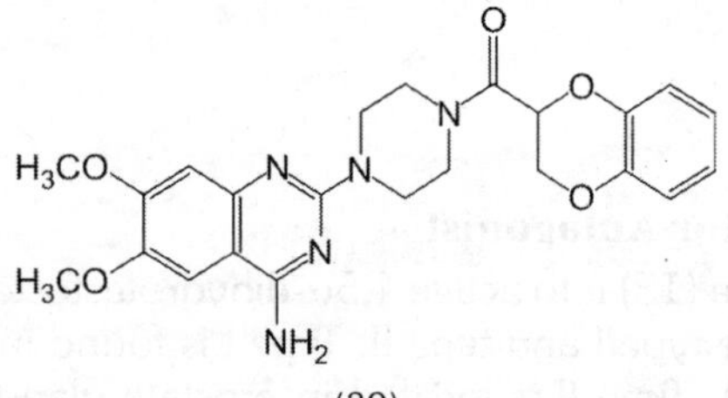

(39)

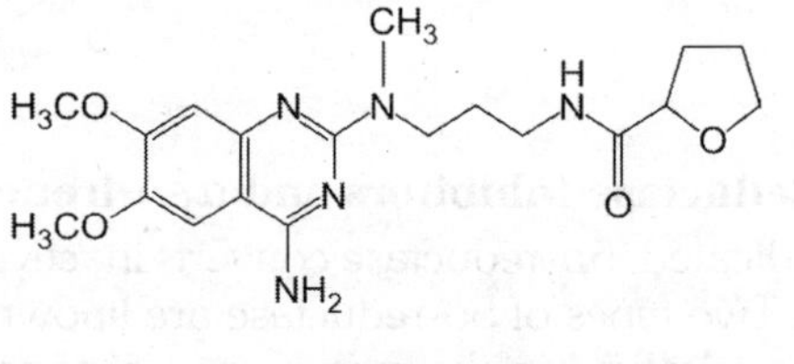

(40)

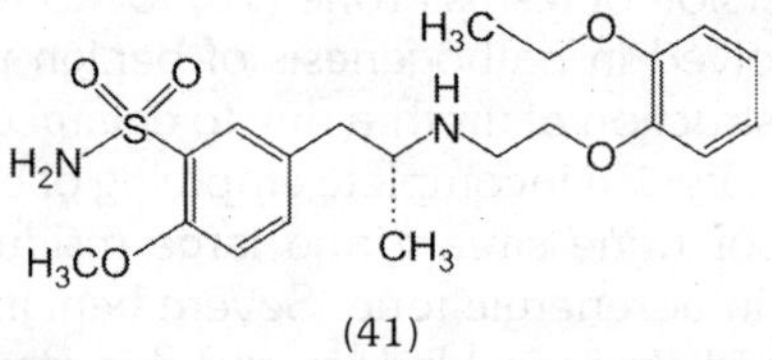

(41)

Antiandrogens

Antiandrogens, block or antagonize the actions of active form of testosterone (15), 4, 5α-dihydro-testosterone (18). They are used in treating hyperandrogenism (hirsutism, acne, and premature baldness) or androgen stimulated cancers, the prostate carcinoma. Two types of antiandrogens have been developed and include steroidal and non-steroidal. Cyproterone (42) and oxendolone (43) constitute the steroidal antiandrogens. The non-steroidal antiandrogens include bicalutamide (44), flutamide (45), and nilutamide (46). Both types of these antiandrogens act by competing with 4, 5α-dihydrotestosterone (18) for the androgen receptor. As the androgen dependent DNA and protein synthesis is inhibited there is arrest of prostate cancer.

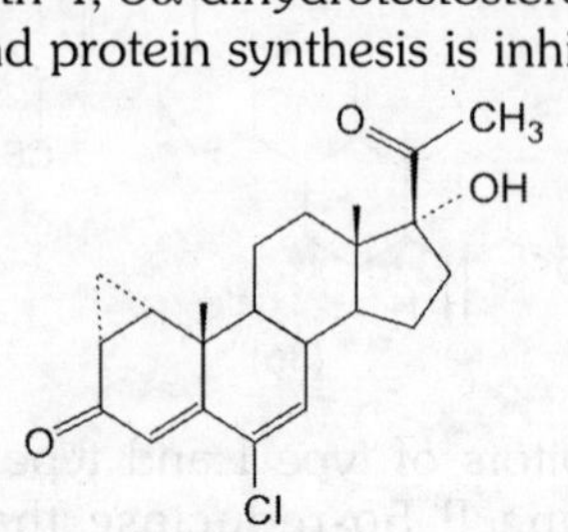

(42)

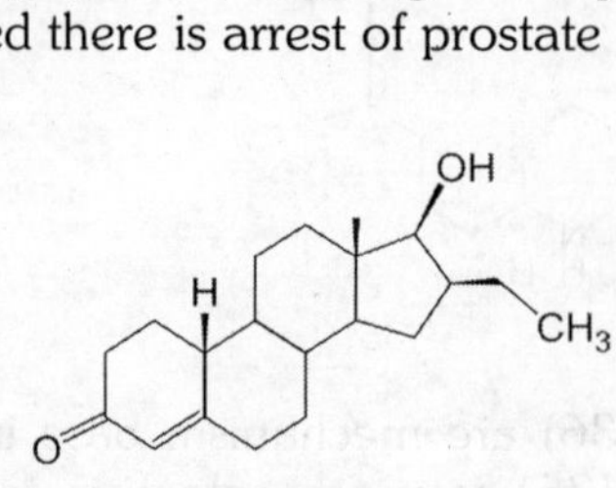

(43)

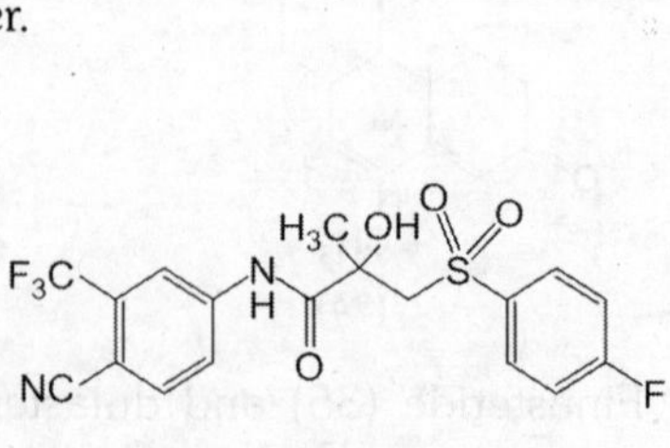

(44)

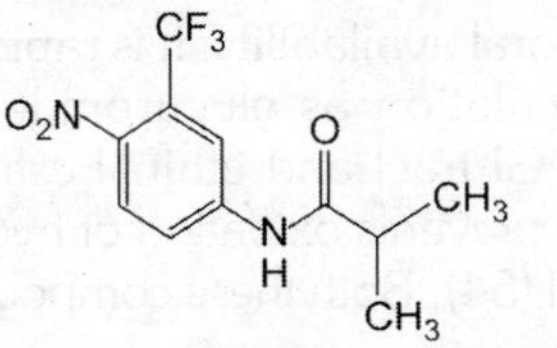

(45) 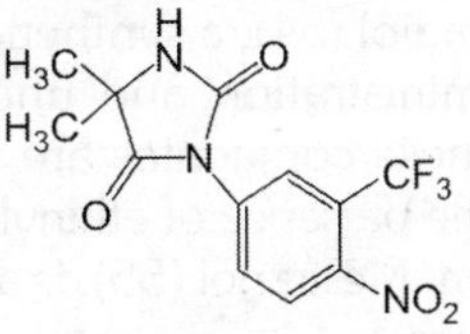 (46)

17α-Hydroxylase/17, 20-lyase Inhibitors

Inhibition of 17α-hydroxylase/17, 20-lyase, leading to inhibition of testosterone (15) biosynthesis, is another line of treating androgen dependent metastatic prostate cancer. Some of the compounds possessing such activity include the antifungal fluconazole (47), liarozole (48), and abiraterone (49).

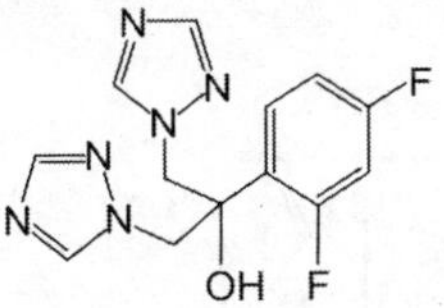

(47) 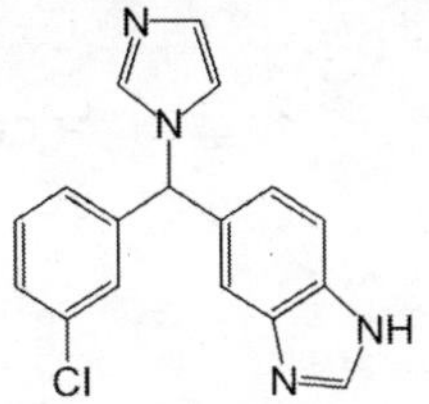 (48) 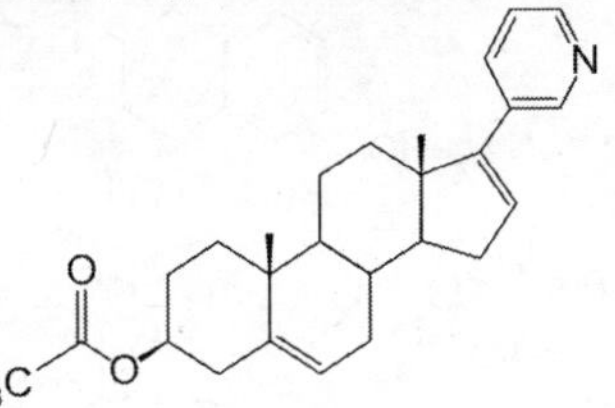 (49)

ESTROGENS

The ovaries of female genital system produce estrogens and progesterone. The principal estrogens produced include estradiol (50), estrone (51), and estriol (52).

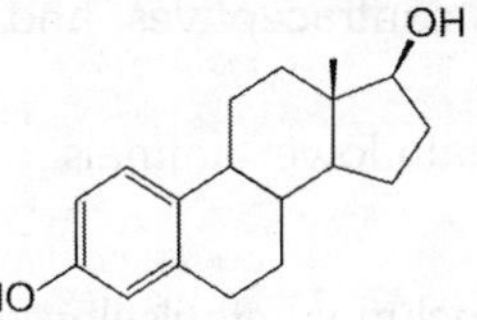

(50) 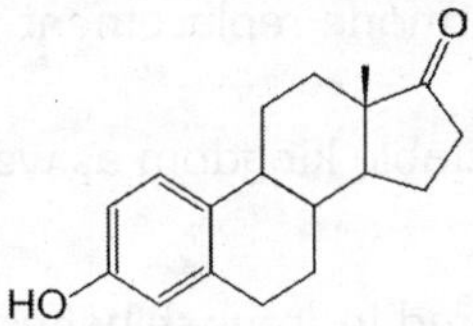 (51) 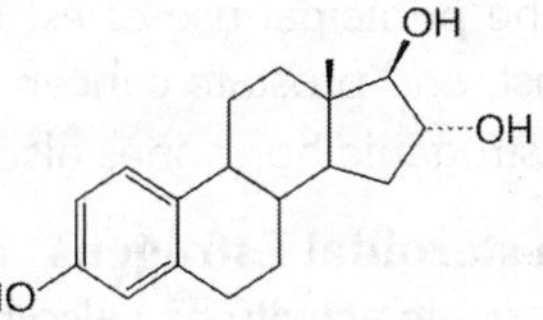 (52)

Estradiol (50) is the most potent of the three endogenous estrogens. It exhibits high potency when administered parenterally. When given orally, it exhibits low bioavailability because of its metabolism in liver to estrone (51) by 17β-hydroxysteroid dehydrogenase.

Estradiol esters like 3-benzoate (53a), dipropionate (53b), 17β-heptanoate [enanthate, (53c)], and 17β-cyclopentylpropionate [cypionate, (53d)] are used as depot preparations and are administered parenterally.

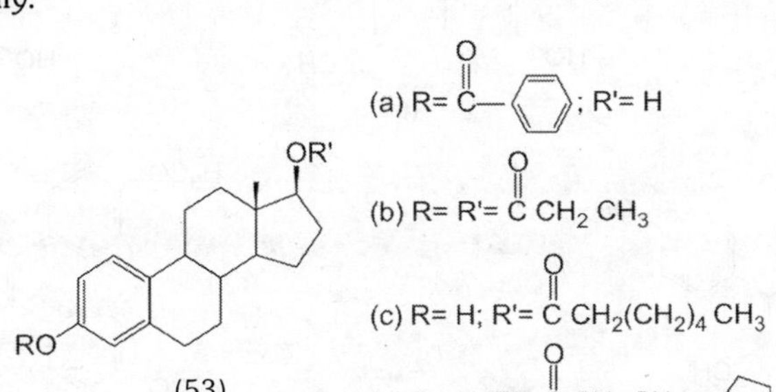

(53)

(a) R= $\overset{O}{\overset{\|}{C}}$—⬡ ; R'= H

(b) R= R'= $\overset{O}{\overset{\|}{C}}$ CH_2 CH_3

(c) R= H; R'= $\overset{O}{\overset{\|}{C}}$ $CH_2(CH_2)_4$ CH_3

(d) R= H; R'= $\overset{O}{\overset{\|}{C}}$ CH_2 CH_2—⬠

Ethinyl estradiol (54), a synthetic analog has shown better oral availability. It is rapidly absorbed after oral administration and undergoes enterohepatic circulation as glucuronide and sulfate conjugates. These conjugates are hydrolyzed by bacteria in GI tract and ethinyl estradiol (54) is reabsorbed. The presence of ethinyl group at 17α-position also prevents oxidation of hydroxyl group. at 17β-position. Mestranol (55), is a prodrug of ethinyl estradiol (54). Both these compounds are used as contraceptives.

Metabolites of estrogens namely equilin (56), its sodium sulphate ester (57), and equilenin (58) have also been used. They have, however, lower activity.

(54)

(55)

(56) R = H
(57) R = SO$_3$Na

(58)

The prinicipal use of estrogens is as hormone replacement therapy, as contraceptives, and in breast, and prostate cancer.

Estrogenic hormones also occur in vegetable kingdom as well as in certain lower animals.

Non-steroidal Estrogens

Estrogenic activity has also been encountered in *trans*-stilbenes (59) and include diethylstilbestrol (60), hexestrol (61)— the *meso*-form of reduced diethylstilbestrol (60), which is less active than diethystilbestrol (60). Dienestrol (62), a diene analog of hexestrol (61), also possesses estrogenic activity. Diethylstilbestrol (60) is used as diphosphate and its sodium salt in therapy. Chlorotrianisene (63) is another weak estrogen.

(59)

(60)

(61)

(62)

(63)

Estrogen Antagonists

Antiestrogens have been found to be useful in estrogen-dependent breast cancers. Some of these include clomiphene (64a and 64b), tamoxifen (65), toremifene (66), raloxifene (67), and fulvestrant (68). Clomiphene (64a and 64b), tamoxifen (65), toremifene (66), and raloxifene (67) possess tissue specific activity. They have tissue specific differential agonist or antagonist activity and accordingly they are classified as tissue specific estrogen receptor modulators. Thus, clomiphene (64a and 64b) which exists as a mixture of geometrical isomers, the *cis*-isomer, zuclomiphene (64a), possesses weak agonist activity on all tissues whereas the *trans*-isomer, the enclomiphene (64b), has antagonist activity in uterine and agonist action on bone tissue. It is used as a mixture of *cis*- and *trans*-isomers as an ovulation stimulant.

(64a)

(64b)

(65)

(66)

(67)

The *Z*-isomer of tamoxifen (65) is an estrogen receptor antagonist in breast tissue but a partial agonist in endometrium and bone. It is used in the treatment and prevention of breast cancer.

Toremifene (66) has similar pharmacological action as tamoxifene and the *Z*-isomer (66) has estrogen receptor antagonist action. It is used for the treatment of metastatic breast cancer in postmenopausal women.

Raloxifene (67) has estrogen receptor agonist activity in bone but is antagonist in both breast and endometrial tissue. The agonist activity of raloxifene (67) in bone decreases bone resorption and is used for prevention and delaying of osteoporosis.

Fulvestrant (68) is a pure antagonist at both ERα- and ERβ-receptors. It is used for the treatemnt of breast carcinoma.

(68)

Aromatase Inhibitors

Another approach to inhibition of growth of estrogen dependent tumors is to block the biosynthesis of estrogens from androgen precursors. This can be achieved by inhibiting the enzyme aromatase. Aromatase inhibitors include steroidal and non-steroidal. The steroidal inhibitors are testolactone (33), exemestane (69), and formestane (70). The non-steroidal inhibitors include aminoglutethimide (71), anastrozole (72), and letrozole (73).

(69)   (70)   (71)

(72)   (73)

Testolactone (33), a D-homosteroid, possesses weak aromatase inhibitory activity. Exemestane (69) and formestane (70) are irreversible inhibitors of aromatase. They bind covalently to aromatase. Formestane (70) lacks oral activity and is administered parenterally Both exemestane (69) and formestane (70) are used for treatment of breast cancer.

All the three non-steroidal aromatase inhibitors, aminogutethemide (71), anastrozole (72), and letrozole (73), are competitive inhibitors of aromatase. Aminoglutethemide (71) is a weak inhibitor of aromatase. It is a first generation aromatase inhibitor. Anastrozole (72) and letrozole (73) are highly effective inhibitors of aromatase.

Aromatase inhibitors produce profound reduction in circulating estrogens. Since estrogens are the major regulators of bone density, women taking aromatase inhibitors are at increased risk of osteoporosis.

Mechanism of Estrogen Action

Estrogens regulate gene expression and subsequent protein biosynthesis via specific high affinity estrogen receptors. Two types of estrogen receptors have been identified and include ERα and ERβ. The predominant estrogen receptor in female reproductive tract and mammary gland is ERα. While ERβ is the estrogen receptor in vascular endothelial cells, bone, and male prostate tissues. Estradiol (50) has similar affinities for both of these receptors while as non-steroidal estrogens and antiestrogens have differing affinities for the two receptors with slightly higher affinity for ERβ receptors.

PROGESTERONE AND PROGESTINS

The hormone which acts on progesterone receptor is progesterone (74). It is produced in the ovaries, testes, and adrenal. It is also secreted by corpus luteum in the second part of menstrual cycle and by placenta during pregnancy.

The physiological effects of progesterone (74) include:

1. Modification of uterine tissue,
2. transport, implant, and development of fertilized ovum,
3. suppression of ovulation in pregnant animals,
4. uterine motility, and
5. development of mammary gland tissue.

Progesterone (74) is not effective orally and has a half-life of only about 5 min. Synthetic substances which act in similar manner as progesterone (74) and commonly known as progestins have been developed.

These include:

(a) Progesterone derivatives,
(b) testosterone and 19-nortestosterone derivatives, and
(c) miscellanous compounds.

The progesterone derivatives include 17α-hydroxyprogesterone caproate (75), medroxyprogesterone acetate (76), and megestrol acetate (77).

(74)

(75)

(76)

(77)

The testosterone and 19-nortestosterone derivatives with progestational activity include ethisterone (78), dimethisterone (79), norethindrone (80), ethynodiol diacetate (81), norethynodrel (82), desogestrel (83), etonogestrel (84), levonorgestrel (85), norelgestromin (86), and norgestimate (87).

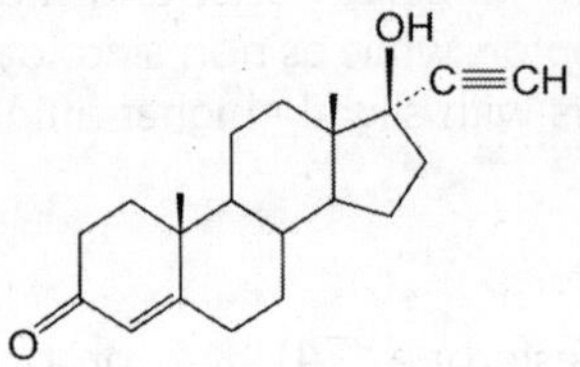

(78)

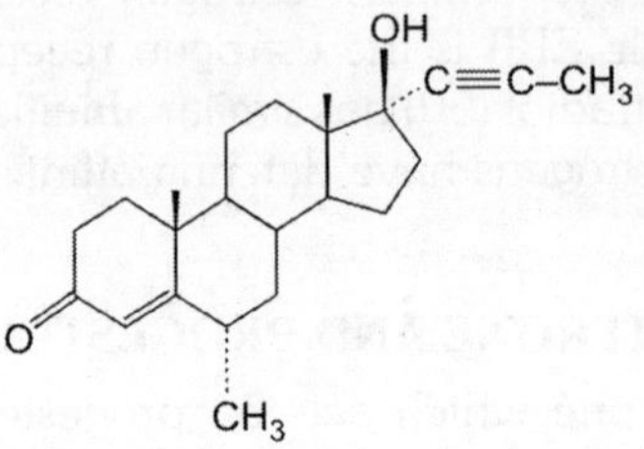

(79)

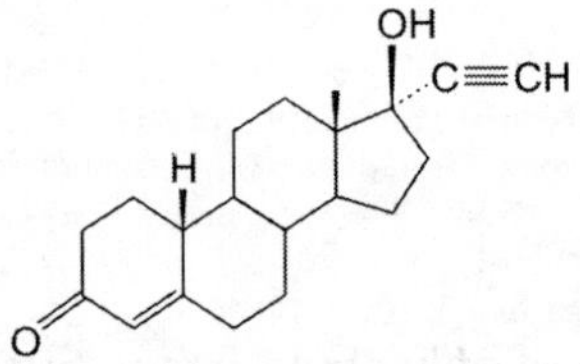

(80)

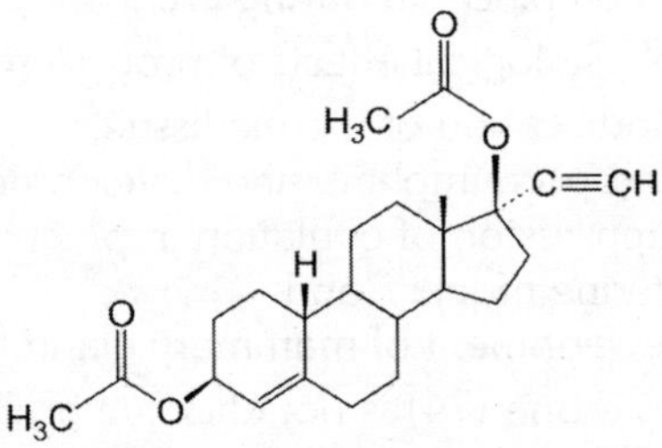

(81)

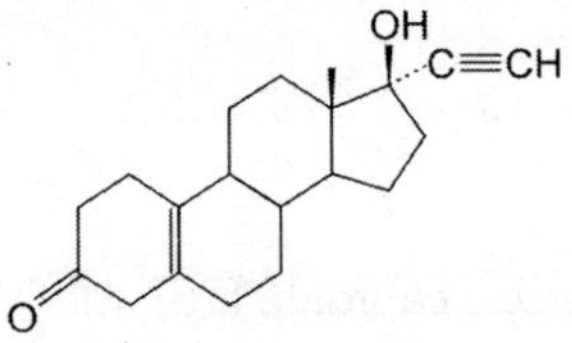

(82)

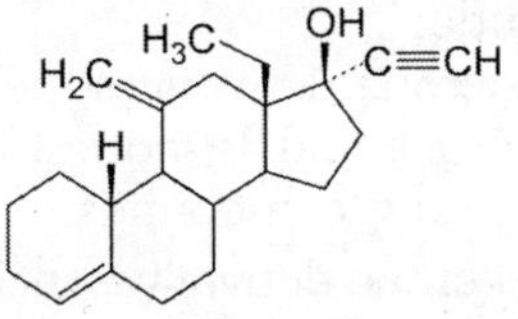

(83)

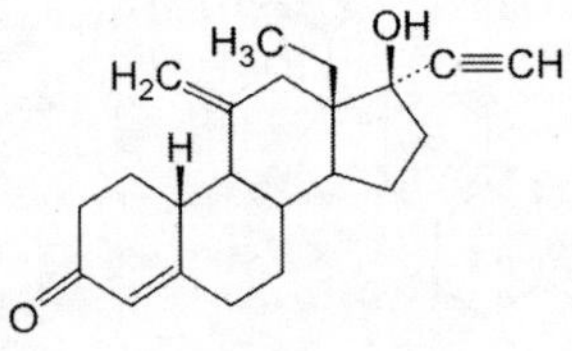

(84)

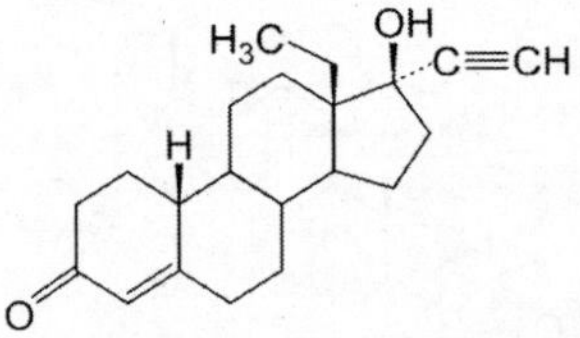

(85)

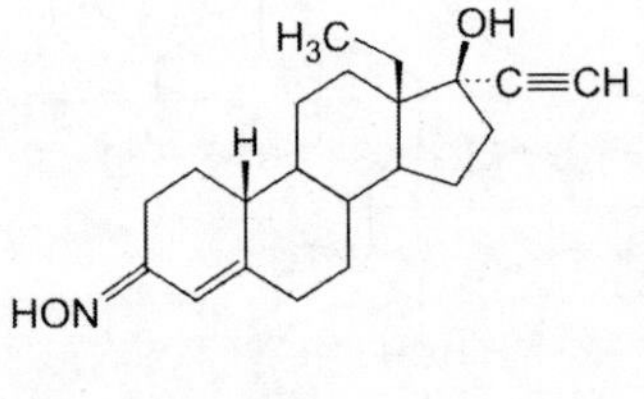

(86)

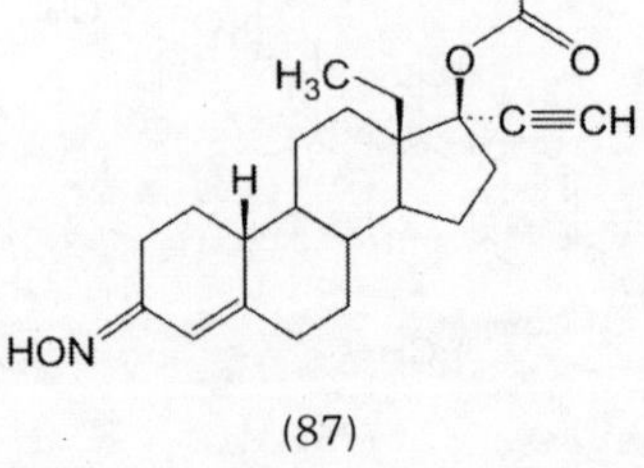

(87)

The miscellanous class of progestins include drospirenone (88) and trimegestone (89).

(88)   (89)

Clinically, progestines are used in combination with estrogens or alone as oral contraceptives. In combination with estrogens, they are also used for long-term estrogen therapy, namely to prevent hyperplasia and carcinoma. They have also found use in breast cancer.

Progestin Antagonists

Compounds that antagonize the action of progesterone (74) by competing with it for the receptor have been developed. These antagonists are useful for termination of pregnancy. Mifepristone (90) is a partial antagonist of progesterone (74). It is used as alternative to surgical termination of pregnancy. It is a 19-norcompound containing an α-propynyl side chain at 17-position. The other compound onapristone (91) is also a 19-nor steroid and contains 17α-hydroxy group, a hydroxypropyl side chain at 17β-position and an α-methyl group at C_{13}. These antiprogestins also possess activity against hormone dependent breast cancers.

(90)   (91)

ORAL CONTRACEPTIVES

With the increase in life-span of an individual, the population control has become important. The unabated growth of population will not be sustainable on the limited sources. Further, the increased population will also hamper the progress and the quality of the human life. It becomes imperative, therefore, to control population by methods which are safe and easy.

Following the observation in 1930 that injection of progesterone (74) in rats, rabbits, and guinea pigs resulted in inhibition of ovulation. Sturgis et al proposed that estrogen and/or progesterone (74) could be used to prevent ovulation in women. In 1955, Pincus reported that progesterone (74) when given from day 5th to day 25th of menstrual cycle, inhibition of ovulation resulted. At the same time, it was found that 19-nortestosterones possessed progestational activity when given orally. Two compounds namely, norethindrone (80) and norethynodrel (82) when tested showed high progestational and ovulation inhibiting activity. These compounds are the most extensively used progestins.

Two types of oral contraceptives are presently available. These include combination tablets and mini-tablet. The combination tablets contain a progestin-like norethindrone (80)/norethynodrel (82), ethynodiol diacetate (81)/levonorgestrel (85)/or desogestrel (83) and an estrogen like ethinyl estradiol (54) or mestranol (55).

The combination tablets act by suppressing the production of luteinizing hormone (LH) and or follicle stimulating hormone (FSH) by a feedback inhibition process (Fig. 17.2). This process is similar to natural inhibition of ovulation due to release of estrogens and progesterone from placenta and ovaries. An additional effect due to progestins is that they cause the cervical mucus to become very thick. The thick cervical mucus acts as a barrier for the passage of sperm through the cervix. These tablets are taken from day 5th to 25th day of menstrual cycle. Use of combination tablets results in weight gain, nausea, mood changes and skin pigmentation. Evidences for and against increased breast cancer have been reported. Further risk of thromboembolism is also there. Combination tablets are safe contraceptives.

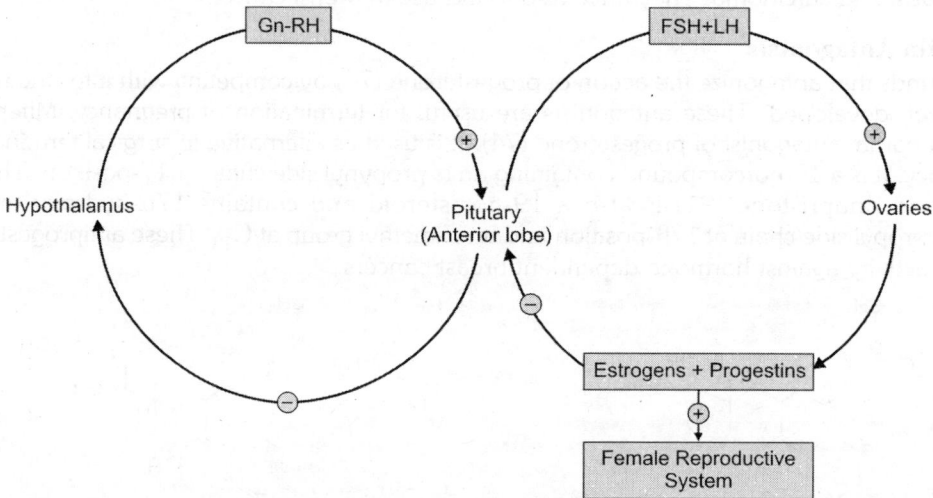

Fig. 17.2: Hormonal control of female reproductive system.

(GnRH–gonadotrophin releasing hormone; FSH–follicle stimulating hormone; LH-lutenising hormone.)

Mini-tablets contain progestins only. These tablets are taken continuously. The progestins cause increase in viscosity of cervial mucus, acting as a barrier to passage of sperm. Further low doses of progestins also increase the rate of ovum transport and then disrupt implantation. Mini-tablets are much less reliable as a contraceptive. Further their use causes irregular bleeding.

LONG-ACTING PROGESTIN-ONLY CONTRACEPTIVES

Medroxyprogesterone acetate (76) given intramuscularly is a safe long-acting (3 months) contraceptive. Some of the side effects in this include menstrual irregularities and infertility, which may continue for many months after the cessation of treatment.

Levonorgestrel (85) has been used as a depot preparation. It is used as subcutaneous implant in non-biodegradable capsule. These capsules release slowly levonorgestrel (85) over a period of 5 years. Side effects include irregular bleeding and headache.

ONCE A WEEK/ONCE A MONTH ORAL CONTRACEPTIVES

Formulation containing quinestrol [17α-ethinylestradiol 3-cyclopentylether (92)] and norethindrone acetate 3-cyclopentyl enol ether (93) was effective when given once a month. However, full protection against conception is achieved only after second month dose has been taken.

(92)   (93)

ADRENAL CORTEX HORMONES

The adrenal gland consists of inner core, the medulla, and the shell, the cortex. The medulla produces epinephrine and the cortex produces cortex hormones.

The cortex hormones are of two types, the mineralocorticoids and glucocorticoids. While the mineralocorticoids regulate the electrolyte and water metabolisms, the glucocorticoids regulate the carbohydrate, fat, and protein metabolisms. There is, however, overlapping of activity with lesser activity of various types in all of them. The major mineralocorticoids are aldosterone (94) and desoxycorticosterone (95). The major glucocorticoids include, hydrocortisone (96) and cortisone (97). The other steroids secreted by cortex are 17α-hydroxydesoxycorticosterone (98), 19-hydroxydesoxycorticosterone (99), corticosterone (100), and 11-dehydrocorticosterone (101).

(94)   (95)   (96)   (97)

(98)   (99)   (100)   (101)

The biosynthetic precursor of adrenocorticoids is cholesterol (5) (Fig. 17.3), which is converted in adrenal gland to pregnenolone by enzymatic cleavage of cholesterol side chain and then to various corticoids.

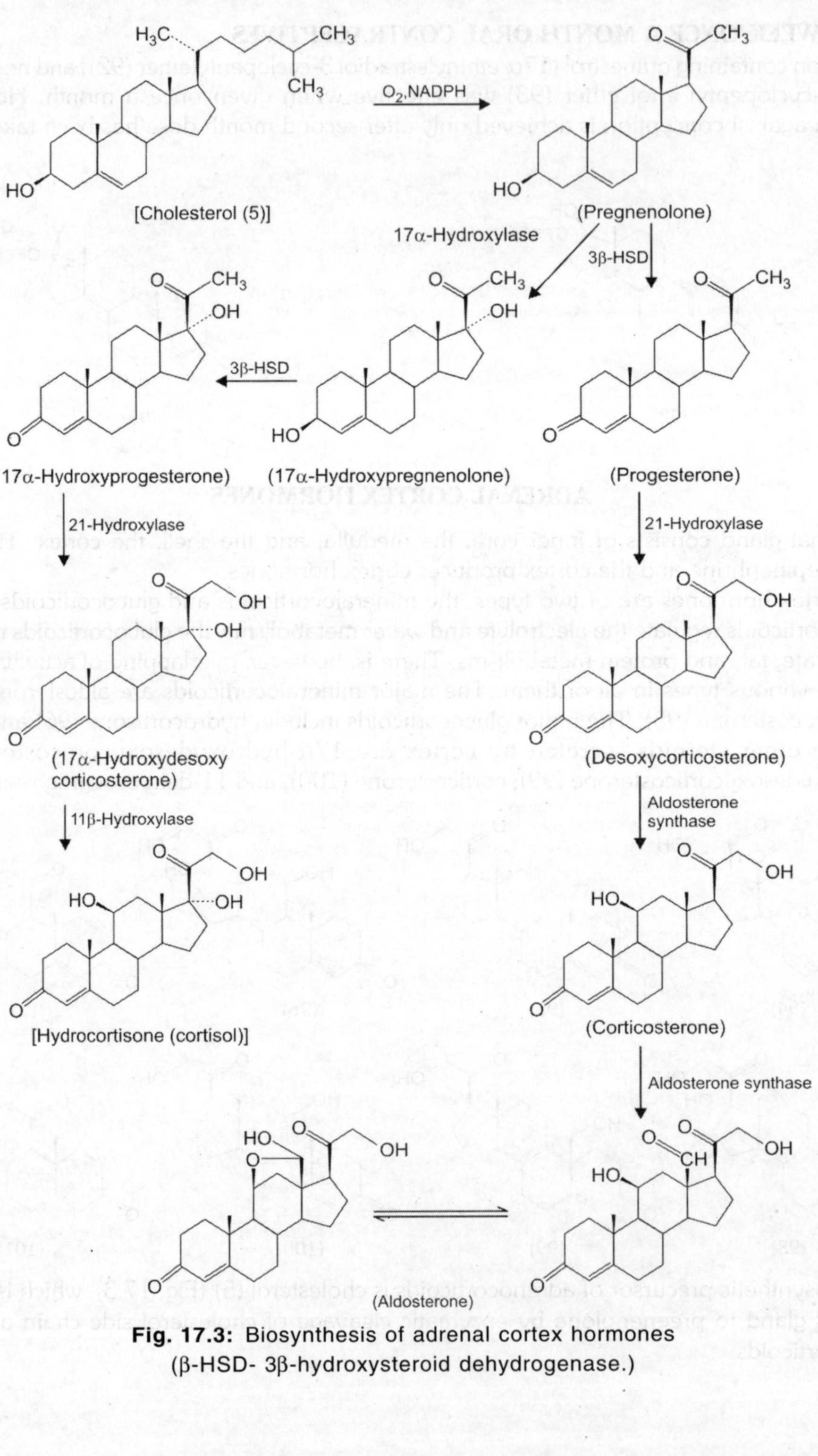

Fig. 17.3: Biosynthesis of adrenal cortex hormones
(β-HSD- 3β-hydroxysteroid dehydrogenase.)

Mineralocorticoids increase Na^+ reabsorption in distal tubule with concomitant increased K^+ and H^+ excretion. In Conn's disease, there is increased aldosterone (94) secretion, which causes increased Na^+ and water retention resulting in increased volume of extracellular fluid, hypokalemia, alkalosis polyurea, and hypertension.

Addison's disease or hypoadrenalism is characterized by increased Na^+ loss, decreased excretion of K^+ resulting in hyperkalemia. The osmotic pressure of extracellular fluid is decreased resulting in shift of fluid into intracellular compartment. In Addison's disease, there is weakness, anorexia, anemia, low blood pressure and vomiting.

Aldosterone (94) like other steroids acts on specific intracellular receptors. Aldosterone (94) receptors occur only in few target tissues, such as in kidney, colon, and in bladder. After binding to receptors, the steroid-receptor complex interacts with DNA, then transcription and protein synthesis takes place.

The main clinical use of mineralocorticoids is in replacement therapy. Desoxycorticosterone acetate (95 a), pivalate (95b), and fludrocortisone acetate (102) are used in Addison's disease.

(95a), R =CCH$_3$

(95b), R =CC(CH$_3$)$_3$

(102)

The effects of glucocorticoids include, decreased uptake and utilisation of glucose, and increased gluconeogenesis resulting in hyperglycemia. Higher glucose levels in blood cause increased insulin secretion which results in increased glycogen formation. The protein breakdown increases while as protein synthesis is decreased. Lipid metabolism and synthesis are significantly increased by glucocorticoids. Glucocorticoids also protect the body from stress. In Cushing's disease which is characterized by overproduction of corticoids, there is wasting of tissue, osteoporosis, and reduced muscle mass.

One of the important effects of glucocorticoids is their anti-inflammatory effect. This action of glucocorticoids is mediated through:

1. Inhibition of transcription of cytokines and other mediators of inflammation.
2. Blockade of synthesis of some cytokine receptors.
3. Inhibition of NK1 receptor involved with inflammatory action of substance P.
4. Increased production of protein lipocortin 1 which inhibits the production of prostaglandin and platelet activating factor in some cells.
5. Inhibition of collagenase, an enzyme involved in inflammation.
6. Inhibition of permeability of capillaries at inflammation site.

The other clinical uses of glucocorticoids are in asthma and in neoplastic diseases in combination with other cytotoxic agents.

Some of the glucocorticoids and their analogs used in clinical practice include prednisolone (103), prednisone (104), 6α-methylprednisolone (105), fluorometholone (106), 16β-methyl-prednisone (107), alclometasone (108), beclomethasone (109), betamethasone (110), dexamethasone (111), clobetasol (112), diflorasone (113), flumethasone (114), paramethasone

(115), amcinonide (116), desonide (117), budesonide (118), fluocinonide (119), flunisolide (120), flurandrenolide (121), triamcinolone acetonide (122), fluticasone propionate (123), halcinonide (124), halobetasol propionate (125), and mometasone furoate (126).

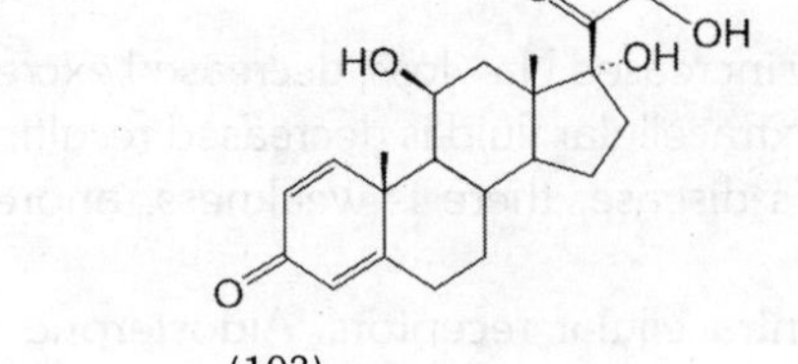

(103)

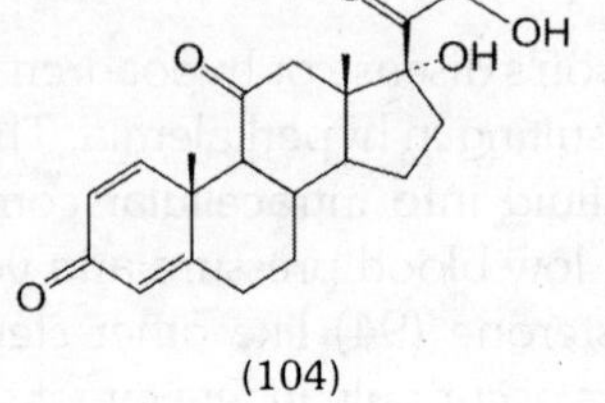

(104)

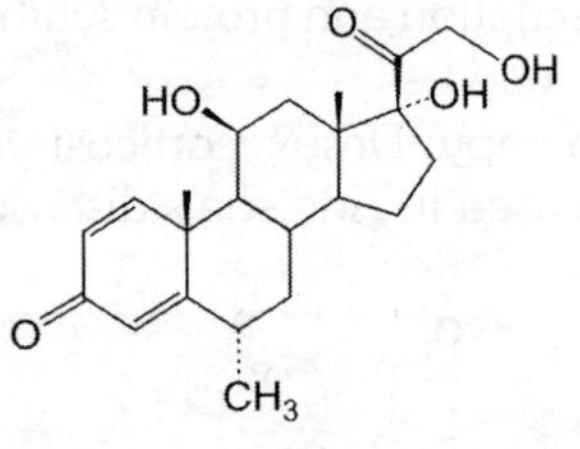

(105)

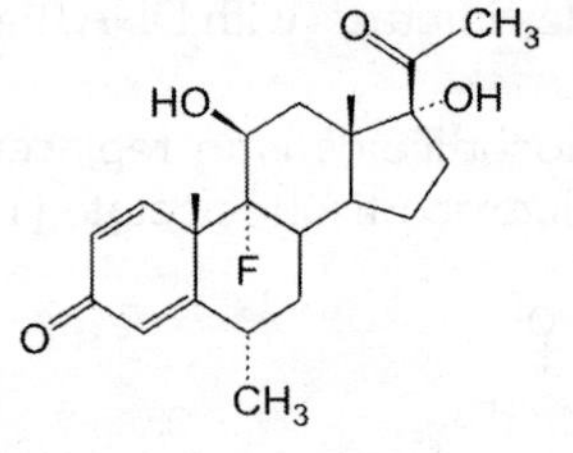

(106)

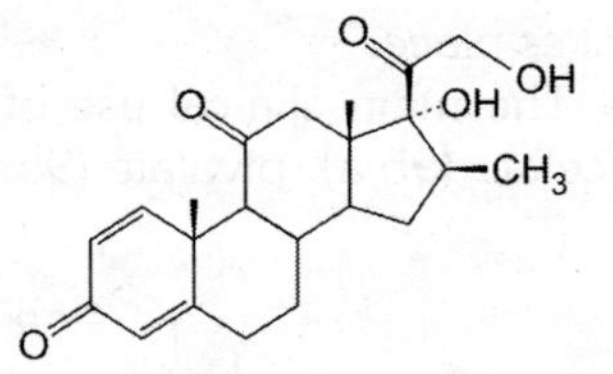

(107)

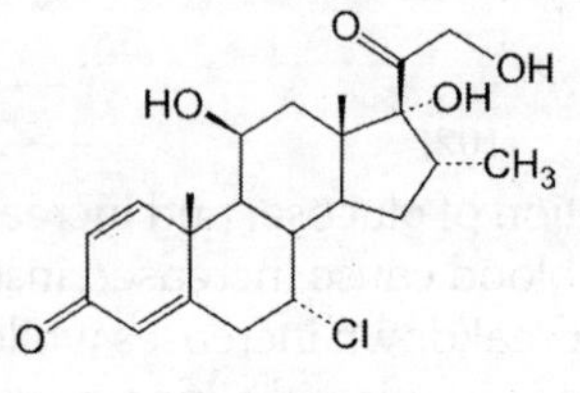

(108)

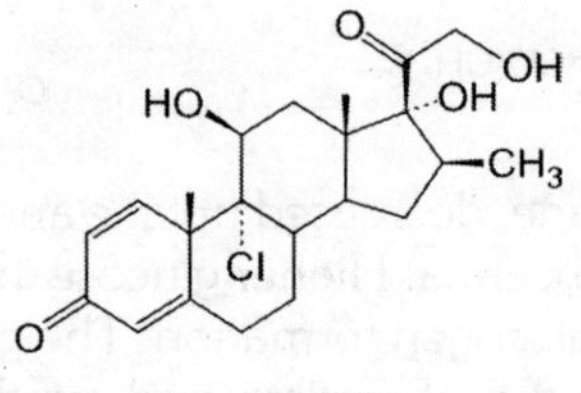

(109)

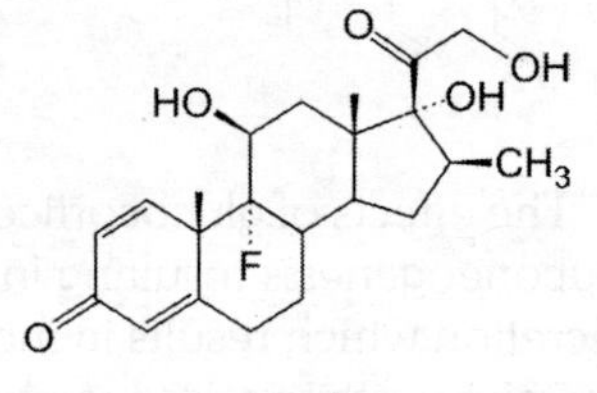

(110)

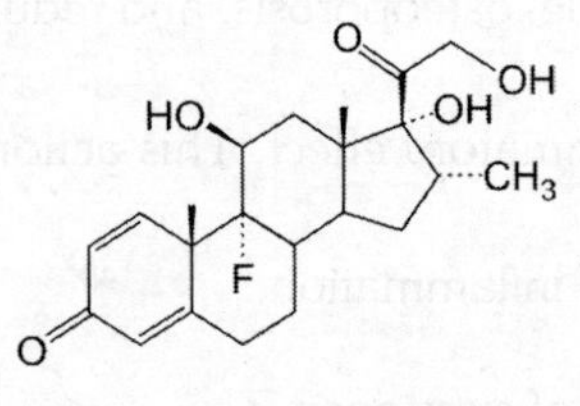

(111)

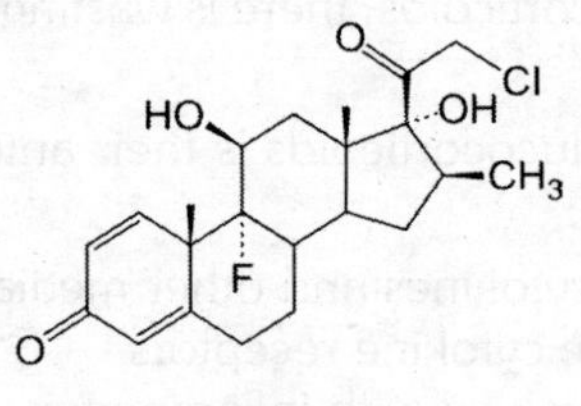

(112)

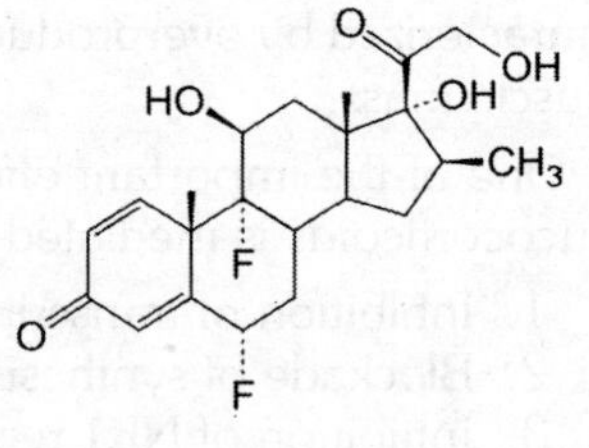

(113)

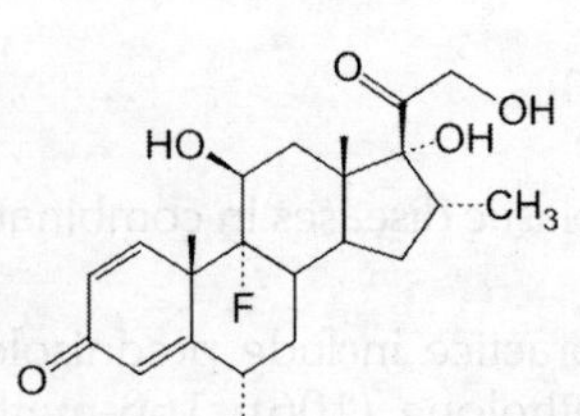

(114)

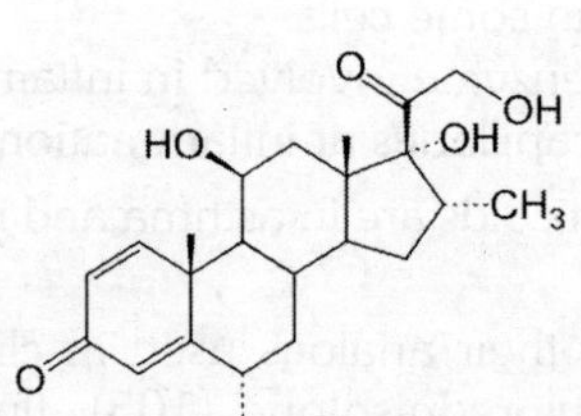

(115)

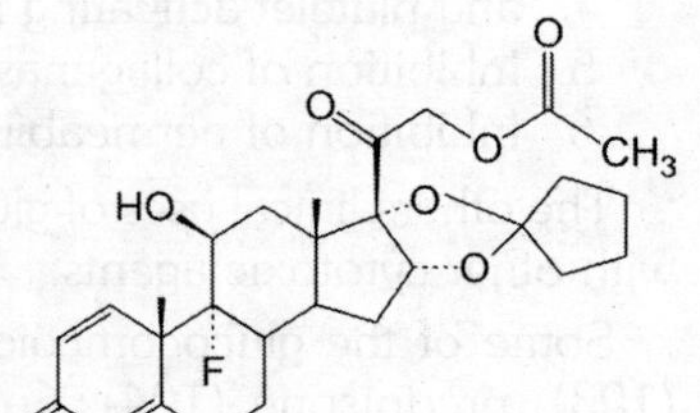

(116)

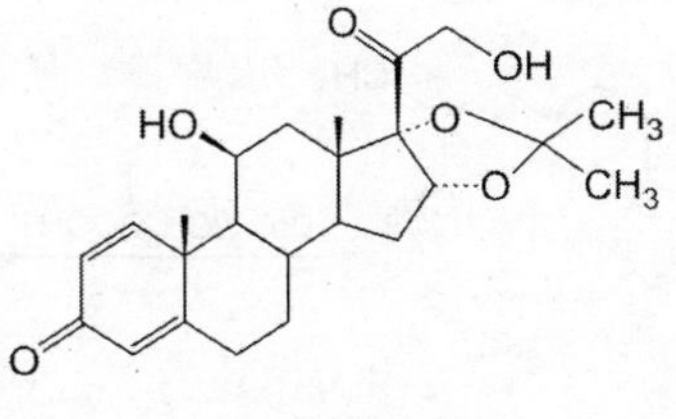

(117)

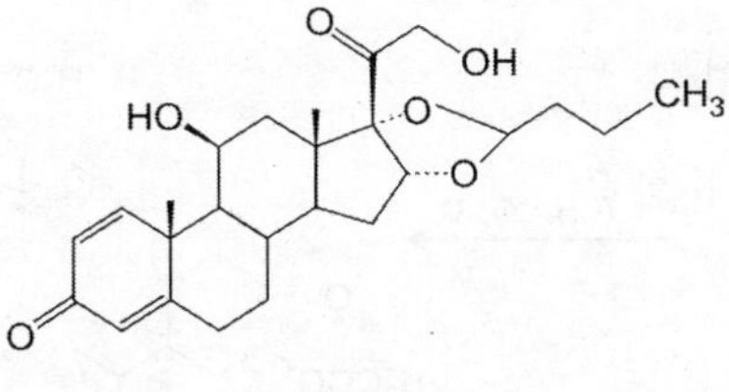

(118)

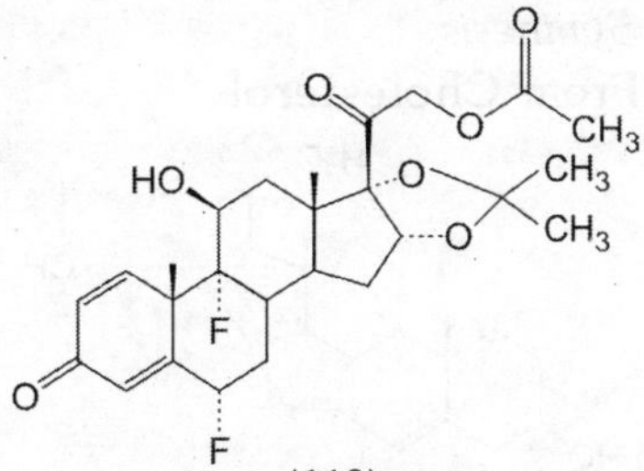

(119)

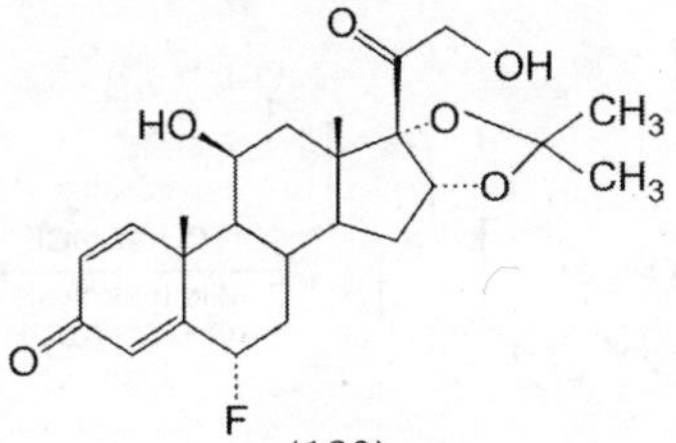

(120)

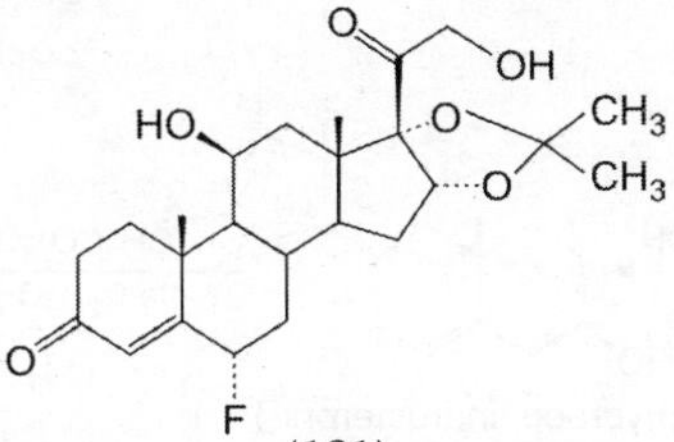

(121)

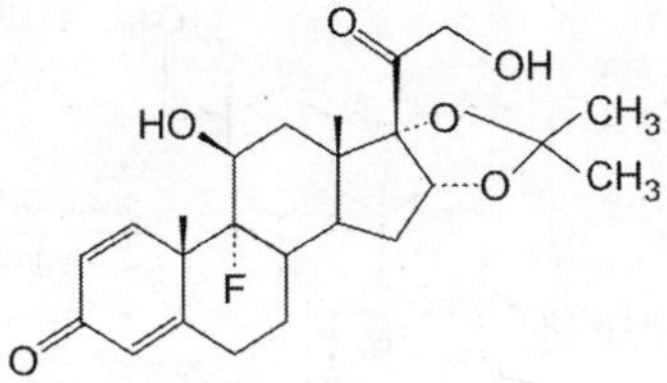

(122)

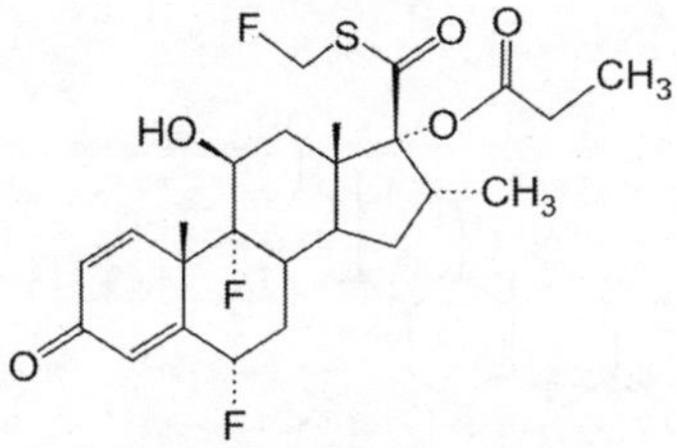

(123)

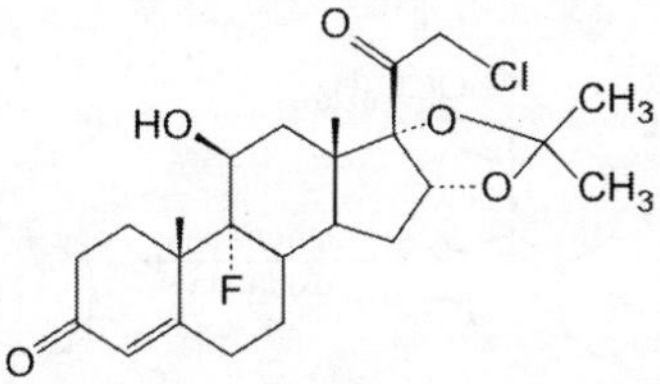

(124)

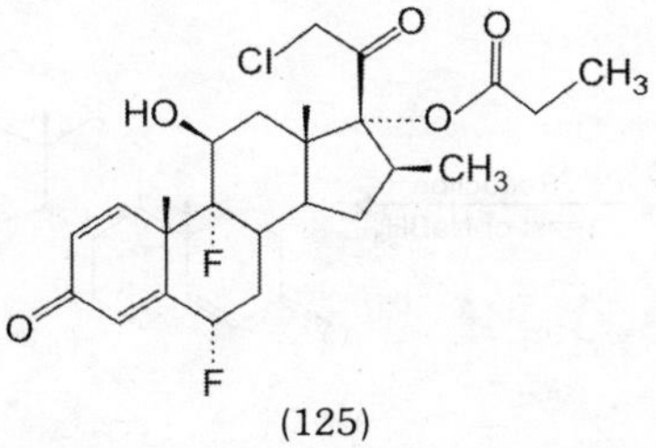

(125)

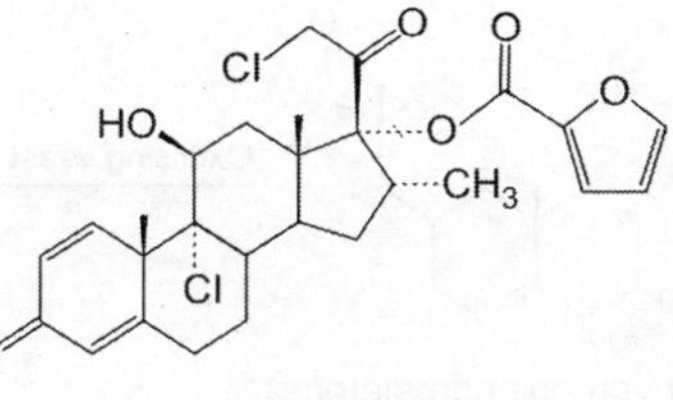

(126)

INDIVIDUAL COMPOUNDS

ANDROGENS : TESTOSTERONE ANALOGS AND ANABOLIC STEROIDS
Testosterone
17β-Hydroxyandrost-4-en-3one.

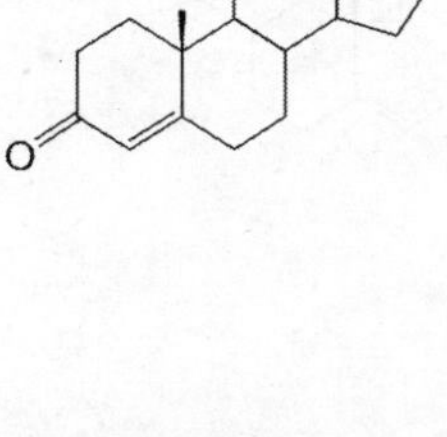

Synthesis
From Cholesterol

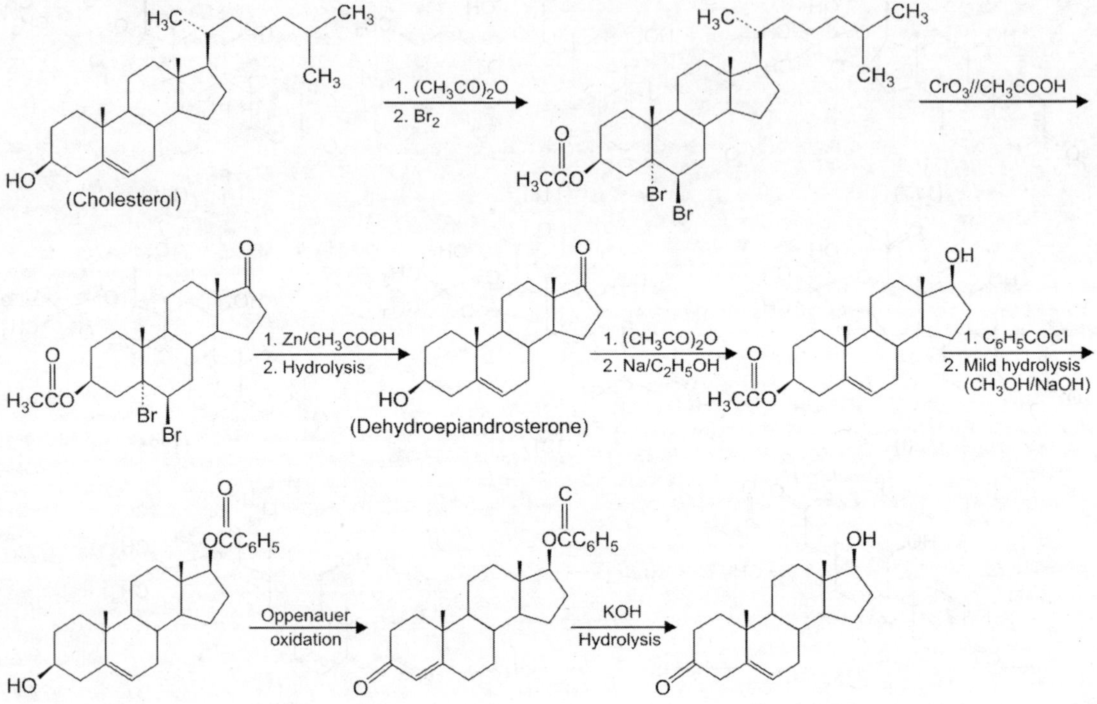

(Cholesterol)

(Dehydroepiandrosterone)

From Dehydroepiandrosterone

(Dehydroepiandrosterone)

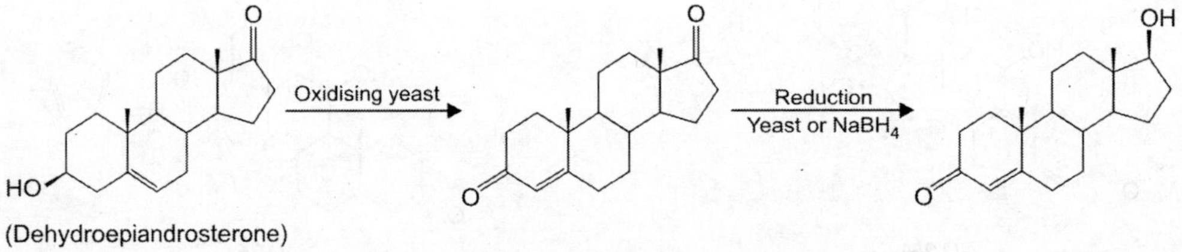

Testosterone is a naturally occurring male sex hormone. It serves as precursor of estradiol (50) in female. Its esters are used as long-acting intramuscular preparation.

Testosterone Propionate

Testosterone 17β-propionate

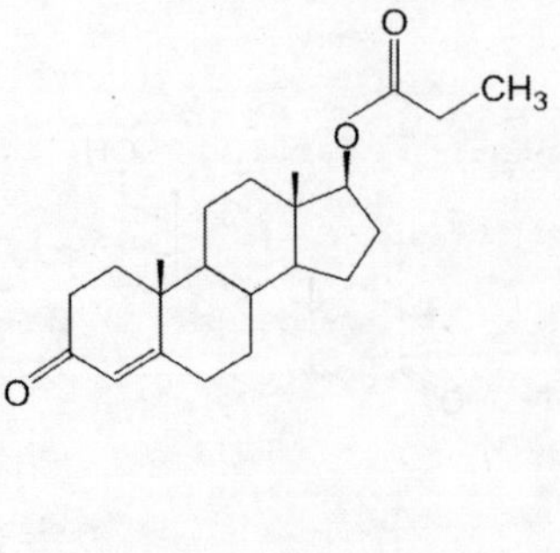

It is prepared by the action of propionyl chloride on testosterone (15) in presence of pyridine. It is used as intramuscular depot preparation.

Testosterone Enanthate
Testosterone 17β-heptanoate

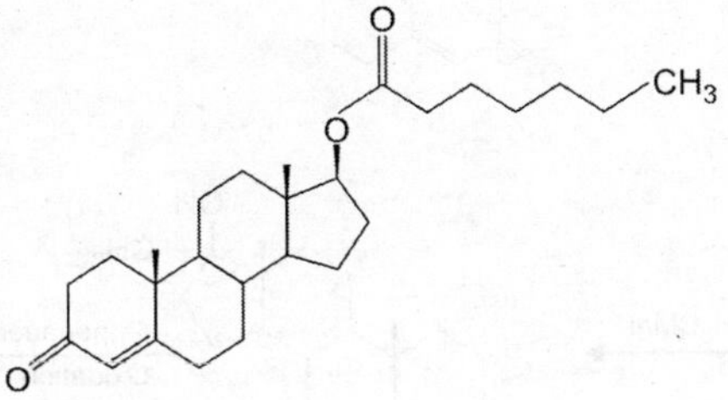

It is prepared by the action of heptanoyl chloride on testosterone (15) in presence of pyridine. It is used as intramuscular depot preparation.

Testosterone Cypionate
Testosterone 17β-cyclopentylpropionate

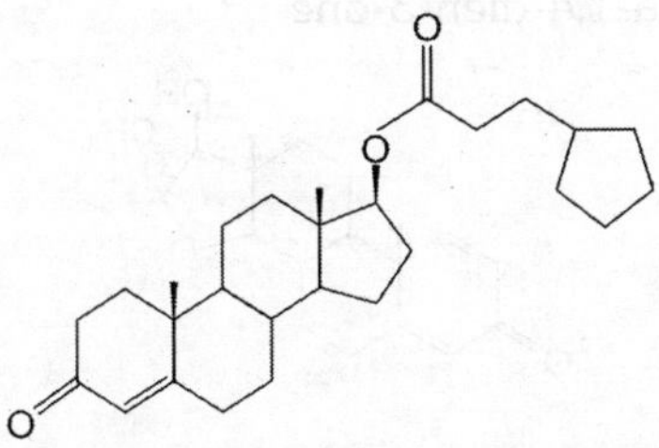

It is prepared by the action of cyclopentylpropionyl chloride on testosterone (15) in presence of pyridine. It is used as intramusciular depot preparation.

Testosterone Phenylpropionate
Testosterone 17β-phenylpropionate

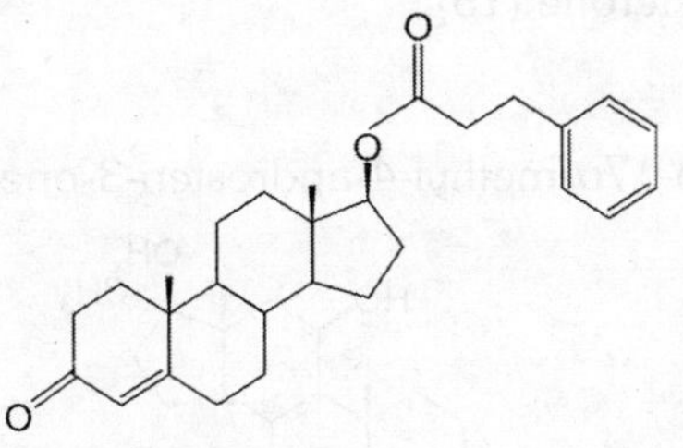

It is used as intramuscular depot preparation.

17α-Methyltestosterone

17β-Hydroxy-17α-methylandrost-4en-3-one

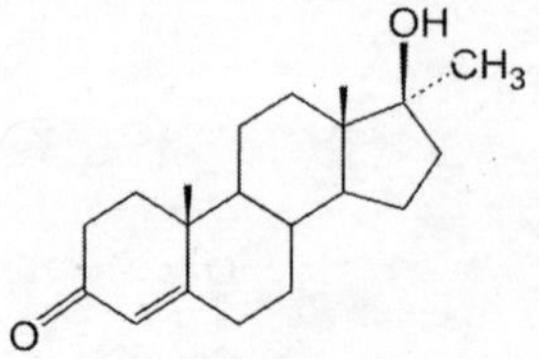

Synthesis

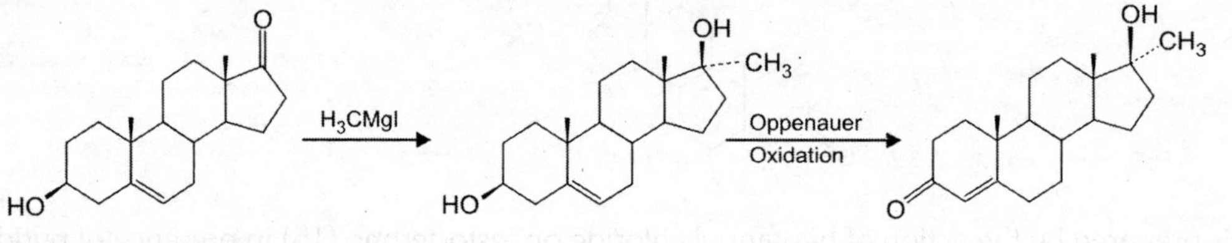

(Dehydroepiandrosterone)

It is half as active as testosterone (15) intramuscularly, but unlike testosterone (15) it can be given orally.

Methandrostenolone

17β-Hydroxy-17α-methylandrosta-1,4-dien-3-one

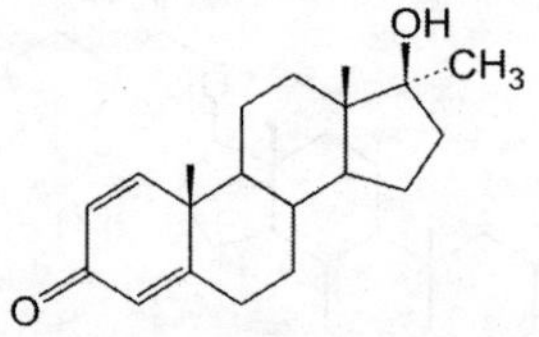

Synthesis

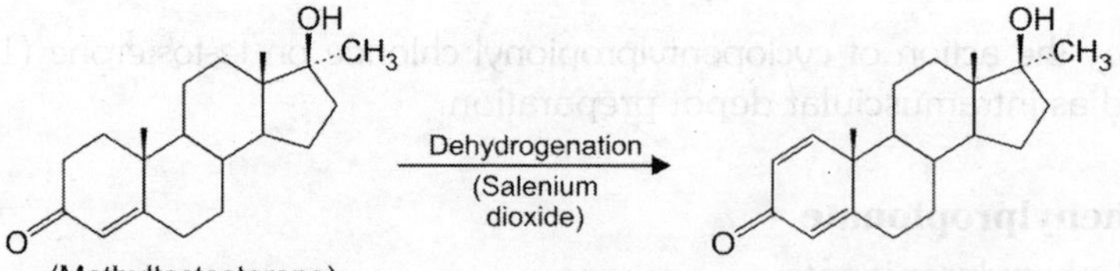

(Methyltestosterone)

It is orally as active as testosterone (15).

Fluoxymesterone

11β, 17β-Dihydroxy-9α-fluoro-17α-methyl-4-androsten-3-one

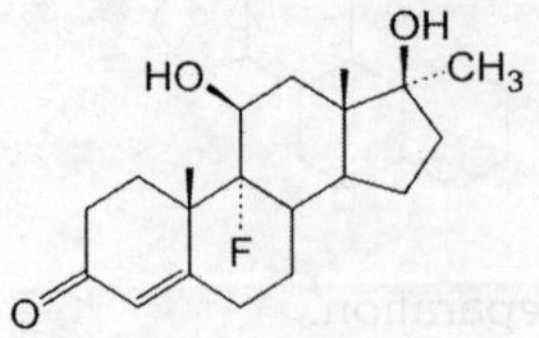

Synthesis

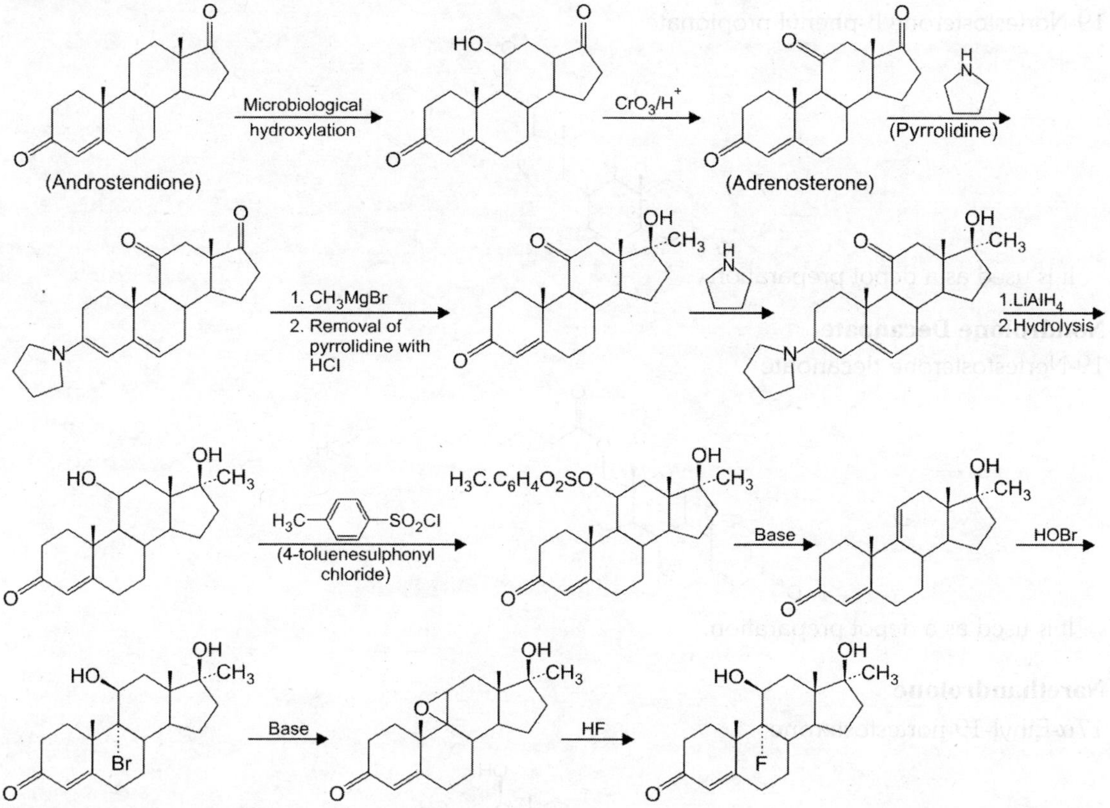

(Androstendione) → Microbiological hydroxylation → CrO₃/H⁺ → (Adrenosterone) → (Pyrrolidine)

1. CH₃MgBr
2. Removal of pyrrolidine with HCl

1.LiAlH₄
2.Hydrolysis

H₃C.C₆H₄O₂SO — (4-toluenesulphonyl chloride) → Base → HOBr

Base → HF

It is a highly potent orally active androgen.

Nandrolone

17β-Hydroxy-4-estren-3-one

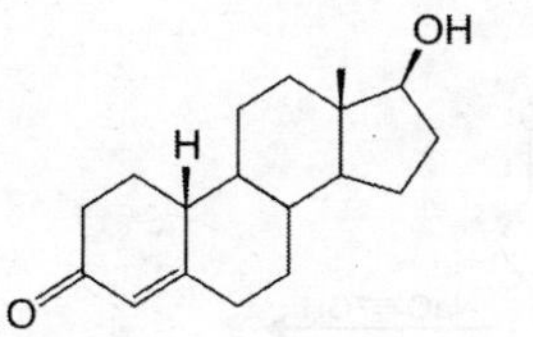

Synthesis

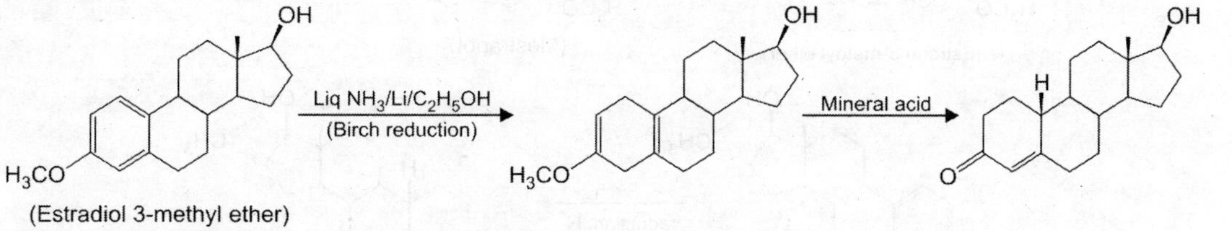

(Estradiol 3-methyl ether) → Liq NH₃/Li/C₂H₅OH (Birch reduction) → Mineral acid

It has a better anabolic/androgenic ratio than testosterone (15).

Nandrolone Phenylproprionate

19-Nortestosterone β-phenyl propionate

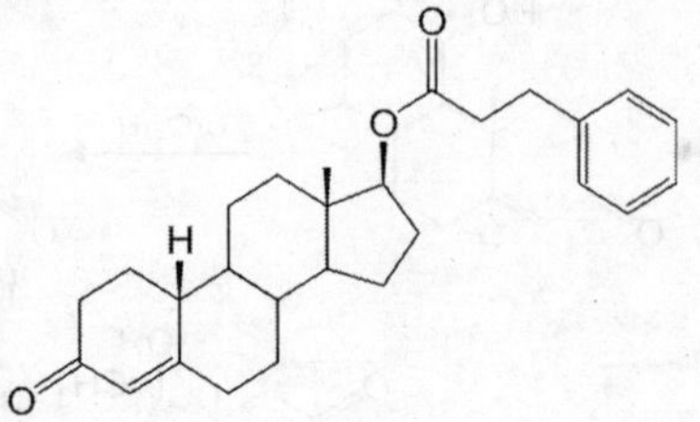

It is used as a depot preparation.

Nondrolone Decanoate

19-Nortestosterone decanoate

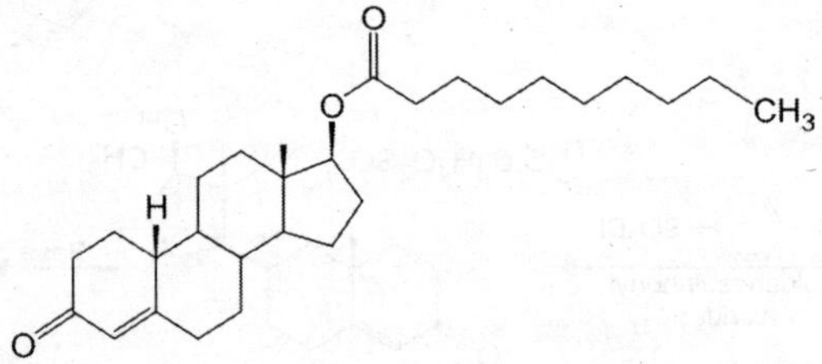

It is used as a depot preparation.

Narethandrolone

17α-Ethyl-19-nortestosterone

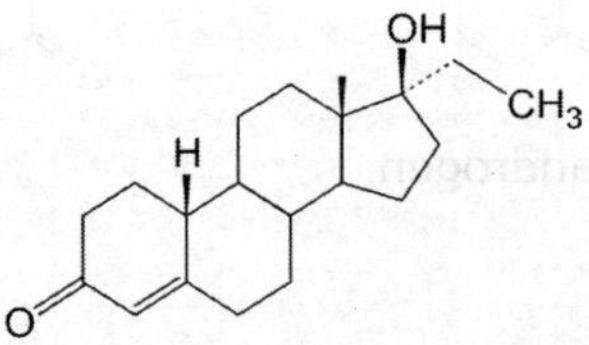

Synthesis

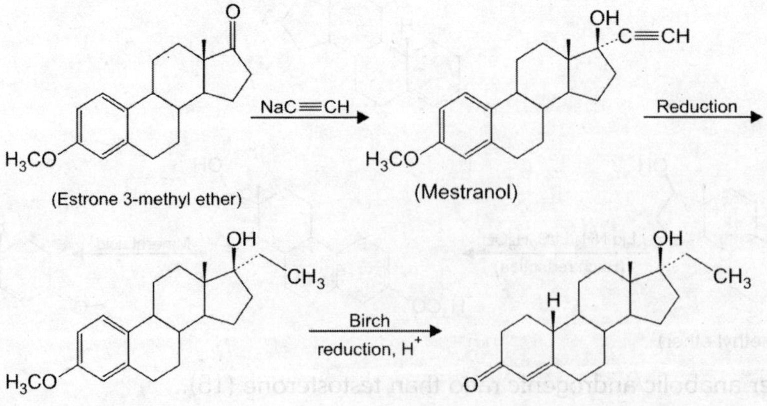

Ethylestrenol

17α-Ethylestr-4-en-17β-ol

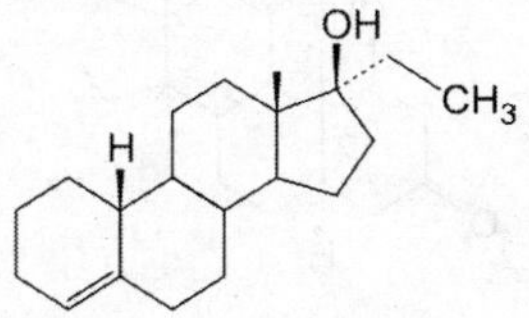

Synthesis

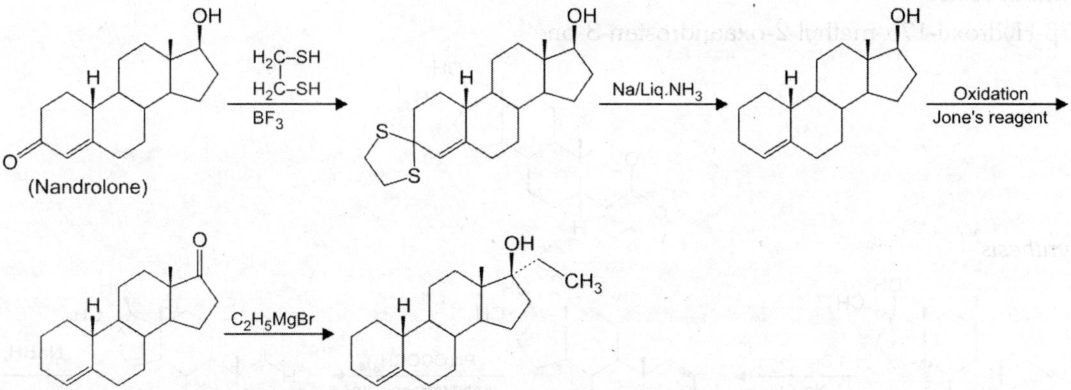

(Nandrolone)

It has an increased anabolic effect in comparison to androgenic effect.

Methenolone Acetate

1-Methyl-1-androsten-3-on-17β-acetate

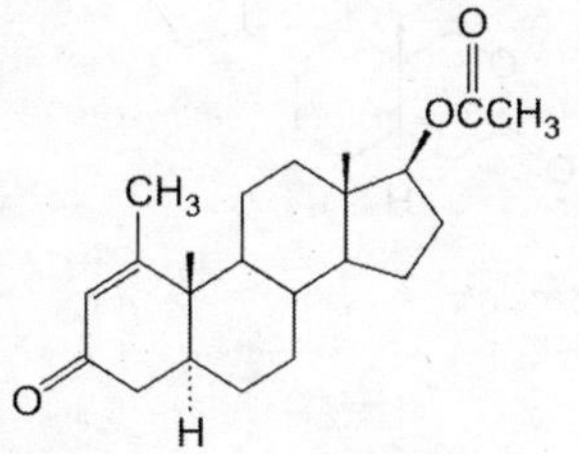

Synthesis

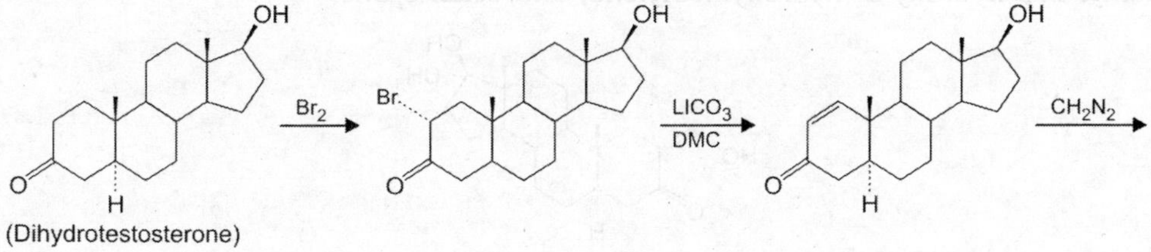

(Dihydrotestosterone)

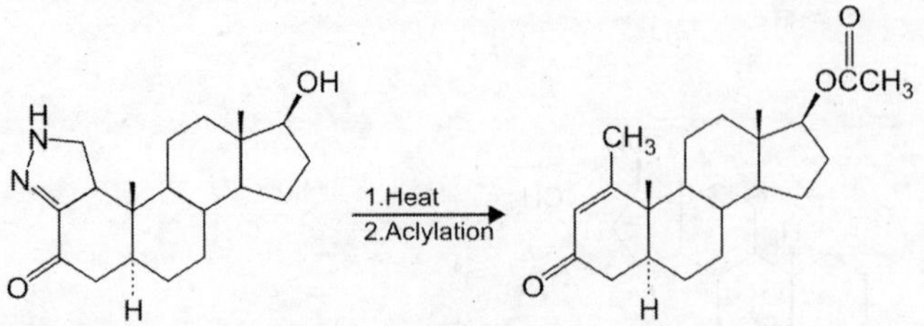

Methenolone acetate has high anabolic activity.

Oxandrolone

17β-Hydroxy-17α-methyl-2-oxaandrostan-3-one

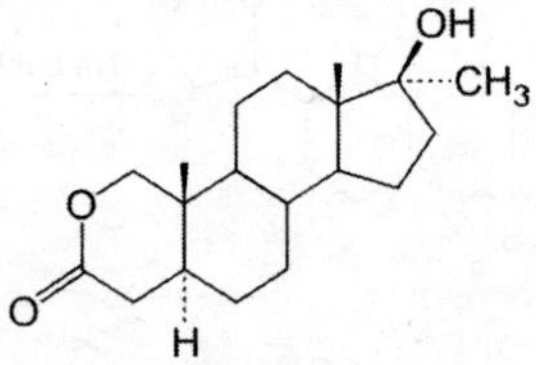

Synthesis

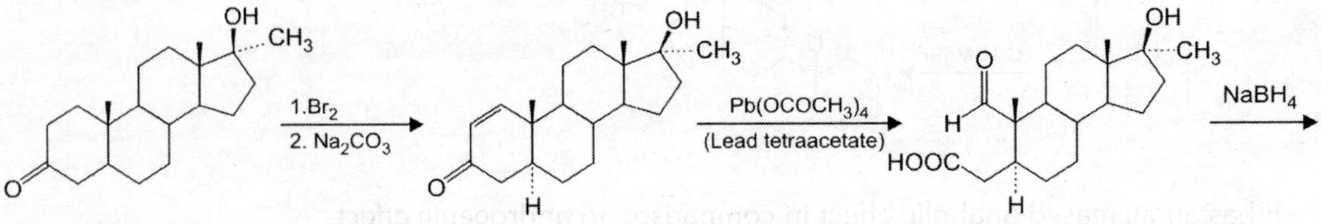

(17α-Methyl dihydro-
testosterone)

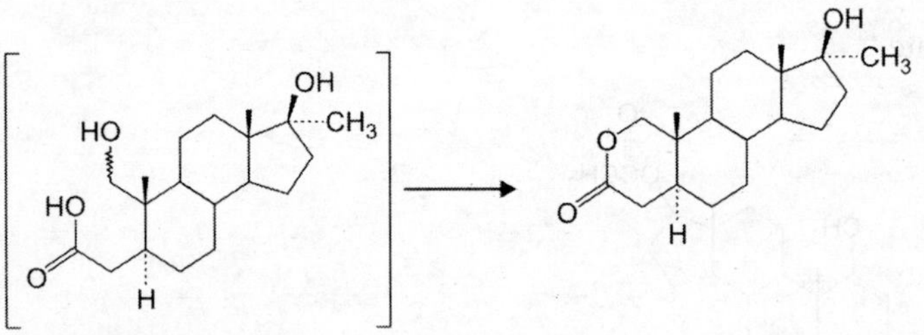

It is a potent anabolic steroid.

Oxymetholone

17α-Methyl-17β-hydroxy-2-(hydroxymethylene)-androstan-3-one

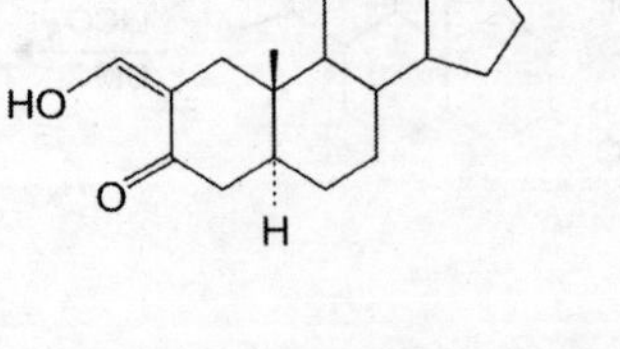

Synthesis

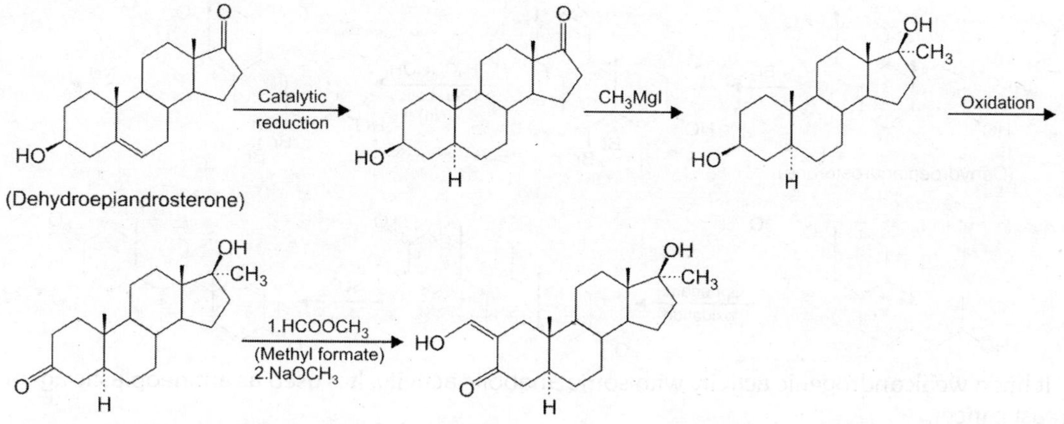

(Dehydroepiandrosterone)

Stanozolol

17α-Methyl-2' *H*-androst-2-eno[3,2-c] pyrazol-17β-ol

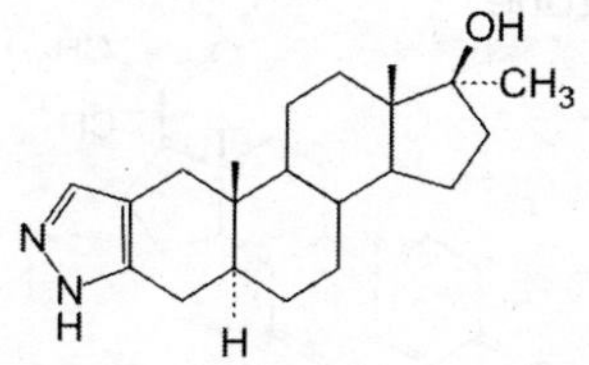

Synthesis

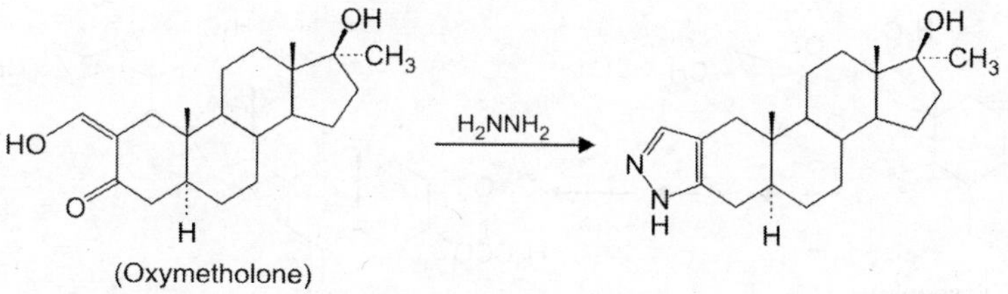

(Oxymetholone)

Testolactone

D-Homo-17α-oxaandrosta-1,4-diene-3,17-dione

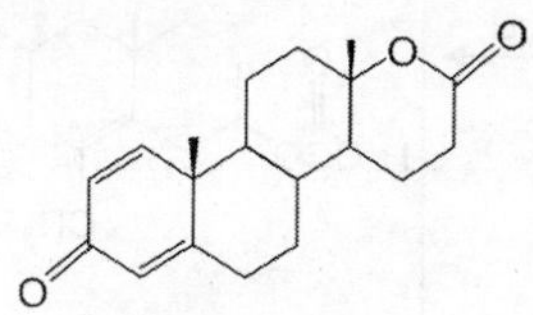

Synthesis

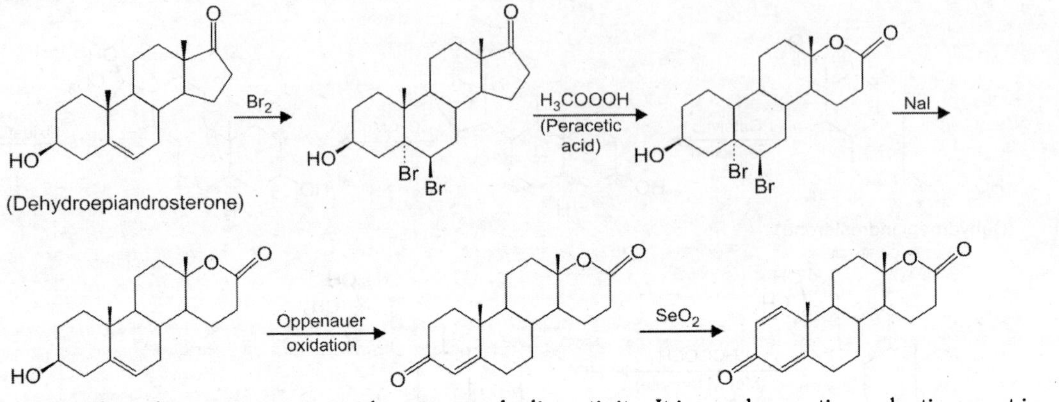

(Dehydroepiandrosterone)

It has a weak androgenic activity with some anabolic activity. It is used as antineoplastic agent in breast cancer.

ANDROGENS : 5α-REDUCTASE INHIBITORS AND α₁-ADRENERGIC RECEPTOR ANTAGONISTS

Medrogestone

6,17α-Dimethyl-6-dehydroprogesterone

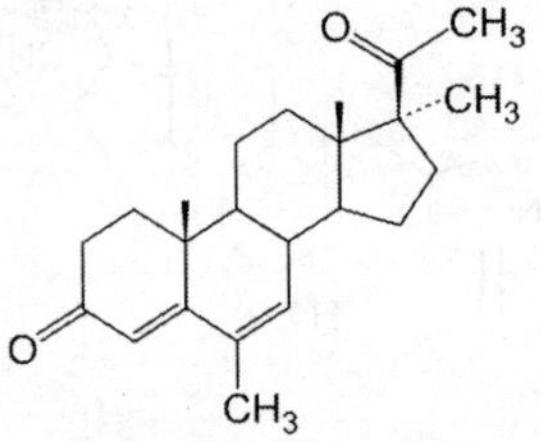

Synthesis

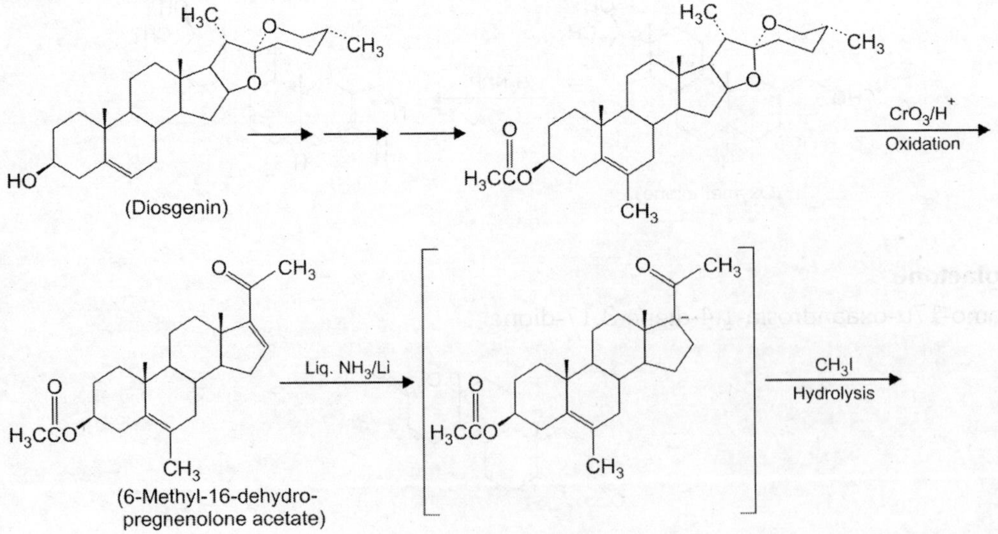

(Diosgenin)

(6-Methyl-16-dehydro-
pregnenolone acetate)

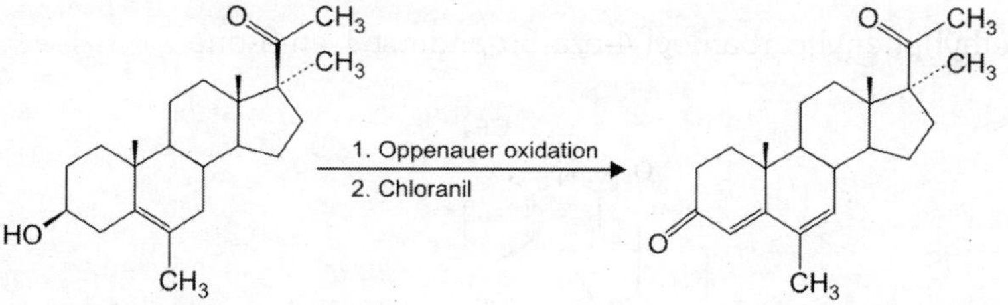

It is used in prostate cancer.

Finasteride

17β-(*N-tert*-Butylcarbamoyl)-4-aza-5α-androst-1-en-3-one

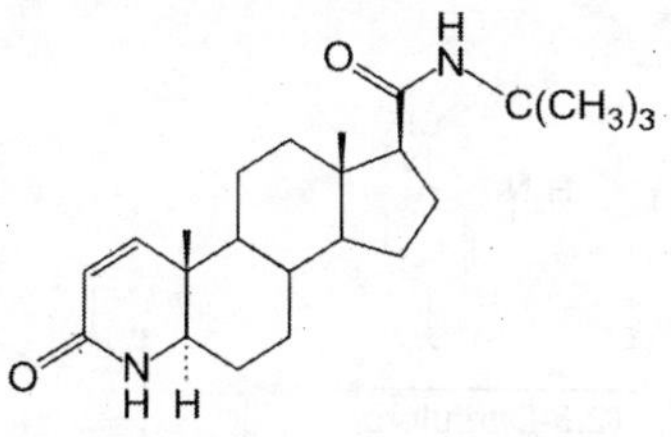

Synthesis

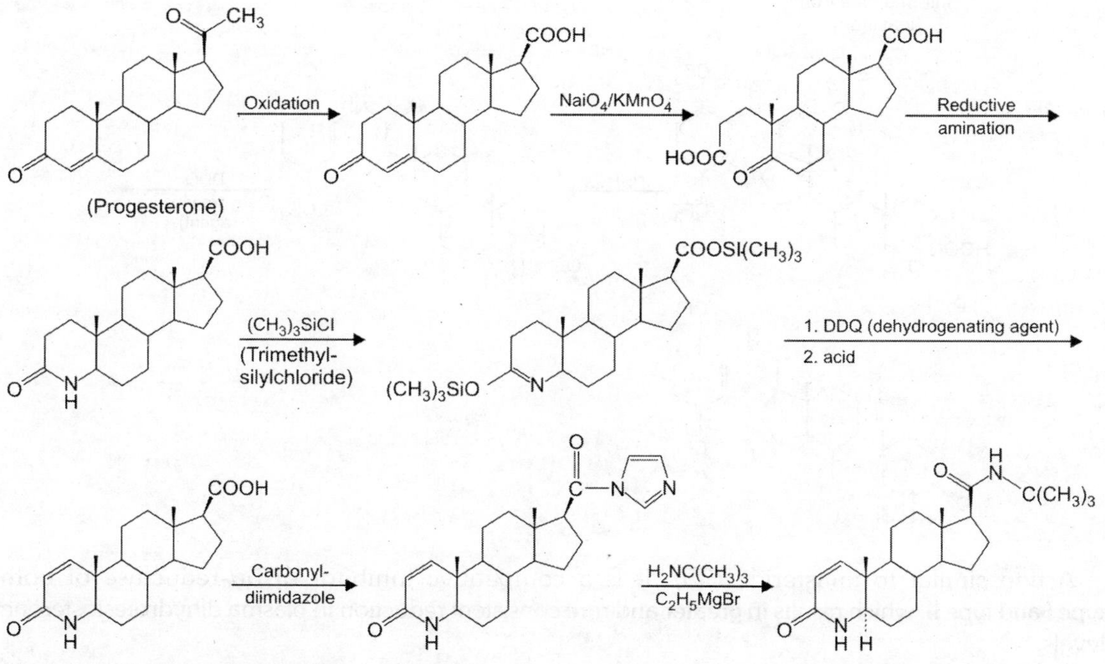

(Progesterone)

(DDQ, 2,3-Dichloro-5,6-dicyanoquinone)

It produces a rapid reduction in plasma dihydrotestosterone through inhibition of 5α-reductase (type II). It is effective in men with large prostrates.

Dutasteride

17β-*N*-[2,5-Bis(trifluoromethyl)phenyl]carbamoyl-4-aza-5α-androst-1-en-3-one

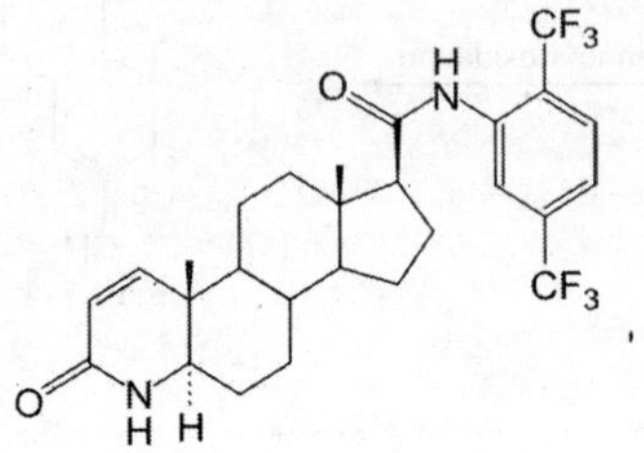
CF3
H
N
O
N
H H
CF3

Synthesis

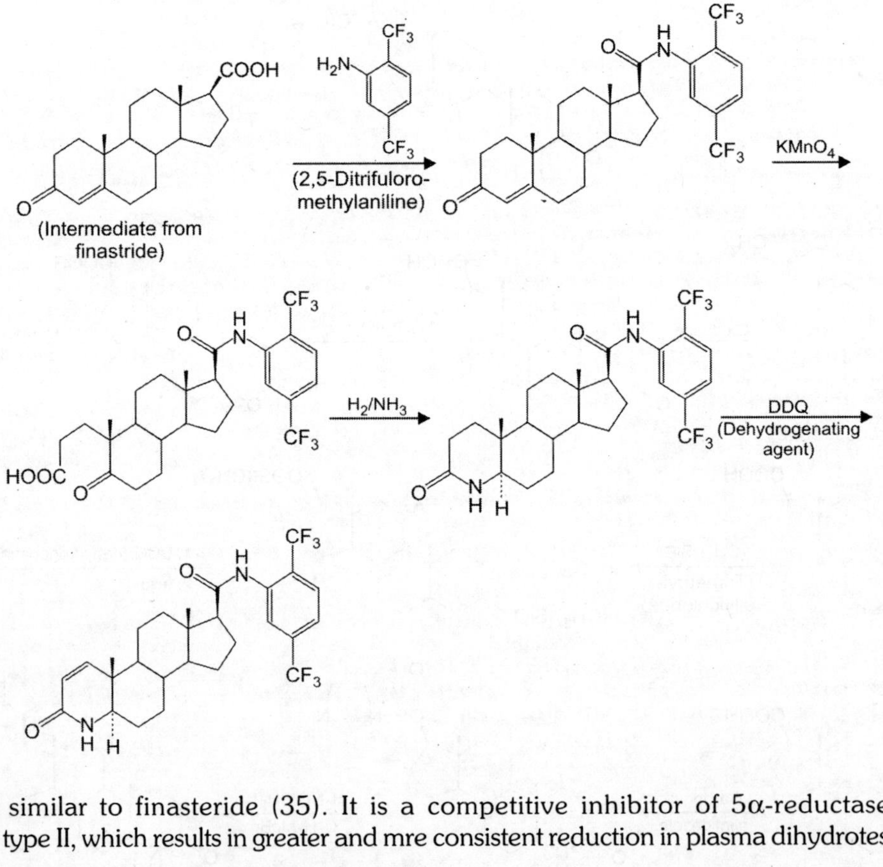
COOH
H2N
CF3
CF3
(2,5-Ditrifuloro-
methylaniline)
(Intermediate from
finastride)
KMnO4
HOOC
H2/NH3
DDQ
(Dehydrogenating
agent)

Action similar to finasteride (35). It is a competitive inhibitor of 5α-reductase of both type I and type II, which results in greater and mre consistent reduction in plasma dihydrotestosterone levels.

Prazosin, Terazosin, and Doxazosin

See ADRENERGIC DRUGS

Alfuzosin

N-[3-[(4-Amino-6,7-dimethoxy-2-quinazolinyl)methylamino]propyl]tetrahydro-2-furancarboxamide

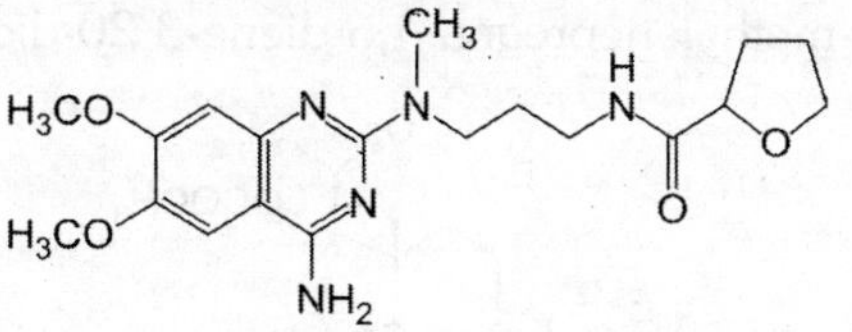

Synthesis

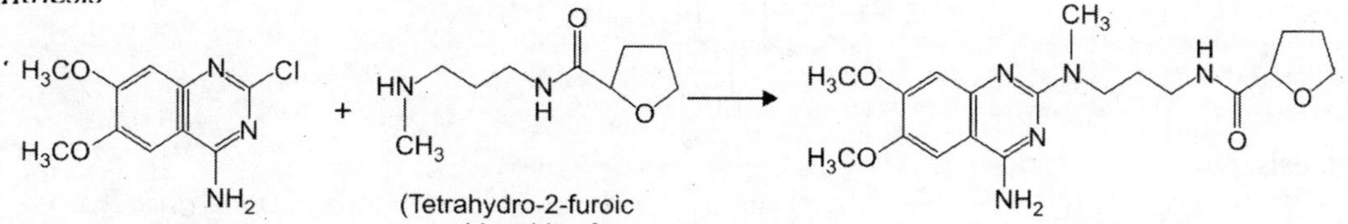

(4-Amino-2-chloro-6,7-dimethoxyquinazoline) (Tetrahydro-2-furoic acid amide of methyl aminopropylamine)

Alfuzosin is the first-line drug for benign prostate hyperplasia.

Tamsulosin

5-[(2*R*)-2-[[2-(2-Ethoxyphenoxy)ethyl]amino]propyl]-2-methoxybenzenesulphonamide

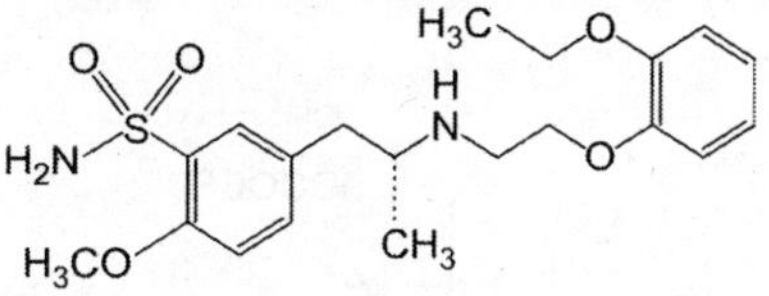

Synthesis

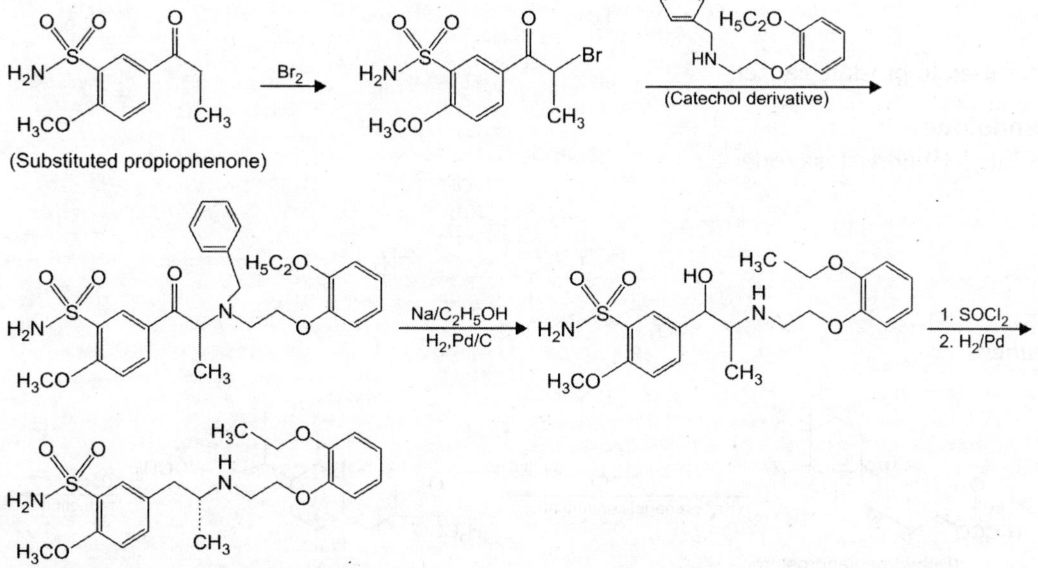
Br2
(Substituted propiophenone)
(Catechol derivative)
Na/C2H5OH
H2,Pd/C
1. SOCl2
2. H2/Pd

Similar action as alfuzosin (40).

ANDROGENS : ANTIANDROGENS

Cyproterone acetate

6-Chloro-17α-hydroxy-1α,2α-methylenepregna-4,6-diene-3,20-dione acetate

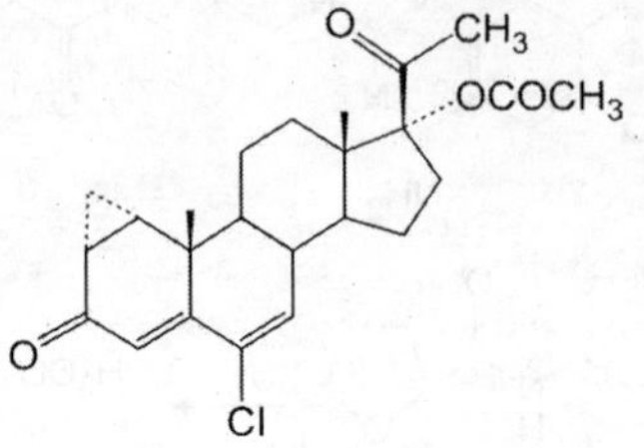

Synthesis

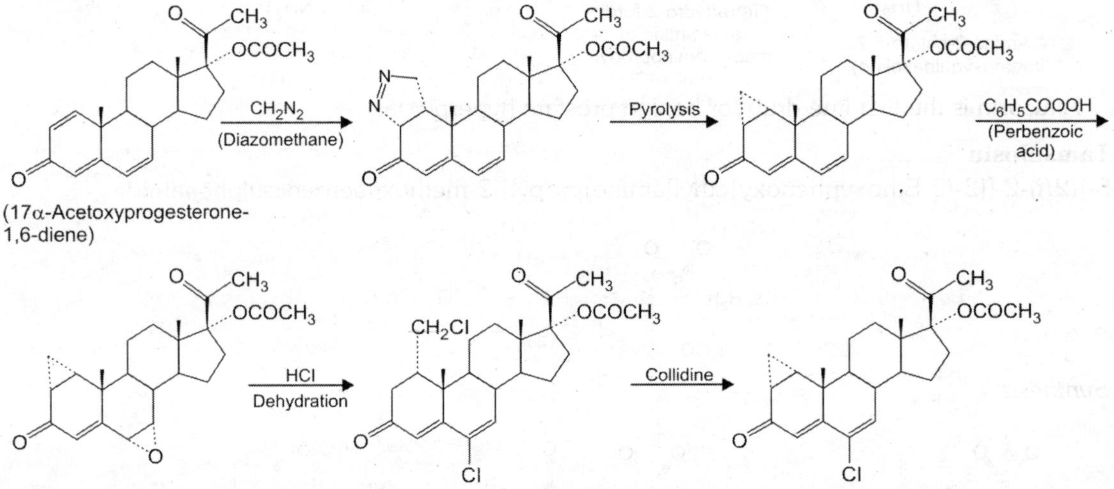

(17α-Acetoxyprogesterone-
1,6-diene)

It is used in prostate cancer.

Oxendolone

16β-Ethyl-19-nortestosterone

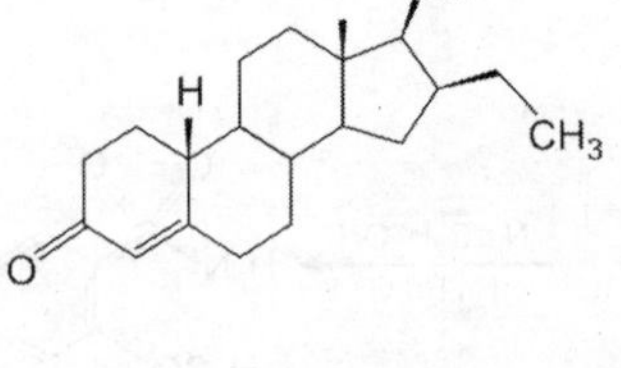

Synthesis

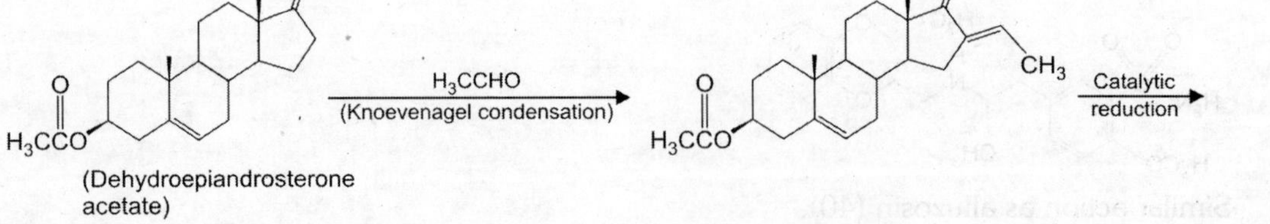

(Dehydroepiandrosterone
acetate)

It is used in prostate cancer.

Bicalutamide

4-Cyano-3-trifluorometyl-N-(3-p-fluorophenylsulphonyl-2-hydroxy-2-methylpropionyl)aniline

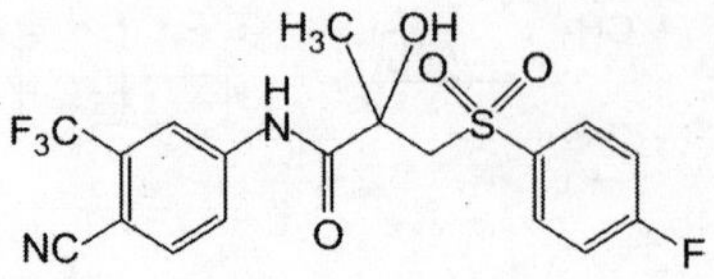

Synthesis

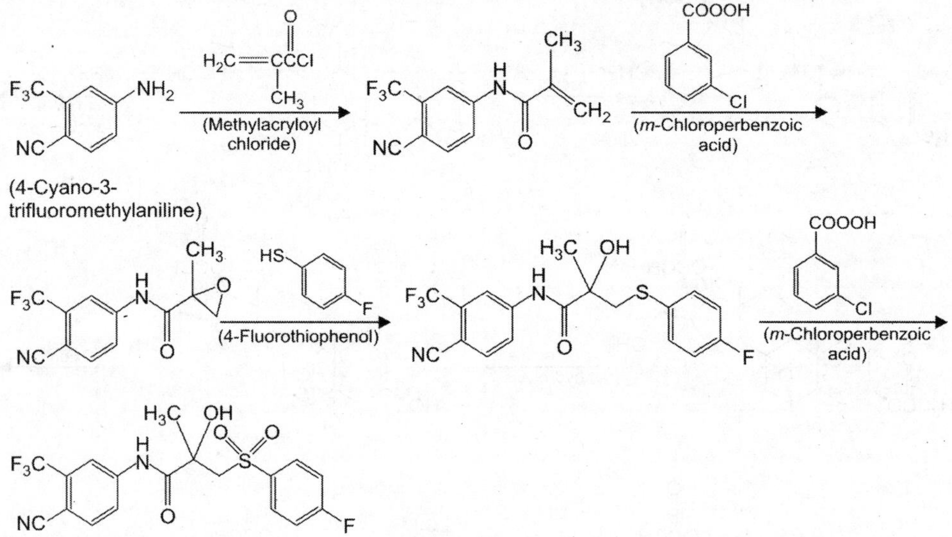

It is used for nonmetastatic prostate cancer. The antiandrogenic activity resides in *R*-enantiomer and *S*-enantiomer has no antiandrogenic activity.

Flutamide

2-Methyl-N-[4-nitro-3(trifluoromethyl)phenyl] propanamide

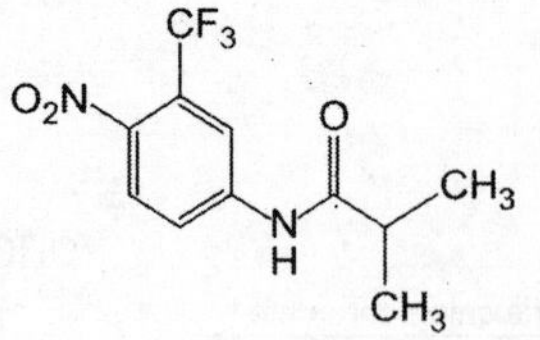

Synthesis

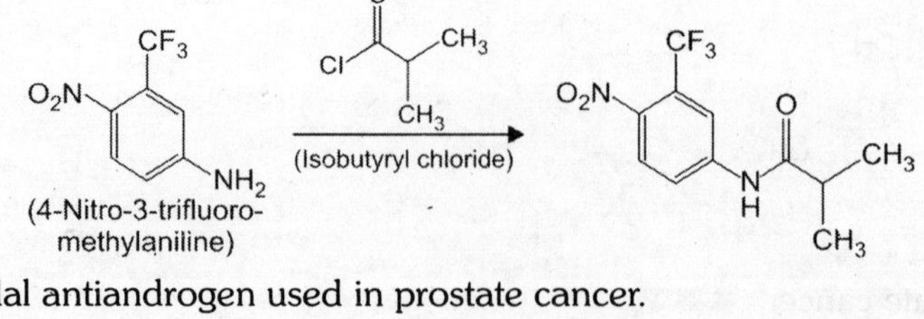

It is a nonsteroidal antiandrogen used in prostate cancer.

Nilutamide

5,5-Dimethyl-3-[4-nitro-3-(trifluoromethyl)phenyl]-2,4-imidazolidinedione

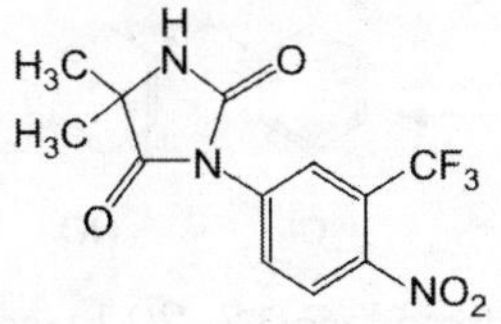

Synthesis

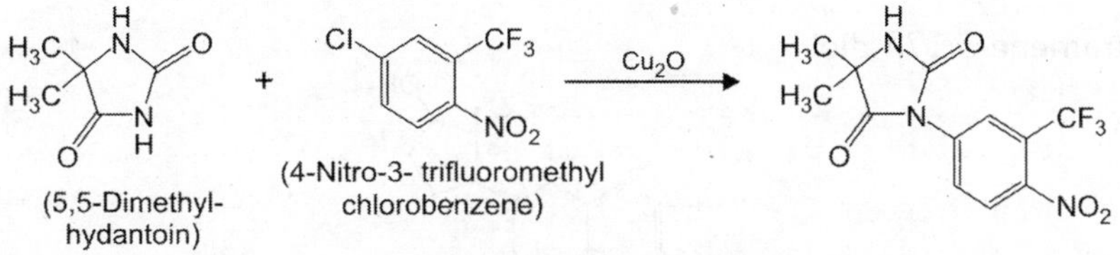

(5,5-Dimethyl-hydantoin)   (4-Nitro-3- trifluoromethyl chlorobenzene)

It is a nonsteroidal antiandrogen used for metastatic prostate cancer.

ANDROGENS : 17α- HYDROXYLASE/17,20 – LYASE INHIBITORS

Fluconazole

See **ANTIFUNGAL AGENTS**

Liarozole

5-[(3-Chlorophenyl)-1*H*-imidazol-1-ylmethyl]-1*H*-benzimidazol

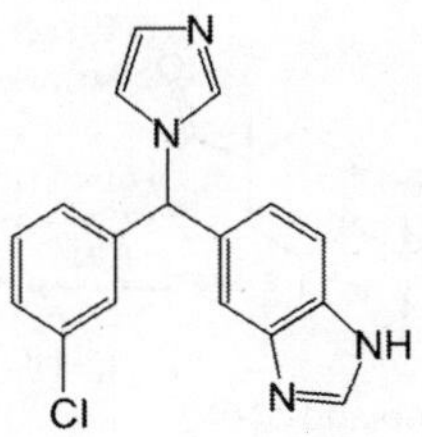

Synthesis

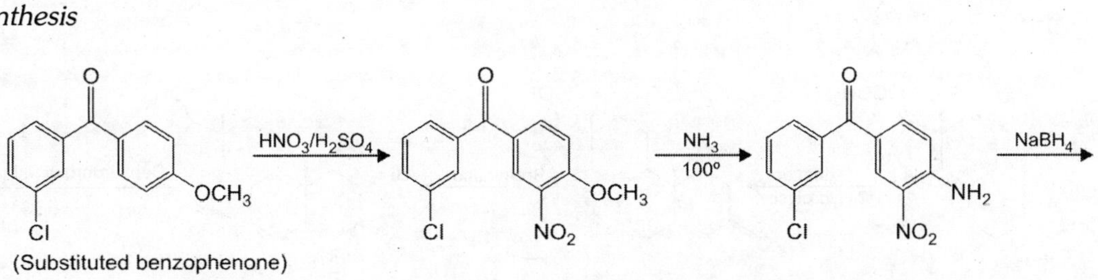

(Substituted benzophenone)

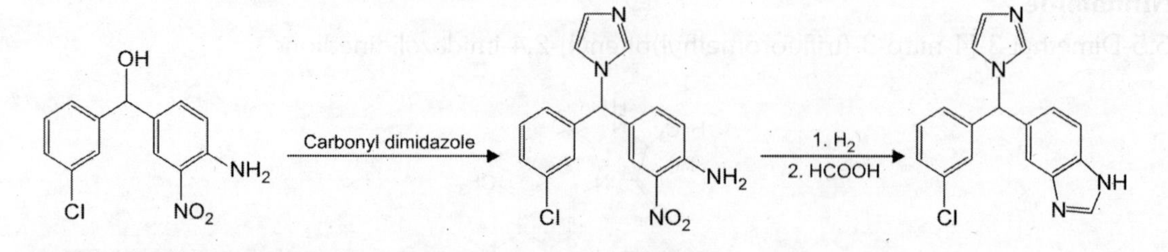

It is a selective inhibitor of 17α-hydroxylase/17, 20-lyase

ESTROGENS : NATURAL

Estradiol

1,3,5-(10)-Estratriene-3,17β-diol

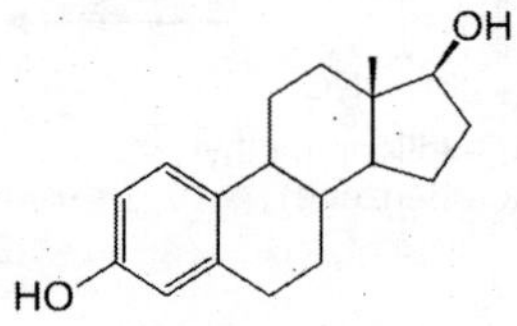

Synthesis

From Estrone

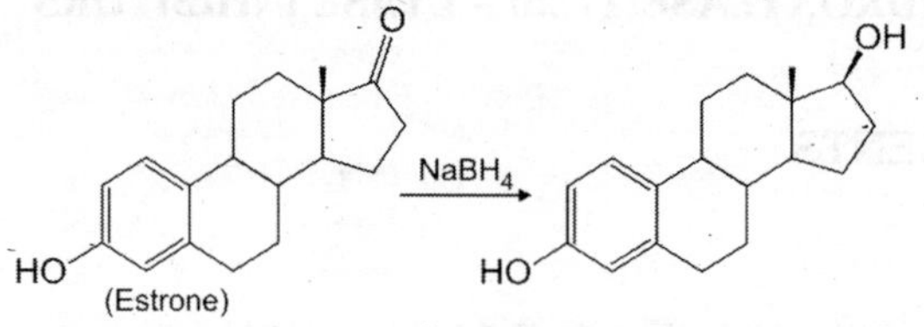

From Cholesterol

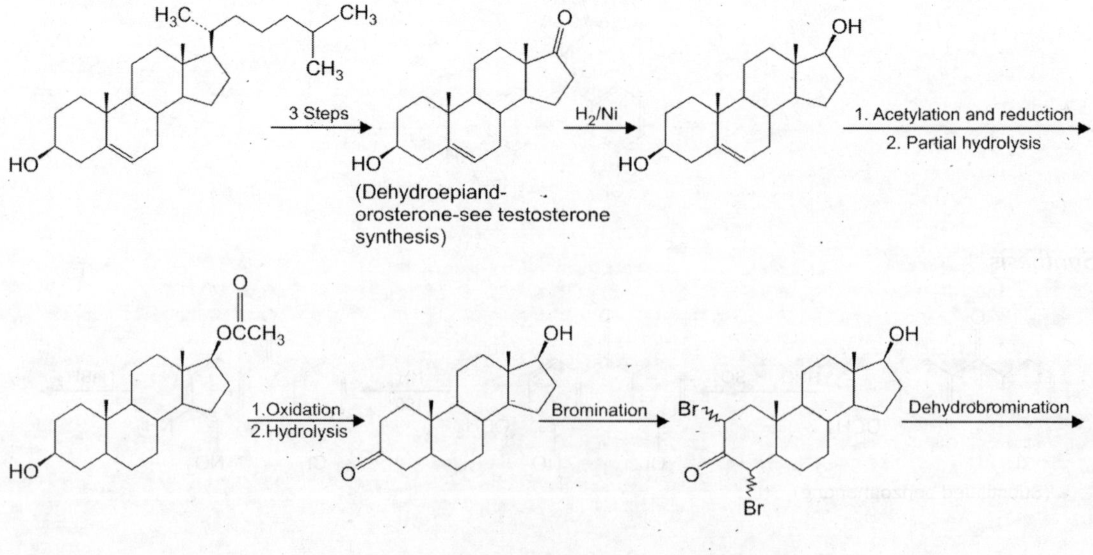

(Dehydroepiand-
orosterone-see testosterone
synthesis)

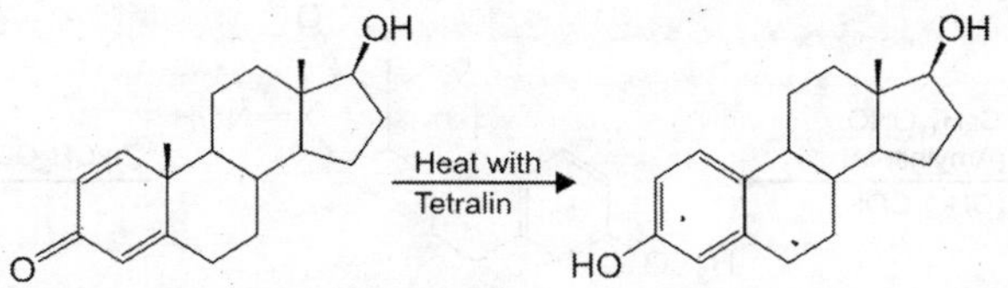

It is used orally and as transdermal cream.

Estrone

3-Hydroxyestra-1,3,5(10)-trien-17-one

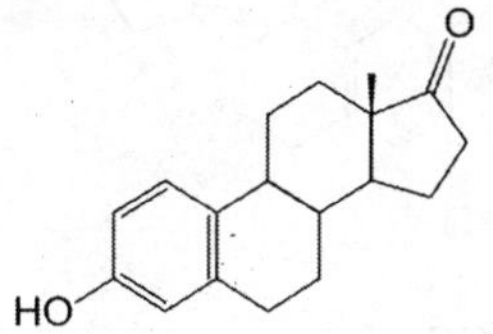

Synthesis

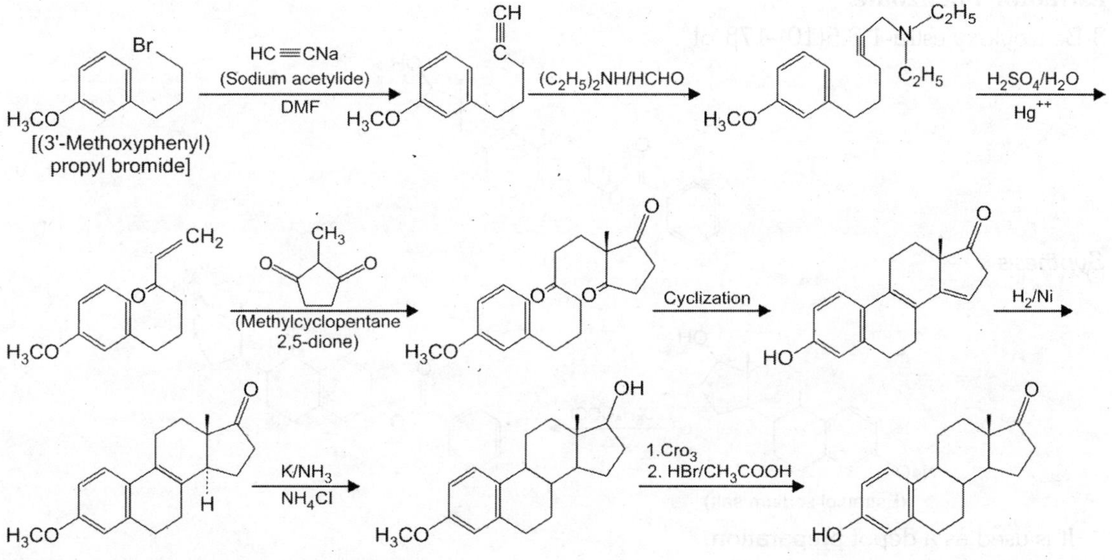

It is used parenterally and topically

Estriol

1,3,5-(10)-Estratriene-3, 16α,17β-triol

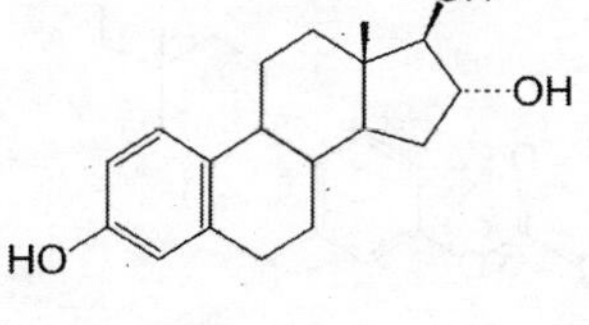

Synthesis

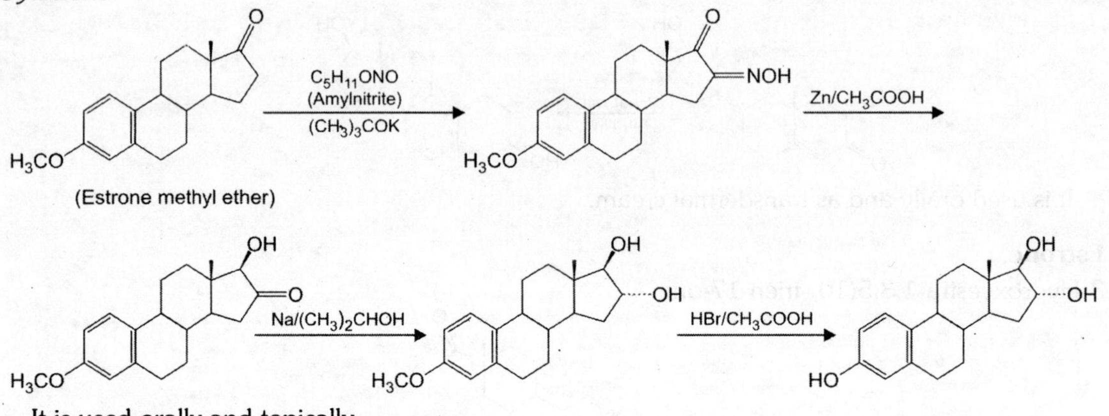

(Estrone methyl ether)

It is used orally and topically.

ESTROGENS : SYNTHETIC ANALOGS

Estradiol 3-Benzoate

3-Benzoyloxy estra-1,3,5(10)-17β-ol

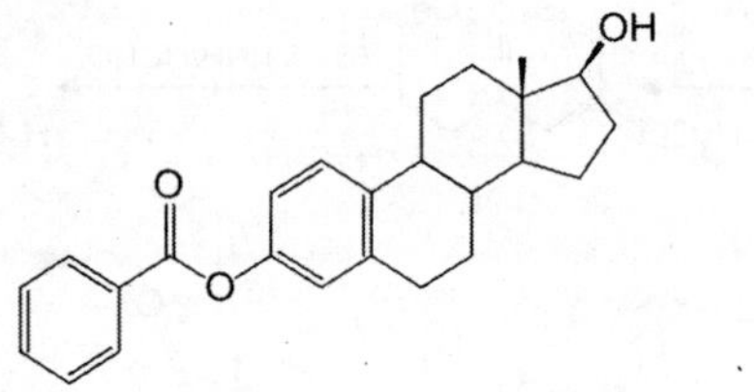

Synthesis

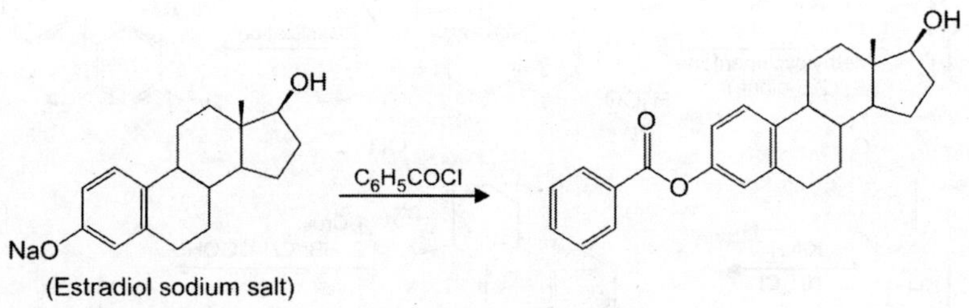

(Estradiol sodium salt)

It is used as a depot preparation.

Estradiol Dipropionate

1,3,5(10) Estratriene-3,17β-diol dipropionate

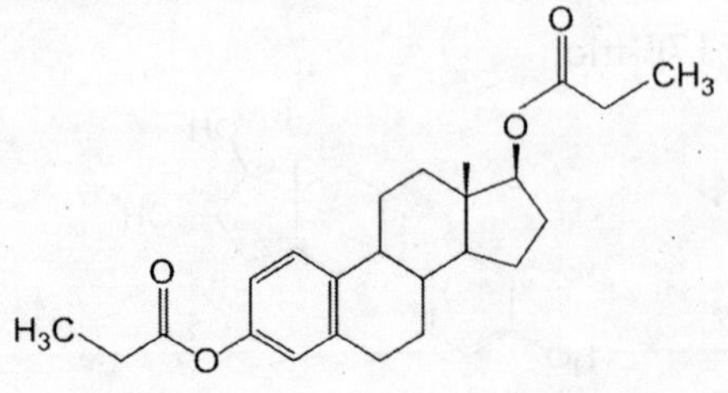

Synthesis

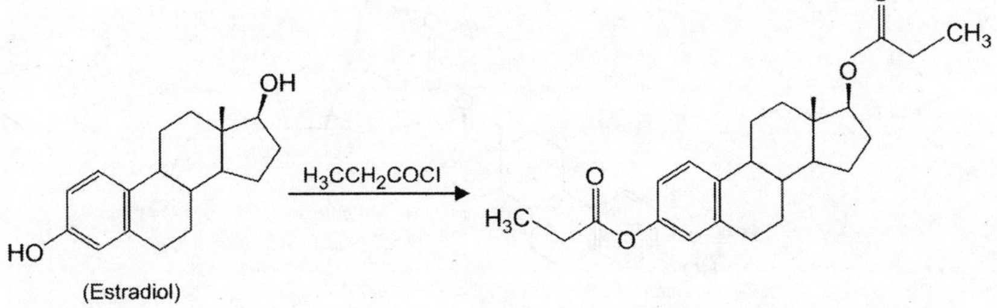
OH
HO
(Estradiol)
H_3CCH_2COCl
O
H_3C
O
O
CH_3

Used as depot preparation.

Estradiol Enanthate

Estradiol 17β-heptanoate

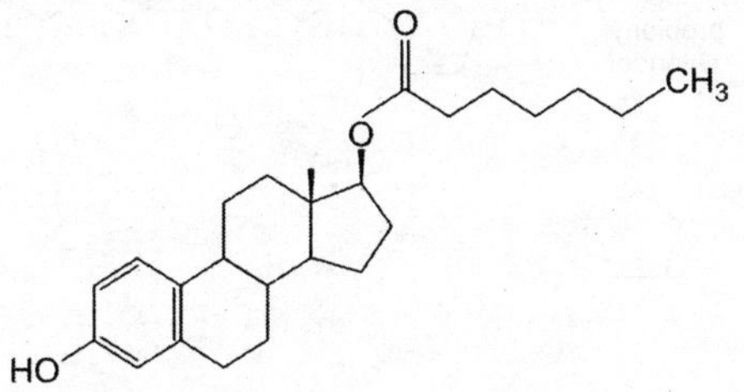
O
CH_3
O
HO

Synthesis

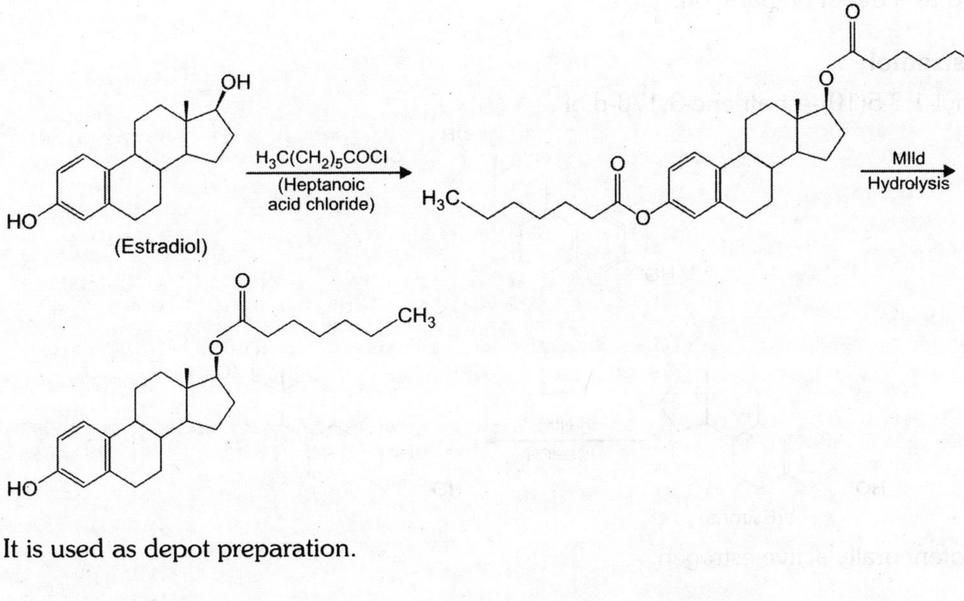
OH
HO
(Estradiol)
$H_3C(CH_2)_5COCl$
(Heptanoic
acid chloride)
H_3C
O
O
CH_3
Mild
Hydrolysis
HO

It is used as depot preparation.

Estradiol Cypionate

Estradiol 17β-cyclopentylpropionate

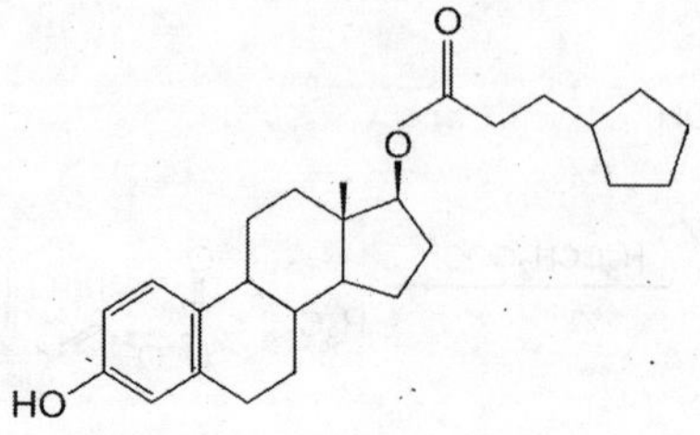

Synthesis

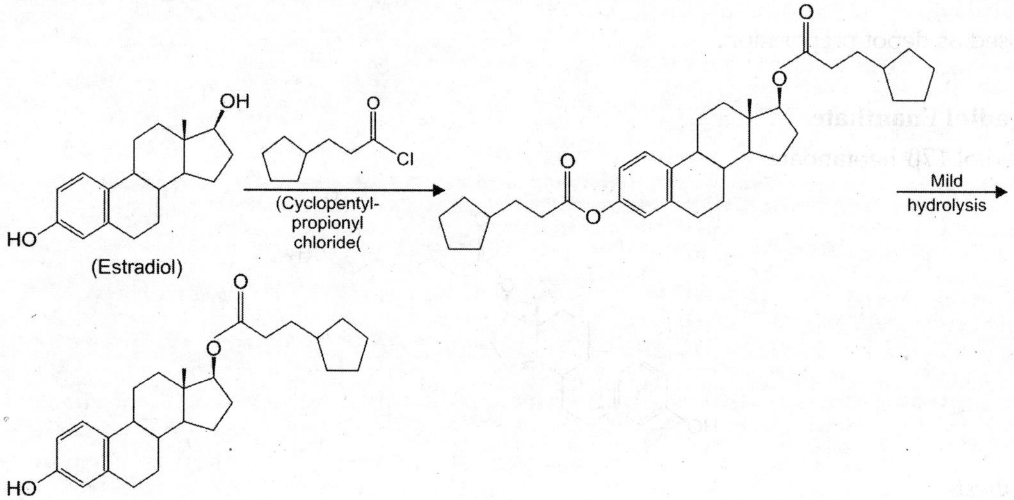

It is used as a depot preparation.

Ethinyl Estradiol

17α-Ethynyl-1,3,5(10)-estratriene-3,17β-diol

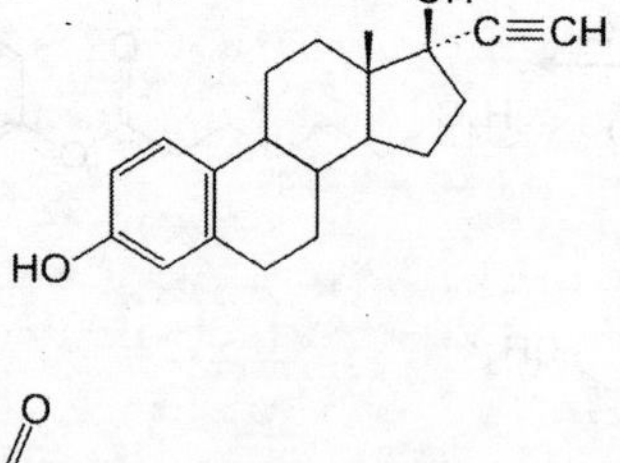

Synthesis

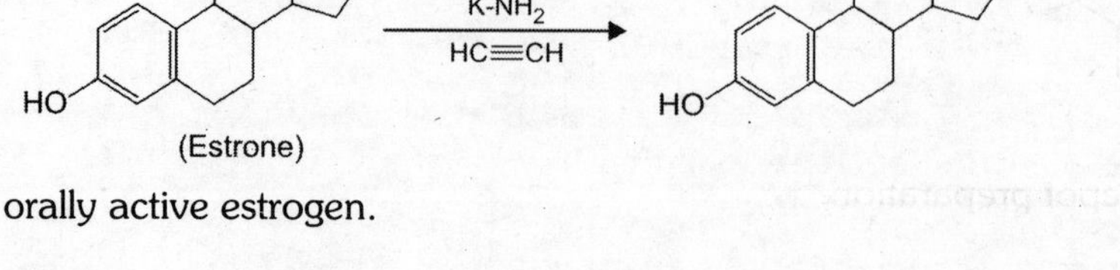

It is a potent orally active estrogen.

Mestranol

17α-Ethynyl-3-methoxy-1,3,5(10)-estratrien-17β-ol

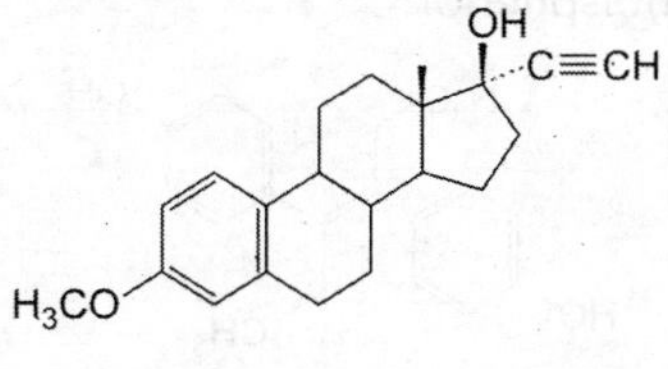

Synthesis

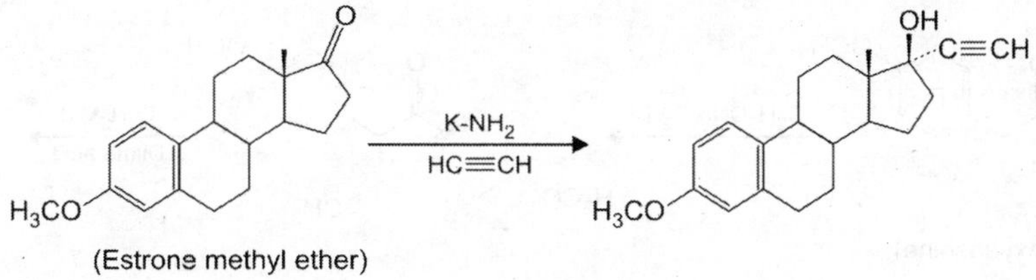

(Estrone methyl ether)

It is prodrug of ethinyl estradiol (54).

Quinestrol

17α-Ethinylestradiol-3-cyclopentyl ether.

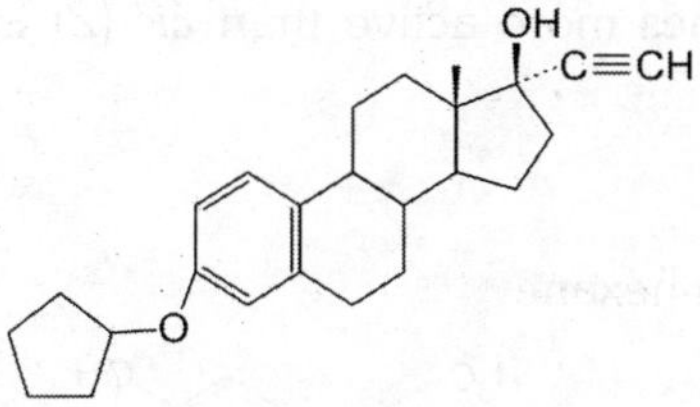

Synthesis

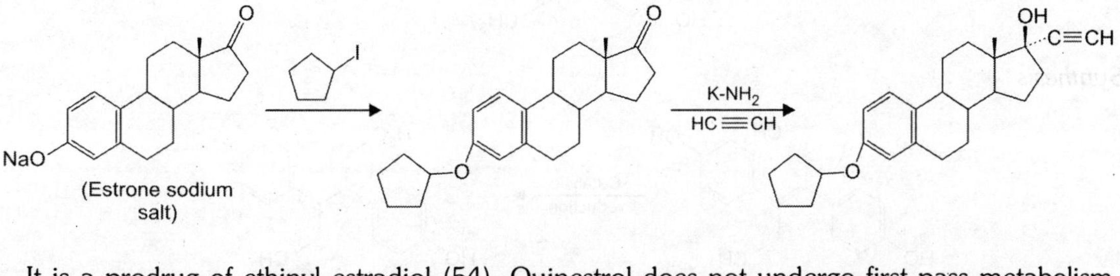

(Estrone sodium
salt)

It is a prodrug of ethinyl estradiol (54). Quinestrol does not undergo first pass metabolism. Ethinyl estradiol (54), on the other hand, undergoes 60% metabolism in intestinal mucosa during first pass metabolism. Cyclopentyl group also enhances its lipid solubility and is thus given weekly.

ESTROGENS : NONSTEROIDAL

Diethylstilbestrol

(*E*)-4,4'(1,2-Diethyl-1,2-ethenediyl)bisphenol

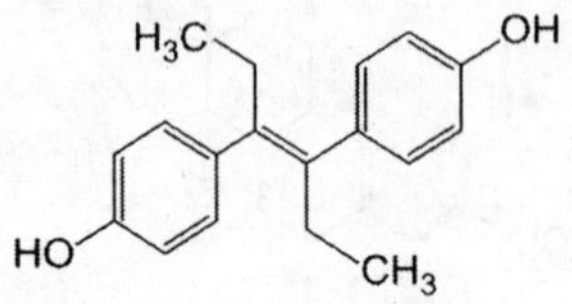

Synthesis

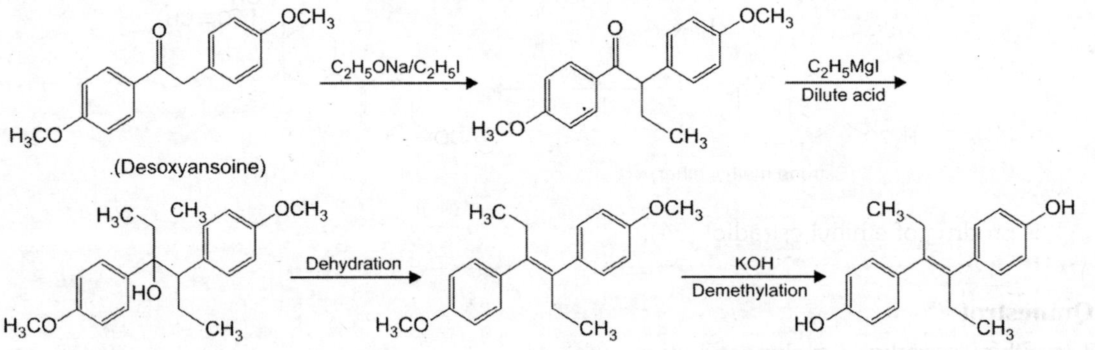

(Desoxyansoine)

The *trans* (*E*) isomer is 10 times more active than *cis* (*Z*) isomer. The *E*-isomer is also well absorbed orally.

Hexestrol

Meso-3,4-bis(*p*-hydroxyphenyl)-*n*-hexane

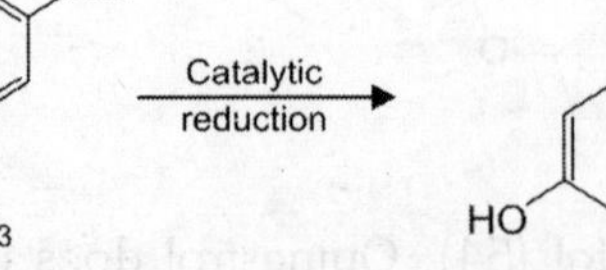

Synthesis

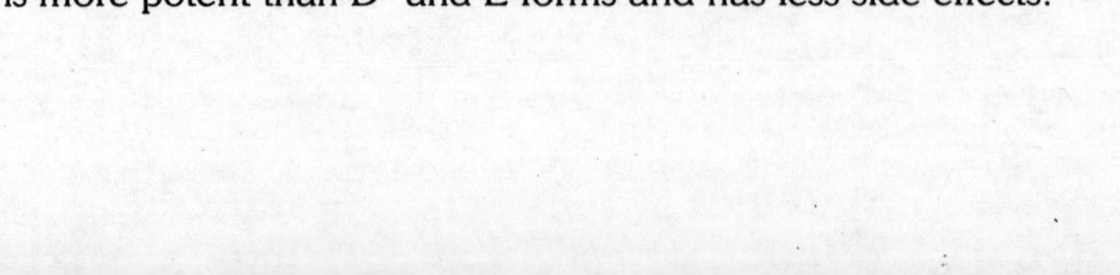

(Diethylstilbestrol)

Meso-isomer is more potent than D- and L-forms and has less side effects.

Dienestrol

3,4-Bis(p-hydroxyphenyl)-2,4-hexadiene.

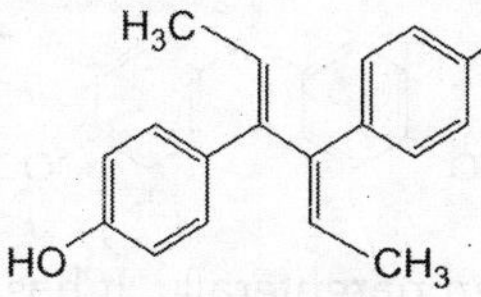

(trans-trans) from

Synthesis

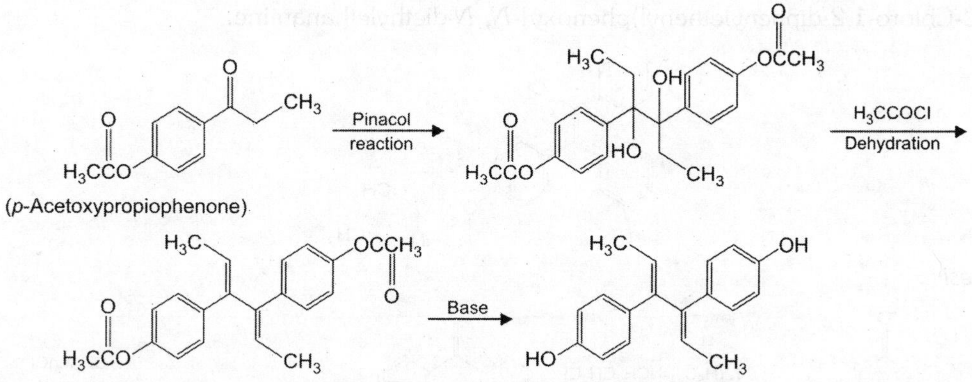

(p-Acetoxypropiophenone)

It has similar activity as that of diethylstilbestrol (60) when used orally.

Chlorotrianisene

Chlorotris(p-methoxyphenyl)ethylene

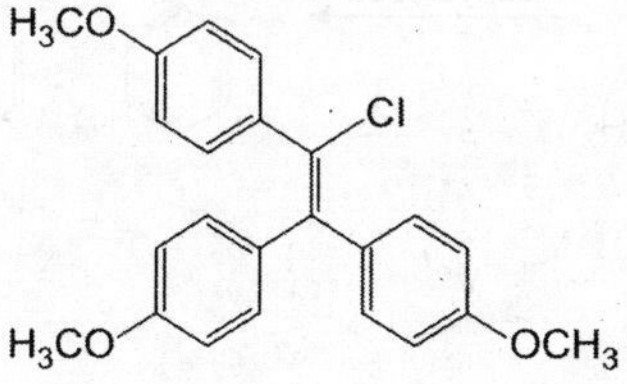

Synthesis

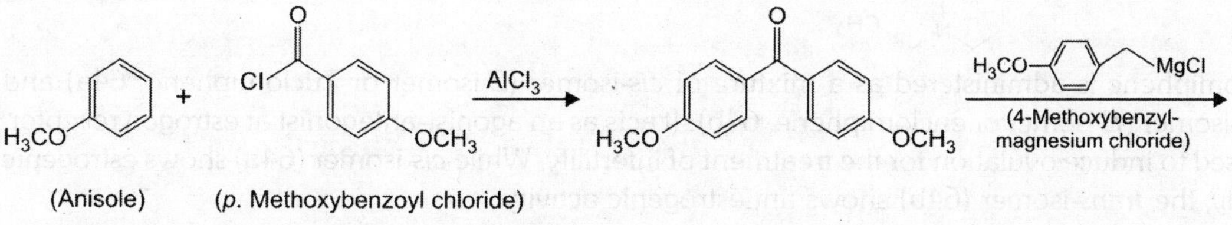

(Anisole) (p. Methoxybenzoyl chloride) (4-Methoxybenzyl-magnesium chloride)

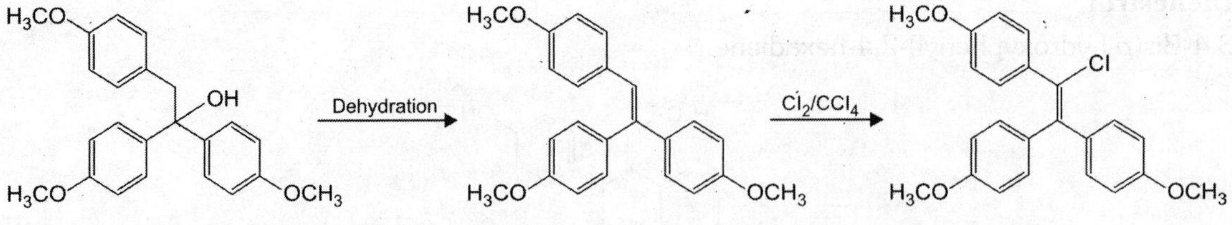

It is more active orally than when given parenterally. It has a longer duration of action because of higher lipid solubility.

ESTROGENS : ESTROGEN ANTAGONISTS

Clomiphene

2-[4-(2-Chloro-1,2-diphenylethenyl)phenoxy]-*N*, *N*-diethylethanamine.

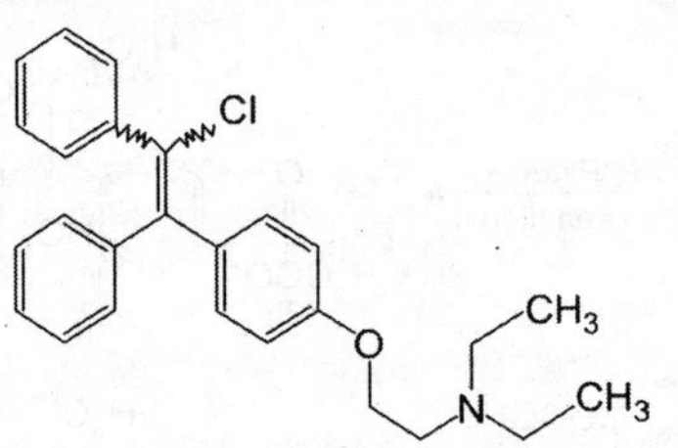

Synthesis

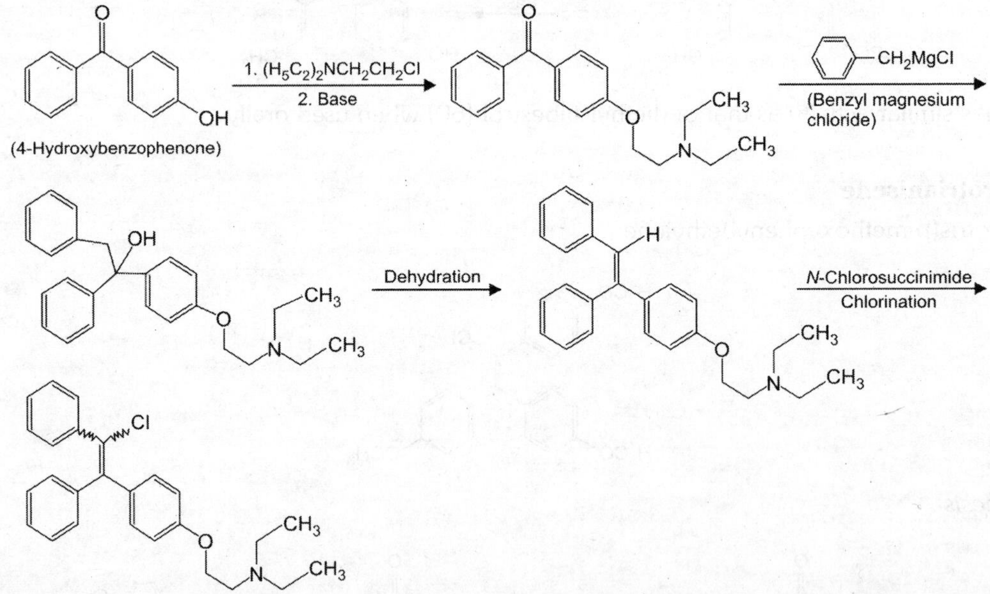

(4-Hydroxybenzophenone)

Clomiphene is administered as a mixture of *cis*-isomer (*Z*-isomer or Zuclomiphene, 64a) and *trans*-isomer (*E*-isomer or enclomiphene, 64b). It acts as an agonist-antagonist at estrogen receptor. It is used to induce ovulation for the treatment of infertility. While *cis*-isomer (64a) shows estrogenic activity, the *trans*-isomer (64b) shows antiestrogenic activity.

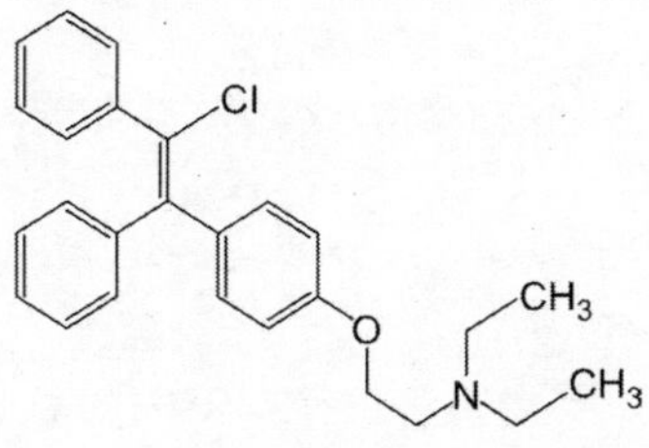

(64a) 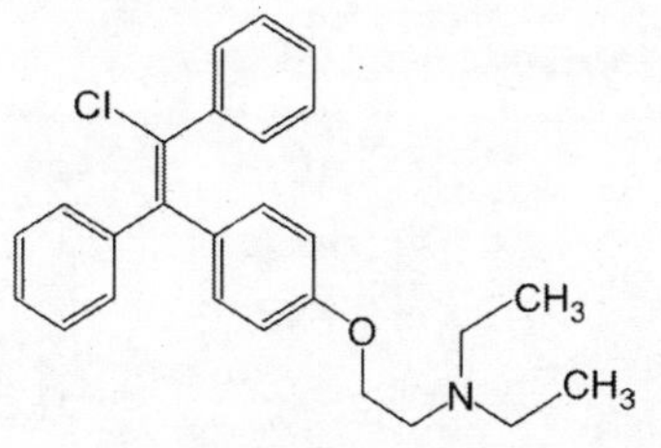   (64b)

Tamoxifen

(*Z*)-2-[4-(1,2-Diphenyl-1-butenyl) phenoxy]-*N, N*-dimethylethanamine.

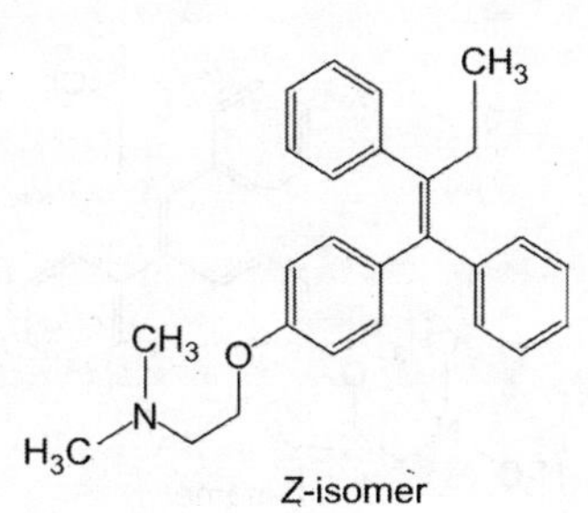

Z-isomer

Synthesis

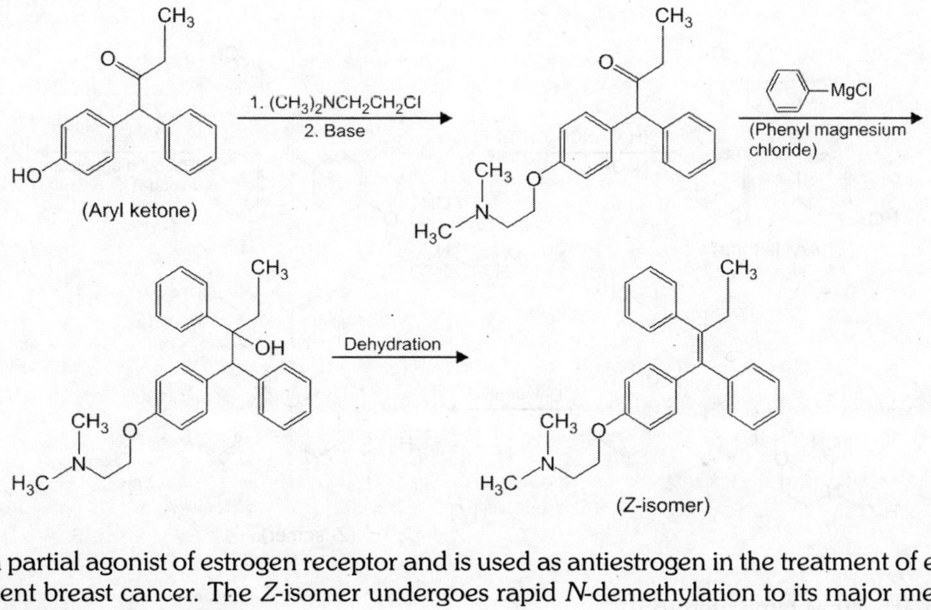

It is a partial agonist of estrogen receptor and is used as antiestrogen in the treatment of estrogen dependent breast cancer. The *Z*-isomer undergoes rapid *N*-demethylation to its major metabolite *N*-demethyltamoxifen (127).

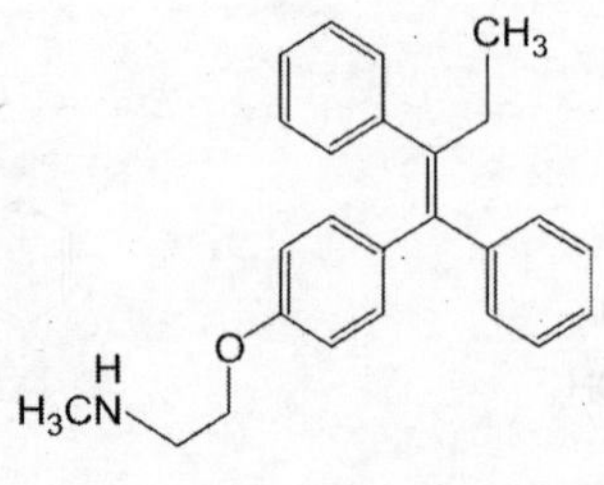

(127)

Toremifene

(Z)-4-Chloro-1,2-diphenyl-1-[4-[2-(N, N-dimethylamino)ethoxy]phenyl]-1-butene

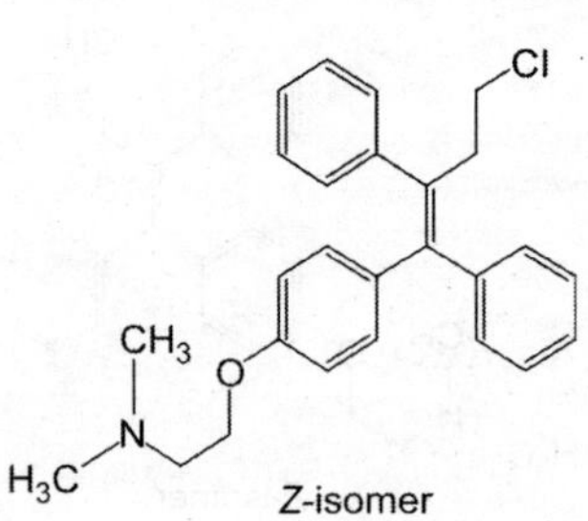

Z-isomer

Synthesis

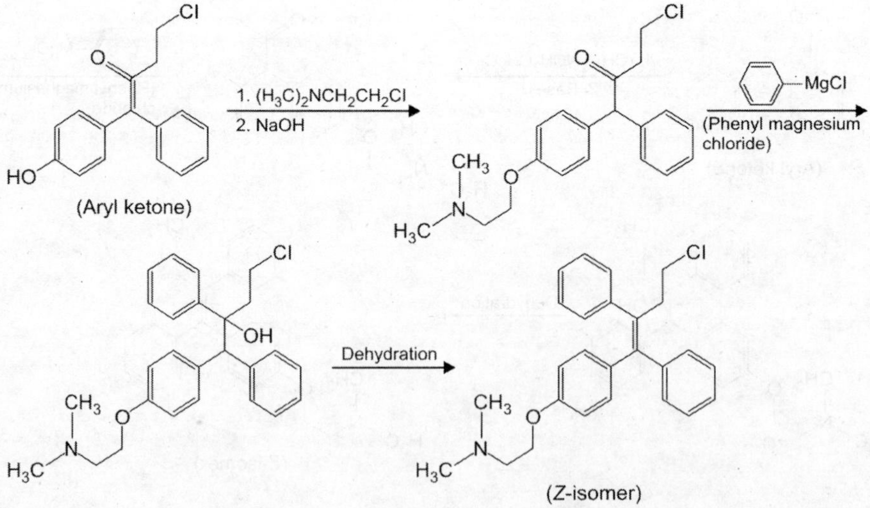

Same activity as tamoxifen (65).

Raloxifene

[6-Hydroxy-2-(4-hydroxyphenyl)benzo[b]thien-3yl][4-[2-(1-piperidinylethoxy]phenyl]methanone

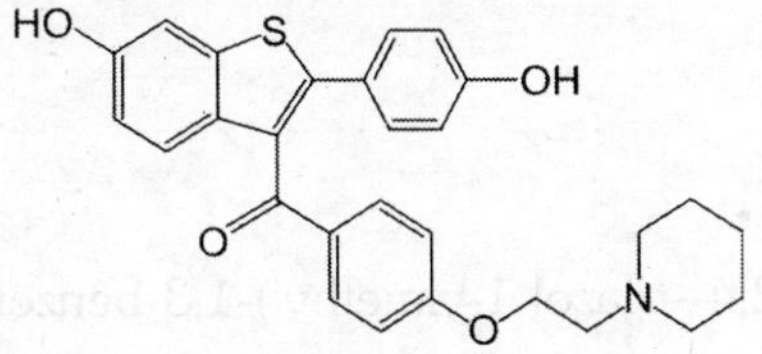

Synthesis

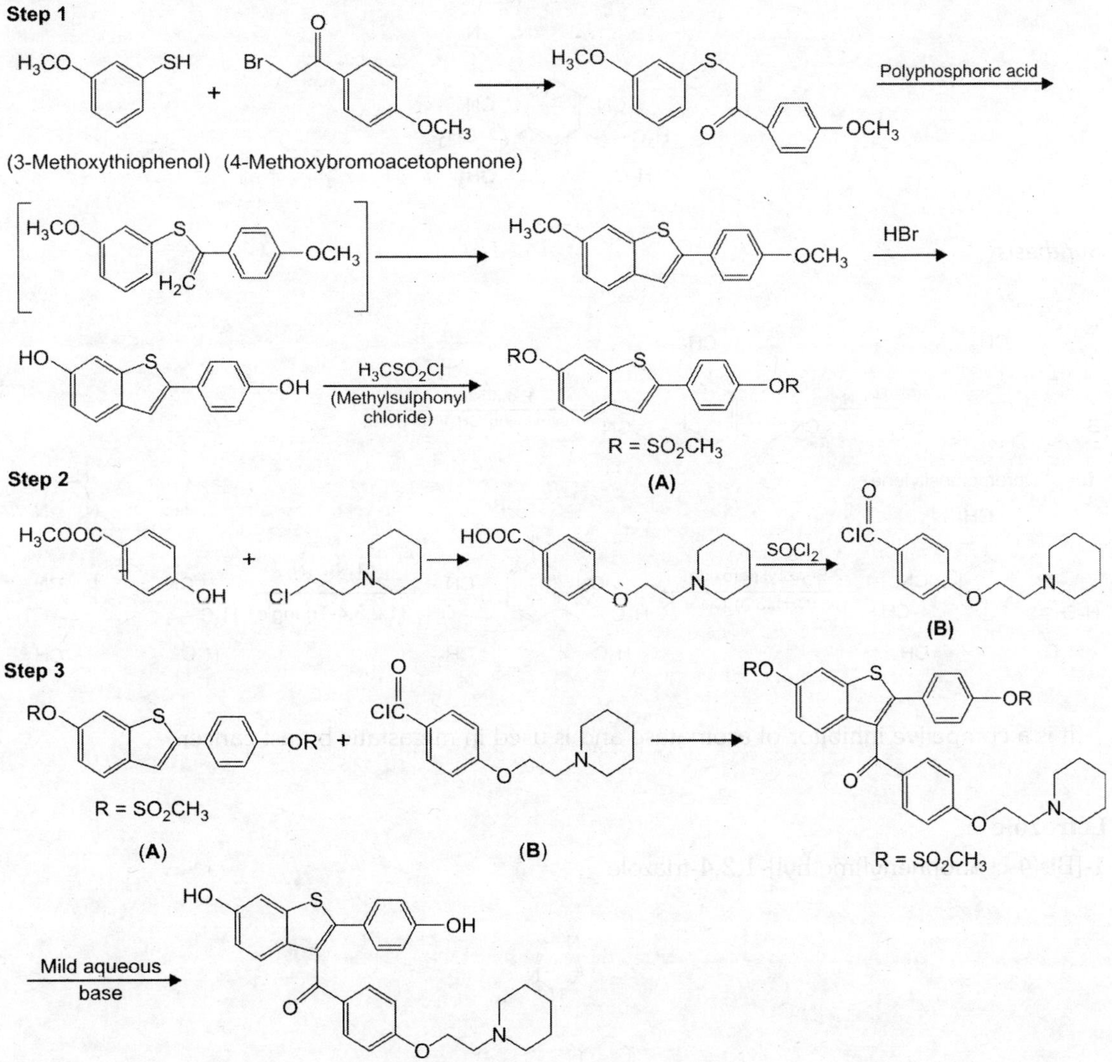

Step 1

(3-Methoxythiophenol)   (4-Methoxybromoacetophenone)

R = SO$_2$CH$_3$

(A)

Step 2

(B)

Step 3

R = SO$_2$CH$_3$

(A)   **(B)**   R = SO$_2$CH$_3$

It is a selective estrogen receptor modulator. It has agonistic activity in bone and antagonistic activity in breast and endometrial tissue. It is used in endometrial hyperplasia and endometrial cancer.

ESTROGENS : AROMATASE INHIBITORS

Testolactone

See ANABOLIC STEROIDS

Anastrozole

α,α,α',α'-Tetramethyl-5-(1H-1,2,4--triazol-1-ylmethyl)-1,3-benzenediacetonitrile

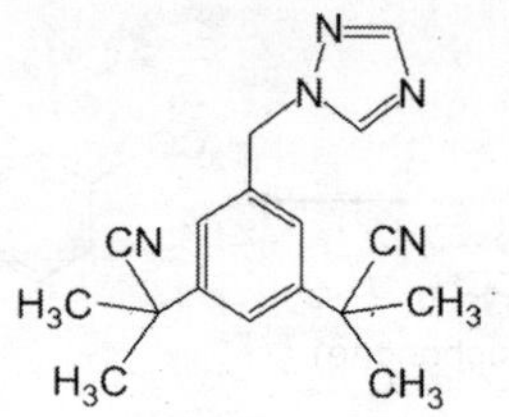

Synthesis

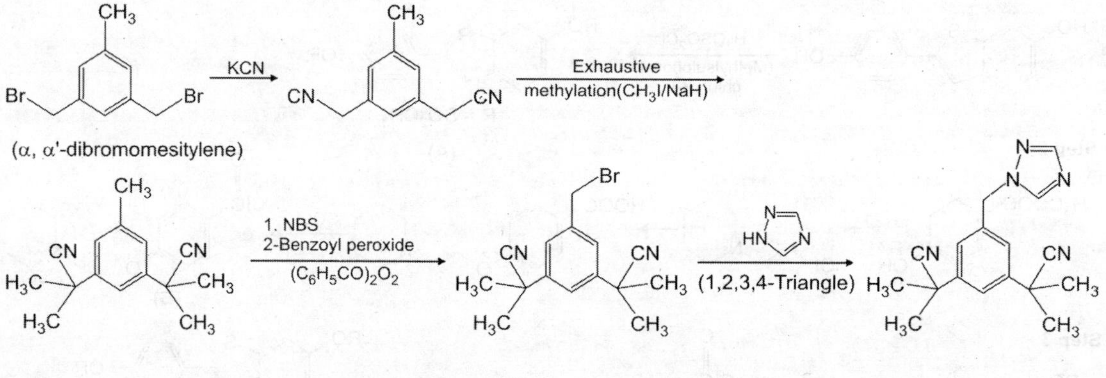

It is a competive inhibitor of aromatase and is used in metastatic breast cancer.

Letrozole

1-[Bis(4-cyanophenyl)methyl]-1,2,4-triazole

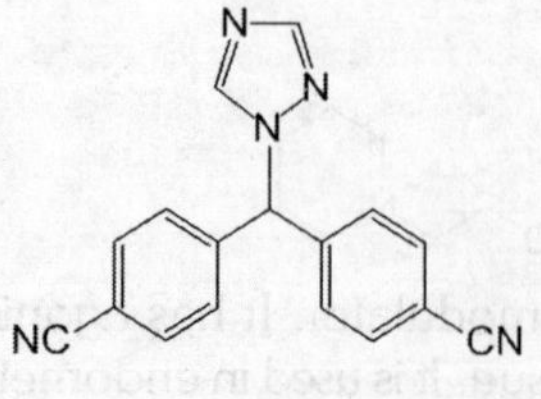

Synthesis

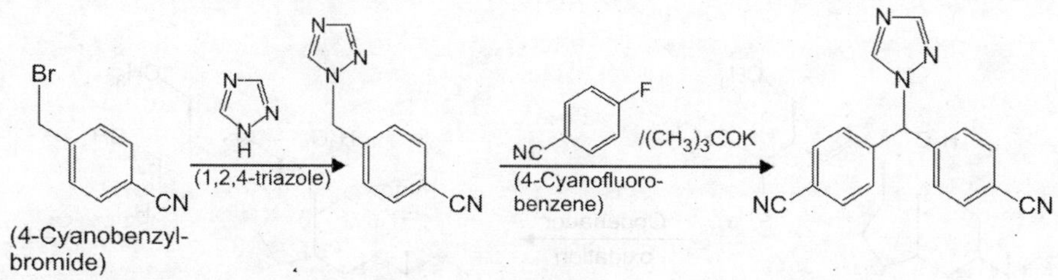

(4-Cyanobenzyl-bromide) → (1,2,4-triazole) → (4-Cyanofluoro-benzene) /(CH₃)₃COK

Same mechanism and activity as anastrozole (72).

PROGESTERONE AND PROGESTINS
Progesterone

Pregn-4-ene-3,20-dione

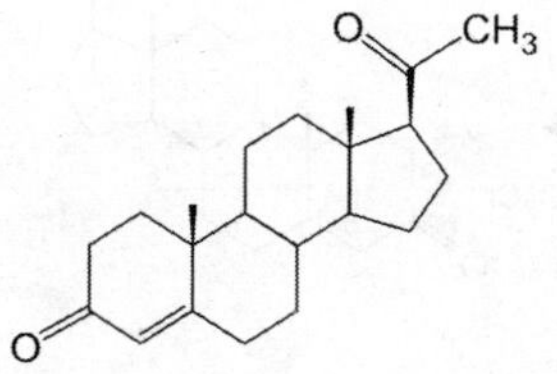

Synthesis
From Diosgenin

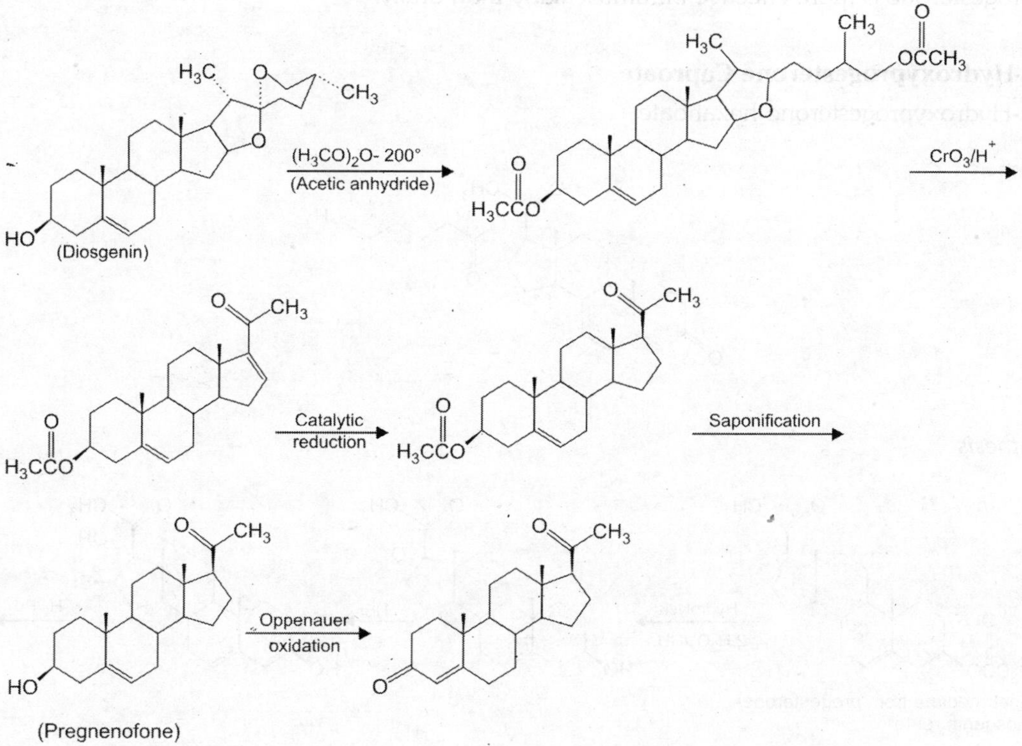

(Diosgenin) → (H₃CO)₂O- 200° (Acetic anhydride) → CrO₃/H⁺

→ Catalytic reduction → Saponification →

(Pregnenofone) → Oppenauer oxidation →

From Stigmasterol

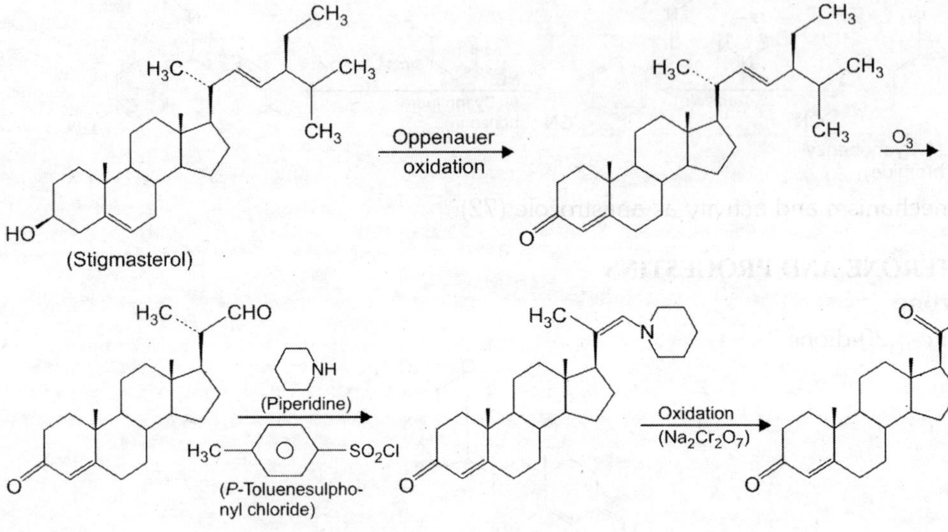

(Stigmasterol)

(Piperidine)

(P-Toluenesulpho-
nyl chloride)

Progesterone is more effective intramuscularly than orally.

17α-Hydroxyprogesterone Caproate

17α-Hydroxyprogesterone hexanoate

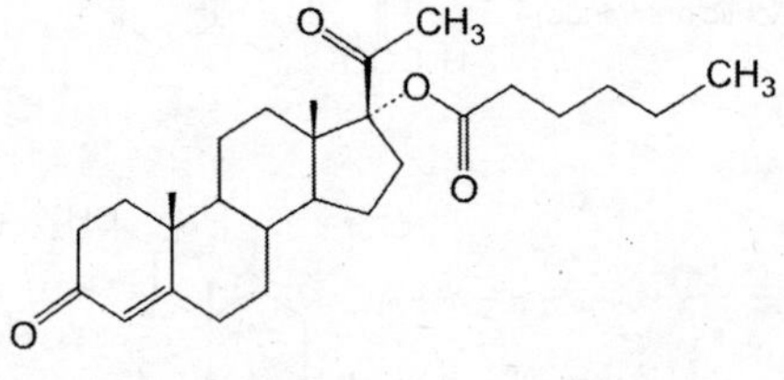

Synthesis

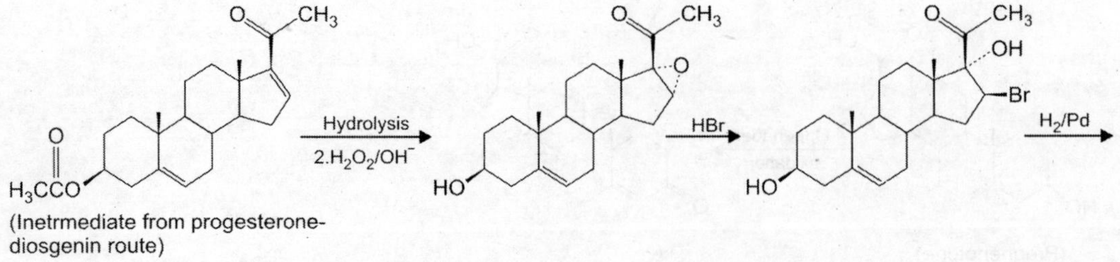

(Inetrmediate from progesterone-
diosgenin route)

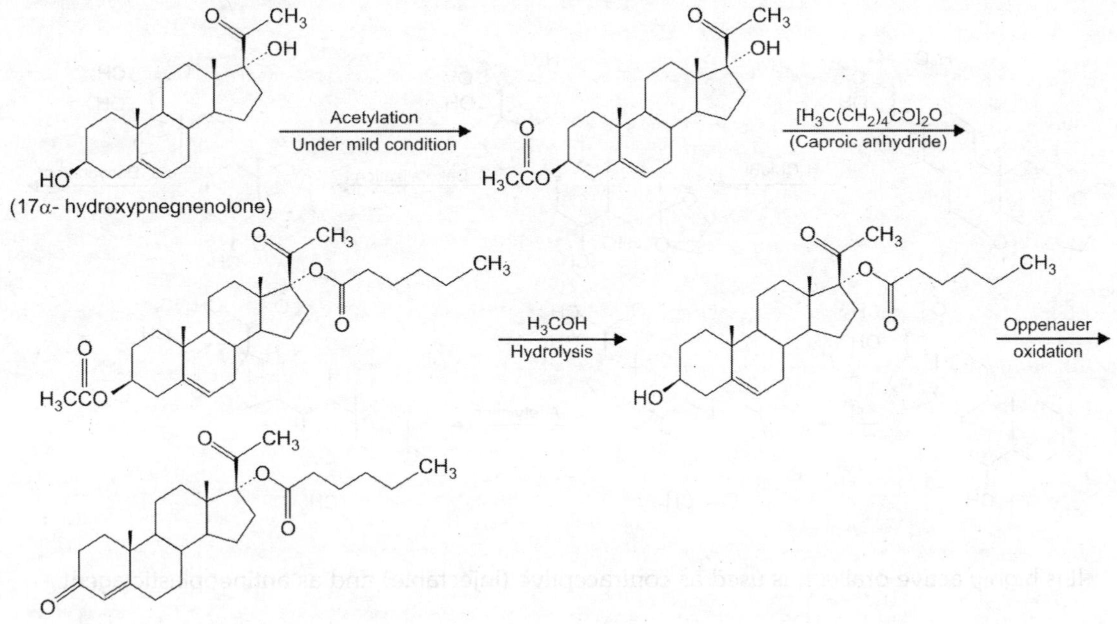

(17α- hydroxypnegnenolone)

It is administered intramuscularly as a depot preparation.

Medroxyprogesterone Acetate

17α-Acetoxy-6α-methylprogesterone

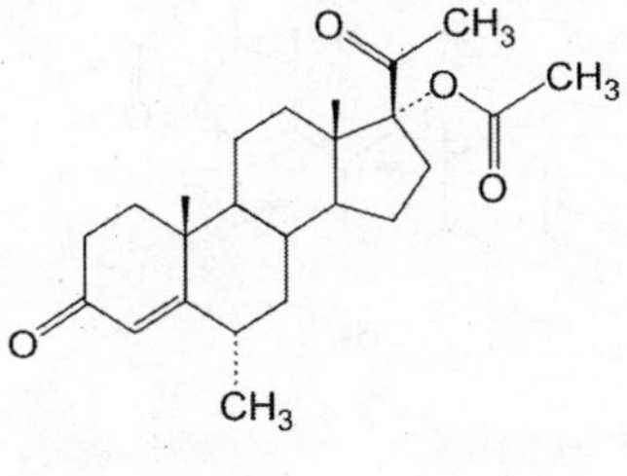

Synthesis

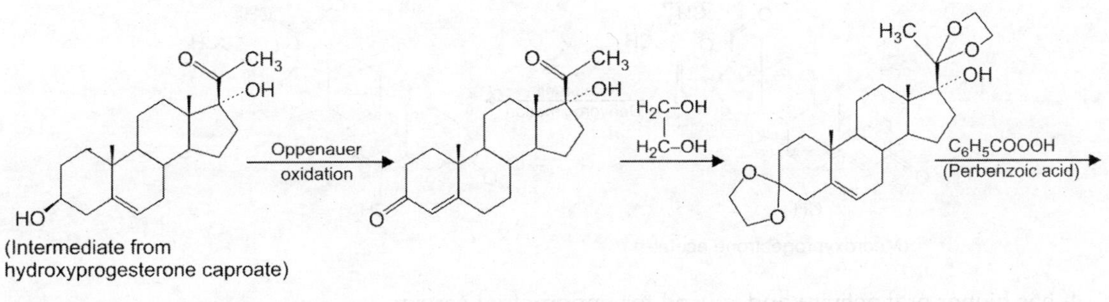

(Intermediate from
hydroxyprogesterone caproate)

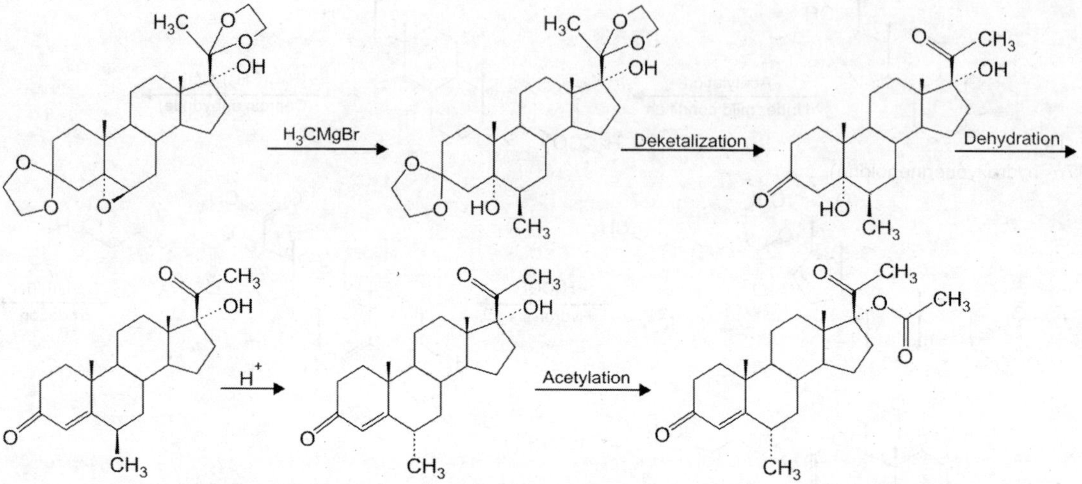

It is highly active orally. It is used as contraceptive (injectable) and as antineoplastic agent.

Megestrol Acetate

17α-Acetoxy-6-methylpregna-4,6-diene-3,20-dione

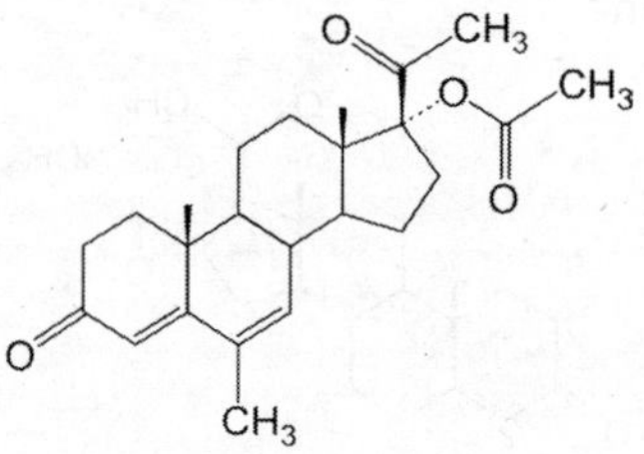

Synthesis

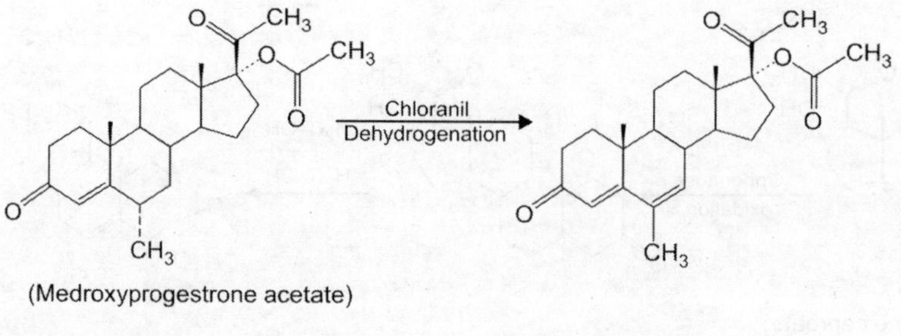

(Medroxyprogesterone acetate)

It has higher oral activity and is used for endometrial cancer.

PROGESTINS : TESTOSTERONE AND 19-NORTESTOSTERONE DERIVATIVES

Ethisterone

17α-Ethynyltestosterone

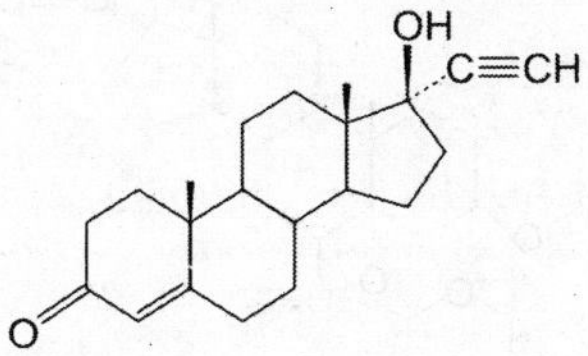

Synthesis

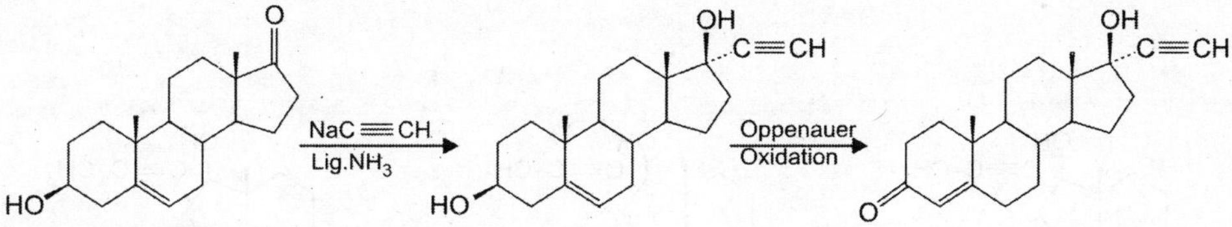

(Dehydroepiandrosterone)

It is an orally effective progestin.

Dimethisterone

6α-Methyl-17α(1-propynyl)testosterone

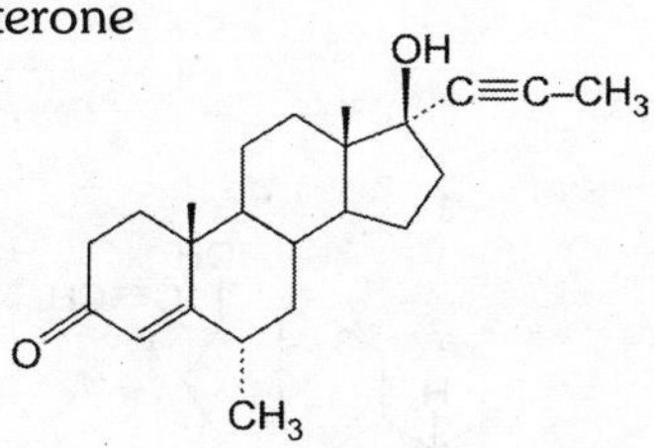

Synthesis

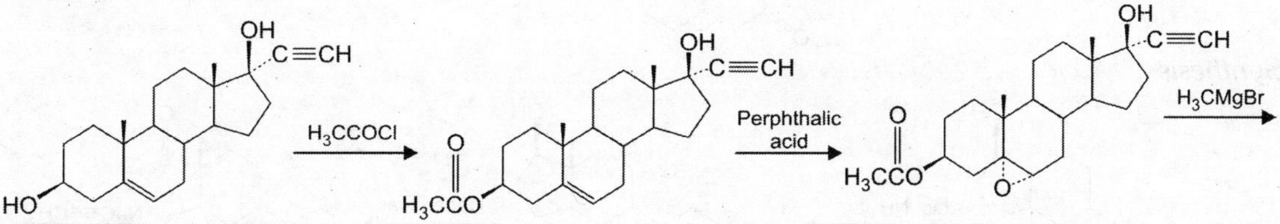

(Intermediate from ethisterone)

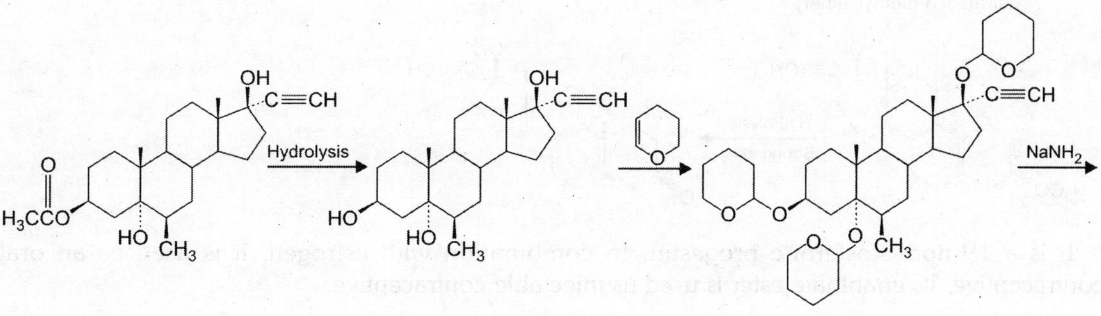

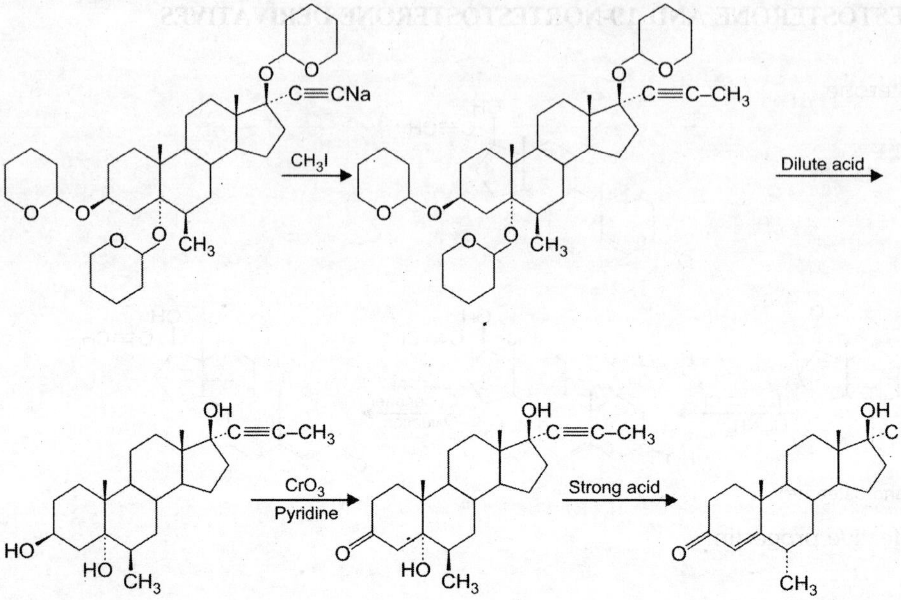

It is a progestin.

Norethindrone

19-Nor-17α-ethynyltestosterone

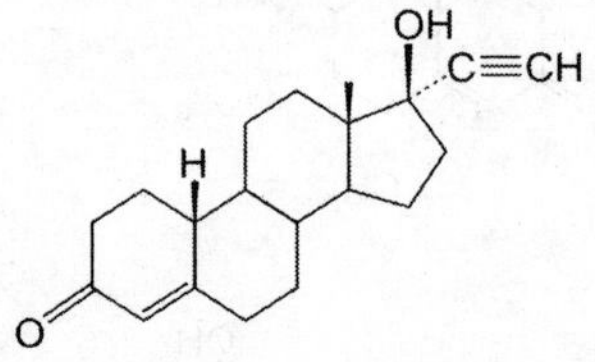

Synthesis

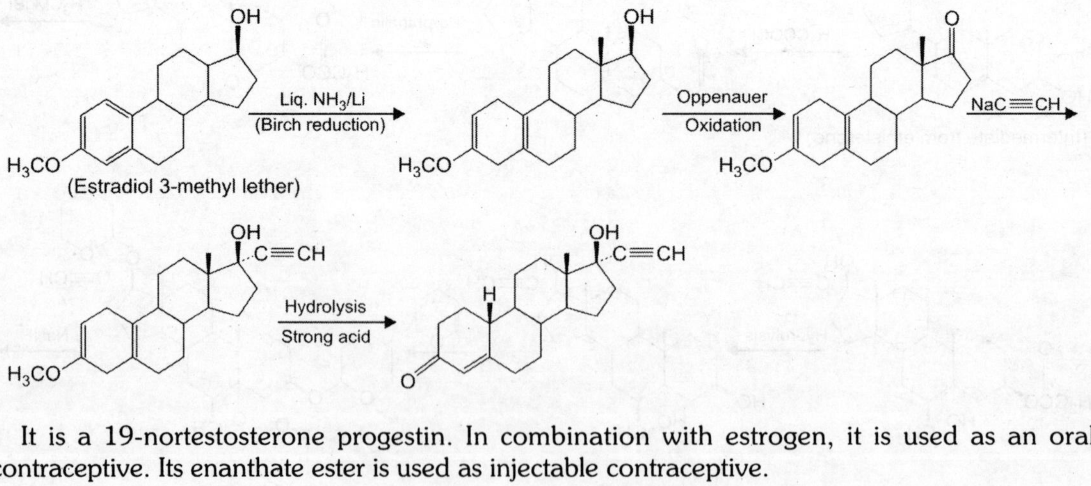

It is a 19-nortestosterone progestin. In combination with estrogen, it is used as an oral contraceptive. Its enanthate ester is used as injectable contraceptive.

Ethynodiol Diacetate

17α-Ethynyl-19-norandrost-4-ene-3β,17β-diol diacetate

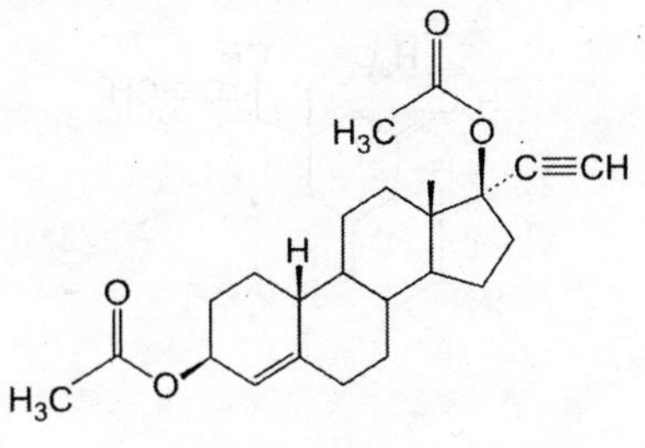

Synthesis

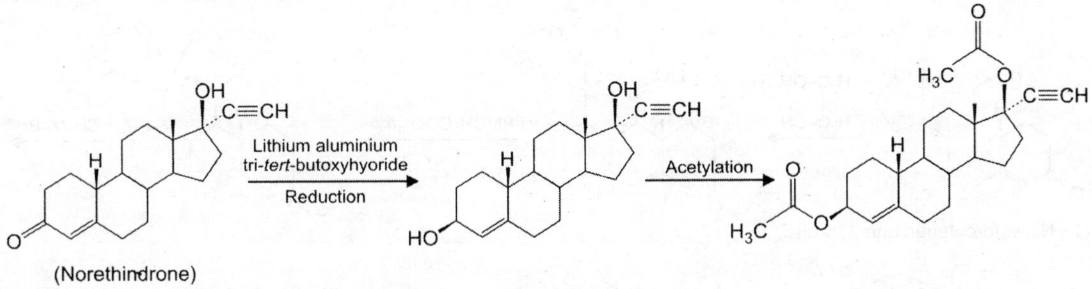

(Norethindrone)

It is a 19-norprogestin and is used as oral contraceptive in combination with estrogens.

Norethynodrel

17α-Ethynyl-17-hydroxy-5(10)-estren-3-one.

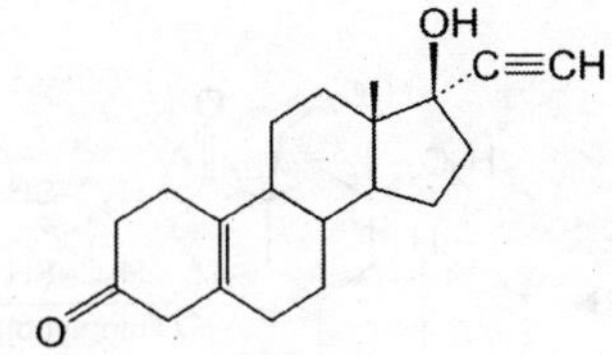

Synthesis

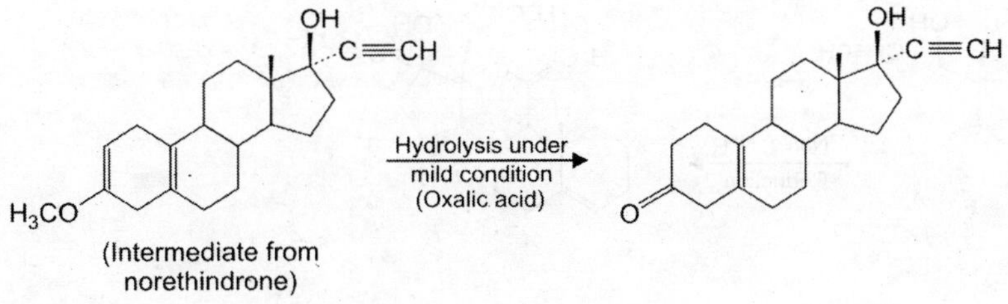

(Intermediate from norethindrone)

Same use as ethynodiol diacetate (81).

Desogestrel

17α-Ethynyl-18-methyl-11-methylene-estr-4-en-17β-ol

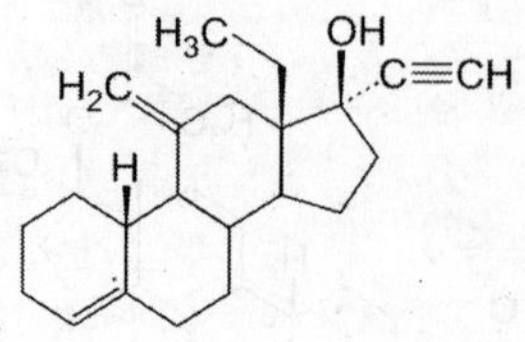

Synthesis

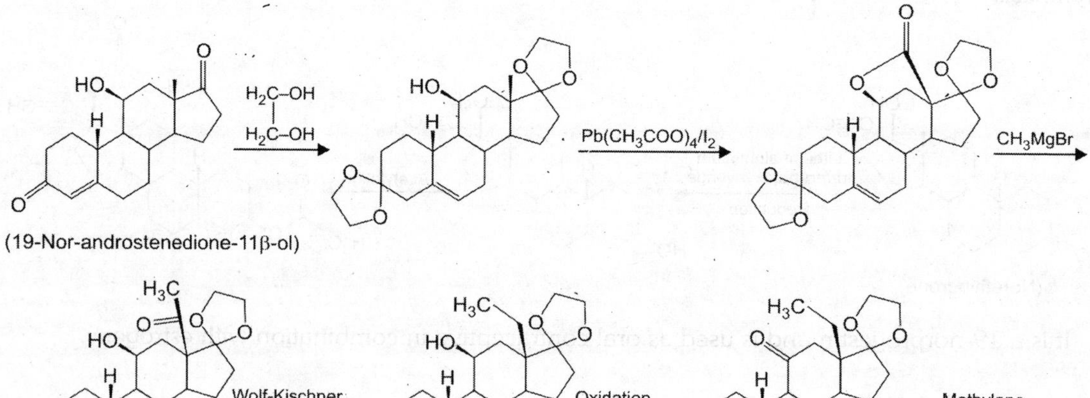

It is orally active progestin and is used in combination with estrogens as an oral contraceptive.

Etonogestrel

17α-Ethynyl-18-methyl-11-methylenestr-4-en-3-one-17β-ol

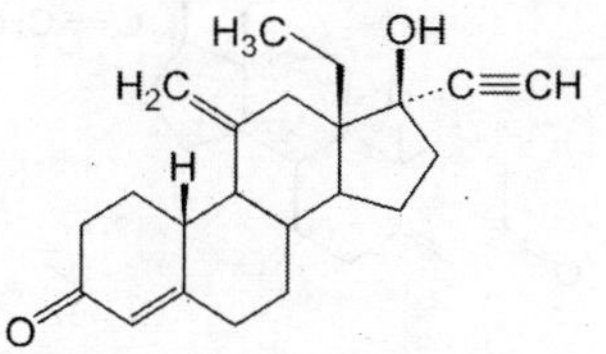

Synthesis

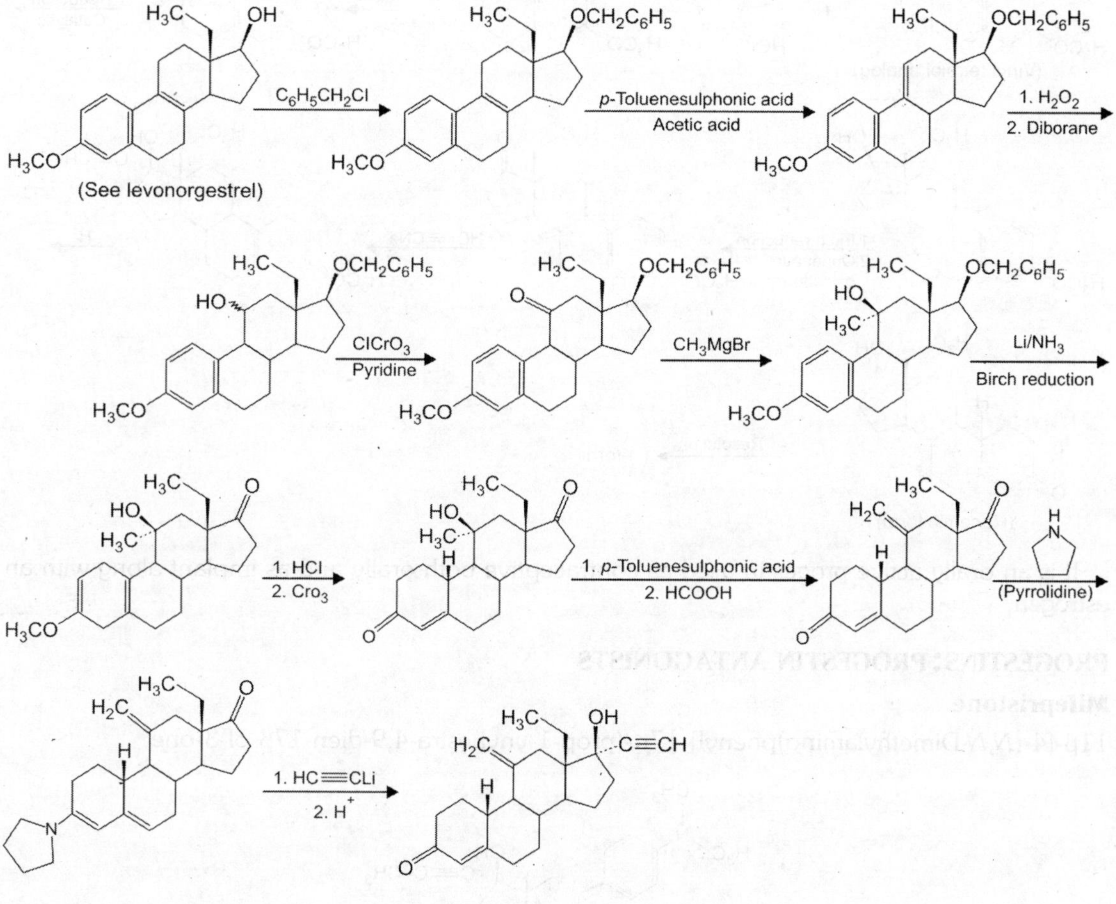

It is used as progestin in implantable contraceptives.

Levonorgestrel

(–)-17α-Ethynyl-18-methyl-19-nortestosterone.

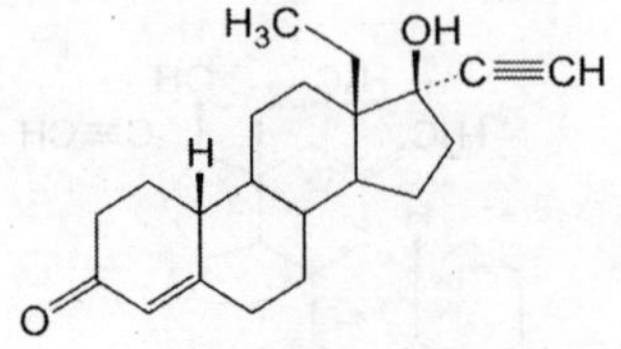

Synthesis

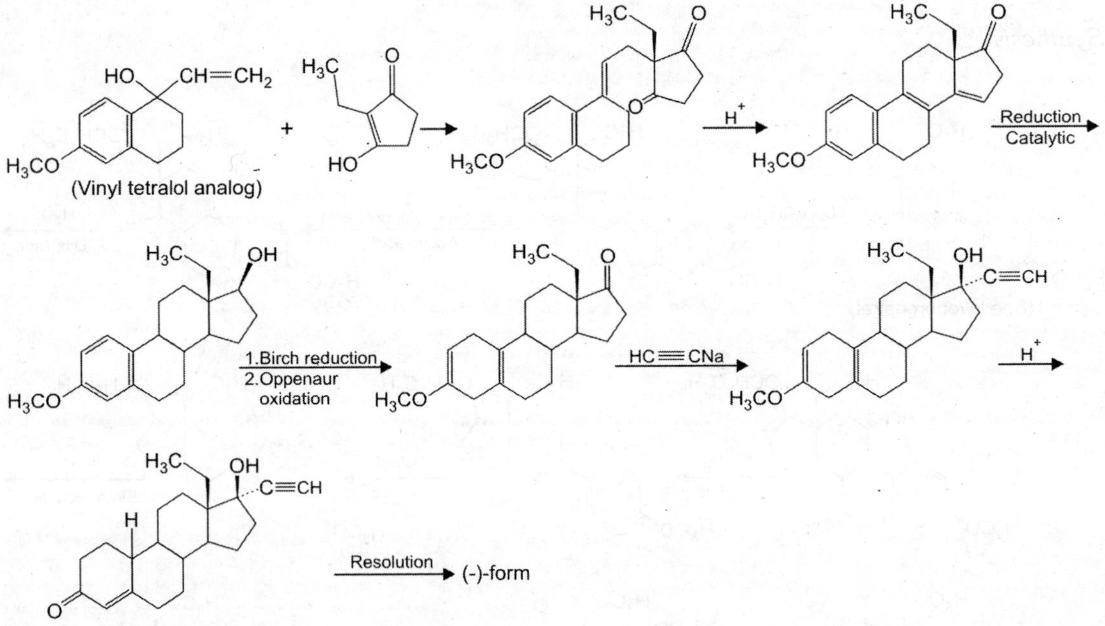

It is an orally active progestin used as contraceptive both orally and as implant along with an estrogen.

PROGESTINS : PROGESTIN ANTAGONISTS

Mifepristone

11β-[4-(N,N-Dimethylamino)phenyl]-17α-(prop-1-ynyl)estra-4,9-dien-17β-ol-3-one

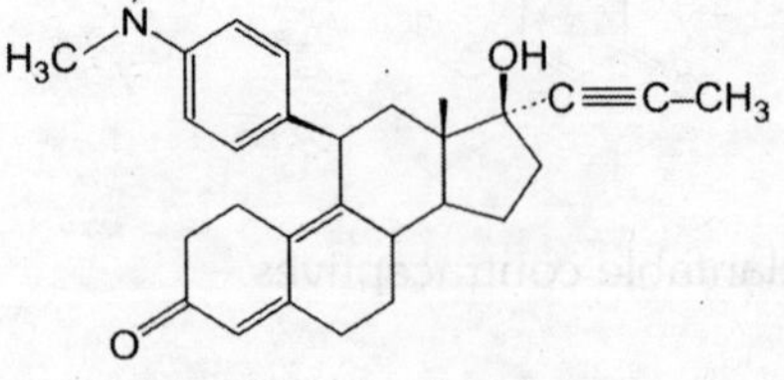

Synthesis

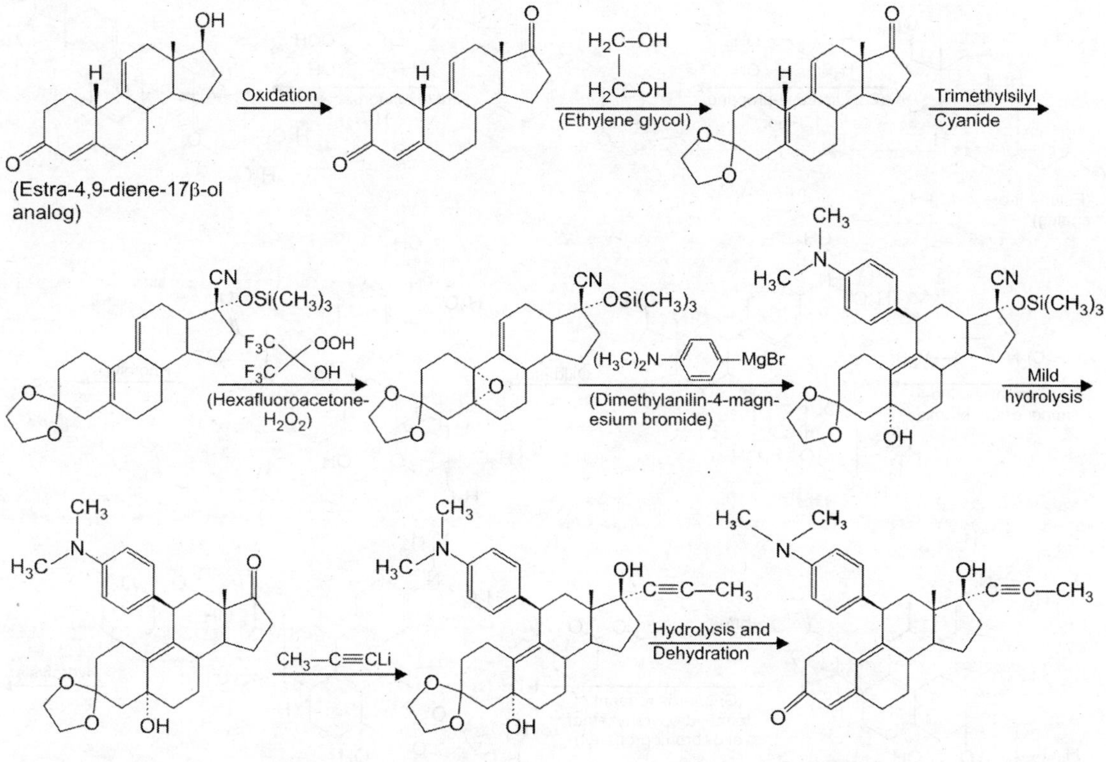

(Estra-4,9-diene-17β-ol analog)

Mifepristone is an orally effective abortifacient in humans. It has minor antagonistic action at corticoid receptor.

Onapristone

11β-(4-Dimethylaminophenyl)-17α-hydroxy-17β-(3-hydroxypropyl)-13α-methyl-4,9-gonadien-3-one

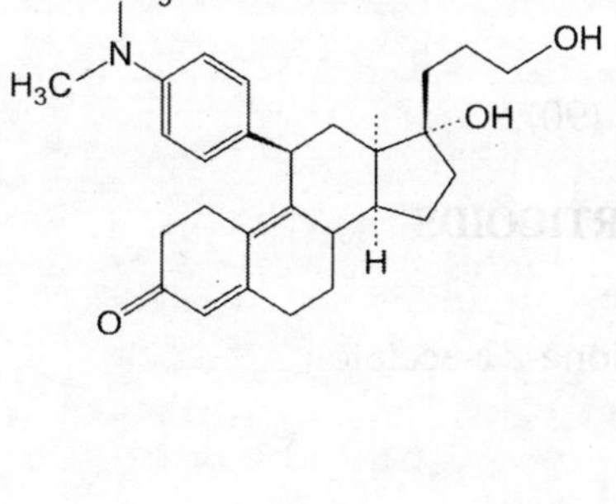

Synthesis

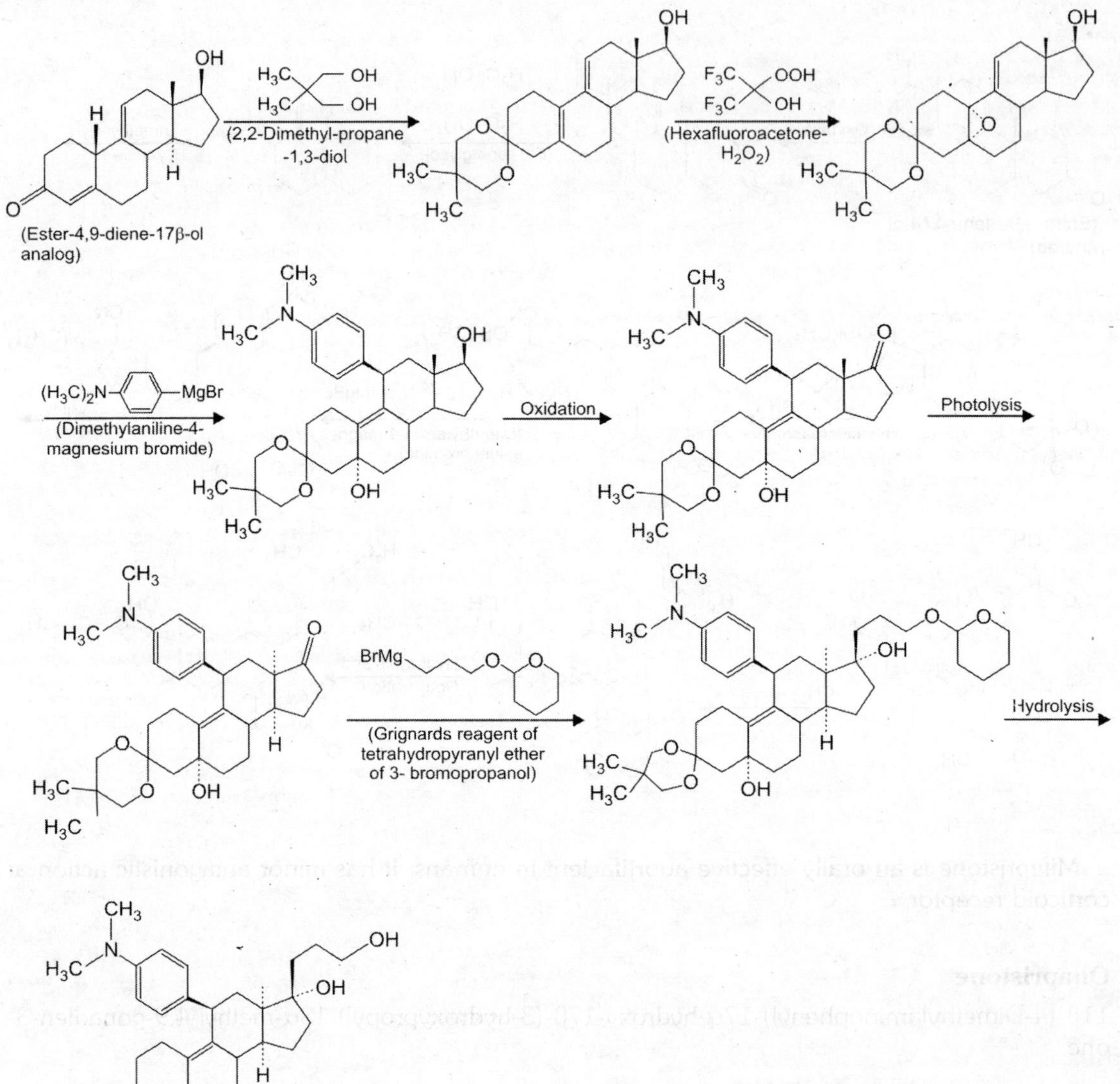

(Ester-4,9-diene-17β-ol analog)

Same activity as mifepristone (90).

CORTICOIDS : MINERALOCORTICOIDS

Desoxycorticosterone Acetate

21-Hydroxypregn-4-ene-3,20 dione-21-acetate

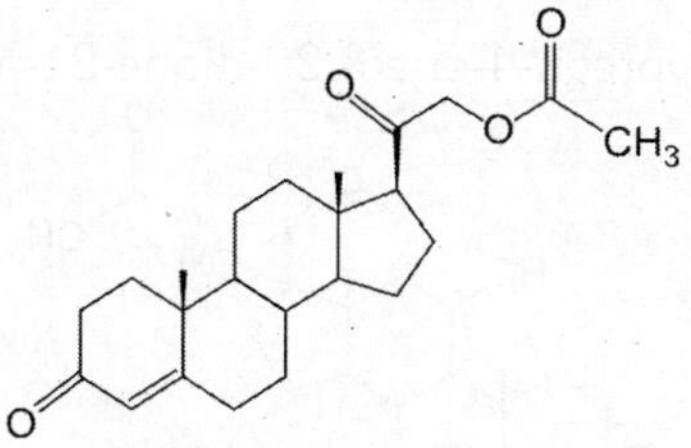

Synthesis

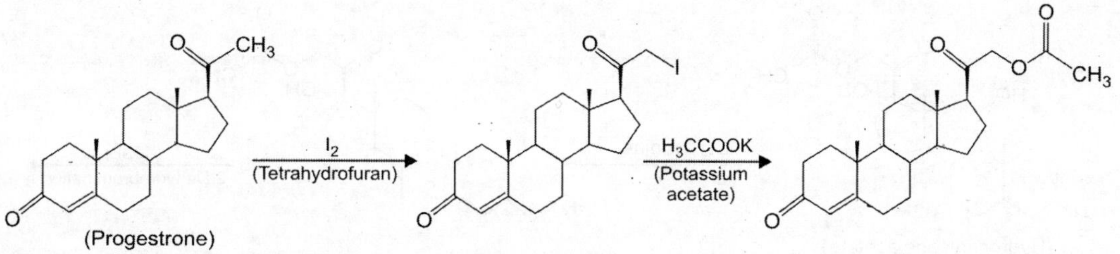

It is a mineralocorticoid used in Addison's diseases.

Desoxycorticosterone Pivalate

21-Hydroxypregn-4-ene-3,20-dione-21-pivalate.

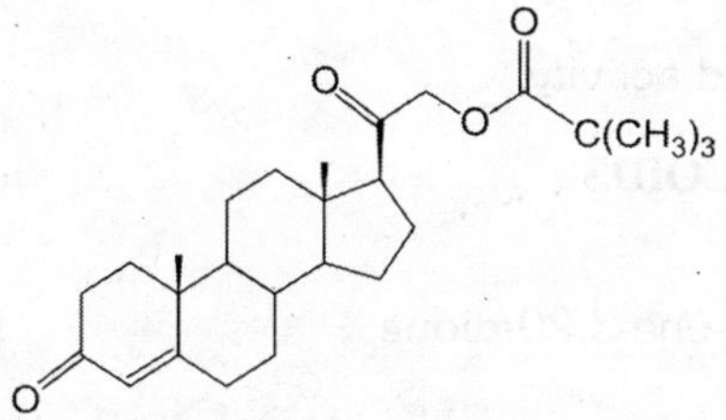

Synthesis

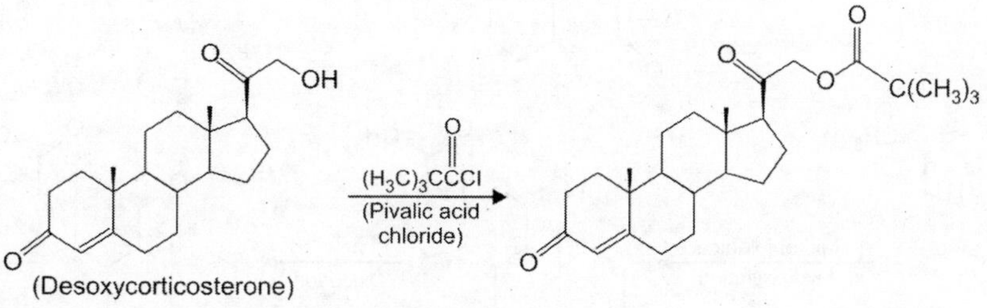

Same use as desoxycorticosterone acetate (95a).

Fludrocortisone Acetate

9α,-Fluoro-11β,17α,21-trihydroxypregn-4-ene-3,20-dione-21-acetate

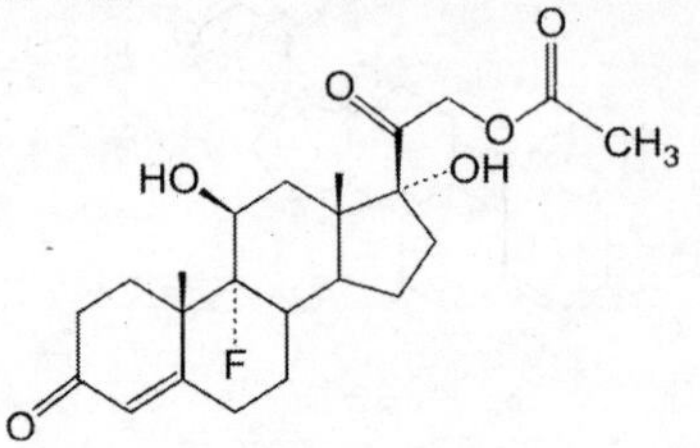

Synthesis

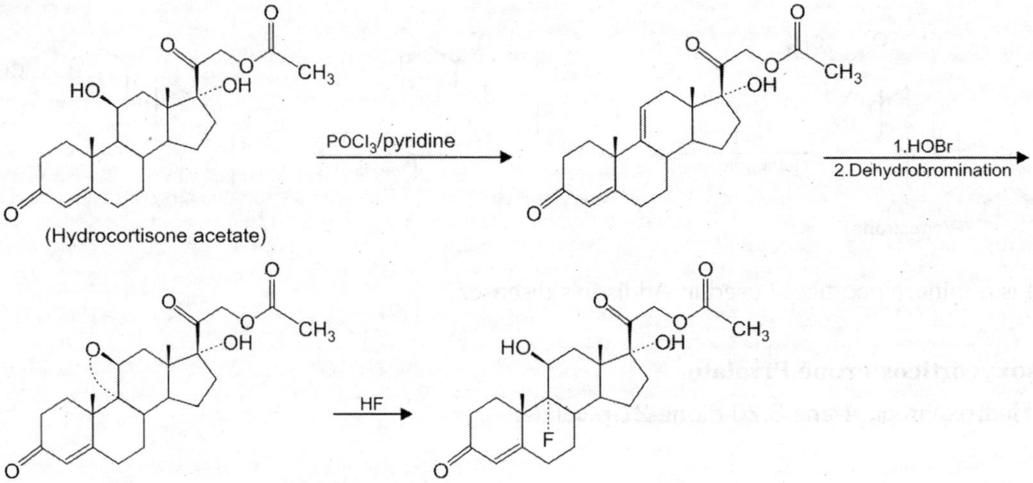

It has a high mineralocorticoid activity.

CORTICOIDS : GLUCOCORTICOIDS

Hydrocortisone

11β,17α,21-Trihydroxy-pregn-4-ene-3,20-dione

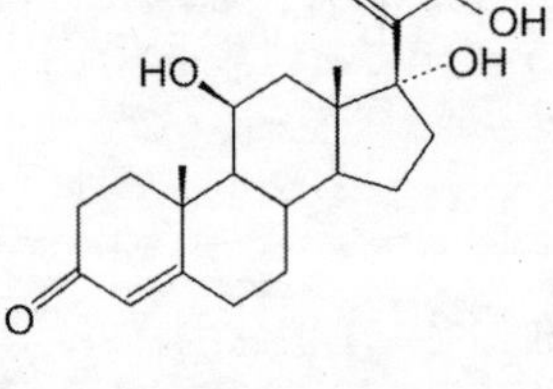

Synthesis

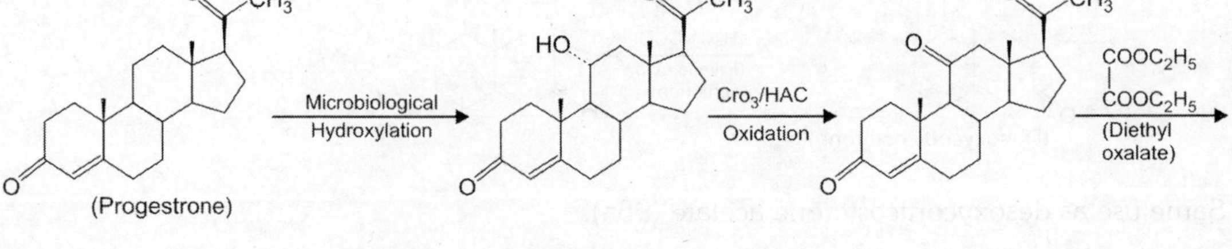

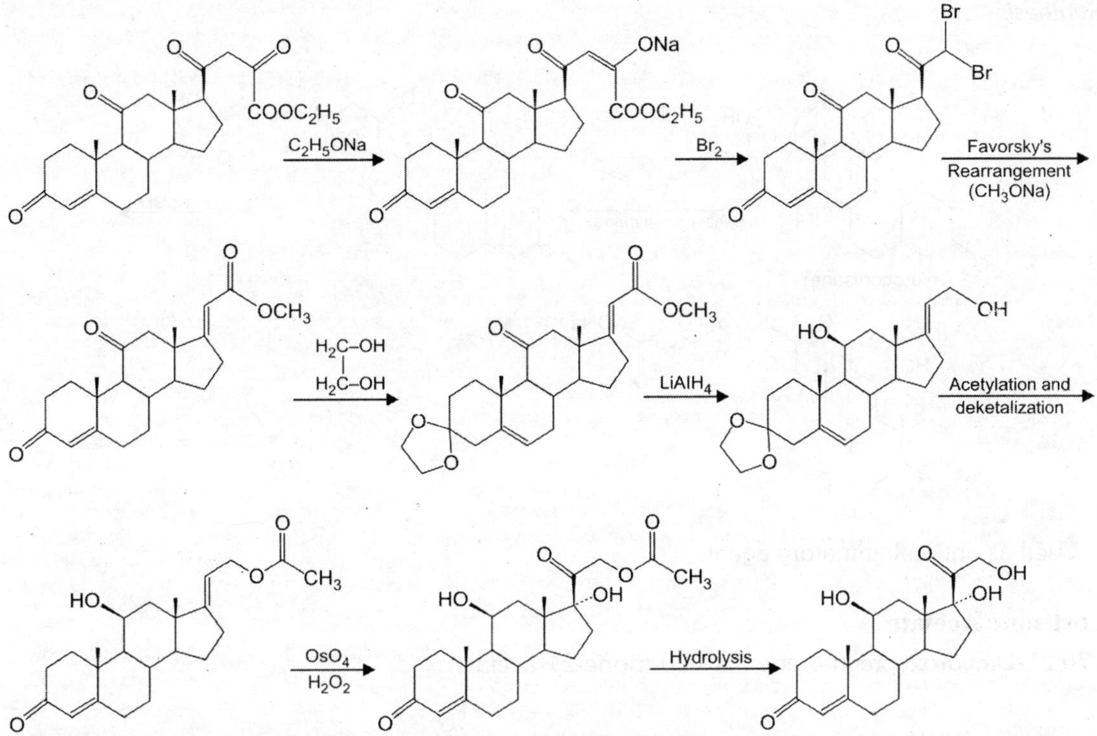

Hydrocortisone and its esters are used as anti-inflammatory agent. It has similar use as cortisone (97).

Hydrocortisone Acetate

11β,17α,21-Trihydroxy-pregn-4-ene-3, 20-dione 21-acetate.

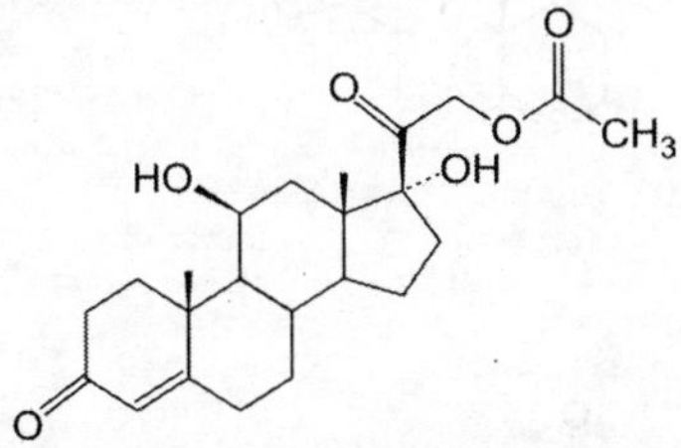

It is obtained by acetylation of hydrocortisone (96). It is used as anti-inflammatory.

Hydrocortisone Sodium Succinate

11β, 17α, 21-Trihydroxy-pregn-4-ene-3, 20-dione-21-hemisuccinate sodium salt

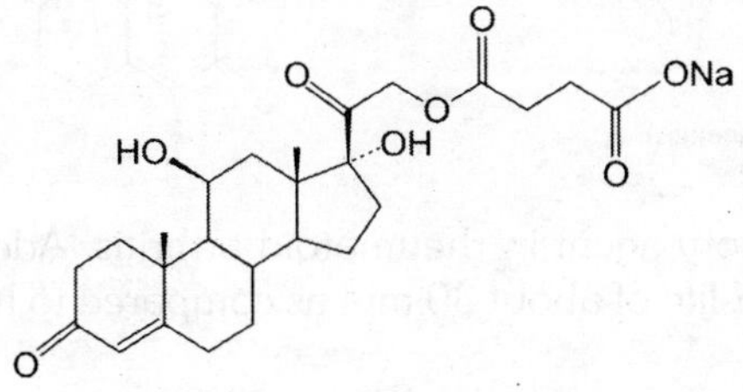

Synthesis

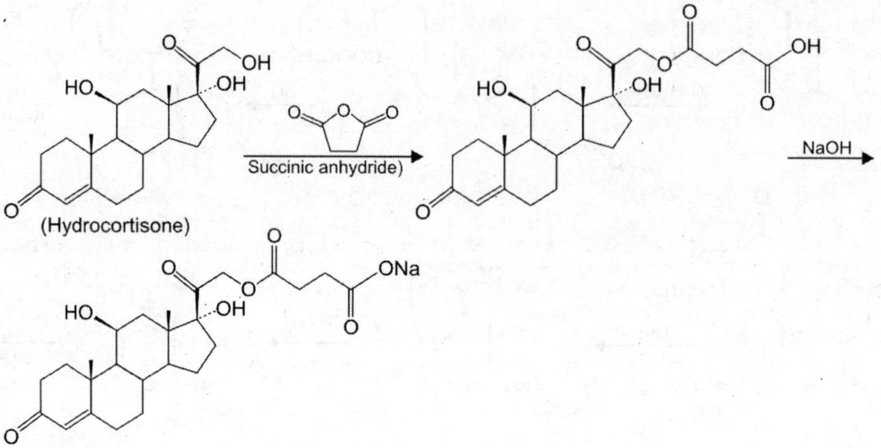

(Hydrocortisone)

Succinic anhydride)

NaOH

Used as anti-inflammatory agent.

Cortisone Acetate

17α,21-Dihydroxypregn-4-ene-3,11,20-trione-21-acetate

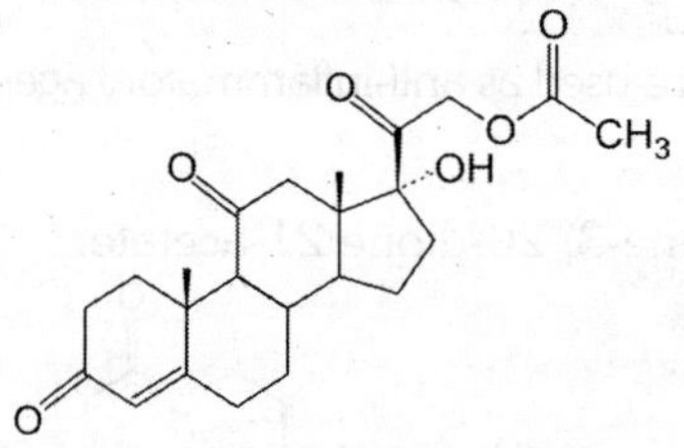

Synthesis

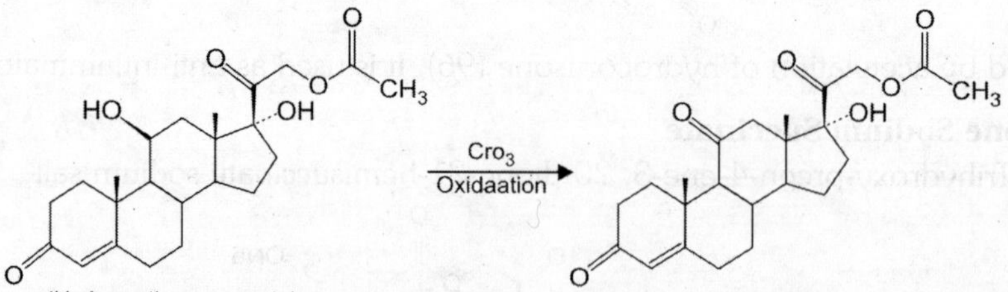

(Hydrocortisone acetate)

Cro₃
Oxidaation

It is used as anti-inflammatory agent in rheumatoid arthritis, Addison's disease and in allergic conditions. It has a shorter half-life of about 30 min as compared to hydrocortisone (96) which has a half-life of 1.5 to 3 hr.

Prednisolone

11β,17α,21-Trihydroxypregna-1,4-diene-3,20-dione

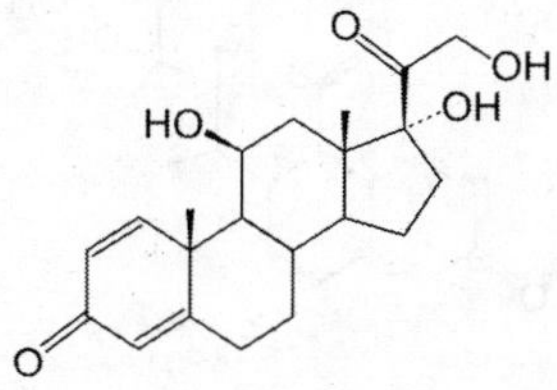

Synthesis

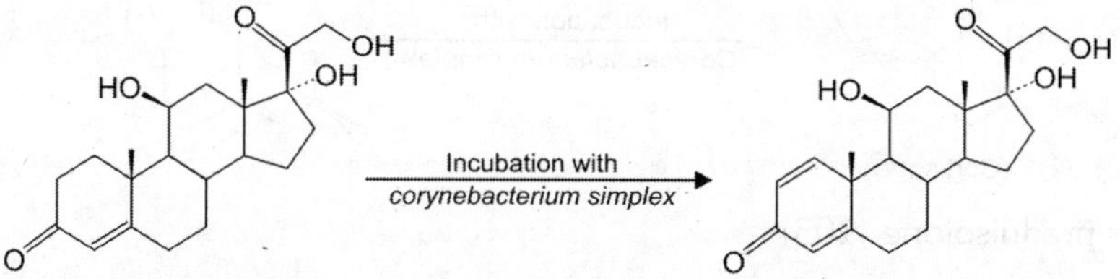

(Hydrocortisone)

It is effective against autoimmune diseases including rheumatoid arthirites, asthama, and lupus erythematosus.

It is used as salt or ester. Some of these include prednisolone sodium succinate (128),prednisolone disodium phosphate (129), prednisolone acetate (130), and prednisolone tebutate (131).

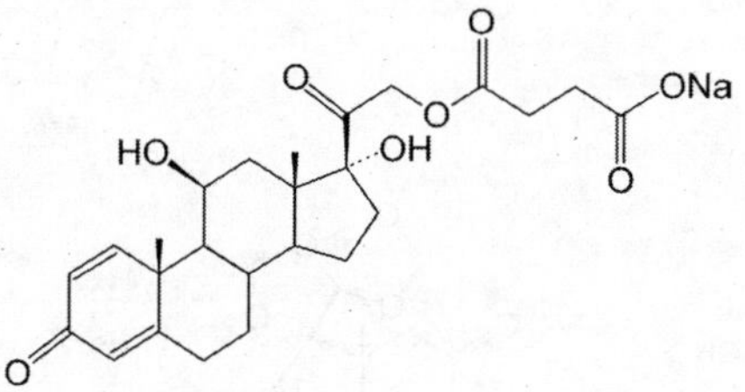

(128)

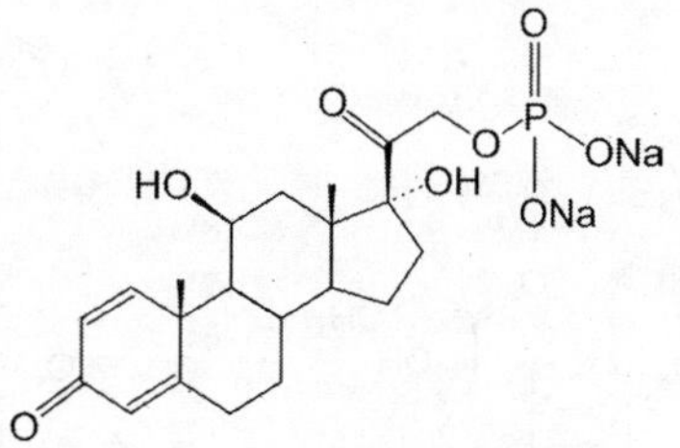

(129)

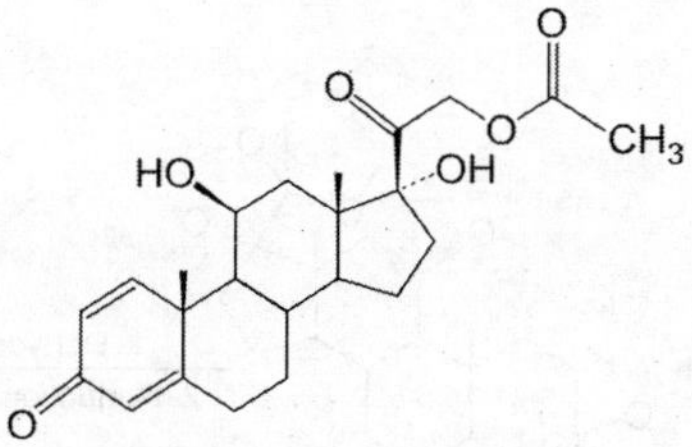

(130)

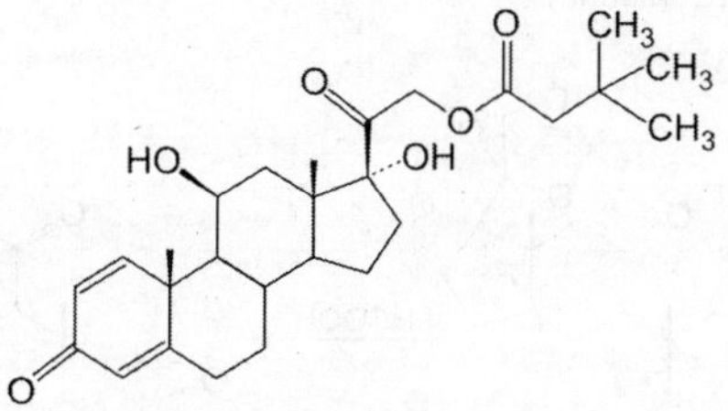

(131)

Prednisone
17α,21-Dihydroxy pregna-1,4-diene-3,11,20-trione

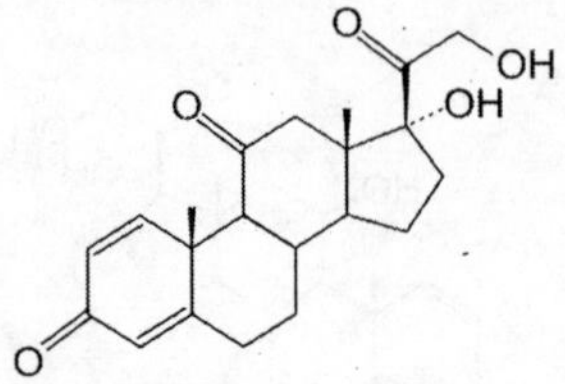

Synthesis

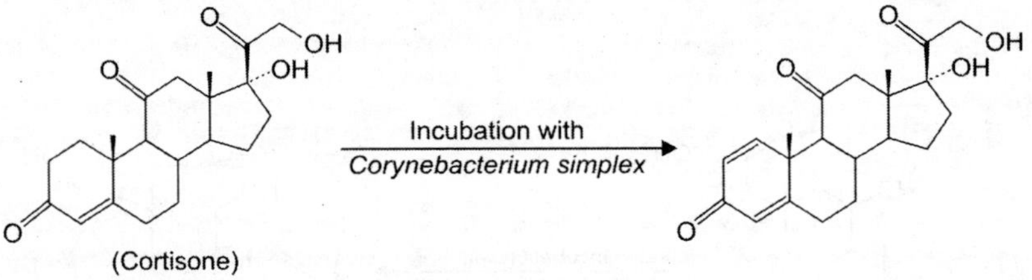

(Cortisone)

Same use as prednisolone (103).

6α-Methylprednisolone
6α-Methyl-11β,17α,21-trihydroxypregna-1,4-diene-3,20-dione

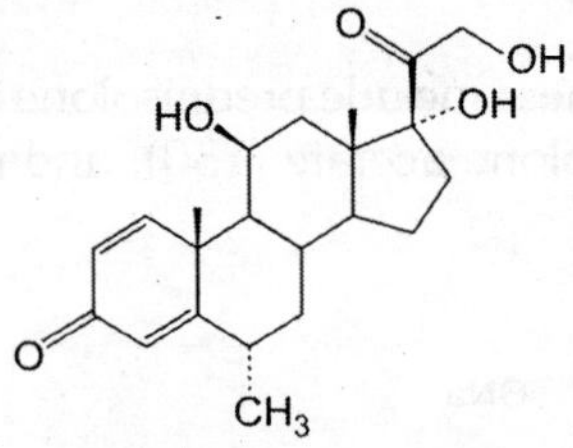

Synthesis

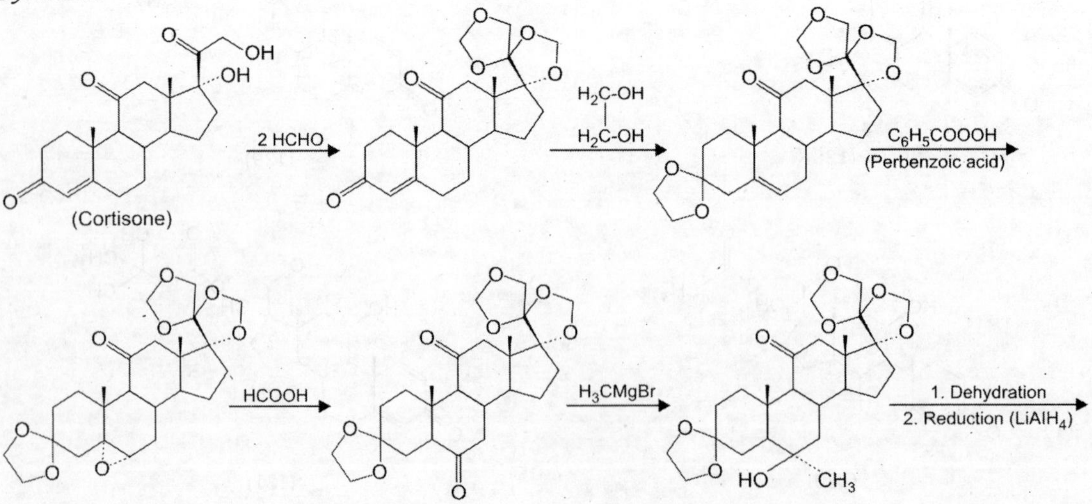

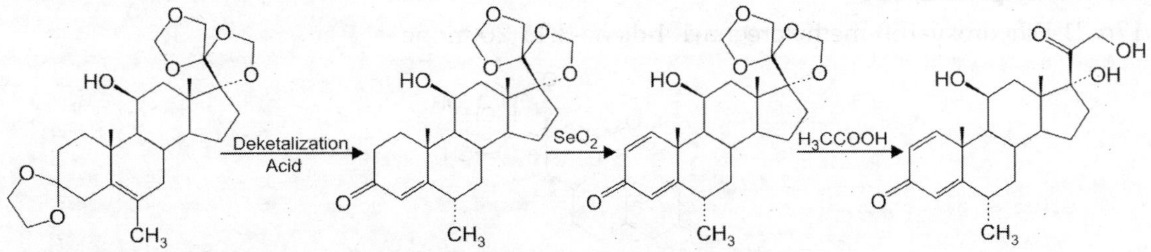

It is used as anti-inflammatory and immunosuppressive agent.

Fluorometholone

21-Deoxy-9α-fluoro-6α-methylprednisolone

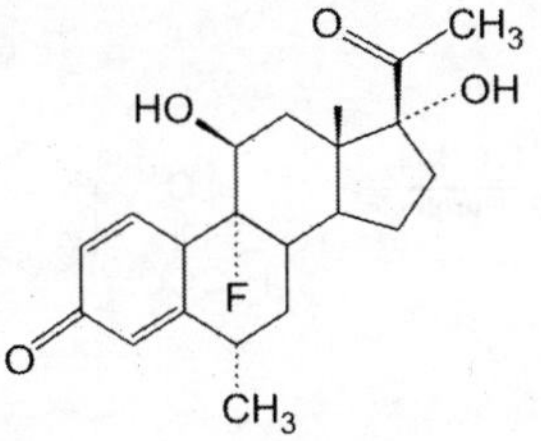

Synthesis

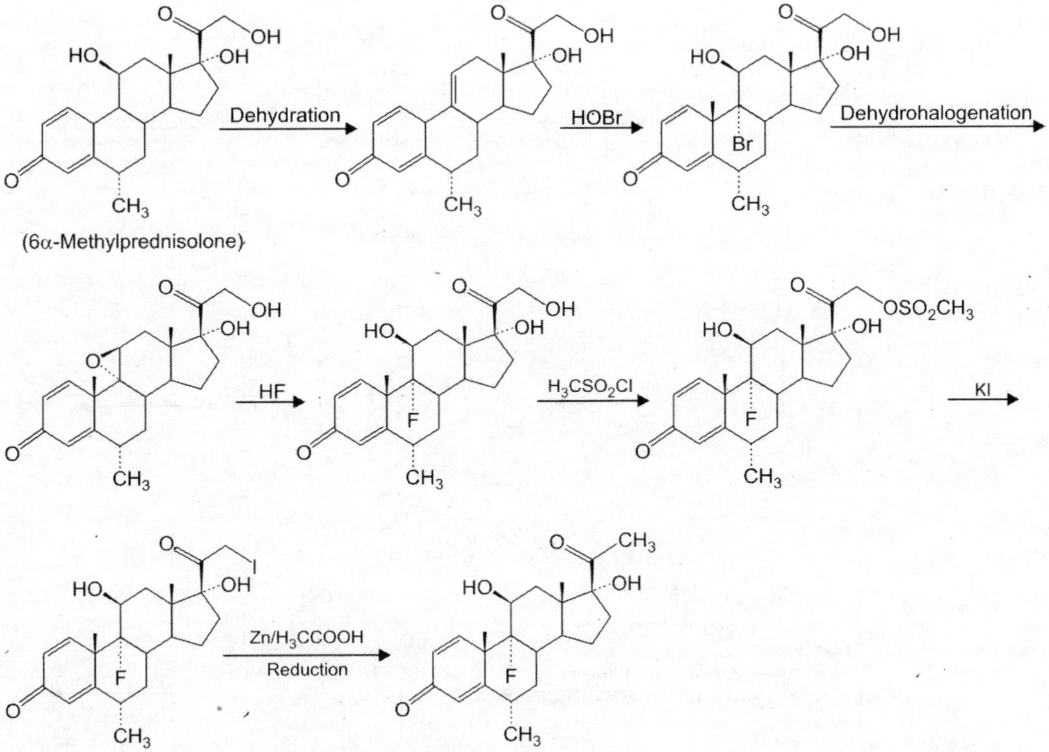

(6α-Methylprednisolone)

Used as ophthalamic suspention.

16β-Methylprednisone
17α,21-Dihydroxy-16β-methylpregna-1,4-diene-3,11,20-trione

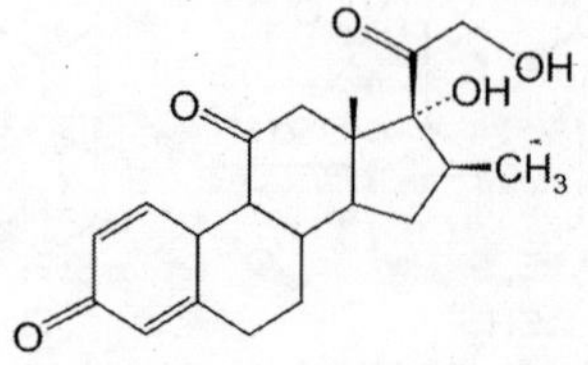

Synthesis

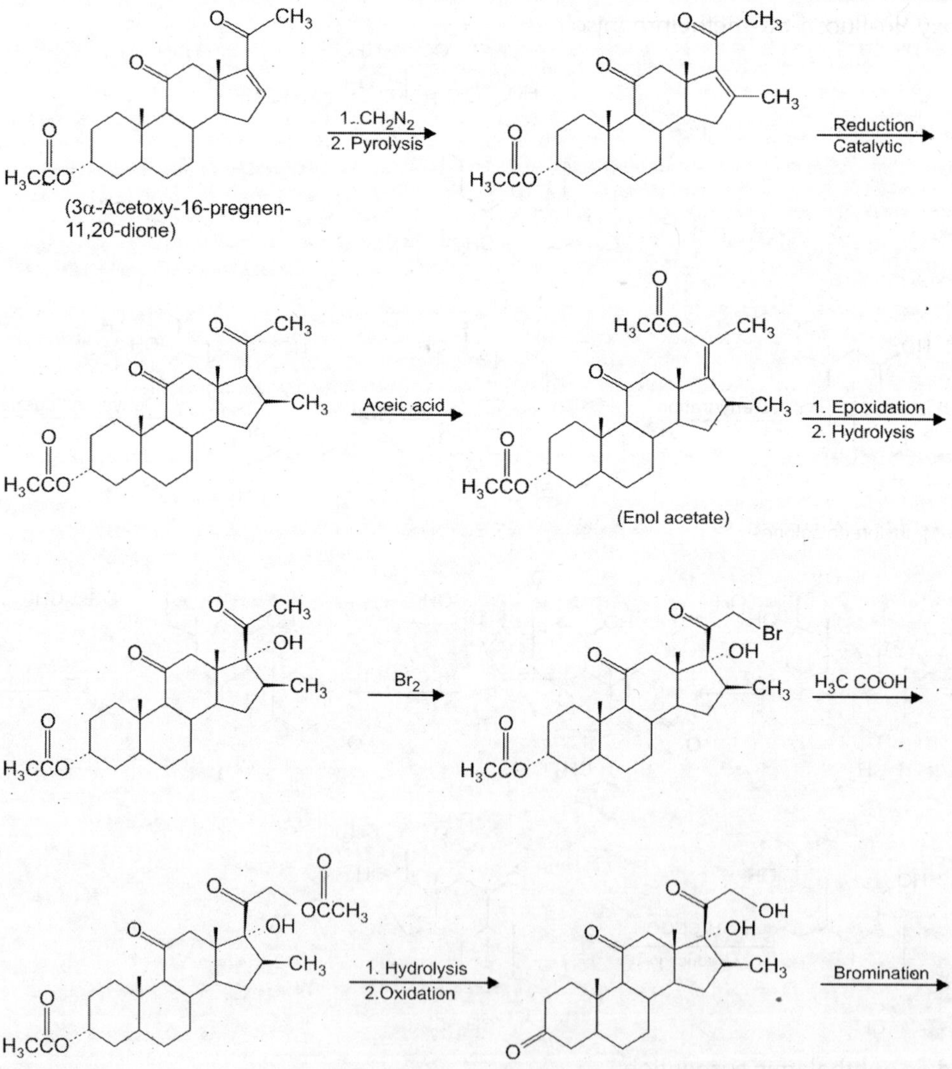

(3α-Acetoxy-16-pregnen-
11,20-dione)

(Enol acetate)

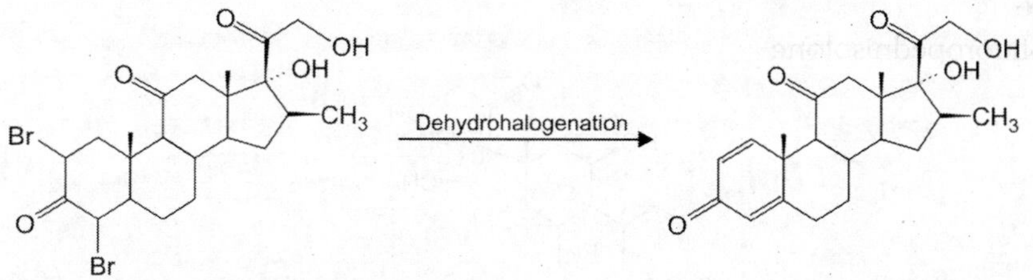

It is used as an anti-inflammatory agent.

Alclometasone

7α-Chloro-16α-methylprednisolone

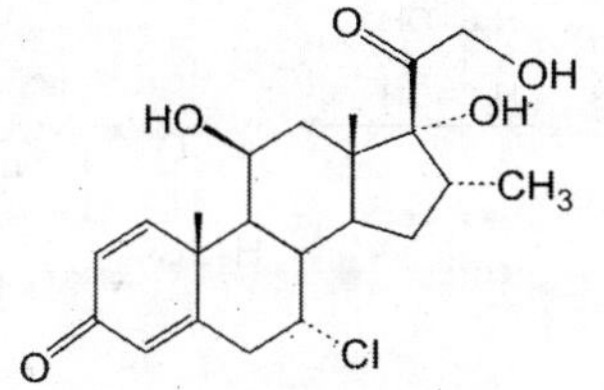

Synthesis

(16α-Methylprednisolone)

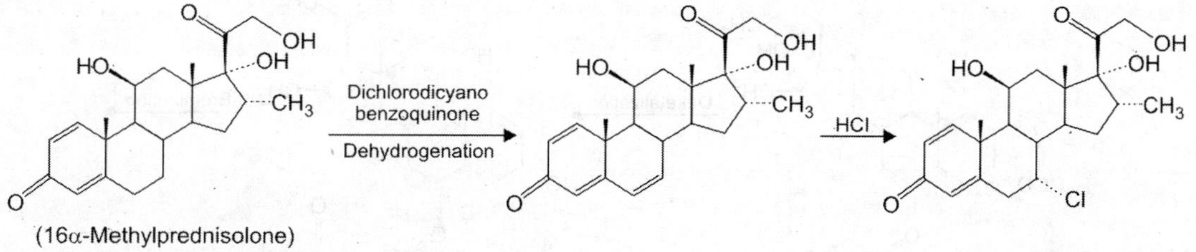

It is anti-inflammatory agent used topically

Beclomethasone

9α-Chloro-16β-methylprednisolone

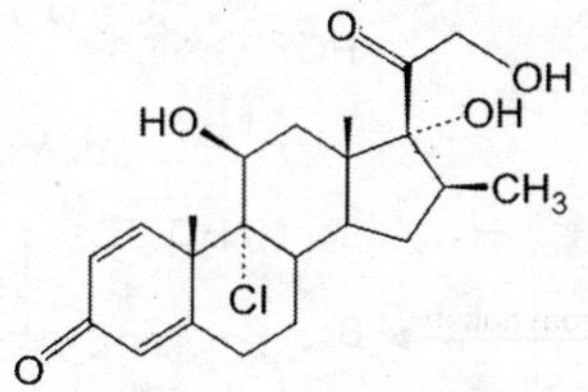

Synthesis

(16β-Methylprednisolone)

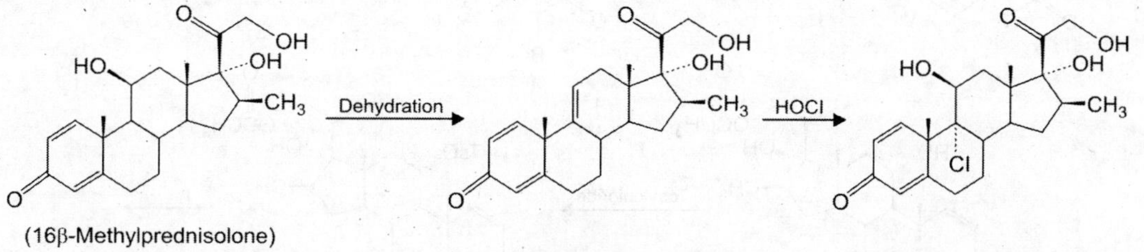

It is used as an antiallergic, inhalation antiasthamatic, and a topical anti-inflammatory agent.

Betamethasone

16β-Methyl-9α-fluoropednisolone

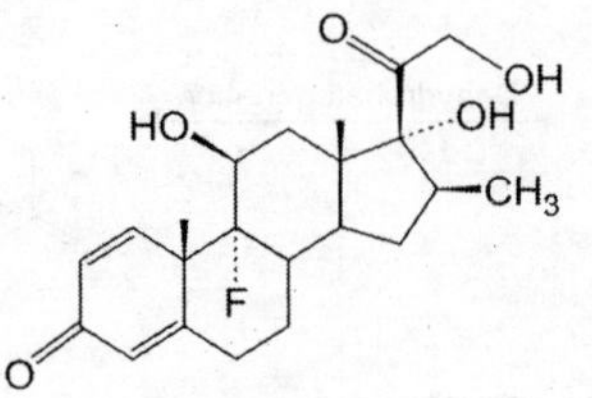

Synthesis

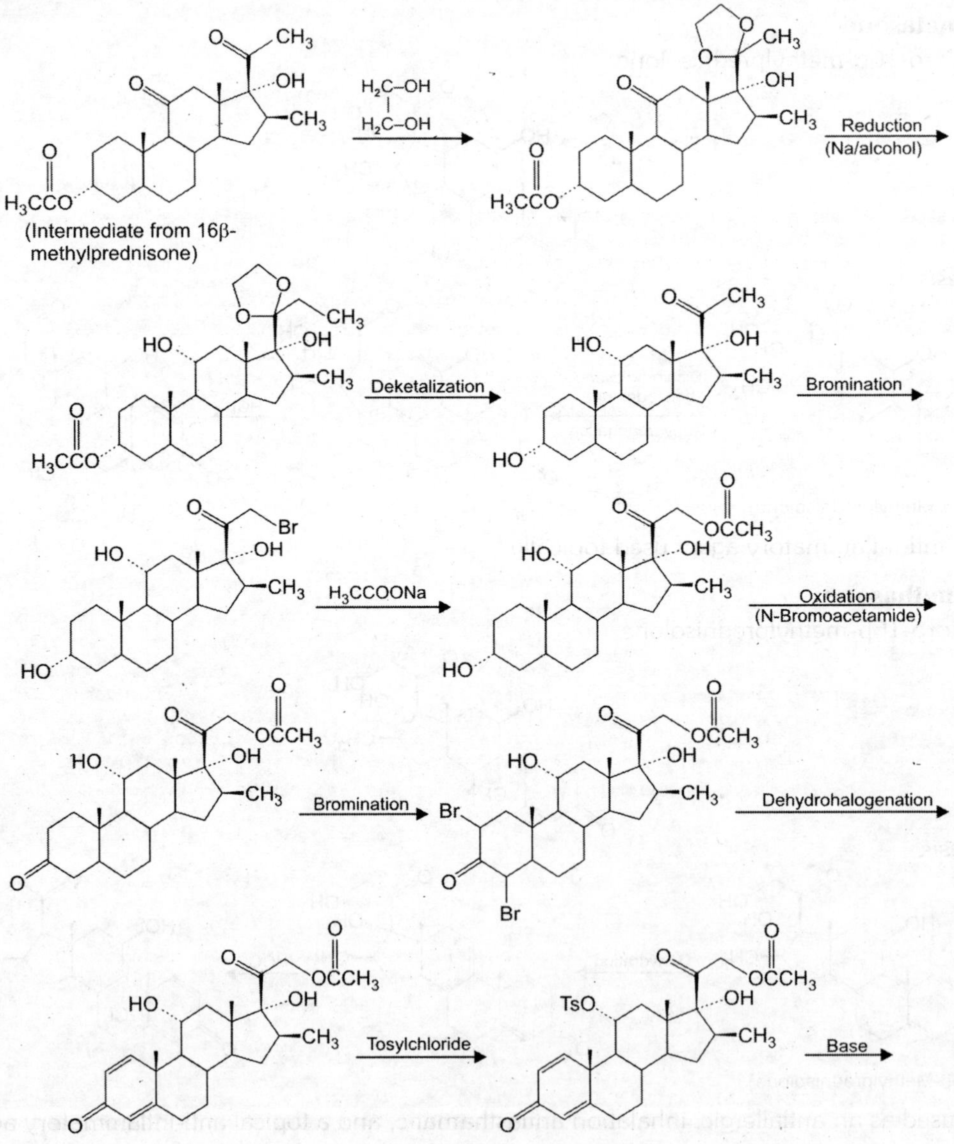

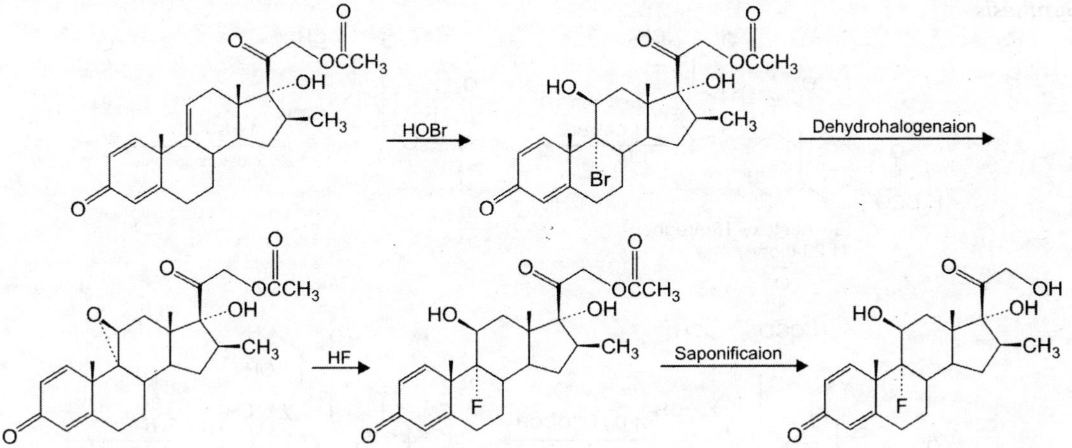

It has lower salt retention and is used as anti-inflammatory agent. Some of its salts and esters used include betamethasone 21-disodium phosphate (132), betamethasone 21-acetate (133), betamethasone 17α-benzoate (134), betamethasone 17α-valerate (135), and betamethasone 17α, 21-dipropionate (136).

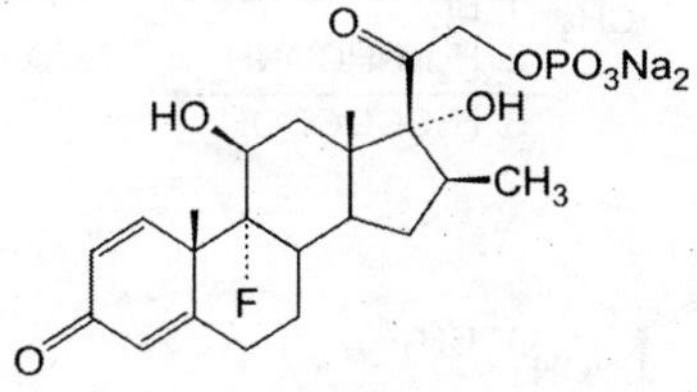

(132)

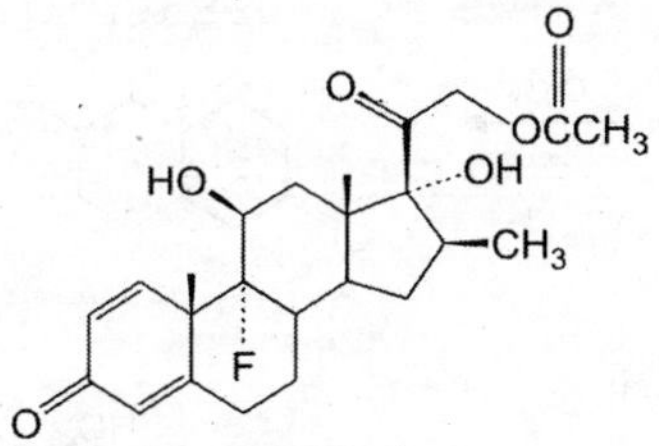

(133)

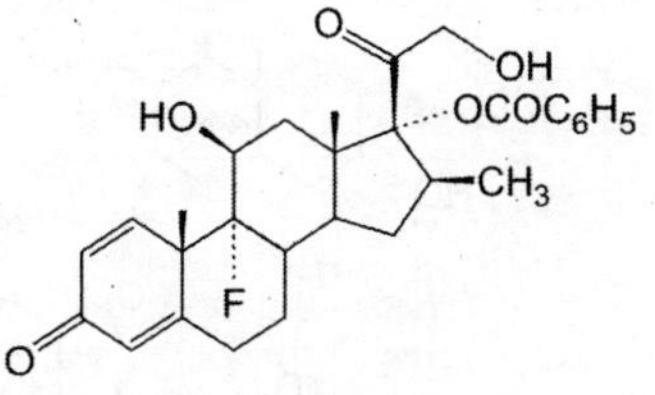

(134)

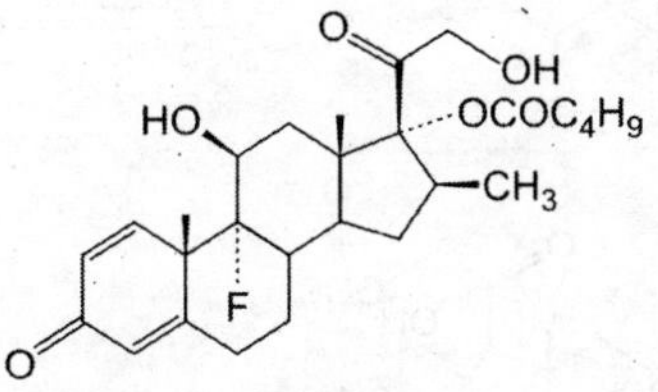

(135)

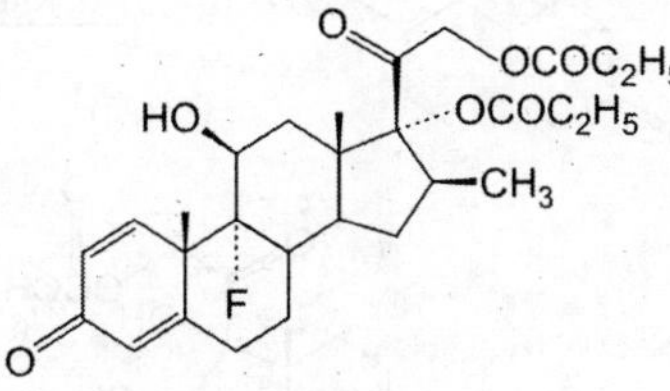

(136)

Dexamethasone Acetate

9α-Fluoro-16α-methylprednisolone 21-acetate

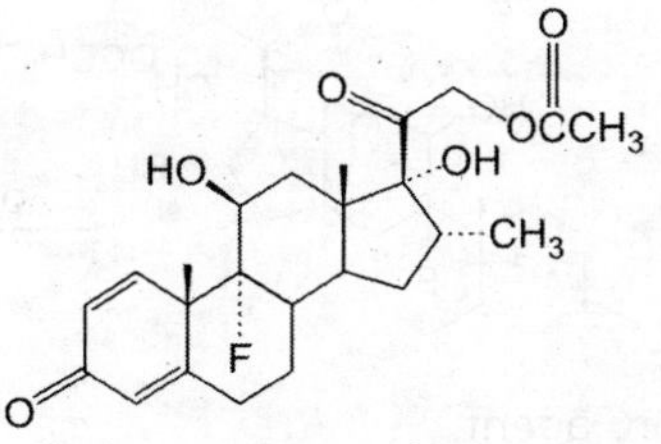

Synthesis

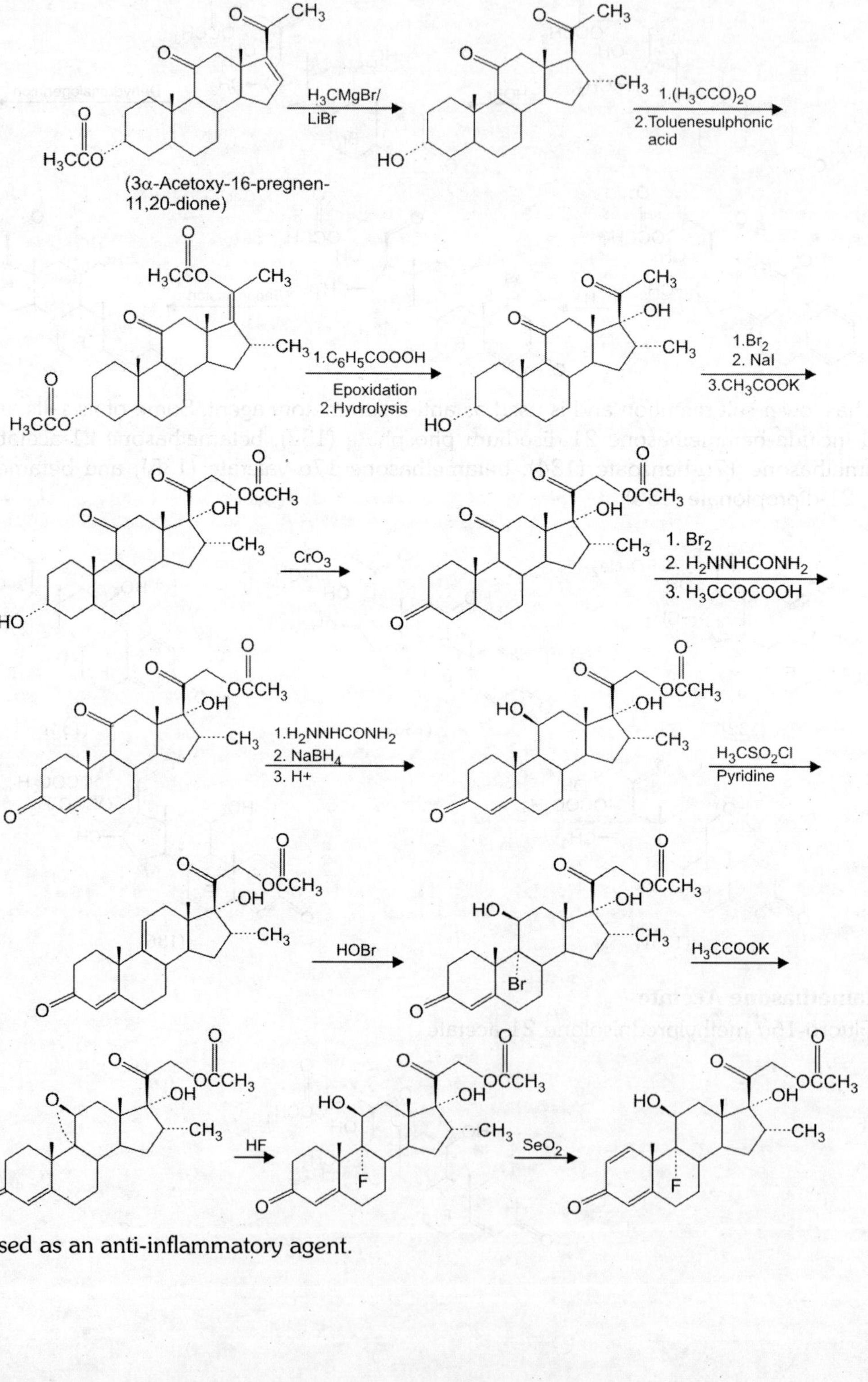

(3α-Acetoxy-16-pregnen-11,20-dione)

It is used as an anti-inflammatory agent.

Clobetasol

21-Chloro-9α-fluoro-11β,17α-dihydroxy-16β-methyl-pregna-1,4-diene-3,20-dione

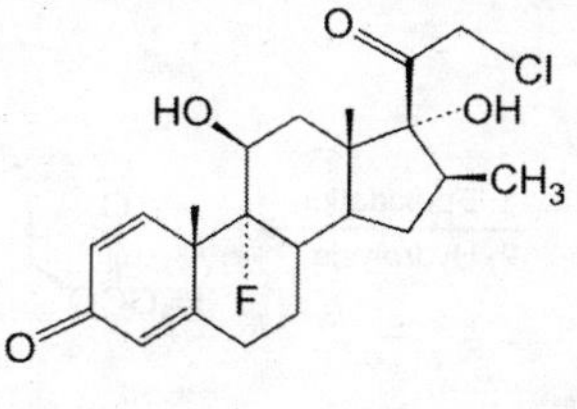

Synthesis

(Betamethasone 17α-propionate)

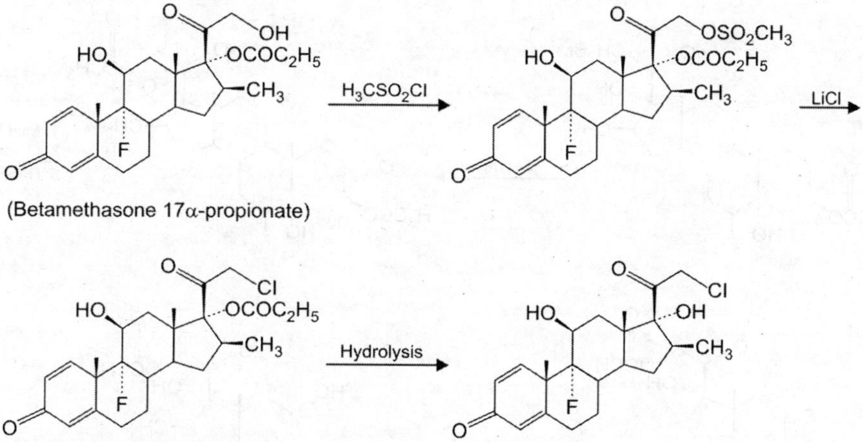

It is as anti-inflammatory agent.

Diflorasone

6α,9α-Difluoro-11β,17α,21-trihydroxy-16β-methylpregna-1,4-diene-3,20-dione.

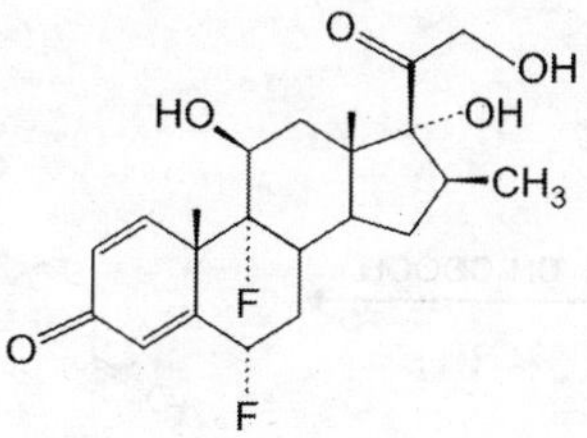

Synthesis

(16β-methylpregnenolone-3-
acetate)

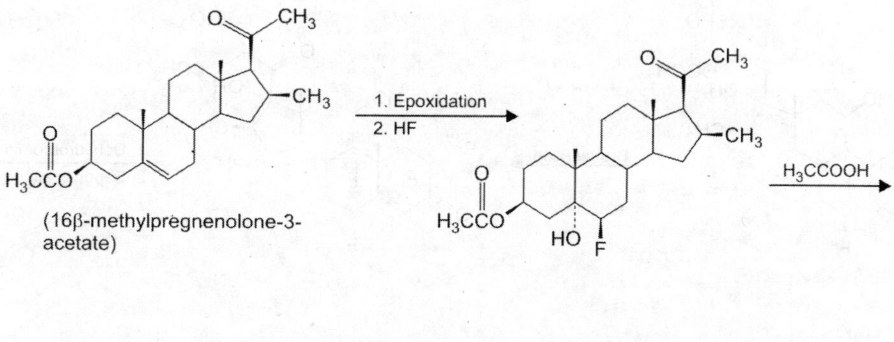

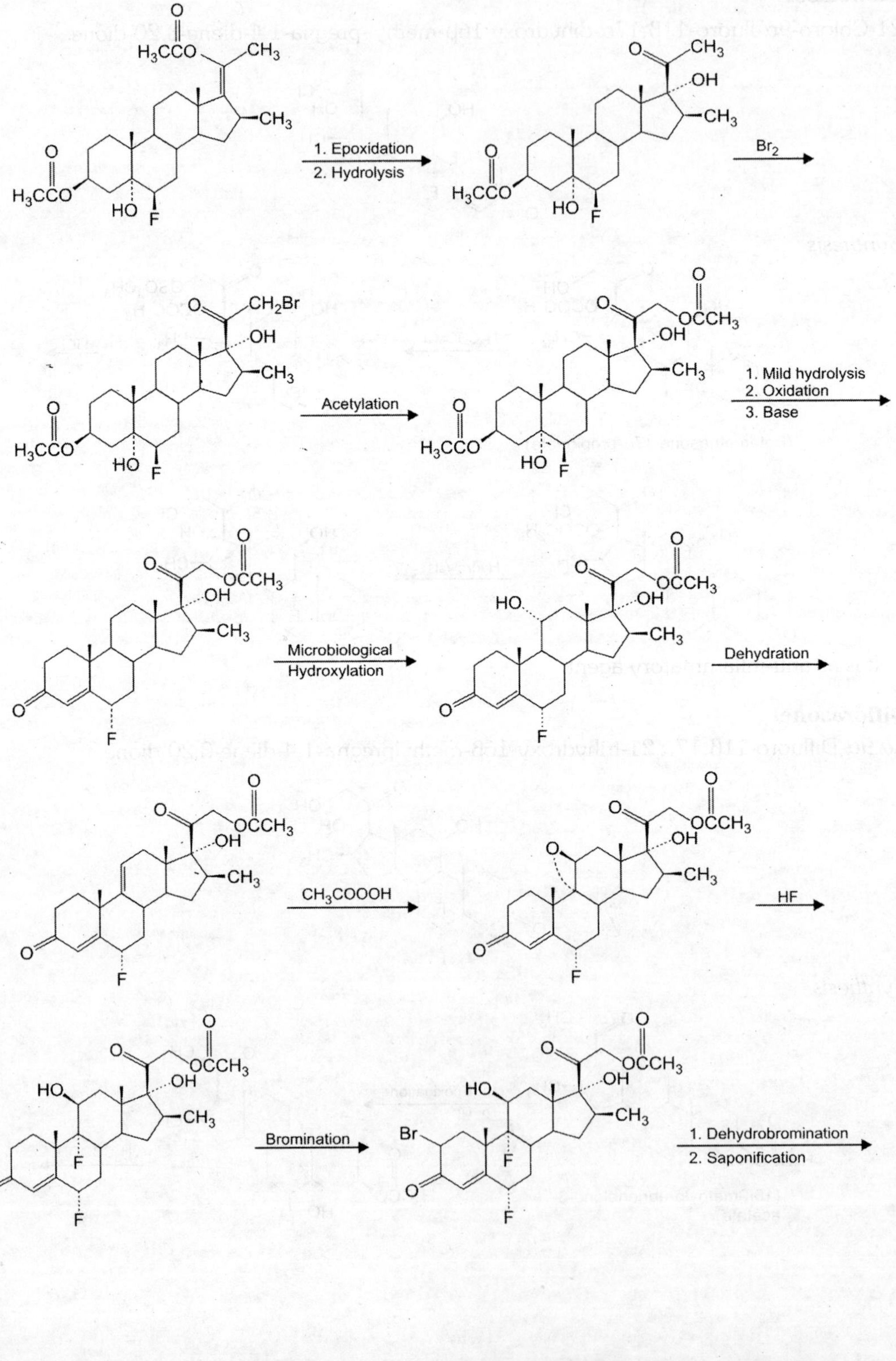

1. Epoxidation
2. Hydrolysis

Br₂

Acetylation

1. Mild hydrolysis
2. Oxidation
3. Base

Microbiological Hydroxylation

Dehydration

CH₃COOOH

HF

Bromination

1. Dehydrobromination
2. Saponification

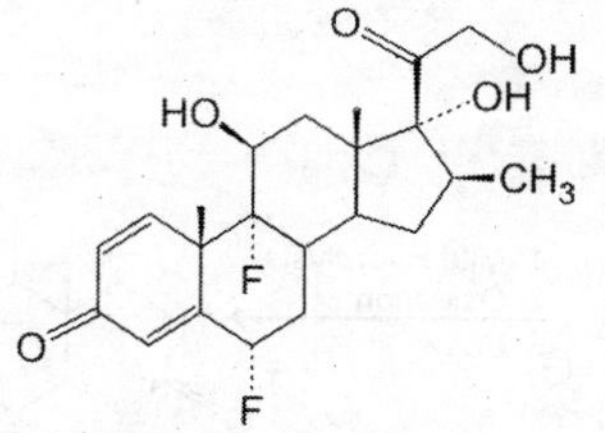

It is used as topical anti-inflammatory agent.

Flumethasone

6α,9α-Difluoro-11β,17α,21-trihydroxy-16α-methylpregna-1,4-diene-3,20-dione.

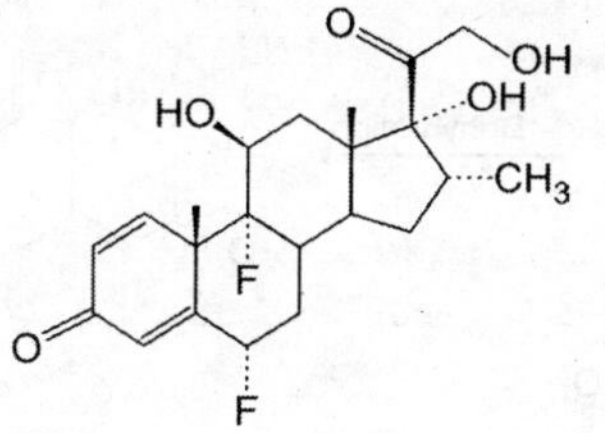

Synthesis

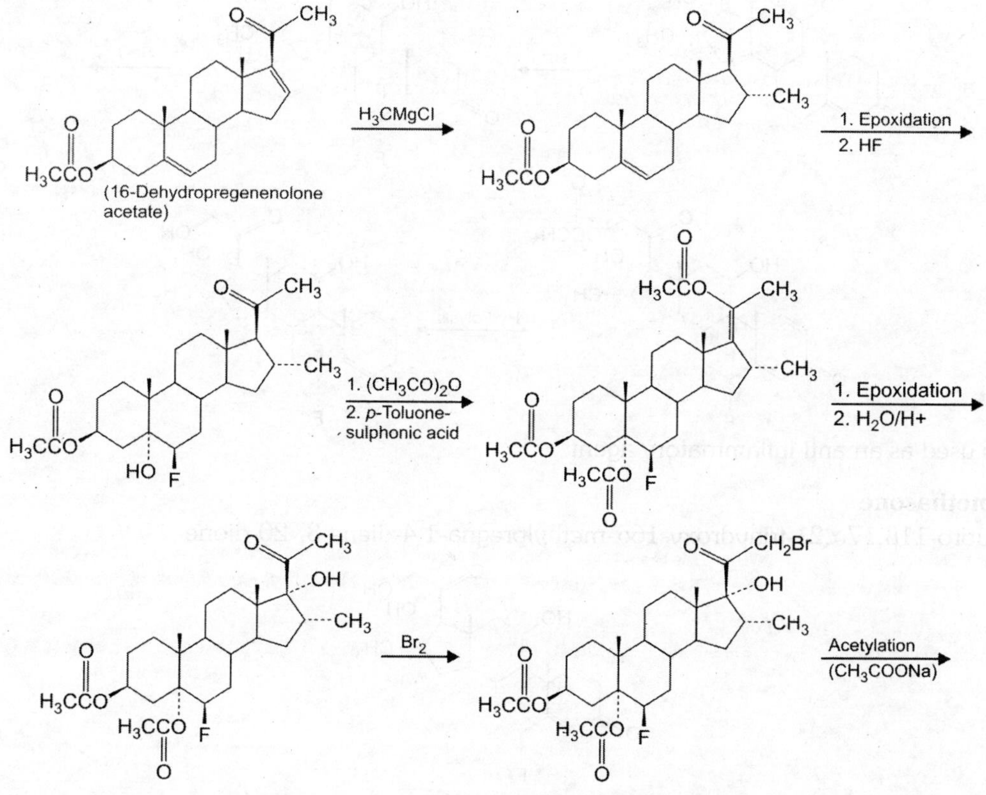

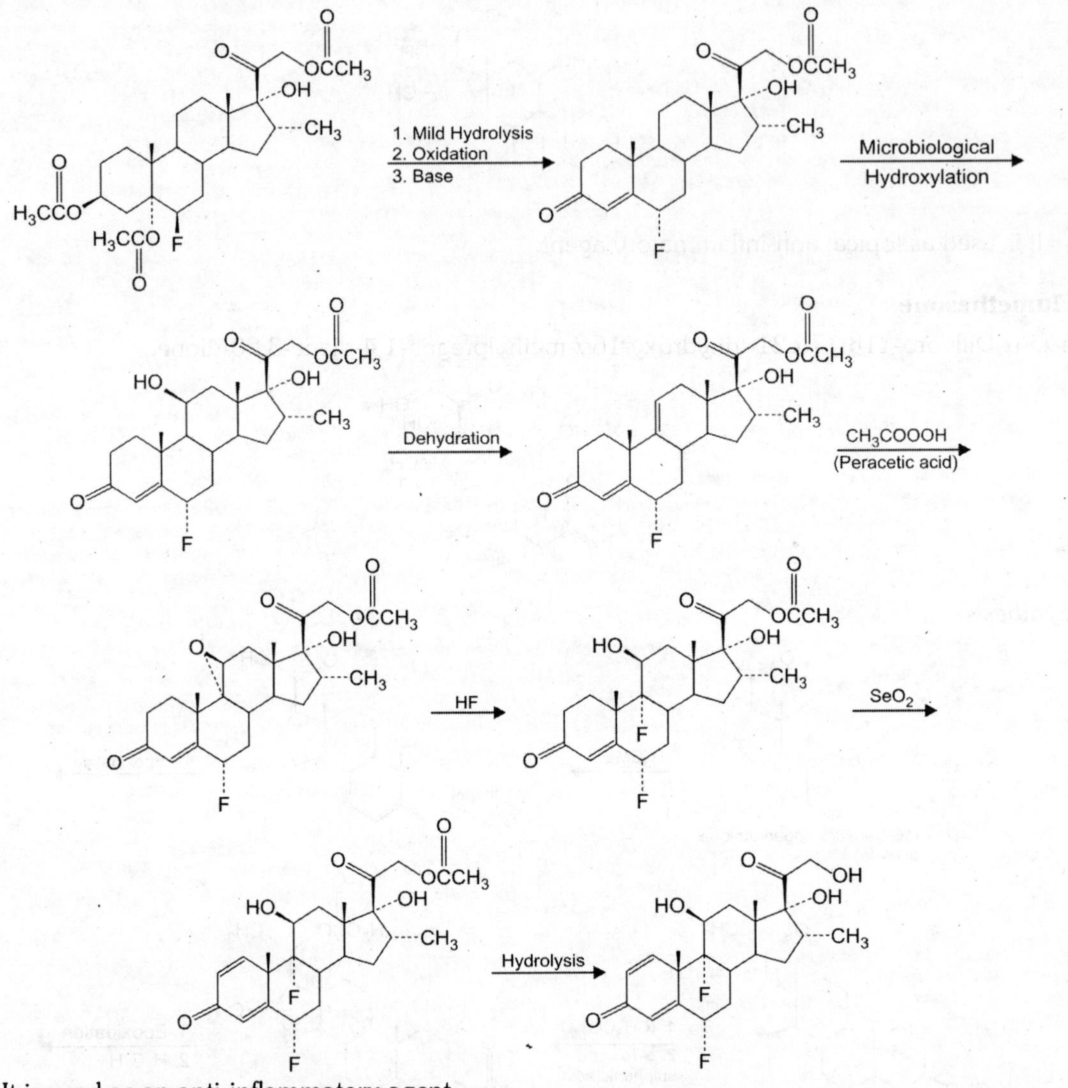

It is used as an anti-inflammatory agent.

Paramethasone

6α-Fluoro-11β,17α,21-trihydroxy-16α-methylpregna-1,4-diene-3, 20-dione

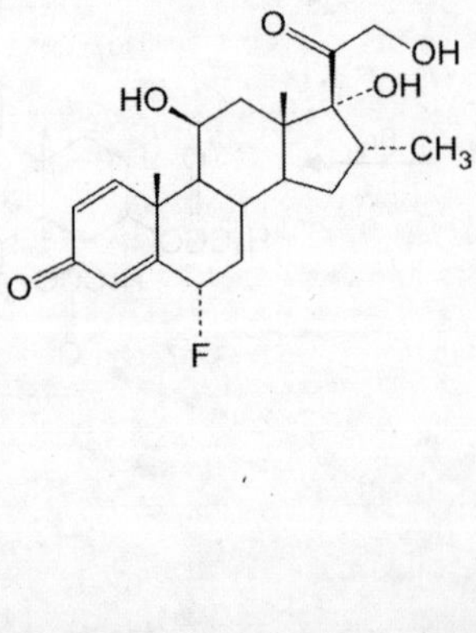

Synthesis

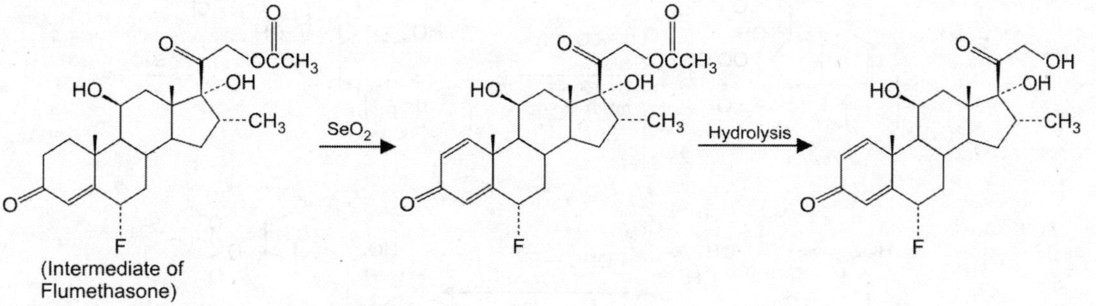
SeO2
Hydrolysis
(Intermediate of
Flumethasone)

It is an anti-inflammatory agent.

Amcinonide

21-(Acetyloxy)-16α,17α-[cyclopentylidenebis (oxy)]-9α-fluoro-11β-hydroxypregna-1,4-diene-3,20-dione.

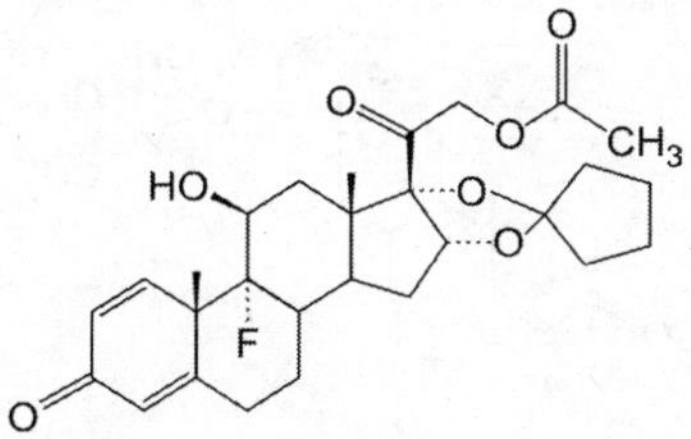

Synthesis

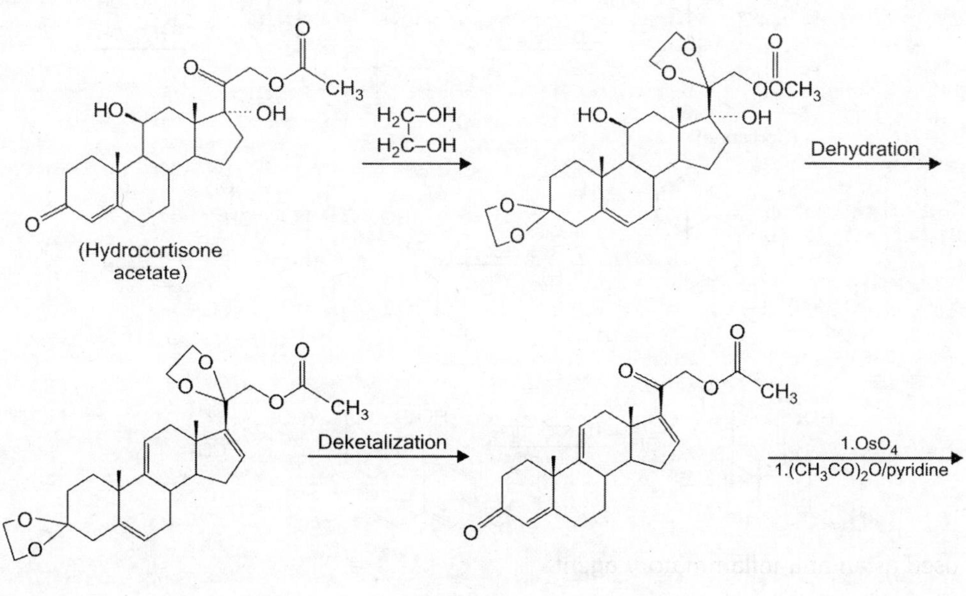
(Hydrocortisone
acetate)
Dehydration
Deketalization
1.OsO4
1.(CH3CO)2O/pyridine

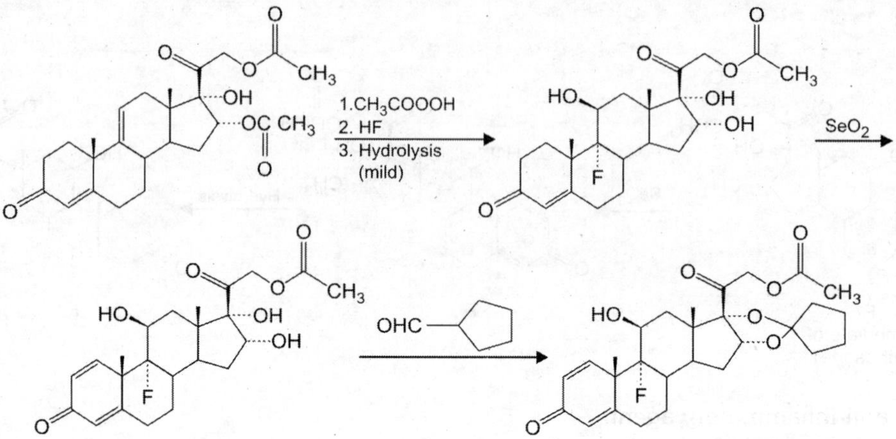

It is used as a glucocorticoid.

Desonide

11β,21-Dihydroxy-16α,17α [(1-methylethylidene)-bis(oxy)]pregna-1, 4-diene-3,20-dione.

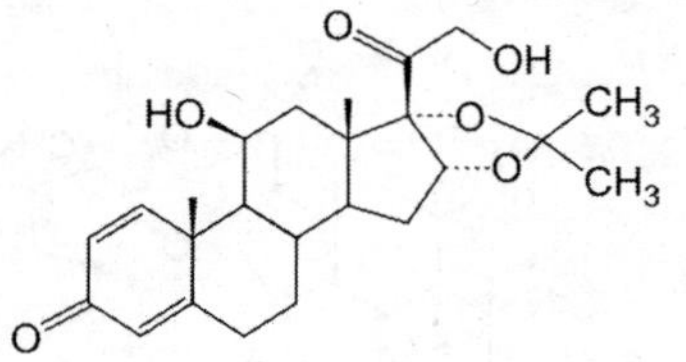

Synthesis

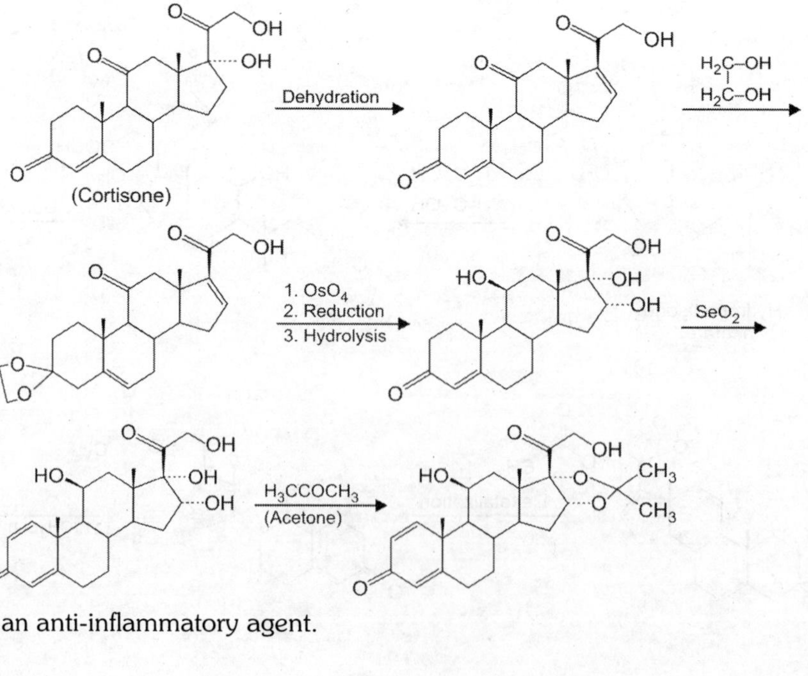

It is used as an anti-inflammatory agent.

Budesonide

(R,S)-11β,16α,17,21-tetrahydroxypregna-1,4-diene-3,20-dione cyclic 16, 17-acetal with butraldehyde.

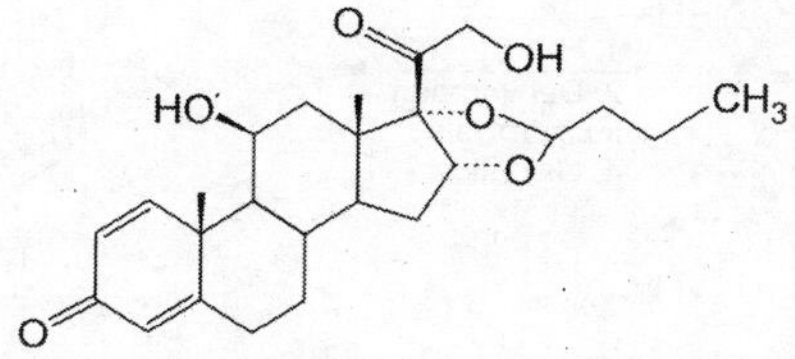

Synthesis

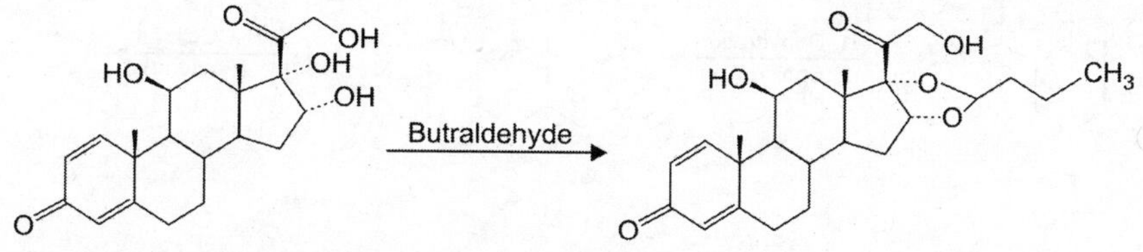

(Intermediate from desonide)

It is used as an anti-inflammatory agent.

Fluocinonide

6α,9α-Difluoro-11β,16α-17α, 21-tetrahydroxypregna-1,4-diene-3,20-dione, cyclic 16,17-ketal with acetone, 21 acetate.

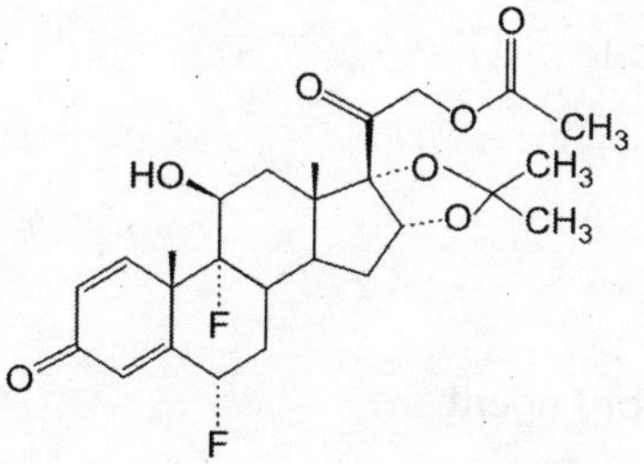

Synthesis

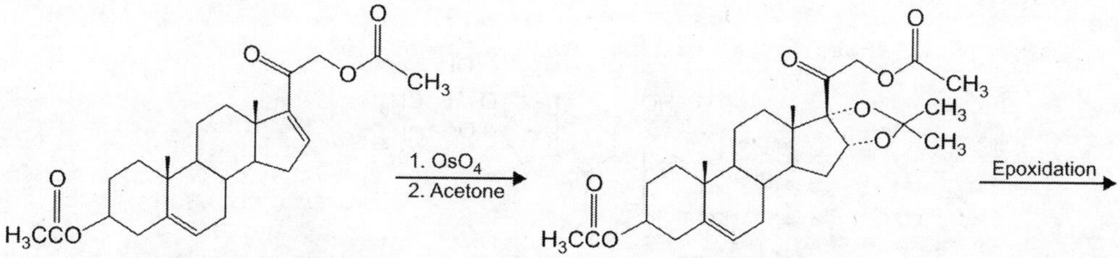

(Enone diacetate)

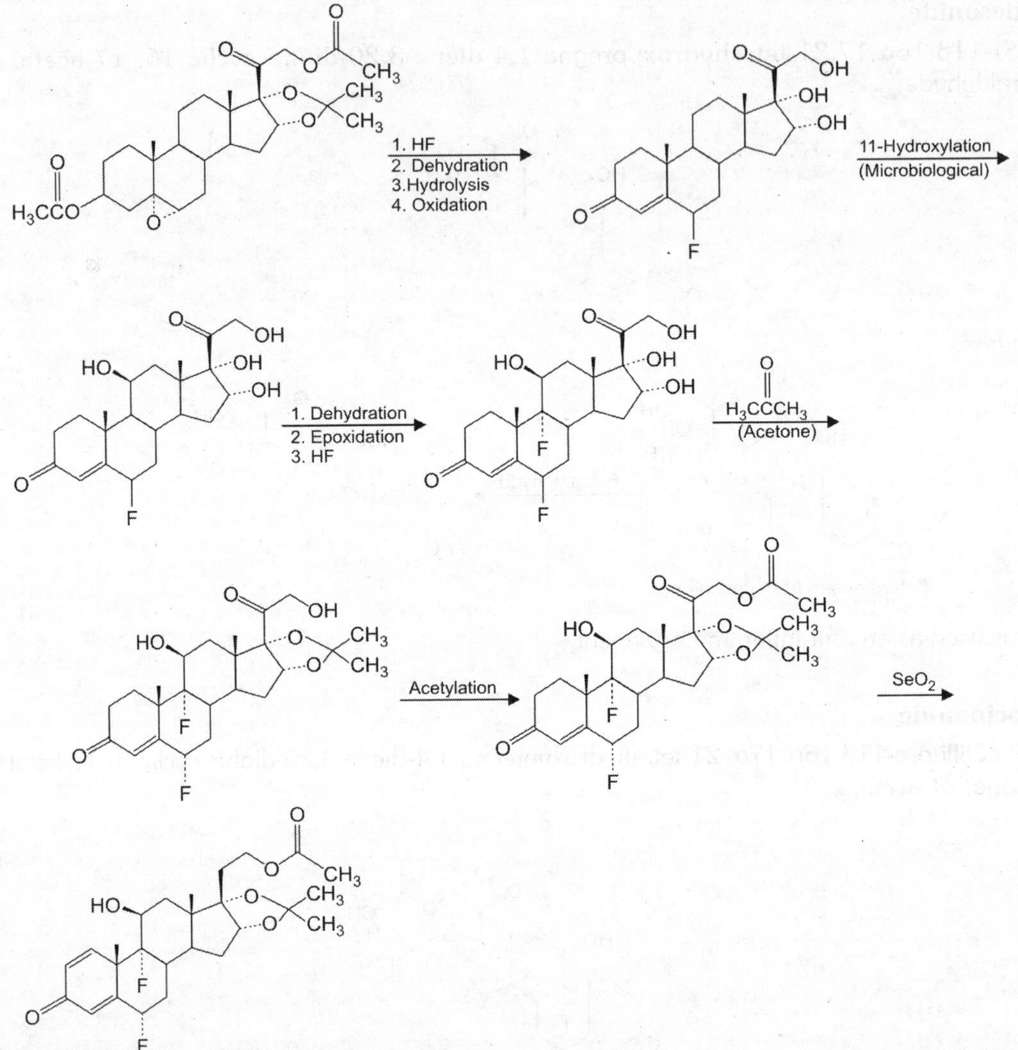

It is used as an anti-inflammatory agent.

Flunisolide

6α-Fluoro-11β,16α,17α, 21-tetrahydroxyprega-1,4-dien-3,20-dione cyclic 16, 17-ketal with acetone

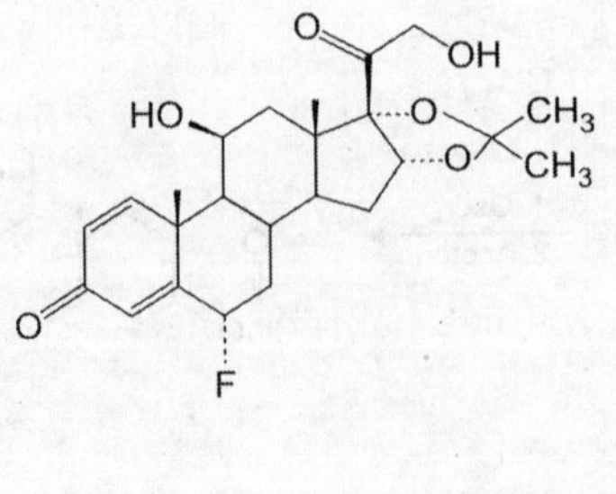

Synthesis

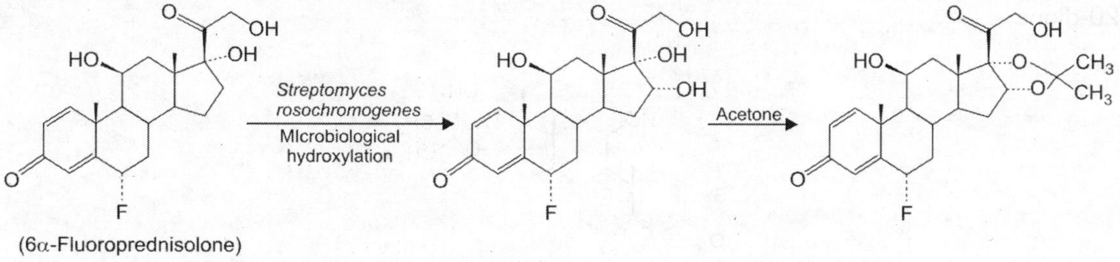

(6α-Fluoroprednisolone)

It is used as antiasthmatic.

Flurandrenolide

6α-Fluoro-11β, 21-dihydroxy-16α,17α [(1-methylethylidene)bis(oxy)]pregn-4-ene-3, 20-dione

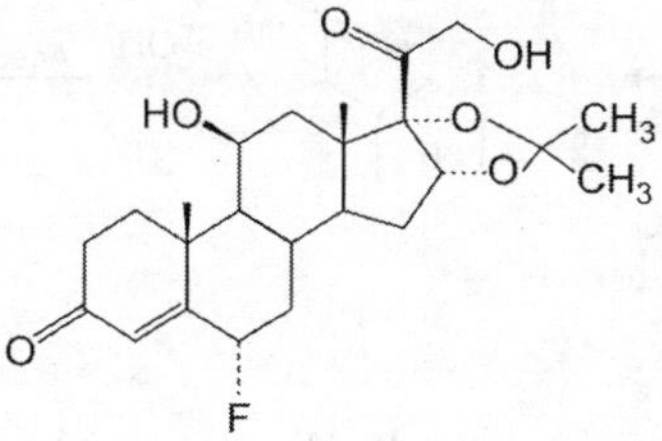

Synthesis

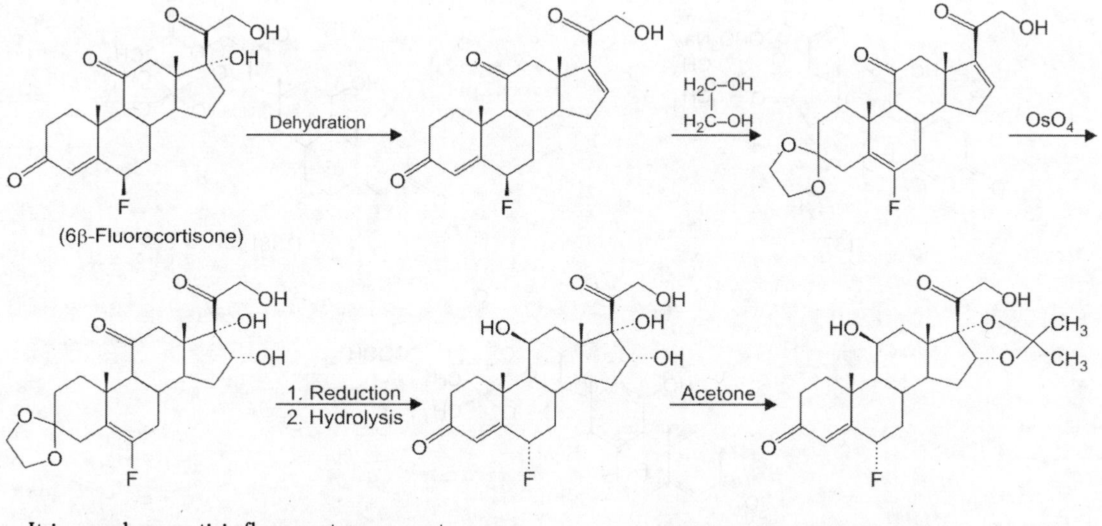

(6β-Fluorocortisone)

It is used as anti-inflammatory agent.

Triamcinolone Acetonide

9α-Fluoro-11β,21-dihydroxy-16α,17α[(1-methylethylidenebis)(oxy)]pregna-1,4-diene-3, 20-dione.

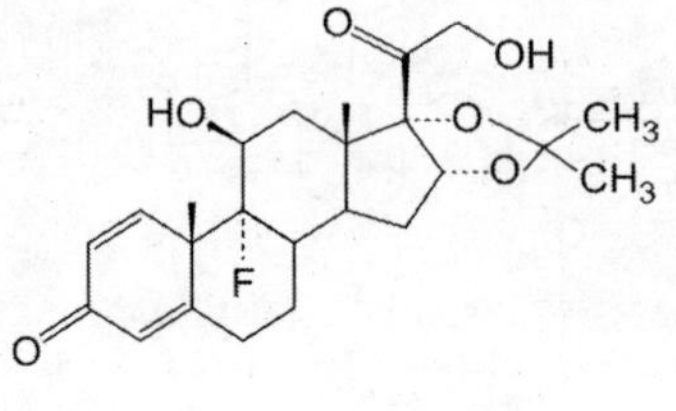

Synthesis

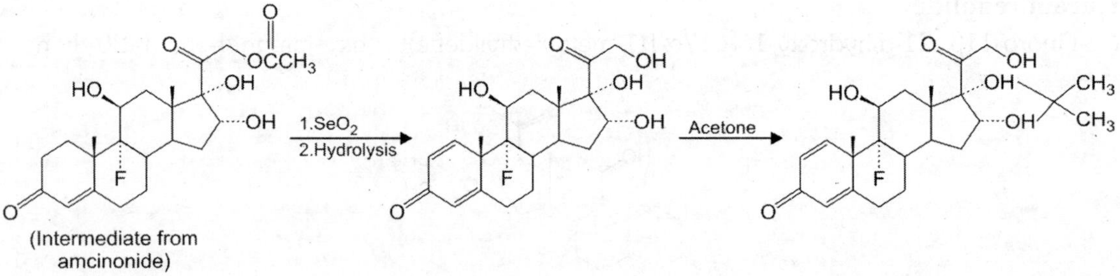

(Intermediate from amcinonide)

It is used as inhalant for asthma and as nasal antiallergic. The other salts and esters used include, 21-disodium phosphate (137), 21-acetate (138), and 21-hemisuccinate (139).

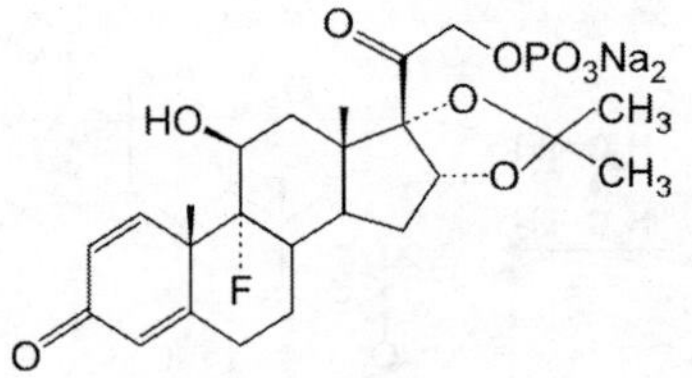

(137)

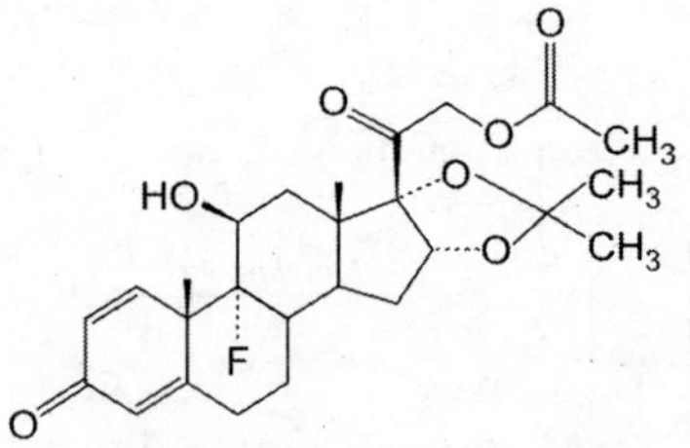

(138)

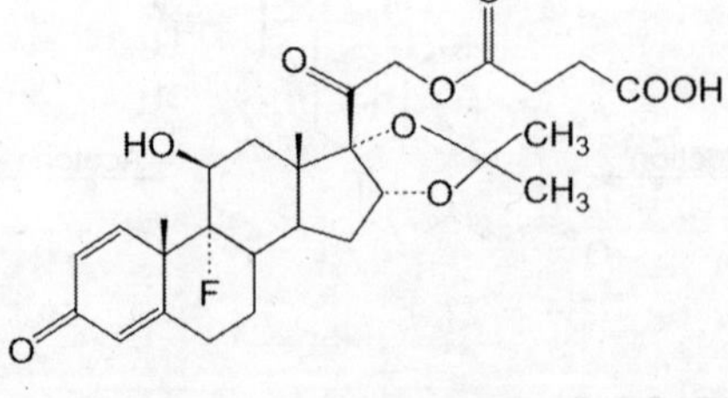

(139)

Fluticasone Propionate

S-Fluoromethyl 6α, 9α-difluoro-11β-hydroxy-16α-methyl-17α-propionyloxy-3-oxoandrosta-1,
4-diene-17β-carbothioate

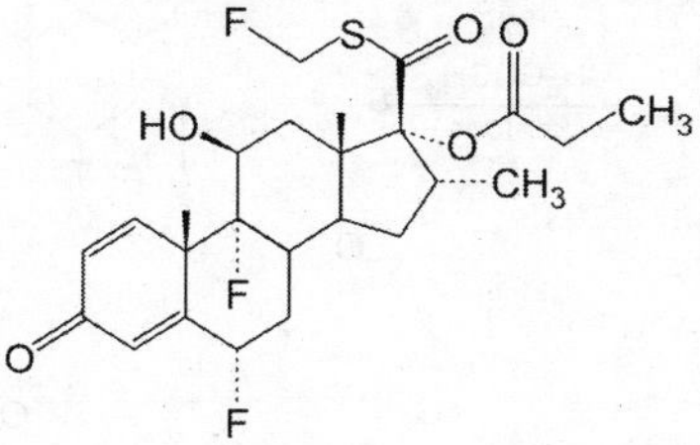

Synthesis

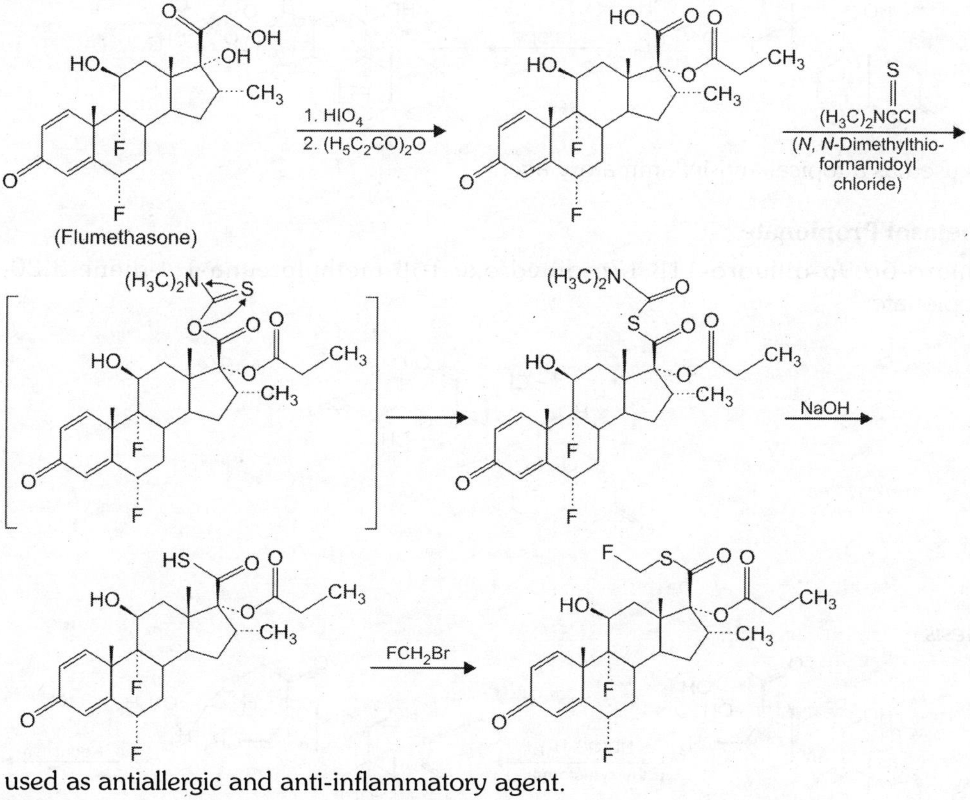

It is used as antiallergic and anti-inflammatory agent.

Halcinonide

21-Chloro-9α-fluoro-11β,16α,17α-trihydroxy-pregn-4-ene-3, 20-dione cyclic 16, 17-ketal with
acetone

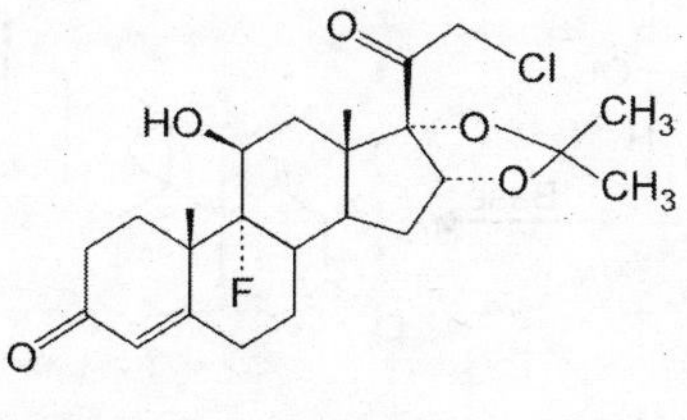

Synthesis

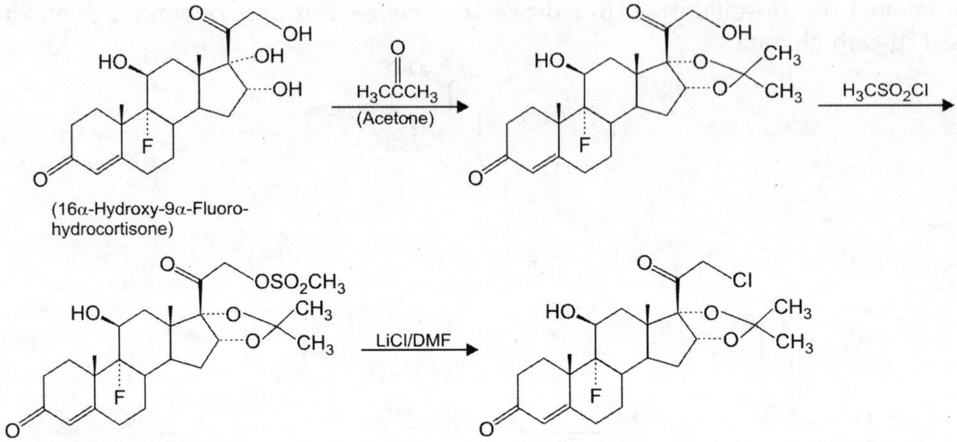

(16α-Hydroxy-9α-Fluoro-
hydrocortisone)

It is used as a topical anti-inflammatory agent.

Halobetasol Propionate

21-Chloro-6α,9α-difluoro-11β,17α-dihydroxy-16β-methylpregna-1,4-diene-3,20-dione 17-propionate

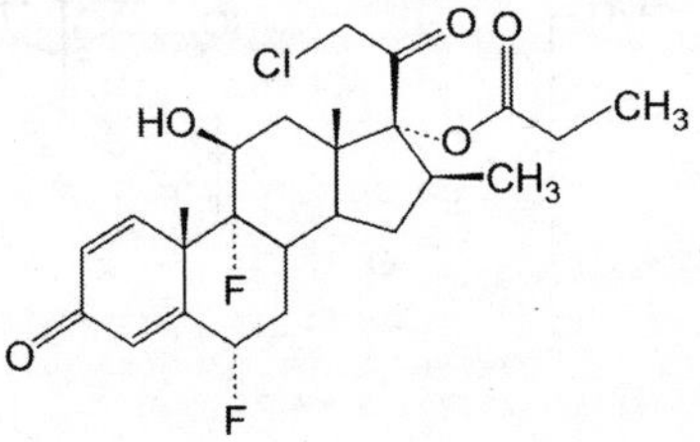

Synthesis

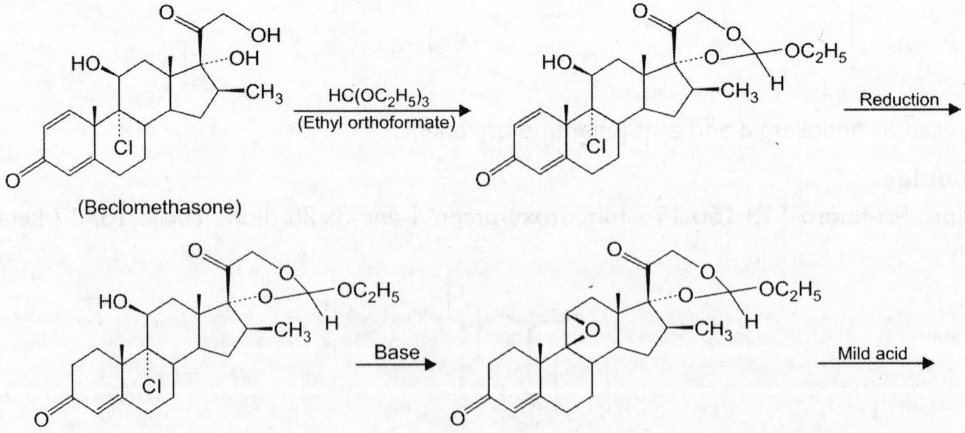

(Beclomethasone)

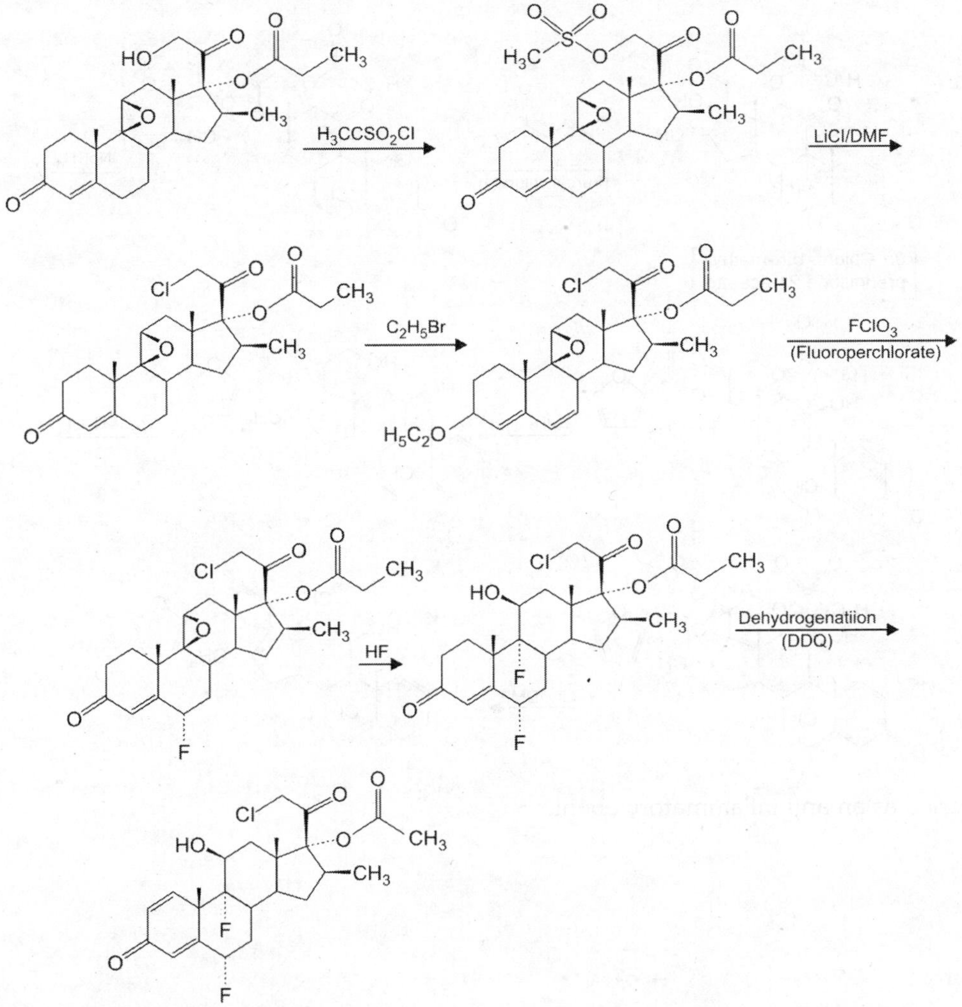

It is used as anti-inflammatory agent.

Mometasone Furoate

9α,21-Dichloro-11β,17α-dihydroxy-16-α-methylpregna-1,4-diene-3,20-dione 17-(2-furoate)

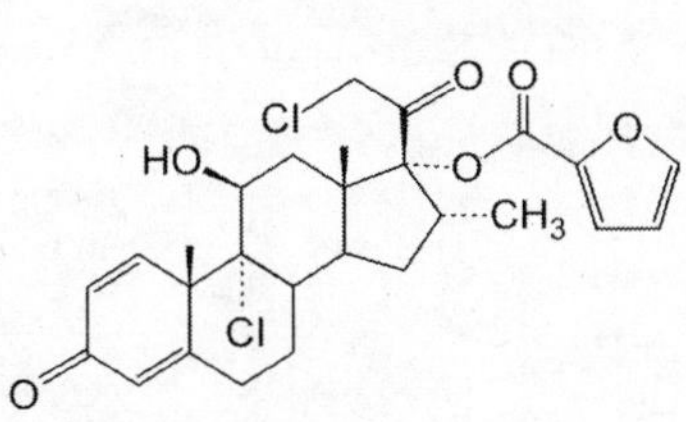

Synthesis

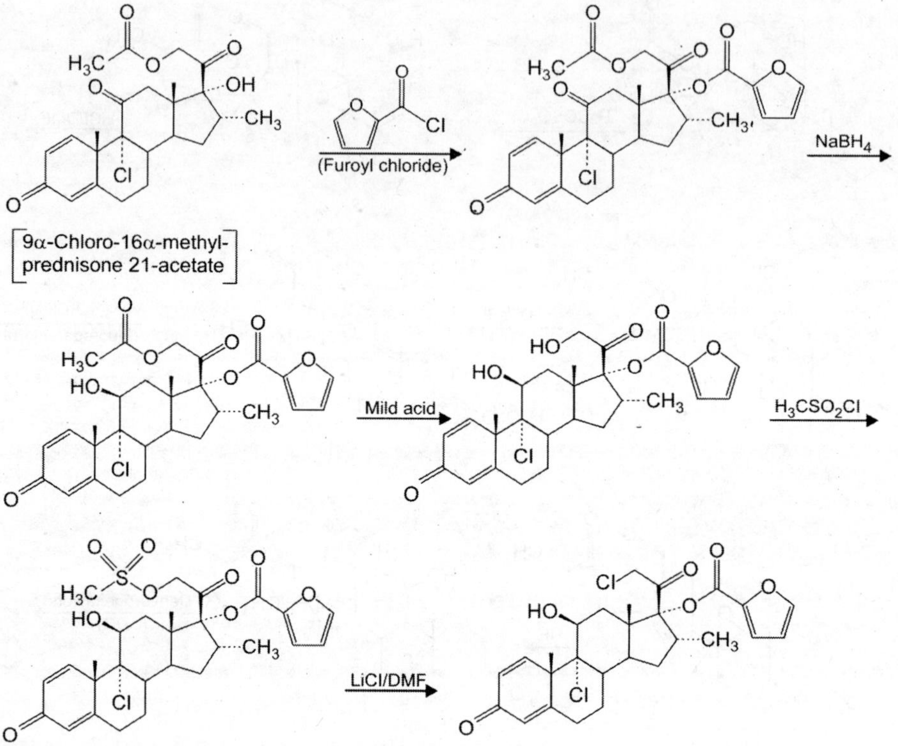

[9α-Chloro-16α-methyl-
prednisone 21-acetate]

It is used as an anti-inflammatory agent.

HYPOGLYCEMIC AGENTS

INSULIN AND RELATED ANALOGS

DIABETES MELLITUS is a disease characterized by high blood sugar levels, hyperglycemia (above 120 mg/100 ml). In hyperglycemia, the renal threshold for glucose is exceeded as a result the glucose is excreted in urine (glucosuria) and this results in osmotic diuresis.

Hyperglycemia occurs because of faulty metabolism of glucose. Two types of diabetes mellitus have been identified and these include: Type 1 diabetes also known as insulin dependent diabetes mellitus (IDDM) and Type 2 diabetes also known as non-insulin dependent diabetes mellitus (NIDDM). In Type 1 diabetes, there is deficiency of insulin (1) which is because of autoimmune destruction of β-cells of Langerhans responsible for secretion of insulin (1). The patient has to be provided with insulin (1). This type of diabetes results from autoimmune process involving interleukin 1. The patient becomes diabetic when 90% of the β-cells are destroyed.

In Type 2 diabetes, there is insulin (1) resistance and impaired regulation of insulin (1) secretion. Type 2 diabetes is usually found in adult and incidence rises with the age as the β-cell function declines. The treatment of Type 2 diabetes is through diet control and use of oral hypoglycemic agents.

The deficiency of insulin (1) not only leads to impaired metabolism of glucose but also to disturbed fat and protein metabolisms. There is incomplete oxidation of fats and fatty acids leading to ketosis (presence of ketone bodies such as acetone, acetoacetic acid, and β-hydroxybutyric acid in blood) and ketonuria (presence of ketone bodies in urine). Similarly, proteins are mobilized and there is increased catabolism of proteins leading to increased amino acid levels which results in gluconeogenesis and formation of ketone bodies. Insulin (1), thus, occupies a central position in intermediary metabolism and acts on liver, muscle and fat.

Insulin (1) is a peptide made up of two chains, called chain A and chain B. These polypeptide chains are joined through sulfur of cysteine amino acids (7 of A & B and 20 of A and 19 of B). A chain is made up of 21 amino acids and B-chain of 30 amino acids.

Insulin (1) influences all the three metabolisms, i.e. carbohydrate, fat, and protein. It stimulates glycogenesis and inhibits glycogenolysis and glyconeogenesis in liver. In the muscle, it stimulates glycogenesis and glycolysis. Metabolism of glucose results in glycerol which is used for formation of triglycerides in adipose tissue. It also inhibits lipolysis. Insulin (1) also causes lipogenesis in liver. The uptake of amino acids and protein synthesis is increased by insulin (1) in muscle. In liver, it inhibits oxidation of amino acids.

```
A 1Gly                                              CHAIN A
    |
  Ile
    |
  Val      S————————————————————S
    |      |                     |
  Glu      |                     |                                              COOH
    |      |  A 7                |                              A 20            |
  Gln — Cys—Cys—Thr — Ser —Ile — Cys—Ser— Leu — Tyr—Gln — Leu —Glu—Asn—Tyr—Cys— Asn
         A 6    \                                                               A 21
                 S                                                       S
                 |                                                       |
                 S                                                       S
                 |                                                       |
  His — Leu —Cys—Gly — Ser —His — Leu —Val — Glu — Ala — Leu —Tyr — Leu —Val — CysB 19
    |          B 7                                                              |
    Gln                                                                        Gly
    |                                                                           |
  Asn                              CHAIN B                                     Glu
    |                                                                           |
  Val                                                                         Arg
    |                                                                           |
 B 1Phe              HOOC — Thr — Lys — Pro — Thr — Tyr — Phe — Phe — Gly
    |                            B 30
  NH₂
                                    (1)
```

Mechanism of Action of Insulin (1)

Insulin (1) regulates metabolism and gene experession. The insulin (1) receptor (Fig. 18.1) is made up of two α-chains and two β-chains joined together through sulphur linkage. The α-chains are entirely extracelluar while as β-chains are transmembrane chains with tyrosine kinase activity. The α-chain contains the site for binding of the insulin (1). Binding of insulin (1) to α-chain causes activation of tyrosine-kinase activity in the β-chain. The tyrosine residues in the chain are phosphorylated. Next, the insulin (1) receptor substrate (IRS-I) gets phosphorylated, which in turn catalyzes the phosphorylation of other enzymes through which the metabolic effects of insulin (1) are mediated.

IRS-I after phosphorylation activates PI-3-Kinase (PI-3K)(Fig. 18.2) which converts phosphatidyl inositol diphosphate (PIP$_2$) to phosphatidyl inositol triphosphate (PIP$_3$), which indirectly activates protein kinase B (PKB). The activated PKB-P triggers the movements of glucose transporter Glu T$_4$ from internal vesicles to plasma membrane, which stimulates the glucose uptake from blood (Fig. 18.2). The glycogen formation takes place through series of steps (Fig. 18.2) in which PKB-P phosphyrlates GSK3 to GSK3-P, thereby, inactivating it. The inactive GSK3-P is unable to convert the active glycogen synthase (GS) to inactive glycogen synthase (GS-P), so it remains active and glycogen synthesis takes place uninterrupted (Fig. 18.2).

Structure-activity relationship studies have shown that:

1. C-terminal amino acid 30-B to be non-essential,

2. The amino groups at the ends of both chains have been found to be unimportant because acylation of these amino groups does not affect the activity,

3. Most of the readily esterfiable carboxyl groups are also not essential since at least two-thirds of these can be esterified without any effect on activity,

4. The disulfide linkage between the two chains is essential because cleavage of this results in loss of activity. It is possible that the disulfide linkage may be responsible for holding the molecule in a particular secondary or tertiary shape.

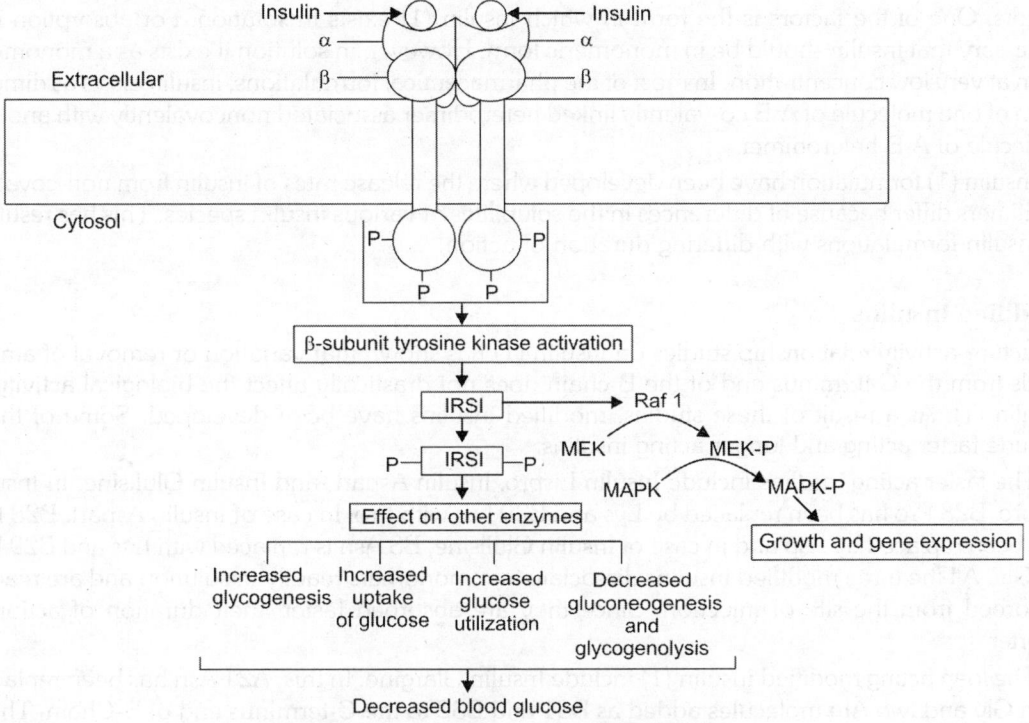

Fig. 18.1: Mechanism of insulin action.

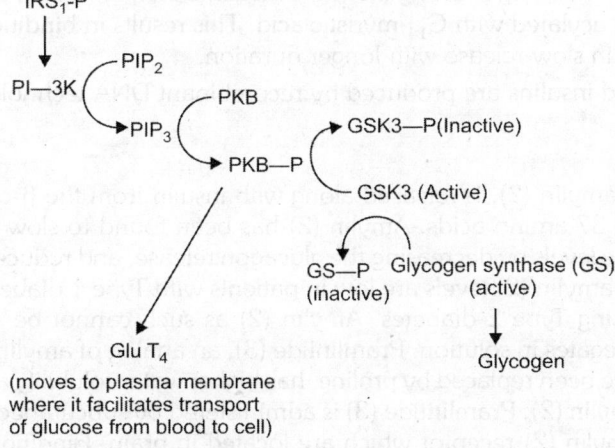

Fig. 18.2: Mechanism of glycogen formation.

Insulin (1) is inactivated in vivo by proteolytic enzyme insulinase that occurs in liver, as well as by pepsin, and chymotrypsin. Accordingly, it is not effective when given orally. It is administered parenterally by subcutaneous route with a fine gauze needle. This results in a small depot of insulin (1) at the site of injection. The absorption of insulin from this site depends upon various factors. One of the factors is the form in which insulin (1) exists in solution. For absorption It is necessary that insulin should be in monomeric form. However, in solution it exists as a monomeric form at very low concentration. In most of the pharmaceutical formulations, insulin exists as dimeric form of one molecule of A-B co-valently linked heterodimer associated noncovalently with another molecule of A-B heterodimer.

Insulin (1) formulation have been developed where the release rates of insulin from non-covalent multimers differ because of differences in the solubilites of various insulin species. This has resulted in insulin formulations with differing duration of action.

Modified Insulins

Structure-activity relationship studies on insulin (1) has shown that variation or removal of amino acids from the C-terminus end of the B-chain does not drastically affect the biological activity of insulin (1). As a result of these studies, modified insulins have been developed. Some of these include faster acting and longer acting insulins.

The faster acting insulins include Insulin Lispro, Insulin Aspart, and Insulin Glulisine. In Insulin Lispro, B28 Pro has been replaced by Lys and B29 Lys with Pro. In case of Insulin Aspart, B28 Pro has been replaced by Asp and in case of Insulin Glulisine, B3 Asn is replaced with Lys and B29 Lys by Glu. All the three modified insulins dissociate into monomers readily in solution and are readily absorbed from the site of injection. Since they are absorbed faster, their duration of action is shorter.

The long acting modified insulin (1) include Insulin Glargine. In this, A21 Asn has been replaced with Gly and two Arg molecules added as B31 and B32 to the C-terminus end of B-Chain. These changes result in change of isoelectric point to 7. The change in isoelectric points results in precipitation of insulin at the site of injection, consequently slow release from the depot and longer duration of action. Another longer acting insulin is Insulin Detemir. In this, the B30 Thr has been removed and B29 Lys acylated with C_{14}-myristic acid. This results in binding of insulin to plasma albumin which results in slow release with longer duration.

All of these modified insulins are produced by recombinant DNA technology.

AMYLIN AGONISTS

Another polypeptide, amylin (2), is released along with insulin from the β-cells of pancreas. This peptide is made up of 37 amino acids. Amylin (2) has been found to slow the gastric emptying, lower the blood glucose levels by decreasing the glucagon release, and reduce food intake. Further, it has been found that amylin (2) levels are low in patients with Type 1 diabetes and insufficient at mealtime in insulin-using Type 2 diabetes. Amylin (2) as such cannot be adminstered because it is insoluble and aggregates in solution. Pramlintide (3), an analog of amylin (2), in which Ala 25, Ser 28, and Ser 29 have been replaced by proline, has higher water solubility and lower aggregation characteristics than amylin (2). Pramlintide (3) is administered by subcutaneous route. Pramlintide (3) is an agonist of amylin (2) receptor which are located in brain. Binding of pramlintide (3) to amylin receptors results in reduced GI motility and reduced food intake.

```
                   2                         7                              15
          Lys—Cys—Asn—Thr—Ala—Thr—Cys—Ala—Thr—Gln—Arg—Leu—Ala—Asn—Phe
                   |                         |                               |
                   S————————————————————————S                              Leu
                                                                            |
  NH2                                                                       Val
   |                                                                        |
  Tyr—Thr—Asn—Ser—Gly—Val—Asn—Thr—AA29—AA28—Leu—Ile—AA25—Gly—Phe—Asn—Asn—Ser—Ser—His
  37                        30             27          24                      19
```

(2), AA_{25} = Ala; AA_{28} = AA_{29} = Ser

(3), AA_{25} = AA_{28} = AA_{29} = Pro

ORAL HYPOGLYCEMIC AGENTS

At present, various classes of orally active hypoglycemic agents, active in type 2 diabetes, are known. These include sulphonylureas, meglitinides, thiazolidinediones, and biguanides

Sulphonylureas

The observation that 5-isopropyl-2-sulphanilamido-1, 3, 4-thiadiazole (4) showed marked hypoglycemic activity led to discovery of sulphonylureas. At present number of sulphonylueas are known. The earlier sulphonylureas, also known as first generation sulphonylureas include carbutamide (5), tolbutamide (6), chlorpropamide (7), tolazamide (8), and acetohexamide (9), possessed low potency. The second generation sulphonylures which have higher potency include glyburide [glibenclamide, (10)], glipizide (11), and glimepiride (12).

First generation sulphonylureas

(4)

(5)

(6)

(7)

(8)

(9)

Second generation sulphonylureas

(10)

(11)

(12)

Structure-activity relationship studies have shown that for hypoglycemic activity the substituent on nitrogen which is not attached to sulphonyl group should carry a bulky aliphatic group. Further, in the first generation sulphonylureas the substituents on aromatic ring were simple atoms or a group of atoms, however, in the second generation sulphonylureas, the compounds with larger substituents on aromatic ring were more potent.

Sulphonylureas act by inhibiting the β-cells K^+/ATP channel at SUR 1 (sulphonylurea receptor 1). This results in blockade of potassium efflux. The resulting depolarization activates voltage gated Ca^{2+} channel thereby, stimulating the influx of Ca^{2+}. Influx of Ca^{2+} mediates fusion of insulin containing secretory vesicles with plasma membrane leading to stimulation of insulin secretion. K^+/ATP Channel is an octamer and is made up of Kir 6.2 and SUR 1 subunits. ATP binds and inhibits Kir 6.2 while as sulphonylureas bind and inhibits SUR 1. Both ATP and sulphonylurea stimulate the insulin secretion.

Meglitinides

Meglitinides are non-sulphonyluras which show their hypoglycemic effect by the same mechanism as sulphonylureas. Some of these include repaglinide (13) and nateglinide (14). Although meglitinides, like sulphonylureas, also act on SUR 1 component of K^+/ATP channel but both of them bind at two distinct region of SUR 1.

(13)

(14)

Biguanides

Biguanides which have gained clinical acceptance include, phenylethylbiguanide or phenformin (15) and dimethylbiguanide or metformin (16).

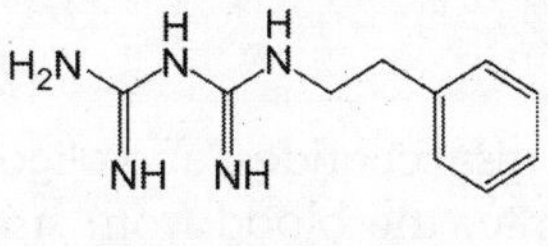

(15) 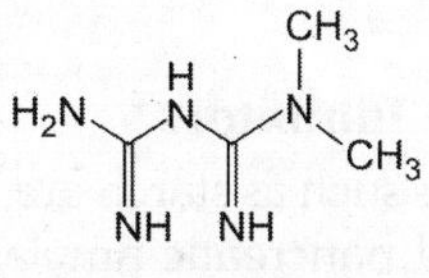   (16)

Biguanides act by increasing sensitivity to insulin and AMP dependent protein kinase (AMPPK) is the target of biguanides. They activate AMPPK to block the breakdown of fatty acid and inhibit hepatic gluconeogenesis and glycogenolysis. Further, there is increased activity of insulin receptor as well as increased insulin action in liver and skeletal muscles. These effects are coupled with inhibition of glucose absorption from intestines. All these effects lead to decreased blood glucose levels.

Thiazolidinediones

Thiazolidinediones or glitazones include ciglitazone (17), troglitazone (18), rosiglitazone (19) pioglitazone (20) rivoglitazone (21) netoglitazone (22), and englitazone (23).

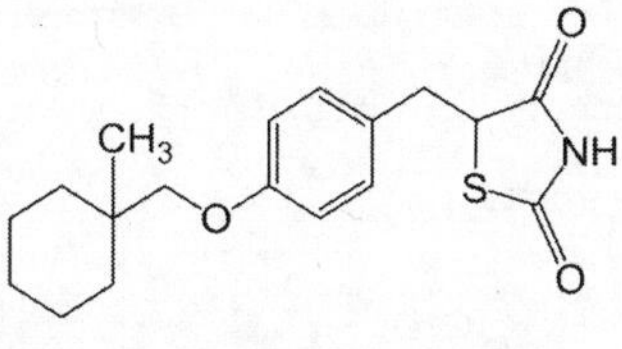

(17) 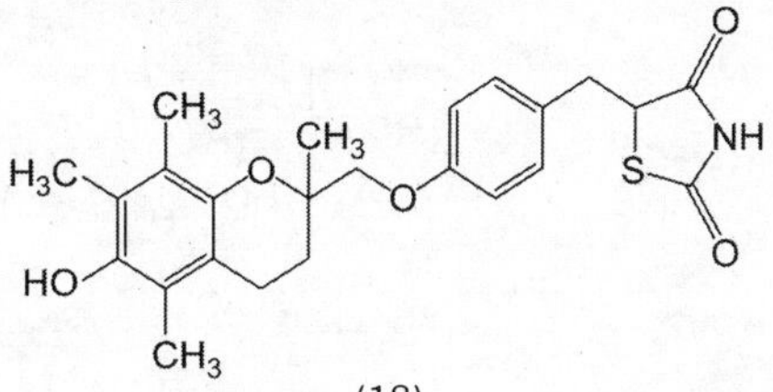   (18)

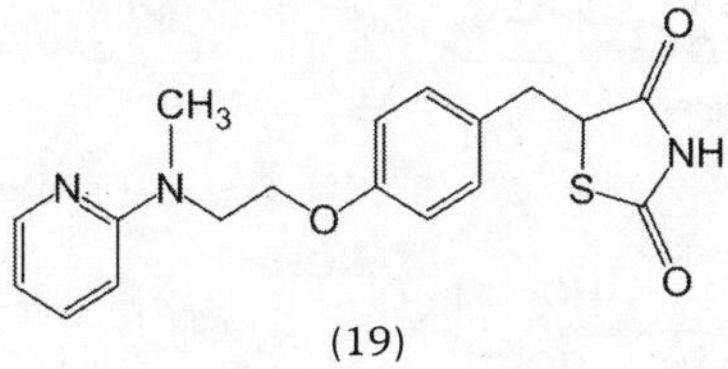

(19) 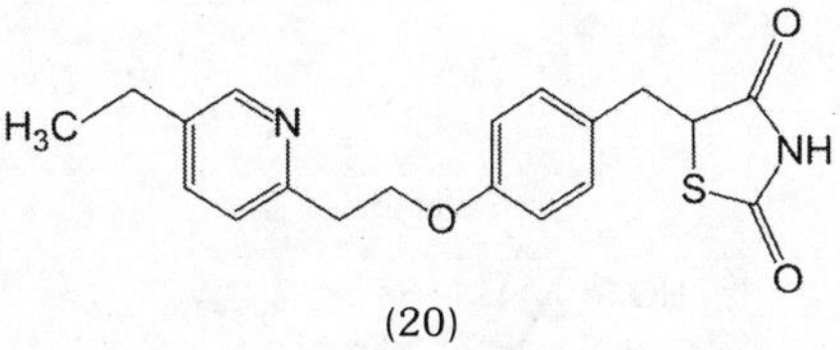   (20)

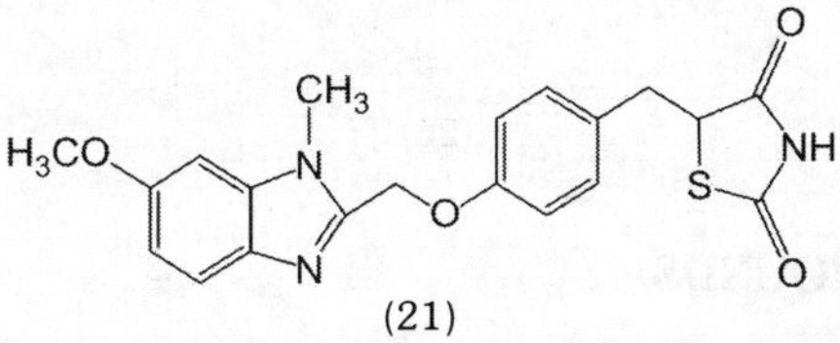

(21) 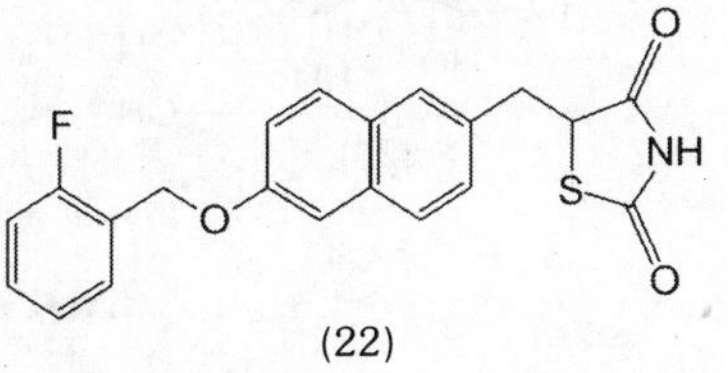   (22)

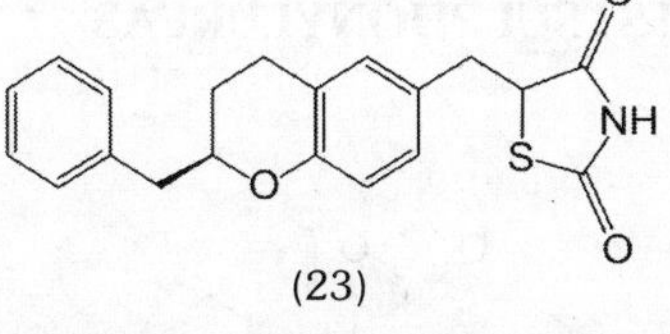

(23)

Like biguanides, thiazolidinediones increase insulin sensitivity not only in adipose tissue but also in liver and muscles. However, their mechanism is different.

Thiazolidinediones are agonists for hormone receptor Peroxisome Proliferator Activator Receptor-γ (PPAR-γ). The activation of PPAR-γ activates transcription of a subset of genes involved in glucose and lipid metabolism. The insulin-sensitivity effect has been found to have beneficial effect on type 2 diabetes.

α-Glucosidase Inhibitors

Polysaccharides such as starch are hydrolyzed to disaccharides, trisaccharides, and oligosaccharides by salivary and pancreatic amylases. The oligosaccharides enter the blood from small intestine after hydrolysis to monosaccharides. The enzymes responsible for hydrolysis to monosaccharides, the α-glucosidases, are located in brush border of small intestines. Use of inhibitors of α-glucosidases could lead to inhibition of hydrolysis of polysaccharides and lower absorption of glucose and consequent lower blood glucose level. The mechanism of action of α-glucosidases is, therefore, not dependent on presence of insulin. One of the α-glucosidase inhibitors is acarbose (24). Studies have shown that acarbose (24) slowed down glucose absorption but not prevented it completely. This could help in lowering of daily insulin dose. Since there is very small absorption of acarbose (24) in blood, its toxicity is almost neglegible. Other α-glycosidase inhibitors include voglibose (25) and miglitol (26).

(24)

(25)

(26)

INDIVIDUAL COMPOUNDS

ORAL HYPOGLYCEMIC AGENTS : SULPHONYLUREAS

Carbutamide
1-Butyl-3-sulphanilylurea

Synthesis

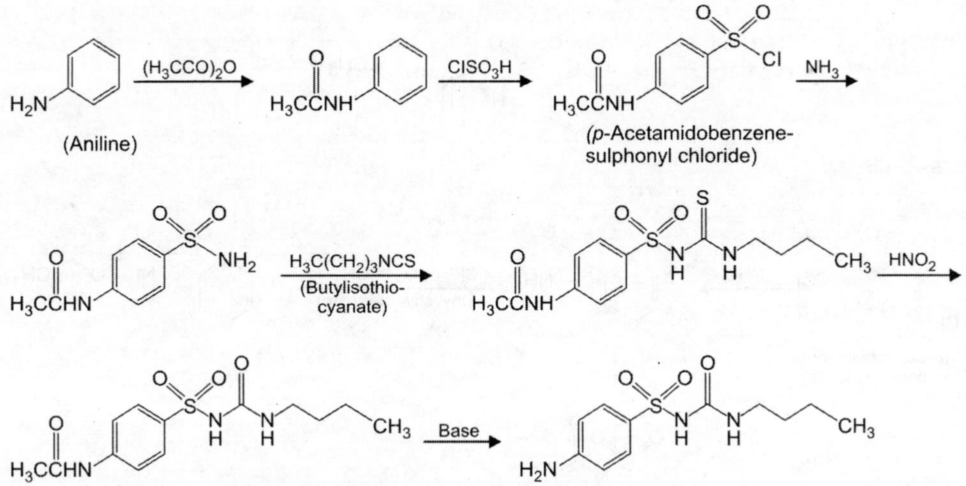

It is a first generation sulphonylurea not used nowadays.

Tolbutamide

1-Butyl-3-(p-tolylsulphonyl)urea

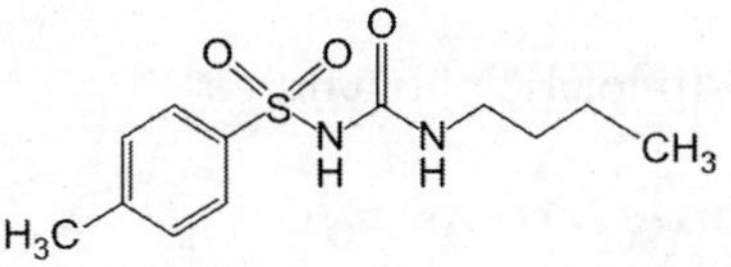

Synthesis

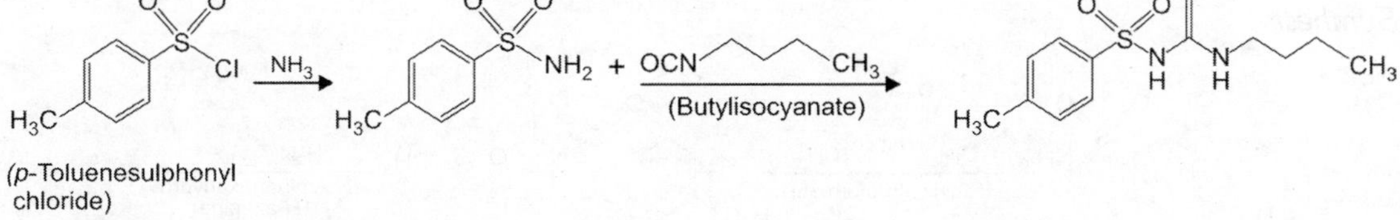

It is a first generation sulphonylurea. It is absorbed rapidly and is oxidized to *p*-carboxy derivative (27) which is inactive.

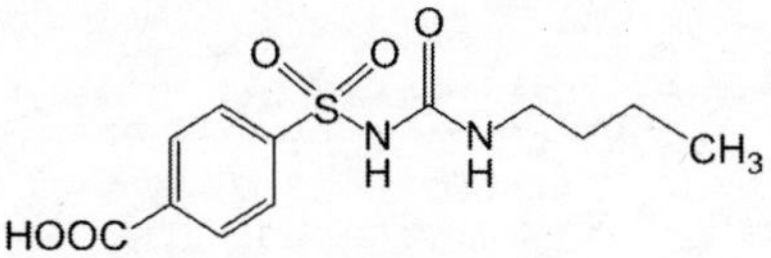

(27)

Chlorpropamide

1-(*p*-Chlorophenylsulphonyl)-3-propylurea

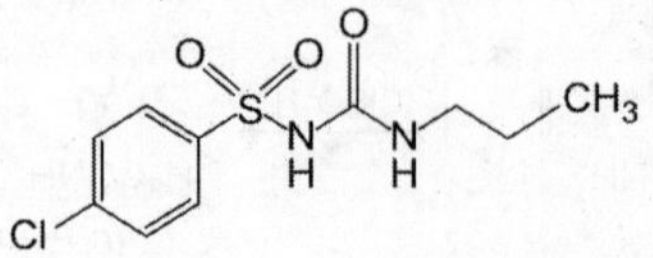

Synthesis

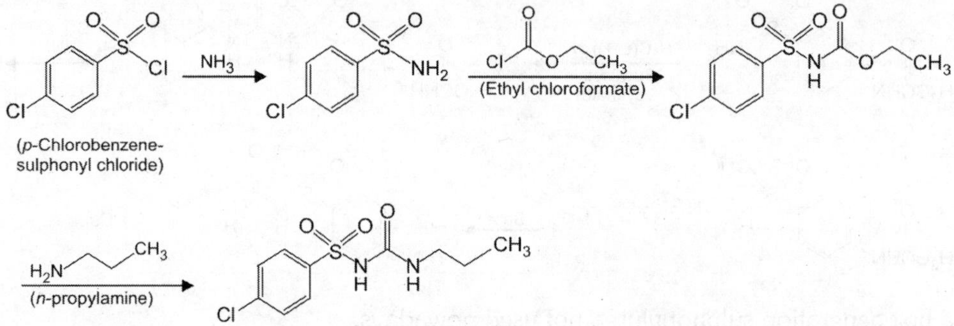

It is a first generation sulphonylurea. It is resistant to metabolic degradation and therefore, has longer duration of action.

Tolazamide

1-(Hexahydro-1*H*-azepin-1-yl)-3-(*p*-tolylsulphonyl)urea

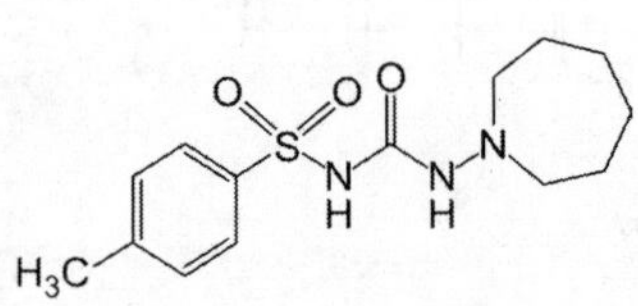

Synthesis

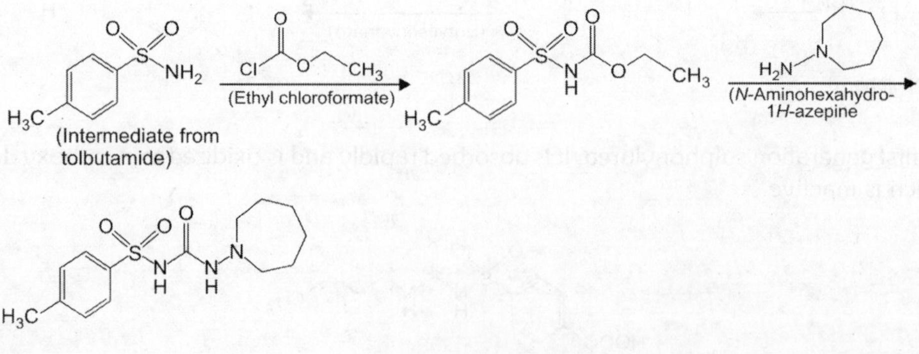

It is a first generation sulphonylurea. It is an analog of tolbutamide (6) but is more active than it.

Acetohexamide

1-[(*p*-Acetylphenyl)sulphonyl]-3-cyclohexylurea

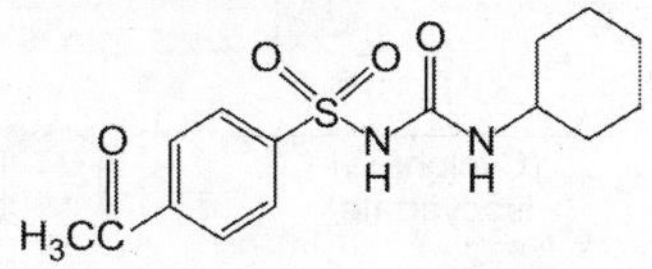

Synthesis

(*p*-Aminoacetophenone)

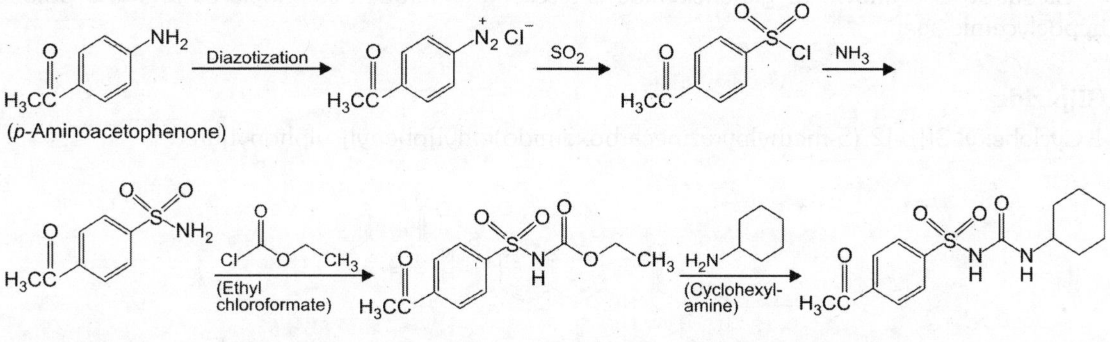

It is a first generation sulphonylurea. It is metabolized to α-hydroxy derivative [(*S*)-form) (28)] which is the active form of the drug.

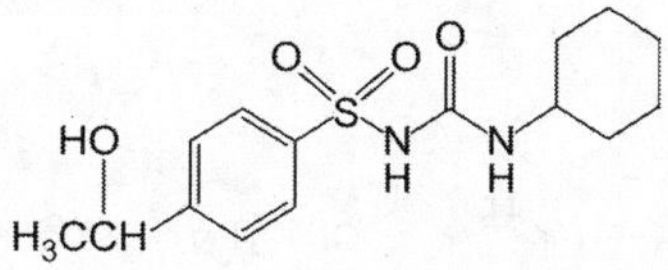

(28)

Glyburide

N-[4-(β-(2-Methoxy-5-chlorobenzamido)ethyl)benzosulphonyl]-*N*′-cyclohexylurea

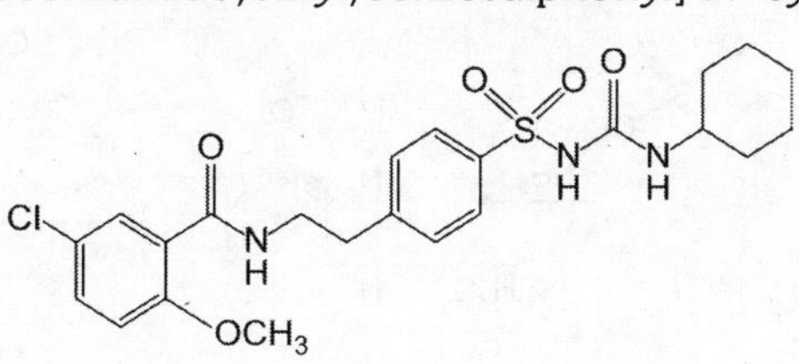

Synthesis

(2-Methoxy-5-
chlorobezoyl chloride)

(2′-Aminoethyl-*p*-benzene
sulphonyl chloride)

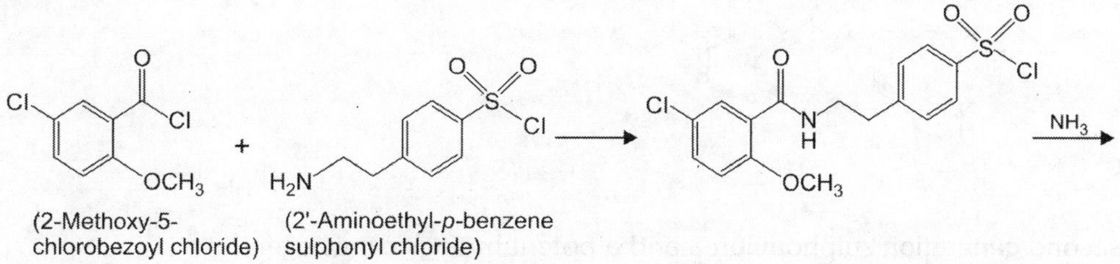

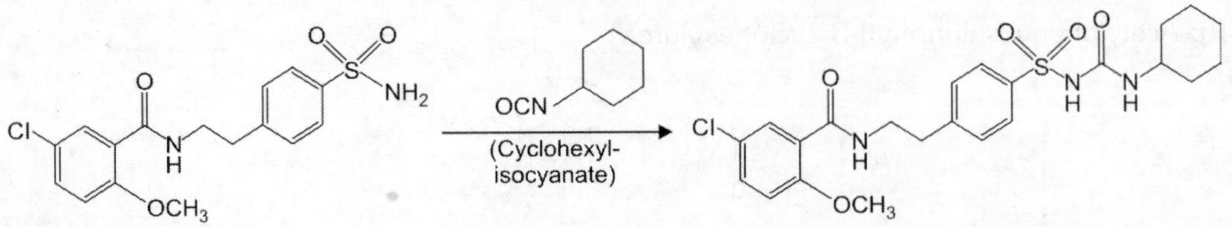

Glyburide also known as glibenclamide is a second generation sulphoylurea and is a potent hypoglycemic agent.

Glipizide

1-Cyclohexyl-3[[p-[2-(5-methylpyrazinecarboxamido)ethyl]phenyl]sulphonyl]urea

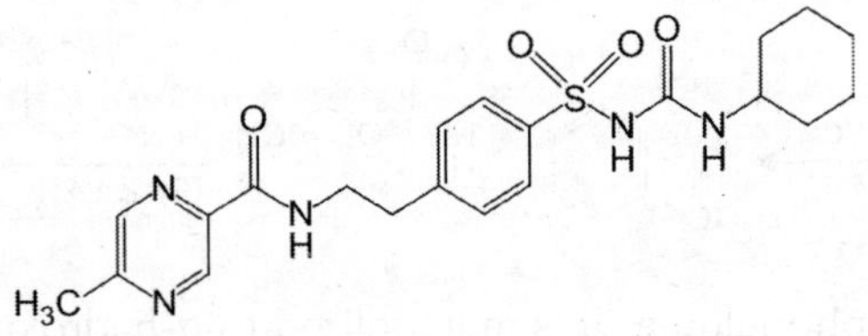

Synthesis

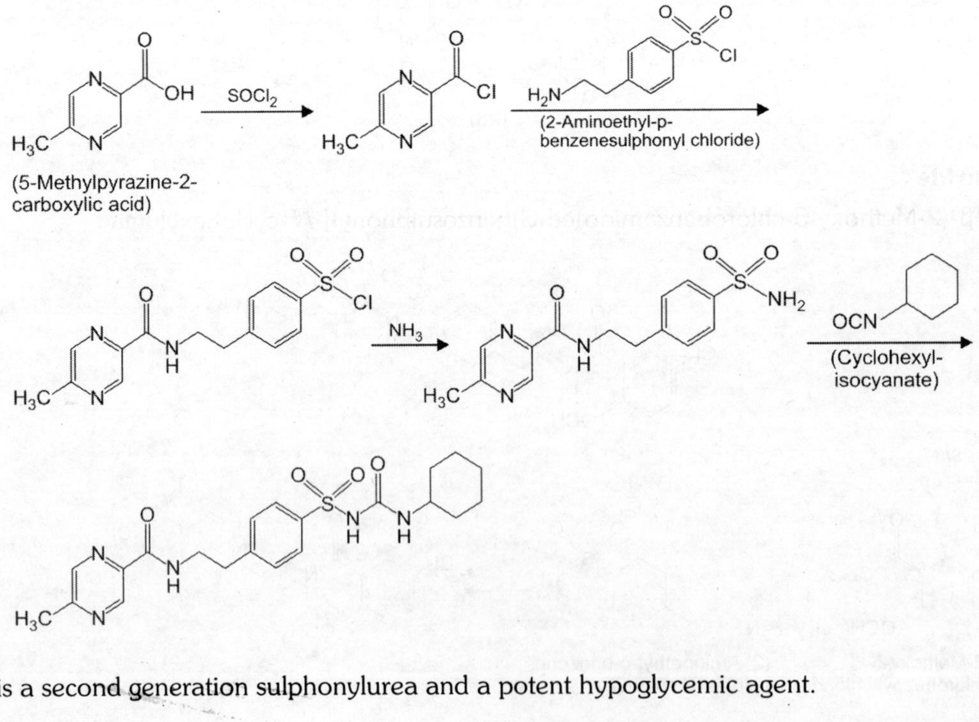

It is a second generation sulphonylurea and a potent hypoglycemic agent.

Glimepiride

1-[4-[2-(3-Ethyl-4-methyl-2-oxo-3-pyrroline-1-carboxamido)ethyl]phenylsulphonyl]-3-(4-methylcyclohexy)urea

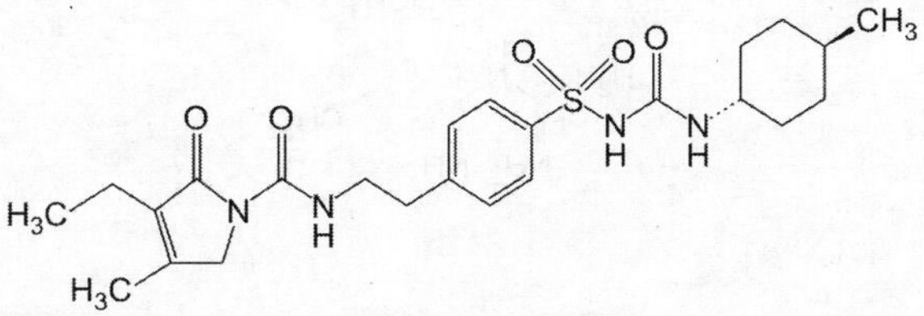

Synthesis

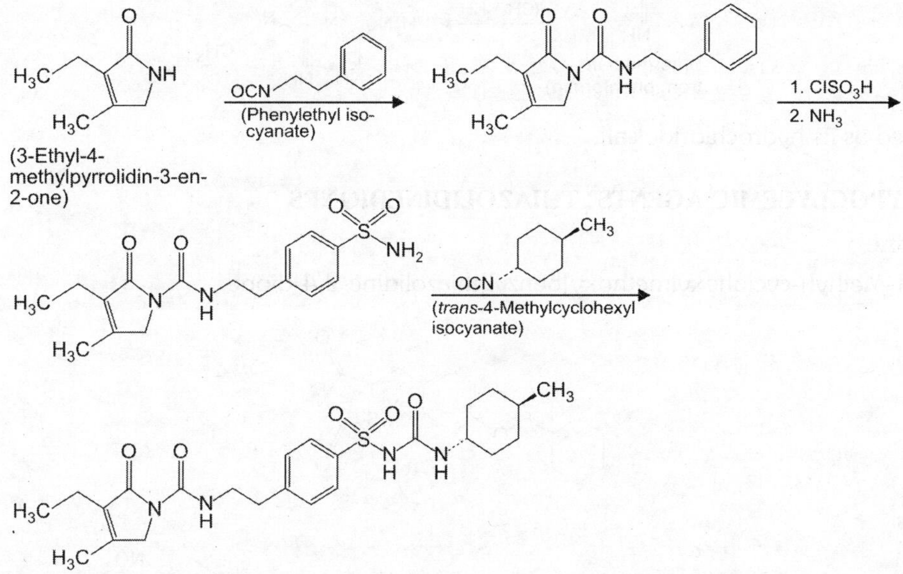

It is a second generation sulphonylurea which has a potent hypoglycemic action.

ORAL HYPOGLYCEMIC AGENTS : BIGUANIDES

Phenformin

1-Phenethylbiguanide

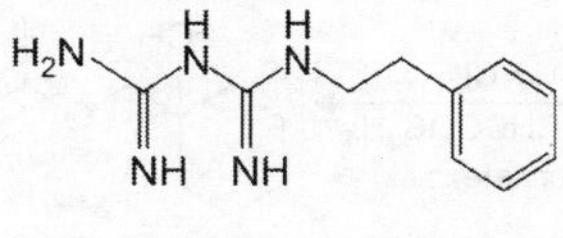

Synthesis

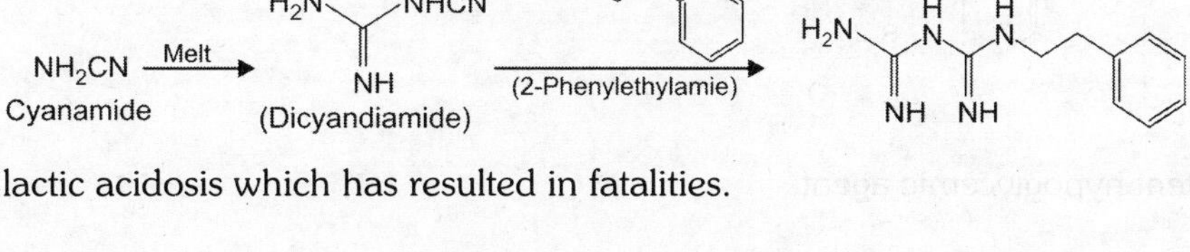

It causes lactic acidosis which has resulted in fatalities.

Metformin

1, 1-Dimethylbiguanide

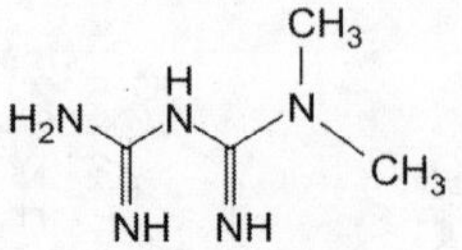

Synthesis

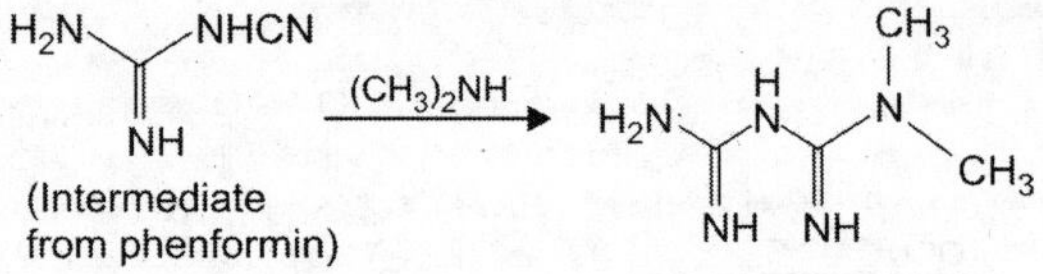

(Intermediate
from phenformin)

It is used as its hydrochloride salt.

ORAL HYPOGLYCEMIC AGENTS : THIAZOLIDINEDIONES

Ciglitazone

5-[4-[1-(1-Methyl)-cyclohexylmethoxy]benzyl]thiazolidine-2,4-dione

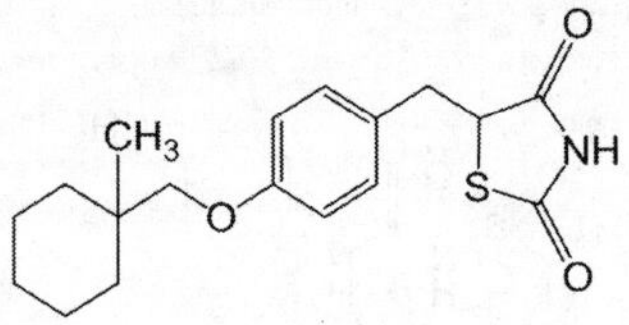

Synthesis

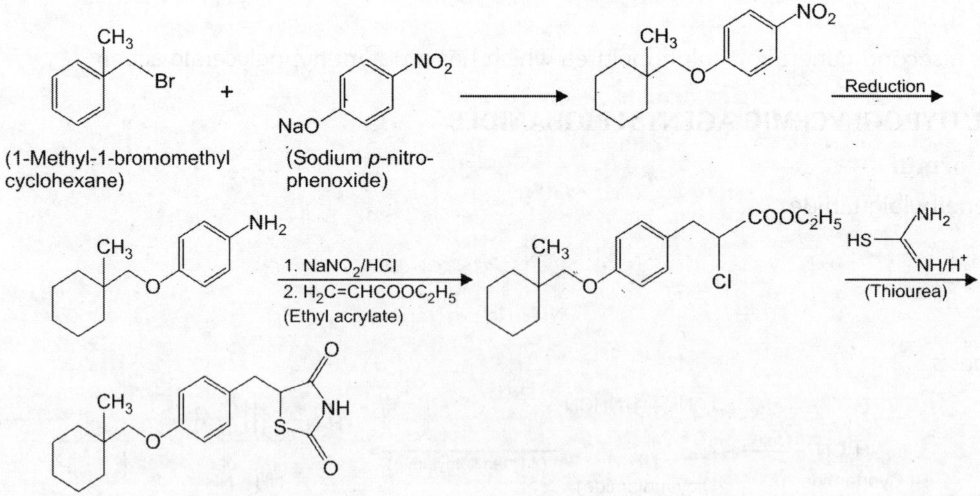

(1-Methyl-1-bromomethyl
cyclohexane)

(Sodium *p*-nitro-
phenoxide)

Reduction

1. NaNO$_2$/HCl
2. H$_2$C=CHCOOC$_2$H$_5$
(Ethyl acrylate)

(Thiourea)

It is a potent hypoglycemic agent.

Troglitazone

5-[4-[2-(2,5,7,8-tetramethyl-6-hydroxy)chromanmethoxy]benzyl]thiazolidine-2,4-dione

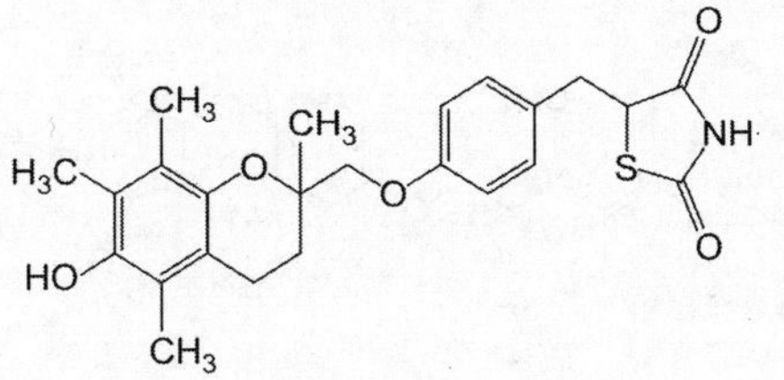

Synthesis

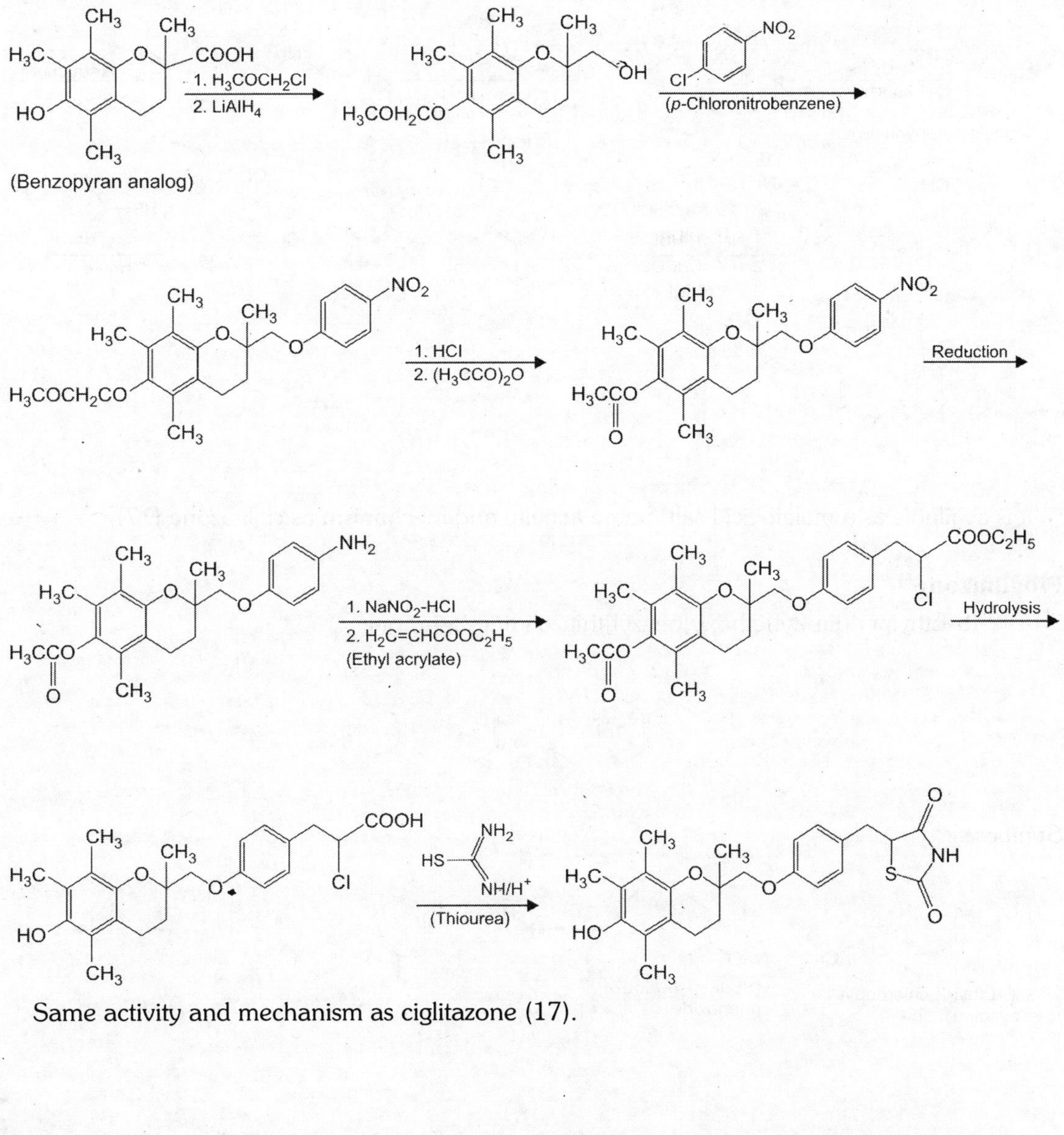

(Benzopyran analog)

Same activity and mechanism as ciglitazone (17).

Rosiglitazone

5-[4-[2-(*N*-methyl-*N*-(2-pyridinyl)amino)ethoxy]benzyl]thiazolidine-2,4-dione

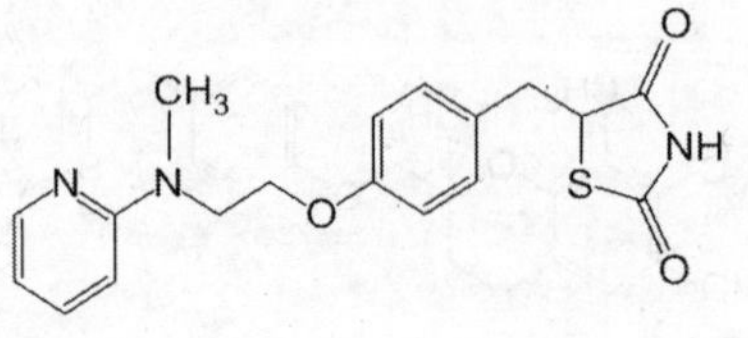

Synthesis

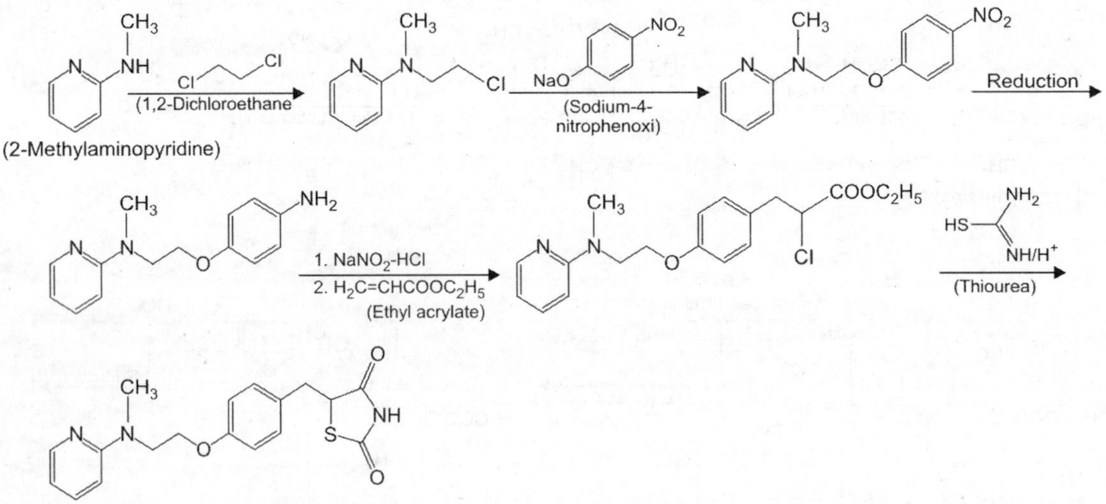

It is available as a maleic acid salt. Same activity and mechanism as ciglitazone (17).

Pioglitazone

5-(4-[2-(5-Ethylpyridin-2yl)ethoxy]benzyl]thiazolidine-2,4-dione

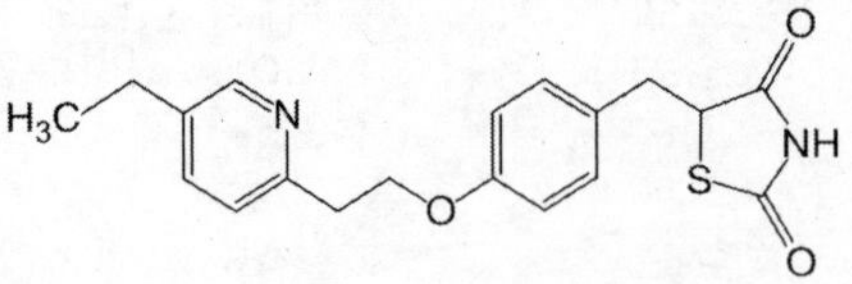

Synthesis

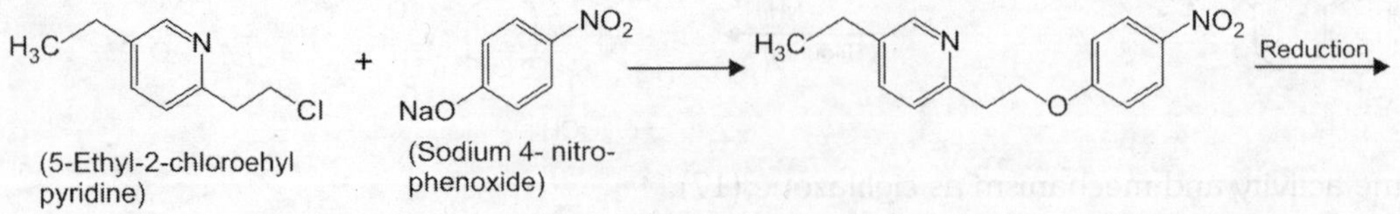

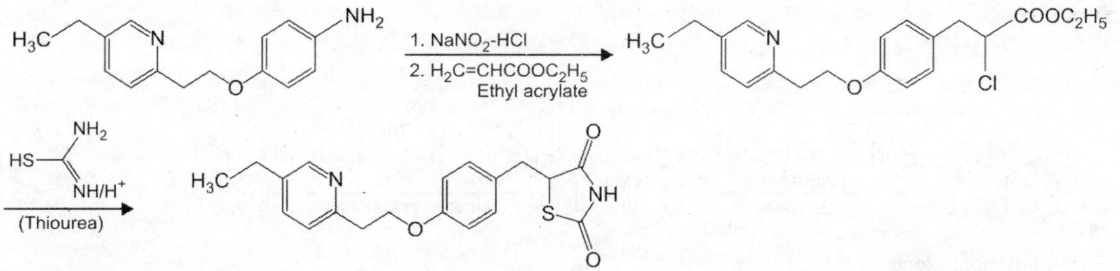

It is available as its hydrochloride salt. Same activity and mechanism as cighiazome (17).

Rivoglitazone

5-[4-[2-(1-Methyl-6-methoxybenzimidazolyl)methoxy]benzyl]thiazolidene-2,4-dione

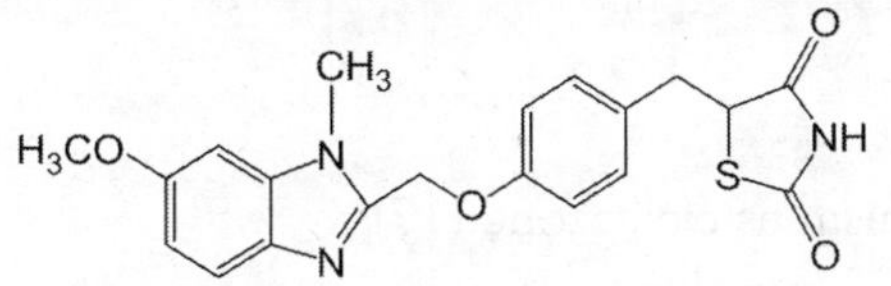

Synthesis

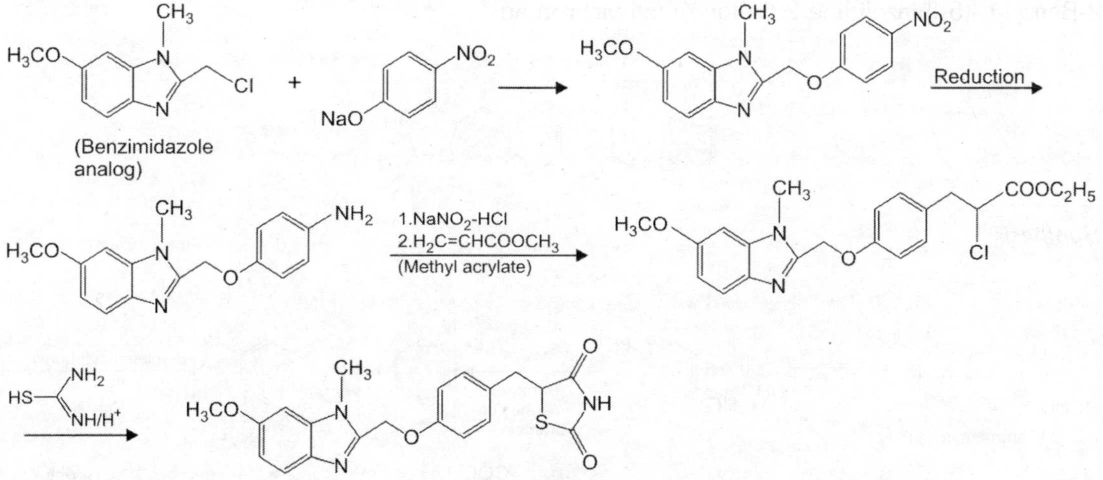

Same activity and mechanism as ciglitazone (17).

Netoglitazone

5-[6-(2-Fluorobenzyloxy)2-naphthylmethyl]thiazolidine-2,4-dione

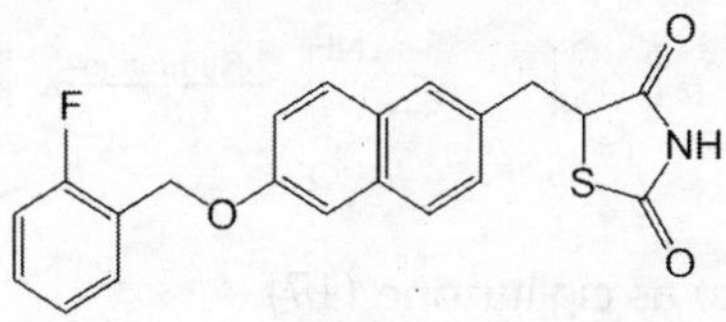

Synthesis

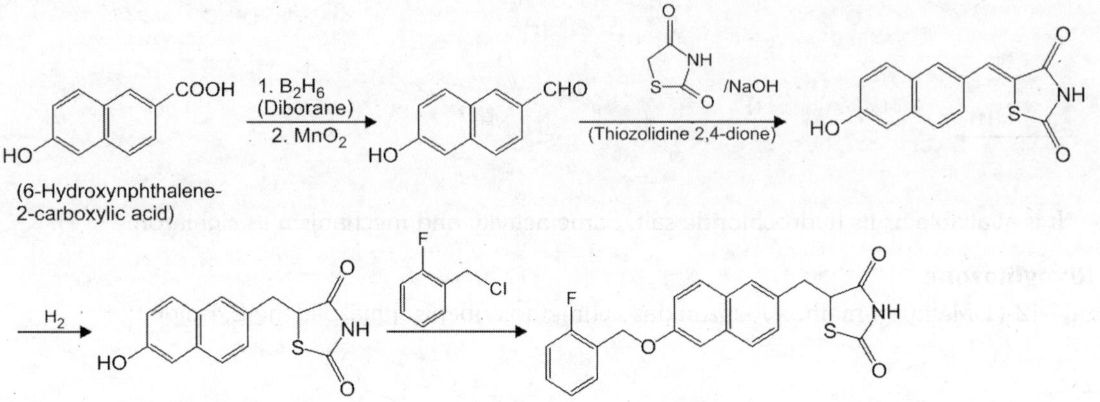

Same activity and mechanism as ciglitazone (17).

Englitazone

2-Benzyl-6-(5-thiazolidine-2,4-dione)methylchroman

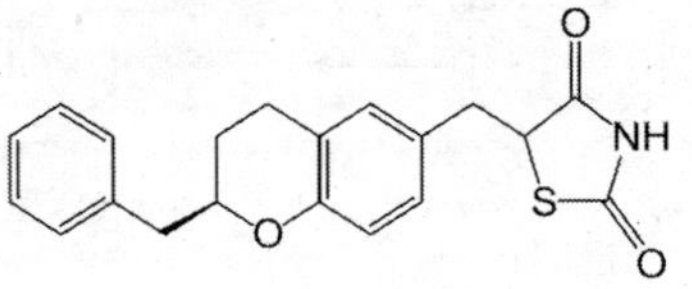

Synthesis

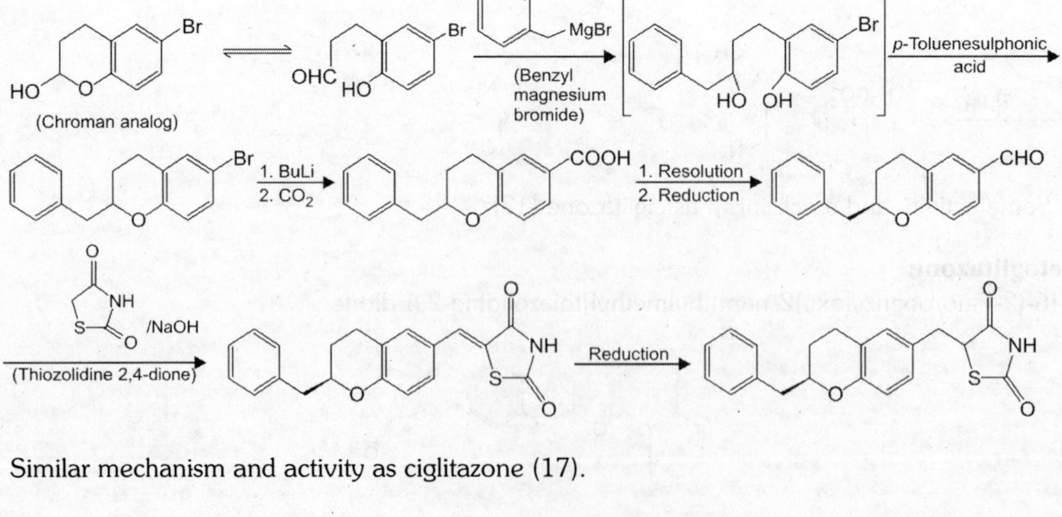

Similar mechanism and activity as ciglitazone (17).

CHAPTER 19

THYROID AND ANTITHYROID DRUGS

THYROID GLAND, which consists of two lobes, is located deep in the neck and close to trachea. Thyroid gland secretes two types of hormones, one of these is associated with energy metabolism and include thyroxine or T_4 (1) and triiodothyronine or T_3 (2). The second type of thyroid hormone is calcitonin, a hormone which regulates the calcium metabolism. The term 'thyroid hormone' is usually associated with thyroxine (1) and triiodothyronine (2).

(1), R = I
(2), R = H

The iodothyronines, thyroxine (1), and triiodothyronine (2), are associated with energy metabolism. Decreased activity of thyroid gland results in decreased production of thyroid hormones, a condition which is known as hypothyroidism. It results in:

(a) Weight gain,
(b) cold and coarse skin,
(c) depressed central nervous system activity resulting in drowsiness and memory impairment, and
(d) slow speech.

Increased activity of thyroid gland results in increased hormone production, a condition known as hyperthyroidism. The clinical symptoms of hyperthyroidism include:

(a) Increased metabolic processes resulting in weight loss, warm and moist skin,
(b) increased central nervous system activity resulting in insomnia, anxiety and nervousness, and
(c) hyperactive tendon reflexes, sensitivity to sympathetic amines, tachycardia, palpitation and increased systolic hypertension.

BIOSYNTHESIS OF THYROID HORMONES

Thyroid hormones are synthesized in the follicle of thyroid gland. Thyroglobulin, a glycoprotein containing tyrosine residues, is synthesized and secreted into the lumen of the follicle where the iodination of the tyrosine residues takes place.

607

Iodine, in form of iodide from food and water, is absorbed from gastrointestinal tract. Once absorbed the thyroid gland removes it from blood and stores it in the gland. The uptake of plasma iodide by thyroid is energy-dependent and is taken up by Iodide pump [(sodium iodide symporter, (NIS)]. The energy being provided by Na^+/K^+-ATPase. The iodide is next oxidized to hypoidous acid (HOI) by TP-O, a radical intermediate formed from thyroperoxidase (TP) and hydrogen peroxide (H_2O_2). The HOI so formed iodinates the tyrosine residues in thyroglobulin. This iodination may result in mono- and di-iodination at the position ortho to the phenolic hydroxyl group of the tyrosine residues. Next, the mono- and di-iodinated residues combine to form triiodothyronine (2) and combination of two di-iodinated residues results in thyroxine (1). These are then cleaved from thyroglobulin by proteases (Fig. 19.1).

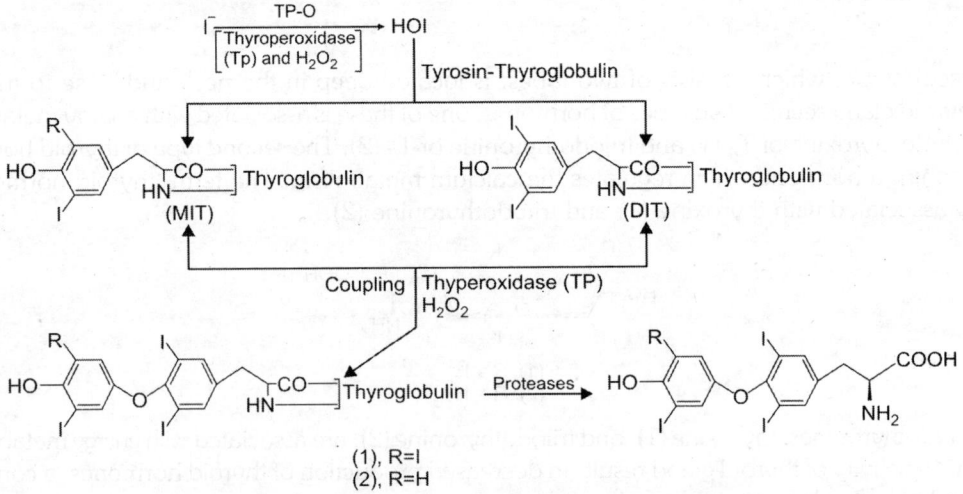

Fig. 19.1: Biosynthesis of thyroid hormones.

(MIT-monoiodothyroglobulin; DIT-diiodothyroglobulin.)

The hormone secretion of thyroid gland is regulated by hypothalamus through thyrotropin releasing hormone (TRH) and somatostatin. TRH stimulates anterior pituitary releasing thyroid stimulating hormone (thyrotropin). While somatostatin inhibits the release of thyrotropin. Release of thyrotropin results in production of thyroid hormones from thyroid gland. The other factors which affect the activity of thyroid gland are:

(a) The release of thyrotropin by anterior pituitary is affected by triiodothyronine (2) and thyroxine (1) through negative feed back mechanism.

(b) Reduced plasma concentrations of iodide has stimulating effect on thyroid gland resulting in increased production of hormone, while higher plasma levels of iodide, excess of exogenous iodide, and thioureylenes reduce the activity of thyroid gland.

MECHANISM OF ACTION OF THYROID HORMONES

Thyroxine (1) is a prohormone. It is first degraded to triiodothyronine (2) which binds to a receptor protein in the cell membrane resulting in increased uptake of glucose and amino acids into the cell.

Triiodothyronine (2) also enters the cell by diffusion and binds to cytosol-binding protein. These interactions of triiodothyronine (2) with the receptors result in increased protein synthesis and stimulation of membrane Na^+/K^+-ATPase which results in increase Na^+ and K^+ transport and oxygen uptake and utilization.

HYPOTHYROIDISM

As indicated earlier hypothyroidism is associated with decreased activity of thyroid gland resulting in deficiency of thyroid hormones. Hypothyroidism can occur with or without enlargement of thyroid gland. Severe hypothyroidism results in myoedema. Deficiency of thyroid hormones due to congenital absence of the gland or incomplete development of the gland results in cretinism. It is characterized by retardation of growth and mental retardation.

The treatment for hypothyroidism is replacement therapy. Thyroxine (1) and triiodothyronine (2) are usually given orally.

HYPERTHYROIDISM

Hyperthyroidism, an increased activity of thyroid gland results in:

(a) Diffuse toxic goiter also called Graves' disease or exophthalmic goiter, and

(b) toxic nodular goiter.

Graves' disease is an autoimmune disease caused by thyroid-stimulating globulin.

Toxic nodular goiter is caused by a benign neoplasm or adenoma and may develop in patients with long-standing simple goiter. A simple non-toxic goiter results because of prolonged dietary deficiency of iodine which causes increased plasma levels of TRH and eventually an increase in the size of the thyroid gland. The enlarged thyroid gland produces normal amounts of thyroid hormones. If the deficiency is severe, it may result in hypothyroidism.

Drugs used in hyperthyroidism include radioiodine and thioureylenes.

Radioiodine, ^{131}I is given orally. It is taken-up in the same way as normal iodine and gets incorporated into thyroglobulin. Radioiodine emits both β- and γ-radiations. The β-radiation which has a shorter duration exerts cytotoxic action resulting in destruction of thyroid follicles. Since the half-life of ^{131}I is 8 days, its radioactivity effectively disappears within a short period.

The treatment with ^{131}I may result in hypothyroidism but it is easily managed with replacement therapy.

Thioureylenes include methimazole (3), carbimazole (4), and propylthiouracil (5). These sustances decrease output of thyroid hormones and cause gradual reduction in signs and symptoms of hyperthyroidism. It is believed that they act by inhibiting the iodination of tyrosyl residues in thyroglobulin.

(3)   (4)   (5)

INDIVIDUAL COMPOUNDS

Thyroxine

3,5,3',5'-Tetraiodo-L-thyronine

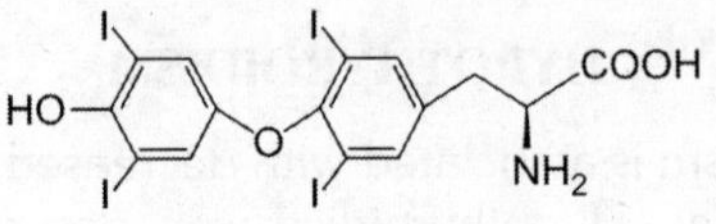

Synthesis

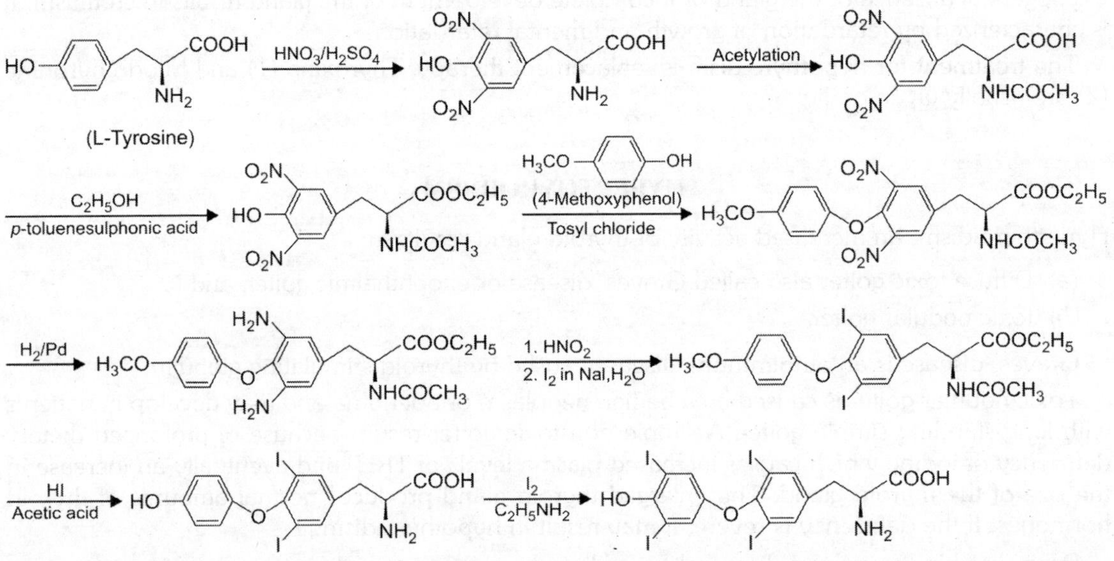

It is a buff coloured solid, soluble in water. It is used as a replacement therapy for decreased thyroid activity.

Methimazole

1-Methylimidazole-2-thiol

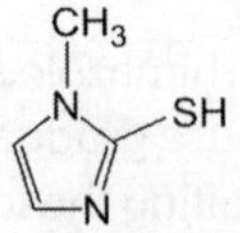

Synthesis

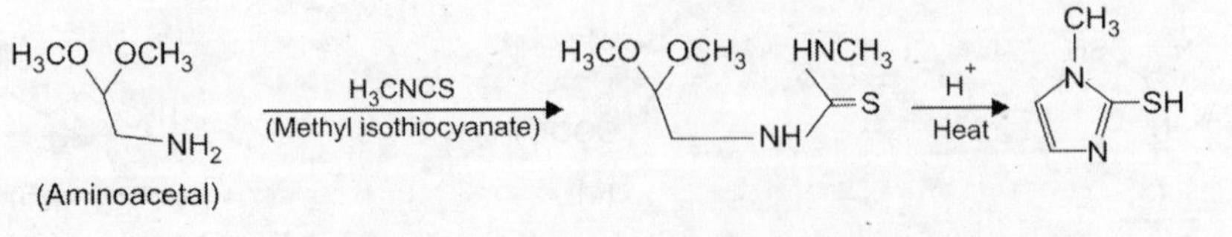

Carbimazole

1-Ethoxycarbonyl-3-methyl-2-thio-4-imidazoline

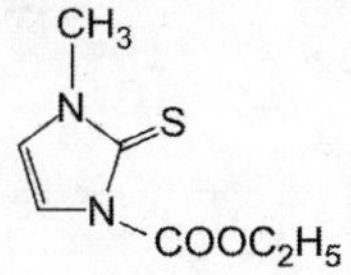

Synthesis

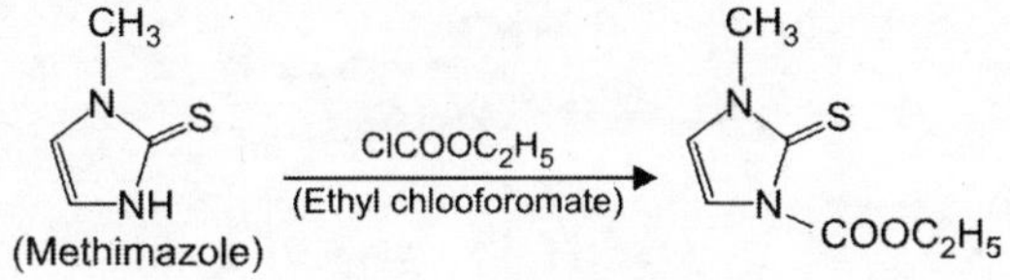

Propylthiouracil

6-Propyl-2-thiouracil

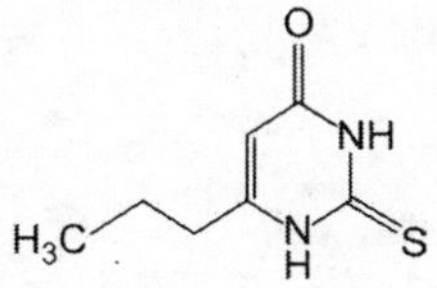

Synthesis

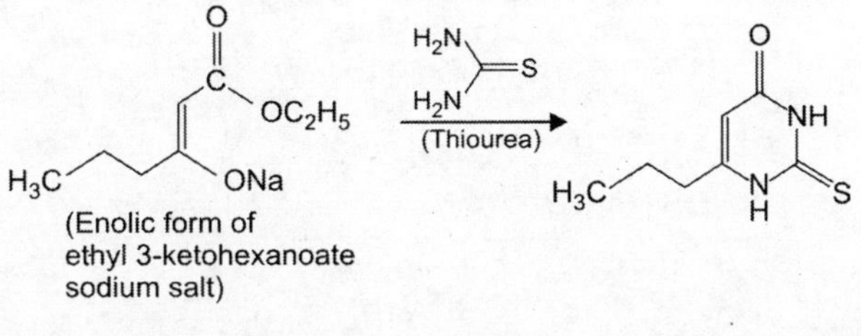

Propylthiouracil is used in Graves' disease and also as an adjunct to radioiodine therapy.

Griseofulvin is used in Onyc... Disease and also as an adjunct to radioiodine therapy.

Section VII
Drugs Affecting Gastrointertinal Functions

Drugs affecting gastrointestinal functions include:

(a) Agents used in control of Acidity and in treatment of Peptic Ulcers,

(b) Agents used as Antiemetics, and

(c) Agents used for the treatment of Constipation, Diarrhea, and Inflammatory Bowl Diseases.

Agents used in control of Acidity and in treatment of Peptic Ulcers have already been covered under Antihistaminics and Antiulcer Agents.

ANTIEMETIC AGENTS

ALTHOUGH vomiting is protective reflex to get rid of toxic substances from stomach and intestines, but certain conditions do need an effective control of emesis and these include motion sickness, pregnancy, hepatitis, and during chemotherapy of cancer. Uncontrolled emesis can also lead to dehydration and depletion of nutrients.

Two sites have been associated with nausea and vomiting and these include Chemoreceptor Trigger Zone (CTZ) and the Vomiting Center.

The CTZ (area postrema) is outside blood-brain barrier and therefore can respond to chemical stimuli in blood or cerebrospinal fluid and relay the information to the vomiting center for triggering nausea or vomiting.

The vomiting center is located in lateral reticular formation of medulla. It receives the information from gut through vagus nerve. The vomiting center also receives information from vestibular system, which functions during motion sickness, the high brain stem, and cortical structures.

The chemotherapeutic agents can activate CTZ or even vomting center. The chemotherapeutic agents also damage the gastrointestinal tract which results in release of serotonin from enterochrmaffin cells. The released serotonin activates 5-HT_3 receptors on vagus which ultimately results in emesis.

ANTIEMETIC AGENTS

The various classes of antiemetic drugs include:

1. Histamine H_1-Receptor Antagonists.
2. Muscarinic Antagonists.
3. Serotonin Receptor Antagonists.
4. Dopamine D_2-Receptor Antagonists.
5. Neurokinin-1 Receptor Blockers.
6. Miscellaneous Agents

Histamine H_1-Receptor Antagonists

These include aminoalkyl ethers like diphenhydramine (1) and its 8-chlorotheophyllinate salt [(dimenhydrinate, (2)]. Piperazine derivatives such as cyclizine (3), meclizine (4), and cinnarizine (5). The phenothiazine derivative include promethazine (6).

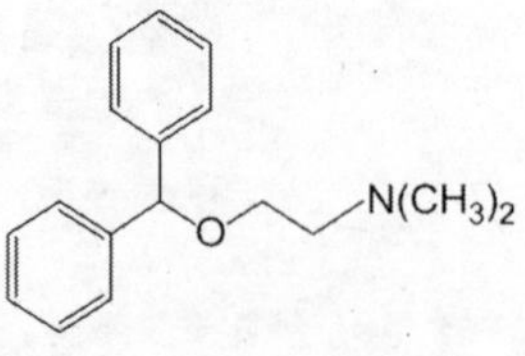

(1)

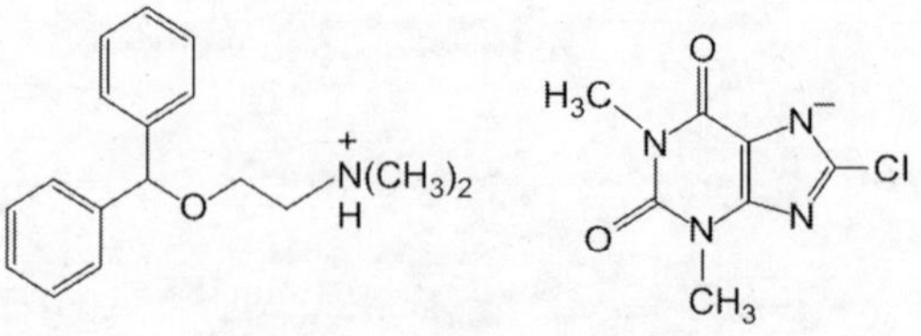

(2)

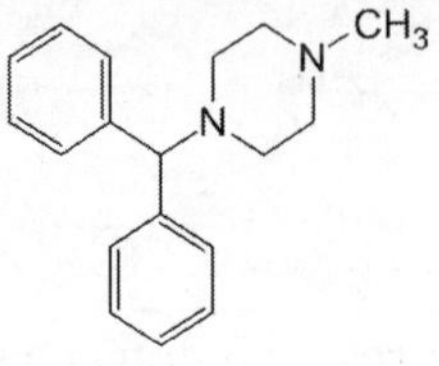

(3)

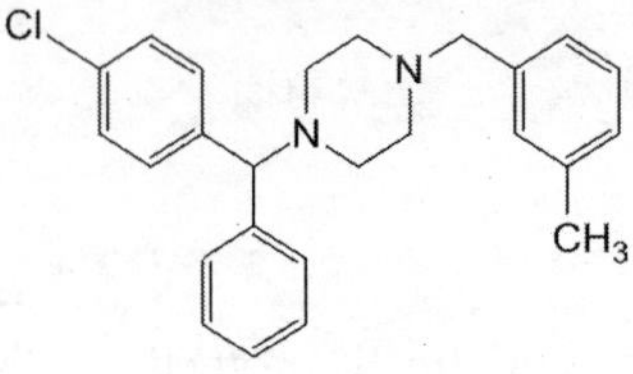

(4)

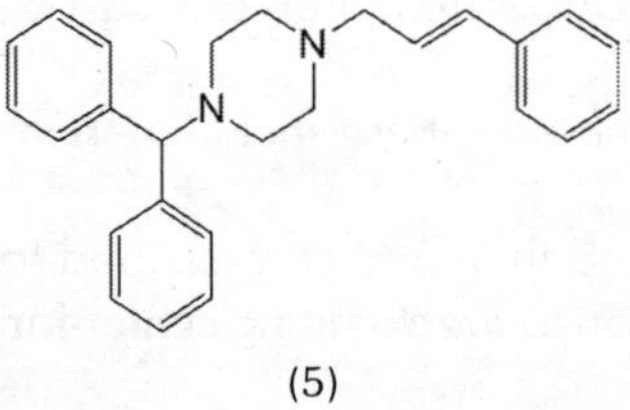

(5)

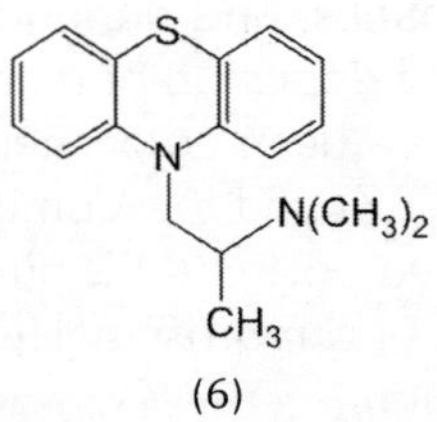

(6)

Antihistaminic H_1-receptor antagonists are effective in motion sickness and postoperative emesis. Promethazine (6) has also been used in morning sickness during pregnancy. They do not have any effect on substances which cause vomiting through action on CTZ.

Muscarinic Antagonists

Among various antimuscarinic agents scopolamine (7) is the most widely used. It is used for prophylaxis and in the treatment of motion sickness as transdermal patches.

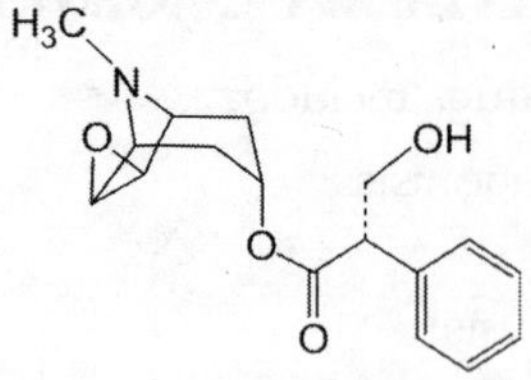

(7)

Serotonin Receptor (5-HT$_3$) Antagonists

These include dolasetron (8), granisetron (9), ondansetron (10), and tropisetron (11). The serotonin receptor antagonists have been found useful in preventing vomiting due to radiation therapy or chemotherapy, particularly by cisplatin. They possess longer duration of action and act primarily at CTZ.

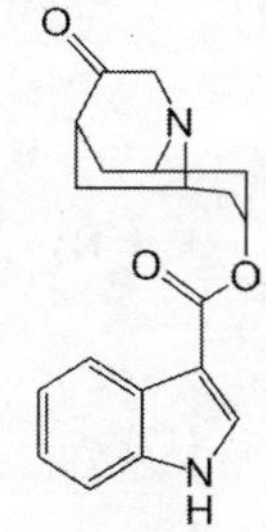

(8)

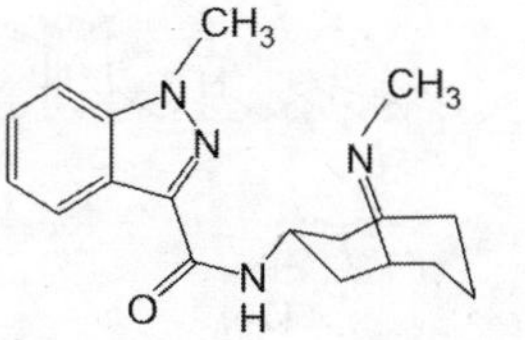

(9)

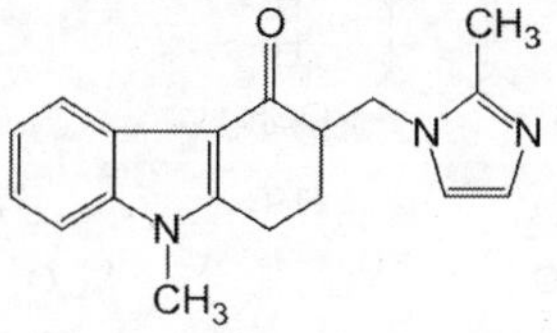

(10)

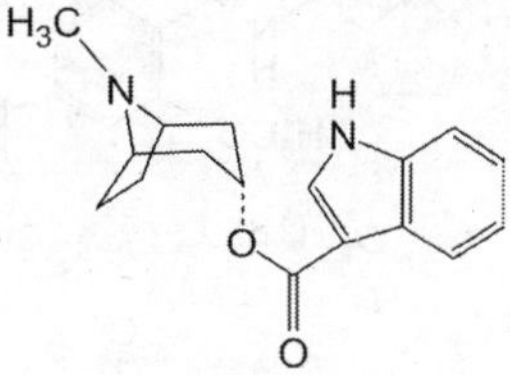

(11)

Dopamine D_2-Receptor Antagonists

The various classes of dopamine D_2-receptor antagonists used as antiemetic agents include phenothiazines, butyrophenones, substituted benzamides, and benzimidazoles.

In addition to their neuroleptic activity, phenothiazines such as chlorpromazine (12), prochlorperazine (13), trifluoperazine (14), and thiethylperazine (15) also possess antiemetic activity. However, out of these, mainly thiethylperazine (15) is used as antiemetic.

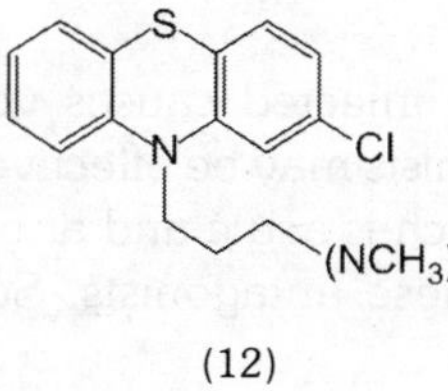

(12)

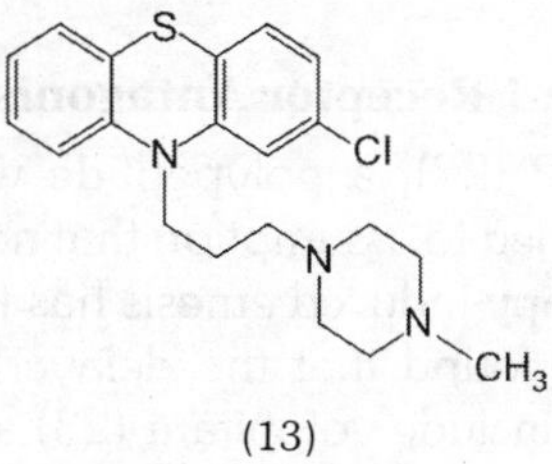

(13)

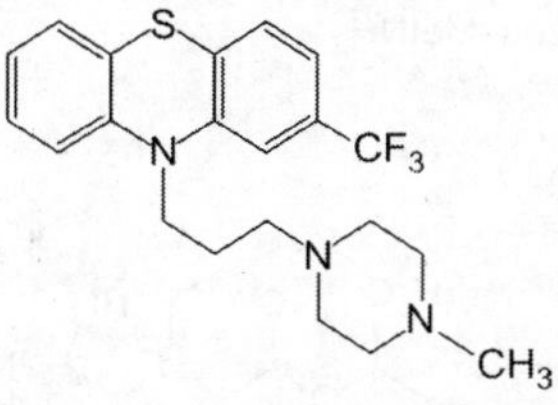

(14)

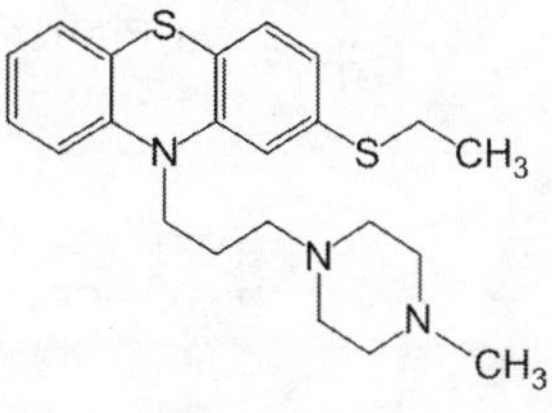

(15)

Neuroleptic butyrophenones such as haloperidol (16) and droperidol (17) have also found use as antiemetic.

The benzamides and benzimidazoles used as antiemetic agents include alizapride (18), metoclopramide (19), trimethobenzamide (20), and domperidone (21).

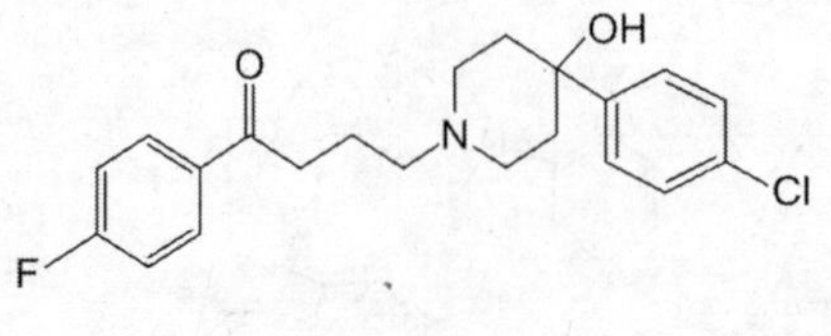

(16)

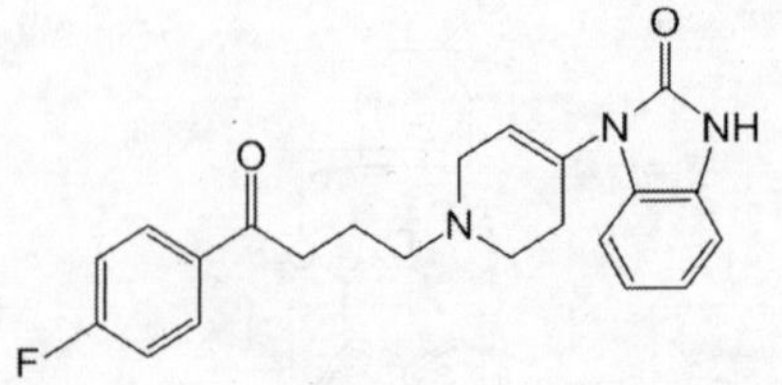

(17)

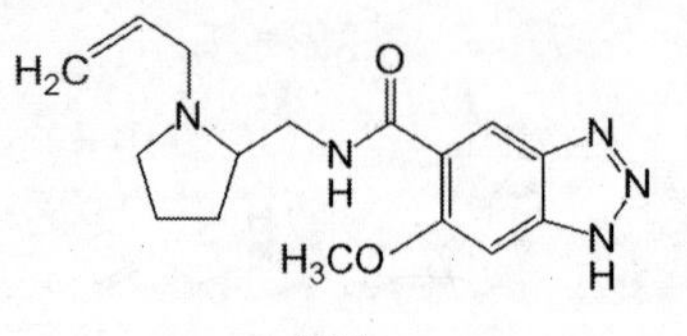

(18)

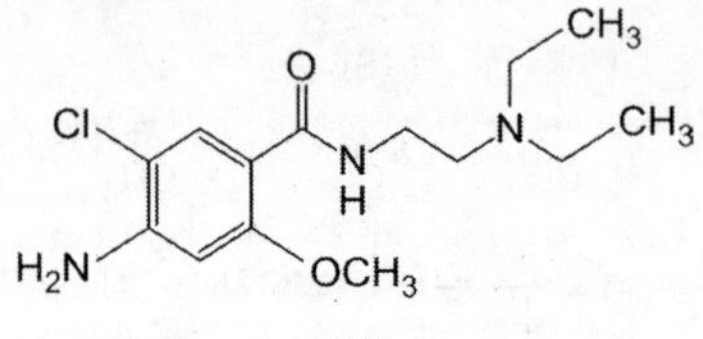

(19)

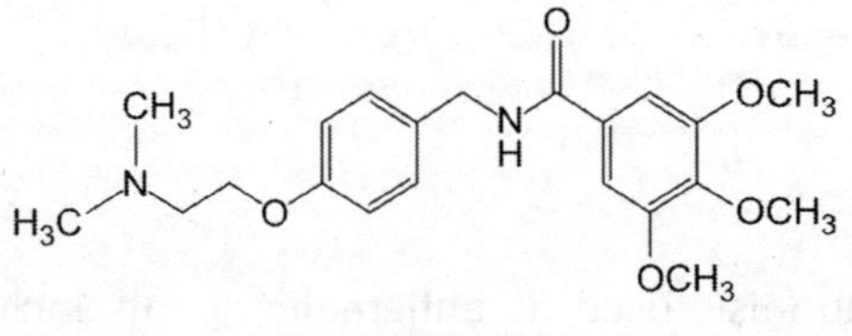

(20)

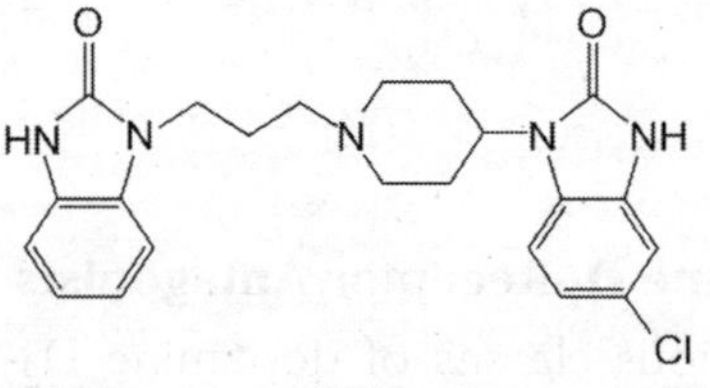

(21)

All these compounds act by blocking dopamine D_2-receptors in CTZ. They have been found to be useful during chemotherapy of cancer. The antidopaminergic side effects include sedation and diarrhea.

Neurokinin-1 Receptor Antagonists

Substance P (22), a polypeptide with 11 amino acids, when injected causes vomiting. This observation led to assumption that neurokinin-1 receptor antagonists may be effective antiemetics. Chemotherapy induced emesis has two components, one of which is acute and another delayed. It has been found that the delayed emesis is prevented by these antagonists. Some of these antagonists include vofopitant (23) and aprepitant (24).

Arg–Pro–Lys–Pro–Gln–Gln–Phe–Phe–Gly–Leu–MetNH$_2$

(22)

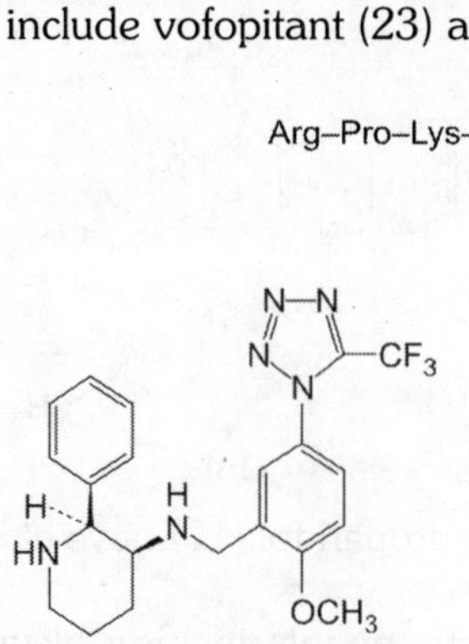

(23)

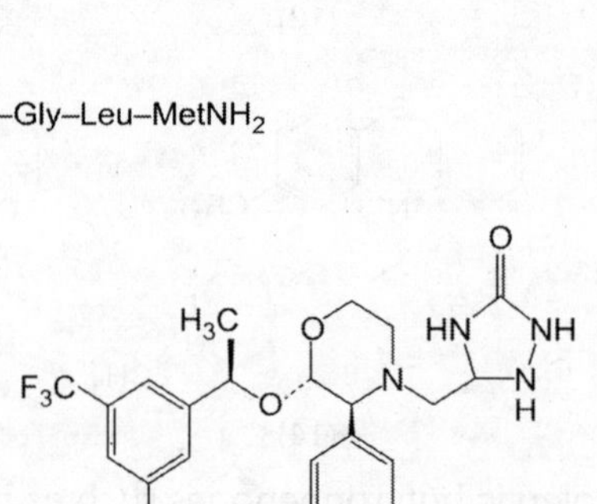

(24)

Miscellaneous Agents

These include benzodiazepines, corticosteroids, and cannabinoids.

Among benzodiazepines, the anxiolytics alprazolam (25) and lorazepam (26) have been used as antiemetics. Their effect may be due to their anxiolytic properties.

Corticosteroids, such as dexamethasone (27) and 6α-methylprednisolone (28), when used alone are effective against mild to moderate chemotherapy induced emesis. They are most frequently used in combination with other agents. They act by blockade of prostaglandin synthesis.

Among the cannabinoids, nabilone (29) and dronabinol (30) have been found to be effective against emesis caused by chemotherapy. Their exact mechanism is not known.

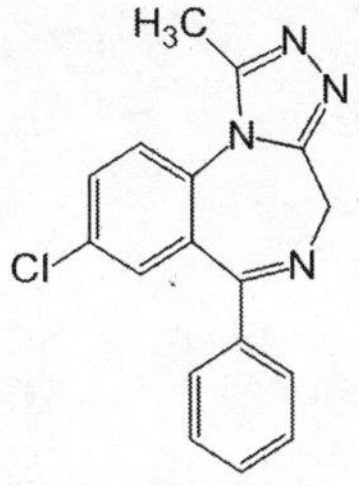

(25) 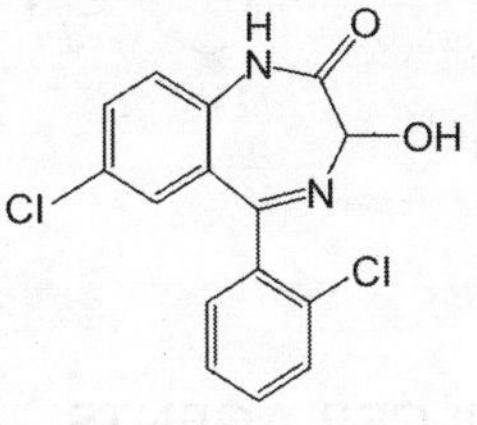   (26) 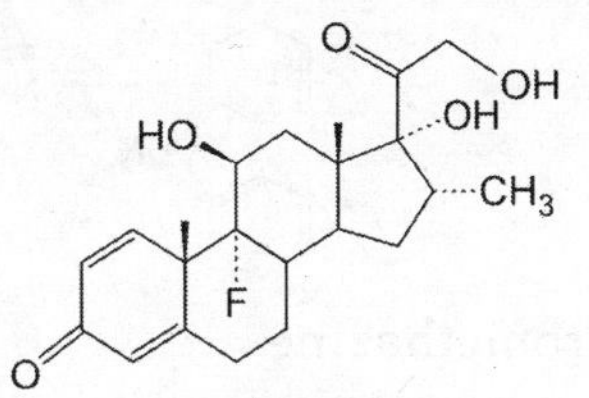   (27)

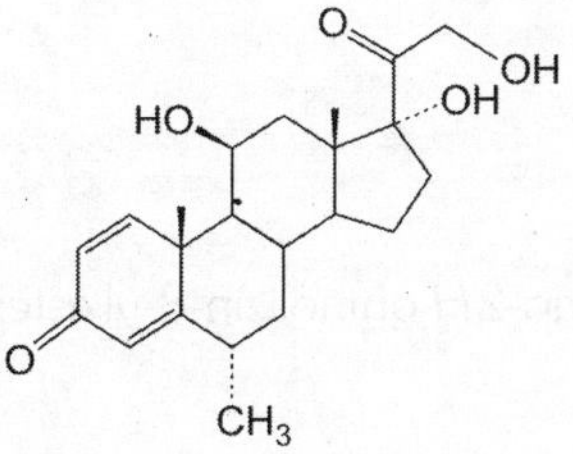

(28) 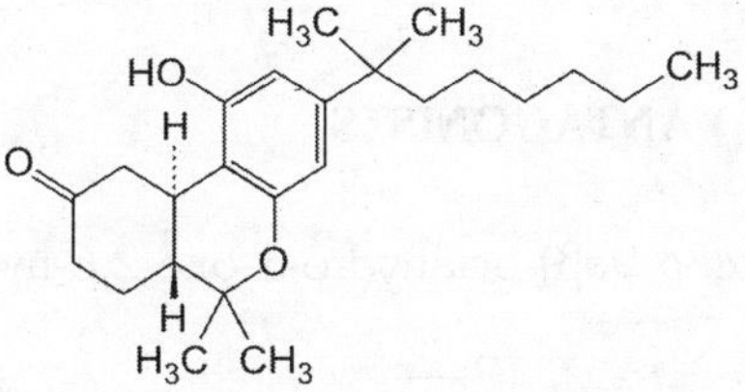   (29) 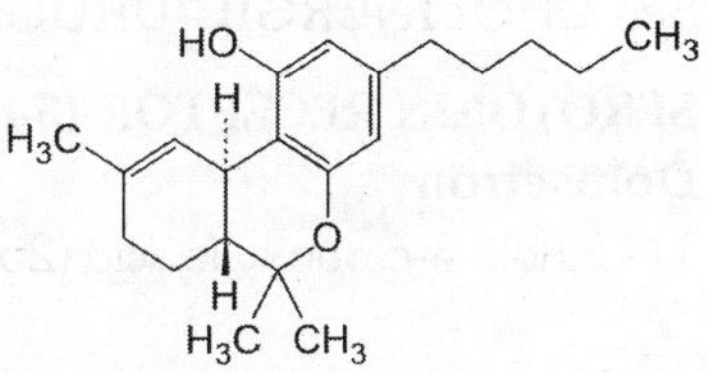   (30)

INDIVIDUAL COMPOUNDS

HISTAMINE H₁-RECEPTOR ANTAGONISTS
Diphenhydramine, Dimenhydrinate, Cyclizine, and Meclizine
See ANTIHISTAMINIC AND ANTIULCER AGENTS

Cinnarizine

1-Diphenylmethyl-4-*trans*-cinnamylpiperazine

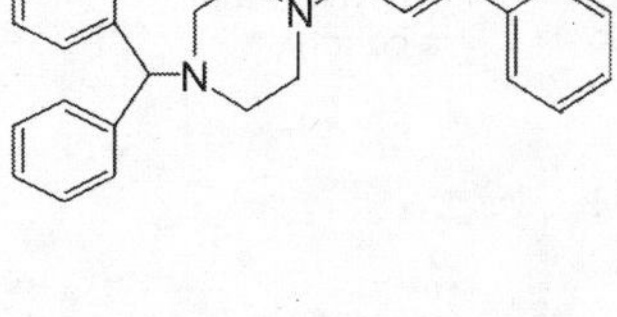

Synthesis

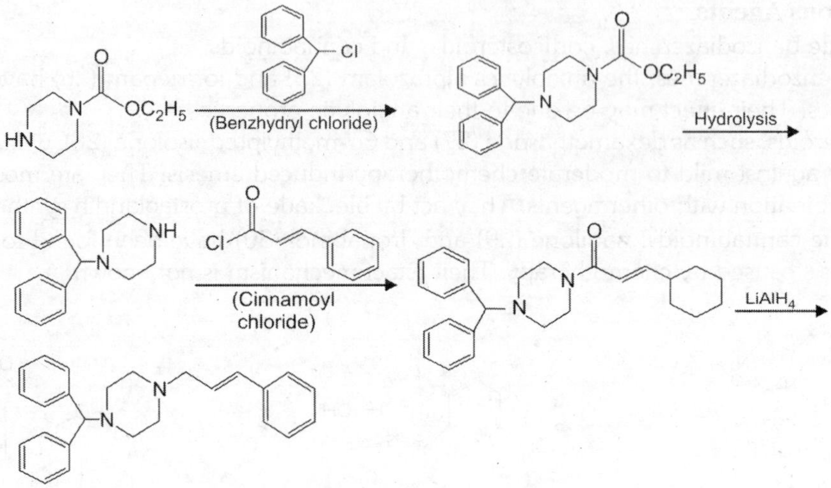

Promethazine

See **ANTIHISTAMINIC AND ANTIULCER AGENTS**

MUSCARINIC ANTAGONISTS

Scopolamine

See **CHOLINERGIC DRUGS**

SEROTONIN RECEPTOR (5-HT$_3$) ANTAGONISTS

Dolasetron

1*H*-Indole-3-carboxylic acid (2α,6α,8α,9aβ)-octahydro-3-oxo-2,6-methano-2*H*-quinolizin-8-yl ester

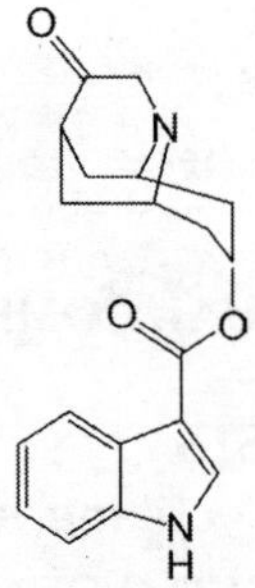

Synthesis

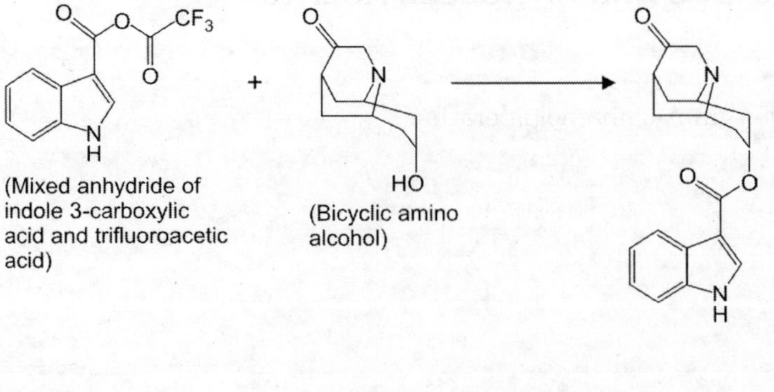

Granisetron

1-Methyl-*N*-(3-*endo*)-9-methyl-9-azabicyclo[3.3.1]non-3-yl]-1*H*-indazole-3-carboxamide

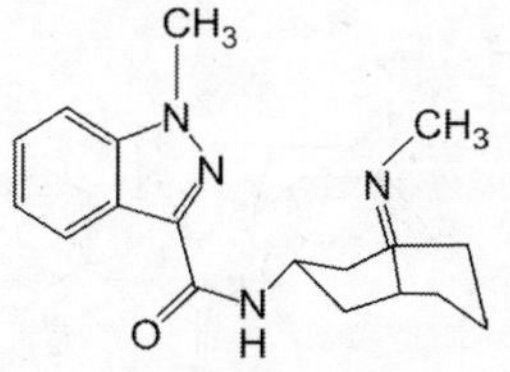

Synthesis

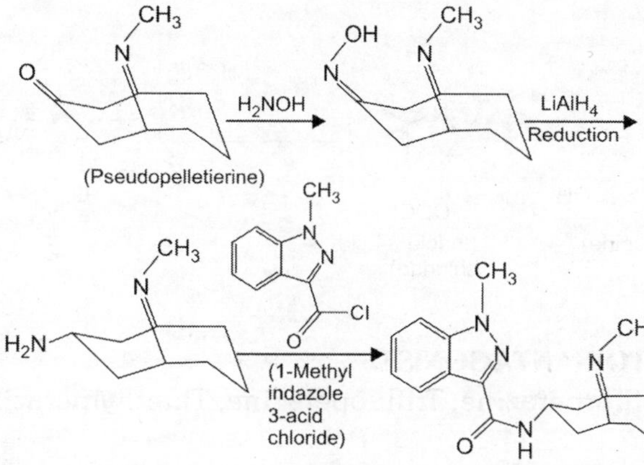
(Pseudopelletierine)
H_2NOH
$LiAlH_4$
Reduction
(1-Methyl indazole 3-acid chloride)

Ondansetron

1,2,3,9-Tetrahydro-9-methyl-3-[(2-methyl-1*H*-imidazol-1-yl-)methyl]-4*H*-carbazol-4-one

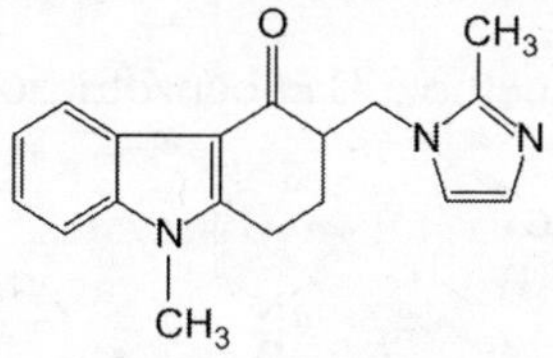

Synthesis

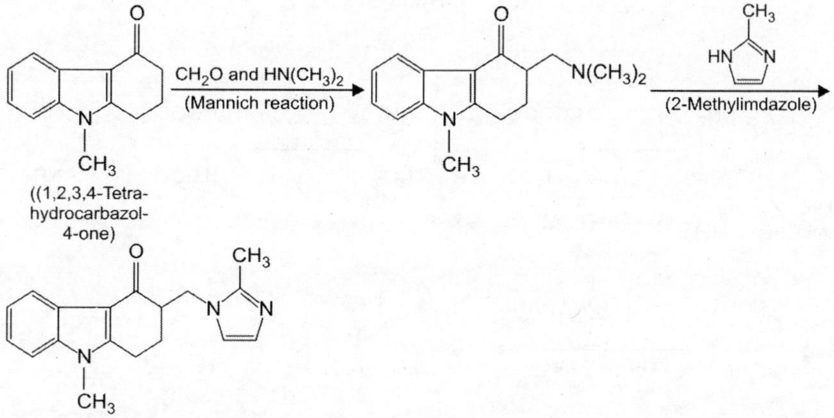
CH_2O and $HN(CH_3)_2$
(Mannich reaction)
(2-Methylimdazole)
((1,2,3,4-Tetra-hydrocarbazol-4-one)

Tropisetron

3α-Tropanyl-1H-indole-3-carboxylic acid ester

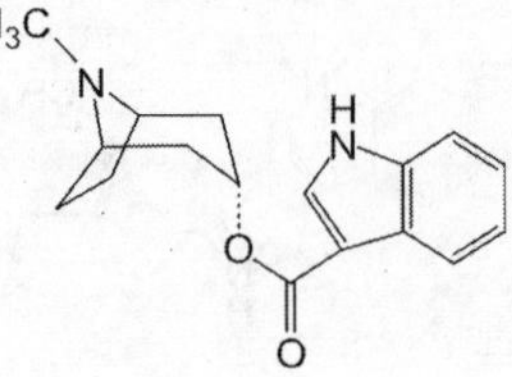

Synthesis

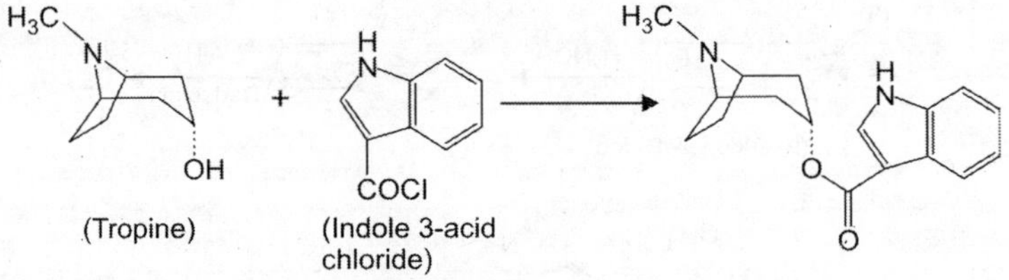

(Tropine) (Indole 3-acid chloride)

DOPAMINE D$_2$-RECEPTOR ANTAGONISTS

Chlorpromazine, Prochlorperazine, Trifluoperazine, Thiethylperazine, Haloperidol, and Droperidol

See NEUROLEPTICS AND ANXIOLYTICS

Alizapride

N-[(1-Allyl-2-pyrrolidinyl)methyl]-6-methoxy-1H-benzotriazole-5-carboxamide

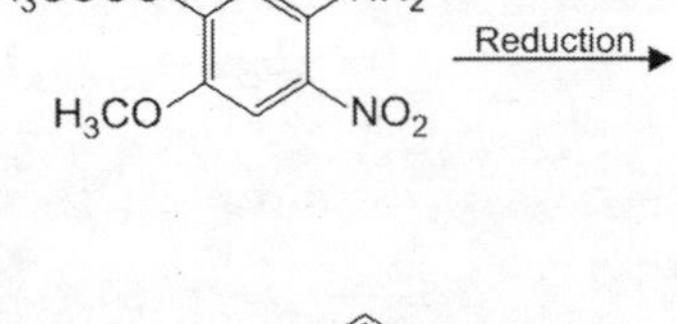

Synthesis

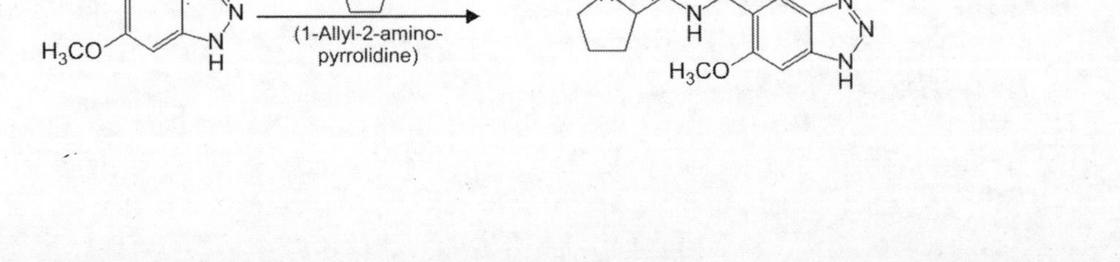

(Methyl 2-methoxy-5-aminobenzoate)

(1-Allyl-2-amino-pyrrolidine)

Metoclopramide
See **CHOLINERGIC DRUGS**

Trimethobenzamide
4-(2-Dimethylaminoethoxy)-N-(3,4,5-trimethoxybenzoyl)benzylamine

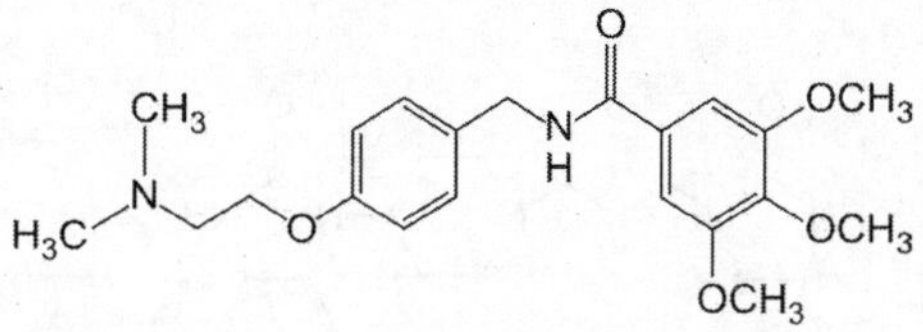

Synthesis

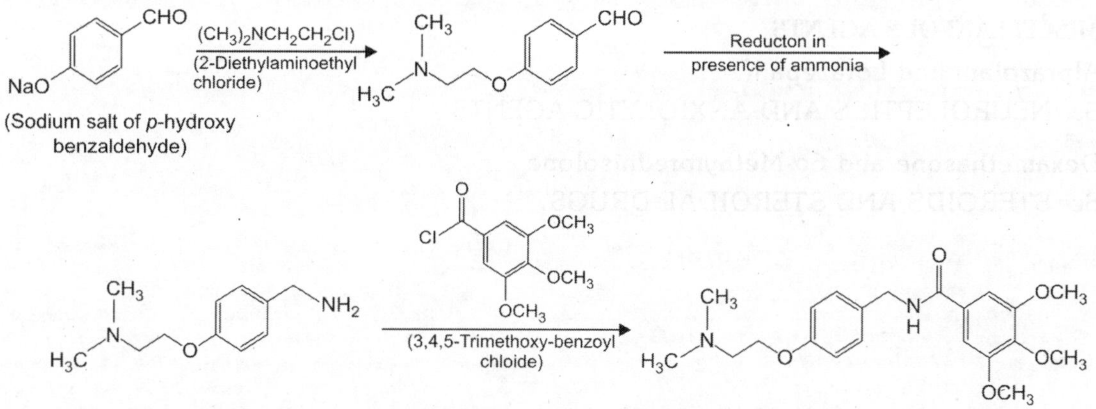

(Sodium salt of *p*-hydroxy benzaldehyde)

Domperidone
5-Chloro-1-[1-[3-(2-oxo-1-benzimidazolinyl)propyl]-4-piperidyl]-2-benzimidazolinone

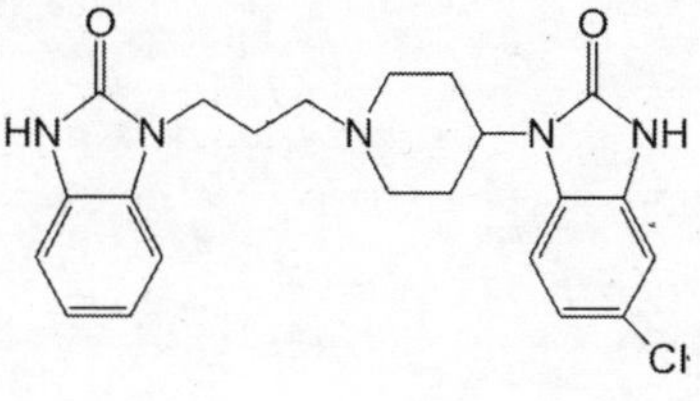

Synthesis

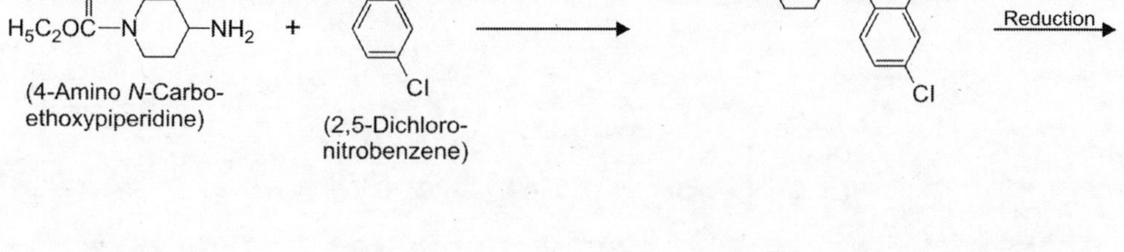

(4-Amino *N*-Carbo-
ethoxypiperidine)

(2,5-Dichloro-
nitrobenzene)

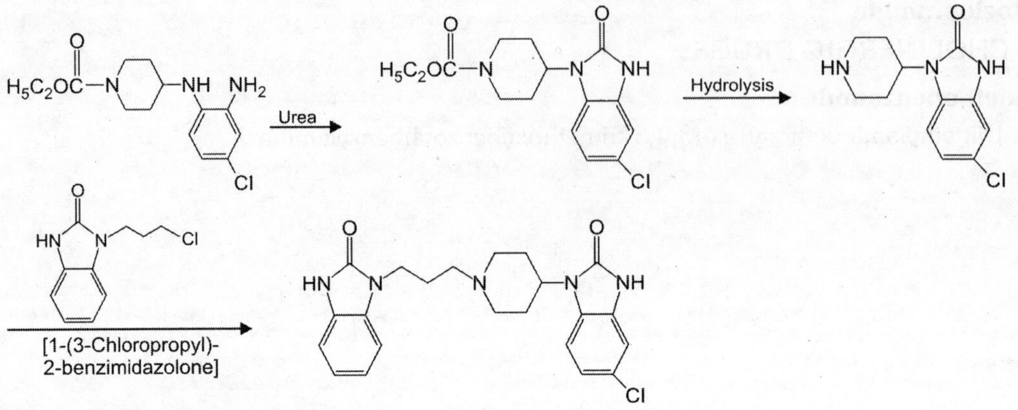

[1-(3-Chloropropyl)-2-benzimidazolone]

MISCELLANEOUS AGENTS

Alprazolam and Lorazepam
See NEUROLEPTICS AND ANXIOLYTIC AGENTS

Dexamethasone and 6α-Methylprednisolone
See STEROIDS AND STEROIDAL DRUGS.

CHAPTER 21

DRUGS USED FOR CONSTIPATION, DIARRHEA, AND IN INFLAMMATORY BOWEL DISEASES

WATER accounts for 70-85% of the stool weight. Normally about 8 to 9 litres of fluid from various sources enter small intestines daily. Most of the absorption of water occurs in small intestine because of osmotic gradient. About 1 to 1.5 litres of water crosses ilececal valve. The colon then extracts most of the remaining fluid leaving about 100 ml of the fecal water daily. Changes in either secretion or absorption of fluid can occur due to neurohumoral mechanisms, pathogens, and drugs. Excess reabsorption of fluids leads to decreased stool volume leading to constipation. On the other hand, lower reabsorption leads to increased stool volume leading to diarrhea.

DRUGS USED FOR CONSTIPATION

Laxative, aperient or a mild purgative, is a substance which helps in evacuation of formed fecal material from the rectum. Cathartics are substances which help in evacuation of unformed, usually watery fecal material, from the colon. In small doses cathartics can act as laxatives.

Depending on the mechanism, drugs used for treatment of constipation can be classified as:

    (a) Luminally active Agents.

    (b) Non-Specific Stimulants or Irritants.

    (c) Prokinetic Agents.

LUMINALLY ACTIVE AGENTS

These include

    (a) Bulk Laxatives,

    (b) Osmotic Agents,

    (c) Stool Softeners and Emollients.

Bulk Laxatives

These include hydrophilic colloids, such as dietary fibre which is resistant to enzymatic digestion. Some of the bulk laxatives are methylcellulose, plant gums such as sterculia, agar, bran, and isphagula. These agents form gels in large intestine causing water retention and intestinal distention.

This results in increased peristaltic movement and evacuation of the stool. These agents do not have any side effects but they take 1 to 3 days to act. They are contraindicated in patients with obstructive symptoms.

Osmotic Agents

Osmotic agents include saline laxatives, nondigestible alcohols, sugars, and polyethylene glycols.

The saline laxatives are those which contain a magnesium cation or a phosphate anion, both of which are nonabsorbable. They hold water by osmosis resulting in increase in the volume of feces, distention of the bowel which results in increased intestinal activity and defecation. They take about 3 to 6 hours for their action. Some of these include magnesium sulphate, magnesium hydroxide, magnesium citrate, and sodium phosphate.

The nondigestible alcohols and sugars include glycerol (1), lactulose (2), sorbitol (3), and mannitol (4).

(1)   (2)   (3)   (4)

Glycerol (1), a trihydroxy alcohol, when given rectally, acts as lubricant. It also possesses hygroscopic properties which results in retention of water and stimulation of peristalsis. It produces bowel movement within an hour.

Lactulose (2), a disaccharide, is hydrolyzed to galactose and fructose by the bacteria in colon. these sugars are not absorbed and undergo fermentation to lactic acid and act as osmotic laxative.

Sorbitol (3) and mannitol (4), which are also nonbsorbable sugars, also undergo fermentation to acids and then act as osmotic laxatives.

Polyethylene glycol (5) with long chain are poorly absorbed, their action is because of retention of water which results in osmotic laxation.

$$H(OCH_2CH_2)nOH$$

[n is > or equal to 4]

(5)

Stool Softeners and Emollients

Anionic surfactants like docusate sodium (6a) and docusate calcium (6b) allow the mixing of aqueous and fatty components of stool and thus making the stool soft. This results in easier defecation. However, these agents also alter the intestinal permeability by stimulating the intestinal secretion and electrolyte secretion.

(a), M=Na+, x = 1
(b), M=Ca^{2+}, x = 2

(6)

Mineral oil which is a mixture of aliphatic hydrocarbons acts as emollient. It is indigestible and is absorbed to limited extent and when taken for 2 to 3 days, it softens the stool which results in easier defecation. However, it cannot be used regularly as it interferes with absorption of fat soluble substances.

NON-SPECIFIC STIMULANTS OR IRRITANTS

These agents cause low grade inflammation of small and large intestines through stimulation of prostaglandin/c-AMP and nitric oxide/c-AMP pathways and inhibition of Na$^+$ K$^+$-ATPase. The inflammation caused results in accumulation of water and electrolyte and stimulation of intestinal motility which ultimately results in laxative action.

The various classes of drugs which act as stimulant or irritant laxatives include:
  (a) Diphenylmethane derivatives,
  (b) anthraquinones, and
  (c) castor oil.

Diphenylmethane Derivatives

This class of compounds includes bisacodyl (7), oxyphenisatin acetate (8), and phenolphthalein (9). Both oxyphenisatin acetate (8) and phenolphthalein (9) are no more used now. Bisacodyl (7) is used as suppositories and enteric coated tablets. Antacids are contraindicated when tablets are used. This is because antacids may cause premature dissolution of the tablets in stomach and this may result in irritation of stomach. The laxative effect in case of suppositories is within 30-60 min while as enteric coated tablets require about 6 hr to show their effect.

(7)

(8)

(9)

Anthraquinones

The leaves, bark, and roots of plants such as senna, cascara, and aloes contain derivatives of anthrone (10a) and anthrol (10b) system. The active agents are the derivatives of anthrol-anthrone system.

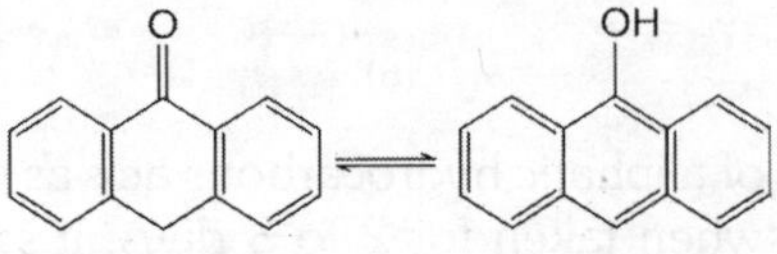

(10a)   (10b)

Some of the anthraquinone derivatives include aloin (11) or barbaloin found in aloes namely *Aloe ferox and Aloe perryi*. The glycosidal anthraquinones include glucofrangulins obtained from *Rhammus frangula* and sennosides found in senna leaflets. Glucofrangulin consists of two isomers namely glucofrangulin A (12) and glucofrangulin B. They differ in linkage to sugar moiety at position 3 of the aglycone.

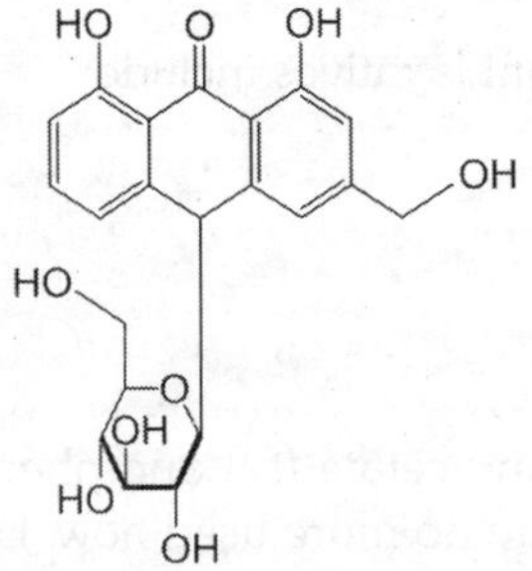

(11) 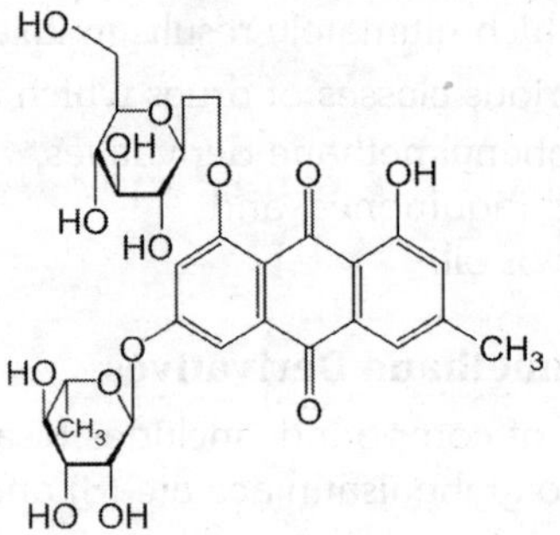   (12)

The sennosides (13) are diglycosides of symmetrical dianthrones and include sennoside A and sennoside B. Sennoside A is made up of dextrorotatory aglycone sennidin A and D-glucose. Sennoside B is built up from meso-sennidin B and D-Glucose.

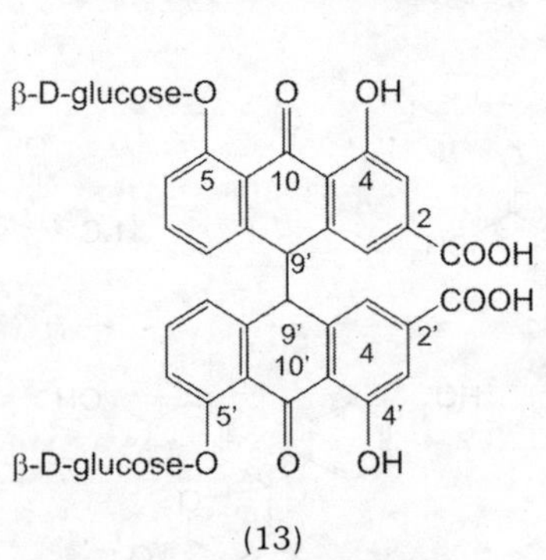

(13)

Both anthrones and anthraquinone glycosides induce water and electrolyte secretion as well clonic contractions. They are poorly absorbed in small bowl.

Castor oil

Castor oil, obtained from beans of castor plant, *Ricinus communis*, contains toxic protein ricin and oil. The principal component of the oil is triglyceride of ricinoleic acid (14).

$$H_3C(CH_2)_5CHCH_2CH=CH(CH_2)_7COOH$$
$$|$$
$$OH$$

(14)

The ricinoleic acid (14), resulting by the action of lipase on triglycerides of castor oil in small bowl, stimulates secretion of fluids and electrolytes which result in the clearing of bowl. Because of its unpleasant taste and toxic effects on intestinal epithelium, castor oil is not used nowadays.

PROKINETIC AGENTS

The luminally active agents and non-specific stimulants stimulate the motility nonspecifically or indirectly. Prokinetic agents are the substances which produce gastrointestinal motility by interacting directly with specific receptors. The synthetic prostaglandin, misoprostol (15), when used as non-steroidal anti-inflammatory agent in high doses, produces diarrhea. This property could be used for the patients with intractable constipation. However, not much clinical data is available for the use of misoprostol (15) as anticonstipative agent.

(15)

DRUGS USED FOR DIARRHEA

Diarrhea is frequent evacuation of liquid faeces. It involves increased motility of gastrointestinal tract, increased discomfort, and increased secretion along with decreased absorption of fluid. This results in loss of electrolytes, mainly Na^+ and water. Diarrhea can be caused by infections, toxins, drugs, and even anxiety.

The treatment of severe and acute diarrhea involves:

1. Maintenance of fluid and electrolyte balance,
2. use of antiinfective agents, and
3. use of antimotility agents, adsorbents, and use of agents that modify fluid and electrolyte transport such as α_2-adrenergic agonists.

Maintenance of Fluid and Electrolyte Balance

Fluid and electrolyte balance is maintained by administration of oral rehydration solutions. These solutions contain electrolytes such as Na^+, K^+, and Cl^- along with glucose. Some preparations contain citrate and bicarbonate also. These preparations are available in ready-to-use powder form. In the ileum there is co-transport of Na^+ along with glucose across epithelial cells. This results in increased Na^+ absorption and thus water uptake. A balanced mixture of glucose and electrolytes prevents the dehydration.

Anti-infective Agents

Campylobacter species is the commonest bacterial species which causes gastroenteritis. Erythromycin (16) and ciprofloxacin (17) are usually used for this purpose. Erythromycin is a mixture of erythromycin A (16a), erythromycin B (16b) and erythromycin C (16c). The commercial preparation is mainly composed of erythromycin A (16a). It is produced by fermentation using *S. erythraeus*.

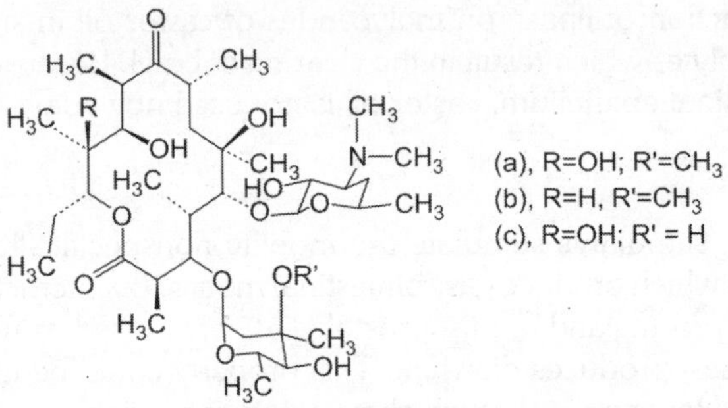

(a), R=OH; R'=CH$_3$
(b), R=H, R'=CH$_3$
(c), R=OH; R' = H

(16)

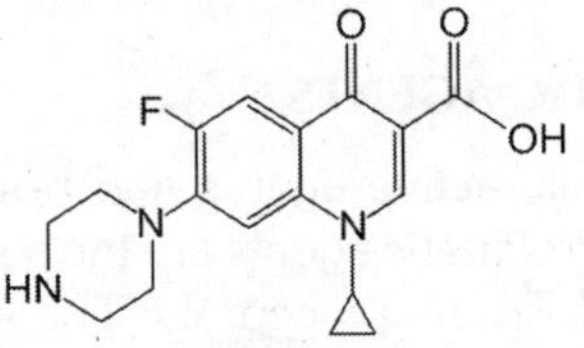

(17)

Antimotility Agents

These include opioids like codeine (18) and the piperidine analogs diphenoxylate (19), difenoxin (20), and loperamide (21). Opioids affect intestinal motility through μ-recepors, intestinal secretion through δ-receptors, or absorption through both μ- and δ-receptors.

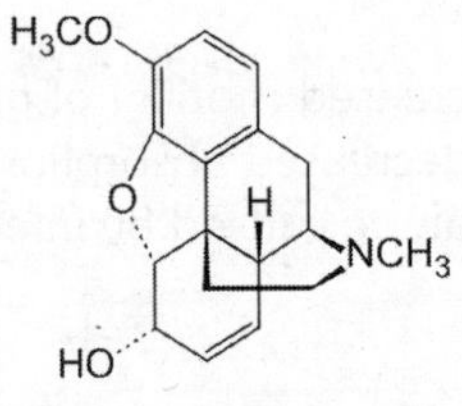

(18)

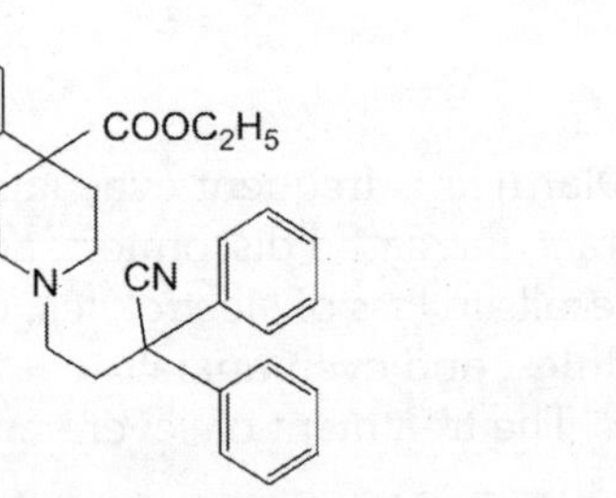

(19)

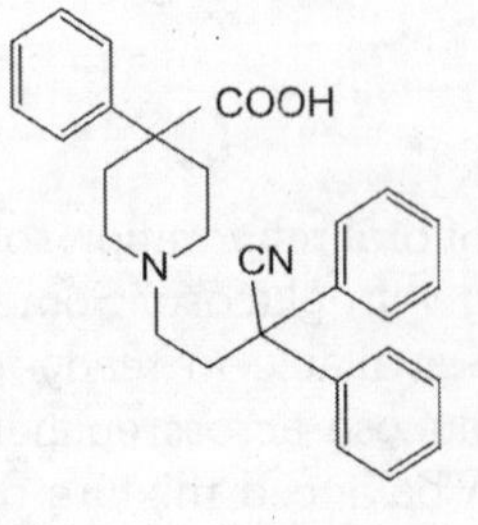

(20)

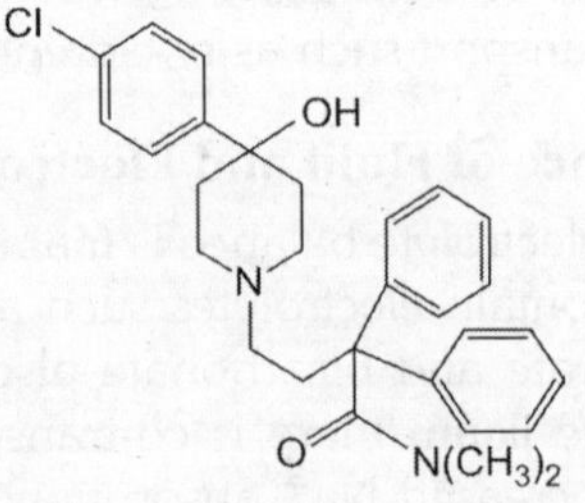

(21)

Codeine (18) is not used nowadays. Diphenoxylate (19), difenoxin (20), and loperamide (21) act on peripheral μ-opioid receptors. Diphenoxylate (19) is a prodrug of difenoxin (20) which is the active from of the drug. All the three piperidine analogs have advantage that they do not penetrate the CNS.

Adsorbents

These include kaolin, pectin, methylcellulose, and activated magnesium aluminium silicates. These agents adsorb intestinal toxins/microorganisms or coat the intestinal mucosa. They are less effective than antimotility agents.

α$_2$-Adrenergic Receptor Agonists

These agents stimulate absorption and inhibit secretion of fluids and electrolytes and also Increase intestinal transit time. They are usually used in diabetics with chronic diarrhea. Drugs in this category include clonidine (22).

(22)

DRUGS USED IN INFLAMMATORY BOWEL DISEASES

Inflammatory bowel diseases include ulcerative colitis and Crohn's disease. Both of these diseases are of uncertain etiology. Ulcerative colitis is confined to colon. It is characterized by chronic inflammation and leukocyte infiltration which leads to progressive mucosal damage.

In Crohn's disease there is damage of both small and large bowl and it is characterized by focal damage, fissuring ulcers and granuloma.

The drugs used in inflammatory bowl diseases include:
1. sulphasalzine and related agents,
2. glucocortcoids, and
3. immunosuppressive agents

Sulphasalazine and Related Agents

These include sulphasalazine (23), olsalazine (24), and balsalazide (25). Reductive cleavage of

(23)

(24)

(25)   (26)   (27)

these drugs results in formation of 5-aminosalicylic acid (26) which inhibits cyclooxygenase and 5-lipoxygenase, thus acting as antiinflammtory agent. The side effects of sulphasalazine (22) are due to sulphapyridine (27), it is not used nowadays.

Glucocorticoids

Among glucocorticoids, prednisolone (28) is given locally by suppository or enema.

(28)

Immunosuppressive Agents

The cytotoxic agents azathioprine (29) and mercaptopurine (30) have been used in severe cases of inflammatory bowl diseases. Azathioprine (29) is a prodrug and yields the active form mrcaptopurine (30) on metabolism. Azathioprine (29) is preferred over mercaptopurine (30) because it yields mercaptopurine (30) slowly which favours immunosuppression. Mercaptopurine (30) is used as antineoplastic agent.

(29)   (30)

Cyclosporins, a mixture of nonpolar cyclic oligopeptides are used as immunosuppressant. The peptide is produced by *Tolypocladium inflatum Gams* and other fungi imperfecti. The major component of this mixture is cyclosporin A (31), the other minor components are cyclosporin B, C, D, and G.

Cyclosporin A (31) has been used in severe ulcerative colitis. It is administered as continuous infusion.

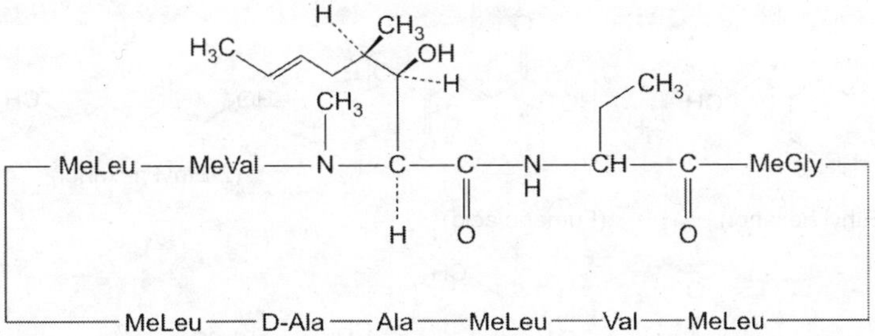

(31)

INDIVIDUAL COMPOUNDS

DRUGS USED FOR CONSTIPATION : LUMINALLY ACTIVE AGENTS — OSMOTIC AGENTS

Glycerol

1,2,3-Propanetriol

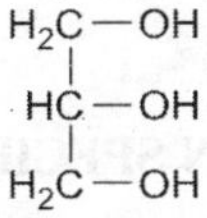

$$H_2C-OH$$
$$HC-OH$$
$$H_2C-OH$$

Synthesis

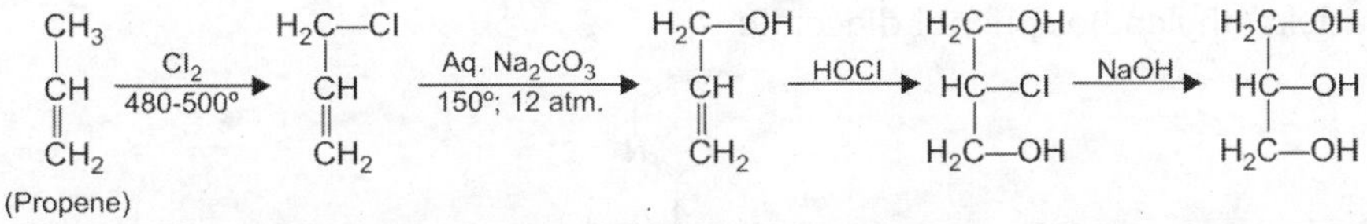

Glycerol occurs in almost in all animal and vegetable oils and fats as glyceryl ester of fatty acids. It is obtained in large quantities as a by-product in the manufacture of soaps.

It is given rectally as suppository. It acts as a lubricant. Since it is hygroscopic, it retains water and stimulates peristalsis. It produces bowel movement within an hour.

DRUGS USED FOR CONSTIPATION : LUMINALLY ACTIVE AGENTS — STOOL SOFTENERS AND EMOLIENTS

Docusate Sodium

Sulphobutanedioic acid 1,4-bis(2-ethylhexyl) ester sodium salt

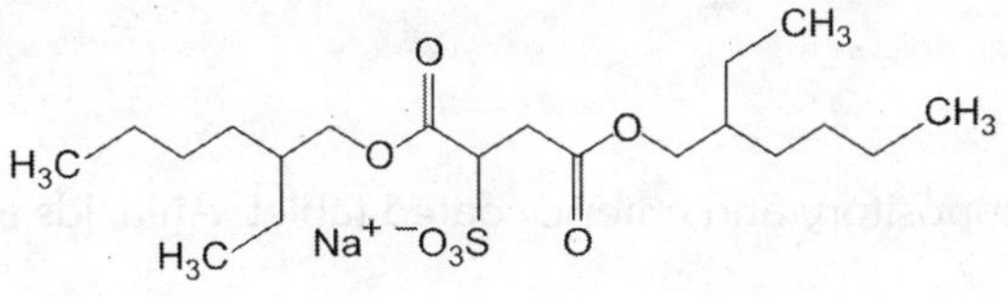

Synthesis

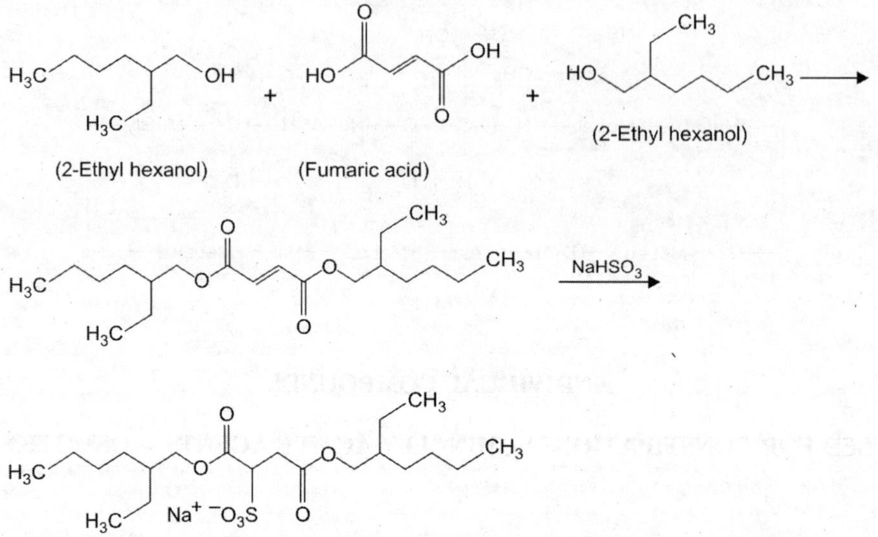

It is anionic surfactant by virtue of which it makes stool soft through mixing of aqueous and fatty components of stool.

DRUGS USED FOR CONSTIPATION : NON SPECIFIC STIMULANTS OR IRRITANTS – DIPHENYLMETHYL DERIVATIVES

Bisacodyl

4,4'-(2-Pyridylmethylene)bisphenol diacetate

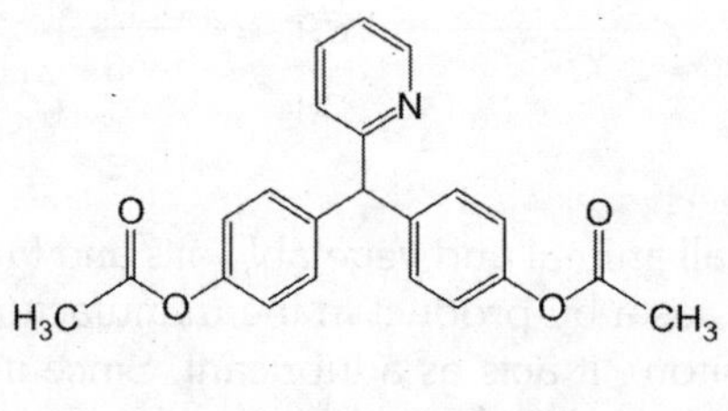

Synthesis

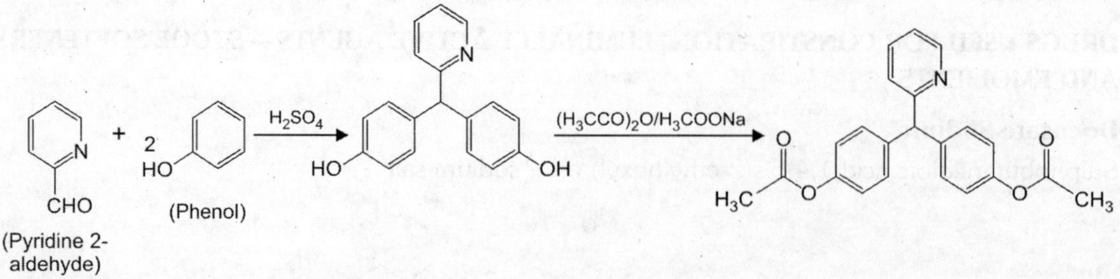

Bisacodyl is used as suppository and enteric coated tablet. Antacids are contraindicated in case of tablets.

Oxyphenisatin Acetate

3,3-Bis(4′-acetoxyphenyl)oxindole

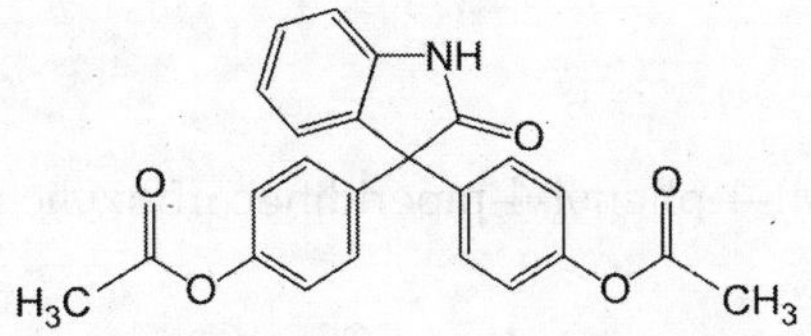

Synthesis

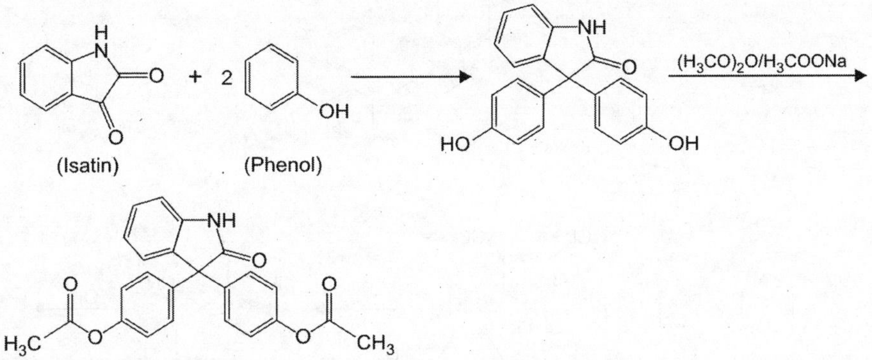

It is a cathartic not used nowadays.

Phenolphthalein

3,3-Bis(4′-hydroxyphenyl)phthalide

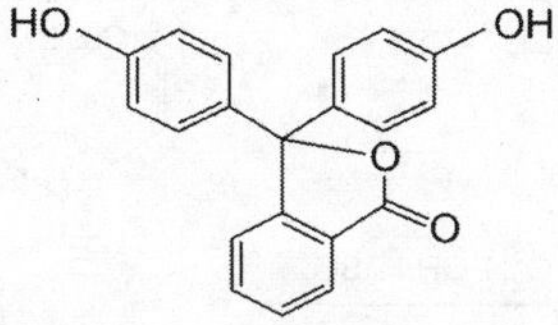

Synthesis

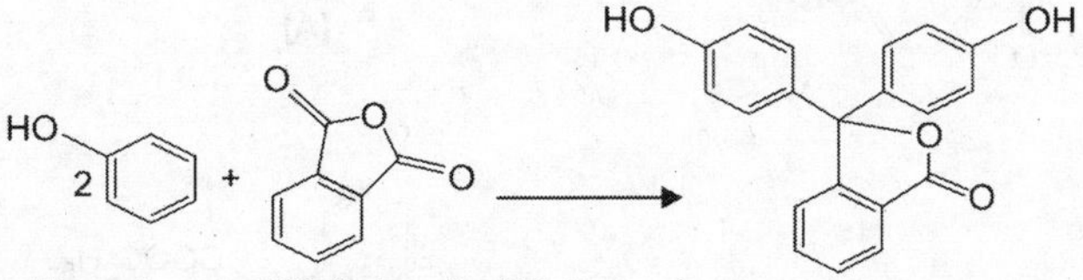

(Phenol) (Phthaic anhydride)

Not used nowadays.

DRUGS USED FOR DIARRHEA : ANTINFECTIVES AGENTS

Erythromycin

See MACROLIDE ANTIBIOTICS

Ciprofloxacin

See SULPHONAMIDES AND QUINOLONES

DRUGS USED IN DIARRHEA : ANTIMOTILITY AGENTS

Codeine

See OPIOID ANALGESICS

Diphenoxylate

1-(3-Cyano-3,3-diphenylpropyl)-4-phenyl-4-piperidinecarboxylic acid ethyl ester

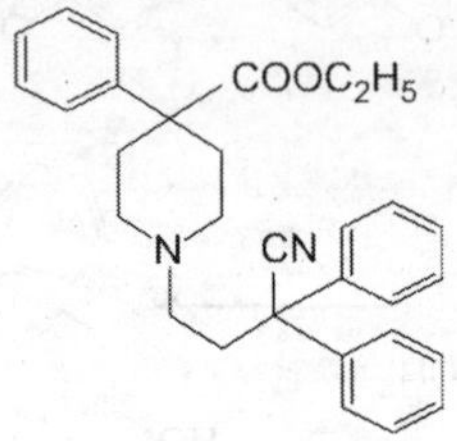

Synthesis

Step 1

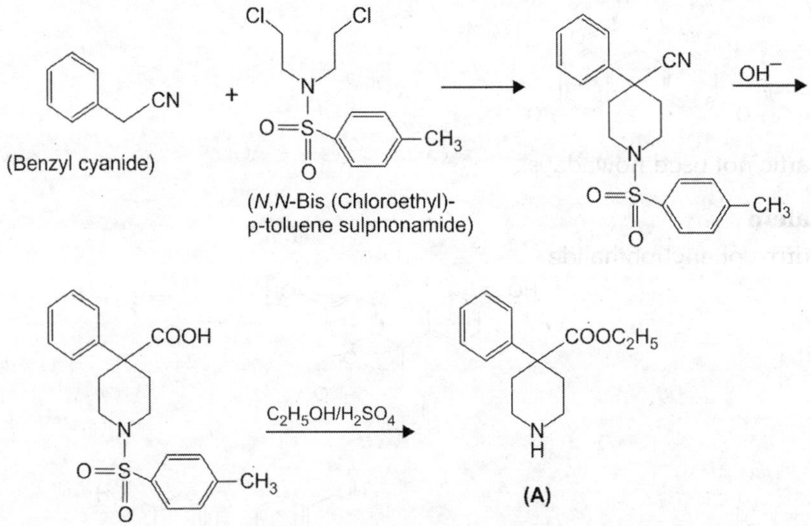

(Benzyl cyanide)

(*N,N*-Bis (Chloroethyl)-
p-toluene sulphonamide)

(A)

Step 2

(1,2-Dibromo-
ethane)

(Diphenyl aceto-
nitrile)

(A)

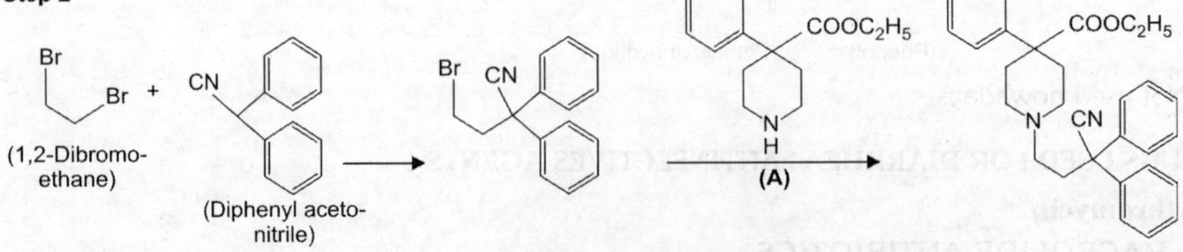

It is the prodrug of difenoxin (20). Acts as antidiarrheal agent by affecting intestinal motility through μ-receptors and intestinal secretion through δ-receptors.

Difenoxin

1-(3-Cyano-3,3-diphenylpropyl)-4-phenyl-4-piperidinecarboxylic acid

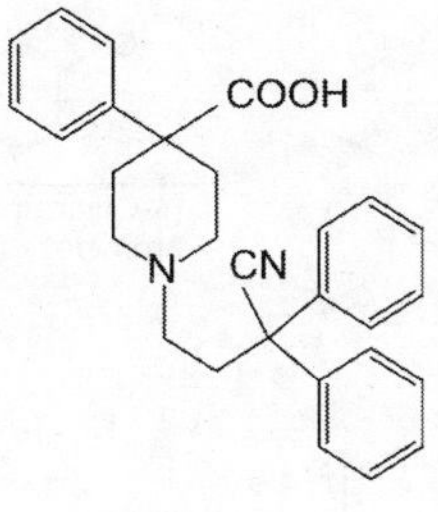

Synthesis

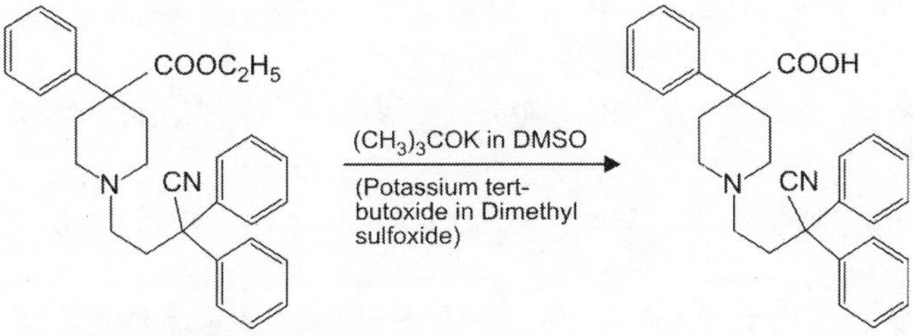

(Diphenoxylate)

It is the active form of diphenoxylate (19).

Loperamide

4-(4-Chlorophenyl)-4-hydroxy-*N,N*-dimethyl-α-α-diphenyl-1-piperidinebutyramide

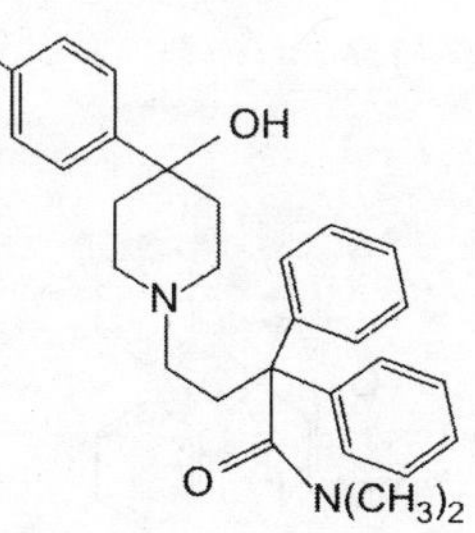

Synthesis

Step 1

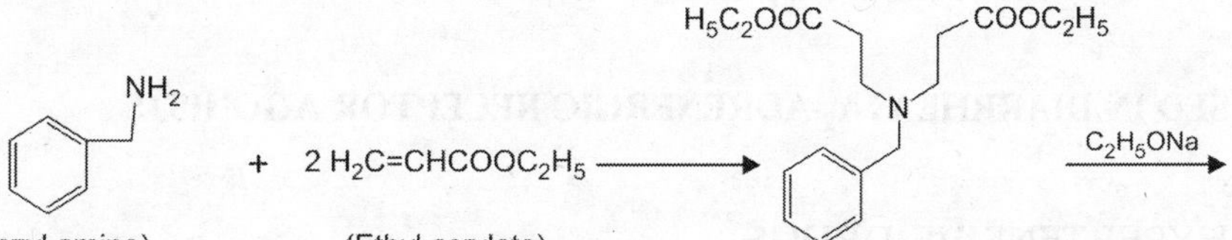

(Benzyl amine)   (Ethyl acrylate)

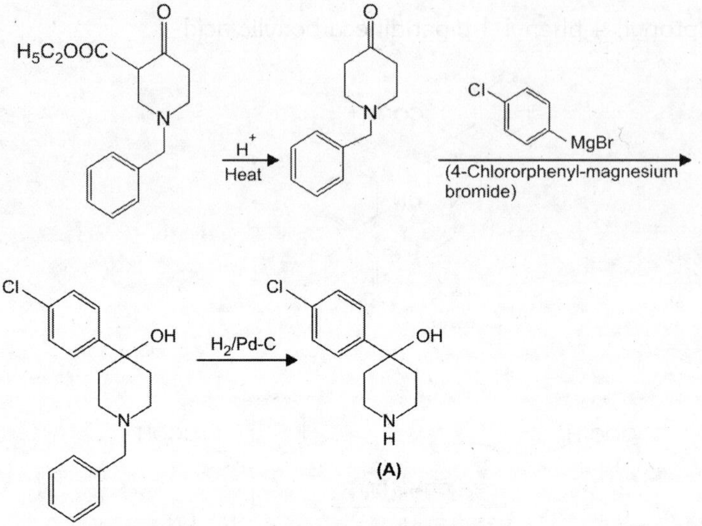

Step 2

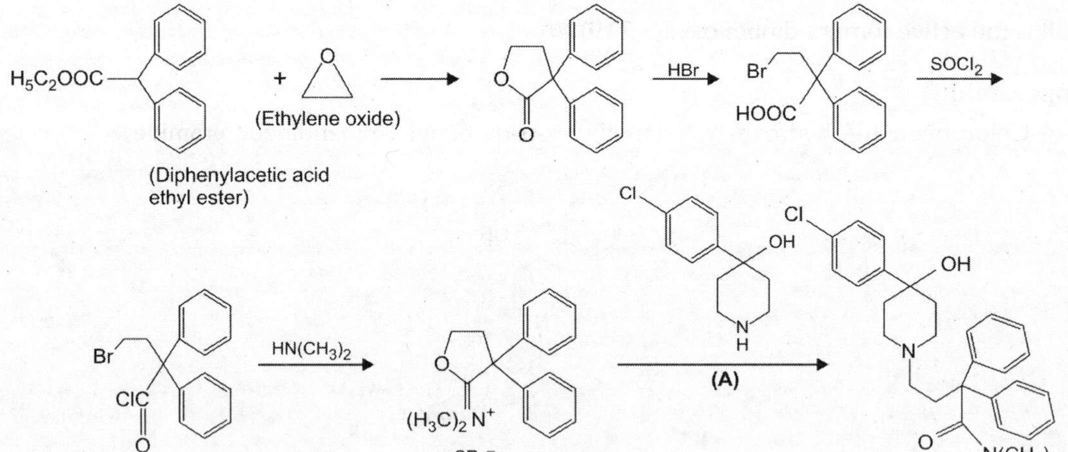

Same action and mechanism as diphenoxylate (19).

DRUGS USED IN DIARRHEA : α_2-ADRENERGIC RECEPTOR AGONISTS

Clonidine
See ANTIHYPERTENSIVE DRUGS

DRUGS USED IN INFLAMMATORY BOWL DISEASES : SULPHASALAZINE AND RELATED COMPOUNDS

Sulphasalazine

5-[p-(2-Pyridylsulphamoyl)phenylazo]salicylic acid

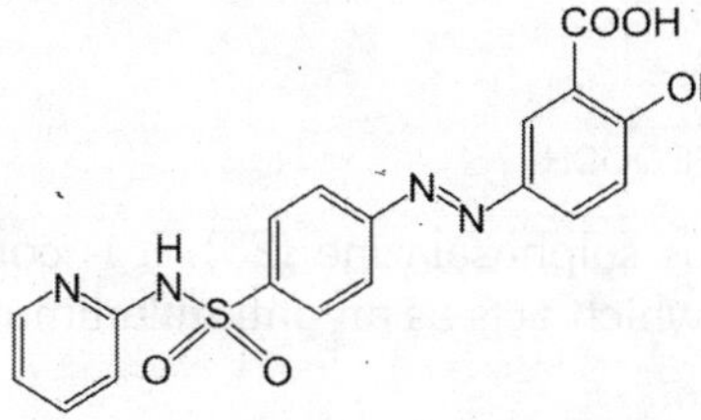

Synthesis

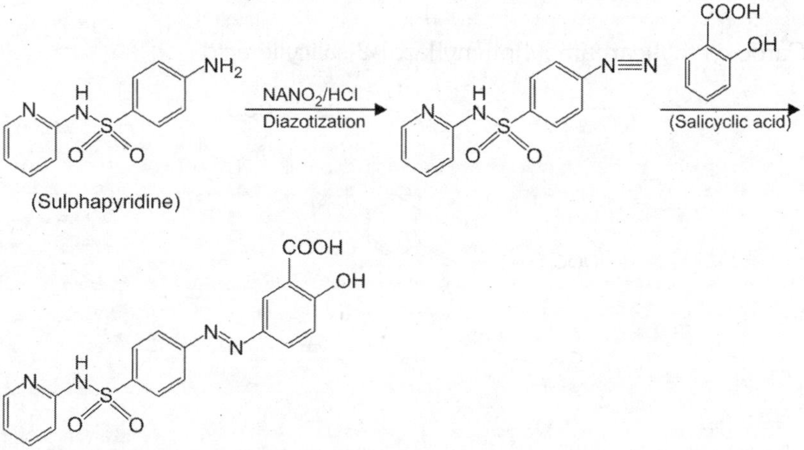

It undergoes reductive cleavage in the gut to give 5-aminosalicylic acid, (26) which acts as an anti-inflammatory agent in ulcerative colitis.

Olsalazine

3,3'-Dicarboxy-4,4'-dihydroxyazobenzene

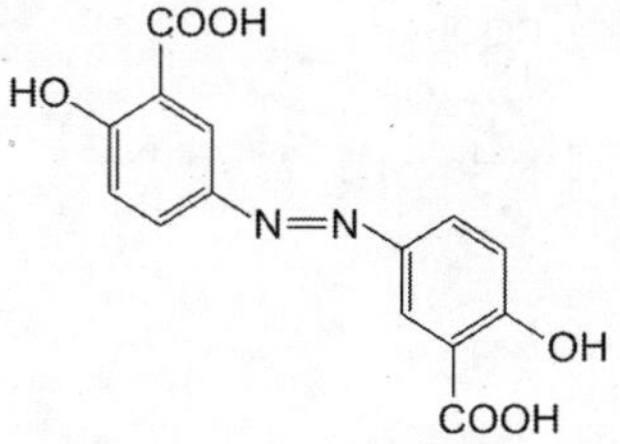

Synthesis

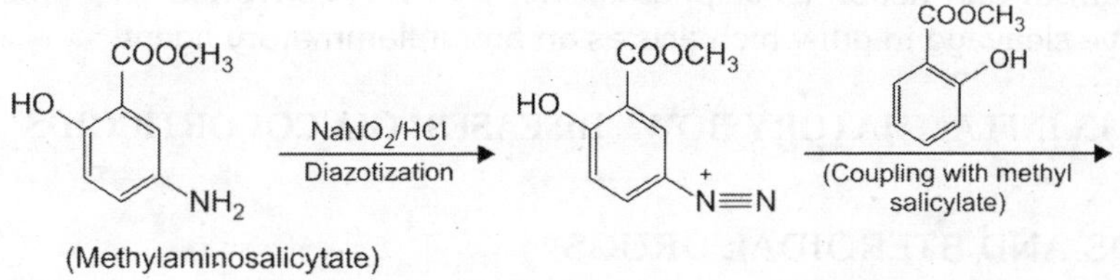

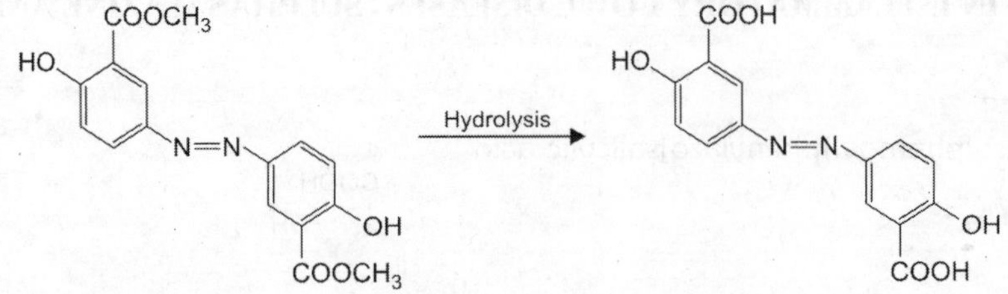

Same mechanism and action as sulphasalazine (23). It is converted to 5-aminosalicylic acid (26) by reductive cleavage in gut which acts as an anti-inflammatory agent.

Balsalazide

(E)-5-[[p-[(2-Carboxyethyl)carbamoyl]phenyl]azo]-2-salicylic acid

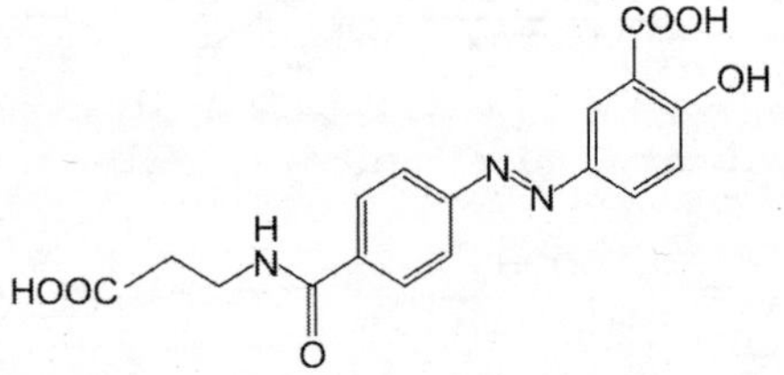

Synthesis

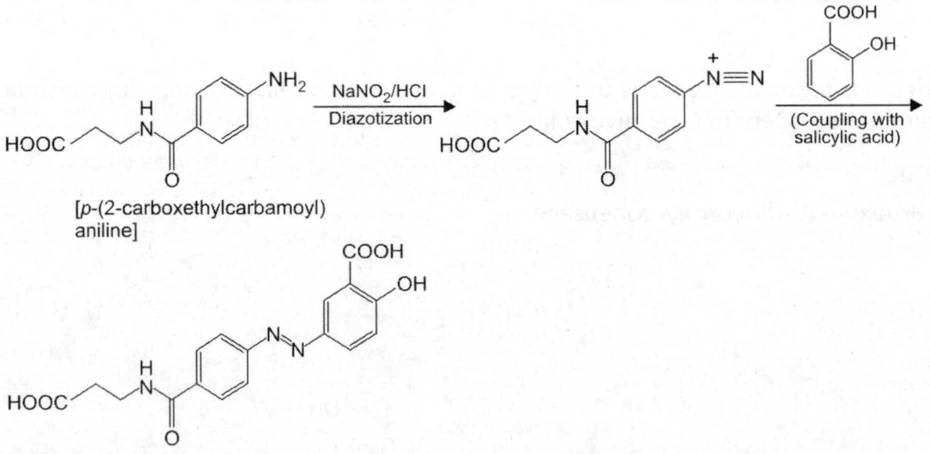

[p-(2-carboxethylcarbamoyl) aniline]

Same mechanism and action as sulphasalazine (23). It is converted to 5-aminosalicylic acid (26) by reductive cleavage in gut which acts as an anti-inflammatory agent.

DRUGS USED IN INFLAMMATORY BOWL DISEASES : GLUCOCORTICOIDS

Prednisolone

See STEROIDS AND STEROIDAL DRUGS

DRUGS USED IN INFLAMMATORY BOWL DISEASES : IMMUNOSUPPRESSIVE AGENTS

Azathioprine

6-(1-Methyl-4-nitro-5-imidazolyl)mercaptopurine

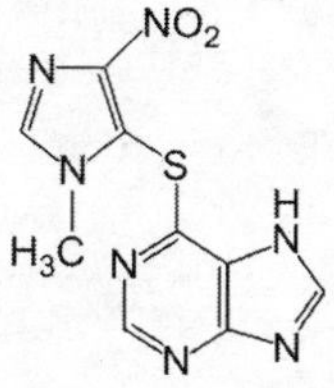

Synthesis

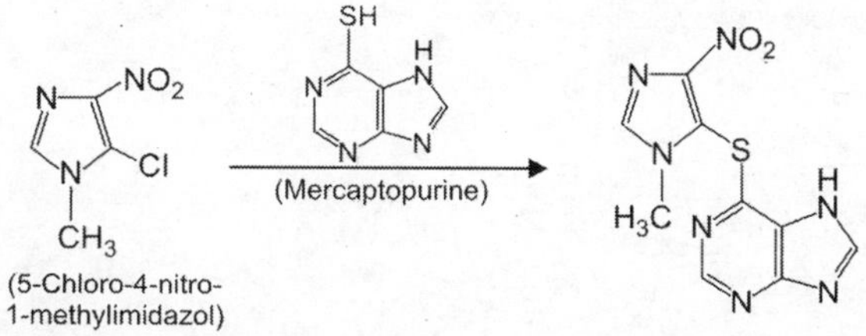

(5-Chloro-4-nitro-
1-methylimidazol)

(Mercaptopurine)

It is a prodrug of mercaptopurine (30). It is preferred over mercaptopurine (30) because it yields small quantities of mercaptopurine (30).

Mercaptopurine

See ANTICANCER AGENTS

Section VIII
Chemotherapy—Drugs Used in Parasitic Infections

ANTIPROTOZOAL DRUGS I: CHEMOTHERARY OF MALARIA

MALARIA is one of the most widespread of all human diseases. Every year millions of people die of this disease. With the emergence of drug resistant strains, the problem has become much more acute.

Contrary to the belief, malaria is not confined to the tropical and subtropical regions. It can occur as far as Arctic circle and a corresponding distance south. The disease has been associated with *miasma* arising from swamps and hence the word malaria–poisonous air arising from marshes.

Malaria is caused by four species of protozoa belonging to the genus *Plasmodium*. The four species implicated include:

1. *Plasmodium vivax*, which is responsible for benign tertian malaria also known as *vivax* malaria.
2. *Plasmodium falciparum*, responsible for malignant tertian or subtertian malaria also known as *falciparum* malaria.
3. *Plasmodium malariae*, causes quartan malaria.
4. *Plasmodium ovale is* responsible for ovale tertian malaria.

The terms "tertian" and "quartan" pertain to the rise of fever. In case of "tertian malaria" the fever rises every 3rd day while as in case of "quartan malaria" it rises every 4th day.

The genus *Plasmodiiae*, belonging to the family *Haemosporidiae*, is defined to include pigment producing parasites that undergo one-cycle of asexual division in RBC and liver of a vertebrate and another cycle of sexual division in the body of mosquito that acts as vector as well as definitive host.

When the female *Anopheles* mosquito bites, it injects sporozoites into the blood of the vertebrate host (Fig. 22.1). After half an hour most of them enter the parenchyma cells of the liver and undergo asexual division from 8th to 12th day after infection. The infected cells rupture and releasing the merozoites into the surrounding tissues. This stage of the development is called pre-erythrocytic or primary tissue stage. At this stage no symptoms of the disease appear. Most of the merozoites enter RBC, while some continue asexual division in the liver.The second asexual division in the liver is called the exoerythrocytic or secondary tissue stage. It is believed that the secondary tissue forms are responsible for the relapse which occurs when they enter the blood at a later stage.

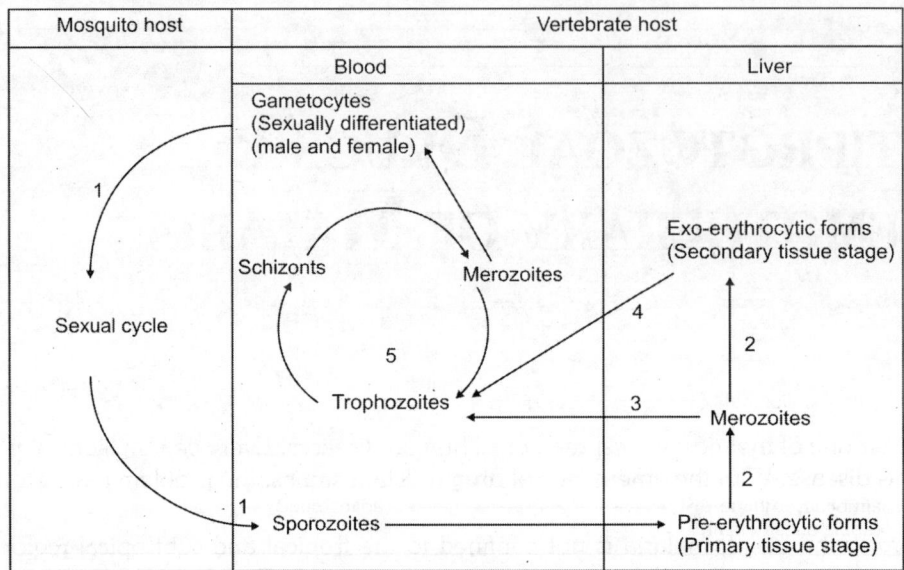

Fig. 22.1: Life cycle of malarial parasite:
(1-mosquito bite; 2-exoerythrocytic stage; 3-initial attack; 4-relapse; 5-erythrocytic schizogony.)

After entering the blood, the young merozoites penetrate the RBC, this stage is known as trophozoite. The parasite grows and it gains pigment which it acquires from the hemoglobin. At this stage, it becomes compact and the nucleus divides. The parasite is now called schizont. Division continues till required number of nuclei are formed. This is the characteristic of species of the parasite. Next, some of the cytoplasm condenses around each of the nucleus and asexual merozoites are formed again. The enlarged red cell ruptures and the merozoites along with pigment and the remains of cytoplasm are set free. The release of the merozoites and the other matter results in rise of the temperature of the host initiating the malarial fever attack.

The merozoites differentiate into male and female parasites and are known as gametocyte. When the vertebrate host is again bitten by the mosquito the gametocytes are sucked along with blood and they undergo sexual cycle, called sporogony, in the gut of female mosquito.

The asexual cycle in vertebrate host may take 2 or 3 days depending on the species. Accordingly, the fever rises on the 3rd or 4th day.

The course of each type of malaria differs according to species of the parasite. In *vivax* malaria, the merozoites entering the blood from liver undergo schizogony for some time, the host showing the typical "tertian" fever. With the building up of the immunity, the schizonts disappear. The immunity, however, does not affect exoerythrocytic forms in the liver which continue to undergo asexual division. As the immunity falls, a new attack or relapse results. Relapses may continue for many years. In general, *vivax* infections are rarely fatal and it is called benign tertian malaria.

In case of the *falciparum* infections, the parasite multiplies rapidly destroying the blood cells forming clumps of cells and cytoplasm. These clumps may localize in internal organs and can also obstruct the circulation. Deaths are common in untreated attacks. This type of attack is known as malignant tertian malaria. *Plasmodium falciparum* does not undergo exoerythrocytic schizogony, thus, no relapses occur once the attack is controlled.

The malarial attack due to *Plasmodium malariae* resembles the benign malaria excepting that the fever rises every 4th day. The *Plasmodium ovale* is relatively uncommon and also causes a mild disease in humans.

According to WHO Report: Malaria Terminology, drugs used in malaria are classified according to what phase of life cycle they affect and include:

1. **Tissue schizontocides:** These are the drugs which act on the asexual form of the parasite in the tissue and these may be:

   (a) **Primary tissue schizontocide:** A drug which acts on the pre-erythrocytic forms of the parasite.

   (b) **Secondary schizontocides:** A drug which acts on exoerythrocytic forms in liver. Drugs of this type are useful as prophylactic.

2. **Blood schizontocides:** Blood schizontocides destroy the erythrocytic stages of the parasites and can cure falciparum infections or suppress relapses.

3. **Gametocyticides:** These kill the sexual form of the parasite which are transmittable to the mosquito, thereby preventing the transmission of the disease.

4. **Sporontocides:** These act on sporozoites and are capable of killing the organisms as soon as they enter the bloodstream following the mosquito bite.

In addition to the above the other terminology used include:

   (a) **Suppression:** It means prevention of clinical symptoms. This can be achieved by action on asexual form of parasite in blood. It can be temporary, i.e. operative only when the drug is being taken or permanent-indicating that no attack will take place even after the drug is withdrawn.

   (b) **Clinical cure:** It indicates that immediate symptoms of an attack have been relieved and the patient has been apparently cured.

   (c) **Radical cure:** It implies that parasite has been eliminated from both blood as well as tissues.

   (d) **Suppressive cure:** It implies that radical cure is achieved while the patient is getting suppressive medication.

ANTIMALARIAL DRUGS

NATURAL DRUGS

Ch'ang Shan

It consists of roots of *Dichroa febrifuga* belonging to the family *Saxifragacea* and has been used against malaria in China for several thousand years. The antimalarial activity of the drug has been attributed to an alkaloid febrifugine (1), a quinazolone alkaloid. Both febrifugine (1) and its 8-chloro analog (2) are active against *Plasmodium falciparum* and *Plasmodium vivax*. However, neither febrifugine (1) nor its chloro analog (2) are used in clinical practice because of their powerful emetic properties.

(1), R = H
(2), R = Cl

Cinchona Alkaloids

The bark of various species of cinchona namely, *Cinchona ledgeriana, C. officinalis, C. succirubra* and other species belonging to the family *Rubiacea*, has been used against malaria. In 1820, Caventou and Pelletier reported the isolation of quinine and cinchonine from cinchona bark. The antimalarial activity of cinchona bark has been attributed to quinine.

Cinchona bark contains about 20 alkaloids. The 4 major alkaloids are the derivatives of rubane (3). All the 4 alkaloids contain a hydroxyl group at position 9 and a vinyl group at position 3. In addition to these two groupings, one pair of alkaloids contain a methoxy group at position 6' while in other pair it is absent. The pair of alkaloids without methoxy group are known as cinchonine group (4) and the pair of alkaloids with 6'-methoxy group are known as quinine group (5). There are four asymmetric centres in the structures of these alkaloids and include C_3, C_4, C_8 and C_9. All the 4 alkaloids have same configuration at C_3 and C_4 and hydrogens are *cis-* to each other. The differences in configuration at C_8 and C_9 results in 4 isomers. Thus, differences in configuration at C_8 lead to cinchonine (4a), cinchonidine (4b), quinidine (5a) and quinine (5b). The differences at C_9 result in epi-series and include epicinchonine (6a), epicinchonidine (6b), epiquinidine (7a) and epiquinine (7b):

(3)

(4)

(5)

(4a), Q = quinolyl
(5a), Q = 6'-methoxyquinolyl

(4b), Q = quinolyl
(5b), Q = 6'-methoxyquinolyl

(6a), Q = quinolyl
(7a), Q = 6'-methoxyquinolyl

(6b), Q = quinolyl
(7b), Q = 6'-methoxyquinolyl

Quinine (5b) is the chief alkaloid of cinchona and is used against malaria. It is absorbed rapidly and nearly completely. The peak blood levels are obtained within 1 to 4 hours. Blood levels fall off very quickly and a single dose of quinine (5b) is excreted within 24 hours. Repeated doses are, therefore, necessary. Quinine (5b) is metabolized first to its 2'-hydroxy carbostyril derivative (8), which is further metabolized to dihydroxy derivative (9).

Quinine (5b) acts on erythrocytic schizonts, the asexual form of malarial parasite. It can cure infections caused by *P. falciparum* since there is no secondary exo-erythrocytic form of this parasite. Quinine (5b) also suppresses the attack due to *vivax* and *falciparum* but not due to *malariae*.

Quinine (5b) also possesses antipyretic activity and this action is due to vasodilation of central temperature regulating centre. In addition to its antimalarial activity, quinine (5b) is also used as a diagnostic agent for myasthenia gravis. It has also some local anesthetic activity but is not used clinically for this purpose. Another major alkaloid, quinidine (5a) has been used in cardiac arrhythmias.

Quinine (5b) causes allergic skin reactions, tinnitus, slight deafness, vertigo, and slight depression. These toxic effects are collectively called "cinchonism". The most serious effect of quinine (5b) is amblyopia, the dimness of vision, which may follow the administration of large doses of quinine (5b). It also produces hemoglobinuria.

In addition to above toxic effects, the other disadvantages associated with quinine (5b) include:

(a) It is contraindicated during pregnancy because it passes from maternal to fetal circulation. This may result in fetal blindness.
(b) It requires frequent administration.

Considering these disadvantages, structure-activity relationship studies were carried out and it was found that:

1. Interference with stereochemistry at C_9 resulting in epi-series leads to loss of activity.
2. Destruction of asymmetry at C_3 by introducing a double bond at C_3 [isoquinine, (10)] or inversion as in epidihydroquinlne (11) results in some loss of activity.

3. Oxidation of the vinyl group to carboxylic acid (12) destroys all the activity, the 3-aldehyde analog (13), however, possesses some activity. The reduction of the aldehydic group to alcoholic group (14) destroys the activity.

4. Replacement of C_9–OH group with H or halogen results in loss of antimalarial activity. Similar loss of activity has been observed in case double beond is introduced between C_8 and C_9.

5. The 6' methoxyl group seems to be essential for the antimalarial activity.

6. Opening of the quinclidine ring results in quinotoxine (15), which is devoid of any activity. Its reduced product (16) is also inactive.

7. The niquine (17) obtained by treating quinine (5b) with hydrogen halide and subsequently with alkalies is active. This demonstrates that the grouping Q-CHOH-CH-N is important for the activity. Based on this 6'-methoxyquinolyl-2-piperidylcarbinol (18) was synthesized and tested. It was found to be active. The compound 2-phenyl-6, 8-dichloro-4-quinolyl-2'-piperidyl carbinol (19) was found to possess high quinine co-efficient. But it has been found to be toxic for human beings.

(12), R = COOH
(13), R = CHO
(14), R = CH₂OH

(15)

(16)

(17)

(18)

(19)

Two mechanisms have been proposed for the antimalarial activity of quinine (5b). One of the mechanisms proposed involves intercalation into the DNA of parasite leading to inhibition of synthesis of nucleic acids.

The other mechanism involves inhibition of detoxification of ferriprotoporphyrin IX. Malarial parasites cannot synthesize their own requirement of amino acids. They depend upon the amino acids released from the hemoglobin of the host after they ingest it. Along with the amino acids, a toxic heme metabolite, ferriprotoporphyrin IX, is also released. The toxic ferriprotoporphyrin IX is detoxified by polymerization to hemozoin by the malarial parasites. Quinine (5b) is a weak base and it readily diffuses across the membrane of food vacuole of malarial parasite, which has an acidic pH. Once inside, it gets protonated and cannot diffuse out. As a result its concentration inside the food vacuole builds up. Quinine (5b) inhibits the conversion of toxic ferriprotoporphyrin IX to nontoxic polymerized heme, hemozoin. Free ferriprotoporphyrin IX forms superoxide (O_2^-) with free oxygen which causes lysosomal membrane damage and toxicity to the malarial parasite.

Artemisnin and its Synthetic Analogs

Artemisinin (20), a sesquiterpene lactone with a peroxide moiety, has been isolated from Chinese herb, *Artemisia annua*, family *Compositae*. The lactone artemisinin (20), its reduced analog dihydroartemisinin (21) and synthetic analogs of dihydroartemisinin (21), artemether (22), arteether (23), and artesunate (24) are some of the compounds of this class presently used in clinical practice.

Artemisnin (20) and its synthetic analogs (21-24) are active against all the species of *Plasmodia* which cause malaria. Adminstration of these results in rapid decrease in malarial parasites in blood. They are not effective as prophylactics.

(20)   (21)   (22)

(23)   (24)

The active form of artemisnin (20) and its derivatives is the carbon centered free radical formed after the activation in presence of iron or heme-bound iron. Next, the artemisnin free radical alkylates heme/proteins (Fig. 22.2) which are toxic to plasmodia. Artemisnin (20) and its analogs (21–24) have specificity for plasmodium infected erythrocytes and plasmodium proteins. Two reasons have been proposed for this specificity and these include requirement of artimisnin (20) and its analogs (21–24) for heme for activation and subsequent formation of a free radical the second being the prefrential accumulation of artemisnin (20) and its analogs (21–24) in plasmodia.

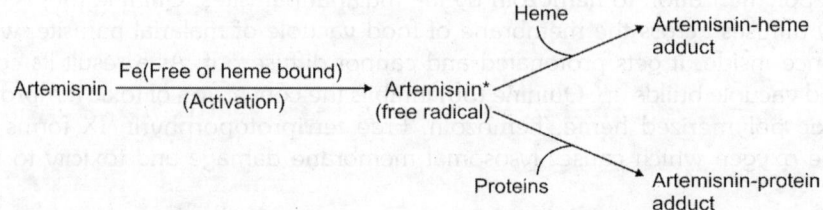

Fig. 22.2: Mechanism of antimaterial action of artemisnin and its analogs.

SYNTHETIC ANTIMALARIALS

8-Aminoquinolines

Methylene blue (25) has been shown to have some beneficial effects on patients suffering from malaria. Based on this, some analogs of methylene blue (25) in which one of the methyl groups on the dimethylamino nitrogen was replaced by dialkylaminoalkyl chain, were synthesized.. Compound (26) was more active than methylene blue but had unfavourable chemotherapeutic index. The compound (27) was active and less toxic. This observation led to belief that dialkylaminoalkyl chain was important for the antimalarial activity. Attempts were made to tag this chain with a wide range of heterocyclic ring system. This led to the first synthetic antimalarial, pamaquin (28), also called plasmochin.

(25), R = CH_3
(26), R = CH_2CH_2N(C_2H_5)_2
(27), R = CHCHCH_2N(C_2H_5)_2
                CH_3CH_3

(28)

The structure activity relationship studies have shown that:

1. Although optimum activity in 8-aminoquinolines is obtained with 6-methoxy group, such a group is, however, not essential. Activity is also encountered in compounds with 6-hydroxy or even with unsubstituted 6-position. Compounds with 6-ethoxy and 6-methyl are having either low activity or are inactive.
2. Additional substitution on quinoline nucleus tends to decrease both activity and toxicity.
3. The reduction of quinoline nucleus to 1, 2, 3, 4-tetrahydro analog is accompanied with reduction in activity.
4. For optimum activity, the basic side chain should be about 4-6 carbon atoms in length.
5. Studies on the effect of branching in the chain showed that branching was disadvantageous.

These studies have resulted in some of 8-aminoquinolines which have proved to be clinically useful and include pamaquine (28), pentaquine (29), isopentaquine (30) and primaquine (31).

(29), R = $CH_2(CH_2)_4NHCH(CH_3)_2$
(30), R = $CH(CH_2)_3NHCH(CH_3)_2$
       |
       CH_3
(31), R = $CH(CH_2)_3NH_2$
       |
       CH_3

Primaquine (31) is the only 8-aminoquinoline presently in use in clinical practice. It is effective against exoerythrocytic forms of *vivax, ovale, falciparum,* and against gametocytes of all four species of *Plasmodia*. It is rapidly metabolized and only small fraction of the administered drug is excreted as such. Four metabolites of it have been identified and include the carboxy metabolite (32), 5-hydroxymetabolite (33), 5-hydroxy-6-desmethyl metabolite (34), and quinone (35).

(32)

(33)

(34)

(35)

The antimalarial activity of primaquine (31) is due to quinone (35). It interferes with the functioning of ubiquinones. Ubiquinones are a group of lipid soluble benzoquinones involved in the electron transfer in respiratory chain. The metabolites of primaquine (31) may also cause non-specific oxidative damage to mitochondria of *Plasmodia*.

8-Aminoquinolines can cause hemolytic anemia in individuals who are deficient in glucose-6-phosphate dehydrogenase (G6PD). G6PD is required to reduce $NADP^+$ to NADPH which is further required for reducing glutathione. The reduced glutathione protects erythrocytes by breaking down the toxic oxidants. Primaquine (31) causes significant oxidative stress because of formation of various oxidized compounds and, therefore, it can cause oxidative damage in G6PD deficient individuals. G6PD is deficient in dark skinned races and, therefore, these subjects should be given 8-aminoquinolines with caution.

Acridines

Since pamaquine (28) was not a good substitute for quinine (5b), search for a good schizontocide continued. In 1932, Mauss and Mietzsch reported the discovery of 6-chloro-2-methoxy-9(1-methyl-4-diethylaminobutylamino) acridine called quinacrine [mepacrine, (36)].

Structure-activity relationship studies have shown that the most favourable position for the methoxy group is 2 and 6 for the chloro. A closely related compound 6-chloro-2-methoxy-9-diethylaminobutylaminoacridine (37) is used in USSR under the name acriquine.

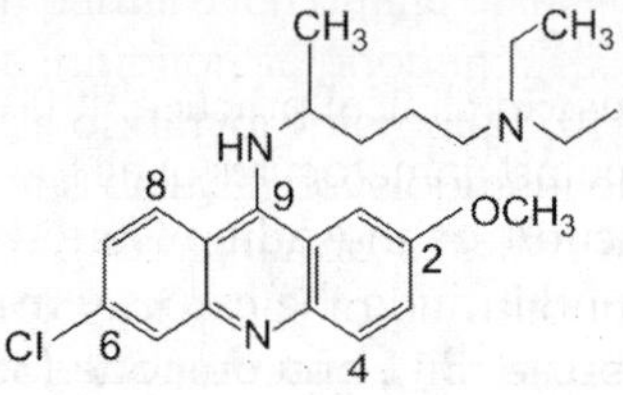

(36) 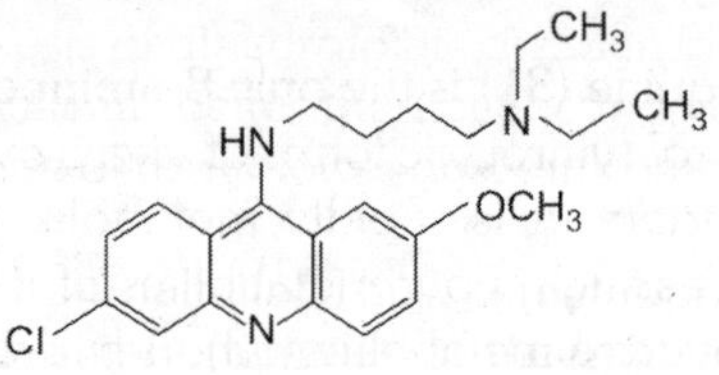   (37)

Quinacrine (36) is an effective suppressive agent and not a radically curative agent. Its antimalarial activity has been attributed to intercalation of DNA strands as well as action at mitochondrial electron transport system.

Quinacrine (36) is not used now because of its higher toxicity which includes mutagenicity as well as carcinogenicity. Further, it has unpleasant property of staining skin and eyes yellow.

4-Aminoquinolines

According to Schoenhoefer the possible positions of basic chain in quinoline nucleus, which can give rise to effective antimalarials, are 4-, 6- and 8-. The quinone formation, involving 6- and 8-positions, can take place only after oxidation (Fig. 22.3). However, in case the basic side chain is at position 4, the the quinone formation can take place by simple prototropy (Fig. 22.3). Such a tautomerism, known as "Schoenhoefer tautomerism", was essential for antimalarial activity. Further,

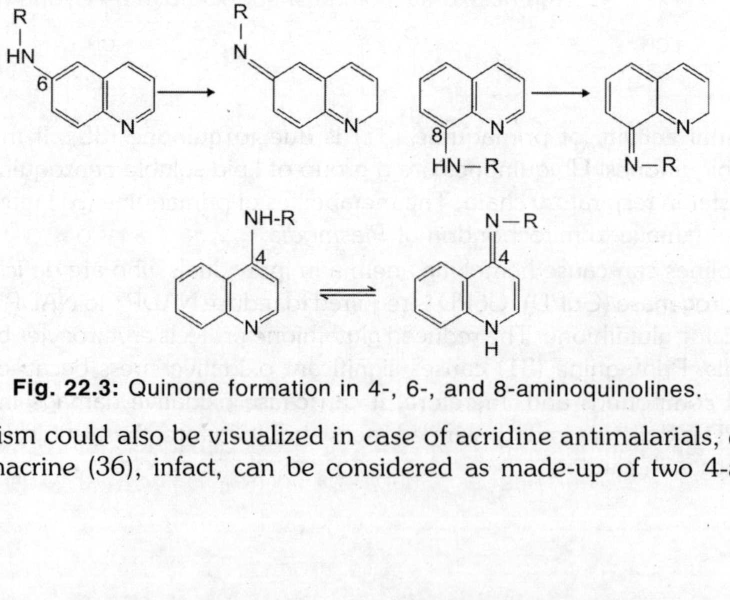

Fig. 22.3: Quinone formation in 4-, 6-, and 8-aminoquinolines.

such a tautomerism could also be visualized in case of acridine antimalarials, quinacrine (36) (Fig. 22.4). Quinacrine (36), infact, can be considered as made-up of two 4-aminoquinoline strucures, one containing rings A and B (38) and another containing rings B and C (38a). Accordingly, compounds corresponding to structures (38) and (38a) were synthesized and tested against avian malarias. They had excellent activity. The most effective compound in this series was 7-chloro-4-(4-diethylamino-1-methylbutylamino) quinoline commonly known as chloroquine (39). Other compounds clinically useful in this series include hydroxychloroquine (40) and sontoquine (41).

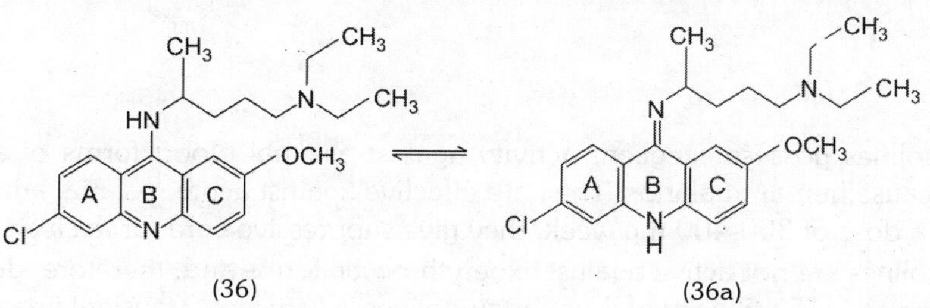

(36) (36a)

Fig. 22.4: Quinone formation in quinacrine (36).

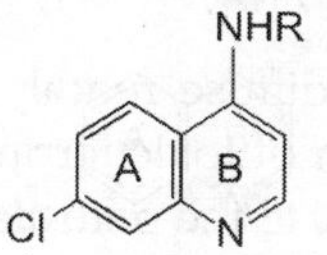

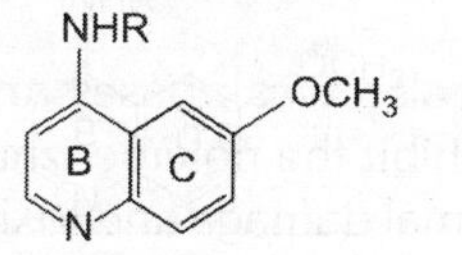

R = dialkylaminoalkyl chain

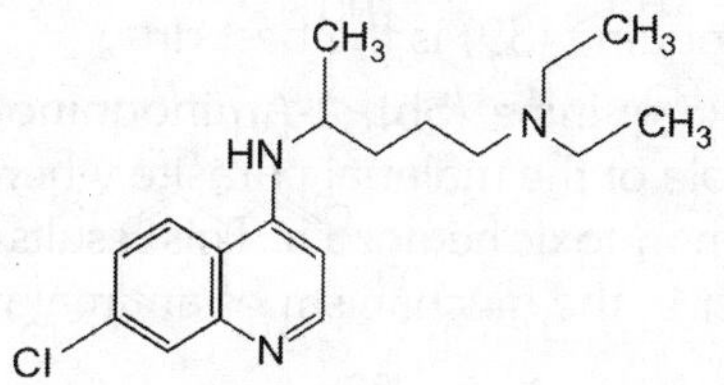

(38) (38a) (39)

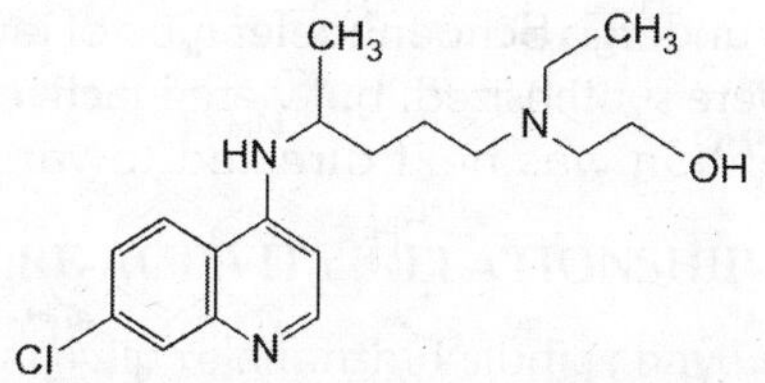

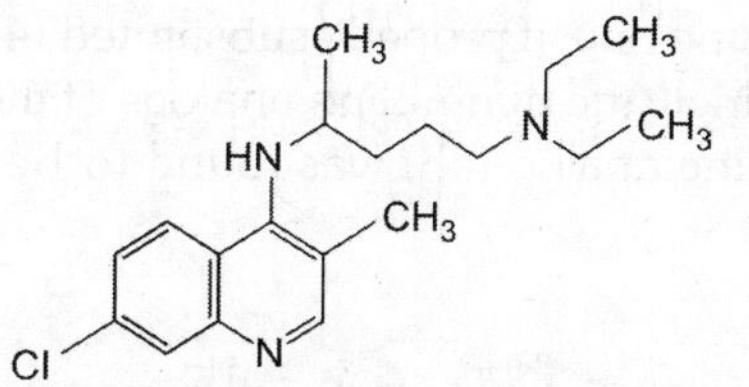

(40) (41)

The observation that certain α-dialkylamino-*o*-cresols (42 and 43) possessed antimalarial activity led to synthesis of 4-aminoquinolines containing such a moiety. Some of the clinically useful compounds in this series include amodiaquine (44) and amopyroquine (45).

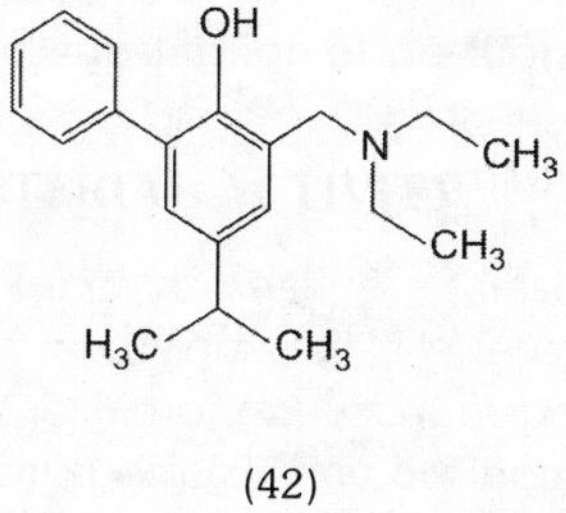

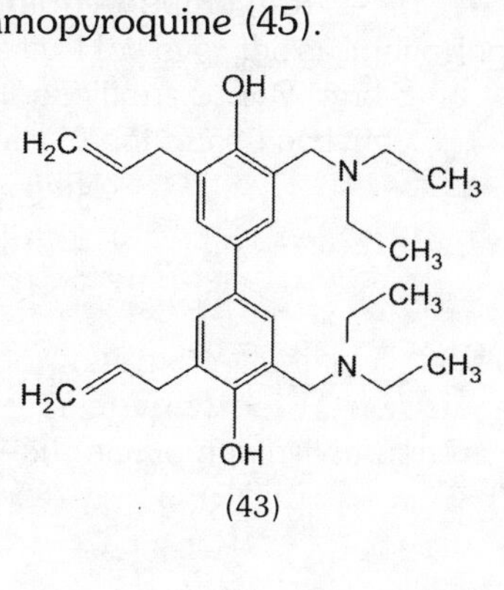

(42) (43)

(44)

(45)

4-Aminoquinolines possess excellent activity against asexual blood forms of all species of plasmodia that cause human malarias. They are effective against acute malarial attack and effect clinical cure. At a dose of 300-400 mg/week, they give suppressive cure for *falciparum* malaria.

4-Aminoquinolines are not active against exoerythrocytic forms and, therefore, do not prevent the relapses of malaria. The toxicity of 4-aminoquinolines is very less. Transient headaches, visual disturbances, and gastrointestinal upsets have been reported with therapeutic doses. None of these is serious and disappear as soon as the drug is withdrawn. Among the 4-aminoquinolines, chloroquine (39) is the best drug.

Like quinine (5b), 4-Aminoquinolines are also weak bases and diffuse readily into the food vacuole of the malarial parasite where they inhibit the polymerization of toxic ferriprotoporphyrin IX to non-toxic hemozoin. This results in lysosomal damage and toxicity to the parasite as mentioned earlier in the mechanism of antimalarial activity of quinine (5b).

Biguanides and 2,4-Diaminopyrimidines

Pyrimidine ring, if properly substituted (46) could also undergo Schoenhoefer type of tautomerism. Accordingly the pyrimidine analogs of the type (47) were synthesized, but were inactive. However, the aniline analog (48) was found to be active. Attention was next directed towards another

(46)

X = 4-Chloro or 3-or 4-Methoxy

(47)

X = 4-Chloro or 3-or 4-Methoxy

(48)

linkage, namely the guanidine group, which could also undergo tautomerism. The compound N^1-(p-chlorophenyl)-N^2-(4-diethylaminoethylamino-6-methyl-2-pyrimidyl)guanidine (49) was synthesized and found to be active against all types of malarias. Further modification of (48) and (49) in which the pyrimidine ring carbons were dispensed off resulted in (48a), which could be considered a derivative of biguanide H_2NC (=NH) NHC (=NH) NH_2 and (49a) a derivative of triguanide, respectively. The biguanide (50) was synthesized but was found to be inactive. Replacement of dialkylaminoalkyl chain in (50) by isopropyl chains resulted in chlorguanide [proguanil (51)] which was found to be active.

(49)

R = $CH_2CH_2N(C_2H_5)_2$

(48)   (48a)

R = $CH_2CH_2N(C_2H_5)_2$

(49)   (49a)

(50)   (51)

The active form of chlorguanide (51) is cycloguanil (52). Chlorguanide (51) is highly active against asexual forms of malarial parasite. Treatment with chlorguanide (51) results in clinical cure of all forms of human malarias and radical cure in most *falciparum* infections. However, it is not suitable for treatment of acute attacks as it acts slowly. The drug can be used as a prophylactic in *falciparum* infections. Chlorguanide (51) has sporontocidal activity rendering plasmodia unable to complete sporogony and preventing transmission of infection. Toxic effects with 100 mg daily dose are rare. However, persons with low nutrition may show deficiency of folic acid which may become serious. The drug is eliminated rapidly from the body so daily administration of the drug is necessary. This factor together with development of resistance has limited the usefulness of the drug.

(51)　→　(52)

The 2, 4-diaminopyrimidine analog (53) was found to be a powerful pteroylglutamic acid inhibitor. An examination of (53) shows that its structure closely resmbles chlorguanide (51). Accordingly, it was predicted that 2, 4-diaminopyrimidine analog (53) and its alkyl derivative might be possessing antimalarial activity. This prediction was found to be true in case of methyl analog (54). Further structure activity relationship studies in 2, 4-diamino-5-arylpyrimidines showed that the 6-ethyl analog, pyrimethamine (55) had the most favourable activity data.

(53),R = H; (54),R = CH₃

(51)

Pyrimethamine (55) and chlorguanide (51) exert nearly similar type of activity against plasmodia excepting that they differ in duration of activity. Pyrimethamine (55) is most powerful suppressive agent and achieves suppressive cure in *falciparum* infections. It also produces clinical cure in case of *falciparum* infections. Pyrimethamine (55) is eliminated from body much less rapidly than chlorguanide (51) and daily administration of drug is unnecessary. Pyrimethamine (55) is blood schizontocide without effect on tissue schizonts. One of the disadvantage of pyrimethamine (55) is its liability to resistance. It is given along with sulphadoxine (56). This combination produces sequential blockade of tetrahydrfolate synthesis. This combination with quinine (5b) is used for chloroquine (39) resistant strains.

(55)

(56)

Chlorguanide (51) and pyrimethamine (55) are powerful inhibitors of dihydrofoliate reductase, the enzyme responsible for reduction of dihydrofoliate to tetrahydrofolate which is later used for one carbon metabolism. Since pyrimethamine has higher affinity for the dihydrofoliate reductase of plasmodium so it binds selectively to it rather than human dihydrfoliate reductase. Combination of pyrimethamine (55) and sulfadoxine (56) results in sequential blockade, first in the incorporation of PABA into guanosine for the synthesis of dihydropteroic acid and then in the reduction of dihydrofolic acid to tetrahydrofolic acid by tetrahydrofolic acid reductase (Fig. 22.5).

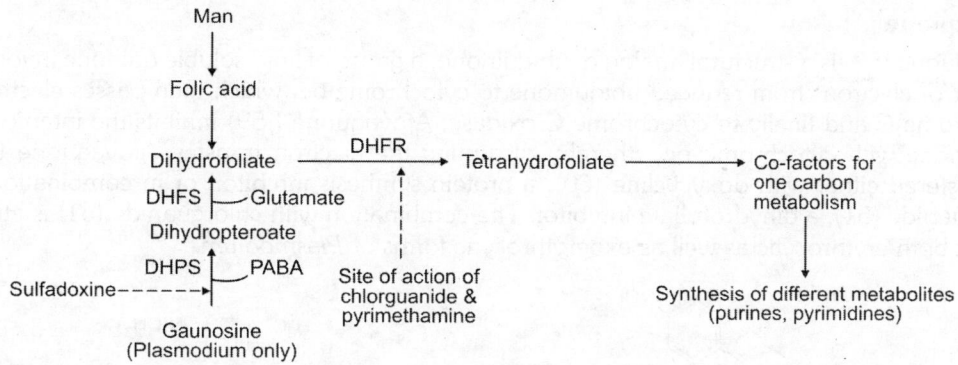

Fig. 22.5: Site of action of chlorguanide (52), pyrimethamine (56) and sulphadoxine (57).

(DHPS-dihydropteroate synthetase; DHFS-dihydrofoliate synthetase;

DHFR-dihydrofoliate reductase; PABA-p-aminobenzoic acid)

Miscellaneous Compounds

This group of synthetic antimalarials comprises of compounds of diverse structures.

Mefloquine

Mefloquine (57) is a 4-quinoline derivative and was introduced in 1989. It has two asymmetric centres and exists in 4-enantiomeric forms. All of these forms have similar activity. Although the drug is active against chloroquine (39) resistant forms yet the cross resistance is not uncommon.

The exact mechanism of mefloquine (57) is not known, however, there is some evidence that it interferes with ability of parasite to process heme.

(57)

Halofantrine

Halofantrine (58) is a phenanthrene analog. It has one asymmetric carbon atom, however, both the enantiomers have similar activity. It is a schizontocide and has no effect on sporozoite, gametocyte, or hepatic stages of the parasite. It is used both against chloroquine (39) sensitive as well as choroquine (39) resistant strains.

(58)

Atovaquone

Atovaquone (59) is a structural analog of ubiquinone, a group of lipid soluble quinone involved in transfer of electrons from reduced ubiquinone to cytochrome bc_1 which then passes electrons to cytochrome C and finally to cytochrome C oxidase. Atovaquone (59) inhibits the interaction of ubiquinone with cytochrome bc_1, thereby disrupting the electron transfer. Atovaquone (59) is administered either with doxycycline (60), a protein synthesis inhibitor, or in combination with chlorguanide (51), a dihydrofoliate inhibitor. The combination with chlorguanide (51) is effective against both erythrocytic as well as exoerythrocytic forms of *Plasmodium*.

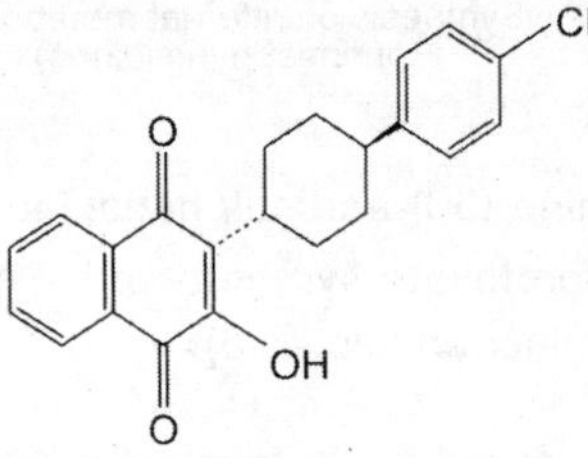

(59) 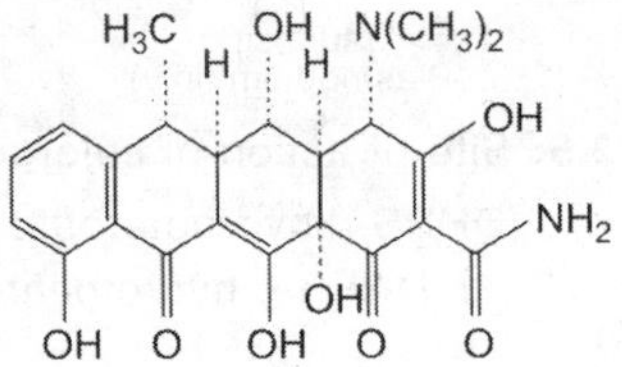   (60)

INDIVIDUAL COMPOUNDS

SYNTHETIC ANTIMALARIALS : 8-AMINOQUINOLINES

Primaquine

8-(4-Amino-1-methylbutylamino)-6-methoxyquinoline

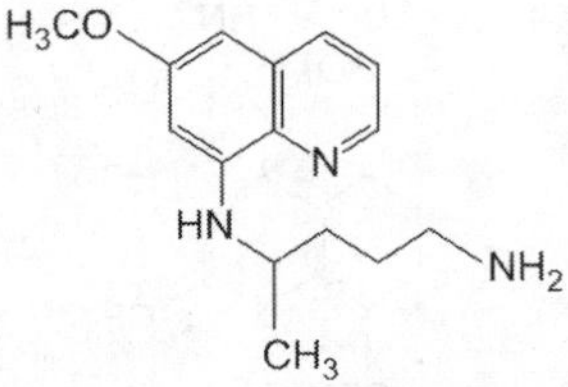

Synthesis

Step 1

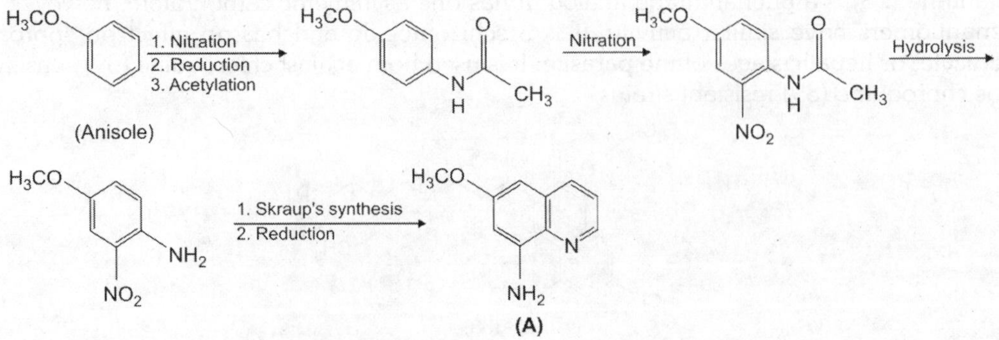

(Anisole)

(A)

Step 2

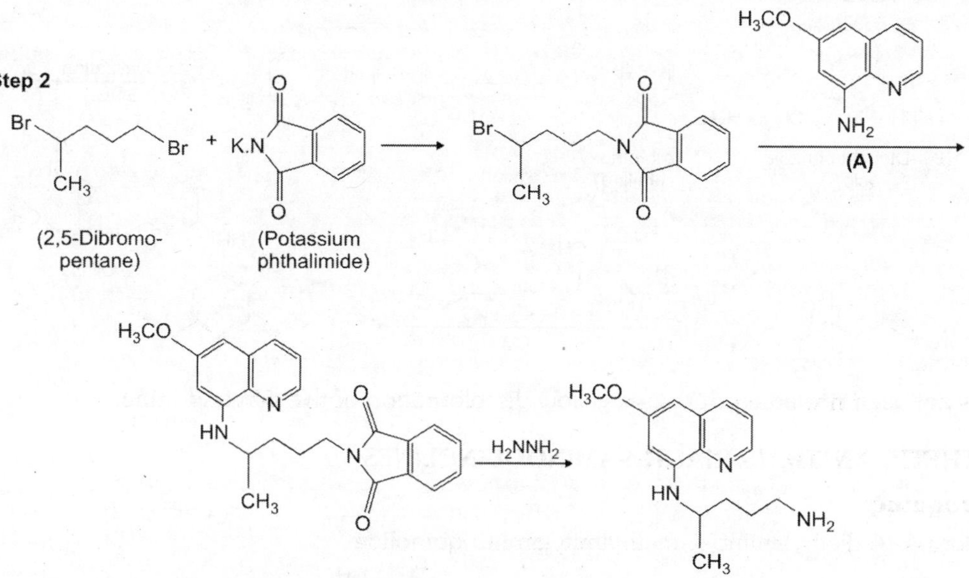

(2,5-Dibromo-
pentane)

(Potassium
phthalimide)

(A)

SYNTHETIC ANTIMALARIALS : ACRIDINES

Quinacrine

6-Chloro-9-[[4-(diethylamino)-1-methylbutyl]amino]-2-methoxyacridine

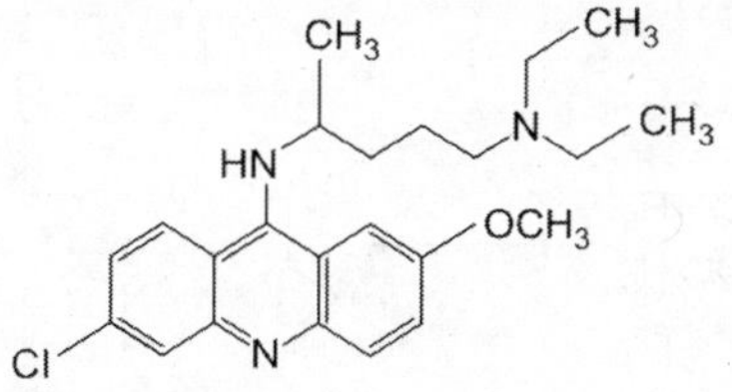

Synthesis

Step 1

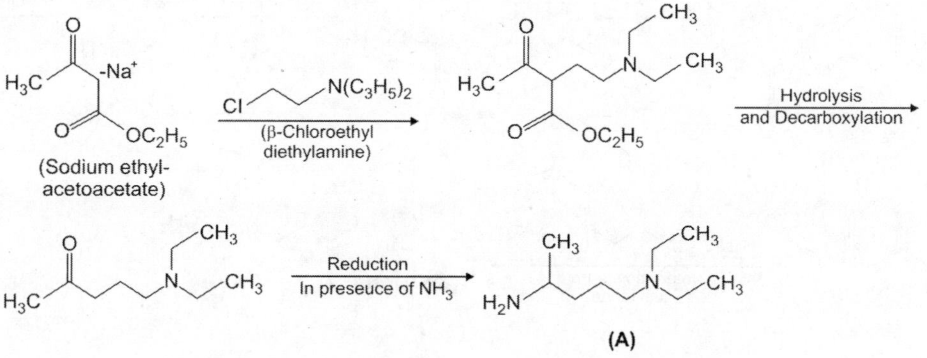

(Sodium ethyl-
acetoacetate)

(β-Chloroethyl
diethylamine)

Hydrolysis
and Decarboxylation

Reduction
In preseuce of NH₃

(A)

Step 2

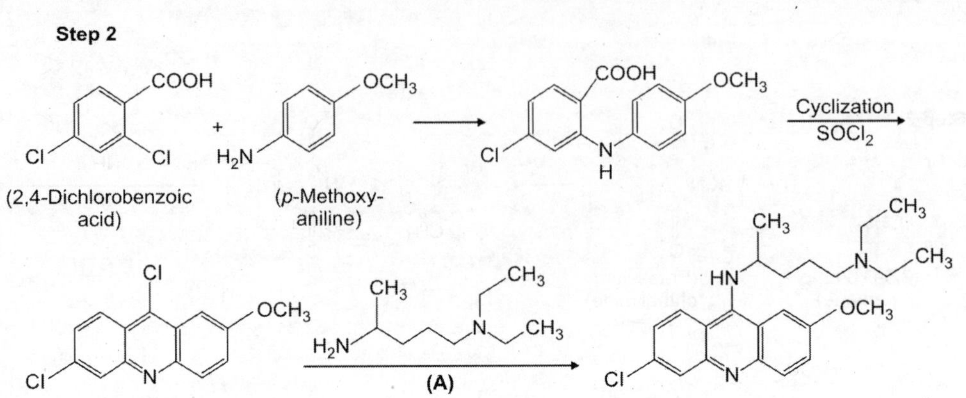
COOH
OCH3
Cl
Cl
H2N
(2,4-Dichlorobenzoic acid)
(p-Methoxy- aniline)
Cyclization
SOCl2
(A)

It is not used nowadays. It causes yellow discolouration of the skin and urine.

SYNTHETIC ANTIMALARIALS: 4-AMINOQUINOLINES

Chloroquine

7-Chloro-4-(4-diethylamino-1-methylbutylamino)quinoline

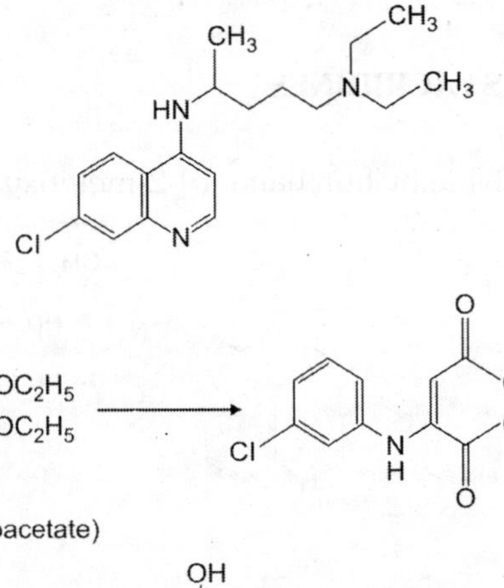

Synthesis

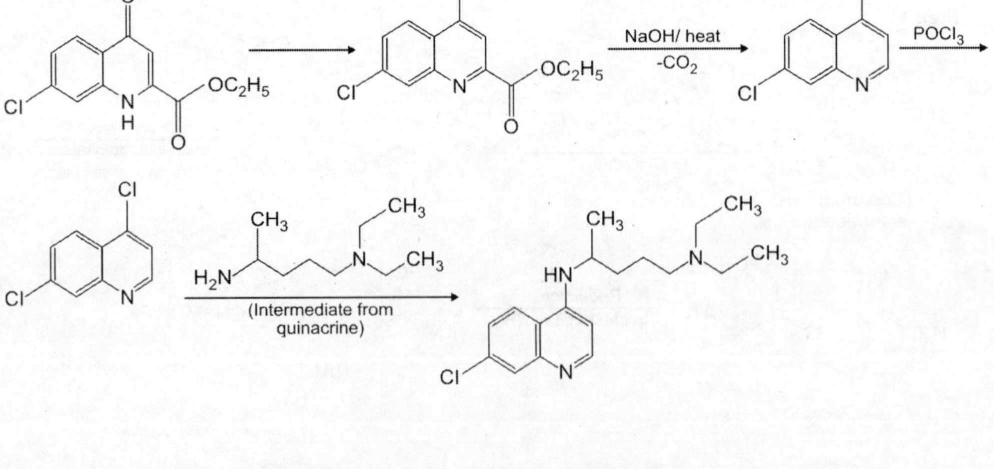
(m-chlroanline)
(Ethyloxaloacetate)
250°
Cyclization
NaOH/ heat
-CO2
POCl3
(Intermediate from quinacrine)

It is one of the commonly used antimalarials. Its other uses include as antiamoebic and antirheumatic agent.

Hydroxychloroquine

7-Chloro-4-[4-[ethyl(2-hydroxyethyl)amino]-1-methylbutylamino]quinoline

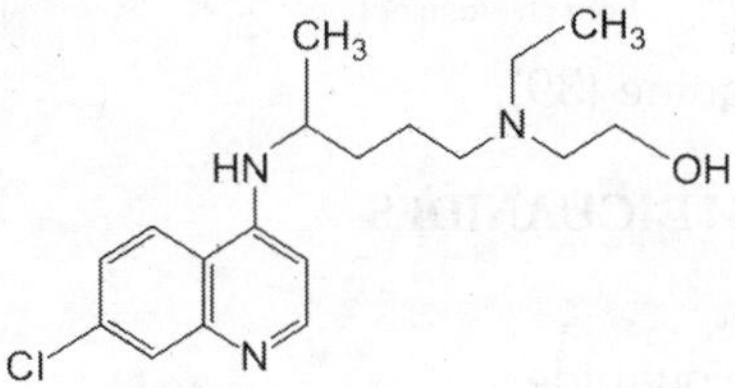
CH3
CH3
HN
N
OH
Cl
N

Synthesis

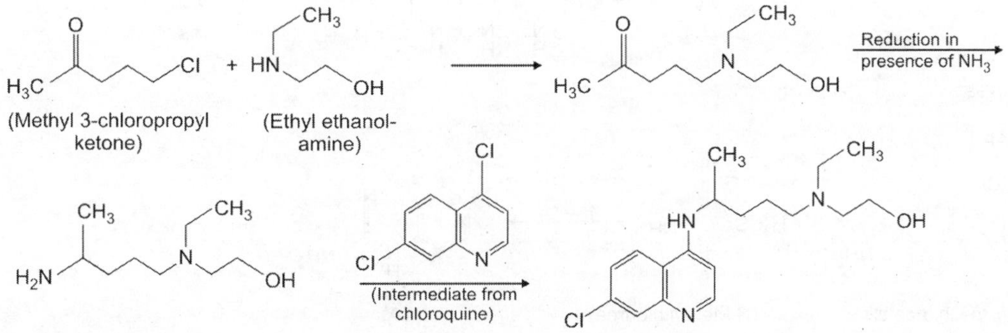
(Methyl 3-chloropropyl ketone)
(Ethyl ethanol- amine)
Reduction in presence of NH3
(Intermediate from chloroquine)

It has similar action as chloroquine (39).

Amodiaquine

7-Chloro-4-(3-diethylaminomethyl-4-hydroxyanilino)quinoline

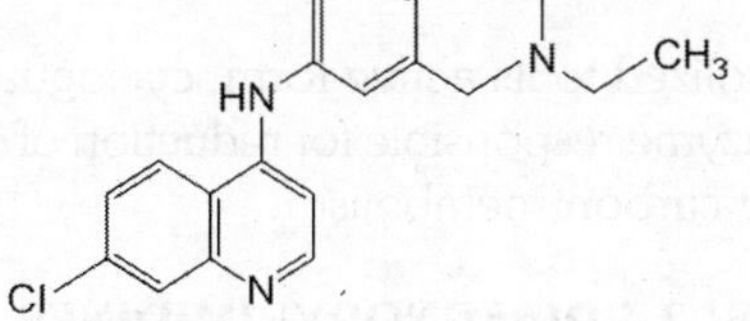
OH
CH3
N
CH3
HN
Cl
N

Synthesis

Step 1

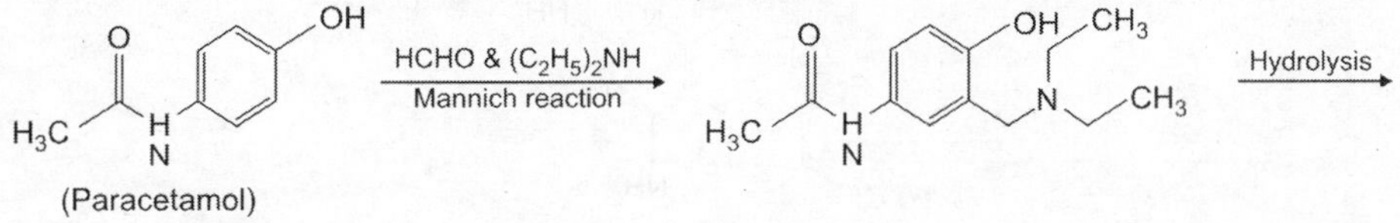
(Paracetamol)
HCHO & (C2H5)2NH
Mannich reaction
Hydrolysis

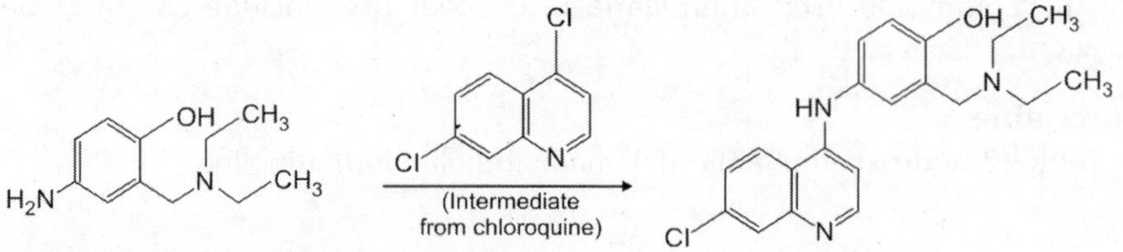

It has similar action as chloroquine (39).

SYNTHETIC ANTIMALARIALS : BIGUANIDES

Chlorguanide

1-(*p*-Chlorophenyl)-5-isopropylbiguanide

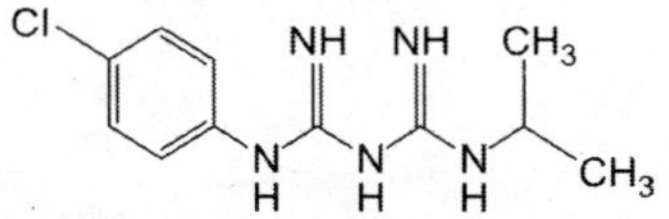

Synthesis

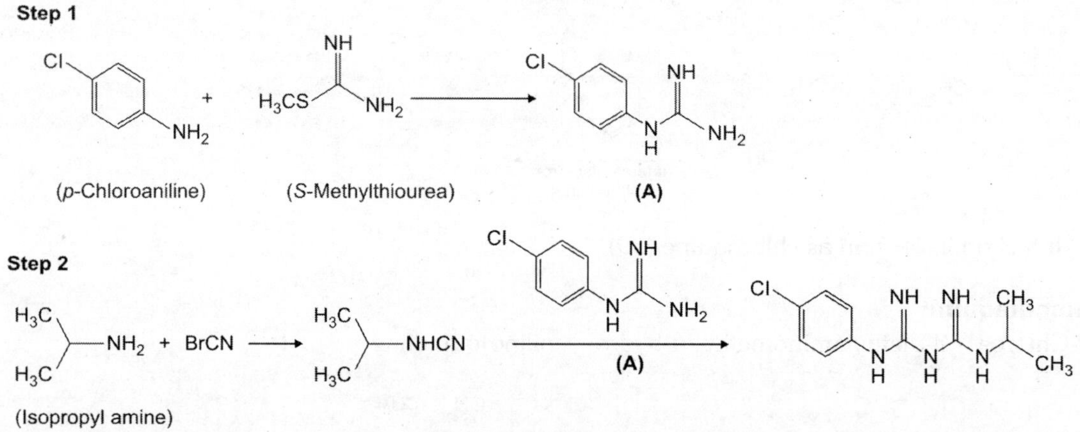

Step 1

(*p*-Chloroaniline)   (*S*-Methylthiourea)   (A)

Step 2

(Isopropyl amine)

It is a prodrug which is metabolized to its active form, cycloguanil (52). It is a powerful inhibitor of dihydrofoliate reductase, an enzyme responsible for reduction of dihydrofoliate to tetrahydrofoliate, a metabolite responsible for one carbon metabolism.

SYNTHETIC ANTIMALARIALS : 2,4-DIAMINOPYRIMIDINES

Pyrimethamine

2,4-Diamino-5-(*p*-chlorophenyl)-6-ethylpyrimidine

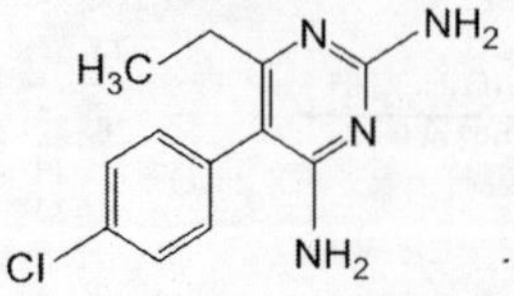

Synthesis

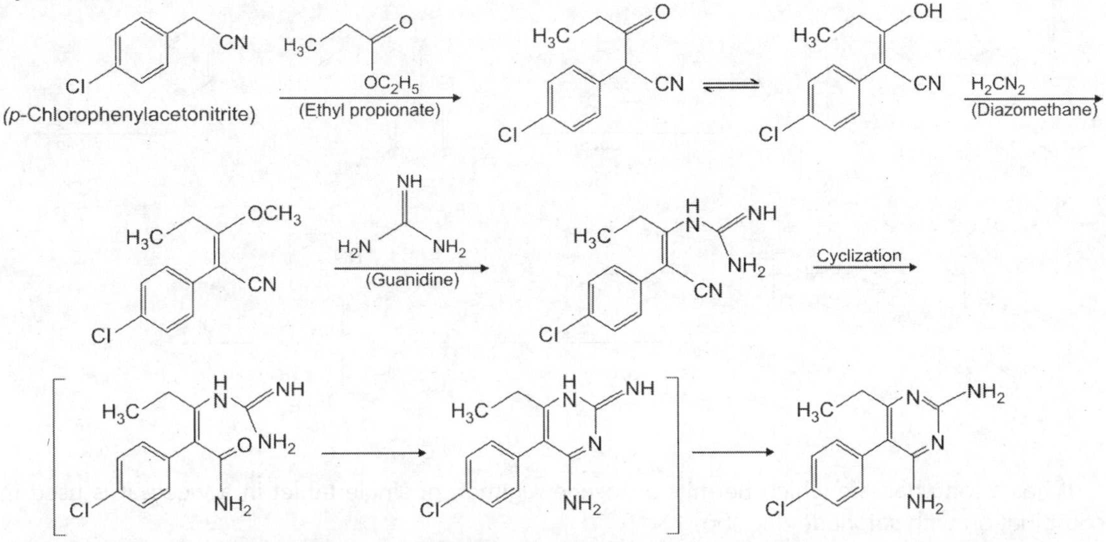

(*p*-Chlorophenylacetonitrite) (Ethyl propionate) (Diazomethane)

(Guanidine) Cyclization

It is a powerful inhibitor of dihydrofoliate reductase, an enzyme responsible for reduction of dihydrofoliate to tetrahydrofoliate. Tetrahydrofoliate is required for one carbon metabolism including synthesis of pyrimidines and purines required for nucleic acid synthesis.

Sulphadoxine

See **SULPHONAMIDES AND QUINOLONES**

SYNTHETIC ANTIMALARIALS : MISCELLANEOUS COMPOUNDS

Mefloquine Hydrochloride

(αS)-(2R)-2-Piperidinyl-2,8-bis(trifluoromethyl)-4-quinolinemethanol monohydrochloide

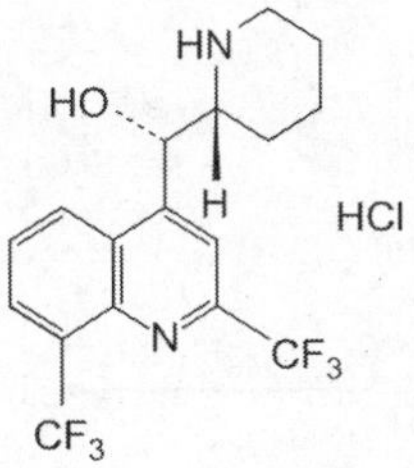

Synthesis

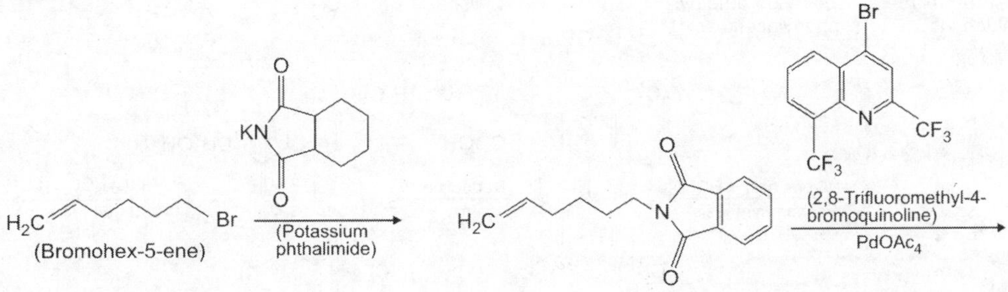

H_2C (Bromohex-5-ene) Br (Potassium phthalimide)

(2,8-Trifluoromethyl-4-bromoquinoline)

$PdOAc_4$

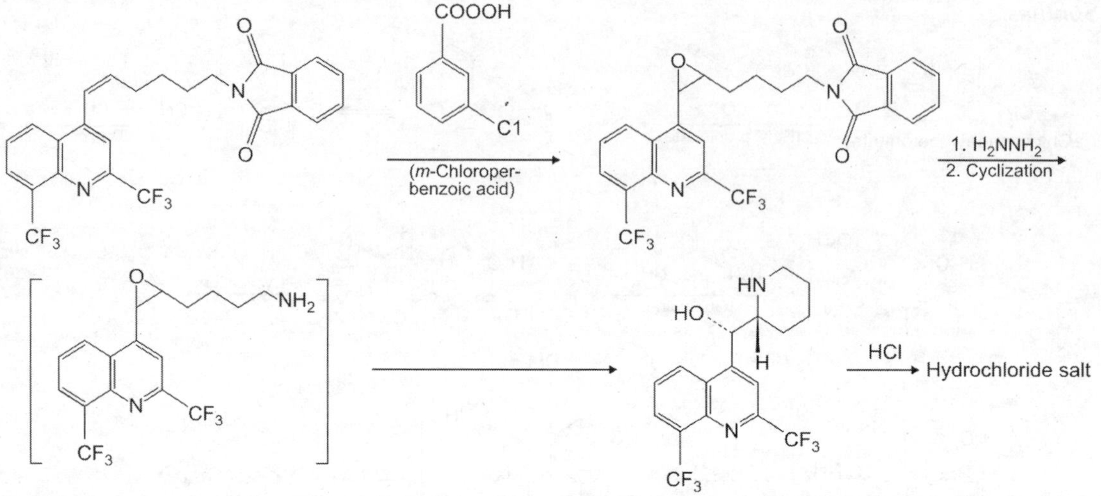

It has a long half-life which permits a dosage regimen of single tablet in a week. It is used in combination with sulphadoxine (56).

Halofantrine

1,3-Dichloro-α-[2-dibutylamino)ethyl]-6-(trifluoromethyl)-9-phenanthrenemethanol

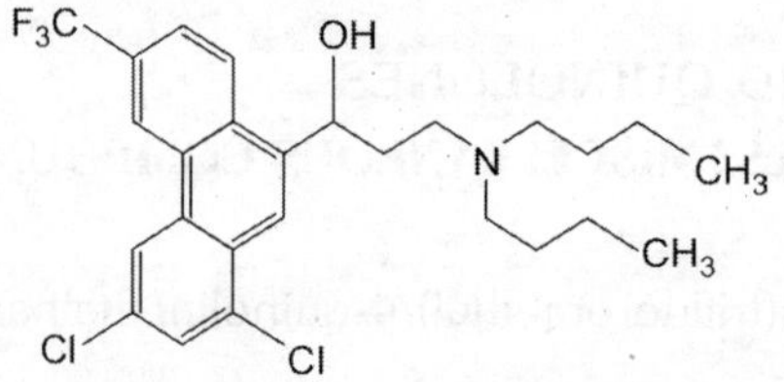

Synthesis

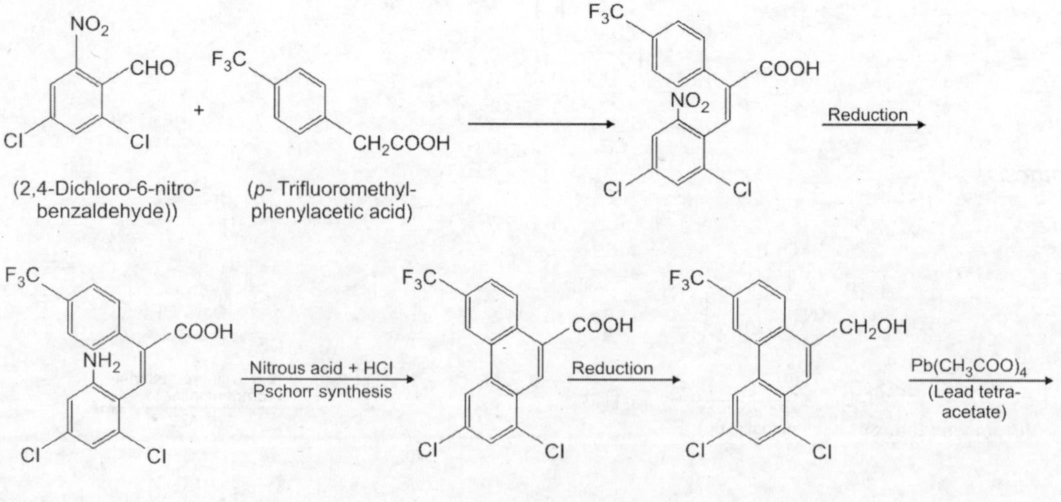

(2,4-Dichloro-6-nitro-benzaldehyde))   (*p*- Trifluoromethyl-phenylacetic acid)

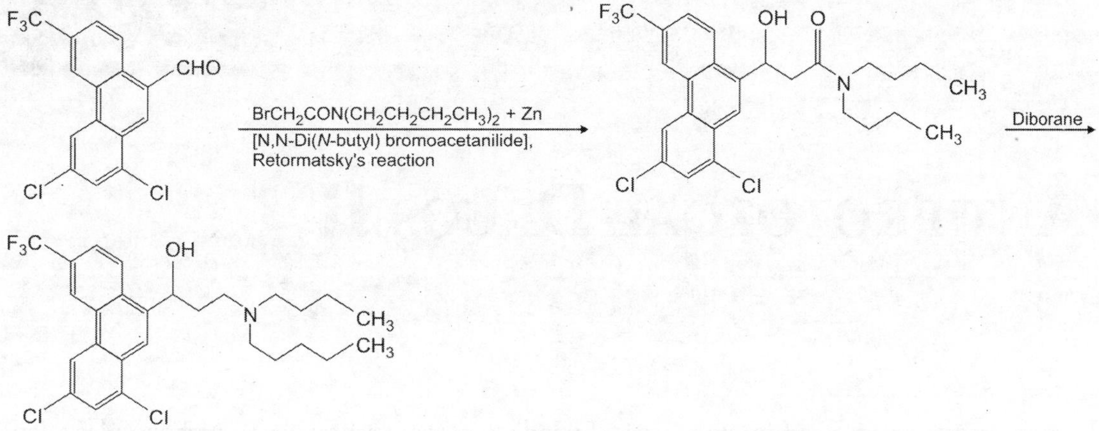

It is a schizontocide and has no effect on sporozoite, gametocyte, or hepatic stages of malarial parasite.

Atovaquone

2-[*trans*-4-(4-Chlorophenyl)cyclohexyl]-3-hydroxy-1,4-naphthalenedione.

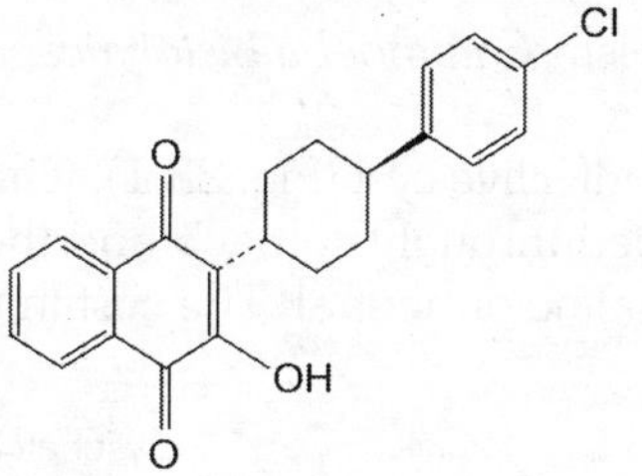

Synthesis

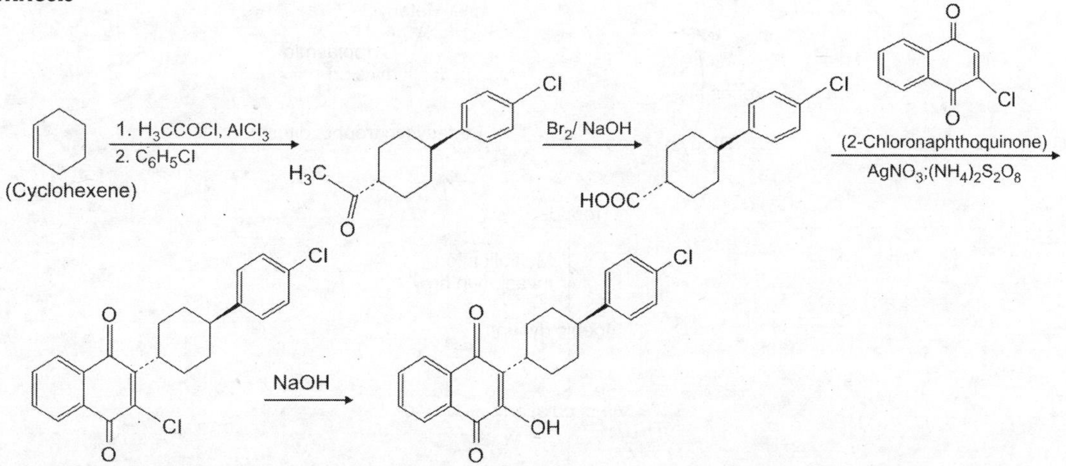

It is administered in combination either with doxycycline (60) or chlorguanide (51).

Doxycycline Hydrate

See **TETRACYCLINE ANTIBIOTICS**

CHAPTER
23

ANTIPROTOZOAL DRUGS II

IN THIS CHAPTER drugs used in amoebiasis, trypanosomiasis, leishmaniasis, trichomoniasis, and giardiasis will be discussed.

CHEMOTHERAPY OF AMOEBIASIS

Amoebiasis is caused by the organism *Entamoeba histolytica*, a microscopic one-celled organism, belonging to family *Amoebidae*.

Infection is aquired by ingesting infective cyst (Fig. 23.1), which is usually found in contaminated food and drink. It passes unchanged through stomach and the proximal portion of intestine and reaches a level where the pH is alkaline or neutral. The cyst in this pH becomes active, ruptures its

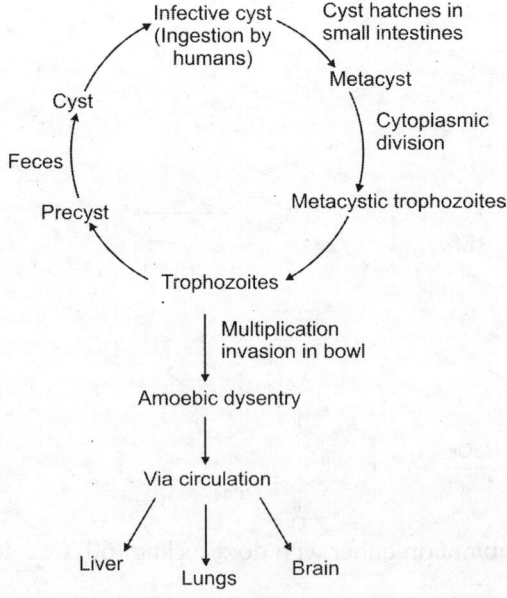

Fig. 23.1: Life cycle of Entamoeba histolytica

envelope to form infective metacyst. The metacyst undergoes cytoplasmic division to form metacystic trophozoites (nuclei in metacyst), this then develops into trophozoite, which is the active, growing, and multiplying stage. It invades tissues and secretes a factor that inhibits IFNr-activated macrophages which would otherwise kill it. It multiplies by binary fission and can exist in trophozoite stage as long as it remains in tissues. The trophozoite stage is also the predominant stage in diarrhoeic or dysenteric stool.

When dehydration of feces takes place in the lower part of colon, the trophozoite expels undigested inclusions and rounds up to form precyst and cyst which after maturation is expelled along with stool.

The parasite may invade other parts of the body such as liver, lungs, or even brain. Amoebiasis may be divided into two classes namely, intestinal amoebiasis and extraintestinal amoebiasis.

DRUGS USED IN AMOEBIASIS – NATURAL

Emetine (1), an alkaloid found in ipecac, is used as hydrochloride. It occurs as a light-sensitive white powder. It is used in hepatic amoebiasis along with chloroquine (2). Dehydroemetine (3), the 2, 3-unsaturated analog is less toxic than emetine (1).

(1)

(2)

(3)

Both emetine (1) and dehydroemetine (3) are protoplasmic poisons that inhibit protein synthesis by preventing protein elongation.

Among the antibiotics, erythromycin (4), paromomycin (5), and some tetracyclines have been used against intestinal amoebiasis. Paromomycin (5) has direct action on amoeba while other antibiotics act by suppressing the intestinal flora which is essential for the growth of amoeba.

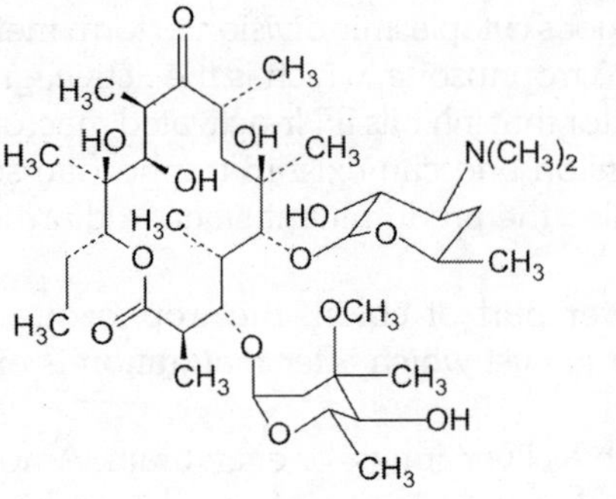

(4) 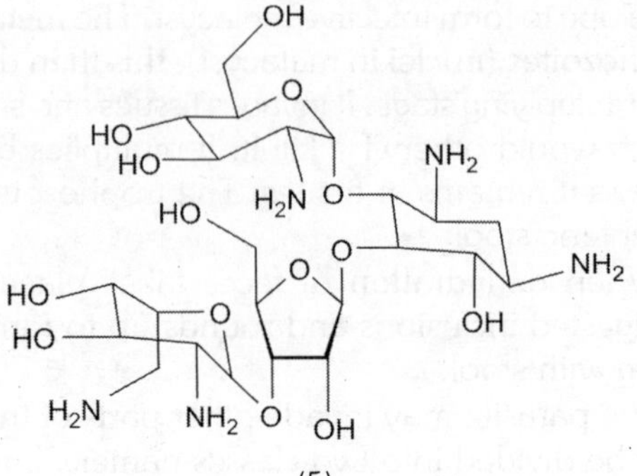 (5)

DRUGS USED AMOEBIASIS – SYNTHETIC

Hydroxyquinolines

Among the hydroxyquinolines, chiniofon (6), iodoquinol (7), and clioquinol (8) have been found to be effective against intestinal amoebiasis. These agents are believed to act through their ability to chelate the metal ions (Fe^{2+}) essential for growth of the parasites. Because of their toxicity they are not used now.

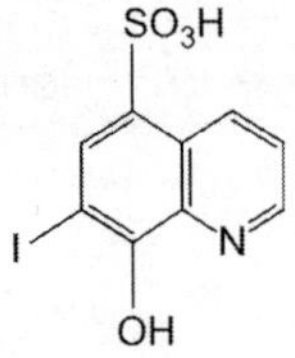

(6) 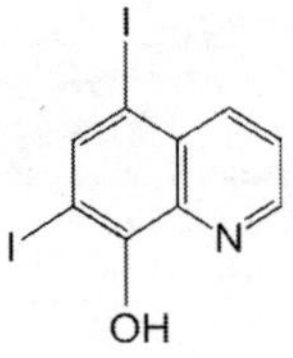 (7) 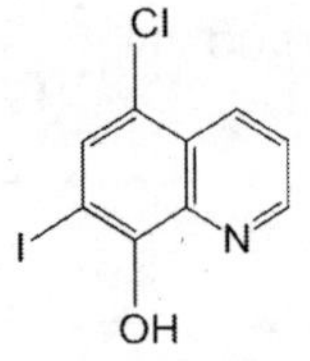 (8)

Aminoquinolines

A number of antimalarials belonging to 4-aminoquinoline group have shown antiamoebic activity. Clinically useful activity, however, has been found in case of chloroquine (2). It is used in hepatic amoebiasis because it is highly concentrated in liver. It is not effective in intestinal amoebiasis probably because it gets absorbed readily and almost completely from small bowl. Chloroquine (2) has a direct action against trophozoites of *E. histolytica*.

Haloacetamides

Among halocacetamides, diloxanide furoate (9a) has been found to be effective. After oral administration, it gets hydrolyzed to diloxanide (9b), the active form, in lumen or mucosa of intestine. It is ineffective in extraintestinal forms of amoebiasis. Little is known about its mechanism of action.

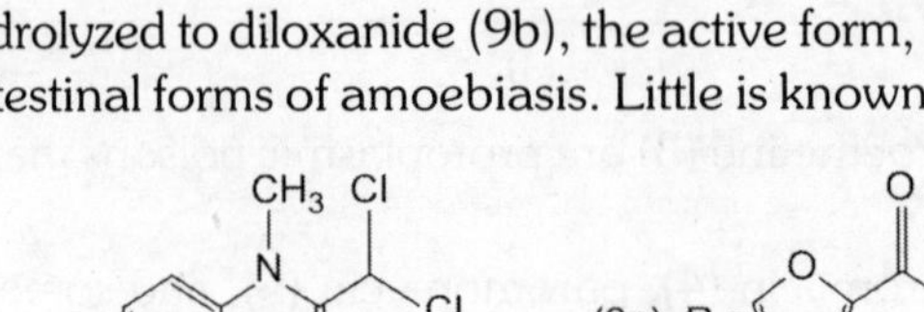

(9a), R =
(9b), R = H

Nitrothiazoles

The discovery of the potent in vitro and systemic trichomonicidal properties of 2-amino-5-nitrothiazole (10) resulted in the synthesis of various analogs of nitrothiazole. The most active compound proved to be 2-acetamido-5-nitrothiazole (11). This compound was effective against intestinal amoebiasis in rats and dogs. Similarly, niridazole (12) was also shown to be active amoebicide. However, these compounds are not used presently in clinical practice.

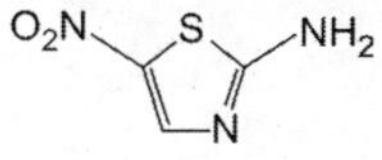

(10) 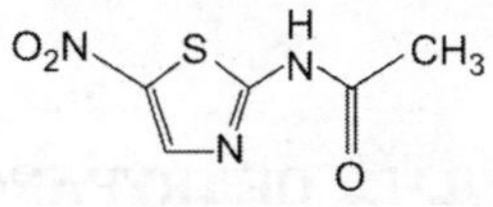   (11) 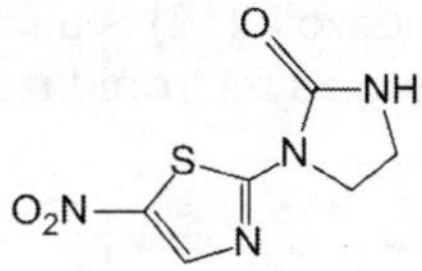   (12)

Imidazole Derivatives

Among the imidazole analogs, metronidazole (13) and tinidazole (14) have shown to be the most effective amoebicidal agents. They are used against both intestinal and extraintestinal amoebiasis. They kill trophozoites but do not have any action on cyst.

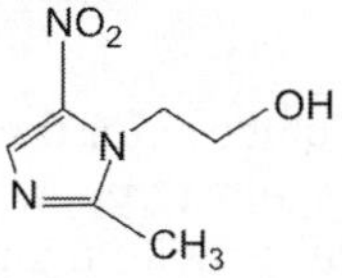

(13) 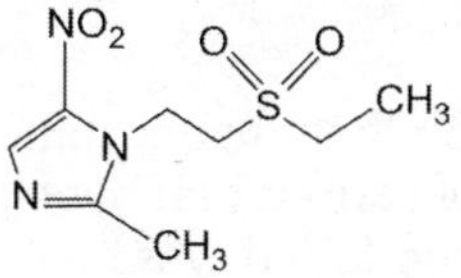   (14)

Metronidazole (13) has selective toxicity towards anaerobic and microphilic organisms such as *E. histolytica, T. vaginalis,* and *G.lamblia.* It requires activation through reduction of nitro group. In anerobic microorganisms the pyruvate is converted to acetyl CoA by the enzyme pyruvate-ferredoxin oxidoreductase (PFOR). The reduced ferredoxin in turn transfers its electron to metronidazole (13). The single electron forms a highly reactive nitro anion radical which on reaction with molecular oxygen generates cytotoxic intermediates such as superoxide and hydrogen peroxide (Fig. 23.2). These cytotoxic intermediates cause damage to DNA, protein, and parasitic cellular membrane. Because PFOR is expressed in protozoa and other anaerobic organisms and is not found in mammalian system, therfore metronidazole is selectively toxic to the anaerobic organisms.

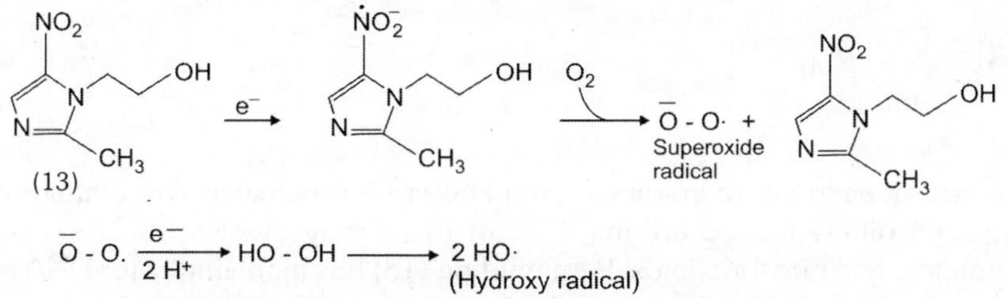

Fig. 23.2: Mechanism of metronidazole action.

Metronidazole (13) has bitter taste, its benzoate ester (15), which is tasteless, is used for the preparation of oral suspensions.

(15)

Tinidazole (14) is a second generation nitroimidazole. It is believed to have similar mechanism of action as metronidazole (13).

CHEMOTHERAPY OF TRYPANOSOMIASIS

Trypanosomiasis which is caused by parasite *Trypanosoma* is transmitted by certain insects. *T. gambiense* and *T. rhodesiense* are responsible for African sleeping sickness and *T. cruzi* causes what is known as Chaga's disease in S. America. Of the two, Chaga's disease is the most serious and generally the more resistant to chemotherapy. Damage to the tissues is caused by release of toxins and the tissues involved include CNS in sleeping sickness and heart, sometimes liver, spleen, bone, and intestine in Chaga's disease.

Diamidines

The observation that trypanosomes require extracellular supply of glucose for their survival led to investigation of various oral hypoglycemic agents for their activity against trypanosomes. The first compound to be tested was synthalin (16). It showed trypanocidal activity against *T. brucei* in mice. However, synthalin (16) was found to be toxic to trypanosomes in vitro in sugar containing medium and at concentrations which would not be hypoglycemic to mammals. Thus, the trypanocidal activity of synthalin was not due to its hypoglycemic activity but due to its direct action. This observation led to investigation of many other diamidines (17–23). Out of these, pentamidine (18) was found to be highly active and has been introduced in clinical practice. It is used for mass prophylaxis against Gambian sleeping sickness and is active against *T. rhodesiense.* Diminazene (23), a related compound is widely used against cattle trypanosomiasis particularly against *T. congolense* and *T. vivax* infections.

(17), $X = CH_2$
(18), $X = O(CH_2)_5O$
(19), $X = O(CH_2)_3O$
(20), $X = CH = CH$
(21), $X = (CH_3)C = C(CH_3)$
(22), $X = O$
(23), $X = N = N – NH$

The mechanism of action of diamidines is not known. It is believed that diamidines may show their effect through different mechanisms. One of these may involve inhibition of synthesis of DNA, RNA, proteins, and phospholipids. Pentamidine (18) has high affinity for DNA in kinetoplasts – a DNA organelle in certain protozoa, and it suppresses kinetoplast replication and function. Pentamidine (18) has also been reported to inhibit dihydrofolate reductase. Some of the strains of *Trypanosoma* have been reported to have high affinity uptake system for pentamidine (18), which contributes towards its selectivity.

Miscellaneous Compounds

This group of trypanocidal agents includes diverse group of compounds and include suramin sodium (24), a nitrofuran analog nifurtimox (25), nitrobenzimidazole analog benznidazole (26), an organarsenic compound, melarsoprol (27), and ornithine analog eflornithine (28).

Among the early drugs were the dyes, but these could not be used in humans and animals. Structure-activity relationship studies led to more effective drug suramin sodium (24). It has been used for more than 50 years for the early cases of trypanosomiasis.

(24)

The mechanism of action of suramin sodium (24) is not established, but the drug is known to interact with many macromolecules and cause their inhibition. Some of these include enzymes, including those involved in energy metabolism. Suramin sodium (24) has also been reported o inhibit RNA polymerase, which results in inhibition of replication in the parasite.

Nifurtimox (25) is trypanocidal against trypomastigote and amastigote forms of *T. cruzi*. Its activity has been attributed to its reduction to anion radical, which later gets oxidized to generate superoxide anion radical and subsequently the formation of hydrogen peroxide (Fig. 23.2, mechanism of metronidazole action). Organisms like trypanosomes are sensitive to hydrogen peroxide because they lack catalase, the enzyme responsible for degradation of hydrogen peroxide. Since mammalian cells contain antioxidants like catalase, superoxide dismutase, and glutathione peroxidase, they therefore, are not affected by nifurtimox (25).

(25)

(26)

(27)

(28)

Unlike other nitroaryl compounds, the nitroimidazole analog benznidazole (26), does not catalyze the formation of reactive oxygen intermediates, like superoxide anion radical and hydrogen peroxide. Its action has been attributed to transfer of one electron to nitro group yielding anion (29). This then dismutates to yield the parent benznidazole (26) and its nitroso analog (30). The nitroso analog (30) then reacts with trypanothione, an essential enzyme for *T. cruzi*, inactivating it and causing its deficiency.

The organoarsenic compound melarsoprol (27) is used as a first-line drug for the treatment of African trypanosomiasis.

For their requirement of ATP, blood trypanosomes are entirely dependent on glycolysis. They lack functional tricarboxylic acid cycle. Melarsoprol (27) inhibits trypanosomal pyruvate kinase, thereby inhibiting glycolysis. This results in decreased ATP production. Affected trypanosomes quickly lose motility and lyse. Melarsoprol (27) also inhibit trypanosomal transporters thereby affecting the uptake of adenine and adenosine. The selectivity of melarsoprol (27) has been attributed to its higher permeability in trypanosomal cells as compared to mammalian cells. However, it is still toxic to humans.

Eflornithine (28), an ornithine (32) analog, has been found to be effective against *T. gambiense* but not against *T. rhodesiense*. It is a selective inhibitor of ornithine decarboxylase which catalyzes the synthesis of putrescine (31) from ornithine (32) and the polyamines spermine (33) and spermidine (34). These are involved in the synthesis of nucleic acids and regulation of protein synthesis. *T. gambiense* is more susceptible to eflornithine (28) as compared to *T. rhodesiense* because of slow turnover of ornithine decarboxylase in former as compared to later.

CHEMOTHERAPY OF LEISHMANIASIS

Leishmaniasis is caused by the protozoa *Leishmania donovani* and *L. tropica*. The disease is spread by sand flies and is known as Kala-azar. The drugs used include pentamidine (18) isethionate and sodium stibogluconate [Sodium antimony gluconate (35)].

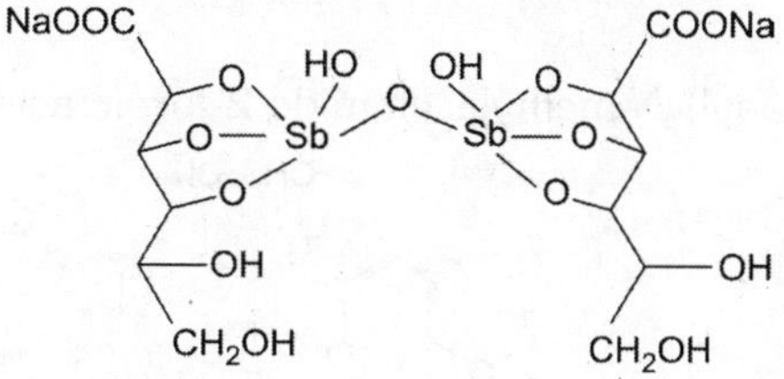

(35)

Sodium stibogluconate (35) suppresses both glycolysis and fatty acid metabolism in glycosomes. It also diminishes the net generation of ATP and GTP.

CHEMOTHERAPY OF TRICHOMONIASIS

Trichomoniasis is caused by *Trichomonas vaginalis* a parasite of human genitourinary tract. Metronidazole (13) and tinidazole (14) are used as trichomonacidal agents. Diiodohydroxyquinoline or iodoquinol (7) is used locally.

CHEMOTHERAPY OF GIARDIASIS

Giardiasis is caused by *Giardia intestinalis* leading to diarrheic or dysentric symptoms. Metronidazole (13), tinidazole (14), and furazolidone (36) have been used for giardiasis. Furazolidone (36) has antibacterial as well as antiprotozoal activity. It is given orally for the treatment of diarrhea and gastroenteritis of bacterial origin. It acts by inhibiting aldehyde dehydrogenase.

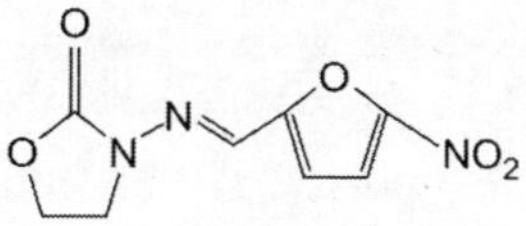

(36)

INDIVIDUAL COMPOUNDS

DRUGS USED IN AMOEBIASIS : NATURAL

Erythromycin

See MACROLIDE ANTIBIOTICS

Paromomycin

See AMINOGLYCOSIDE ANTIBIOTICS

DRUGS USED IN AMOEBIASIS : SYNTHETIC — AMINOQUINOLINES

Chloroquine

See ANTIPROTOZOAL DRUGS I: CHEMOTHERAPY OF MALARIA

DRUGS USED IN AMOEBIASIS : SYNTHETIC — HALOACETAMIDES

Diloxanide furoate

2,2-Dichloro-*N*-(4-hydroxyphenyl)-*N*-methylacetamide 2-furoic acid ester

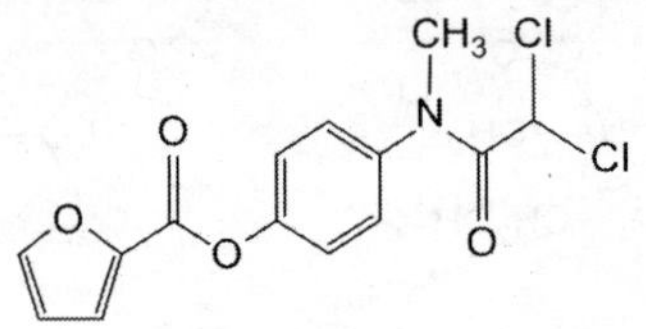

Synthesis

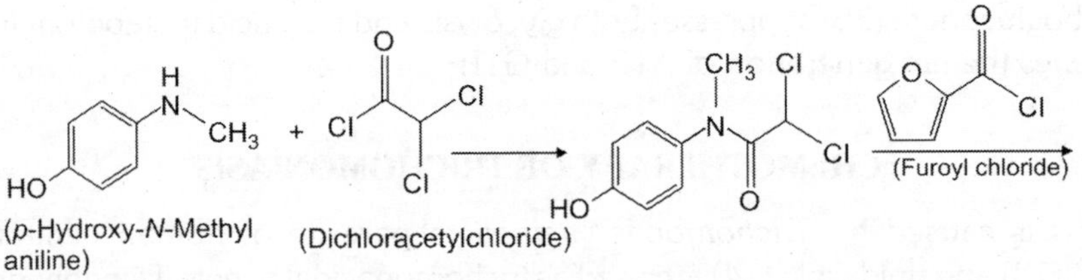

Diloxanide furoate is highly insoluble. It is used for intestinal amoebiasis.

DRUGS USED IN AMOEBIASIS : SYNTHETIC — IMIDAZOLE DERIVATIVES

Metronidazole

2-Methyl-5-nitroimidazol-1-ethanol

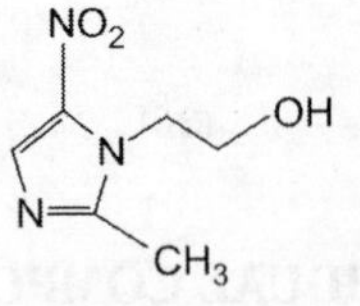

Synthesis

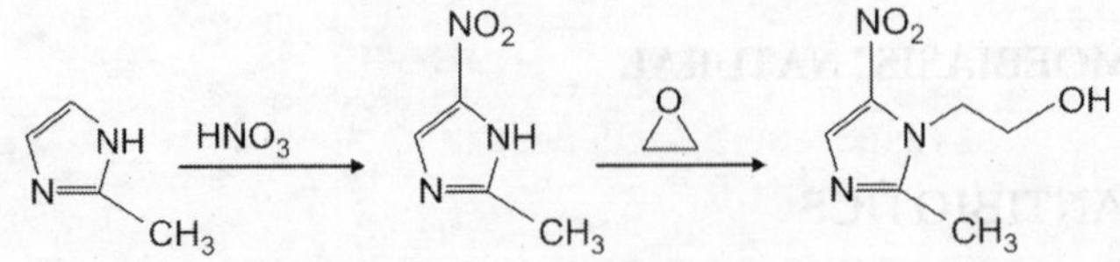

It is effective against both intestinal and hepatic amoebiasis. It has a bitter taste.

Metronidazole Benzoate
Benzoic acid ester of metronidazole

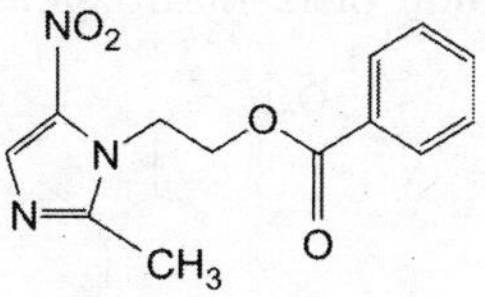

Synthesis

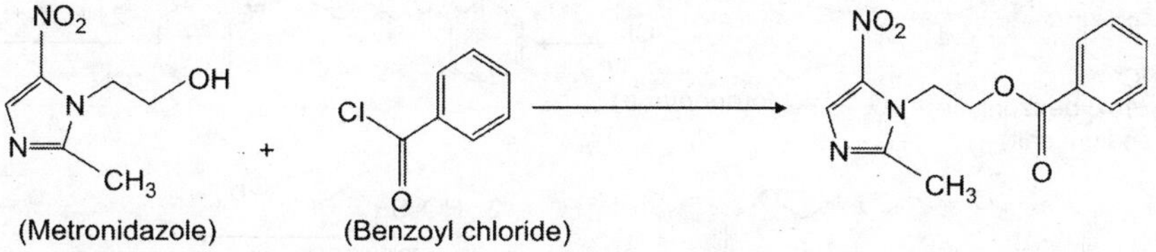

(Metronidazole)   (Benzoyl chloride)

It is tasteless and is used for the preparation of oral suspension.

Tinidazole
1-[2-(Ethylsulphonyl)ethyl]-2-methyl-5-nitro-1*H*-imidazole

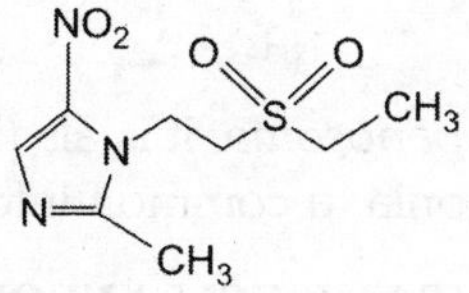

Synthesis

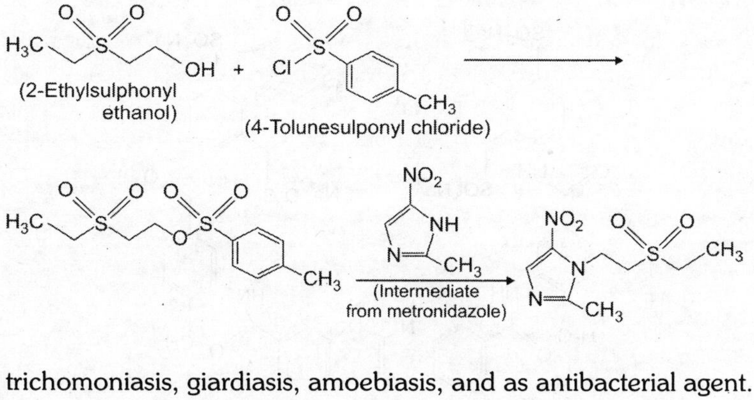

(2-Ethylsulphonyl
ethanol)   (4-Tolunesulponyl chloride)

(Intermediate
from metronidazole)

It is used for trichomoniasis, giardiasis, amoebiasis, and as antibacterial agent.

DRUGS USED IN TRYPANOSOMIASIS : DIAMIDINES

Pentamidine isethionate

4, 4'-(Pentamethylenedioxy)dibezamidine bis(2-hydroxyethylsulphonate)

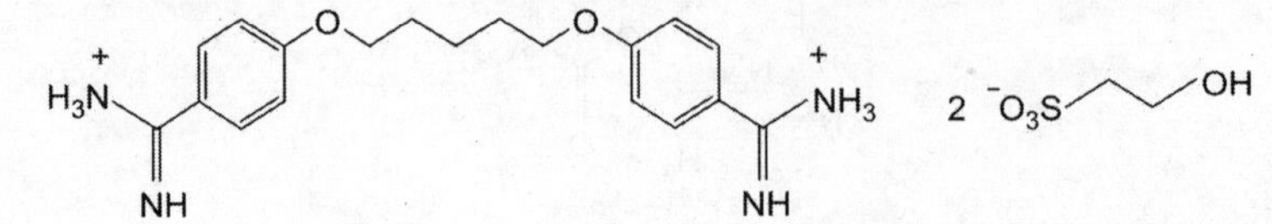

Synthesis

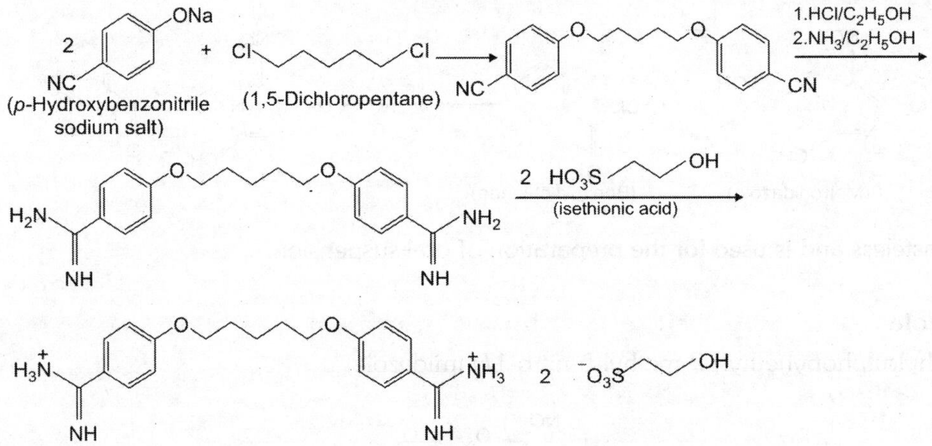

In addition to its activity against *Trypanosoma*, it is also used as second-line treatment against *Pnemocystic jiroveci* (*P. carinii*) pneumonia, a common infection in patients with AIDS.

DRUGS USED IN TRYPANOSOMIASIS : MISCELLANEOUS COMPOUNDS

Suramin Sodium

8, 8'-[Carbonylbis-[imino-3, 1-phenylenecarbonylimino(4-methyl-3, 1-phenylene) carbonylimino]]-bis-1, 3, 5-naphthalenetrisulphonic acid hexasodium salt

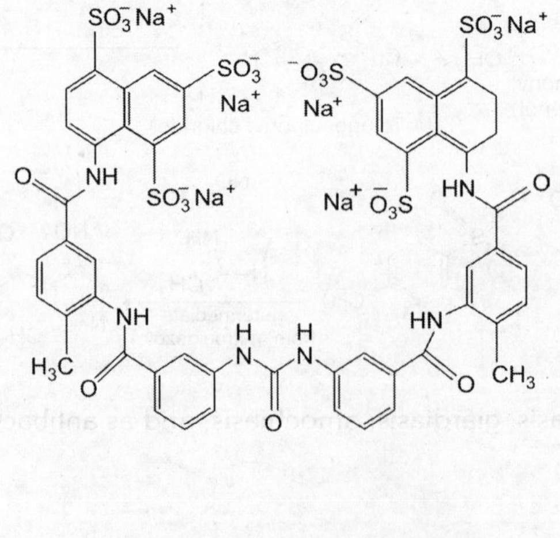

Synthesis

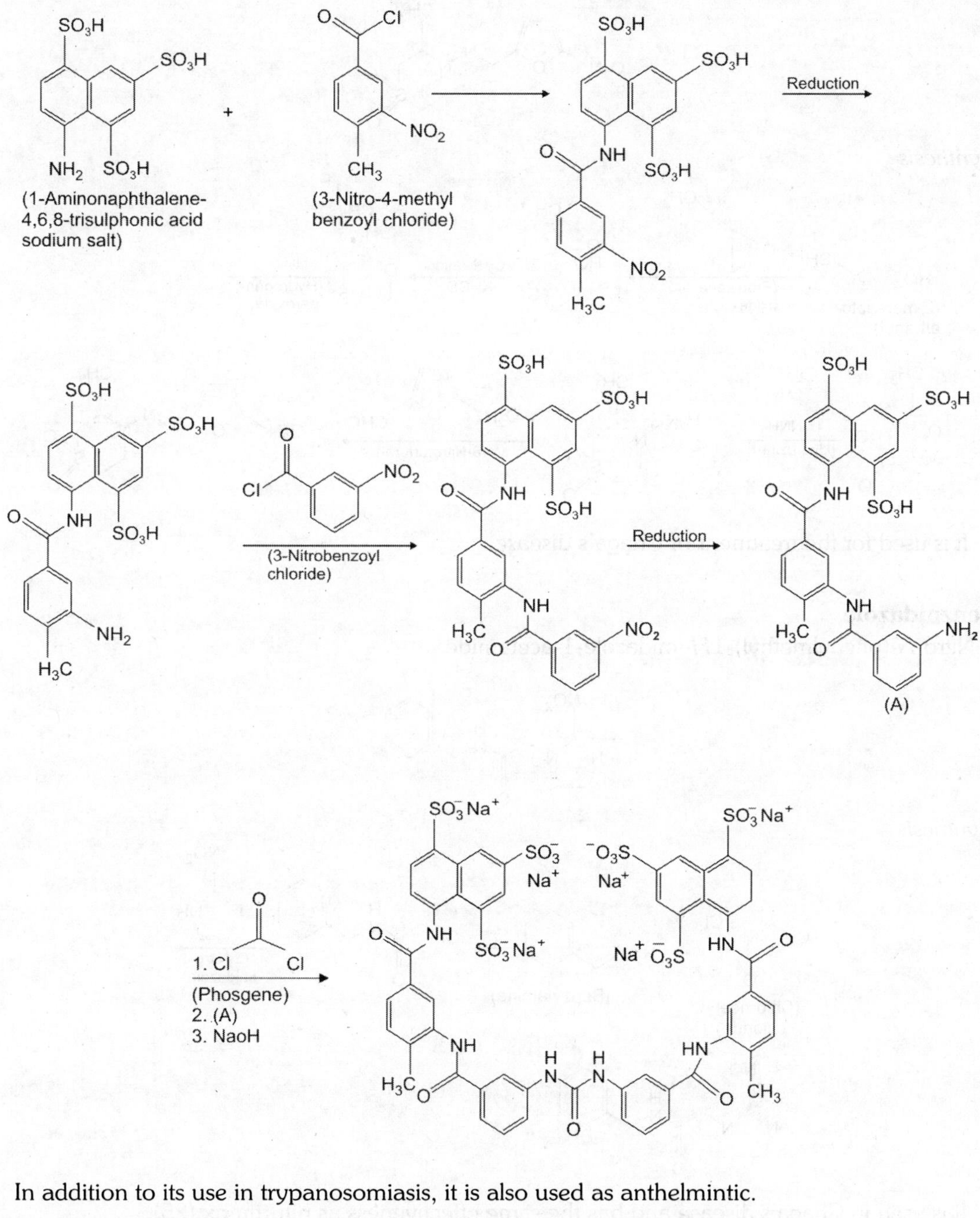

(1-Aminonaphthalene-4,6,8-trisulphonic acid sodium salt) + (3-Nitro-4-methyl benzoyl chloride) → Reduction →

(3-Nitrobenzoyl chloride) → Reduction → (A)

1. Cl—Cl (Phosgene)
2. (A)
3. NaoH →

In addition to its use in trypanosomiasis, it is also used as anthelmintic.

Nifurtimox

3-Methyl-N-[(5-nitro-2-furanyl)methylene]-4-thiomorpholinamine 1, 1-dioxide

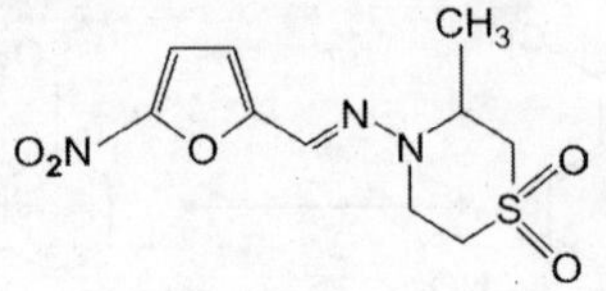

Synthesis

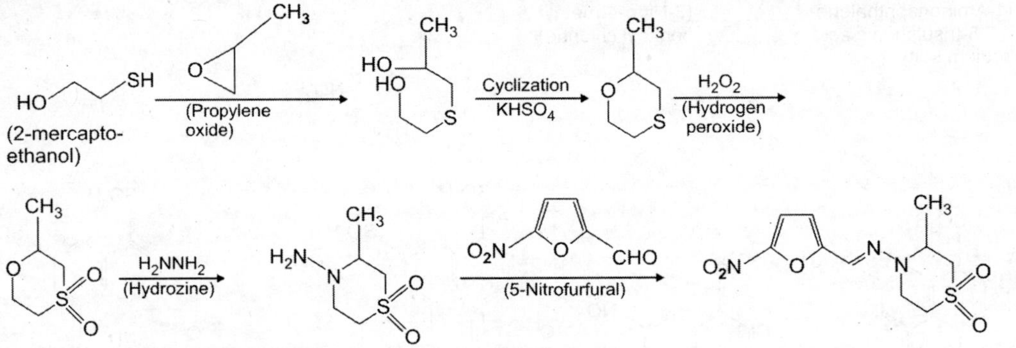

It is used for the treatment of Chaga's disease.

Benznidazole

2-Nitro-N-(phenylmethyl)-1H-imidazole-1-acetamide

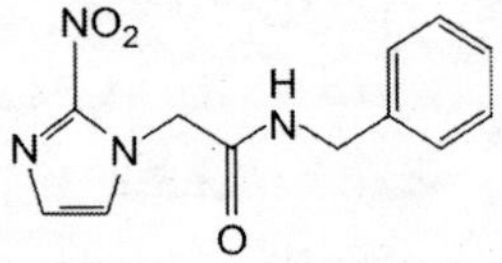

Synthesis

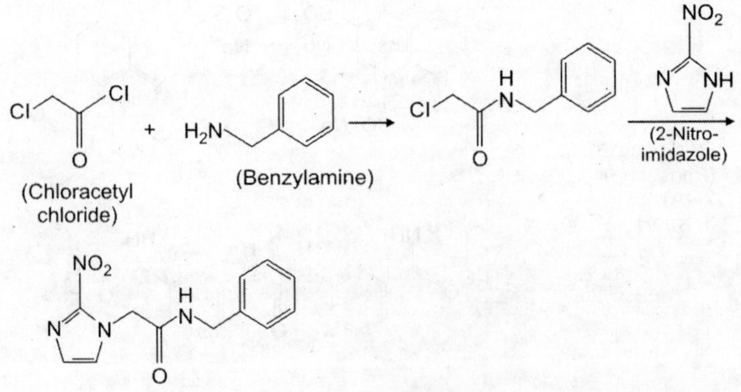

It is used in Chaga's disease and has the same effectiveness as nifurtimox (25).

Eflornithine

2-(Difluoromethyl)-DL-ornithine

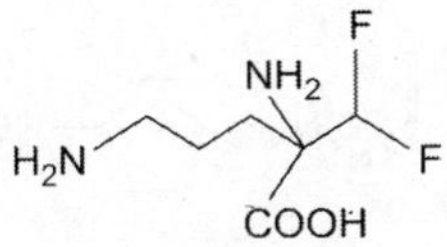

Synthesis

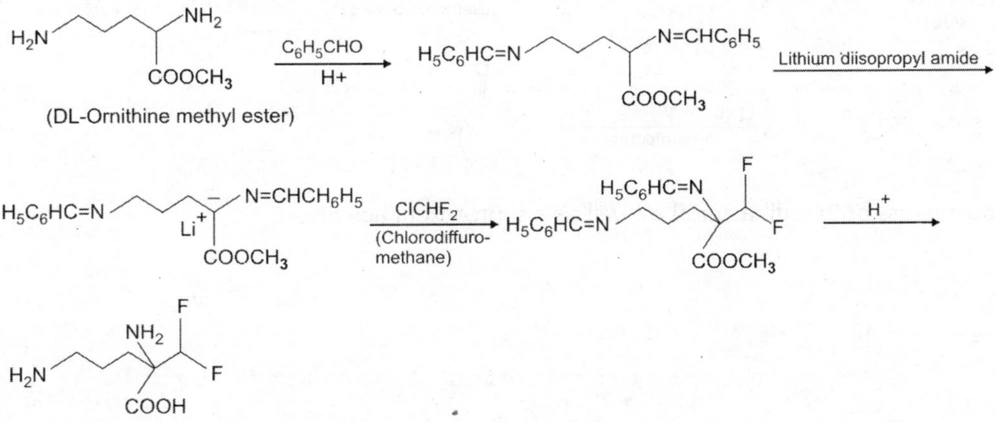

(DL-Ornithine methyl ester)

It is less toxic than melarsoprol (27) for the treatment of African trypanosomiasis. It is also highly effective against the early and late stages of African sleeping sickness.

DRUGS USED IN LEISHMANIASIS

Sodium Stibogluconate

Sodium antimony gluconate

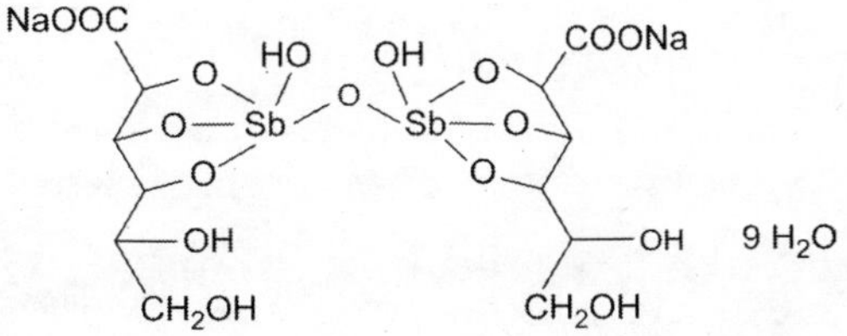

It is prepared by treating antimony pentachloride with gluconic acid and sodium hydroxide. It is used for kala-azar.

DRUGS USED IN GIARDIASIS

Furazolidone

3-[[(5-Nitro-2-furanyl)-methylene]amino]-2-oxazolidinone

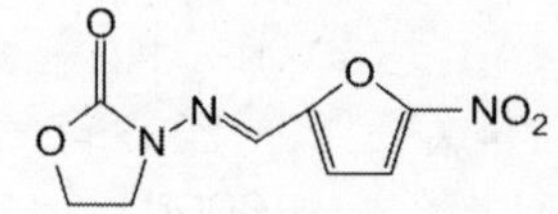

Synthesis

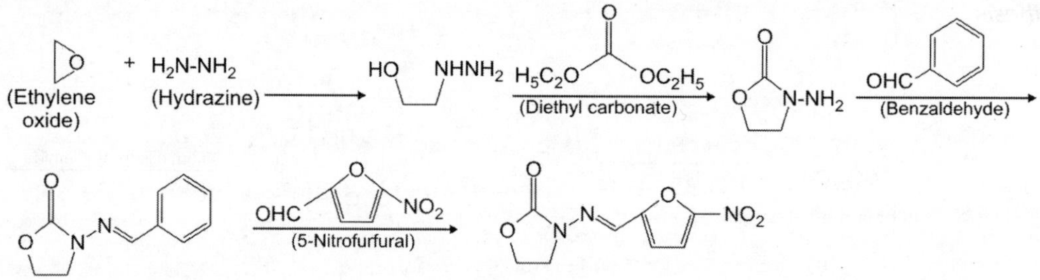

It possessess both antibacterial as well as antiprotozoal activity.

DRUGS USED IN HELMINTHIASIS

HELMINTHIASIS or worm infestation is the most common disease world over. Anthelmintics are the drugs that destroy or remove the worms from the infested host. Helminths, that are parasite to both humans and cattle, are divided into two categories:

1. The phylum Platyhelminths with classes Cestoda (*tapeworm*) and Trematoda (*flukes or Schistosoma*).
2. The phylum Nemathelminthes with the class Nematoda (roundworms).

Clinically there are two important types of worm infections and these include:

1. Those that live in host's alimentary canal, and
2. Those that live in tissue other than alimentary canal.

Alimentary Canal Infections

These include:

1. Cestoda infections, caused by
   (a) Beef tapeworm (*Taenia saginata*),
   (b) Pork tapeworm (*T. solium*), the infection is caused by eating of raw or uncooked meat which contains the larvae, and
   (c) Fish tapeworm (*Diphyllobothrium latum*), these tapeworms attach themselves to the intestinal walls and deplete the host of the nutrients.

2. Nematoda infections, caused by
   (a) Common roundworm (*Ascaris lumbricoides*),
   (b) Threadworm or pinworm in USA (*Enterobius vermicularis*),
   (c) Whipworm (*Trichuris trichiura*),
   (d) Threadworm in USA (*Strongyloides stercorali*), and
   (e) Hookworm *(Necator americanus* and *Ancylostoma duodenale*).

Other Tissue Infections

These include:

1. Trematoda (flukes) infections, caused by
   (a) *Schistosoma haematobium,*

(b) *S. mansoni*, and

(c) *S. japonicum.*

The cercaria develop to preadult forms in lungs and skin. Then the parasite travels in pairs via the bloodstream and invade other tissues. Untreated worms can live from 5-10 years within the host.

2. Nematoda infections, caused by

   (a) *Trichinella spiralis*

   (b) *Dracunculus medinensis* (guinea worm)

   (c) Filariae which include *Wuchereria bancrofti*, *Loa loa*, *Onchocerca volvulus*, and *Brugia malayi.*

The adult filariae live in lymphatic tissue or mesentry of host and produce embryo or microfilaria which find their way to bloodstream. This may be ingested when mosquito bites. After a development in secondary host, they are injected in the humans. Major filarial diseases are caused by *Wuchereria* or *Brugia* and include elephantiasis (obstruction of lymphatic vessels), infection in eye (river blindness) and inflammation of skin and other tissues.

3. Cestoda infections, caused by *Echinococcus* species. These are cestodes for which canines are primary hosts. The primary intestinal stage does not occur in human but humans can function as hosts.

ANTHELMINTIC DRUGS

Anthelmintics may act by paralyzing the worm or by damaging its cuticle, or by interfering with metabolism of the worm. Since the metabolic requirement of these parasites vary greatly, drugs that are effective against one parasite may be ineffective against the other parasite.

BENZIMIDAZOLES

Benzimidazoles possess a broad spectrum of activity against gastrointestinal helminths. Some of the useful benzimidazoles include thiabendazole (1), mebendazole (2), and albendazole (3). Thiabendazole (1), however, is not used now because of its higher toxicity.

   Two mechanisms have been proposed for benzimidazole action. One of the mechanism involves inhibition of tubulin polymerization by binding of benzimidazoles to β-tubulin. This results in disruption of nematodal motility and DNA replication causing immobilization and death of the parasite. Since these agents are selective for nematodal isoform of β-tubulin, the toxicity to the host is much less.

(1)

(2)

(3)

Another mechanism involves inhibition of fumarate reductase, the enzyme responsible for oxidation of NADPH to NAD$^+$. This inhibition results in uncoupling of oxidative phosphorylation which is necessary for ATP synthesis.

PIPERAZINES

Piperazines include piperazine citrate (4) and diethylcarbamazine citrate (5). Both these piperazine salts are still in use for the treatment of roundworm and pinworm infections. Diethylcarbamazine citrate (7) has been found to be effective against all type of lymphatic filariasis.

Piperazine salts acts by blocking the acetylcholine regeneration in ascaris resulting in paralysis of the worm and subsequent dislodging of the parasite from the intestinal wall.

(4)

(5)

MISCELLANEOUS COMPOUNDS

Niclosamide and Dichlorophen

The earlier drugs used for tapeworm were niclosamide (6) and dichlorophen (7). Both of these drugs have been replaced by newer drugs. Niclosamide (6) interferes with respiration and glucose uptake of the parasite. It also inhibits the uptake of inorganic phosphate into ATP.

(6)

(7)

Ivermectin

Ivermectin (8) is a 80:20 mixture of dihydroavermectin B_{1a} and B_{1b}, respectively. It is obtained by reducing the 22-23 double bond of naturally occurring avermectin, an antibiotic, isolated from soil actinomycetes *Streptomyces avermitilis*. The naturally occurring avermectin has very low activity as compared to the dihydroavermectin mixture of B_{1a} and B_{1b} (8). Ivermectin (8) has been found to be effective against various nematodes, particularly *Oncocerca volvulus*. It acts by binding irreversibly to glutamate gated chloride channel when it is in open conformation. This allows the ions to cross the membrane which leads to paralytic action.

Another mechanism which has been proposed involves degeneration of microfilariae in utero. This results in fewer microfilariae to be released from the female worms. Further, the degenerated microfilariae in utero prevents further fertilization and production of microfilariae.

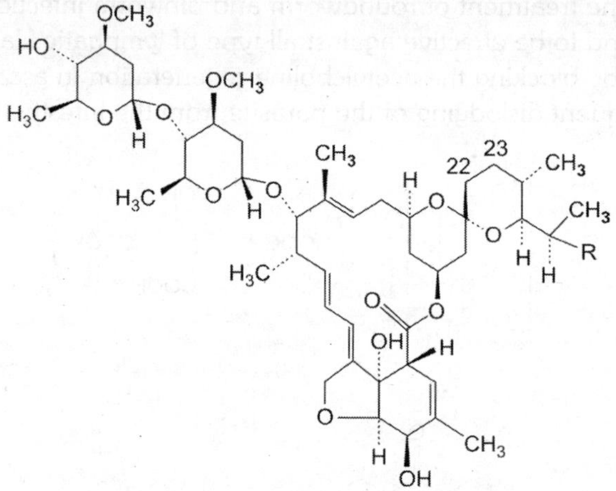

Component B_{1a}, R = CH_2CH_3 (80%)
Component B_{1b}, R = CH_3 (20%)

(8)

Praziquantel

Praziquantel (9) is an isoquinoline analog. It is active against cestodes and trematodes. Depending upon the parasite, different mechanisms are operative. In case of cestodes infection in alimentary canal of the host, the mechanism involves Ca^{2+} redistribution. This leads to muscle contraction, paralysis of pathogen, and ultimately the expulsion.

In case of intravascular trematode infection, praziquantel (9) acts by damaging the tegument of the worm. This is followed by interaction between the antigen of the parasite and antibodies of the host leading to death of the parasite. Praziquantel (9) has also been reported to affect the glycogen content and energy metabolism of the parasite.

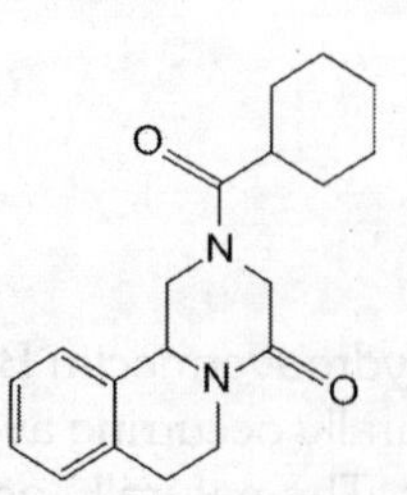

(9)

Oxamniquine

Oxamniquine (10) has been found to be effective against trematode infection caused by *Schistosoma mansoni*. The mechanism of action of oxamniquine (10) involves its activation through esterification to a sulphate/phosphate ester (11). This activated ester then alkylates the DNA of parasite which leads to irreversible inhibition of nucleic acid metabolism. Helminths which are resistant to oxamniquine (10) do not esterify it, therefore no activation takes place.

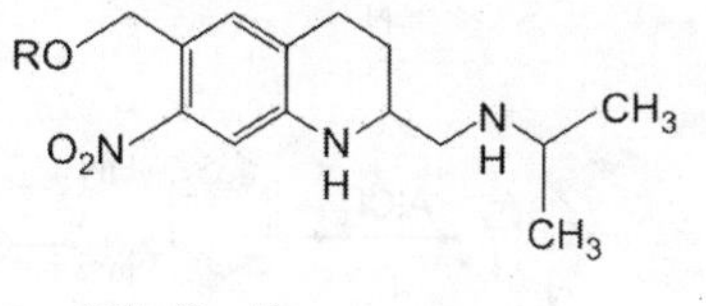

(10), R = H
(11), R = OSO$_3$H/OPO$_3$H$_2$

Metrifonate

Metrifonate (12) is an organophosphorus compound which was used earlier for trematode infections. It is a prodrug and acts through its metabolite, phosphoric acid 2,2-dichlorovinyldimethyl ester, dichlorvos, (13). Dichlorvos (13) is an inhibitor of acetylcholinesterase of *Scistosomes*, resulting in paralysis and subsequent death of the worms. The drug is, however not used now.

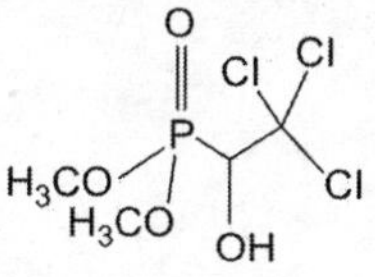

(12)

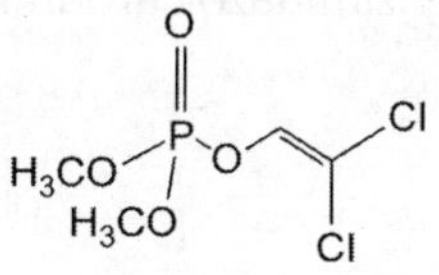

(13)

Pyrantel Pamoate

Pyrantel pamoate (14) is used against intestinal nematode infections. It is a drug of choice in case of pinworm infection. The pamoate salt of pyrantel is highly insoluble and is not readily absorbed. It acts as a neuromuscular blocking agent, activating nicotinic receptors and inhibiting cholinesterase which leads to paralysis and subsequent death of the worm.

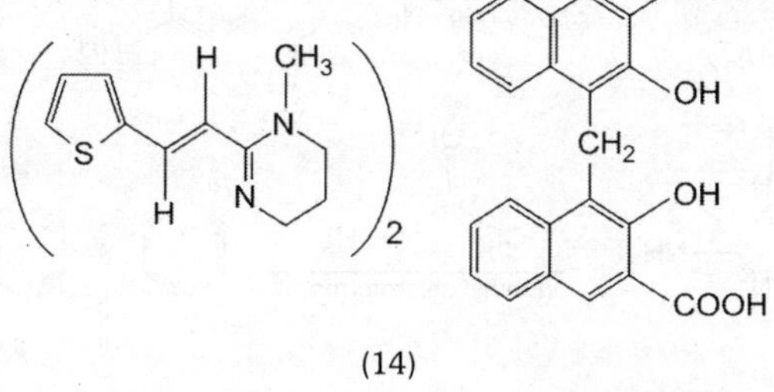

(14)

INDIVIDUAL COMPOUNDS

BENZIMIDAZOLES

Thiabendazole

4-(2-Benzimidazolyl)thiazole

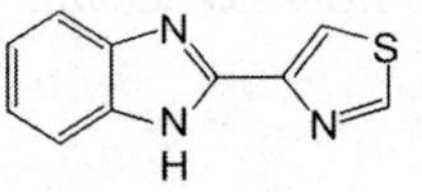

Synthesis

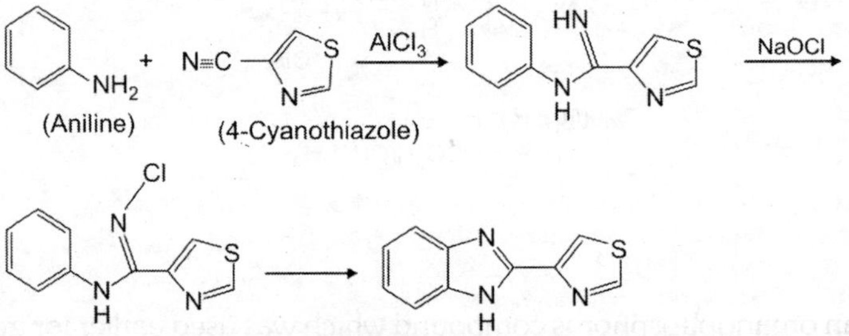

It has broad-spectrum of activity and is effective against threadworm, hookworm, and whipworm. It is also used for control of helminth infections in livestock.

Mebendazole

5-Benzoyl-2-benzimidazolcarbamic acid methyl ester

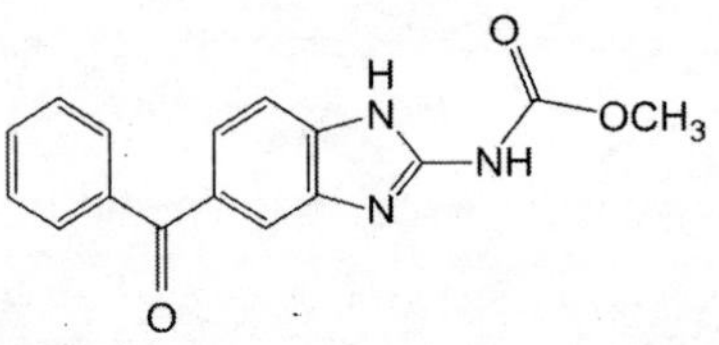

Synthesis

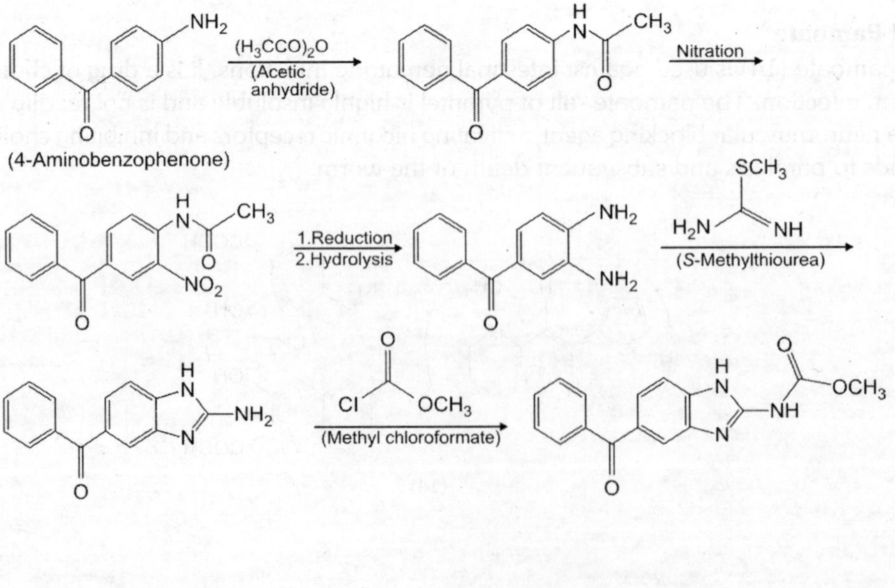

It has a broad spectrum of activity against nematodes including whipworm, pinworm, roundworm, and hookworm. It is poorly absorbed by oral route.

Albendazole

Methyl 5-(propylthio)-2-benzimidazolecarbamate

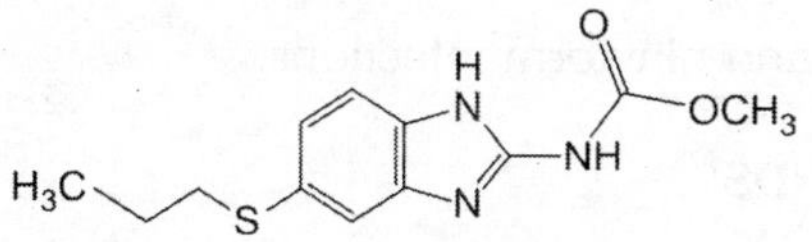

Synthesis

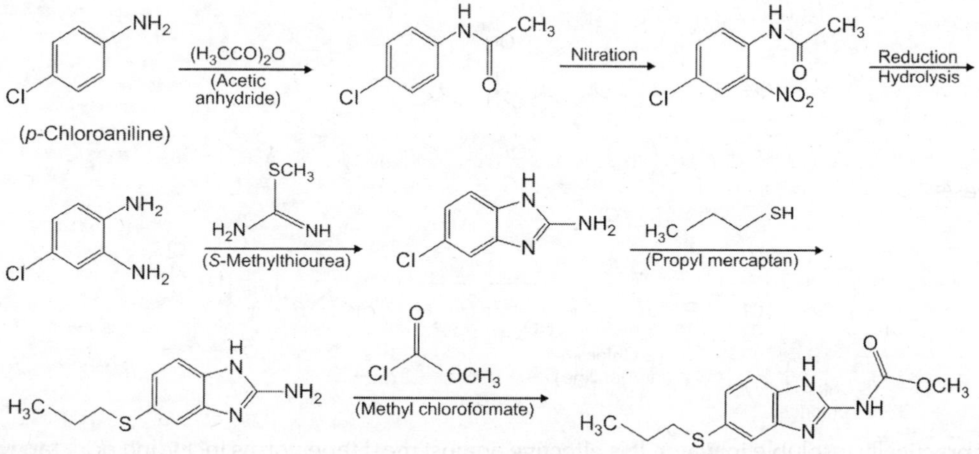

It is a white crystalline powder that is insoluble in water. It undergoes extensive first-pass metabolism to sulphoxide which is the active form in plasma. It is active against hookworm, pinworm, and threadworm.

PIPERAZINES

Diethylcarbamazine Citrate

N, N-Diethyl-4-methyl-1-piperazinecarboxamide citrate salt

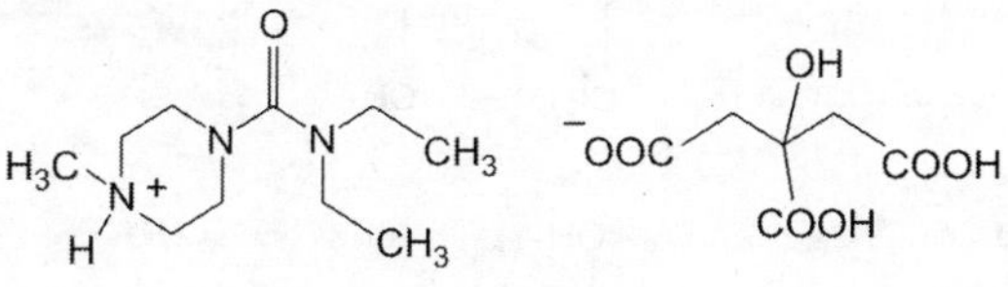

Synthesis

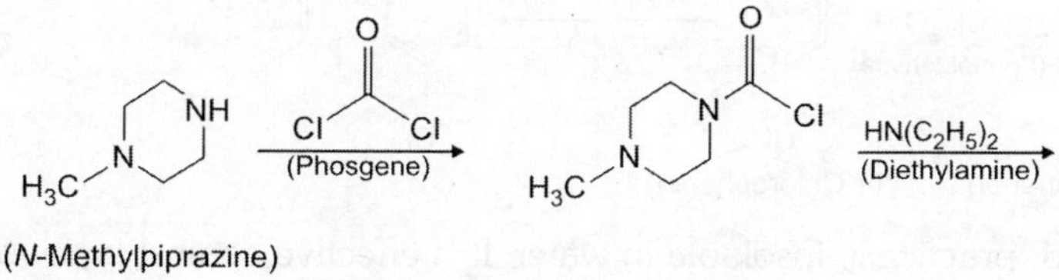

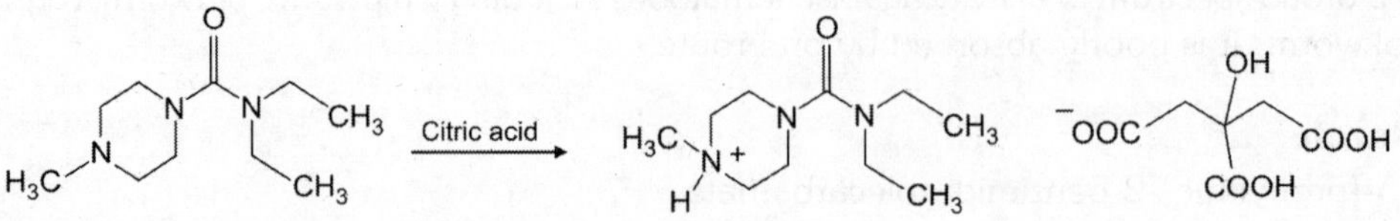

It is effective in roundworm and pinworm infections.

MISCELLANEOUS COMPOUNDS

Niclosamide

5-Chloro-*N*-(2-chloro-4-nitrophenyl)-2-hydroxybenzamide

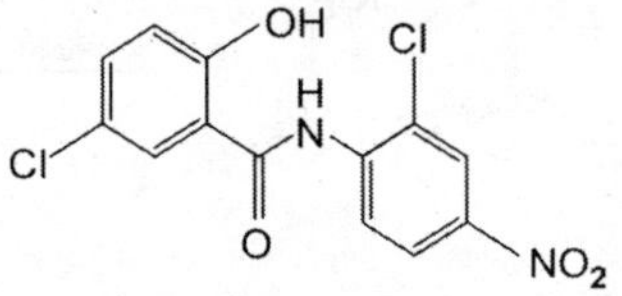

Synthesis

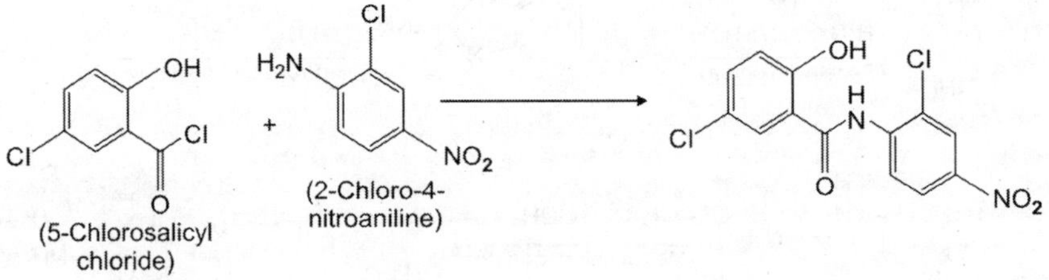

It is practically insoluble in water. It is effective against most tapeworms including pork tapeworm, beef tapeworm, and fish tapeworm.

Dichlorophen

2, 2'-Methylenebis[4-chlorophenol]

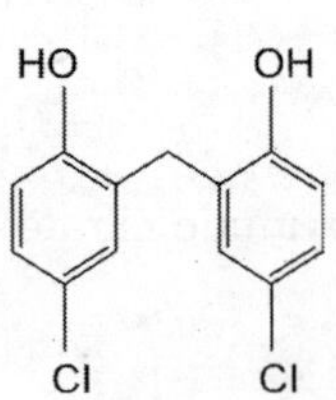

Synthesis

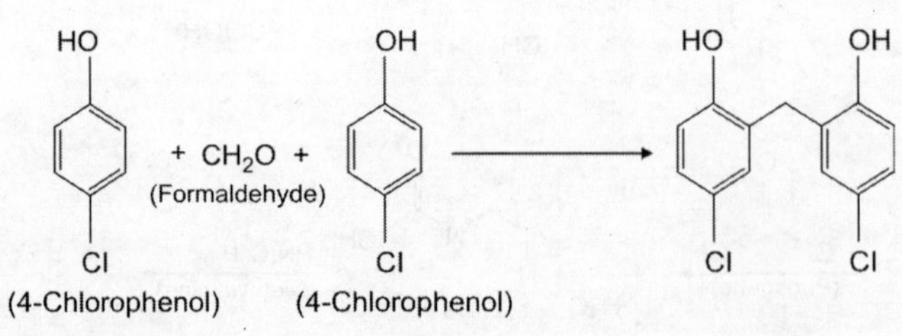

It is a white crystalline solid, practically insoluble in water. It is effective against tapeworms.

Praziquantel

2-(Cyclohexylcarbonyl)-1,2,3,6,7,11b-hexahydro-4*H*-pyrazino[2,1-a]isoquinoline-4-one

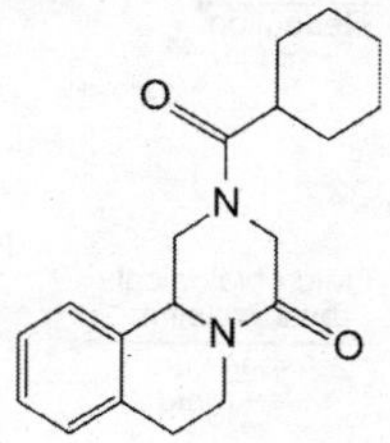

Synthesis

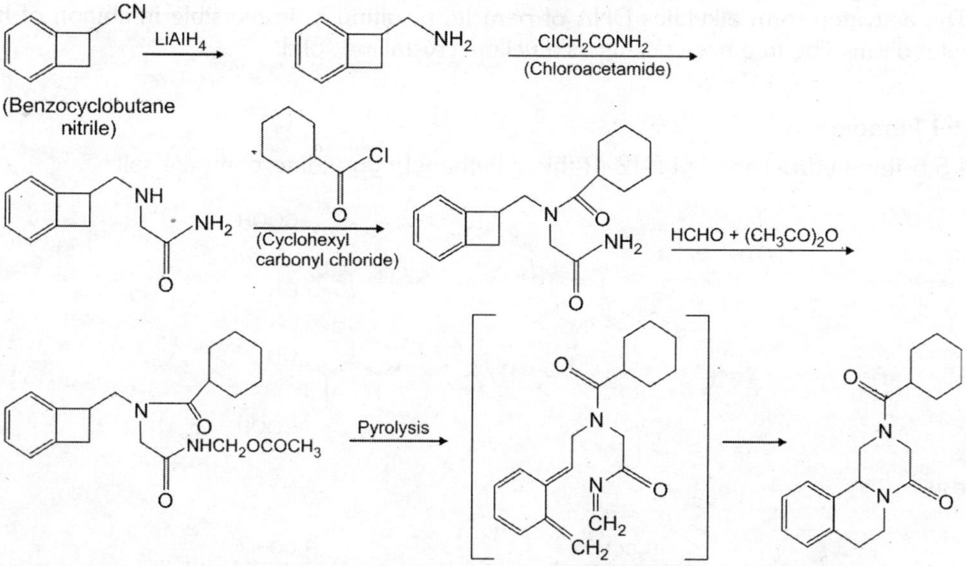

(Benzocyclobutane nitrile)

(Cyclohexyl carbonyl chloride)

It has a broad spectrum of activity against a variety of cestodes and trematodes.

Oxamniquine

6-Hydroxymethyl-2-isopropylaminomethyl-7-nitro-1,2,3,4-tetrahydroquinoline

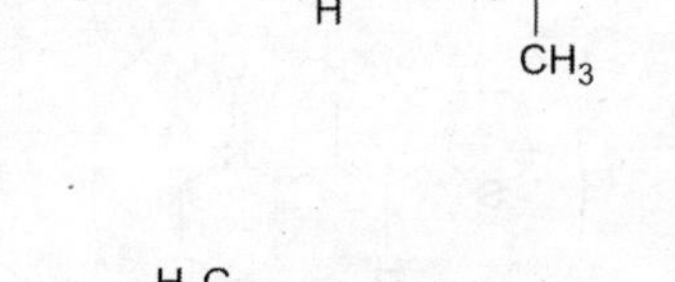

Synthesis

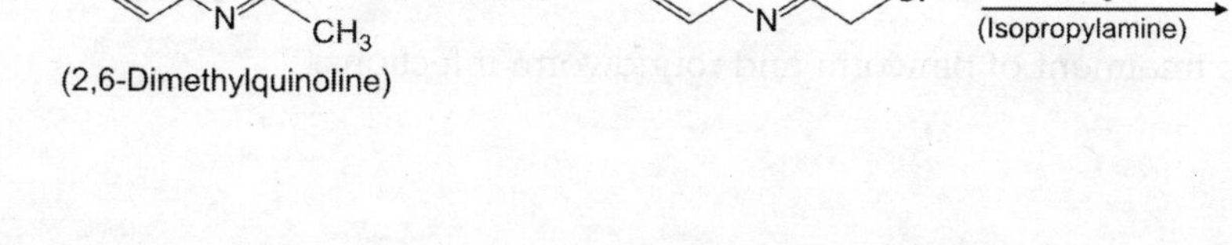

(2,6-Dimethylquinoline)

(Isopropylamine)

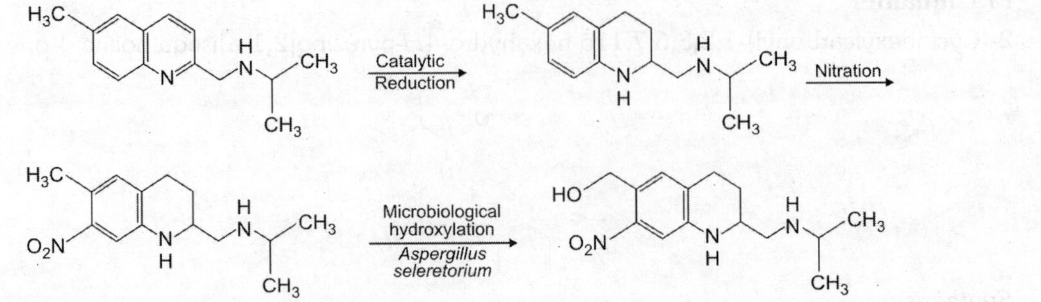

It is active against Schistosomes and acts by alkylating DNA through its activated form, the ester. The activated form alkylates DNA of parasite resulting in irreversible inhibition of nucleic acid metabolism. The free base occurs as a yellow crystalline solid.

Pyrantel Pamoate

(*E*)-1,4,5,6-Tetrahydro-1-methyl-2-[2-(2-thienyl)ethenyl]pyrimidine pamoate salt

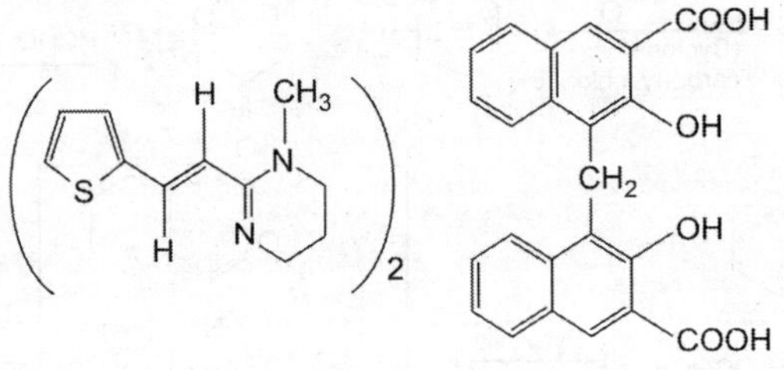

Synthesis

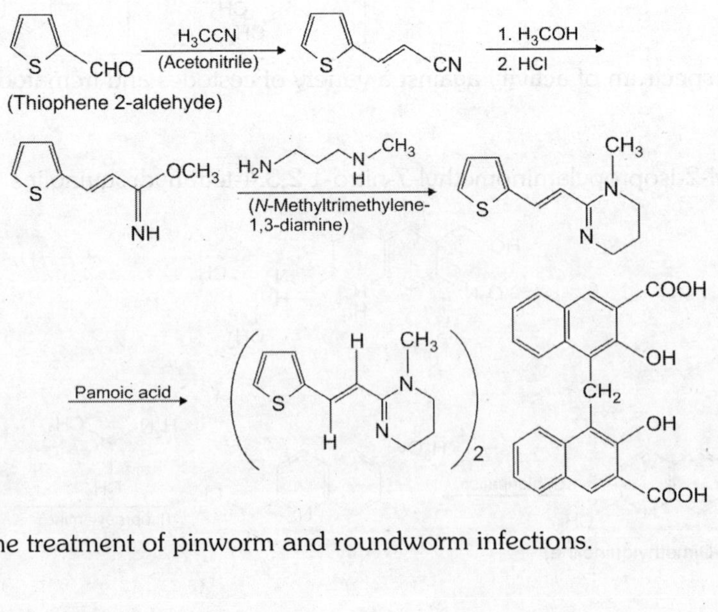

It is used for the treatment of pinworm and roundworm infections.

Section IX
Chemotherapy—Drugs Used in
Microbial Infections

SULPHONAMIDES AND QUINOLONES

T HE DISCOVERY that the antibacterial activity of prontosil (1), a brilliant red dye, was due to its metabolite sulphanilamide (2), marked the beginning of the chemotherapeutic era. Since then thousands of sulphonamides have been synthesized with a wide-spectrum of activity. This includes sulphonamides active against acute and chronic Gram-positive and Gram-negative bacterial infections through tuberculosis and leprosy to malaria and coccidioides. In addition to their antibacterial activity, sulphonamides have also shown oral hypoglycemic as well as diuretic activity. Here we shall consider sulphonamides which are used in chemotherapy.

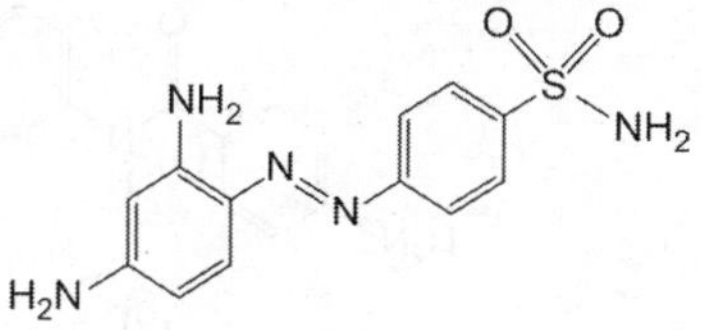

(1)

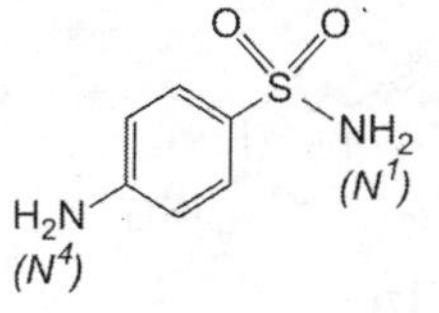

(2)

NOMENCLATURE

The general structure of sulphonamides is (3). Structure (2) is sulphanilamide, while as group (4) is sulphanilamido. The group (5) constitutes sulphanilyl and the group (6) is sulphamido. The sulphonamide nitrogen is designated as N^1, and the aromatic nitrogen as N^4 (2).

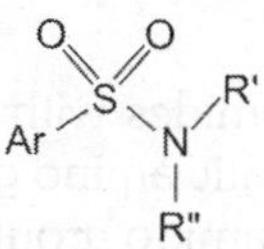

(3) 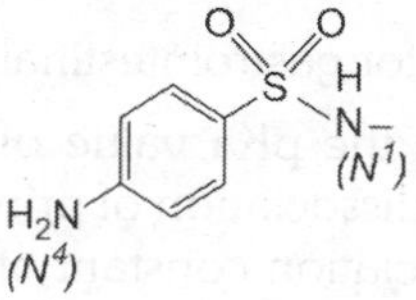   (4) 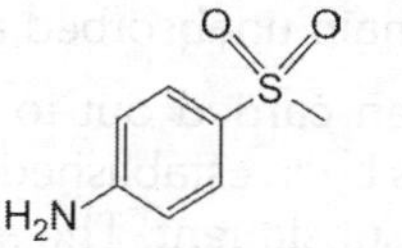   (5) 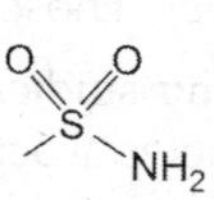   (6)

ANTIBACTERIAL ACTIVITY

Sulphonamides have a wide and varied spectrum of antimicrobial activity. This includes activity against Gram-positive and Gram-negative bacteria, *Nocardia*, *Chlamydia trachomatis*, some protozoa, enteric bacteria such as *E. coli* and *Klebsiella, Salmonella, Shigella,* and *Enterobacteria* species. Sulphonamides are usually used in combination with trimethoprim and pyrimethamine.

STRUCTURE-ACTIVITY RELATIONSHIPS

A wide variety of sulphonamides have been synthesized and tested for their biological activity. From these studies, the following conclusions with regard to structure and activity have been drawn:

(2)

1. In order to show the activity, the sulphamido and the amino groups should be in 1 and 4 positions.
2. The amino (N^4) group should be unsubstituted or should be substituted by a group which can be readily removed.
3. Substitution of benzene nucleus at other positions leads to loss of activity.
4. Exchange of $-SO_2NH_2$ by $-SO_2-C_6H_4-p-NH_2$ (7) leads to retention of activity, whereas exchange by $-CONH_2$ (8), $CONHC_6H_4-p-NH_2$ (9) markedly reduces the activity.
5. N^1–monosubstitution results in more active compounds. N^1–disubstitution in general leads to inactive compounds.

(7)   (8)   (9)

Sulphonamides have varied rate of absorption and plasma half-lives (2.5 to 150 hr). Based on this, they have found use in different types of infections, thus:

(a) Sulphonamides that have high solubility, quick absorption and rapid excretion with a half-life of 10 hr are used for urinary tract infections.

(b) Those that are absorbed rapidly but excreted slowly with a half-life of 10-24 hr, are used for general infections.

(c) Those which remain unabsorbed are used for gastrointestinal infections.

Many studies have been carried out to correlate the pKa value of sulphonamides with their antibacterial activity. It has been established that the dissociation of primary aromatic amino group is not affected by the N^1- substituent. The acid dissociation constant of sulphanilamido group, on the other hand varies greatly from 3 to 11, it stabilizes itself by losing a proton (Fig. 25.1). A plot of log 1/MIC vs pKa has been found to be parabolic, with highest point between pKa 6.0 and 7.4. The maximum activity of the compound, therefore, lies at physiological pH. It has been postulated that sulphonamides penetrate the bacterial cell in unionized form and once inside, they show their action due to ionized form. Thus, for their optimum activity, they should have pKa which will give proper balance between the penetration and activity.

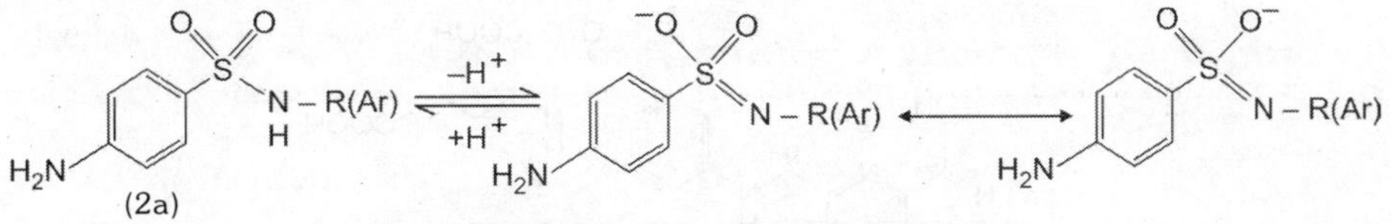

Fig. 25.1: Ionization of sulphonamides.

Sulphonamides and their metabolites, the N^1-acylated products are excreted entirely through urine. The pKa of the sulphanilamido group is 10.4, so the pH at which the drug is 50% ionized is 10.4. Unless the pH is above the pKa, little of water-soluble salt is present. Because the pH of urine is usually about 6 and lower during the bacterial infections, therefore essentially all the sulphonamide is relatively present in insoluble nonionized form in kidneys and this results in crystalluria. To overcome this, some of the earlier approaches were:

1. To increase the water intake, this would result in increased glomerular filtration rate resulting in less opportunity for seed crystals to form in the renal tubules.
2. Increasing the pH of urine, which would increase the solubility of the sulphonamides or their acylated products. Sodium bicarbonate has been used occasionally for this purpose.
3. Another way is to prepare sulphonamides with a pKa value closer to the pH of urine. Some of the examples of these types of sulphonamides are:

    Sulphadiazine with a pKa value of 6.5
    Sulphamerazine with a pKa value of 7.1
    Sulphmethazine with a pKa value of 7.4
    Sulphisoxazole with a pKa value of 5.0
    Sulphamethoxazole with a pKa value of 6.1.

The lower pKa values of these sulphonamides are because of the electron-withdrawing heterocyclic rings attached to N^1.

MECHANISM OF ACTION

Folic acid (10) is an essential growth factor for humans. Intracellularly, it is reduced to dihydrofolic acid (11) and then to tetrahydrofolic acid (12) by the enzyme folic acid reductase. Tetrahydrofolic acid is converted to N^5-formyltetrahydrofolate (13), N^{10}-formyl-tetrahydrofolate (14), N^5, N^{10}-methenyltetrahydrofolate (15), and N^5, N^{10}-methylenetetrahydrofolate(16), the cofactors for one-carbon-transfer enzymes required for the syntheses of purine nucleotides in both humans and microbes. Since folic acid (10) is an essential metabolite for humans, it has to be supplied from outside. However, microbes synthesize their own requirement of dihydrofolic acid (11). This is then converted to tetrahydrofolic acid (12) which is then converted to various cofactors of one carbon transferases.

Microbes are not able to utilize the preformed folic acid (10) of the host because it requires an enzyme for its transport across the bacterial cell wall which it lacks. The microbes utilize hydroxymethyldihydropterin (17) for the synthesis of dihydrofolic acid (11). Hydroxymethyldihydropterin (17) is converted to its pyrophosphate (18) which after reaction with p-aminobenzoic acid [PABA, (19)] is converted to dihydropteroate (20). This in presence of dihydrofolate synthetase reacts with glutamic acid (21) to give dihydrofolate (11). The dihydrofolate is then converted to tetrahydrofolic acid (12) by the dihydrofoliate reductase and the tetrahydrofolic acid (12) to various cofactors.

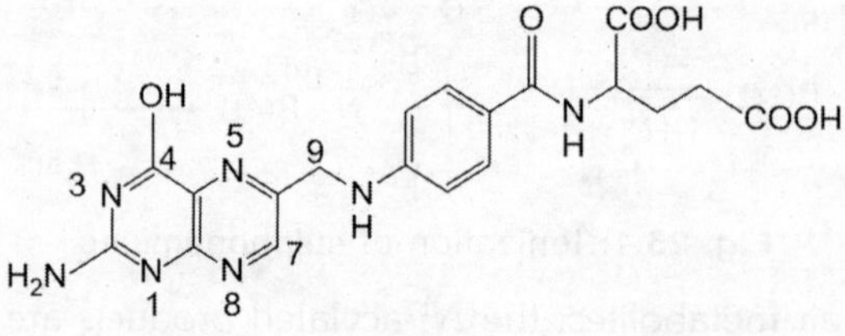

(10)

Folic acid reductase

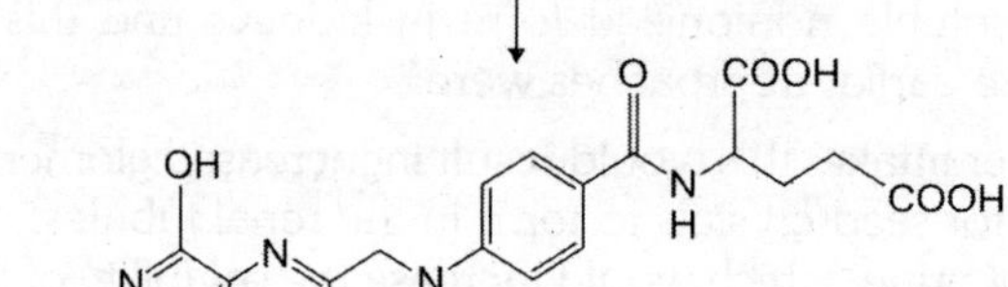

(11)

Folic acid reductase

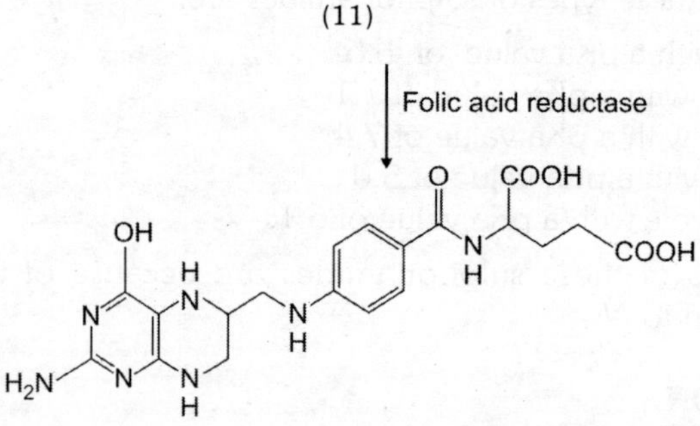

(12)

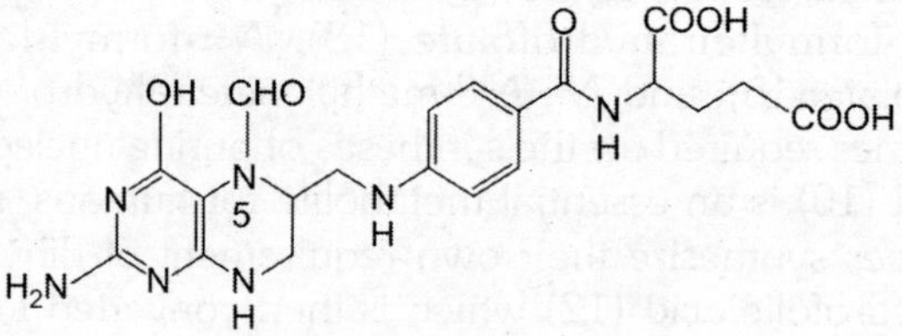

(13)

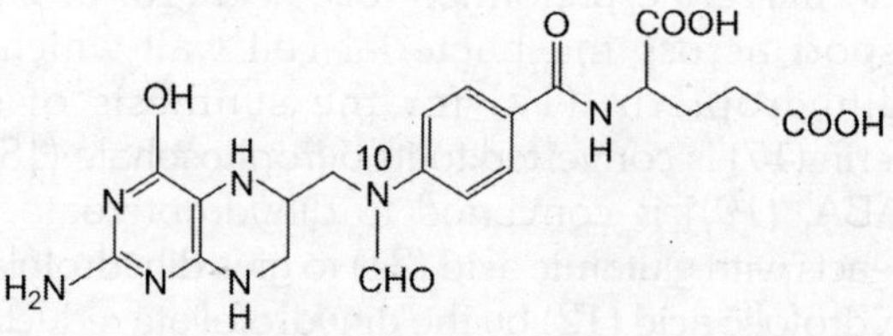

(14)

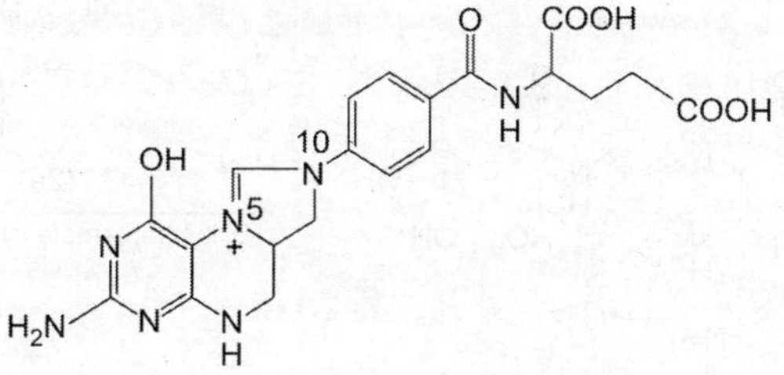

(15)

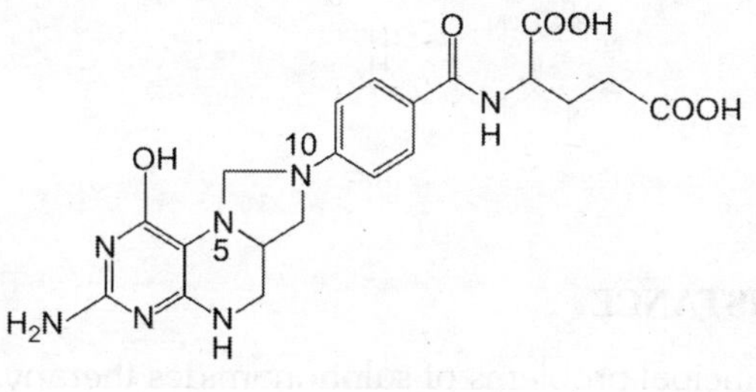

(16)

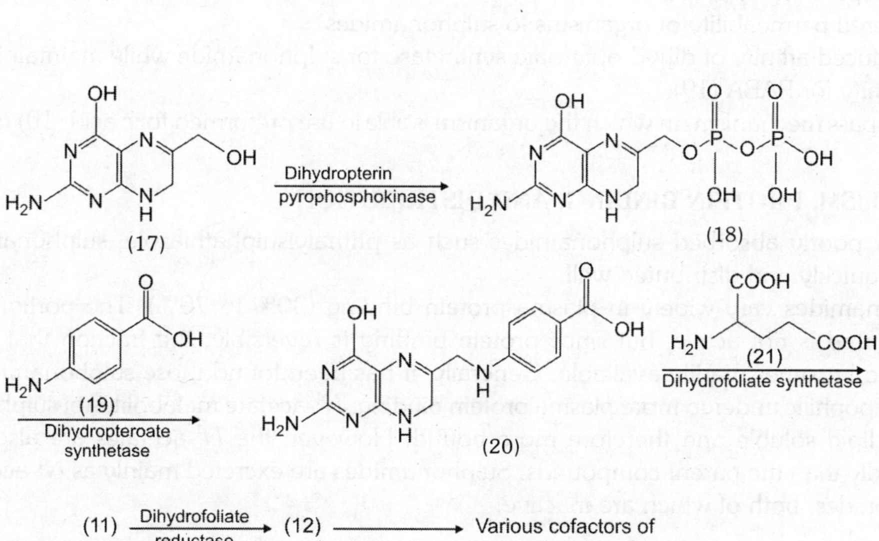

(11) $\xrightarrow[\text{reductase}]{\text{Dihydrofoliate}}$ (12) $\longrightarrow$ Various cofactors of one carbon transferases

The sulphonamides (2a) act by competing with PABA (19) for incorporation into pteridine pyrophosphate (18) resulting in (22) which acts as false metabolite and cannot be further converted to dihydrofoliate (11). Further, they also inhibit dihydropteroate synthetase and dihydrofoliate synthetase for which direct evidence has been obtained on bacterial cell cultures and cell-free enzymes of bacteria.

(18)

(22)

DEVELOPMENT OF RESISTANCE

Resistance is one of the principal problems of sulphonamides therapy. It develops because of:

(a) Overproduction of PABA (19).

(b) Altered permeability of organisms to sulphonamides.

(c) Reduced affinity of dihydropteroate synthetase for sulphonamide while maintaining the affinity for PABA (19).

(d) By-pass mechanism, in which the organism is able to use preformed folic acid (10) of the host.

METABOLISM, PROTEIN BINDING, AND DISTRIBUTION

Except for poorly absorbed sulphonamides such as phthalylsulphathiazole, sulphonamides are absorbed quickly and distributed well.

Sulphonamides vary widely in plasma protein binding (30% to 70%). The portion which is protein bound is not active, but since protein binding is reversible, the fraction that is protein bound also becomes readily available. Generally, it has been found those sulphonamides which are more lipophilic undergo more plasma protein binding. N^4-acetate metabolites of sulphonamides are more lipid soluble and therefore more bound. However, the N^4-acetates are also excreted more rapidly than the parent compounds. Sulphonamides are excreted mainly as N^4-acetates and as glucuronides, both of which are inactive.

DIHYDROFOLATE REDUCTASE INHIBITORS

The observation that folic acid (10) analogs, aminopterin (23) and methotrexate (24), inhibited dihydrofolic acid reductase, led to further investigations of this class of inhibitors. This led to discovery of substituted 2, 4-diaminopyrimidines as the inhibitors of dihydrofolic acid reductase. These inhibitors, unlike aminopterin (23) and methotrexate (24), lack glutamic acid residue, and are known as non-classical dihydrofolic acid reductase inhibitors. Some of these include trimethoprim

(25) used as antibacterial and pyrimethamine (26) used as antiprotozoal (against malaria). Another compound chlorguanide [proguanil, (27)] which is also active against malaria, acts after it is metabolized to its cyclic analog, cycloguanil (28).

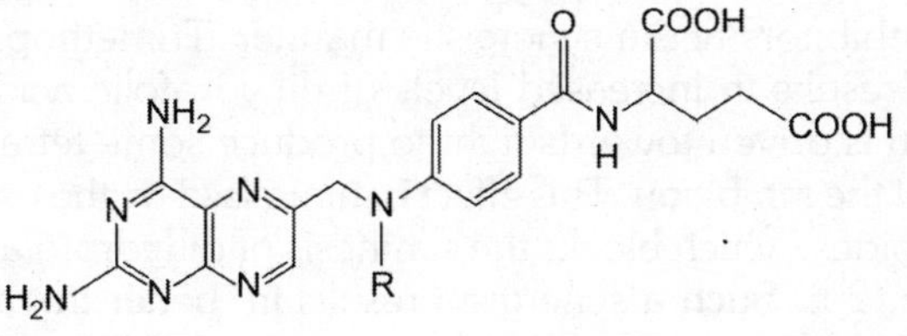

(23), R = H
(24), R = CH₃

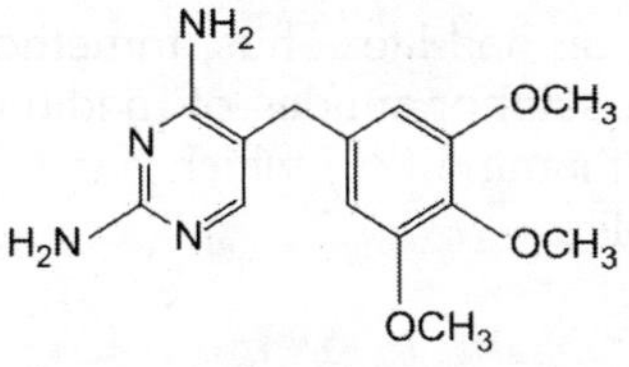

(25)

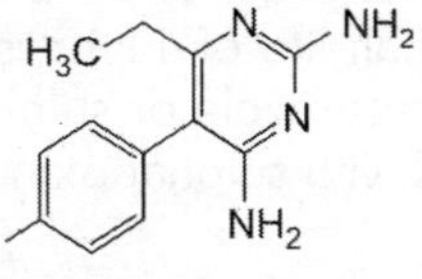

(26)

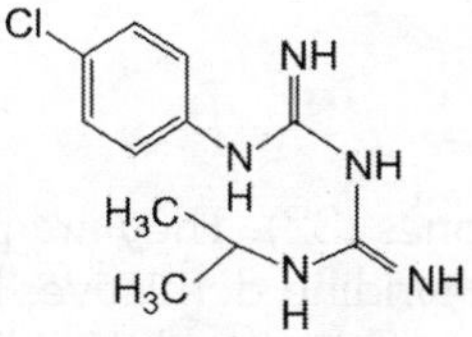

(27)

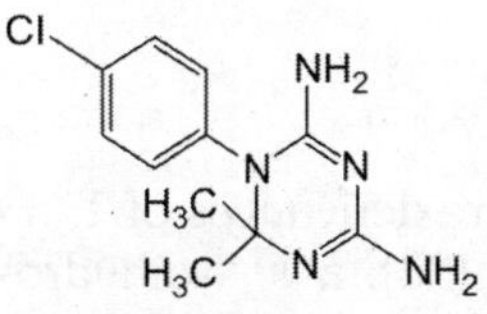

(28)

The differences in the activity of various dihydrofolate reductase inhibitors has been attributed to the differences in the affinity of these compounds to dihydrofolate reductases of bacteria, protozoa, and the reductases of mammalian origin. This difference in the affinity explains the differences in the potency and selectivity of these inhibitors. For example, methotrexate (24) binds tightly to all types of dihydrofolate reductases, thus it has no selectivity and is toxic to any cell it can enter. Trimethoprim (25) and pyrimethamine (26), on the other hand, show selectivity and are active against bacterial and protozoal dihydrofolate reductases, respectively.

Some of the second generation non-classical dihydrofolate reductase inhibitors include trimetrexate (29) and piritrexim (30). They are used in cancer and antiprotozoal chemotherapy. They have superior spectrum of activity.

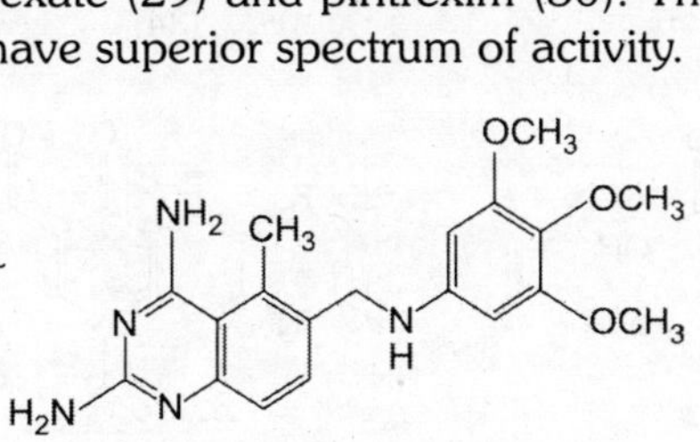

(29)

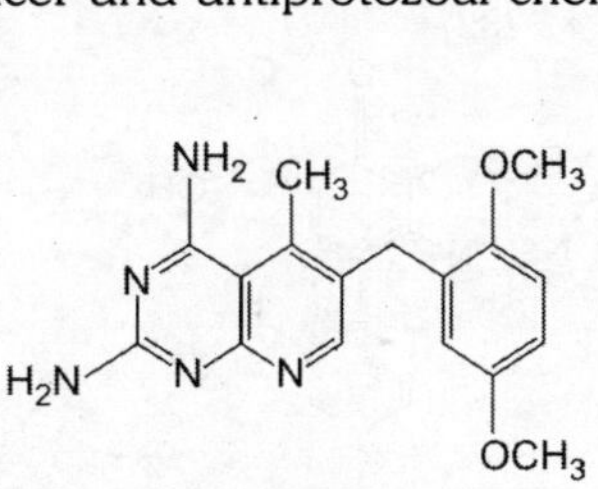

(30)

SYNERGISM OF DIHYDROFOLATE REDUCTASE INHIBITORS (DHFRI) AND SULPHONAMIDES

The sulphonamides and dihydrofolic acid reductase inhibitors act at two different sites of folic acid pathway, the dihydropteroate synthetase and dihydrofoliate reductase, respectively. It has been suggested that two classes of inhibitors act in synergistic manner. Trimethoprim (25) inhibits the dihydrofolate reductase which results in increased levels of dihydrofolic acid (11). According to law of mass action, this reaction is driven towards right to produce some tetrahydrofolic acid (12) resulting in partial overcoming of the inhibition. This effect is minimized by the use of dihydropteroate synthetase inhibitor, sulphonamides, which blocks the synthesis of dihydrofolate through blockade of synthesis of dihydropteroate (20). Such a synergism results in, better therapeutic index, better tolerance and delay in development of resistant strains, because of use of lower doses in combination as compared to higher doses when used individually.

The choice of drugs to be used in combination is based on half-life. Thus, trimethoprim (25) which has a half-life of 11 hr is used in combination with sulphonamides of medium half-life, e.g. sulphamethoxazole or sulphadiazine. Similarly, pyrimethamine (26) which has a half-life of 130 hr is used with sulphadoxine (31) which has same half-life.

(31)

QUINOLONES

Quinolones are derivatives of 1, 4-dihydro-3-carboxy-4-quinolones (32). They are patterened on nalidixic acid (33), a 1, 4-dihydro-3-carboxy-4-one-1, 8-naphthyridine derivative. Nalidixic acid (33) was introduced in clinical practice for urinary tract infection. Other naphthyridine derivative used as antibacterial include enoxacin (34) and trovafloxacin (35). The naphthyridine derivatives have been largely replaced by dihydroquinolones (32) and include norfloxacin (36), ciprofloxacin (37), lomefloxacin (38), gatifloxacin (39), sparfloxacin (40), moxifloxacin (41), oxolinic acid (42), ofloxacin (43) and 1,4-dihydrocinnoline analog, cinoxacin (44).

(32)   (33)   (34)

(35)   (36)   (37)

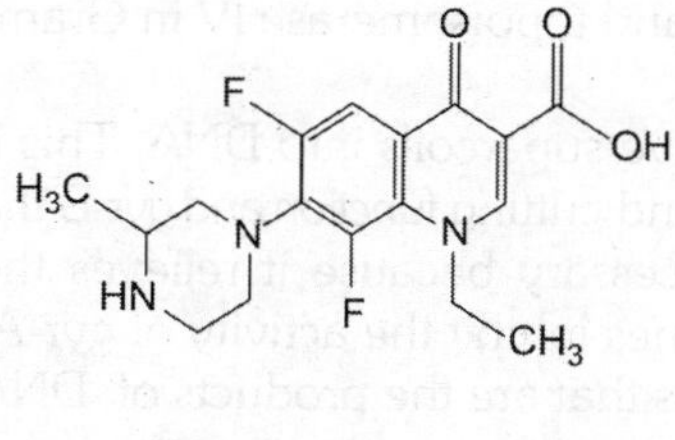

(38) 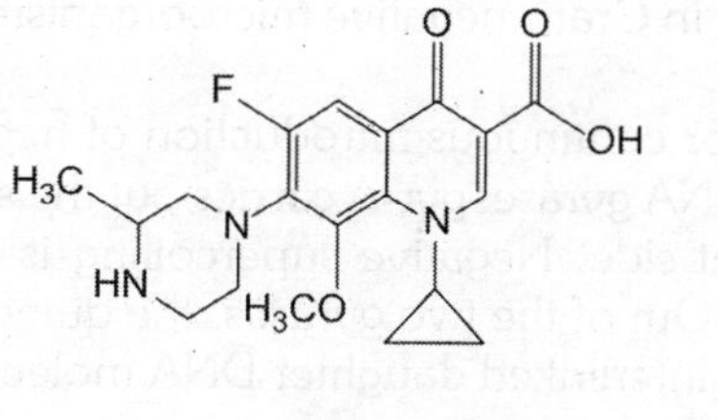   (39) 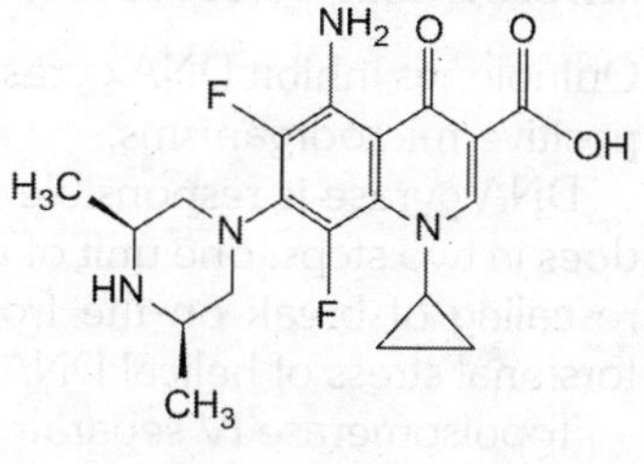   (40)

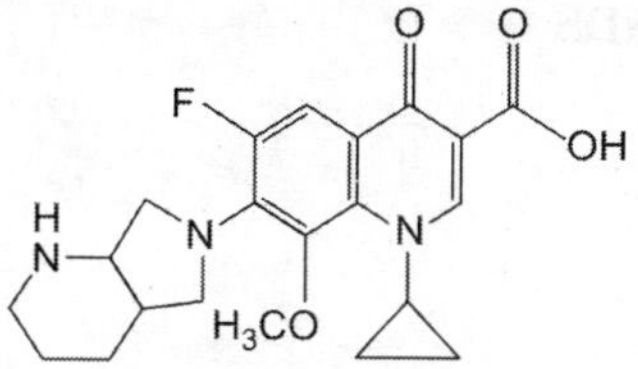

(41) 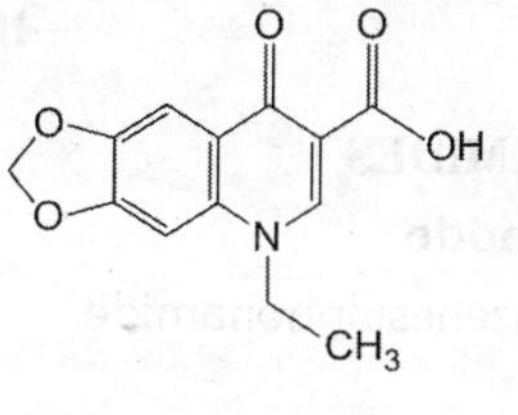   (42)

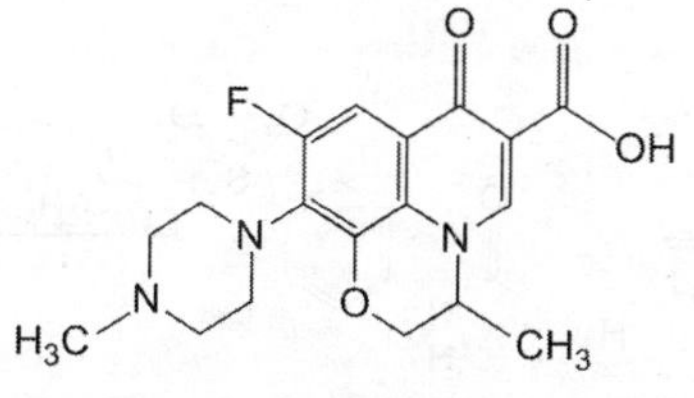

(43) 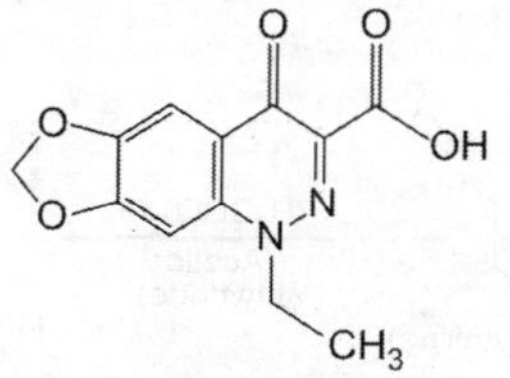   (44)

STRUCTURE-ACTIVITY RELATIONSHIP

Structure-activity relationship studies have shown that:

1. 1,4-Dihydro-4-oxo-3-carboxylic acid system fused to an aromatic system is essential for antibacterial activity.
2. The antibacterial activity is retained when -CH- at position 2, 5, 6, or 8 is replaced isosterically with nitrogen.
3. Substitution at position 2 usually results in loss of activity. However, the aromatic ring annulated with the dihydropyridone ring can be substituted at positions 5, 6, 7, and 8.
4. Fluoro substitution at position 6 and 8 usually results in enhanced activity.
5. Alkyl substitution at position 1 is essential for the activity.

ANTIBACTERIAL ACTIVITY

The quinolones are active against Gram-negative microorganisms including *E. coli, Klebsiella, Enterobacter, Citrobacter, Proteus, Shigella, Salmonella, H. influenzae, P. aeroginosa,* and *N. gonorrhoeae.* Among the Gram-positive organisms, they are active against *S. aureus,* and some *Streptococci* species. They are not active against anaerobes.

MECHANISM OF ACTION

Quinolones inhibit DNA gyrase in Gram-negative microorganisms and topoisomerase IV in Gram-positive microorganisms.

DNA gyrase is responsible for continuous introduction of negative supercoils into DNA. This it does in two steps, one unit of DNA gyrase, gyr-A carries out the strand cutting function and gyr-B the resealing of break on the front side. Negative supercoiling is necessary because it relieves the torsional stress of helical DNA. Out of the two gyrases, the quinolones inhibit the activity of gyr-A.

Topoisomerase IV separates interlinked daughter DNA molecules that are the products of DNA replication

INDIVIDUAL COMPOUNDS

SULPHONAMIDES

Sulphanilamide

4-Aminobenzenesulphonamide

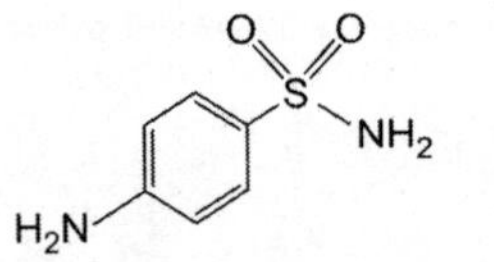

Synthesis

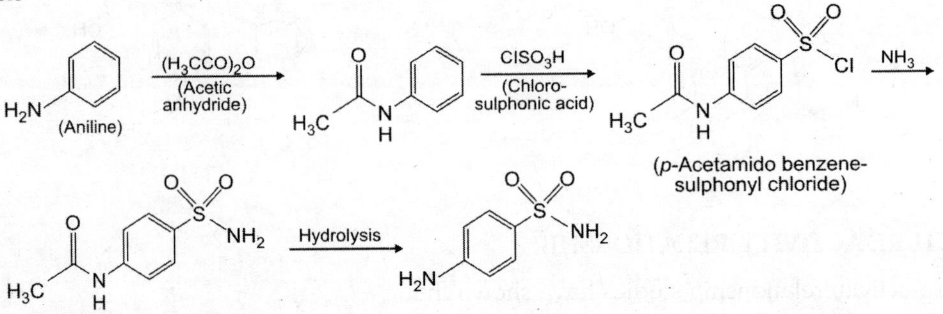

Sulphathiazole

4-Amino-*N*-2-thiazolylbenzenesulphonamide

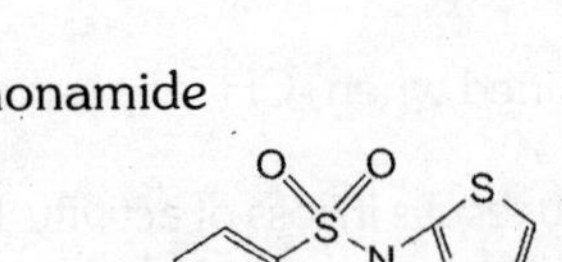

Synthesis

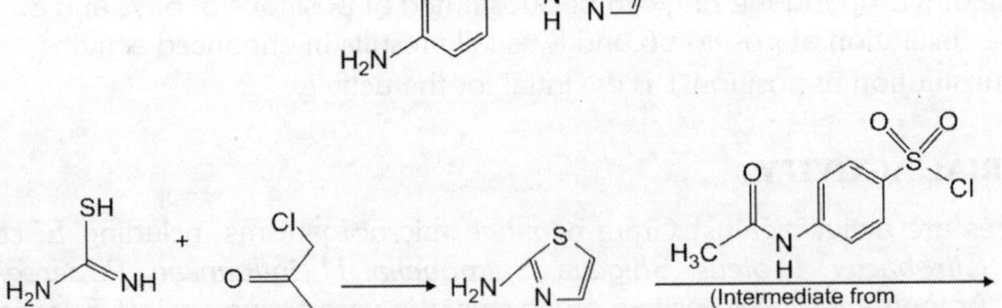

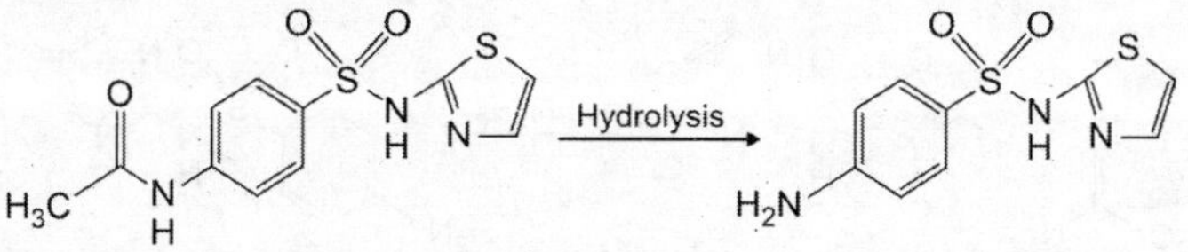

It is specially useful against *staphylococcal* infections. Its succinyl derivative, succinylsulphathiazole (45) is absorbed poorly from gastrointestinal tract and is therefore used for intestinal infections.

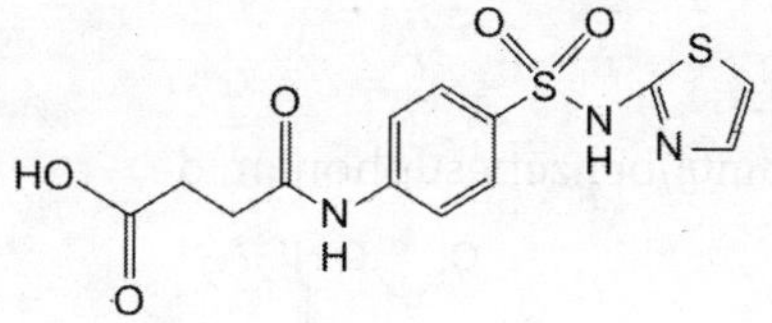

(45)

Synthesis

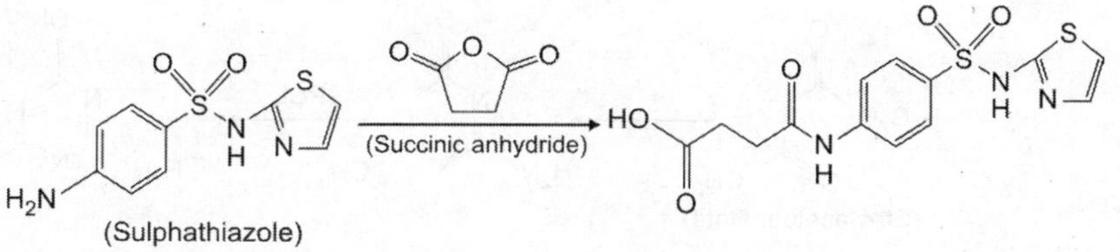

Sulphadiazine

4-Amino-*N*-2-pyrimidinylbenzenesulphonamide

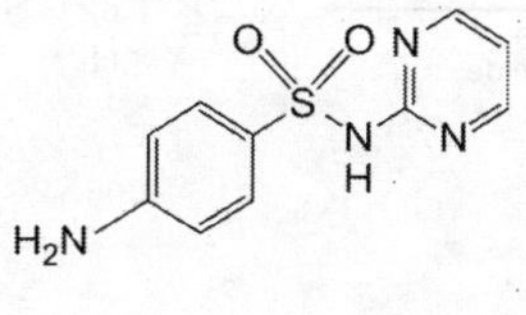

Synthesis

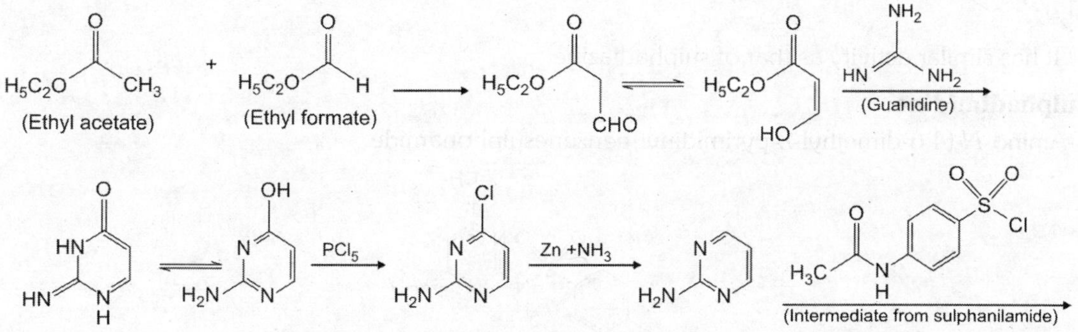

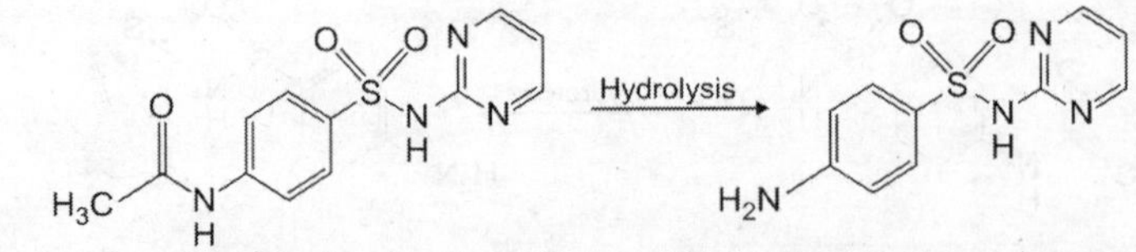

In vivo, it is about 8-times as active as sulphanilamide (2). It is absorbed slowly. It is medium acting (12-16 hr) and is effective against pneumococcal, meningococcal, *Shigella*, and *H. influenzae* infections.

Sulphamerazine

4-Amino-*N*-(4-methyl-2-pyrimidinyl)benzenesuphonamide

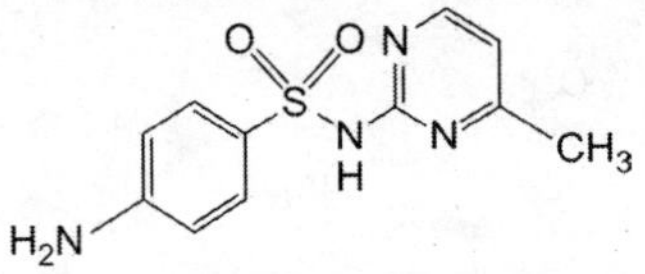

Synthesis

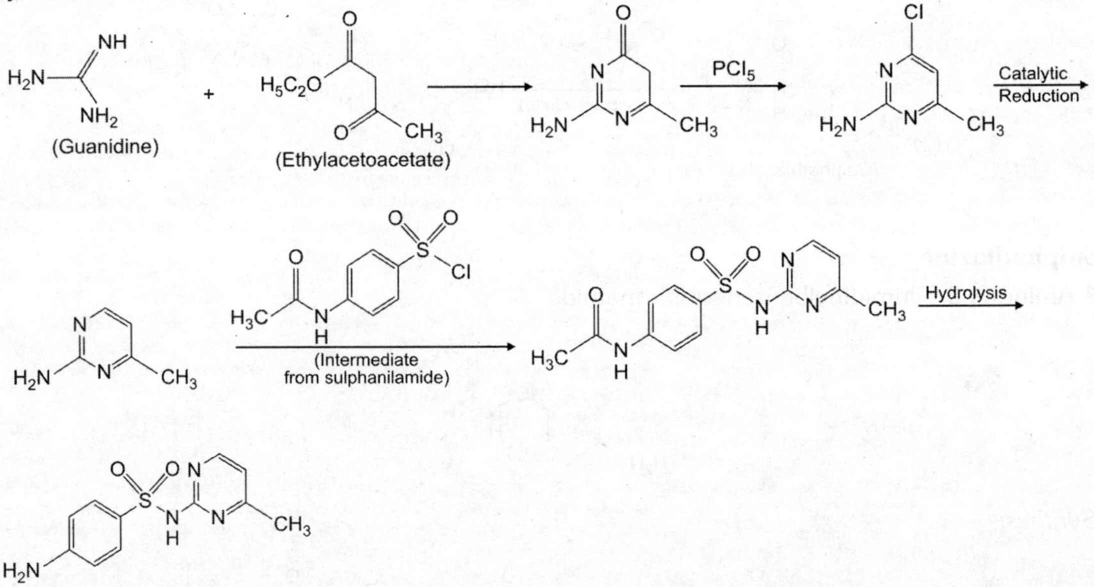

It has similar activity as that of sulphadiazine.

Sulphadimidine

4-Amino-*N*-(4,6-dimethyl-2-pyrimidinyl)benzenesulphonamide

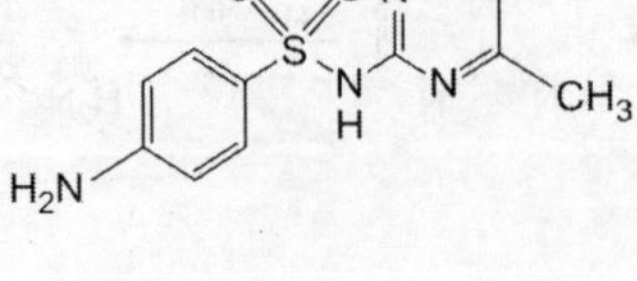

Synthesis

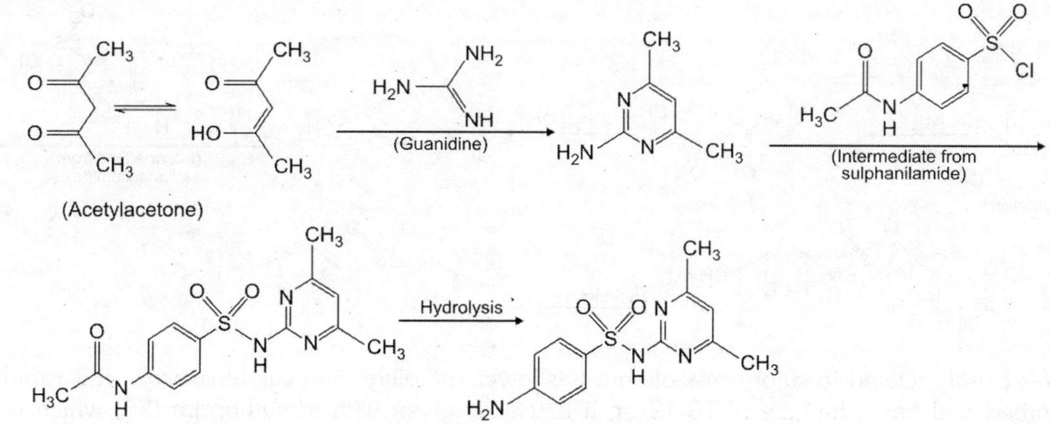

(Acetylacetone)   (Guanidine)   (Intermediate from sulphanilamide)

Hydrolysis

It has similar action as that of sulphamerazine and sulphadiazine but has higher solubility than either of them. Thus, crystalluria problems are less. It is a short-acting (7hr) sulphonamide.

Sulphamethizole

4-Amino-*N*-(5-methyl-1,3,4-thiadiazol-2-yl)benzenesulphonamide

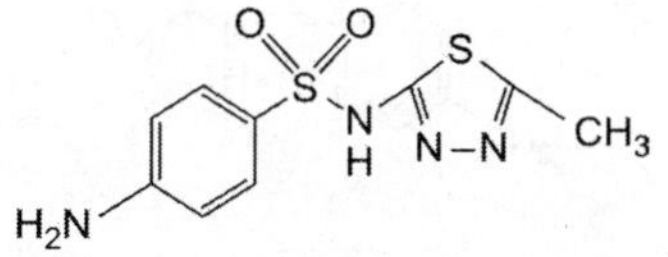

Synthesis

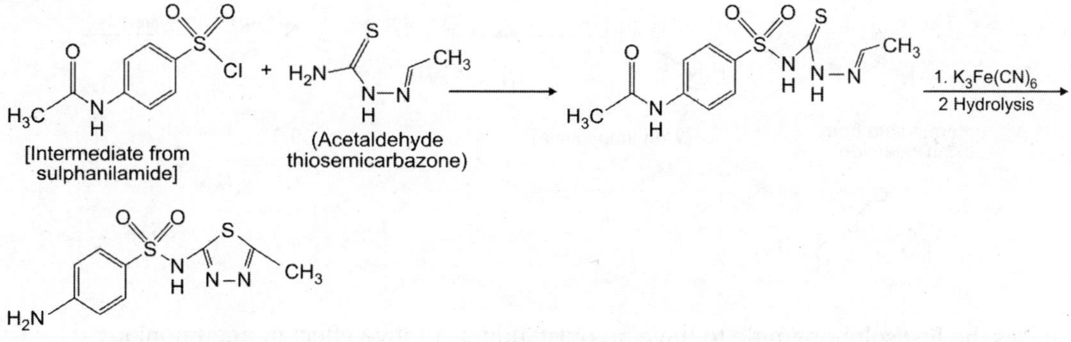

[Intermediate from sulphanilamide]   (Acetaldehyde thiosemicarbazone)   1. K$_3$Fe(CN)$_6$ 2 Hydrolysis

It has high solubility in water and is used for the treatment of urinary tract infections.

Sulphamethoxazole

4-Amino-*N*-(5-methyl-3-isoxazolyl)benzenesulphonamide

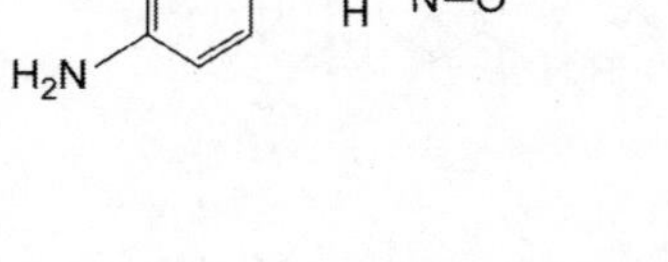

Synthesis

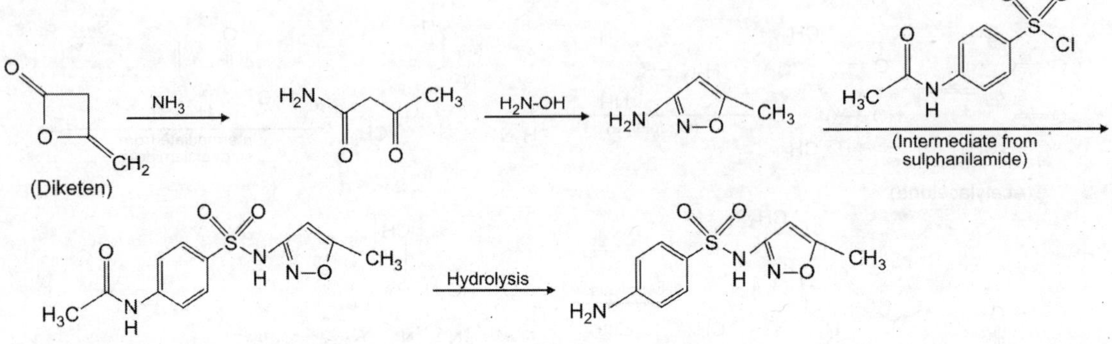

It is closely related to sulphisoxazole but has lower solubility than sulphisoxazole. It is rapidly absorbed and has a half-life of 10-12 hr. It is usually given with trimethoprim (25) which is a dihydrofolate reductase inhibitor.

Sulphapyridine

4-Amino-*N*-2-pyridinylbenzenesulphonamide

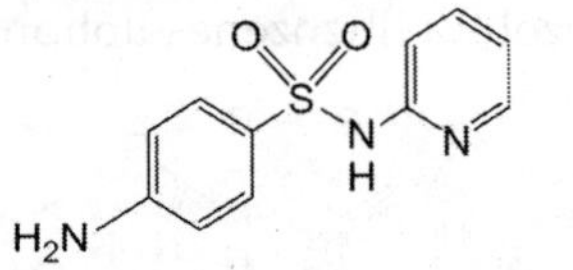

Synthesis

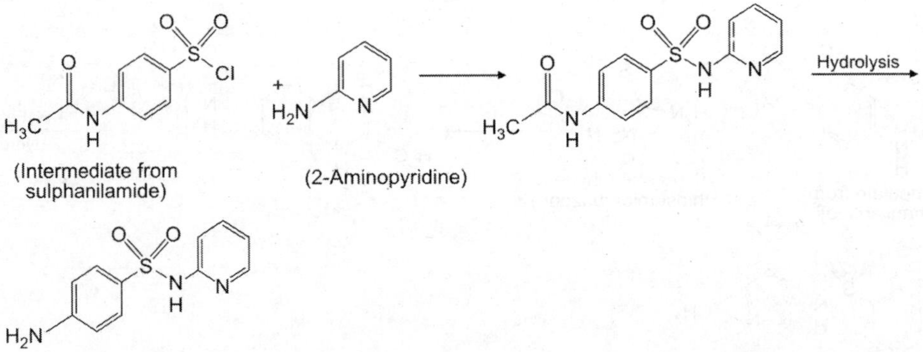

It was the first sulphonamide to have an outstanding curative effect in pneumonia.

Sulphisoxazole

4-Amino-*N*-(3,4-dimethyl-5-isoxazolyl)benzenesulphonamide

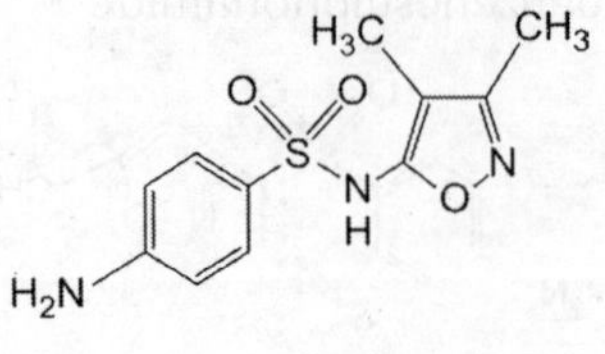

Synthesis

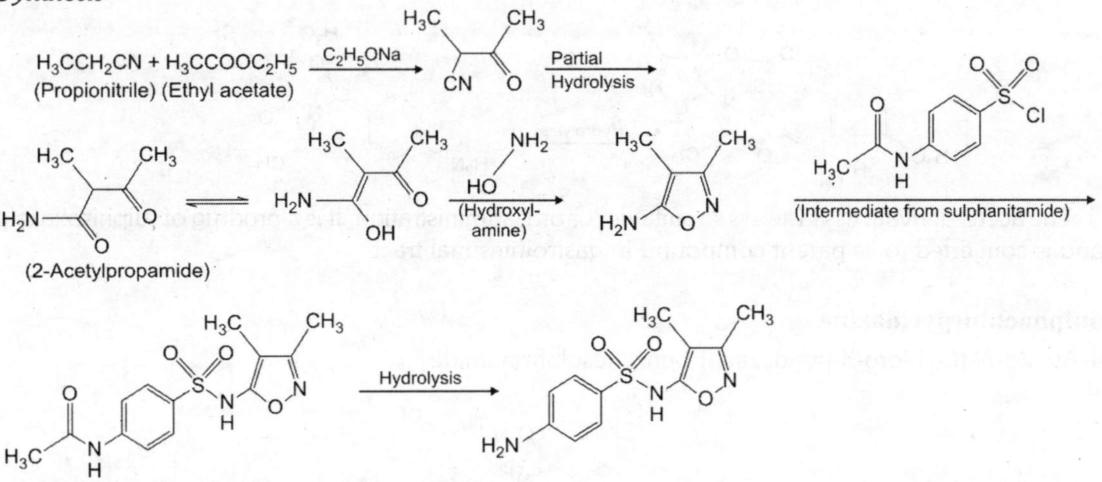

It has a pKa of 5.0. It is claimed to be effective in treatment of Gram-negative urinary tract infections.

Sulphisoxazole Diolamine

Sulphisoxazole diethanolamine salt

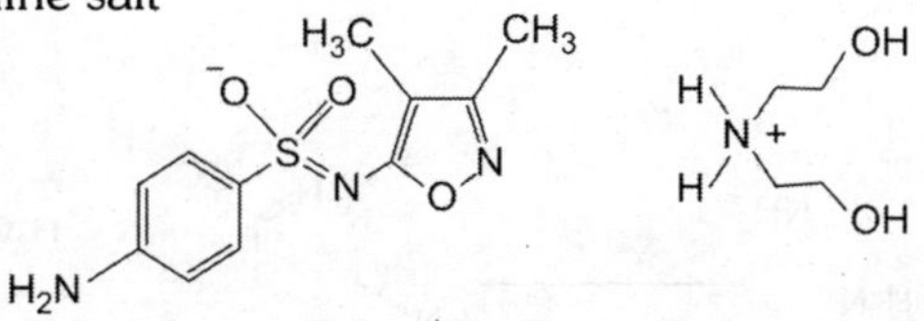

It is prepared by adding diethanolamine to solution of sulphisoxazole. This salt is more soluble at physiological pH and is used for slow administration of the drug by IV, IM, or subcutaneous routes when high blood levels cannot be maintained by oral administration.

Acetyl Sulphisoxazole

N-[(4-Aminophenyl) sulphonyl]-N-(3,4-dimethyl-5-isoxazolyl) acetamide

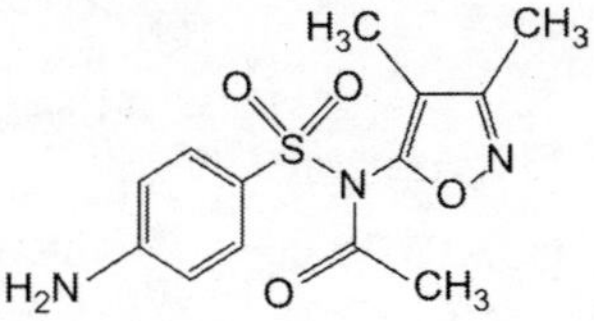

Synthesis

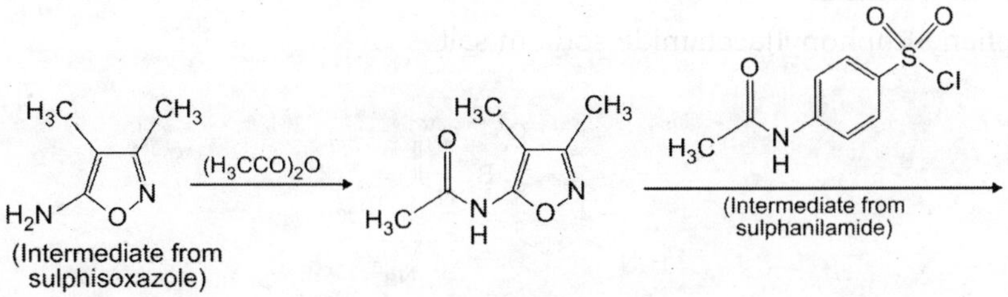

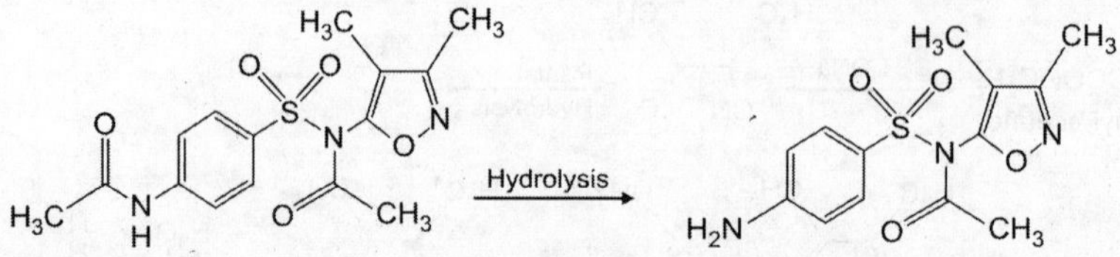

The acetyl derivative is tasteless so suitable for oral administration. It is a prodrug of sulphisoxazole and is converted to its parent compound in gastrointestinal tract.

Sulphachlorpyridazine

4-Amino-*N*-(6-chloro-3-pyridazinyl) benzenesulphonamide

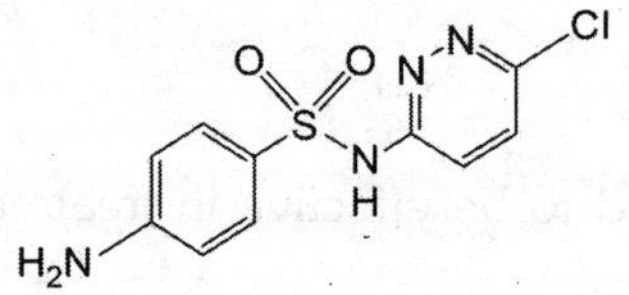

Synthesis

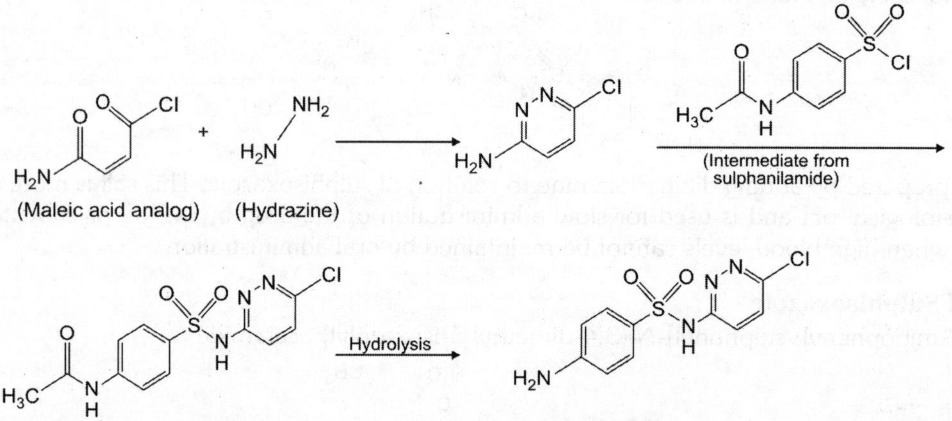

It has a plasma half-life of 8 hr.

Sulphacetamide Sodium

N-[(4-Aminophenyl)suphonyl]acetamide sodium salt

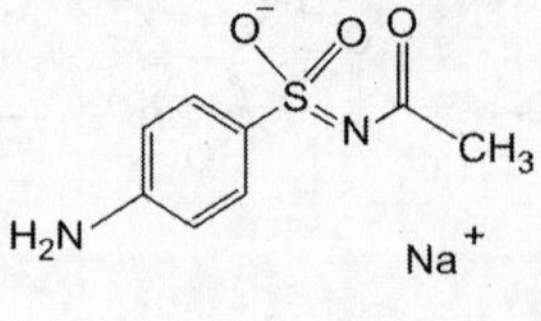

Synthesis

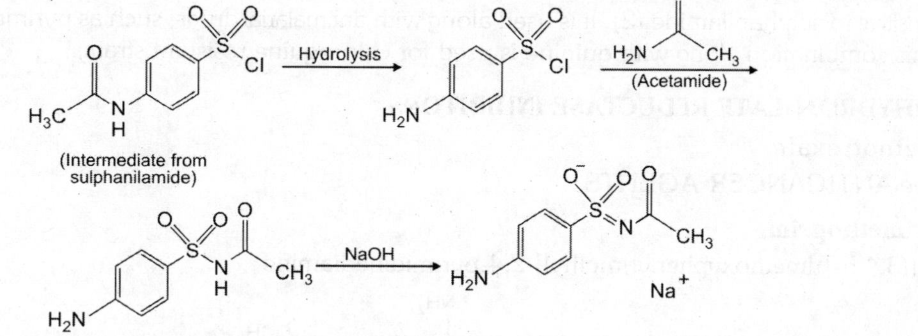

Because of its high solubility and ready elimination, it has found considerable use in urinary tract infections and as ophthalmic preparations.

Sulphadoxine

4-Sulphanilamido-5,6-dimethoxypyrimidine

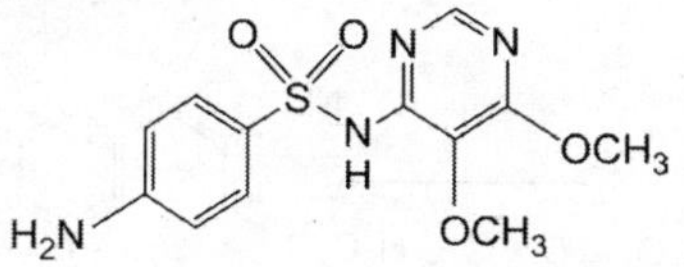

Synthesis

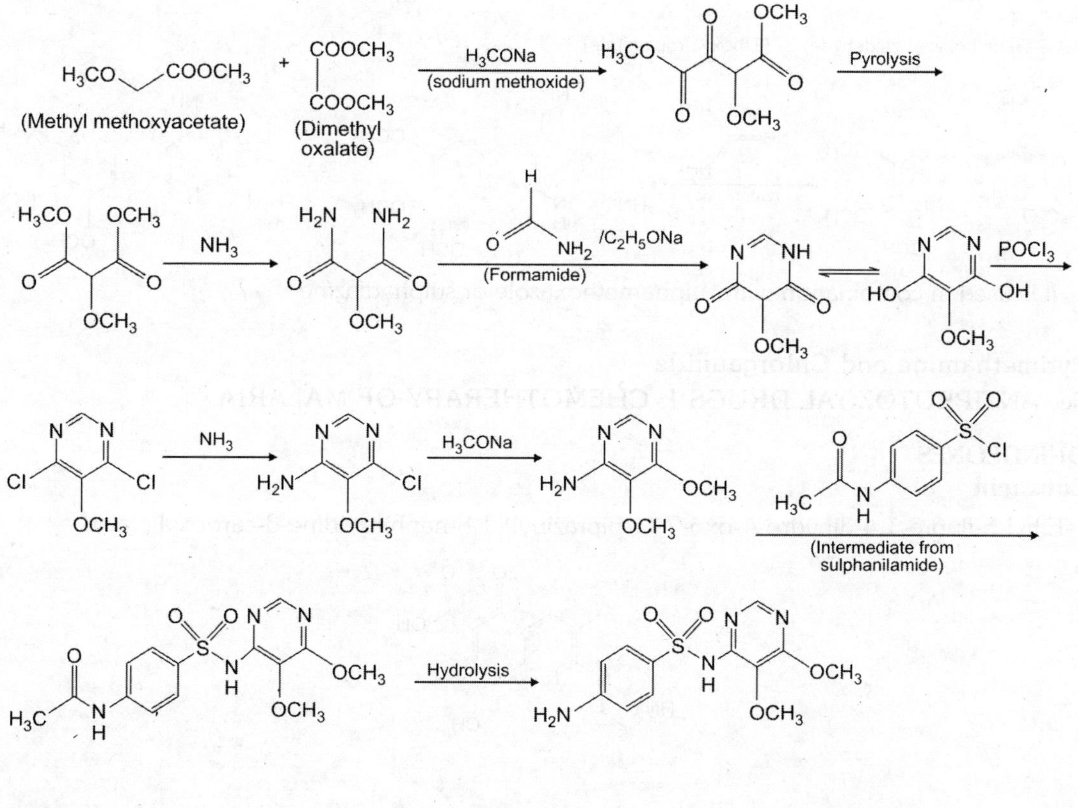

It has a very long half-life about 120 hr to 200 hr and effective in microorganisms which are sensitive to sulphanilamide (2). It is used along with antimalarial drugs, such as pyrimethamine (26). This combination along with quinine is used for chloroquine resistant strains.

DIHYDROFOLATE REDUCTASE INHIBITORS

Methotrexate
See **ANTICANCER AGENTS**

Trimethoprim
5-[(3,4,5-Trimethoxyphenyl)methyl]-2,4-pyrimidinediamine

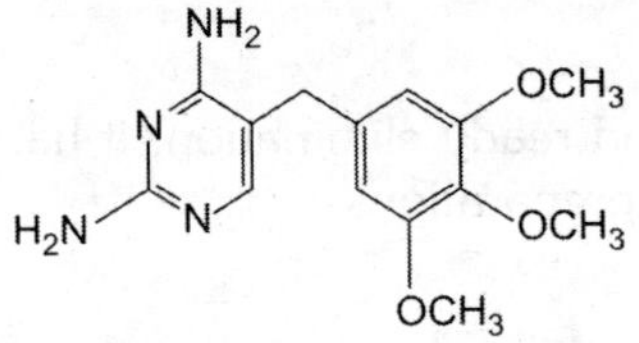

Synthesis

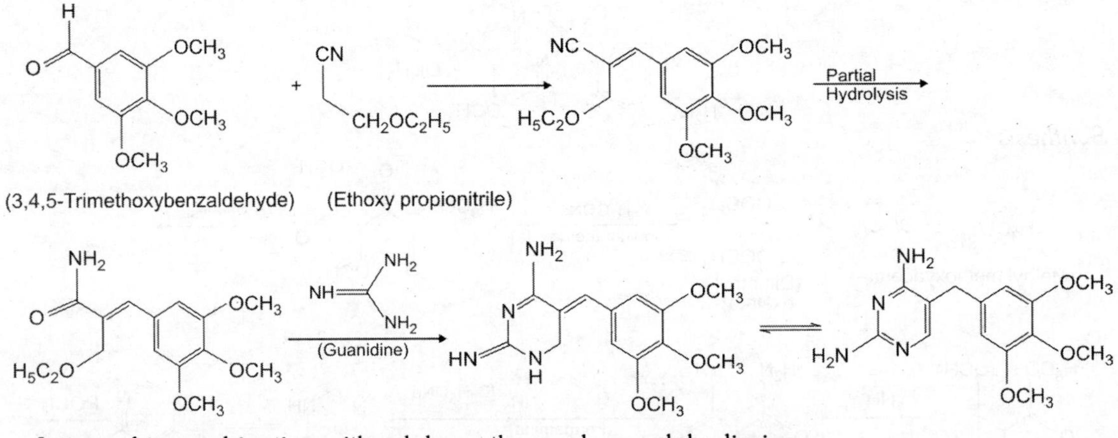

(3,4,5-Trimethoxybenzaldehyde)   (Ethoxy propionitrile)

(Guanidine)

It is used in combination with sulphamethoxazole or sulphadiazine.

Pyrimethamine and Chlorgaunide
See **ANTIPROTOZOAL DRUGS I: CHEMOTHERAPY OF MALARIA**

QUINOLONES
Enoxacin
1-Ethyl-6-fluoro-1,4-dihydro-4-oxo-7-(1-piprazinyl)-1,8-naphthyridine-3-carboxylic acid

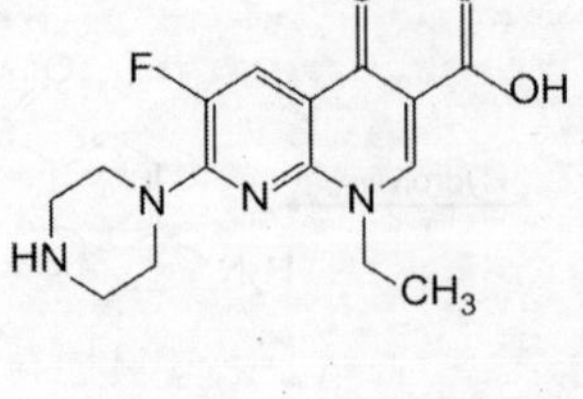

Synthesis

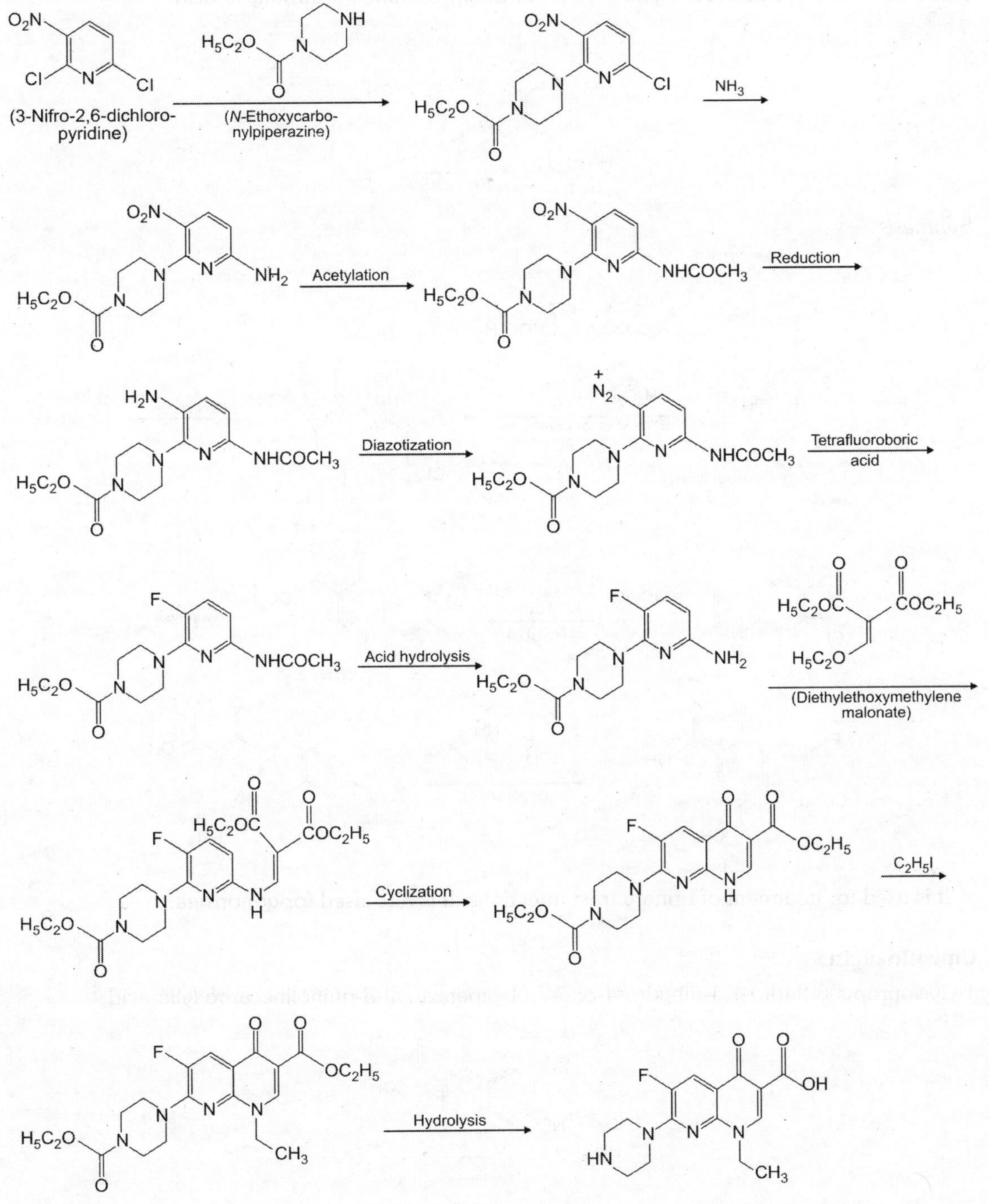

(3-Nifro-2,6-dichloro-pyridine) + (N-Ethoxycarbo-nylpiperazine) → NH₃ →

Acetylation → Reduction →

Diazotization → Tetrafluoroboric acid →

Acid hydrolysis → (Diethylethoxymethylene malonate) →

Cyclization → C₂H₅I →

Hydrolysis →

Norfloxacin

1-Ethyl-6-fluoro-1,4-dihydro-4-oxo-7-(1-piperazinyl)-3-quinolinecarboxylic acid

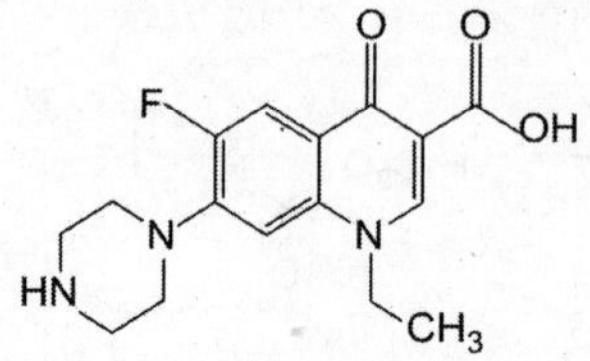

Synthesis

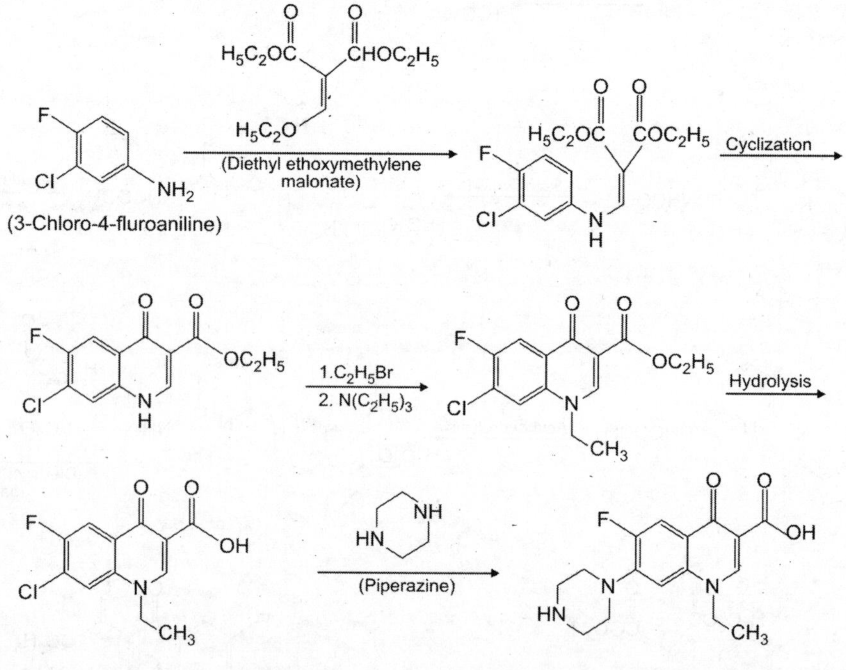

It is used for treatment of urinary tract infections. It is also used for gonorrhea.

Ciprofloxacin

1-Cyclopropyl-6-fluoro-1,4-dihydro-4-oxo-7-(1-piperazinyl)-3-quinolinecarboxylic acid

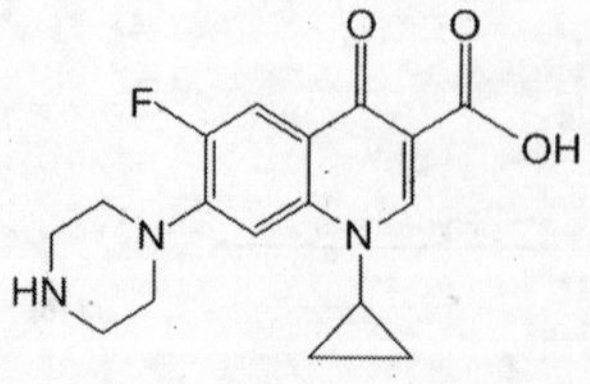

Synthesis

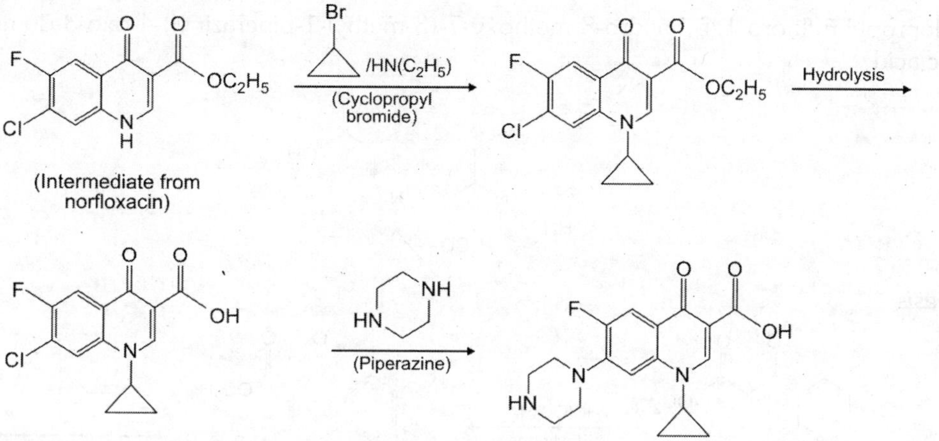

(Intermediate from norfloxacin)

(Cyclopropyl bromide)

Hydrolysis

(Piperazine)

It is used for the treatment of bacterial gastroenteritis caused by Gram-negative bacilli and the treatment of respiratory tract infections, particularly for bronchitis and pneumonia.

Lomefloxacin

1-Ethyl-6,8-difluoro-1,4-dihydro-4-oxo-7-(3-methyl-1-piperazinyl)-3-quinolinecarboxylic acid

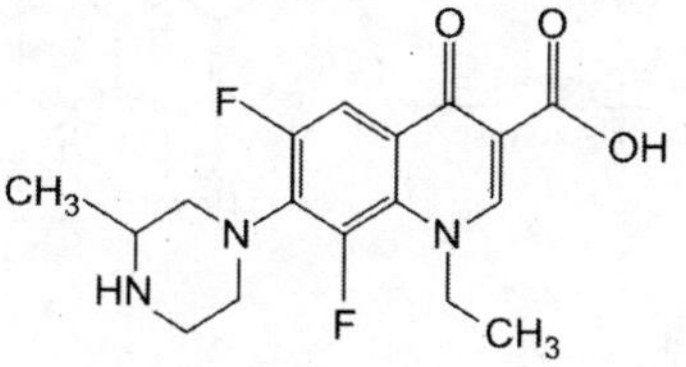

Synthesis

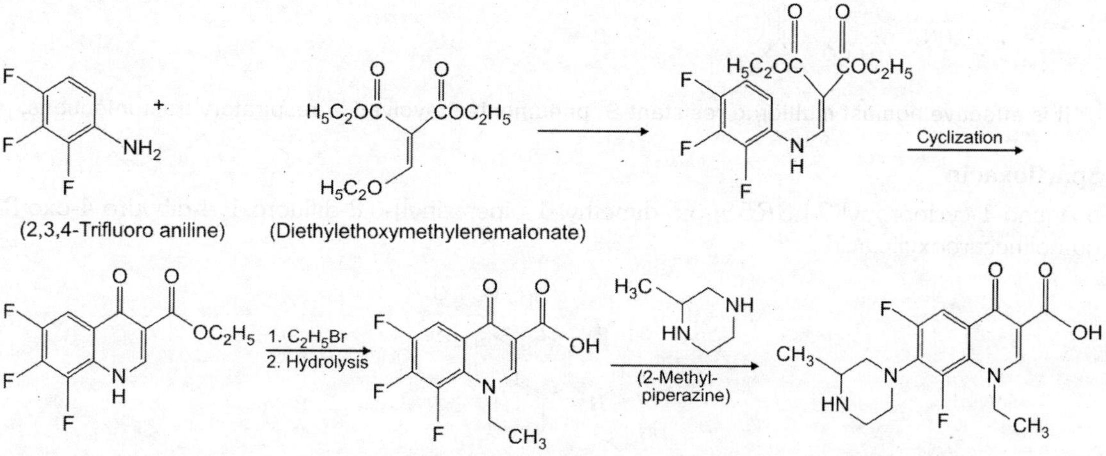

(2,3,4-Trifluoro aniline)　(Diethylethoxymethylenemalonate)

Cyclization

1. C_2H_5Br
2. Hydrolysis

(2-Methyl-piperazine)

It is indicated for acute and chronic bronchitis, acute cystitis, and chronic urinary tract infections.

Gatifloxacin

1-Cyclopropyl-6-fluoro-1,4-dihydro-8-methoxy-7-(3-methyl-1-piperazinyl)-4-oxo-3-quinolinecarboxylic acid

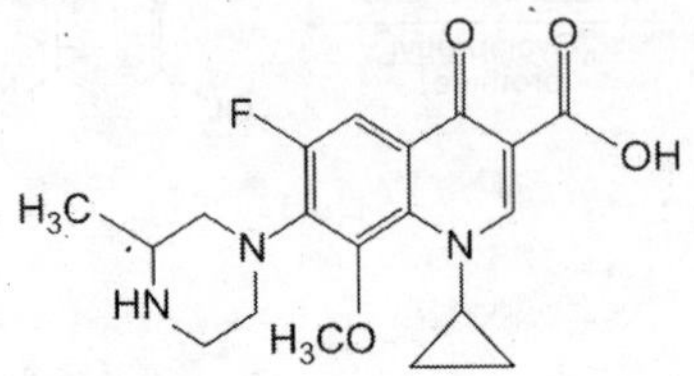

Synthesis

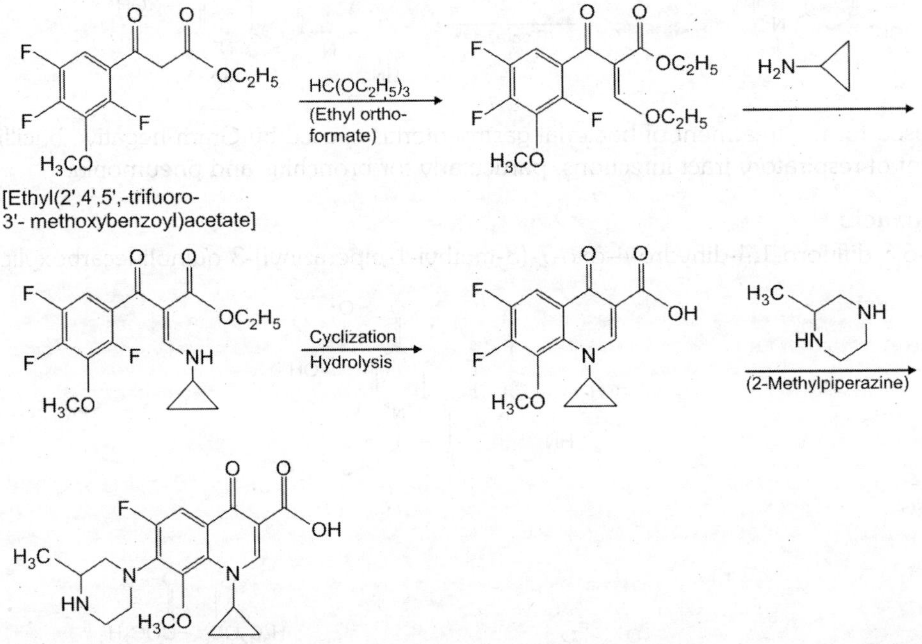

[Ethyl(2',4',5',-trifuoro-3'- methoxybenzoyl)acetate]

It is effective against multidrug resistant S. pneumoniae involved in respiratory tract infections.

Sparfloxacin

5-Amino-1-cyclopropyl-7-[(3R,5S)-3,5-dimethyl-1-piperazinyl]-6,8-difluoro-1, 4-dihydro-4-oxo-3-quinolinecarboxylic acid

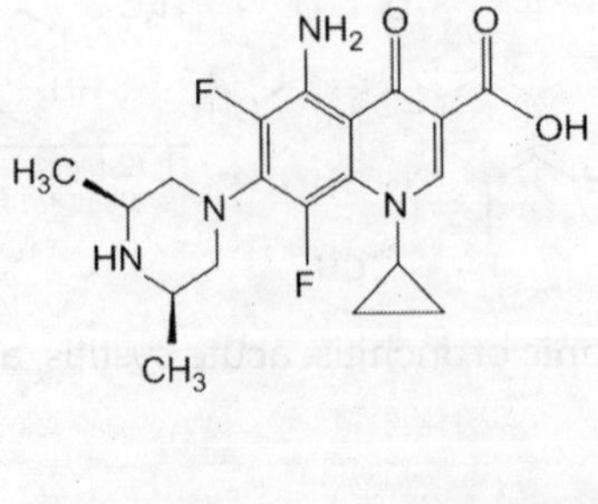

Synthesis

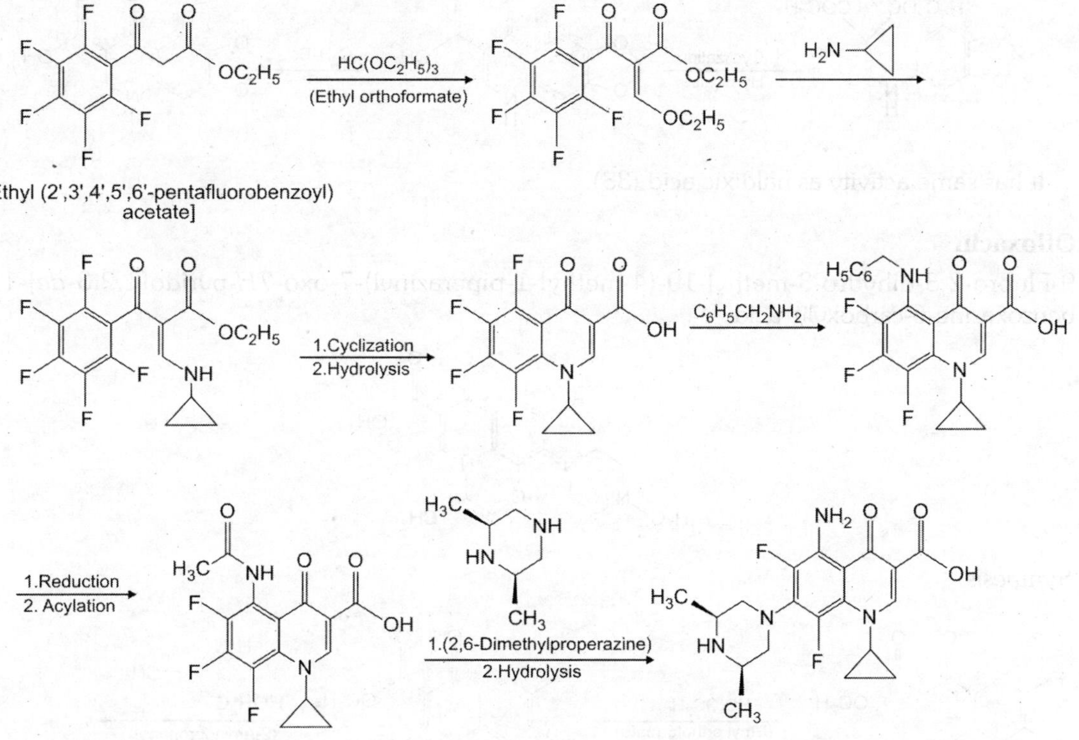

[Ethyl (2',3',4',5',6'-pentafluorobenzoyl) acetate]

It has high potency against Gram-positive and Gram-negative bacteria. It is used for gastroenteritis.

Oxolinic Acid

1-Ethyl-1,4-dihydro-6,7–methylenedioxy-4-oxo–3–quinolinecarboxylic acid

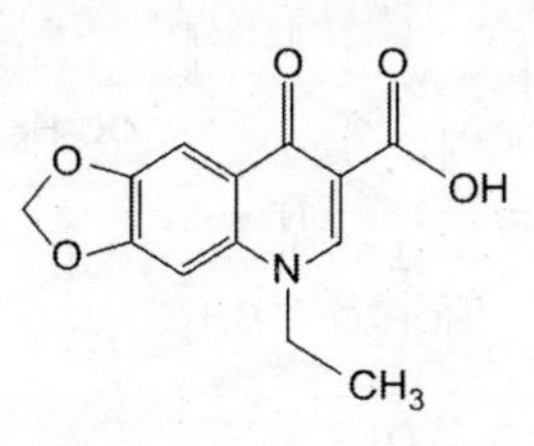

Synthesis

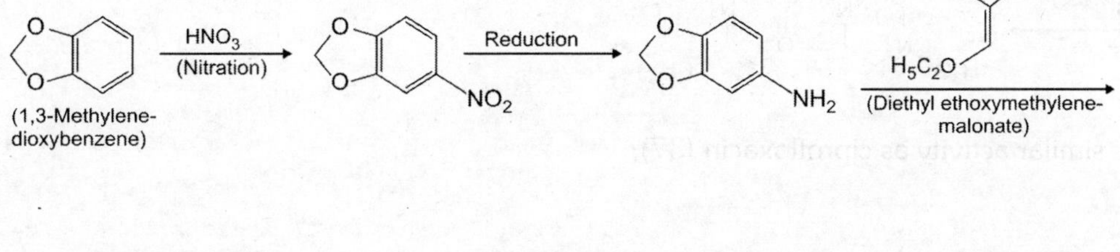

(1,3-Methylene-
dioxybenzene)

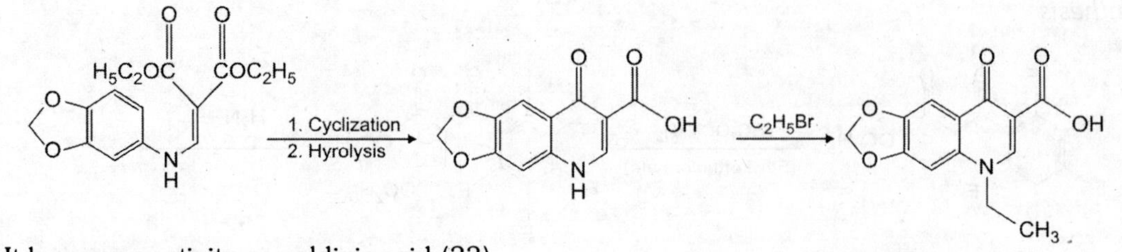

It has same activity as naldixic acid (33).

Ofloxacin

9-Fluoro-2,3-dihydro-3-methyl-10-(4-methyl-1-piperazinyl)-7-oxo-7H-pyrido[1,2,3-de]-1,4-benzoxazine-6-carboxylic acid

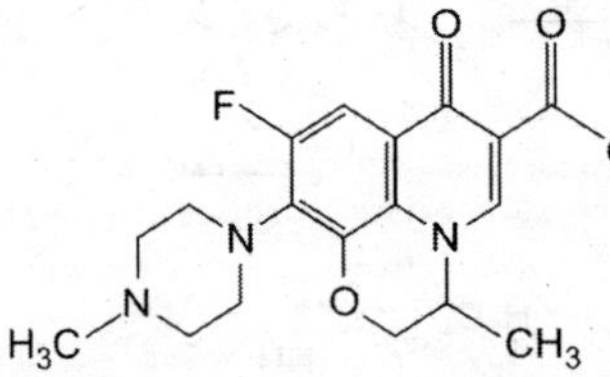

Synthesis

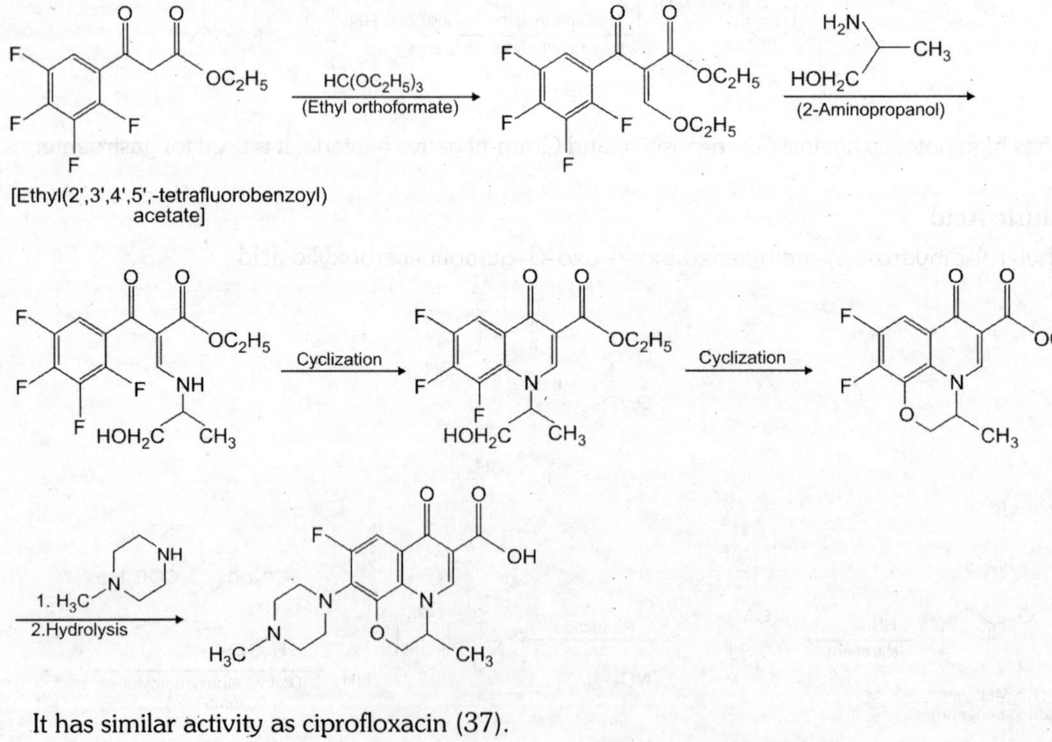

[Ethyl(2',3',4',5',-tetrafluorobenzoyl) acetate]

It has similar activity as ciprofloxacin (37).

Cinoxacin

1-Ethyl-1,4-dihydro-4-oxo[1,3]-dioxolo[4,5-g]cinnoline-3-carboxylic acid

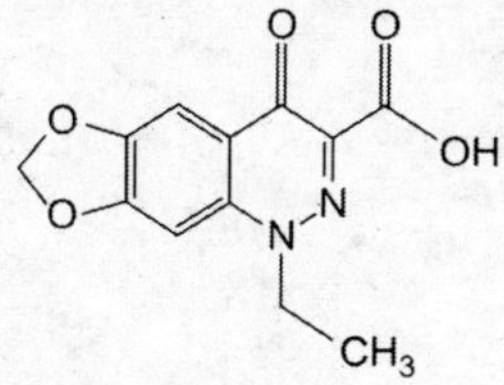

Synthesis

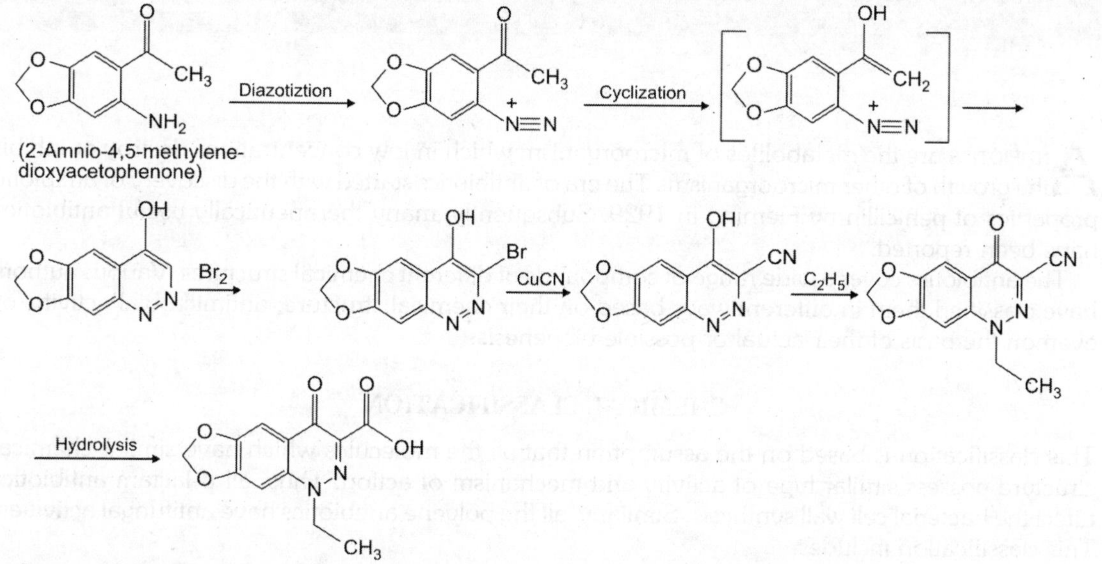

(2-Amnio-4,5-methylene-
dioxyacetophenone)

It is used for urinary tract infections caused by Gram-negative organisms.

ANTIBIOTICS

A NTIBIOTICS are the metabolites of microorganism which in low concentrations destroy or inhibit the growth of other microorganisms. The era of antibiotics started with the discovery of antibiotic properties of penicillin by Fleming in 1929. Subsequently, many therapeutically useful antibiotics have been reported.

The antibiotics cover a wide range of compounds of different chemical structures. Various authors have classified them in different ways based on their chemical structure, antimicrobial activity, or even on the basis of their actual or possible biogenesis.

CHEMICAL CLASSIFICATION

This classification is based on the assumption that all the molecules which have similar chemical structure possess similar type of activity and mechanism of action. Thus, all β-lactam antibiotics affect the bacterial cell wall synthesis. Similarly, all the polyene antibiotics have antifungal activities. This classification includes:

1. β-Lactam antibiotics.
2. Peptide antibiotics.
3. Polyene antibiotics.
4. Macrolide antibiotics.
5. Aminoglycoside antibiotics.
6. Antibiotics with fused rings/tetracyclines.
7. Miscellaneous antibiotics.

β-LACTAM ANTIBIOTICS

Antibiotics belonging to this class include penicillins (1), carbapenems (2), cephalosporins (3), carbacephems (4), oxacephems (5), and monobactams (6).

(1)   (2)   (3), X = S
(4), X = C
(5), X = O

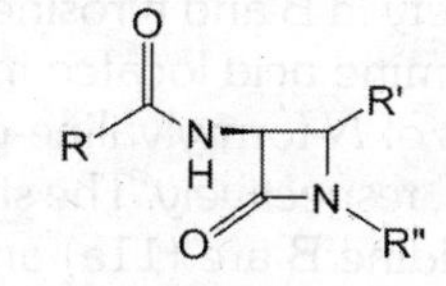

(6)

All of these antibiotics contain a β-lactam ring. While in case of penicllins (1) the β-lactam ring is fused to a heterocyclic, thiazolidine ring, in case of carbapenems (2), the β-lactam ring is fused to a five membered unsaturated ring. Further, carbapenems (2) do not contain an acylamino side chain. In cephalosporins (3), the β-lactam ring is fused with heterocyclic dihydrothiazine ring. The carbacephems (4) and oxacephems (5) are analogs of cephalosporins in which the sulphur of the six-membered ring is substituted by carbon and oxygen, respectively. The monobactams (6) include antibiotics without any fused bicyclic structure.

PEPTIDE ANTIBIOTICS

As the name indicates, they have a peptide moiety with unusual amino acids attached to non-amino acid moiety. They have been further classified as:

(*i*) **Actinomycin group:** This group of antibiotics is produced by *Streptomyces* species. The actinomycins are active against Gram-positive bacteria. They are also cytotoxic and form reversible complexes with DNA and inhibit DNA polymerization. All of the actinomycins contain a 3-phenoxazone-1,9-dicarboxylic acid [actinocin (7)] moiety. Each of the carboxylic acid group is bonded to a pentapeptide lactone ring. Those actinomycins which have similar pentapeptide lactone ring are called isoactinomycins and those which have different pentapeptide lactone rings are known as anisoactinomycins. Example, dactinomycin (8) is an isoactinomycin.

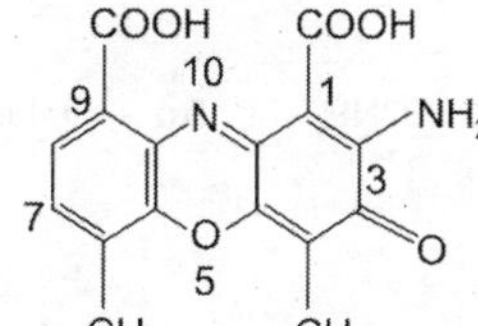

(7)

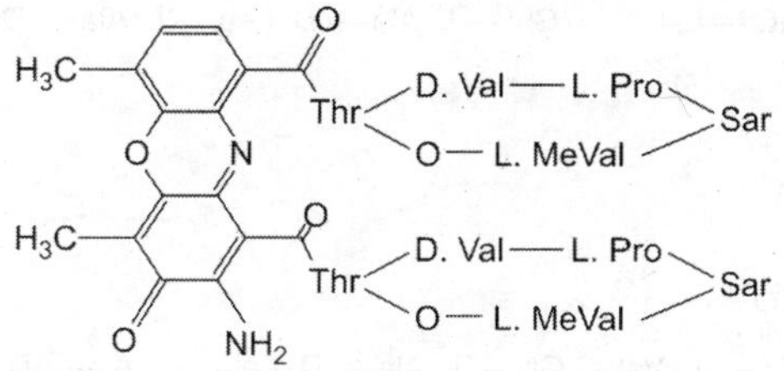

(8)

(*ii*) **Bacitracin group:** This group of antibiotics is produced by *Bacillus licheniformis* and *B.subtilis*. The commercial grade of bacitracin is a mixture of six components namely, A, B, C, D, E, and F. Of this bacitracin A(9) forms 80%. Bacitracin is mainly used as topical application. It possesses bactericidal activity against Gram-positive bacteria including hemolytic and non-hemolytic *streptococci*, *staphylococci*, and *pneumococci*.

(*iii*) **Linear gramicidins:** Gramicidins are components of tyrothricin which is a mixture of gramicidin and tyrocidine. Of the two components, gramicidin is more active. Five gramicidins have been isolated and include A_2, A_3, B_1, B_2, and C. They differ in having tryptophan moiety in A, L-phenylalanine moiety in B and tyrosine moiety in C. In both gramicidin A and B pairs, the difference lies in the amino acid located in the beginning of chain and carrying a formyl group. Thus, the structures of *N*-formylvaline-gramicidine A and *N*-formylisoleucine-gramicidine A are (10a) and (10b), respectively. The structures of *N*-formylvaline-gramicidine B and *N*-formylisoleucine-gramicidine B are (11a) and (11b), respectively.

Tyrocidine is a mixture of tyrocidine A (12), tyrocidine B (13), tyrocidine C (14), and tyrocidine D (15).

$$
\begin{array}{c}
\text{CH}_3 \\
\text{H}_3\text{C} \qquad \text{S} \\
\text{H}_2\text{N} \qquad \text{N} \\
\qquad\qquad \text{O} \\
\text{L. Leu} \\
\text{L. His-D. Asp-Asn. D. Glu} \\
\text{D. Phe} \qquad\qquad | \qquad | \\
\text{L. Ile-D. Orn-L. Lys-}\alpha\text{-Ile}
\end{array}
$$

(9)

O
‖
HC — L. Val — Gly — L. Ala — D. Leu — L. Ala — D. Val — L. Val — D. Val — L. Trp — D.Leu — **L. Trp** — D. Leu

HOH₂CH₂CNH — L. Trp — D.Leu — L. Trp

(10a)

O
‖
HC — L. Ileu — Gly — L. Ala — D. Leu — L. Ala — D. Val — L. Val — D. Val — L. Trp — D. Leu — **L. Trp** — D. Leu

HOH₂CH₂CNH — L. Trp — D. Leu — L. Trp

(10b)

O
‖
HC — L. Val — Gly — L. Ala — D. Leu — L. Ala — D. Val — L. Val — D. Val — L. Trp — D. Leu — **L. Phe** — D. Leu

HO₂CH₂CNH — L. Trp — D. Leu — L. Trp

(11a)

O
‖
HC — L. Ileu — Gly — L. Ala — D. Leu — L. Ala — D. Val — L. Val — D. Val — L. Trp — D. Leu — **L. Phe** — D. Leu

HOH₂CH₂CNH — L. Trp — D. Leu — L. Trp

(11b)

L. Val → L. Orn → L. Leu → X → L. Pro

L. Tyr ← Glu ← L. Asp ← Z ← Y
　　　　　|　　　　|
　　　　NH$_2$　　NH$_2$

	X	Y	Z
(12),	D. Phe	D. Phe	D. Phe
(13),	D. Phe	L. Tyr	D. Phe
(14),	D. Tyr	L. Tyr	D. Phe
(15),	D. Tyr	L. Tyr	D. Tyr

(*iv*) **Polymyxin group:** This group of peptide antibiotics was isolated from *Bacillus polymixia* and consists of polymyxin B$_1$ (16), polymyxin B$_2$ (17), polymyxin D$_1$ (18), polymyxin D$_2$ (19), and polymyxin E$_1$ (20). Polymyxin group of antibiotics have a wide spectrum of activity against Gram-negative bacteria.

γ-NH$_2$
|
DAB → D.X → Y
|
R → DAB → Thr — Z — DAB
|　　　　　　　　　Thr ← DAB ← DAB
γ-NH$_2$　　　　　　|　　　|
　　　　　　　　γ-NH$_2$　γ-NH$_2$

	R	X	Y	Z
(16),	MOC	Phe	Leu	DAB
(17),	MHP	Phe	Leu	DAB
(18),	MOC	Leu	Thr	D—Ser
(19),	MHP	Leu	Thr	D—Ser
(20),	MOC	Leu	Leu	DAB

DAB = L–α,γ-Diaminobutryl
MHP = 6-Methylheptanoyl
MOC = (+)-6-Methyloctanoyl

POLYENE ANTIBIOTICS

This group of antibiotics contain a macrocyclic lactone ring which is highly unsaturated. The lactone ring contains alternate double bonds and is linked to a desoxy amino sugar. These antibiotics which are produced by *Streptomyces* species are highly active against fungi. They are classified according to the number of alternate double bonds present, i.e. tri-, tetra-, penta-, hexa-, and heptaenes. Examples of this class of antibiotics include nystatin A$_1$ (21) and amphotericin B (22).

(21)

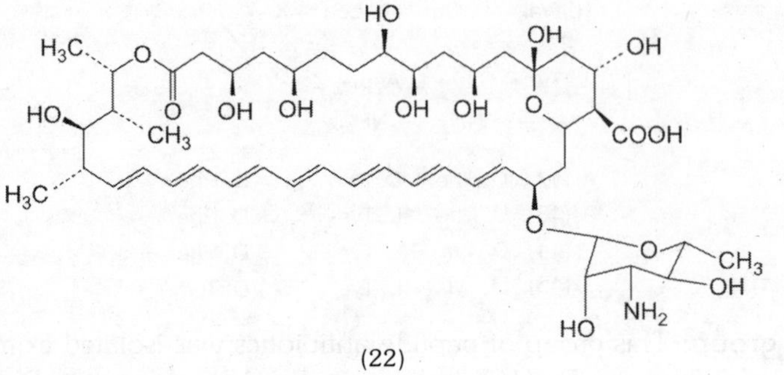

(22)

MACROLIDE ANTIBIOTICS

These antibiotics contain a macrocyclic lactone ring linked glycosidically to a desoxy sugar. Examples of these include erythromycin A (23), clarithromycin (24), azithromycin (25), oleandomycin (26), etc.

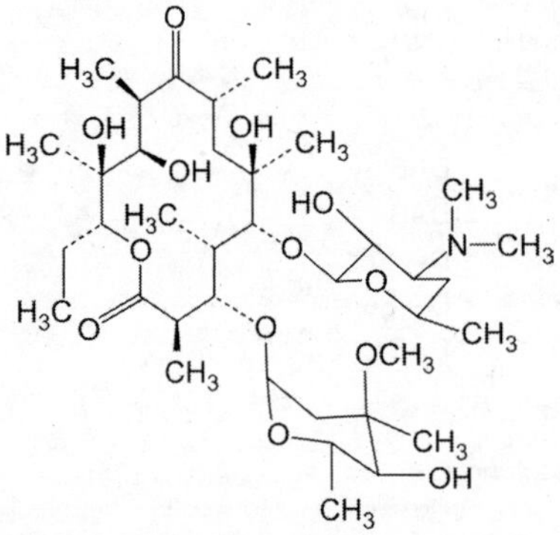

(23)

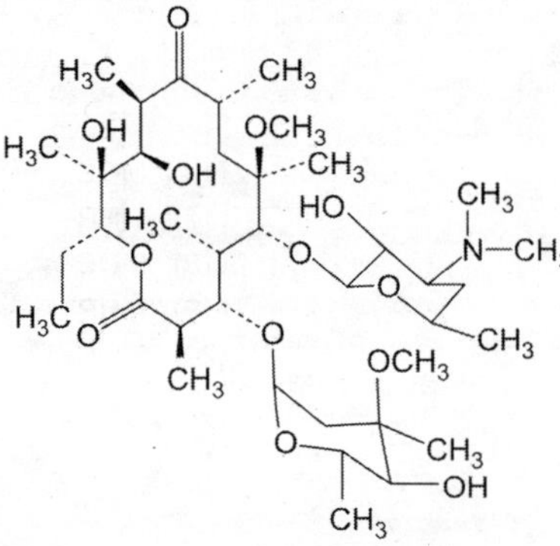

(24)

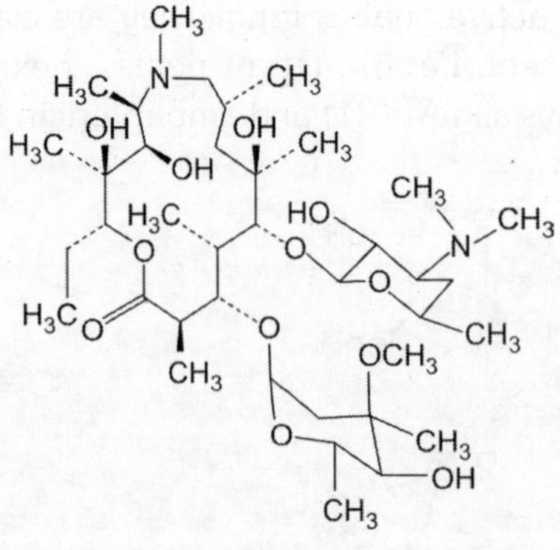

(25)

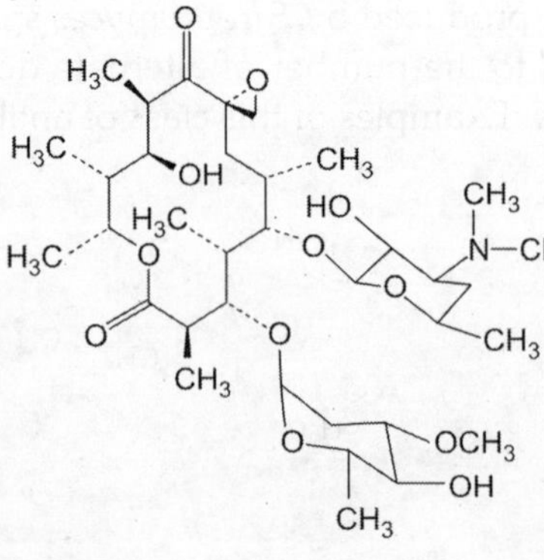

(26)

AMINOGLYCOSIDE ANTIBIOTICS

Aminoglycoside antibiotics contain aminosugars which are glycosidically linked. They also contain a substituted 1, 3-diaminocyclohexane moiety. Amnioglycoside antibiotics are highly basic in nature. Examples of this class of antibiotics include streptomycin (27), neomycin B (28), amikacin (29), etc.

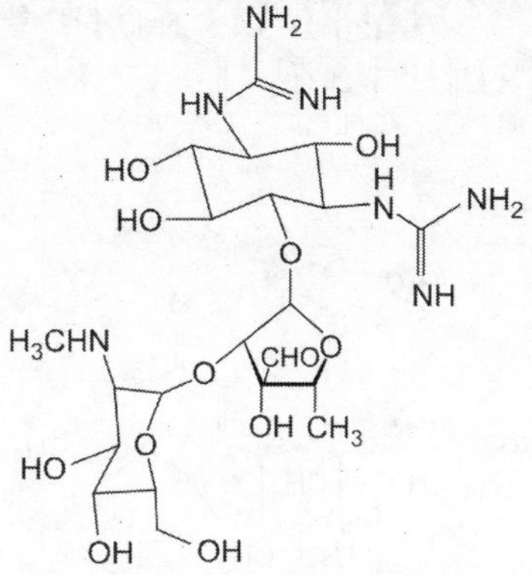

(27)

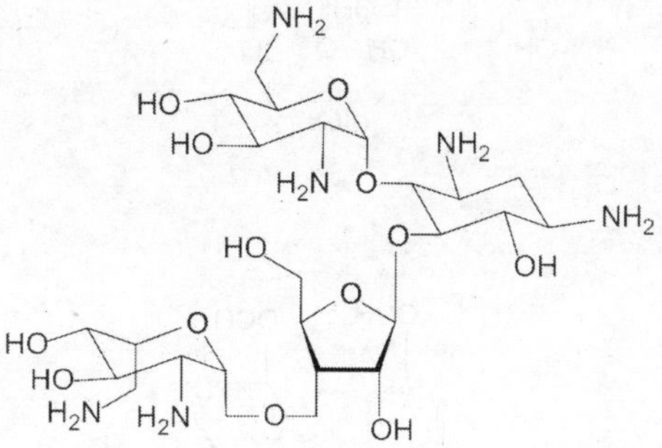

(28)

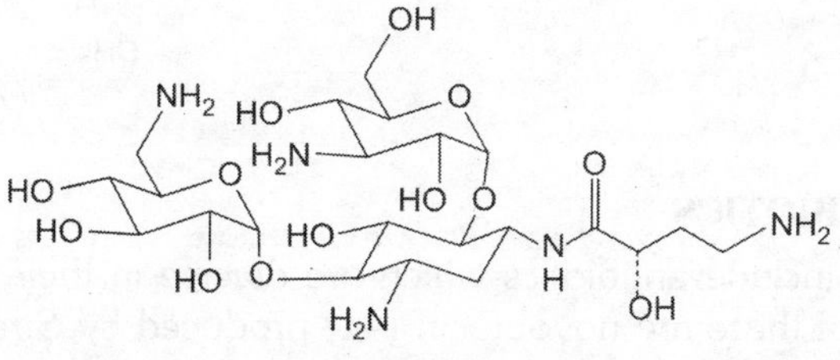

(29)

ANTIBIOTICS WITH FUSED RINGS/TETRACYCLINES

Some of the members of this class of antibiotics possess broad-spectrum of activity and include tetracycline (30), chlortetracycline (31), oxytetracycline (32), demeclocycline (33), doxycycline (34), minocycline (35), rolitetracycline (36), methacycline (37), and meclocycline (38). The other groups include antifungal antibiotic griseofulvin (39) and antibacterial antibiotic fusidic acid (40).

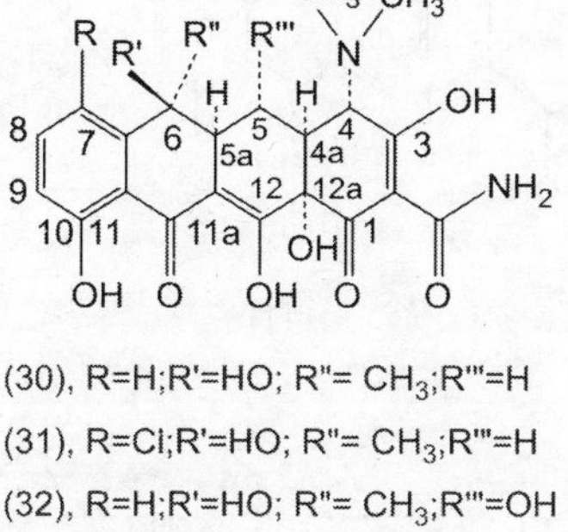

(30), R=H;R'=HO; R"= CH_3;R'''=H

(31), R=Cl;R'=HO; R"= CH_3;R'''=H

(32), R=H;R'=HO; R"= CH_3;R'''=OH

(33), R=Cl;R'=HO; R"= R'''=H

(34), R=R'=H; R"= CH_3;R'''=OH

(35), R=$N(CH_3)_2$, R'=R"=R'''=H

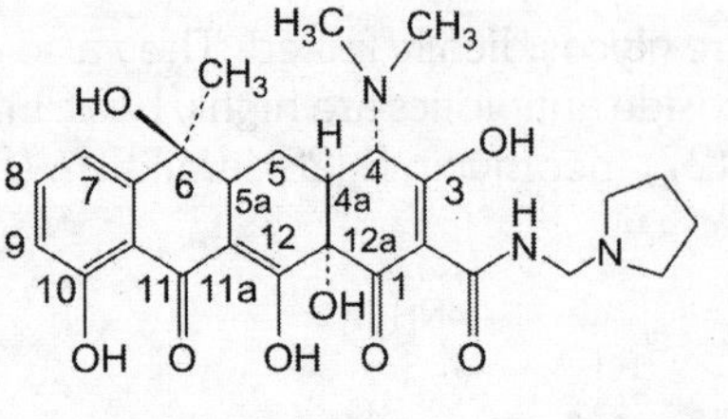

(36)

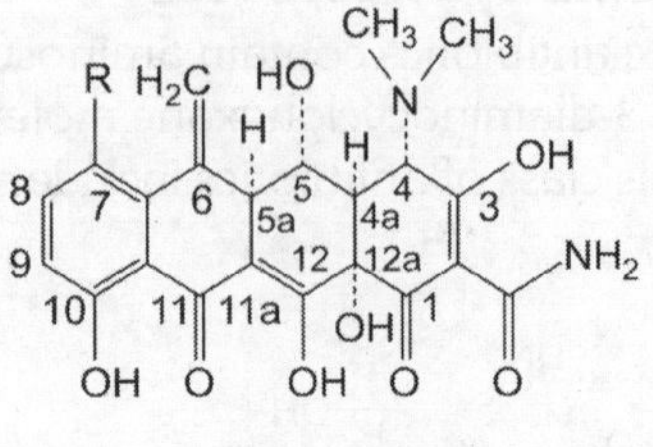

(37), R=H
(38), R=Cl

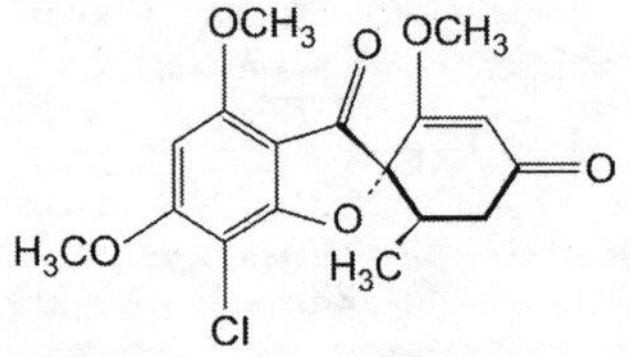

(39)

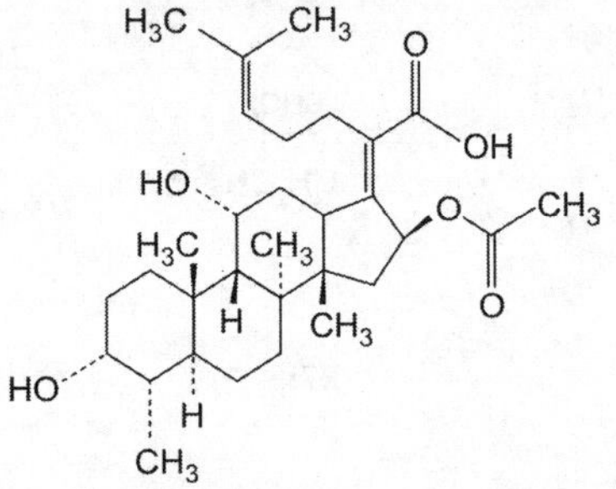

(40)

MISCELLANEOUS ANTIBIOTICS

This group of antibiotics include antibiotics which are diverse in their structures and cannot be clubbed together. Some of these are novobiocin (41) produced by *Streptomyces spheroids*. It is active against Gram-positive bacteria.

Chloramphenicol (42) produced by *Streptomyces venezeulae* was the most widely used antibiotic earlier.

Fosfomycin tromethamine (43) produced by *Streptomyces* species is a broad-spectrum bactericidal antibiotic.

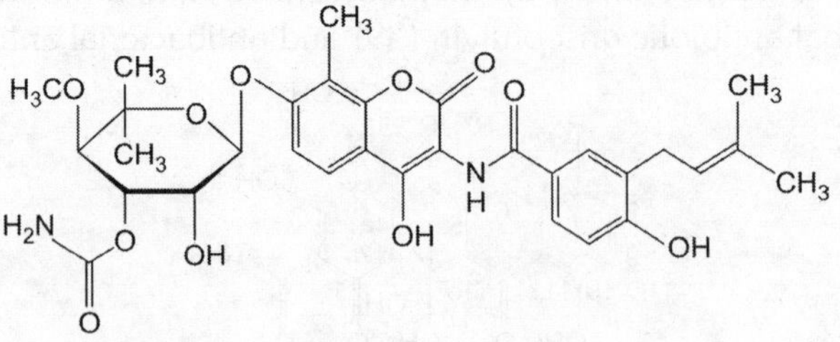

(41)

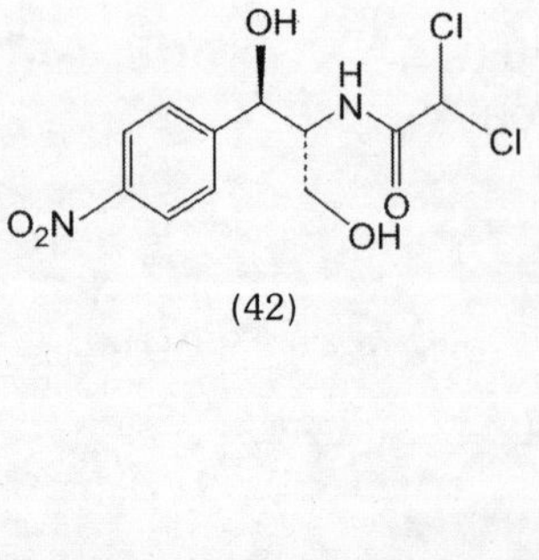

(42)

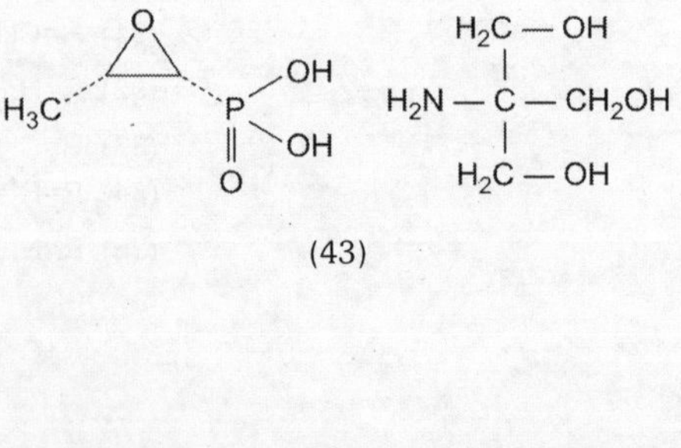

(43)

β-LACTAM ANTIBIOTICS

The β-lactam antibiotics include penicillins, carbapenems, cephalosporins, carbacephems, oxacephems, and monobactams.

PENICILLINS

Penicillins (1) constitute the most widely used antibiotics. They may be produced in whole or in part by fermentation process using various species of the mould *Penicillium*. Some of the penicillins obtained by fermentation process and commonly known as natural penicillin are given in Table 27.1.

Table 27.1: Some natural penicillins.

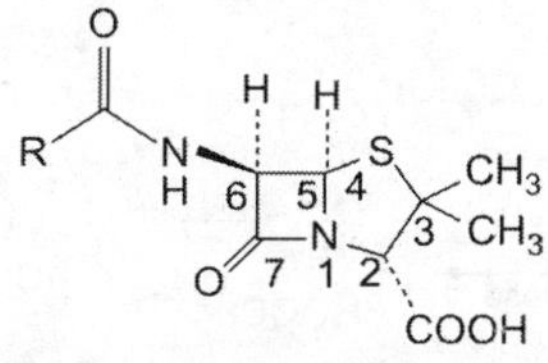

(1)

Name	R
Penicillin F or I or pent-2-enylpenicillin	$H_3CCH_2CH = CHCH_2$
Penicillin G or II or Benzylpenicillin	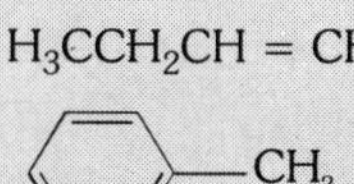 ⟨benzyl⟩—CH_2
Penicillin X or III or *p*-Hydroxybenzyl penicillin	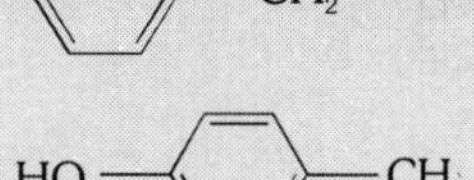 HO—⟨phenyl⟩—CH_2
Penicillin K or IV or *n*-Heptylpenicillin	$H_3C(CH_2)_5CH_2$
Dihydro F penicillin or *n*-Amylpenicillin	$H_3C(CH_2)_3CH_2$
Penicillin V or Phenoxymethylpenicillin	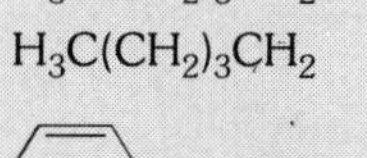 ⟨phenyl⟩—OCH_2

Before the structure of the natural penicillins was elucidated, the American and British workers used the designations such as "F", "G" and the Roman numerals such as "I" and "II", respectively.

As can be seen all the natural penicillins (1) are derivatives of 6-aminopenicillanic acid (2) and they are obtained by addition of side-chain precursors such as phenylacetic acid, phenylacetamide, etc. to the culture media to yield the corresponding penicillins. The commercial penicillins so obtained contain one or more penicillins in varying proportions.

(2)

The penicillin (1) molecule contains 3 chiral centres, namely C-2, C-5 and C-6. The absolute configuration at these centres are 2S, 5R, and 6R.

Penicillin (1) molecule undergoes degradation in both alkaline as well as in acid medium. In alkaline pH, the β-lactam ring is cleaved resulting in formation of penicilloic acid (3). Since β-lactam ring is essential for the antimicrobial activity, penicilloic acid (3) is inactive. Further, degradation of penicilloic acid (3) leads to penilloic acid (4). which further decomposes to penicillamine (6) and penilloaldehyde (8).

Under acidic conditions, penicillins (1) are degraded to penaldic acid (5), penicillamine (6), and penillic acid (7). Penaldic acid (5) further decomposes to penilloaldehyde (8). Thus, for the stability of aqueous solutions of penicillins (usually sodium or potassium salts) pH becomes an important factor. The aqueous solutions of soluble penicillins can be stored at a pH of 6 to 6.8 under refrigeration for several weeks.

In addition to sodium and potassium salts, salts with organic bases have also been used. These salts are usually water insoluble and they are used as depot preparations.

The naturally occurring penicillin G is active against Gram-positive microorganism. It has least toxicity and daily doses as high as 60 g of its sodium/potassium salts have been administered without any side effects. The only adverse effect observed has been allergic in nature and includes urticaria and anaphylactic shock. The other drawbacks of penicillin G include:

(a) Its poor absorption from gastrointestinal tract as a result it has to be administered by parenteral route.

(b) Its rapid excretion which necessitates its frequent administration.

(c) Its susceptibility to hydrolysis by β-lactamases.

SEMISYNTHETIC PENICILLINS

The resistance to penicillins had become a serious problem by late fifties. At the same time, the fermentation process, used for the manufacture of penicillins, allowed only limited introduction of side chain in the penicillin molecule. This coupled with sensitivity of β-lactam ring did not allow modifications in other parts of the penicillin molecule. A major breakthrough was achieved with the isolation of 6-aminopenicillanic acid (2) from the fermentation tanks when no side chain precursors were added. Although 6-aminopenicillanic acid (2) was biologically inactive but it could be converted to various amides by reacting it with various acylating agents. Further, the 6-amino group could also be converted to various other derivatives namely ureas, thioureas, carbamates, etc. thus providing an opportunity for preparing newer analogs which could have better antimicrobial activity.

Next, methods were developed to prepare 6-aminopenicillanic acid (2) in good yields. One of these methods involved deacylation of a natural penicillins by the enzyme penicillinacylases. Two types of penicillinacylases have been described. The penicillinacylase obtained from actinomycetes and fungi splits aliphatic side chain. On the other hand, the penicillinacylase of bacterial origin splits benzyl group of penicillin G but acted slowly on the penicillins with aliphatic side chain.

Another method involved splitting of the side chain by chemical method. The method involves conversion of natural penicillins to trimethylsilyl ester (9). The ester (9) on treatment with phosphorus pentachloride gave the intermediate (10) which on treatment with an alcohol yielded the iminoether (11). The iminoether (11) on hydrolysis yielded the desired 6-aminopenicillanic acid (2).

The isolation of 6-aminopenicillanic acid (2) provided means of preparing number of semisynthetic penicillins with:

(a) penicillinase resistant properties,
(b) broad-spectrum of activity, and
(c) increased acid resistant properties.

Semisynthetic Penicillins with Penicillinase Resistant Properties

Penicillinase resistant semisynthetic penicillins are effective against staphylococcal infections. The resistance to penicillinase can be achieved by multiple substitution on the carbon adjacent to amide carbonyl. This is achieved by incorporating the α-carbon atom of side chain into an aromatic/ heterocyclic ring and placing appropriate substituent at ortho-position. Some of the examples of the penicillinase resistant penicillins include methicillin (12), nafcillin (13), oxacillin (14 a), cloxacillin (14b), and dicloxacillin (14c).

(14)

The penicillinase resistant penicillins need not be resistant to acid hydrolysis. Thus, methicillin (12) is rapidly inactivated by acid and is poorly absorbed when given orally. It is also ineffective against Gram-negative microorganisms. Nafcillin (13) is about 2 to 4 times more effective than methicillin (12) and is well absorbed when given orally. The most promising of the penicillinase resistant penicillins are oxacillin (14a), cloxacillin (14b), and dicloxacillin (14c).

Semisynthetic Penicillins with Broad-spectrum of Activity

Broad-spectrum semisynthetic penicillins are those which possess activity against Gram-negative microorganisms and these include penicillin N (15), ampicillin (16), amoxicillin (17), carbenicillin (18), carindacillin (19), ticarcillin (20), mezlocillin (21), piperacillin (22), and hetacillin (23). Out of these, ampicillin (16) has proved to be one of the best semi-synthetic penicillins. Some of the advantages of ampicillin (16) include:

(a) Its Gram-negative activity is comparable to that of chloramphenicol and tetracyclines,
(b) It is more active than chloramphenicol and tetracycline against Gram-positive microorganisms,

(c) It is also stable towards acids and can be given orally, and

(d) It has low toxicity.

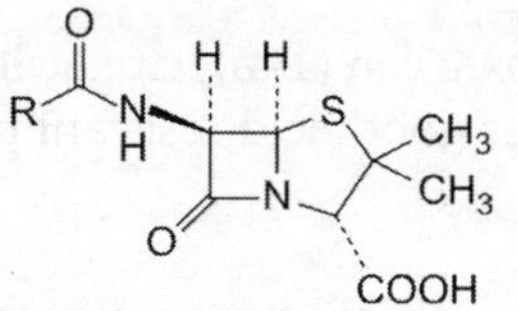

(15), R = D - HOOCCHCH$_2$CH$_2$CH$_2$

(16), R =

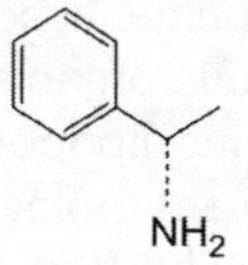

(17), R =

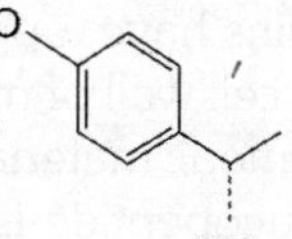

(18), R =

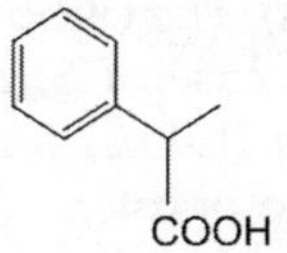

(19), R =

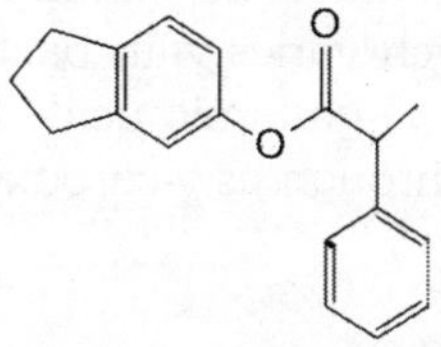

(20), R =

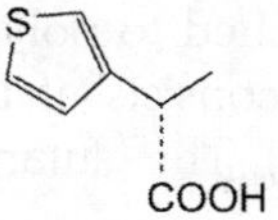

(21), R =

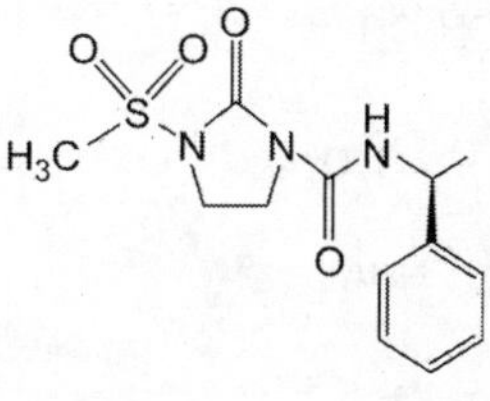

(22), R =

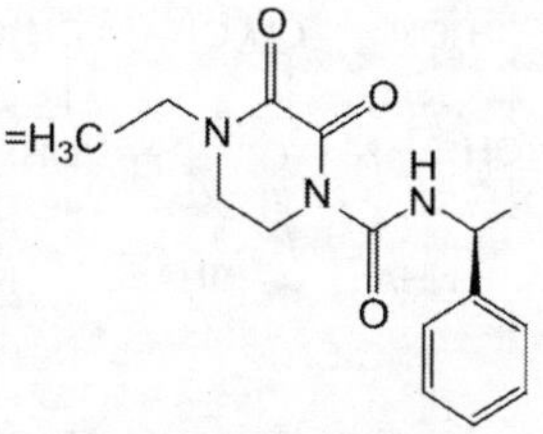

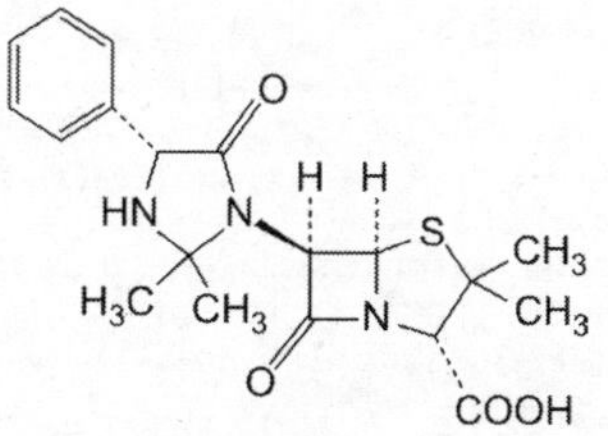

(23)

Some of the disadvantages of ampicillin (16) are that it produces allergic reactions and its susceptibility to penicillinase. As a result, it is not active against penicillinase producing microorganisms.

Semisynthetic Penicillins with Acid Resistant Properties

Incorporation of α-aryloxyalkyl moiety in the amide portion imparts acid-resistant property to the penicillin molecule. Infact they were the first semisynthetic penicillins to be prepared from 6-aminopenicillanic acid (2). Some of these include penicillin V [phenoxymethylpenicillin, (24)], phenethicillin [α-phenoxyethylpenicillin, (25)], propicillin [α-phenoxypropylpenicillin, (26)], and clometicillin [3, 4-dichloro-α-methoxybenzylpenicillin, (27)].

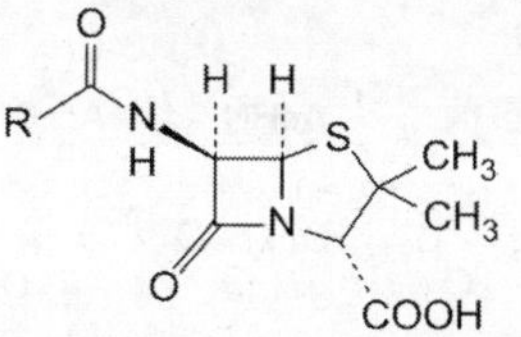

(24), R = 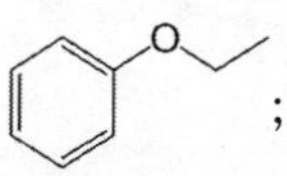 ; (25), R = 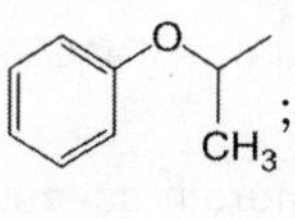 ; (26), R = 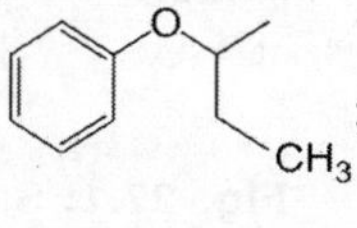 ; (27), R =

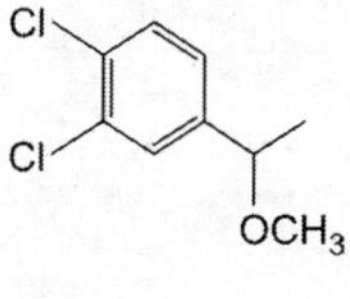

With the exception of penicillin V (24), all of these contain an asymmetric carbon atom in the side chain.The commercial preparations are usually racemic mixtures.

In addition to these, nafcillin (13) oxacillin (14a), cloxacillin (14b), dicloxacillin (14c), ampicillin (16), and amoxicillin (17) also possess good acid resistant properties.

MECHANISM OF ACTION

Penicillins have a potent and rapid bactericidal action against growing bacteria.

The cell wall of most of the Gram-positive organisms is a complex structure made-up of variety of polymeric materials including lipoproteins, lipopolysaccharides, teichoic acid and mucopeptide. The mucopeptide is highly cross-linked giant molecule that provides rigidity to the cell wall. This cross-linked structure is called murein saccullus (Fig. 27.1). The mucopeptide consists of alternating units of D-N-acetylglucosamine (NAG) and N-acetylmuramic acid (NAMA). The carboxyl of NAMA is attached to polypeptide chain which varies with bacterial species. In case of *S. aureous*, this chain consists of L-alanine (L-Ala), D-glutamic acid (D-Glu), L-lysine (L-Lys) and D-alanine (D-Ala). The glutamic acid is linked through its γ-carboxyl to the α-amino of L-Lys.

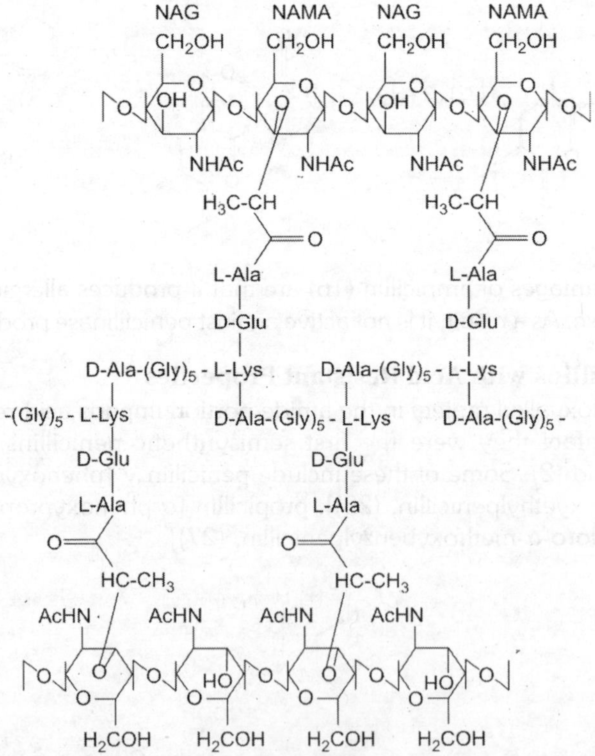

Fig. 27.1: Structure of murein sacculus

The murein strands are cross-linked by bridges of 5-glycine units to form murein sacculus (Fig. 27.1). These bridges link the ε-amnio of L-Lys with carboxyl terminal of D-Ala. This cross-linking is carried out by transpeptidase.

Before the cross-linking by pentaglycyl units takes place, the peptide strands from lactate carboxyl of muramic acid unit terminates in D-Ala-D-Ala. The terminal D-Ala unit of this strand is cleaved by transamidase-which is one of the penicillin-binding protein (PBP). The PBPs differ from bacterium to bacterium and several of them have been identified. In order to cleave the terminal D-Ala residue from the pentapeptide attached to muramic acid, the transamidase (PBP) uses its serine-OH group. After the terminal D-Ala unit is cleaved, it diffuses away. Next, the tetrapeptide is attached by the free amnio end of the pentaglycyl unit in presence of transpeptidase to crosslink the different strands (Fig. 27.2A).

The penicillins and other β-lactam antibiotics act by acylating the serine-OH of the transamidases. This acylation is irreversible as a result the terminal D-Ala unit of the pentapeptide strand is not cleaved and consequently the cross-linking does not take place. This results in the lysis (Fig. 27.2B).

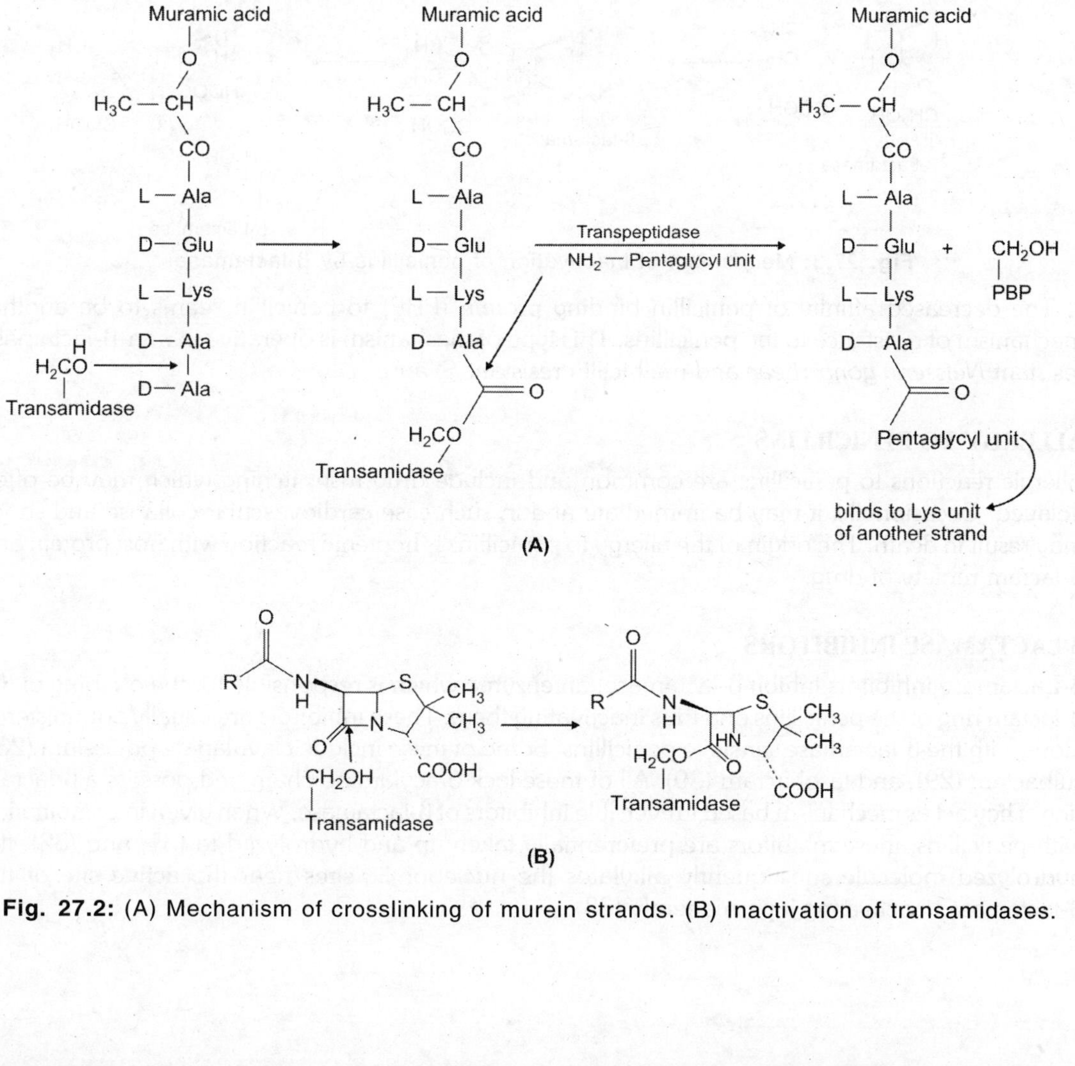

Fig. 27.2: (A) Mechanism of crosslinking of murein strands. (B) Inactivation of transamidases.

RESISTANCE TO PENICILLINS

Number of mechanisms have been proposed for resistance to the penicillins. One of the mechanisms of resistance is through inactivation of penicillin. This inactivation is by the enzyme penicillinase, which is non-specific. Penicillinases are of two types, β-lactamases and acylases. β-Lactamases catalyze the inactivation of penicillin through opening of the β-lactam ring. This hydrolysis takes place through nucleophilic attack by the hydroxyl of serine residue of the β-lactamase, converting penicillin into penicilloic acid [(3), Fig. 27.3)]. The β-lactamase is regenerated and this can thus inactivate large amount of drug. The acylases hydrolyze the acylamino side chain. Specific acylases have been obtained from many Gram-negative bacteria. Their specific role in bacterial resistance is not known.

Another mechanism of bacterial resistance is decreased permeability to penicillin. The decreased permeability to penicillins is particularly found in Gram-negative bacteria. These microorganisms contain an outer membrane which acts as a barrier to penetration of the antibiotic.

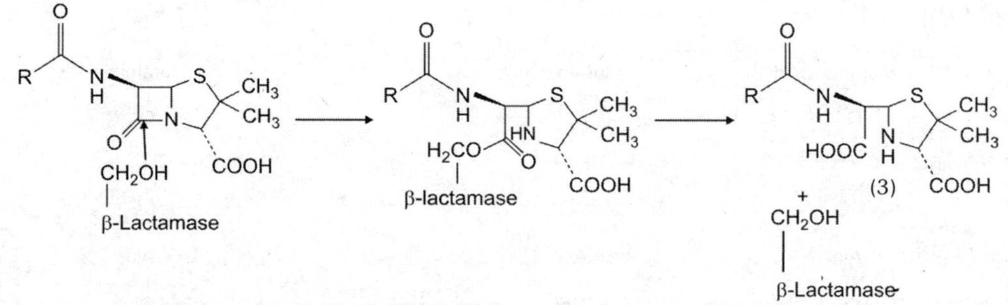

Fig. 27.3: Mechanism of inactivation of penicillins by β-lactamases.

The decreased affinity of penicillin binding protein (PBP) to penicillin seems to be another mechanism of resistance to the penicillins. This type of mechanism is operative in non-β-lactamase resistant *Neisseria gonorrheae* and methicillin resistant *S. aureus*.

ALLERGY TO PENICILLINS

Allergic reactions to penicillins are common and include drug rash, itching which may be often delayed. Occasionally, it may be immediate and in such case cardiovascular collapse and shock may result in death. The origin of the allergy to penicillins is heptenic reaction with host protein and β-lactam moiety of drug.

β-LACTAMASE INHIBITORS

β-Lactamase inhibitors inhibit β-lactamase, an enzyme which is responsible for the opening of the β-lactam ring of the penicillins and thus inactivating them. These inhibitors are usually administered along with the β-lactamase sensitive penicillins. Some of these include clavulanate potassium (28), sulbactam (29), and tazobactam (30). All of these lack 6-acylamino chain and possess a β-lactam ring. They act as mechanism based irreversible inhibitors of β-lactamase. When given in combination with penicillins, these inhibitors are preferentially taken up and hydrolyzed to (31) and (32). the hydrolyzed molecule subsequently alkylates the nucleophilic sites near the active site of the β-lactamase, inactivating it permanently (33).

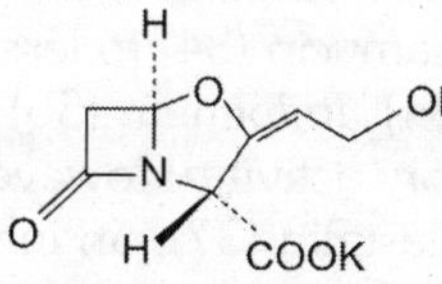

(28) 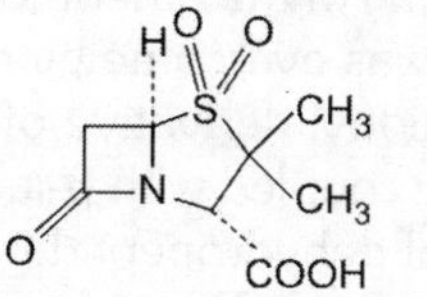 (29) 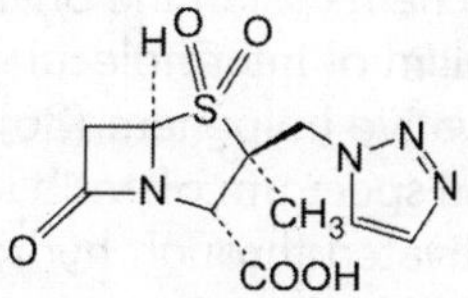 (30)

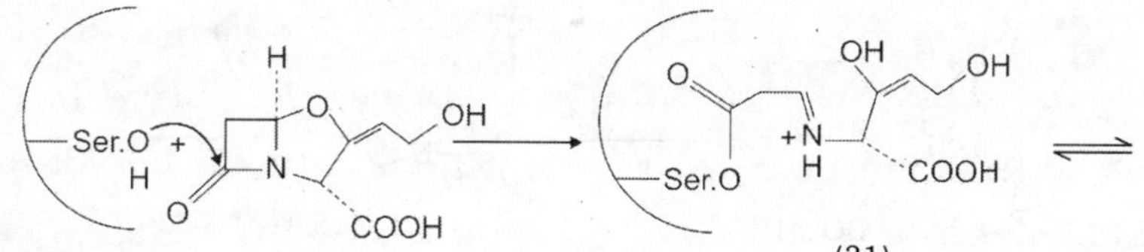

(β-Lactamarse active site) (31)

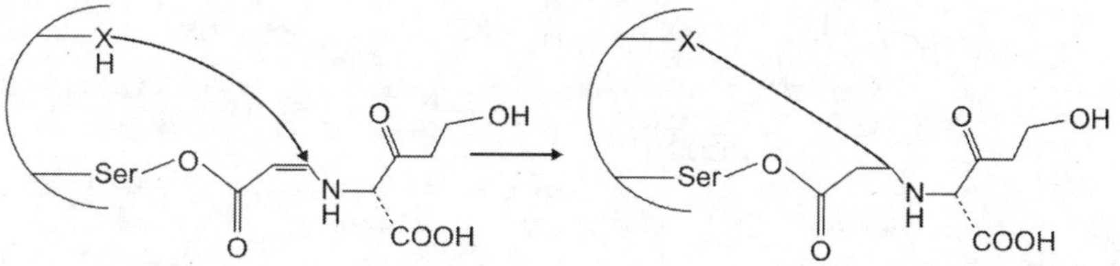

(32) (33)

CARBAPENEMS

Thienamycin (34), a carbapenem, was isolated from the *Streptomyces cattleya*. It has a broad spectrum of activity against most of aerobic, anaerobic, Gram-postive, and Gram-negative bacteria. It also possesses inhibitory activity against β-lactamases of Gram-negative and Gram-positive bacteria.

Thienamycin (34) differs from penicillins (1) in having a methylene carbon instead of sulphur atom. It also has a double bond in five membered ring. Further, there is no acylamino-side chain at position 6.

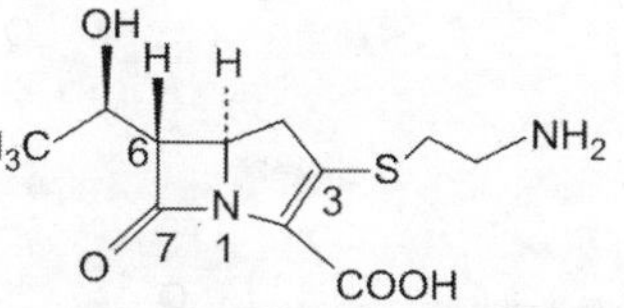

(34)

Although thienamycin (34) possesses a broad spectrum of activity coupled with β-lactamase inhibitory activity, it is highly ustable and is more susceptible to hydrolysis in both acidic and basic solutions which is because of highly strained fused ring system. Further, it undergoes inactivation at pH 6-7 through intermolecular reaction involving a nucleophilic attack by the amino group of the side chain cystamine on the β-lactam ring of the other molecule resulting in formation of (35). This problem of intermolecular interaction was overcome by converting thienamycin (34) to less basic derivative imipenem (36), a *N*-formimidoyl derivative of thienamycin (34). Imipenem (36) has a broad spectrum of antibacterial activity coupled with β-lactamase inhibitory activity. However, it is inactivated through hydrolysis by renal dehydropeptidase-1 (DHP-I). Cilastatin (37), an inhibitor of DHP-I, administered along with imipenem (36), is a potent combination for treatment of urinary tract infections caused by Gram-negative bacilli, anaerobes, and *Staphylococcus aureus*. Imipenem (36) is also used in bacterial infections of skin, tissues, respiratory tract, bones, and joints.

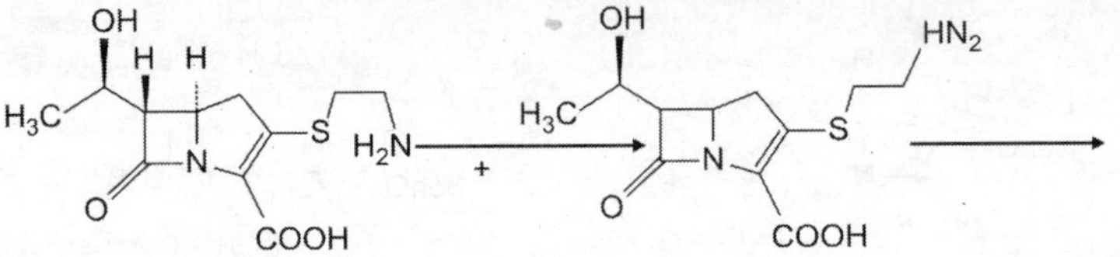

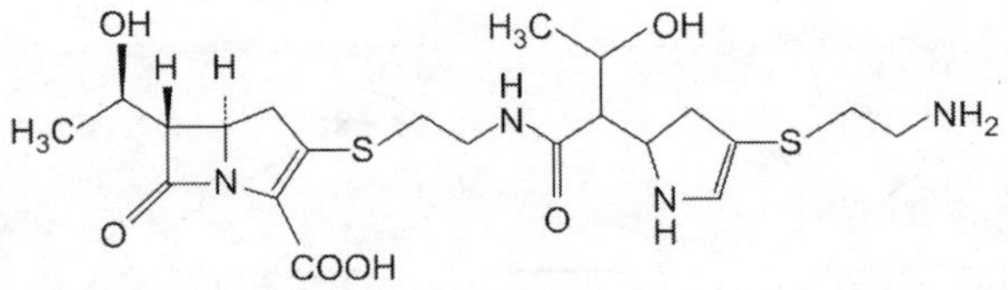

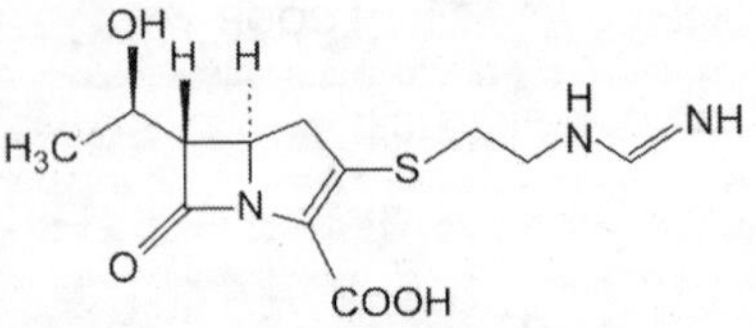

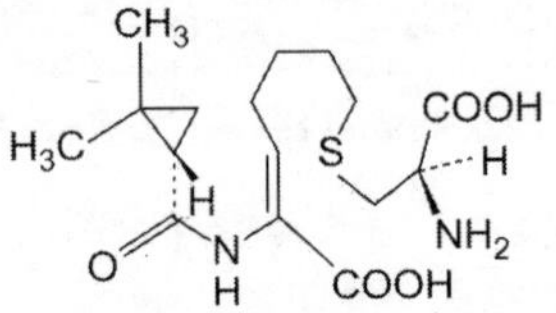

Some of the totally synthetic second generation carbapenem include biapenem (38), meropenem (39), and ertapenem (40). The β-methyl group at position 4 confers stability towards DHP-1.

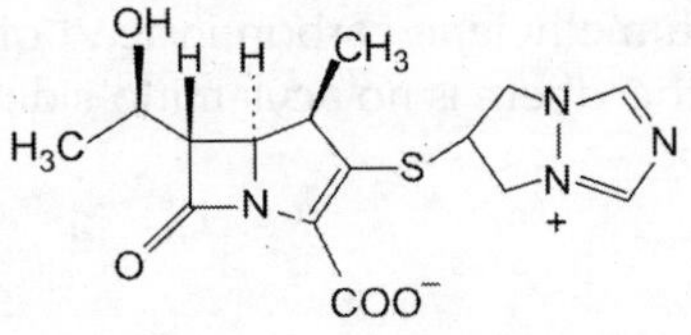

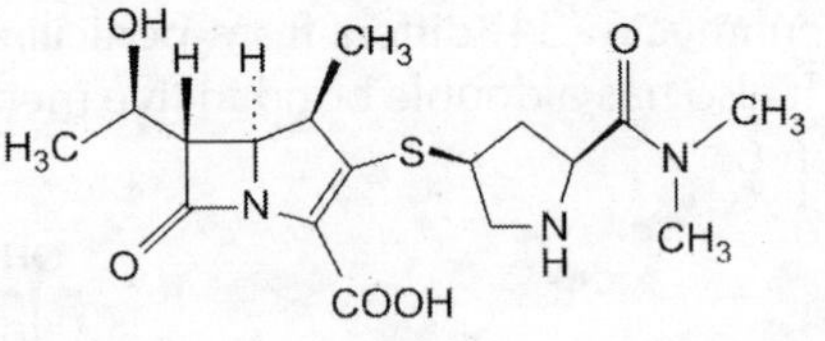

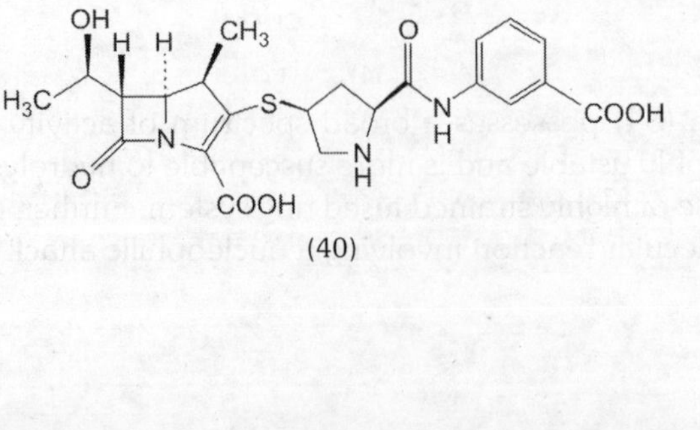

CEPHALOSPORINS

The fungus *Cephalosporium acremonium* was isolated from sewage fall in Sardinia by Brotzu in 1945. The cultures of this fungus inhibited the growth of a wide variety of Gram-positive and Gram-negative bacteria. Abraham and Newton in 1961 reported the isolation of three substances from the cultures of *C. acremonium* and these included a steroid which was devoid of any antibacterial activity and other substances namely penicillin N (15) and cephalosporin C (41). Penicillin N (15), which is not an approved drug, is more active against Gram-negative bacteria but less active against Gram-positive microorganisms than penicillin G. Cephalosporin C (41) which has similar side chain as penicillin N (15), however, differs from it in that the β-lactam ring in cephalosporin C (41) is fused to a dihydrothiazine ring instead of thiazolidine ring in penicillins. This confers some stability to the β-lactam ring because of less strain. Cephalosporin C (41) is resistant to β-lactamases but has less activity than penicillin N (15). Like 6-aminopenicillanic acid, 7-aminocephalosporanic acid (42) has been obtained by degradation of cephalosporin C (41) with NOCl. This coupled with modification of substituents at position 3 and introduction of substituents at position 7 has led to synthesis of newer analogs.

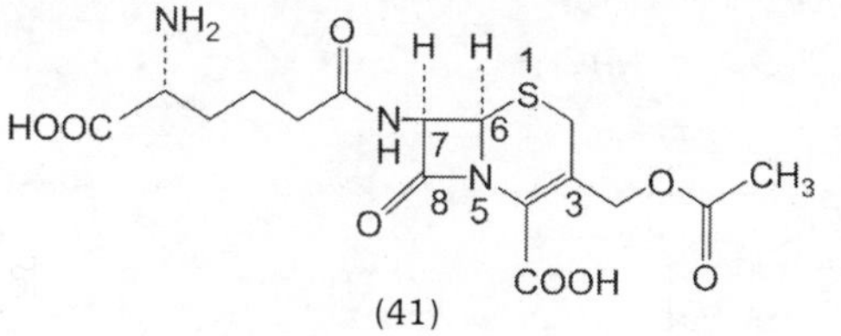

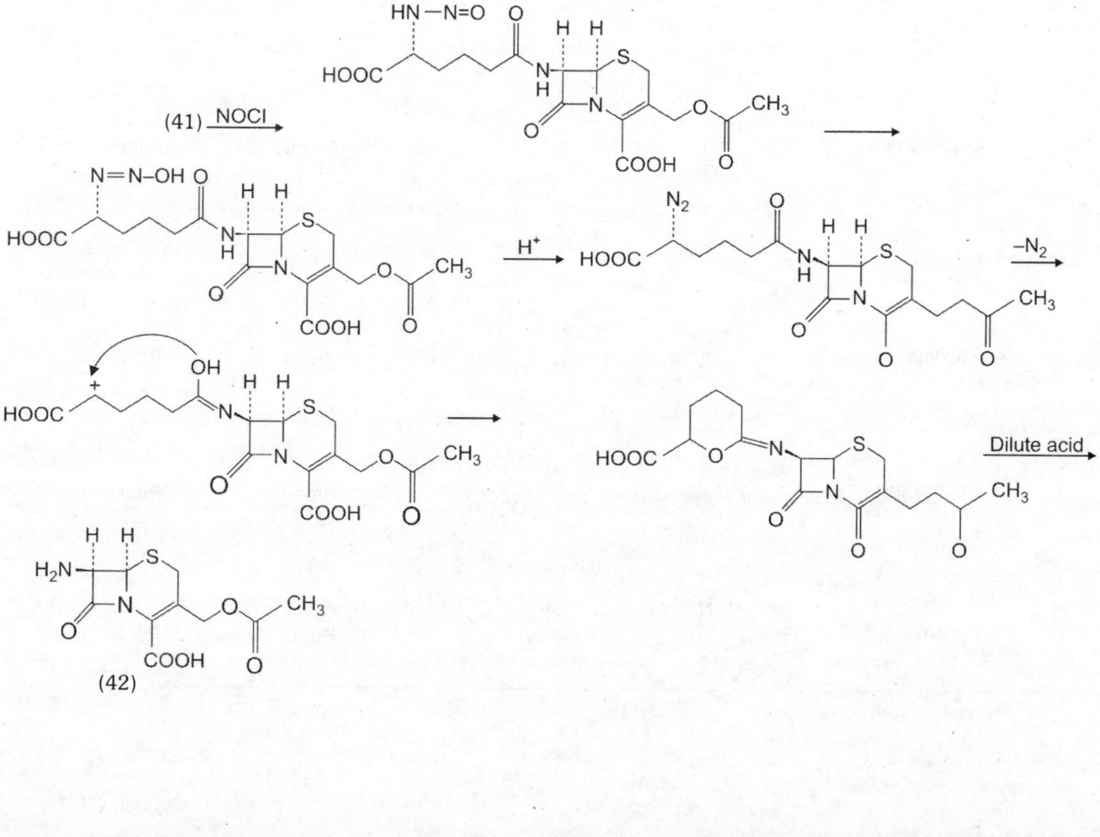

Cepalosporins have been classified into first-, second-, third-, and fourth-generation. Such a classification not only reflects the time of their descovery but also an increase in Gram-negative activity as well as resistance to β-lactamase. Some of these are listed in Table 27.2 to Table 27.5.

Table 27.2: First generation cephalosporins

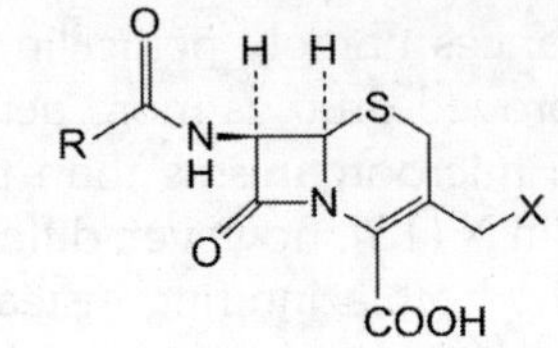

Name	R	X	Spectrum of activity	β-Lactamase resistance
1. Cephalexin	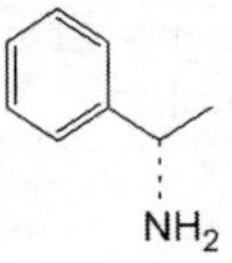	H	Broad	Poor
2. Cefadroxil	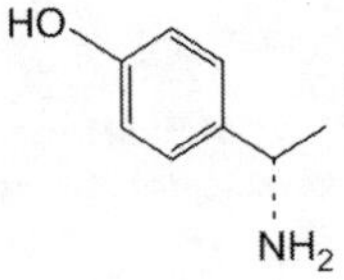	H	Broad	Poor
3. Cephradine	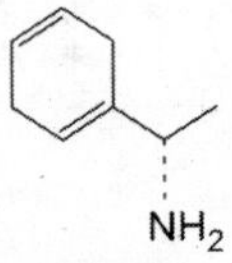	H	Broad	Poor
4. Cephapirin	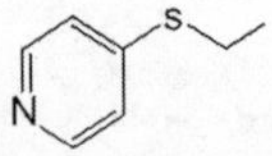	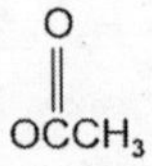 OCCH₃	Broad	Poor
5. Cephalothin	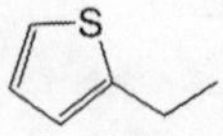	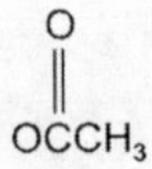 OCCH₃	Broad	Poor
6. Cefazolin	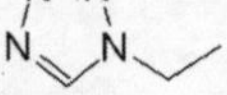	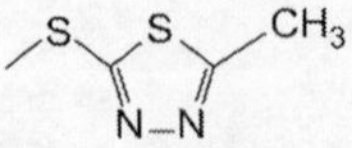	Broad	Poor

Table 27.3: Second generation cephalosporins.

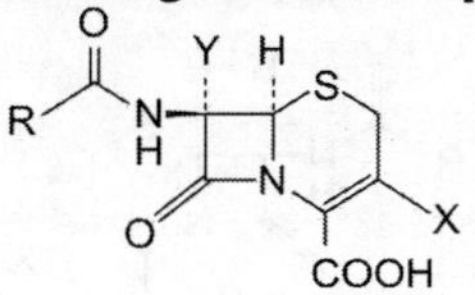

Name	R	X	Y	Spectrum of activity	β-Lactamase resistance
1. Cefaclor	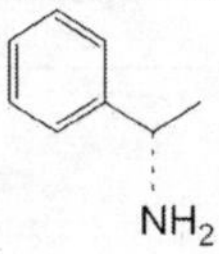	Cl	H	Broad	Poor
2. Cefprozil	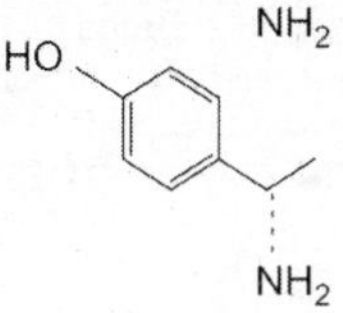	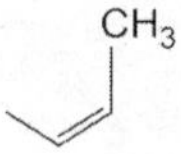 CH_3	H	Broad	Poor
3. Cefamandole	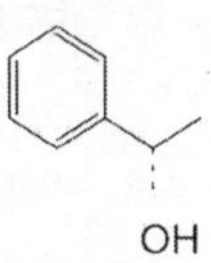	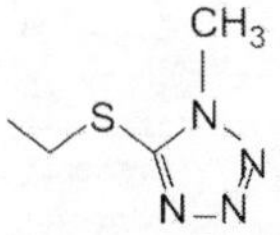	H	Broad	Poor
4. Cefonicid	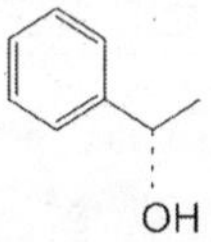	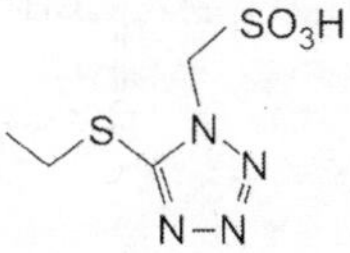	H	Broad	Good
5. Cefpodoxime	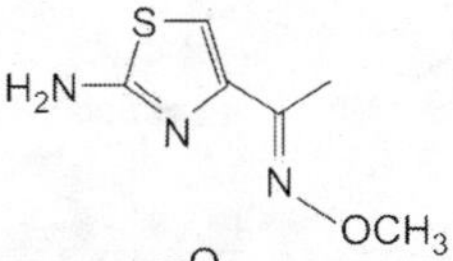	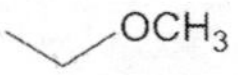 OCH_3	H	Broad	Good
6. Cefuroxime	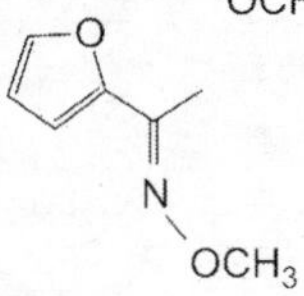	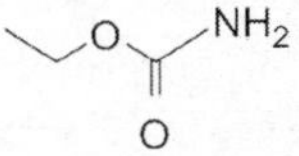 NH_2	H	Broad	Good
7. Cefoxitin	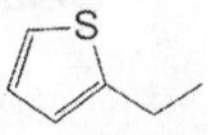	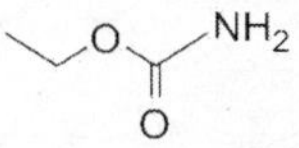 NH_2	OCH_3	Broad	Good
8. Cefmetazole	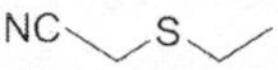	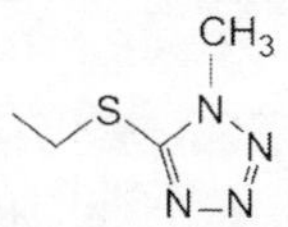	OCH_3	Broad	Good
9. Cefotetan	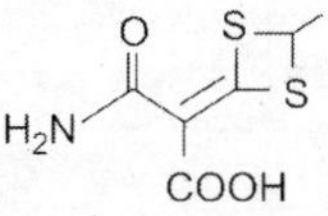	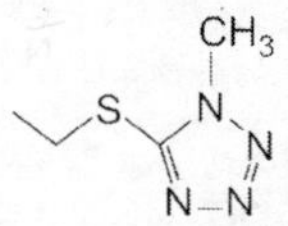	OCH_3	Broad	Good

Table 27.4: Third generation cephalosporins.

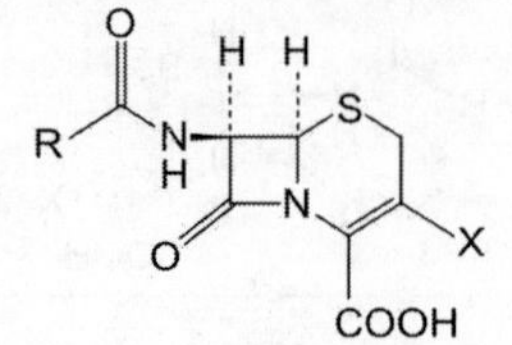

Name	R	X	Spectrum of activity	β-Lactamase resistance
1. Ceftibuten	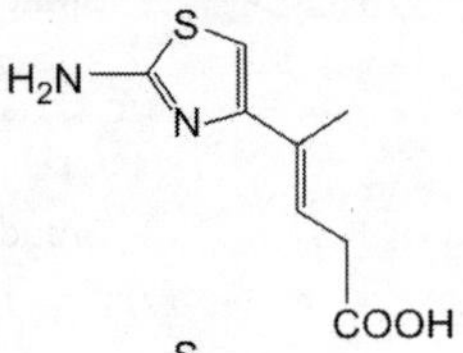	H	Broad	Good
2. Ceftizoxime	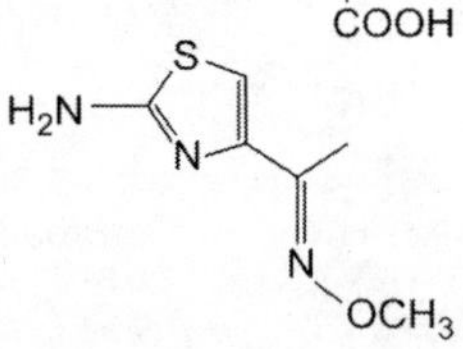	H	Broad	Good
3. Cefotaxime	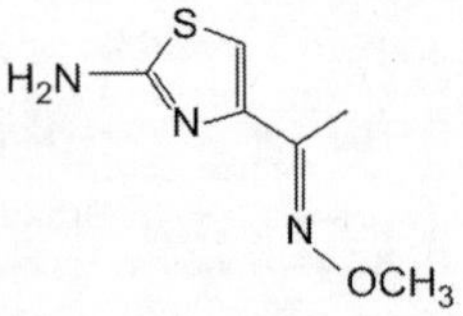	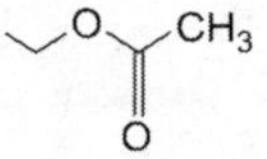	Broad	Good
4. Cefixime	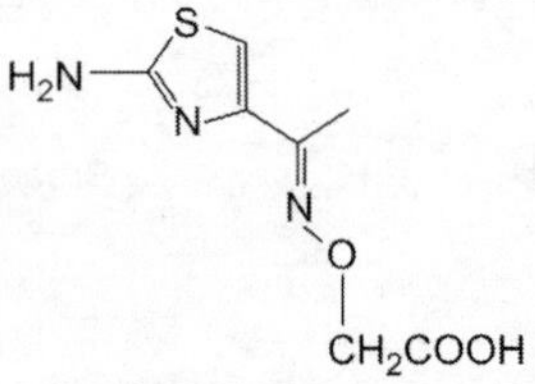	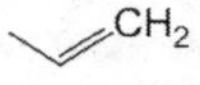	Broad	Good
5. Ceftazidime	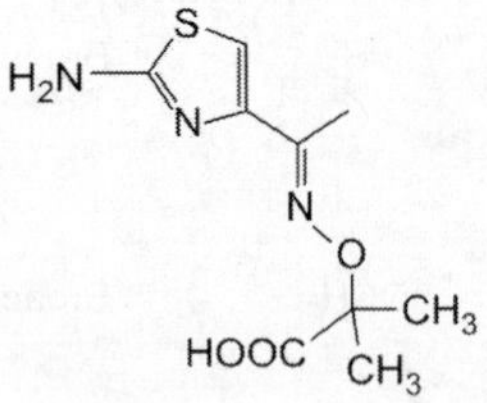	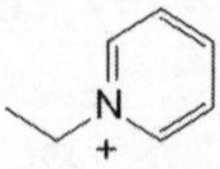	Broad	Good
6. Cefoperazone	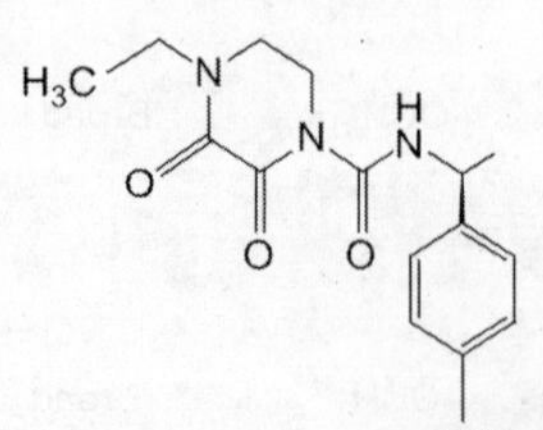	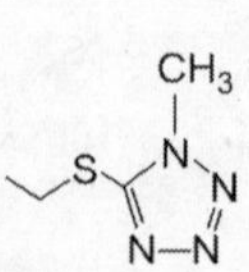	Broad	Good

Table 27.5: Fourth generation cephalosporins.

Name	R	X	Spectrum of cavity	β-Lactamase resistance
1. Cefepime			Broad	Good
2. Cefpirome			Broad	Good

DEGRADATION

Cephalosporins undergo a variety of hydrolytic degradations and these are given in Fig. 27.4.

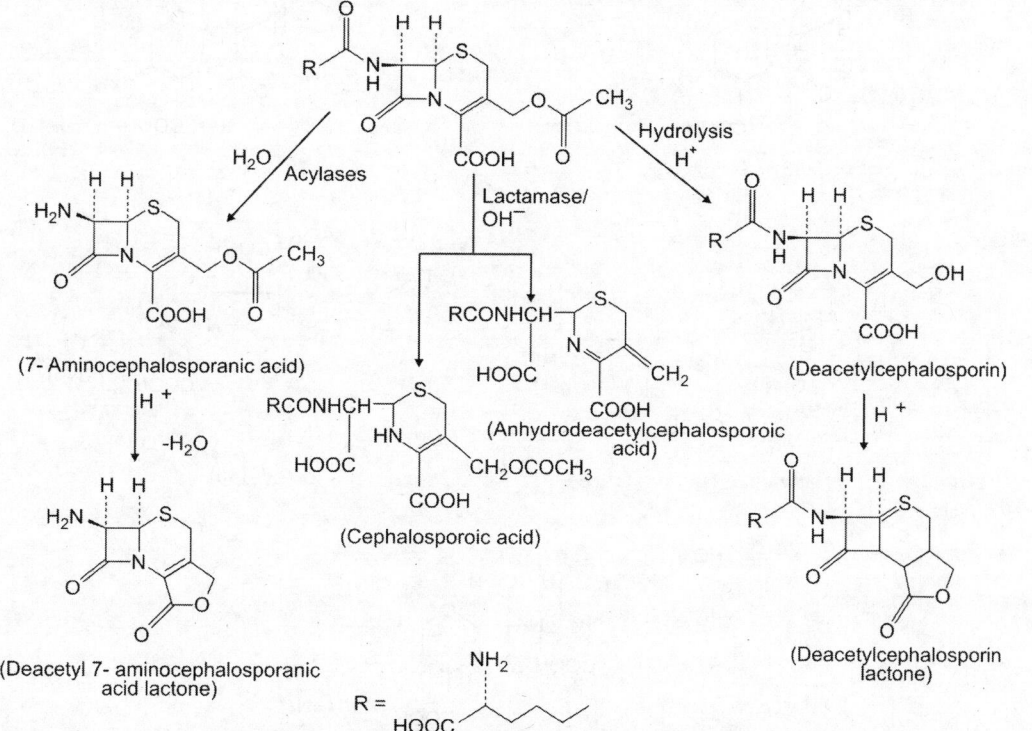

Fig. 27.4: Degradation products of cephalosporin C.

SPECTRUM OF ACTIVITY

Cephalosporins are broad-spectrum antibiotics. Their activity is comparable to that of ampicillin (16). However, as compared to ampicillin (16), they are much more resistant to β-lactamases particularly that produced by Gram-positive bacteria. The better activity of cephalosporins as compared to penicillins has been attributed to:

(a) Resistance to inactivation by β-lactamases and
(b) better permeability of cell wall.

MECHANISM OF ACTION

Cephalosporins are believed to act in a manner similar to that of penicillins by binding to penicillin binding protein (PBP) followed by cell lysis. In clinical terms, cephalosporins are bactericidal.

CARBACEPHEMS AND OXACEPHEMS

Analogs of cephalosporins in which the sulphur of six-membered ring has been substituted by carbon and oxygen, commonly known as carbacephem (43) and oxacephem (44), respectively, have been reported. Some of these include loracarbef (45) flomoxef (46), and moxalactam (47). All of them have shown good antibacterial activity as well as good resistance to β-lactamase.

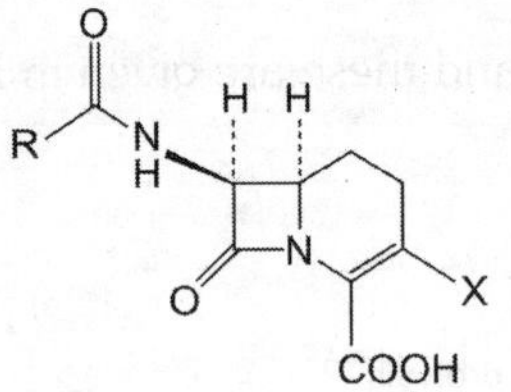

(43)

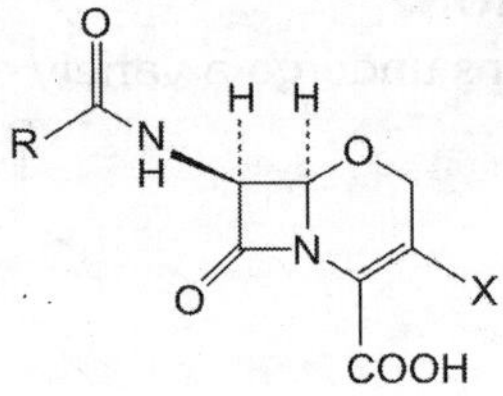

(44)

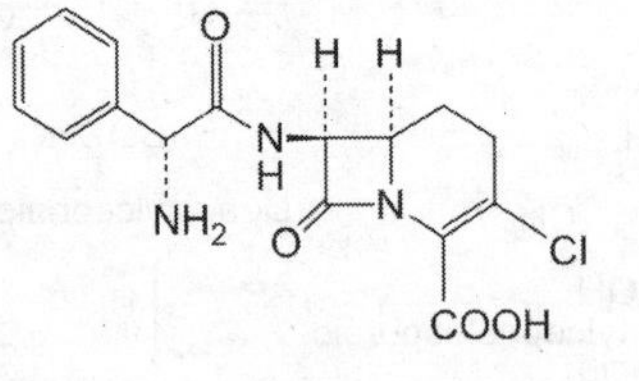

(45)

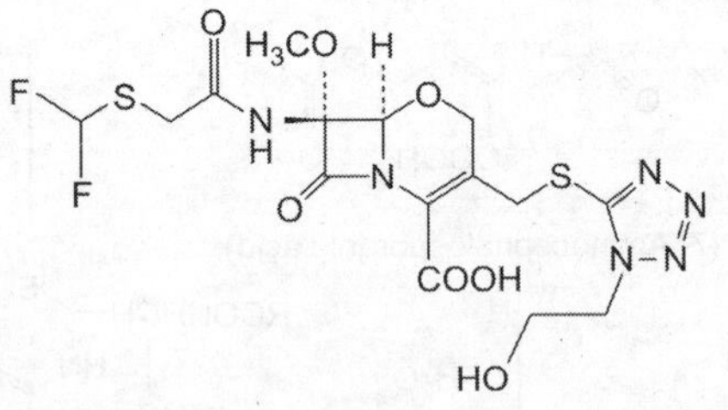

(46)

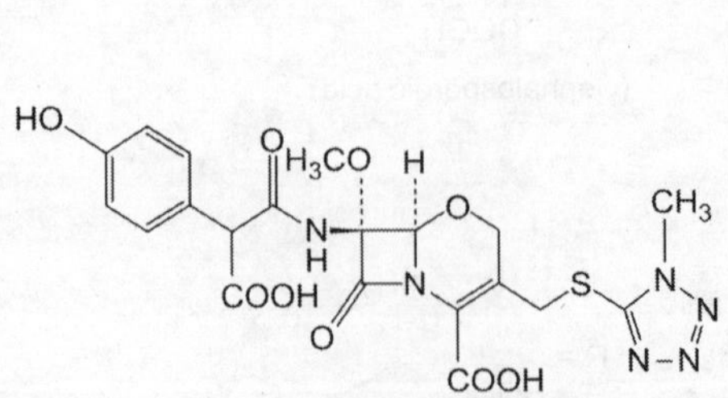

(47)

MONOBACTAMS

The monocyclic β-lactam antibiotic sulfazecin (48) was isolated from cultures of *Pseudomonas acidophila* and *P. mesoacidophila*. It had, however very weak antibacterial activity. Structure-activity relationship studies led to a totally synthetic antibiotic, aztreonam (49). Aztreonam (49) was found to be active against Gram-negative microorganisms as well as had high stability towards β-lactamases. It is used as disodium salt parenterally. The other monobactams include tigemonam (50) and carumonam (51). Both of them have similar antibacterial spectrum as aztreonam (49) and are also stable towards β-lactamases.

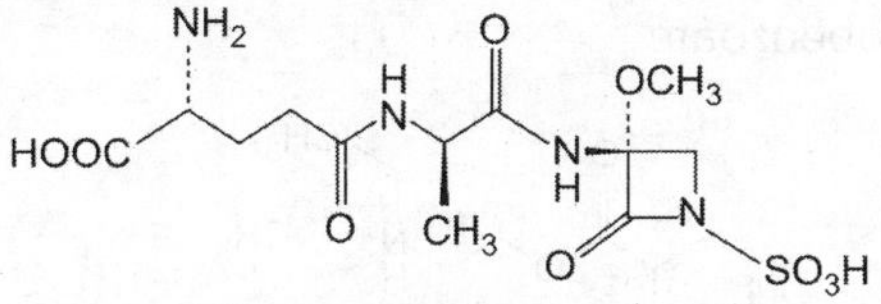

(48)

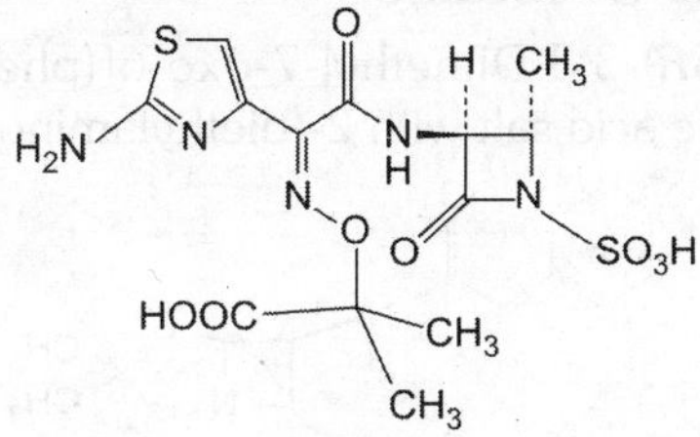

(49)

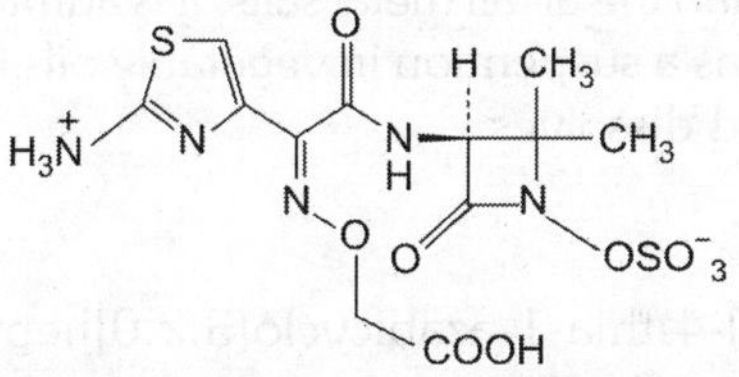

(50)

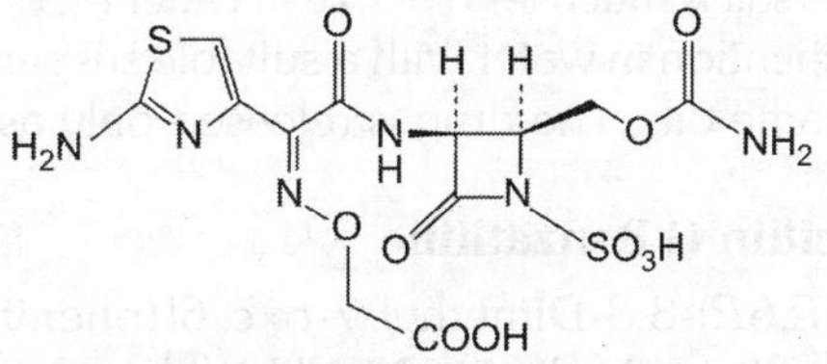

(51)

The finding of antibacterial activity in monobactams shows that fused bicyclic ring system is not necessary for antibiotic activity. Monobactams act by the same mechanism as penicillins and cephalosporins.

INDIVDIUAL COMPOUNDS

PENICILLINS

Penicillin G Sodium

(2S,5R,6R)-3,3-Dimethyl-7-oxo-6-[(phenylacetyl)amino]-4-thia-1-azabicyclo[3.2.0]heptane-2-carboxylic acid monosodium salt

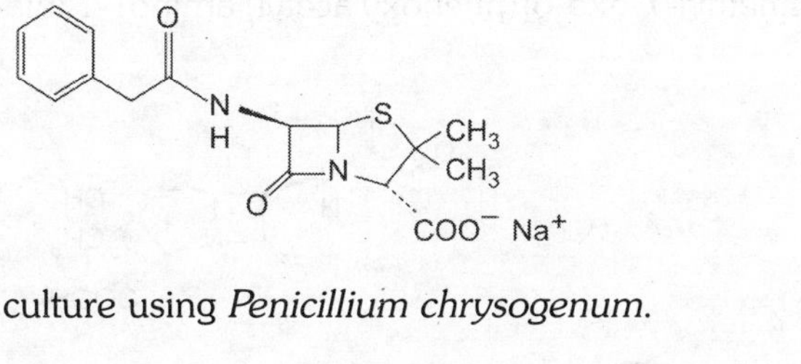

It is obtained by submerged culture using *Penicillium chrysogenum*.

Pencillin G is used as water soluble sodium, potassium, or calcium salt. It cannot be given orally because it is inactivated by acidic pH of the stomach and also its oral absorption is poor. It is administered parenterally. Penicillin G is eliminated rapidly through kidney. So in order to maintain the blood levels, frequent administration of the drug is necessary. Many 'repository' formulations of the drug have been developed to overcome this problem. Suspension of penicillin in peanut oil with white beeswax was used earlier to prolong the duration of injected forms of penicillin. Another formulation consisted of suspension of penicillin in vegetable oil with aluminium monostearate. Salts of penicillin with high molecular weight amines are also used to overcome this problem.

Penicillin G Procaine

(2S,5R,6R)-3,3-Dimethyl-7-oxo-6[(phenylacetyl)amino]-4-thia-1-azabicyclo[3.2.0]heptane-2-carboxylic acid salt with 2-(diethylamino)ethyl 4-aminobenzoate

This salt is much less soluble in water (about 1g/250 ml) than the alkali metal salts. It is administered as suspention in water with a suitable suspending agent or as a suspension in vegetable oils (peanut or sesame oil). The drug is released only as the compound dissolves.

Penicillin G Benzathine

(2S,5R,6R)-3,3-Dimethyl-7-oxo-6[(phenylacetyl)amino]-4-thia-1-azabicyclo[3.2.0]heptane-2-carboxylic acid salt with N, N'-bis(phenylmethyl)-1,2-ethanediamine

It is highly insoluble, more stable, and has prolonged duration of action. It is also stable at gastric pH.

Penicillin V

(2S,5R,6R)-3, 3-Dimethyl-7-oxo-6[(phenoxy acetyl) amino]-4-thia-1-azabicyclo[3.2.0]heptane-2-carboxylic acid

It is obtained by fermentation process using the fungus *Penicillium chrysogenum* as the organism and phenoxyacetic acid as the precursor. It was the first acid resistant penicillin to be used in clinical practice. The free acid and its salt are highly insoluble. The salt with ethylenediamine is a very long acting penicillin.

SEMISYTHETIC PENICILLINS : PENICILLINASE RESISTANT

Methicillin Sodium

(2S,5R,6R)-6-[(2,6-Dimethoxybenzoyl)amino]-3, 3-dimethyl-7-oxo-4-thia-1-azabicyclo[3.2.0]-heptane-2-carboxylic acid monosodium salt

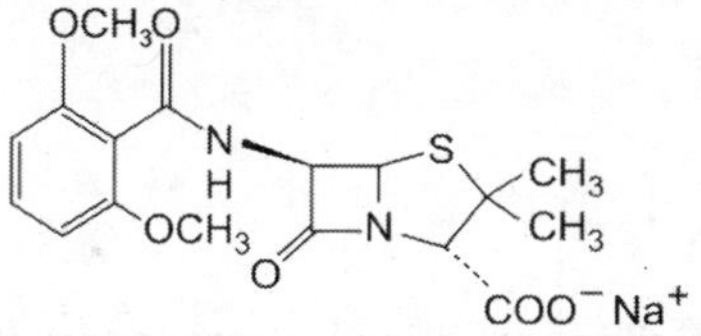

Synthesis

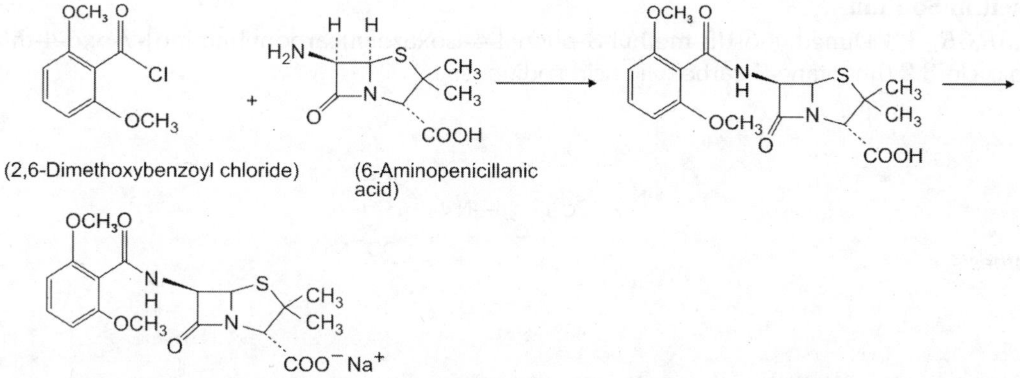

(2,6-Dimethoxybenzoyl chloride)   (6-Aminopenicillanic acid)

It is a penicillinase resistant penicillin. Penicillinase resistant penicillins are used in clinical practice to avoid the development of resistant strains.

Nafcillin Sodium

(2S,5R,6R)-6-[[(2-Ethoxy-1-naphthalenyl)carbonyl]amino]-3,3-dimethyl-7-oxo-4-thia-1-azabicyclo[3. 2. 0]heptane-2-carboxylic acid sodium salt

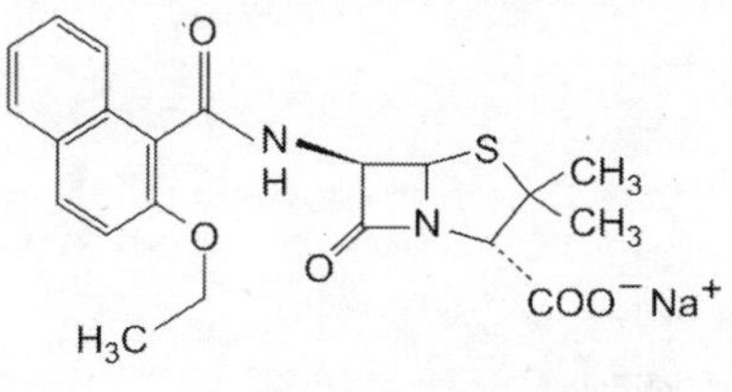

Synthesis

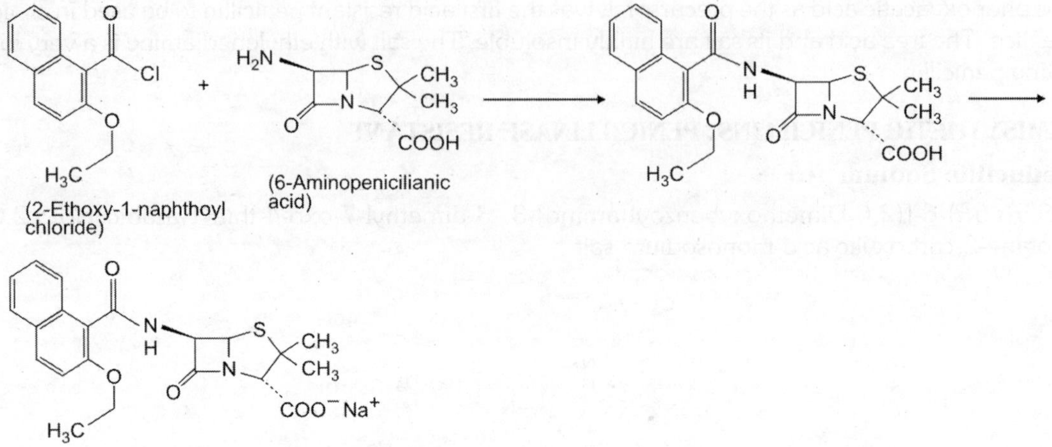

In addition to resistance to penicillinase, it is also stable towards acid. Because of this it can be given orally. Its absorption is slow and satisfactory plasma levels are obtained within 1 hr.

Oxacillin Sodium

(2S,5R,6R)-3,3 Dimethyl-6[[(5-methyl-3-phenyl-4-isoxazolyl)carbonyl]amino]-7-oxo-4-thia-1-azabicyclo[3.2.0]heptane-2-carboxylic acid sodium salt

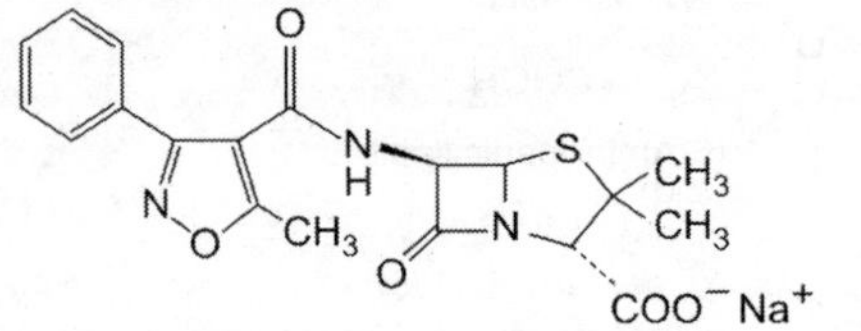

Synthesis

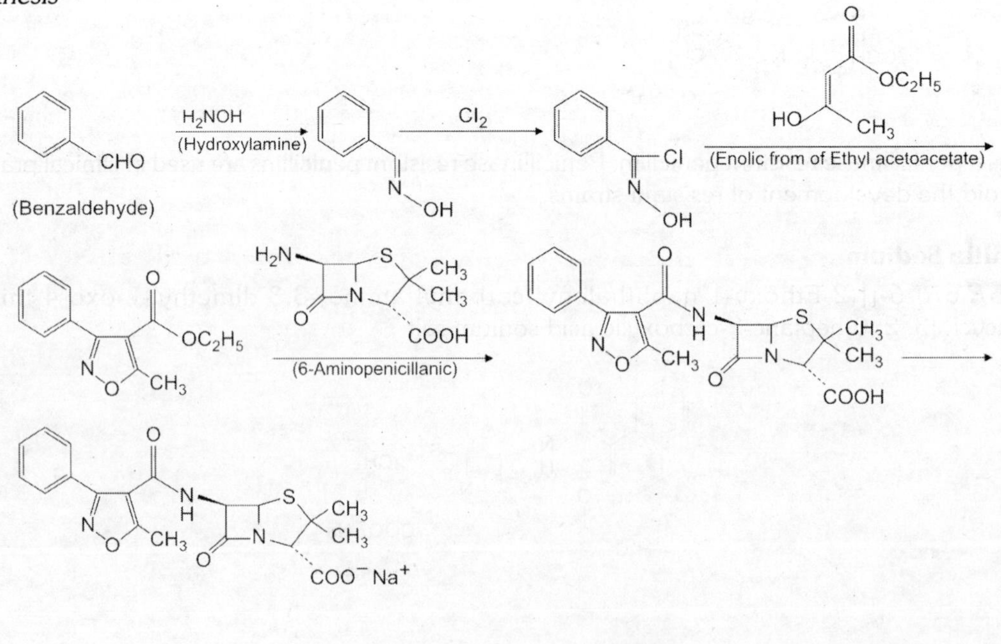

It is highly resistant to hydrolysis by penicillinase because of steric effects of 3-phenyl and 5-methyl group of isoxazolyl ring which prevent its binding to β-lactamase active site. It undergoes first-pass metabolism to 5-hydroxymethyl derivative (52). This metabolite has activity comparable to oxacillin.

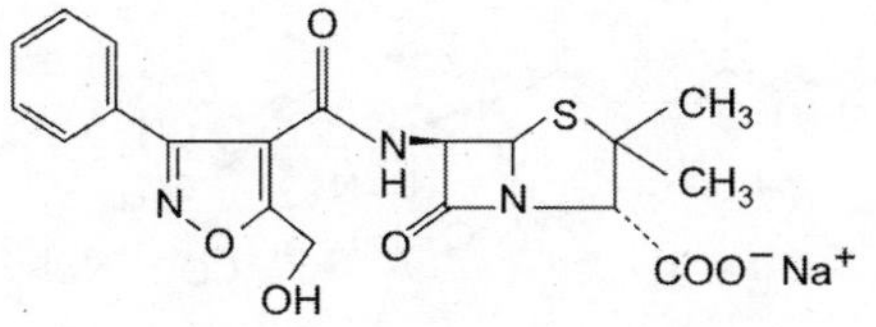

(52)

Cloxacillin Sodium

(2S,5R,6R)-6-[[[3-(2-Chlorophenyl)-5-methyl-4-isoxazolyl]carbonyl]amino]-3, 3-dimethyl-7-oxo-4-thia-1-azabicyclo[3. 2. 0]heptane-2-carboxylic acid sodium salt

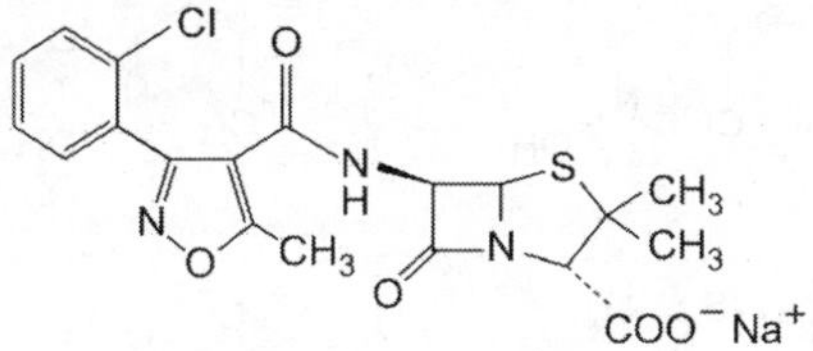

Synthesis

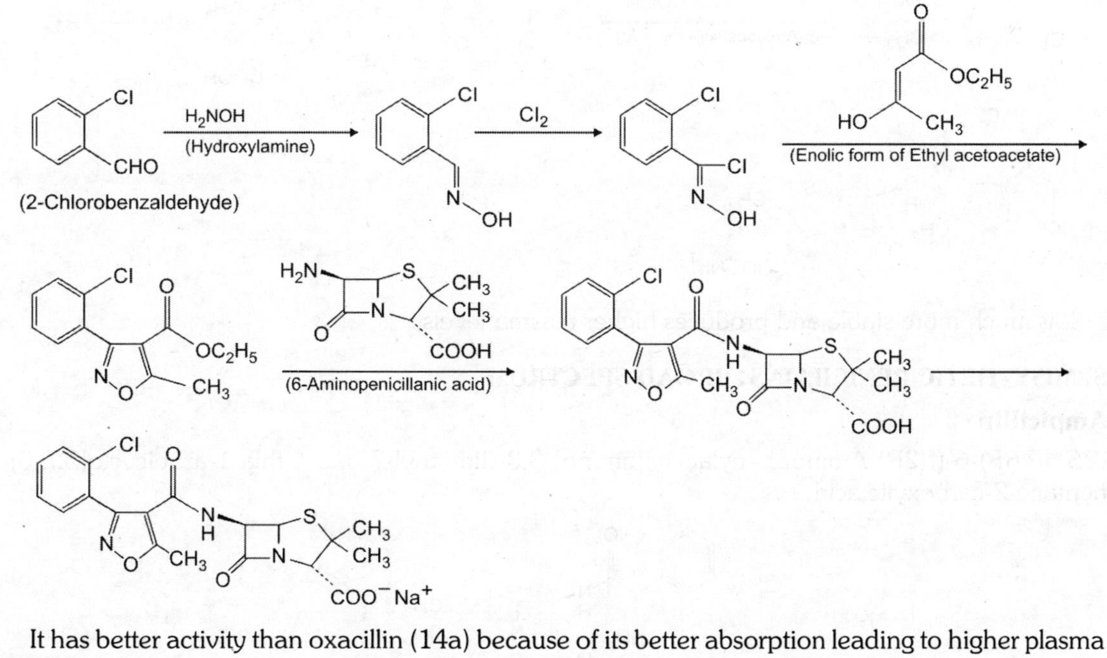

It has better activity than oxacillin (14a) because of its better absorption leading to higher plasma levels.

Dicloxacillin Sodium

(2S,5R,6R)-6-[[[3-(2, 6-Dichlorophenyl)-5-methyl-4-isoxazolyl]carbonyl]amino]-3,3-dimethyl-7-oxo-4-thia-1-azabicyclo[3. 2. 0]heptane-2-carboxylic acid sodium salt

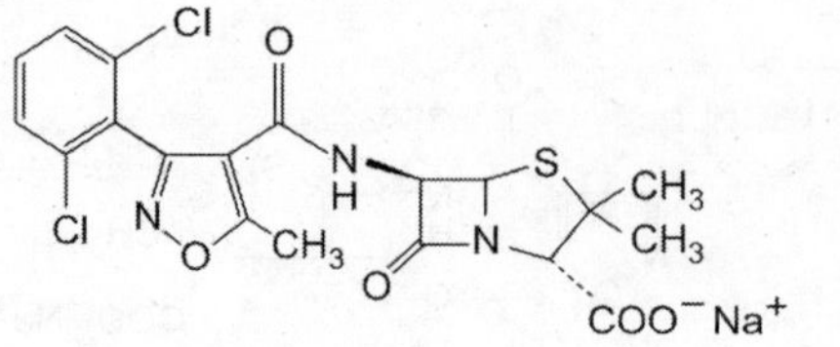

Synthesis

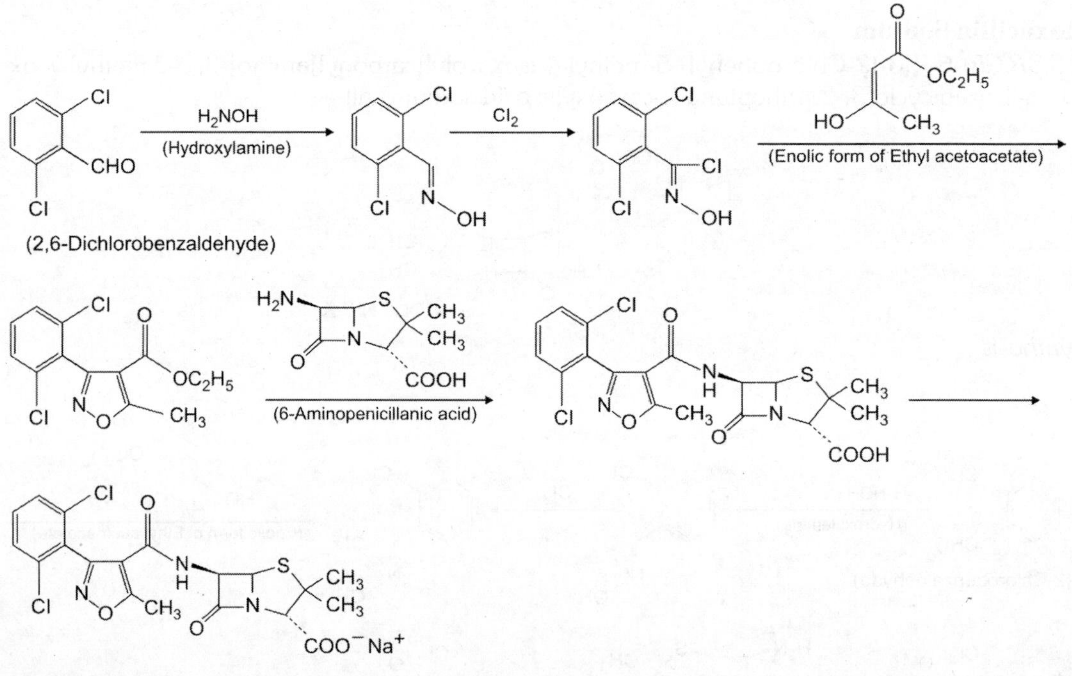

It is much more stable and produces higher plasma levels.

SEMISYTHETIC PENICILLINS : BROAD SPECTRUM

Ampicillin

(2S,5R,6R)-6-[[[(2R)-Aminophenylacetyl]amino]-3,3-dimethyl-7-oxo-4-thia-1-azabicyclo[3.2.0]-heptane-2-carboxylic acid

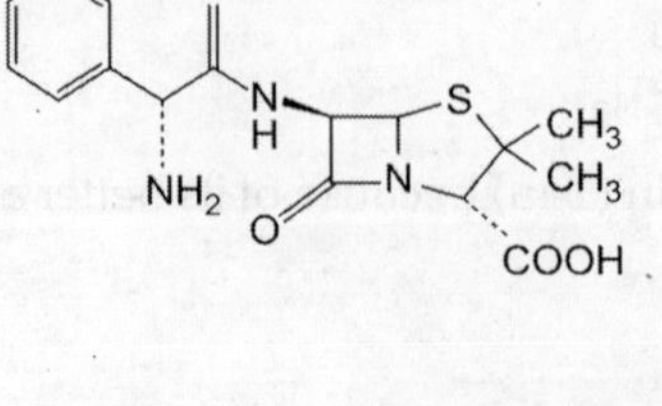

Synthesis

Route I

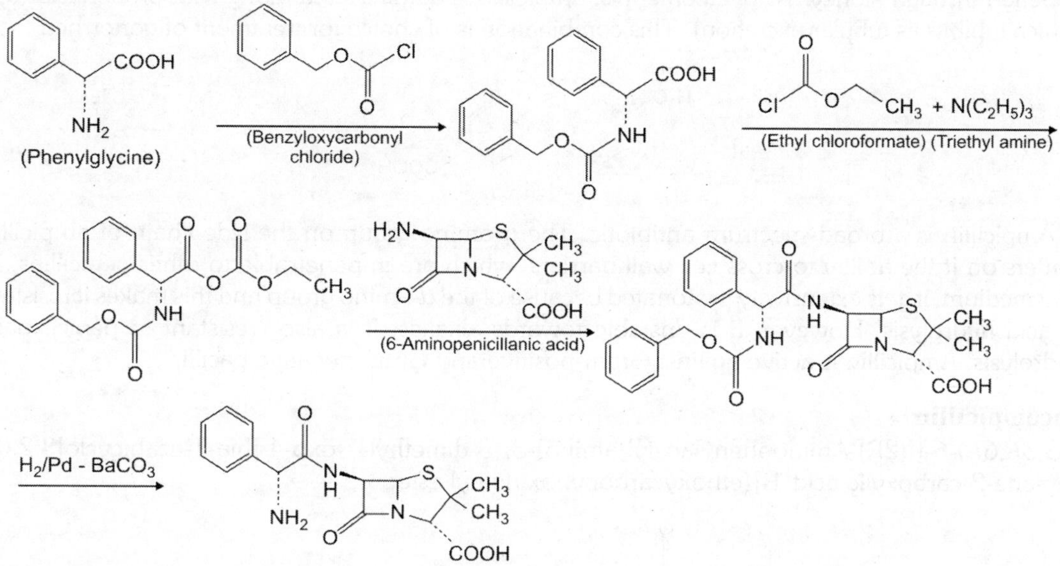

Route II

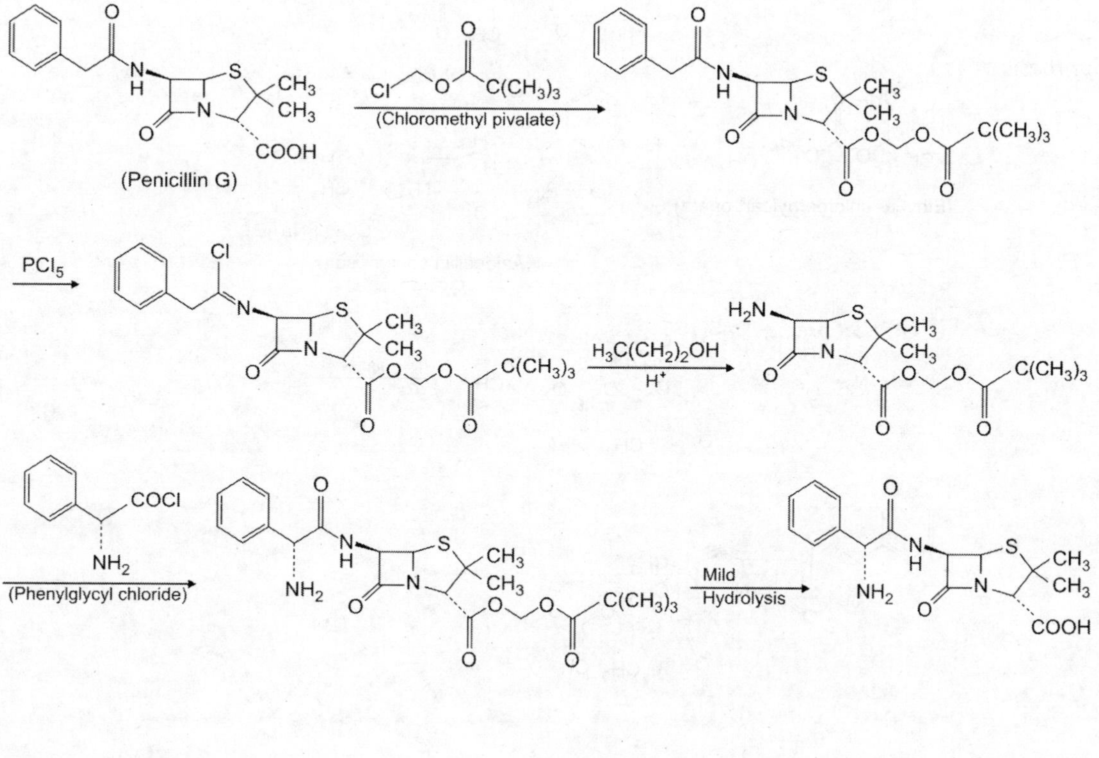

Ampicillin is water soluble. It is administered orally and is absorbed from intestinal tract to produce peak plasma levels in about 2 hours. Oral doses have to be repeated every 6 hr because of its excretion through kidney. To overcome this, ampicillin is administered along with probenecid (53) (which inhibits its tubular excretion). This combination is of choice for treatment of gonorrhea.

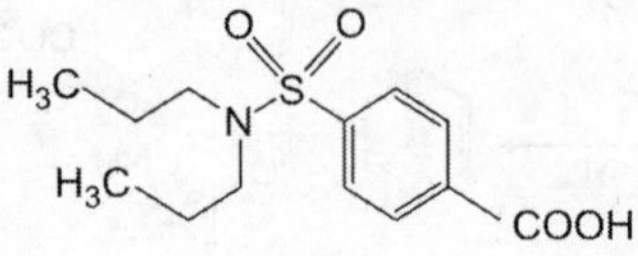

(53)

Ampicillin is a broad-spectrum antibiotic. The α-amino group on the side chain of ampicillin confers on it the ability to cross cell wall barriers which are impenetrable to other penicillins. In acid medium, it gets extensively protonated because of the α-amino group and this makes it resistant to acid hydrolysis. However, it is unstable towards alkalies. It is also resistant to penicillinase hydrolysis. Ampicillin is active against Gram-positive and Gram-negative bacilli.

Bacampicillin

(2S,5R,6R)-6-[[(2R)-Aminophenylacetyl]amino]-3, 3-dimethyl-7-oxo-4-thia-1-azabicyclo[3.2.0]-heptane-2-carboxylic acid 1-[(ethoxycarbonyl)oxy]ethyl ester

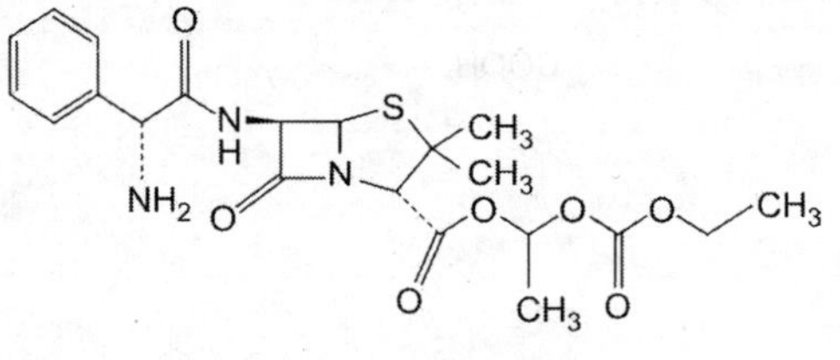

Synthesis

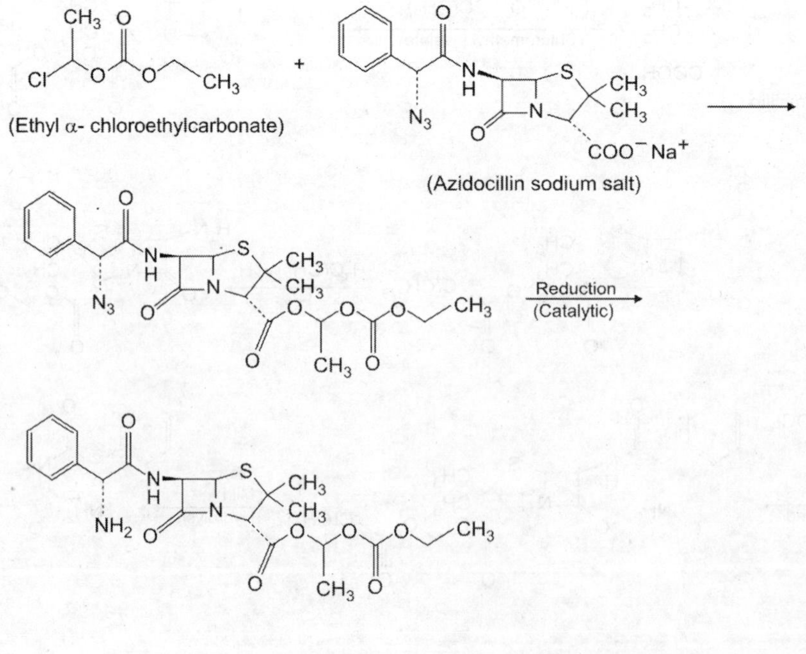

(Ethyl α- chloroethylcarbonate)

(Azidocillin sodium salt)

Reduction
(Catalytic)

It is a prodrug of ampicillin (16). It has rapid absorption than ampicillin (16). After oral absorption, it is hydrolysed by the esterase to ampicillin (16).

Amoxicillin

(2S,5R,6R)-6-[[(2R)-Amino(4-hydroxyphenyl)acetyl]amino]-3,3-dimethyl-7-oxo-4-thia-1-azabicyclo[3. 2. 0]heptane-2-carboxylic acid

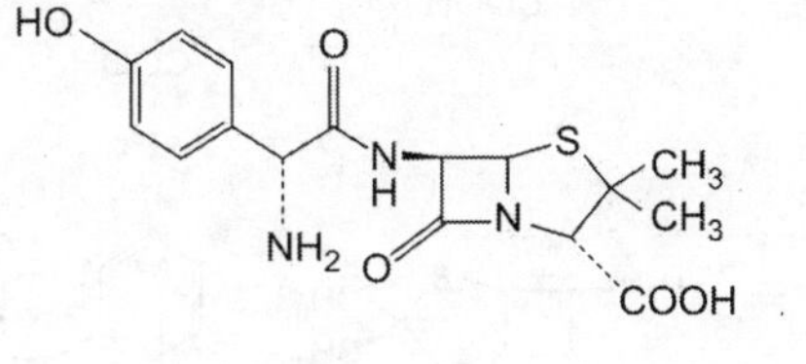

Synthesis

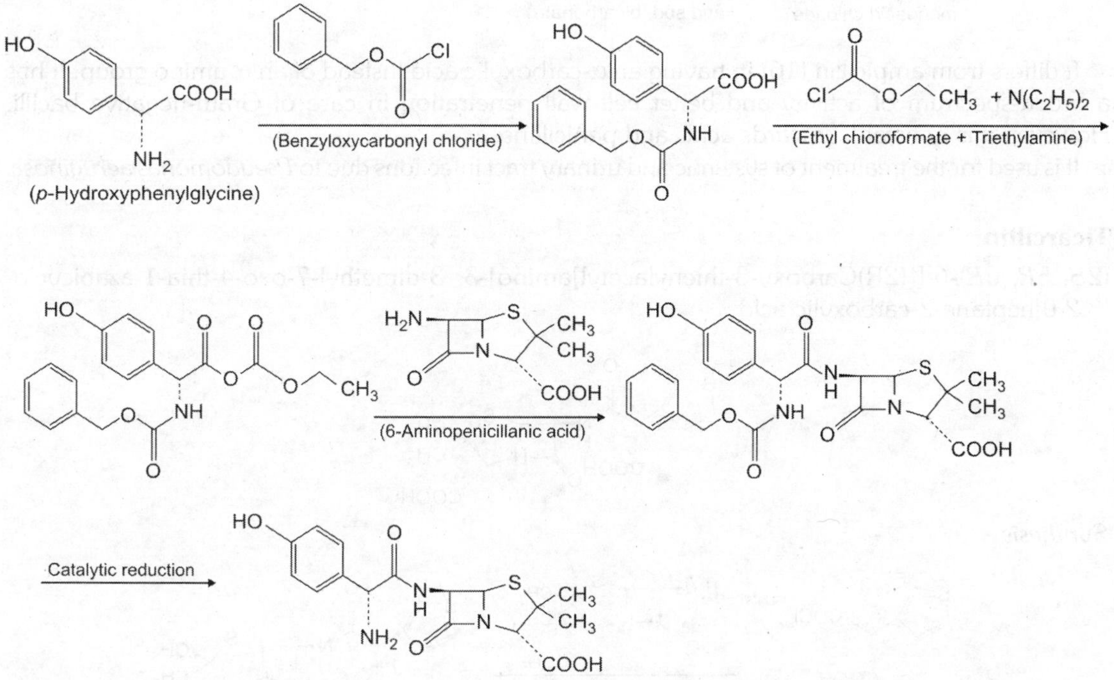

The antibacterial spectrum of amoxicillin is similar to ampicillin (16). It has more complete gastrointestinal absorption, so less of diarrhea and there is no effect of food on its absorption. It is preferred over ampicillin (16) but is less effective than ampicillin (16) in the treatment of bacillary dysentery. Like ampicillin (16), it is resistant to acid hydrolysis but is susceptible to alkaline and β-lactamase hydrolysis.

Carbenicillin

(2S,5R,6R)-6-[(Carboxyphenylacetyl)amino]-3,3-dimethyl-7-oxo-4-thia-1-azabicyclo[3.2.0]-heptane-2-carboxylic acid

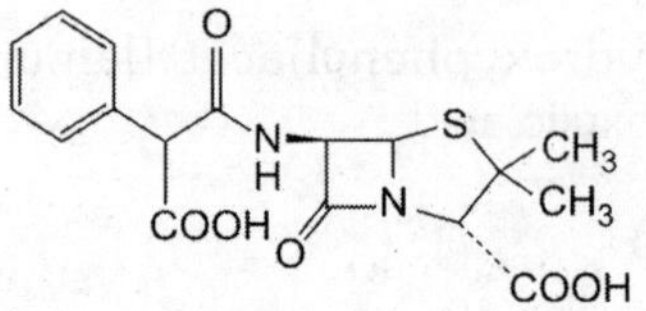

Synthesis

(Phenylmalonic acid monoacid chloride)   (6-Aminopenicillanic acid and sod. bicarbonate)

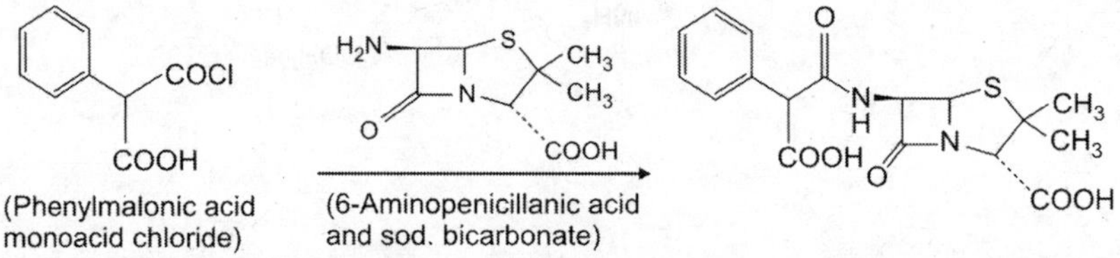

It differs from ampicillin (16) in having an α-carboxylic acid instead of an α-amino group. It has a broad-spectrum of activity and better cell wall penetration in case of Gram-negative bacilli. However, it is not stable towards acids and penicillinase.

It is used for the treatment of systemic and urinary tract infections due to *Pseudomonas aeruginosa*.

Ticarcillin

(2S, 5R, 6R)-6-[[(2R)Carboxy-3-thienylacetyl]amino]-3, 3-dimethyl-7-oxo-4-thia-1-azabicyclo-[3.2.0]heptane-2-carboxylic acid

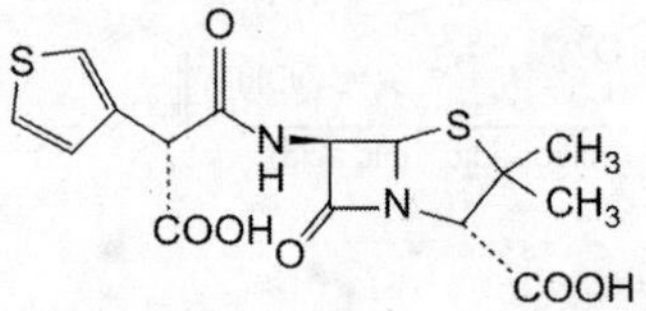

Synthesis

(Thienylmalonic acid monoacid chloride)   (6-Aminopenicillanic acid and sod. bicarbonate)

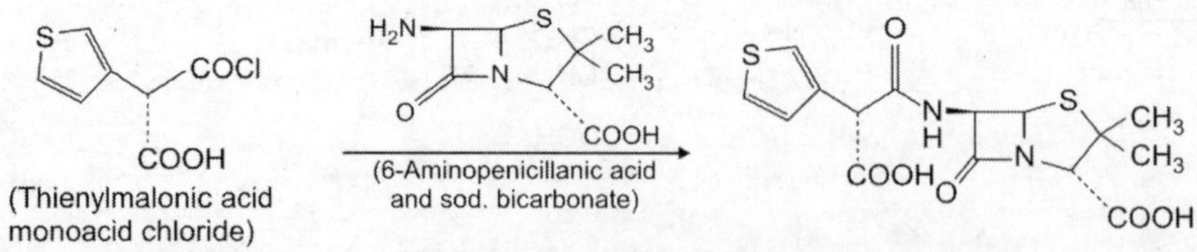

It is an isostere of carbenicillin (18), in which phenyl ring has been replaced by thienyl ring. Like carbenicillin (18), it is not stable towards acids and its antibacterial spectrum is similar to that of carbenicillin (18). However, it has better pharmacokinetic property including higher serum levels and longer duration of action and greater in vitro potency against several Gram-negative bacilli, particularly *Peudomonas aeruginosa* and *Bacteroides fragilis*.

Mezlocillin

(2S,5R,6R)-3, 3-Dimethyl-6-[[(2R)-[[[3-(methylsulphonyl)-2-oxo-1-imidazolidinyl]carbonyl] amino]-phenylacetyl]amino]-7-oxo-4-thia-1-azabicyclo[3.2.0]heptane-2-carboxylic acid

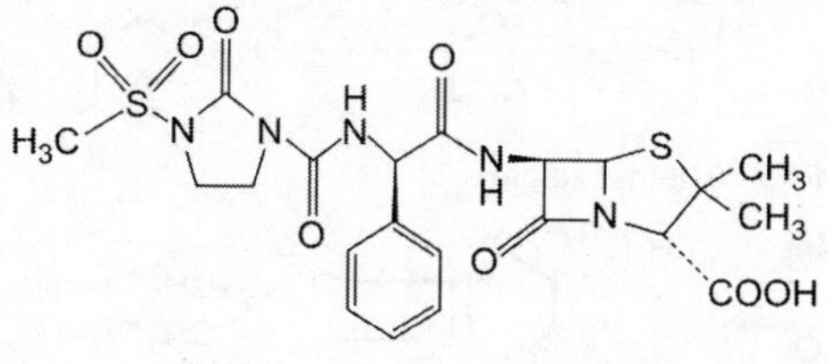

Synthesis

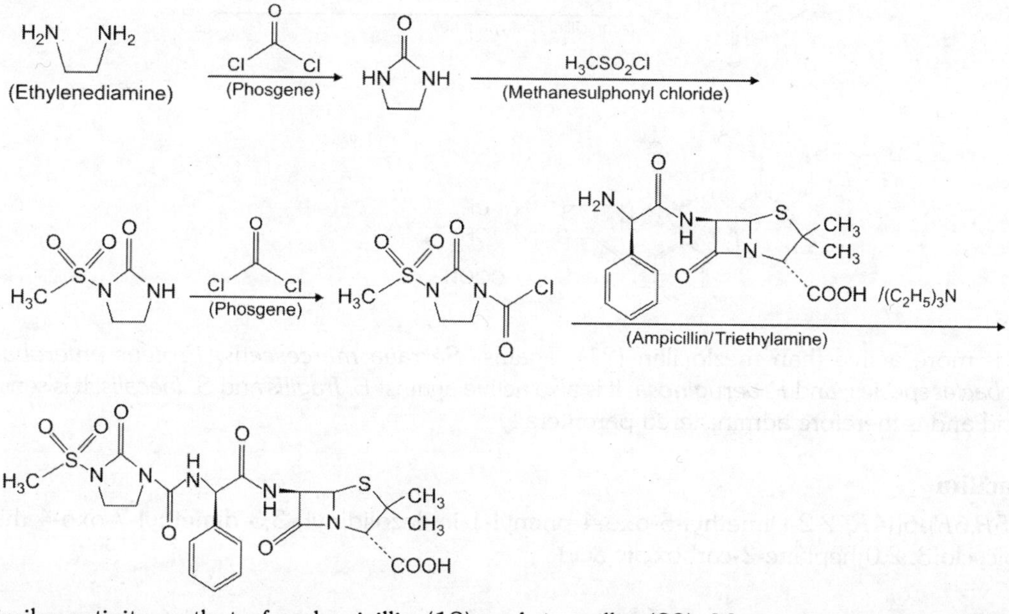

Similar activity as that of carbenicillin (18) and ticarcillin (20). More active against *Klebsiella* species. and *Pseudomonas aeruginosa*, anaerobic bacteria *Streptococcus faecalis*, *Bacillus fragilis*, and *H. influenzae*.

Piperacillin

(2S,5R,6R)-6-[(R)-2-(4-Ethyl-2,3-dioxo-1-piperazinecarboxamido)-2-phenylacetamido]-3,3-dimethyl-7-oxo-4-thia-1-azabicyclo[3.2.0]heptane-2-carboxylic acid

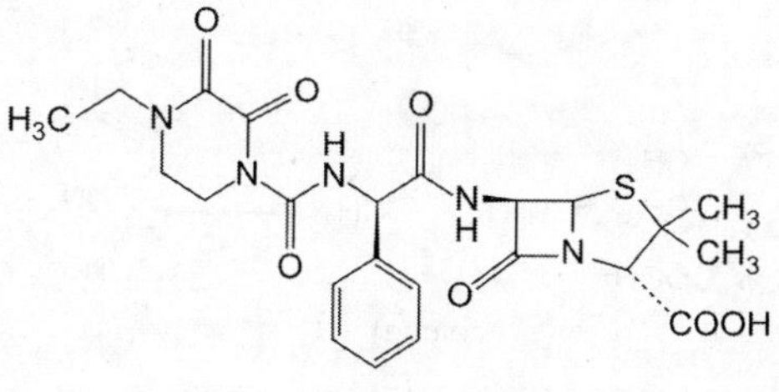

Synthesis

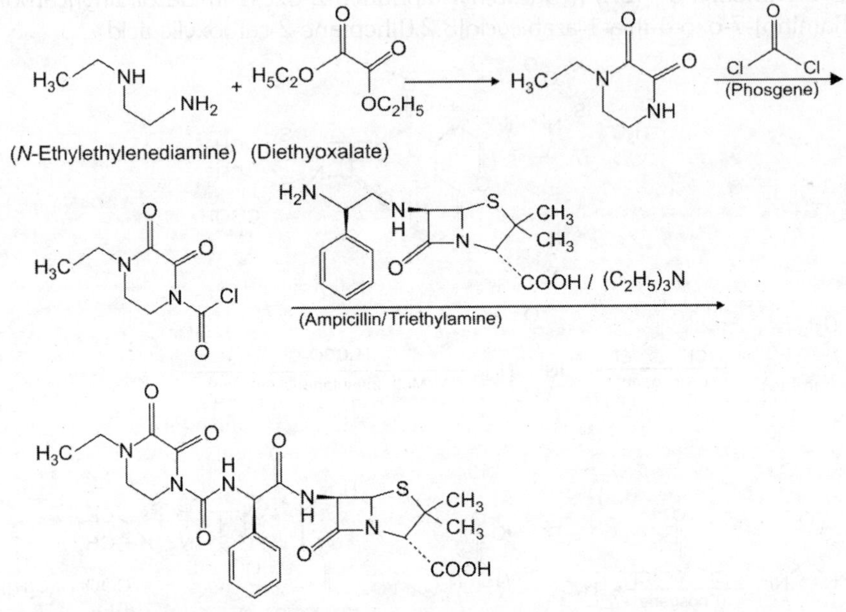

It is more active than mezlocillin (21), against *Serratia marcescens*, *Proteus enterobacter*, *Citrobacter* species, and *P. aeruginosa*. It is also active against *B. fragilis* and *S. faecalis*. It is sensitive to acid and is therefore administered parenterally.

Hetacillin

(2S,5R,6R)-6[(4R)-2,2-Dimethyl-5-oxo-4-phenyl-1-imdazolidinyl]-3,3-dimethyl-7-oxo-4-thia-1-azabicyclo[3..2.0]heptane-2-carboxylic acid

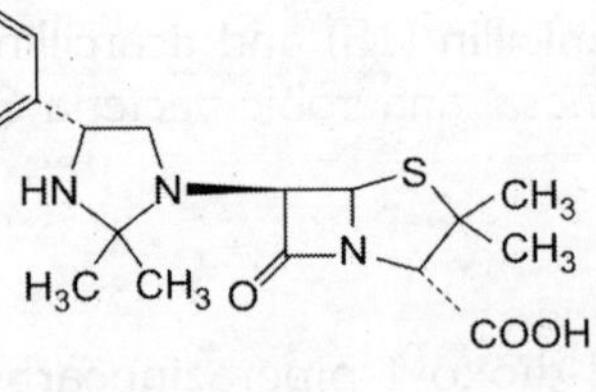

Synthesis

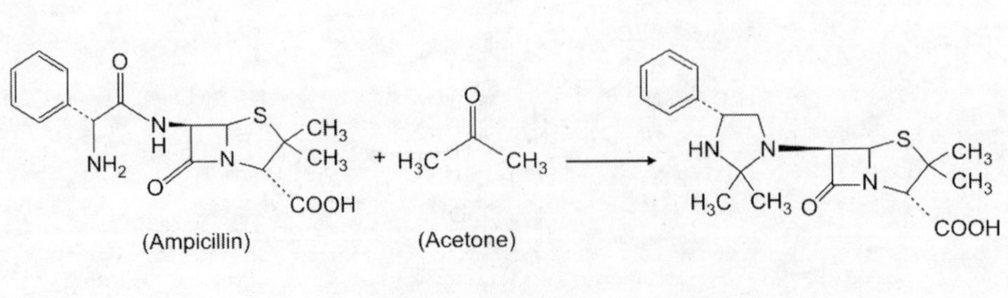

It is a produrg of ampicillin (16) and is obtained by latentiation of ampicillin by tying the amino and amide function with actone. It is hydrolyzed to ampicillin (16).

SEMISYTHETIC PENICILLINS : ACID RESISTANT

Phenethicillin

(2S,5R,6R)-3,3-Dimethyl-7-oxo-6[(1-oxo-2-phenoxypropyl)amino]-4-thia-1-azabicyclo[3.2.0]-heptane-2-carboxylic acid

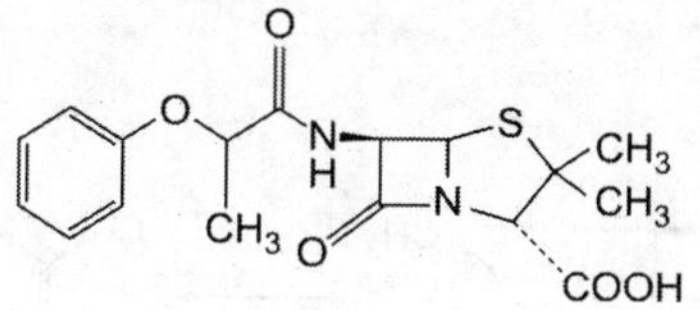

Synthesis

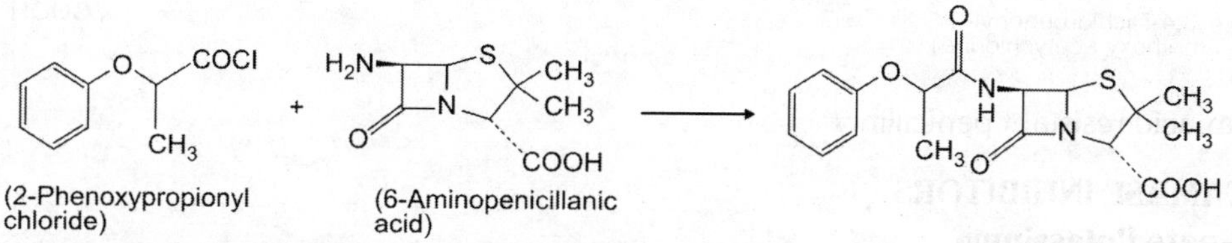

(2-Phenoxypropionyl chloride) + (6-Aminopenicillanic acid)

It is an acid resistant penicillin. Its potassium salt is used.

Propicillin

(2S,5R,6R)-3,3-Dimethyl-7-oxo-6-[(1-oxo-2-phenoxybutyl)amino]-4-thia-1-azabicyclo[3.2.0]-heptane-2-carboxylic acid

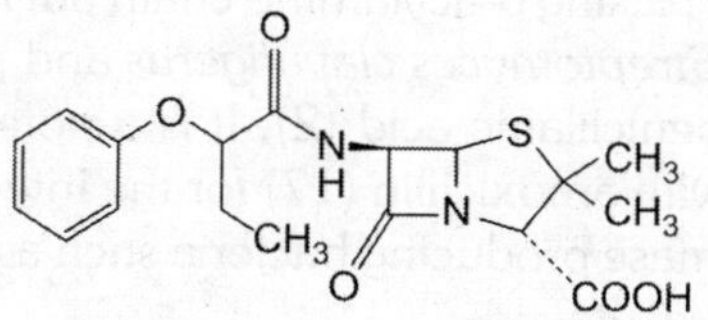

Synthesis

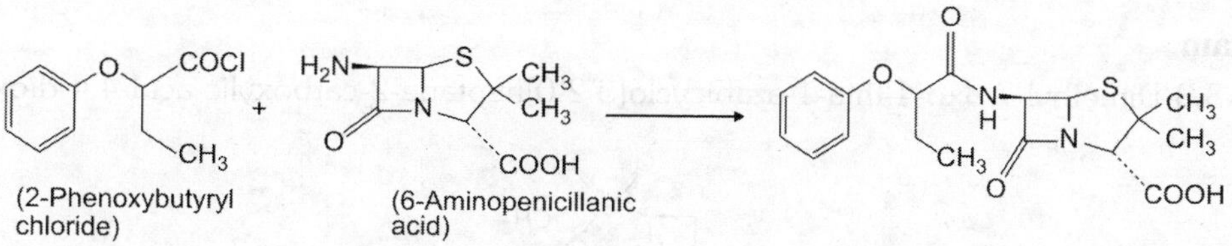

(2-Phenoxybutyryl chloride) + (6-Aminopenicillanic acid)

It is an acid resistant penicillin.

Clometocillin

(2S,5R,6R)-6[[(3,4-Dichlorophenyl)methoxyacetyl]amino]-3,3-dimethyl-7-oxo-4-thia-1-azabicyclo[3.2.0]heptane-2-carboxylic acid

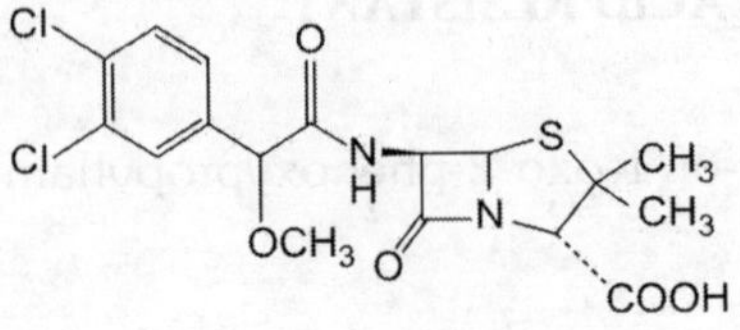

Synthesis

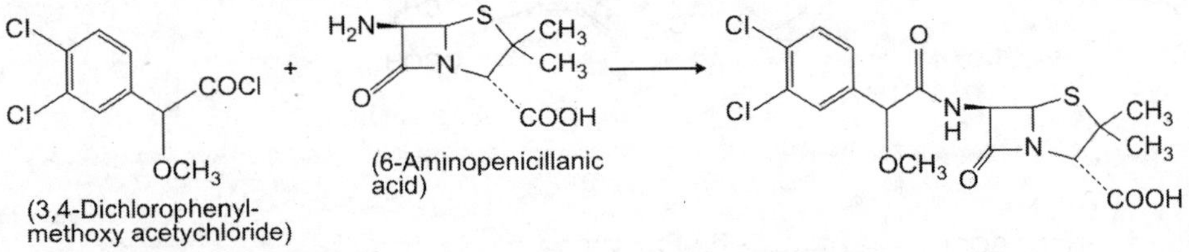

(3,4-Dichlorophenyl-methoxy acetychloride)

(6-Aminopenicillanic acid)

It is an acid resistant penicillin.

β-LACTAMASE INHIBITORS

Clavulanate Potassium

[2R-(2α,3Z,5α-)]3-(2-Hydroxyethylidene-7-oxo-4-oxa-1-azabicyclo[3.2.0]heptane-2-carboxylic acid potassium salt

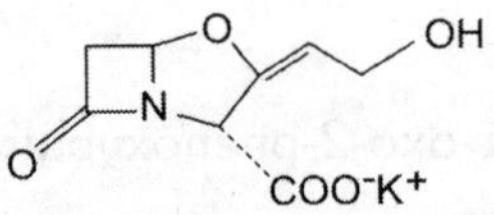

Clavulanic acid is an oxapenam lacking 6-acylamino chain but has a 2-hydroxyethylidene moiety at position 3. It is obtained from *Streptomyces clavuligerus* and possesses weak antibiotic activity which is comparable to 6-aminopenicillanic acid (2). It is a potent inhibitor of β-lactamase of *S. aureus*. It is used in combination with amoxicillin (17) for the infection of skin, ear, respiratory, and urinary tract caused by the β-lactamase producing bacteria such as *S. aureus*, *E. coli*, *K. pneumonia*, *Enterobacter* species, *H. influenzae*, etc.

It has also been used in combination with tricarcillin (20) against β-lactamase producing bacteria.

Sulbactam

(2S,5R)-3,3-Dimethyl-7-oxo-4-thia-1-azabicyclo[3.2.0]heptane-2-carboxylic acid 4,4-dioxide

Synthesis

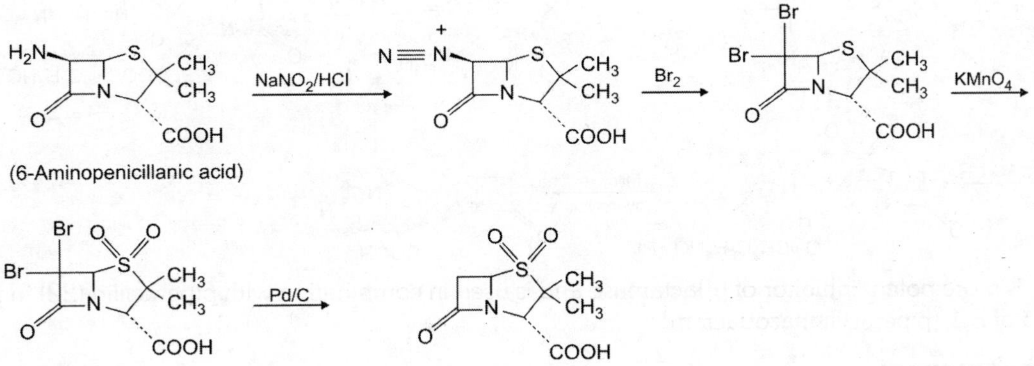

(6-Aminopenicillanic acid)

It is an inhibitor of β-lactamase of *S. aureus* as well as β-lactamases elaborated by Gram-negative bacilli. It has weak intrinsic activity but potentiates the activity of ampicillin (16) and, carbenicillin (18) against β-lactamase producing *S. aureus* and members of *Enterobacteriacea* family.

Tazobactam

(2S,3S,5R)-3-Methyl-7-oxo-3-(1*H*-1, 2, 3-triazol-1-ylmethyl)-4-thia-1-azabicyclo[3. 2. 0]heptane-2-carboxylic acid 4,4-dioxide

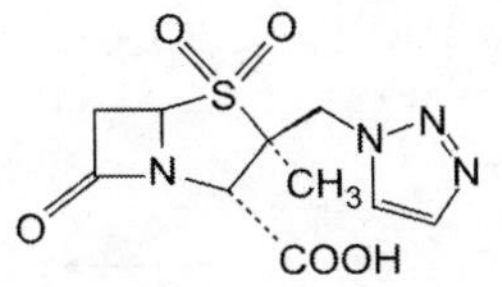

Synthesis

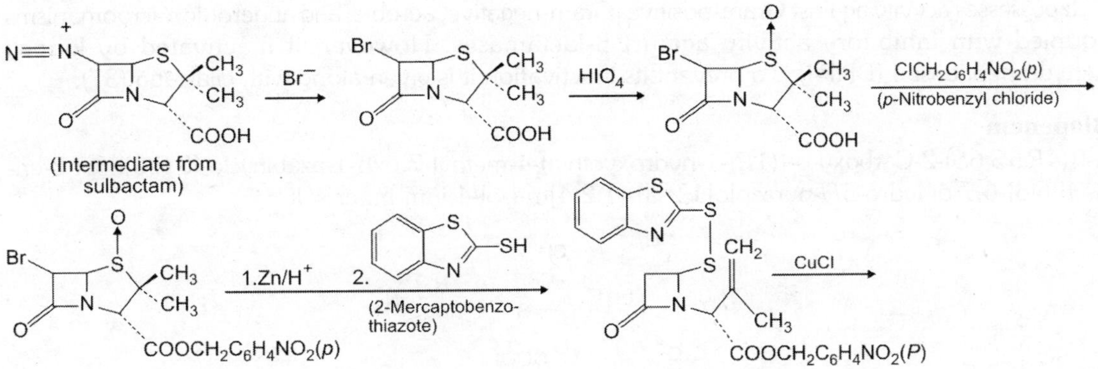

(Intermediate from sulbactam)

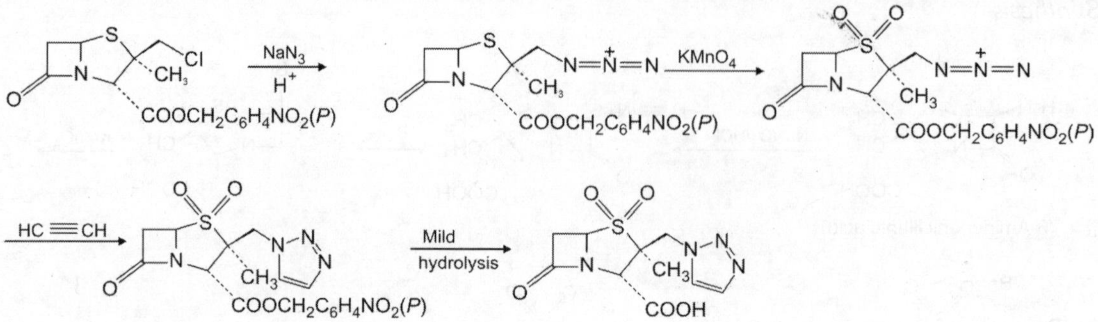

It is more potent inhibitor of β-lactamase and is used in combination with piperacillin (22) in the ratio of 8:1 (piperacillin:tazobactam).

CARBAPENEMS

Imipenem

[5*R*-[5α,6α(*R*)]]-6-(1-Hydroxyethyl)-3-[[2-[(iminomethyl)amino]ethyl]thio]-7-oxo-1-azabicyclo[3.2.0]hept-2-ene-2-carboxylic acid

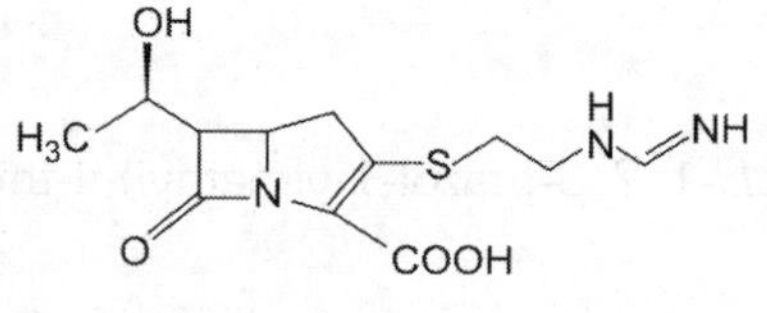

Synthesis

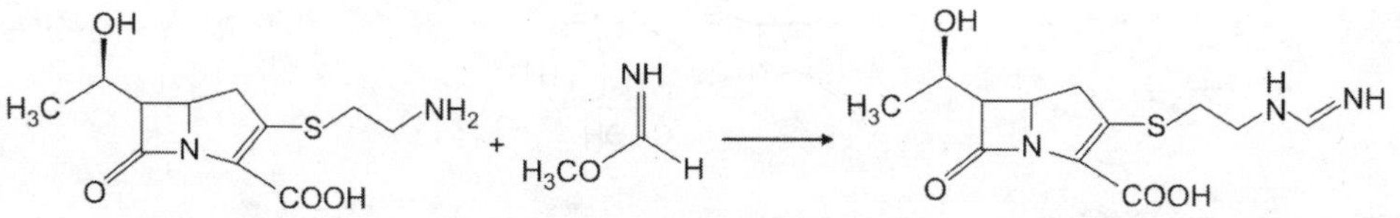

It possesses activity against Gram-positive, Gram-negative, aerobic, and anaerobic microorganisms coupled with inhibitory activity against β-lactamases. However, it inactivated by kidney dehydropeptidase-I (DHP-I). To prevent its inactivation it is given along with cilastatin (37).

Biapenem

6-[[[(4*R*,5*S*,6*S*)-2-Carboxy-6-((1*R*)-1-hydroxyethyl)-4-methyl-7-oxo-1-azabicyclo-[3.2.0]hept-2-en-3-yl]thio]-6,7-dihydro-5*H*-pyrazolo[1,2-a]-[1,2,4]triazol-4-ium inner salt

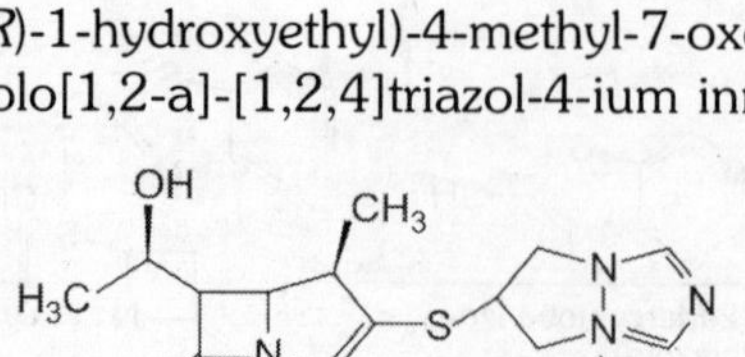

Synthesis

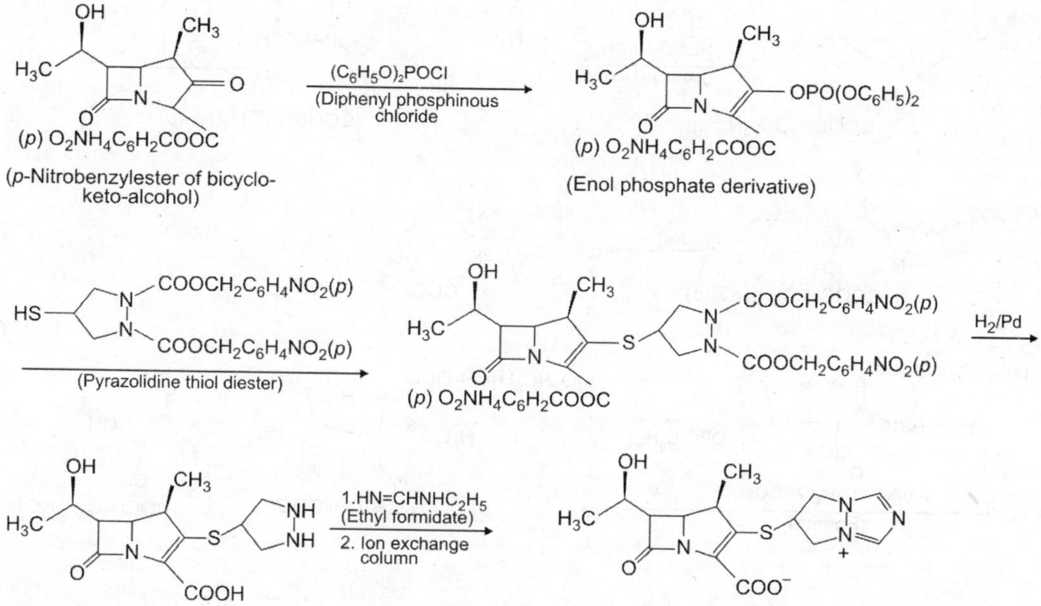

(p) O₂NH₄C₆H₂COOC

(p-Nitrobenzylester of bicyclo-
keto-alcohol)

(C₆H₅O)₂POCl
(Diphenyl phosphinous
chloride)

(p) O₂NH₄C₆H₂COOC

(Enol phosphate derivative)

HS
(Pyrazolidine thiol diester)

(p) O₂NH₄C₆H₂COOC

H₂/Pd

1. HN=CHNHC₂H₅
(Ethyl formidate)
2. Ion exchange
column

Biapenem is a second generation carbapenem having a broad spectrum of antimicrobial activity which includes activity against Gram-positive, Gram-negative, and anaerobes. It is also resistant to DHP-I and β-lactamases.

Meropenem

(4R,5S,6S)-3-[[3S,5S)-5-[(Dimethylamino)carbonyl]-3pyrrolidinyl]thio]-6[1R)-1-hydroxyethyl]-4-methyl-7-oxo-1-azabicyclo[3.2.0]hept-2-ene-2-carboxylic acid

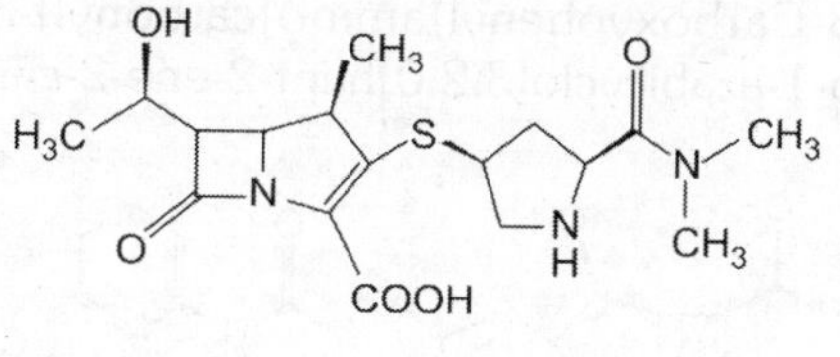

Synthesis

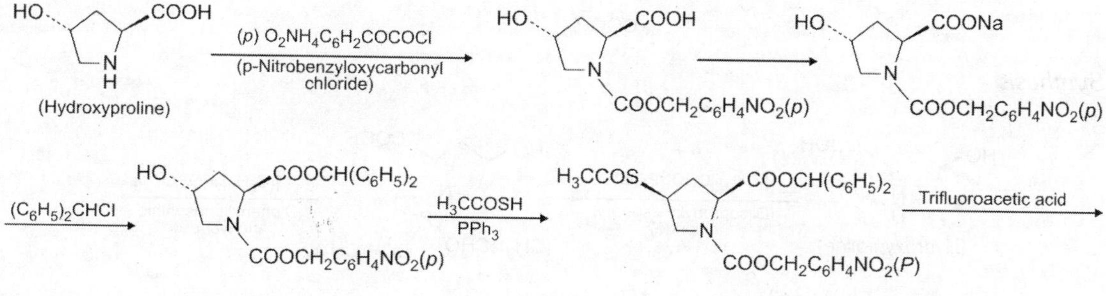

(Hydroxyproline)

(p) O₂NH₄C₆H₂COCOCl
(p-Nitrobenzyloxycarbonyl
chloride)

(C₆H₅)₂CHCl

H₃CCOSH
PPh₃

Trifluoroacetic acid

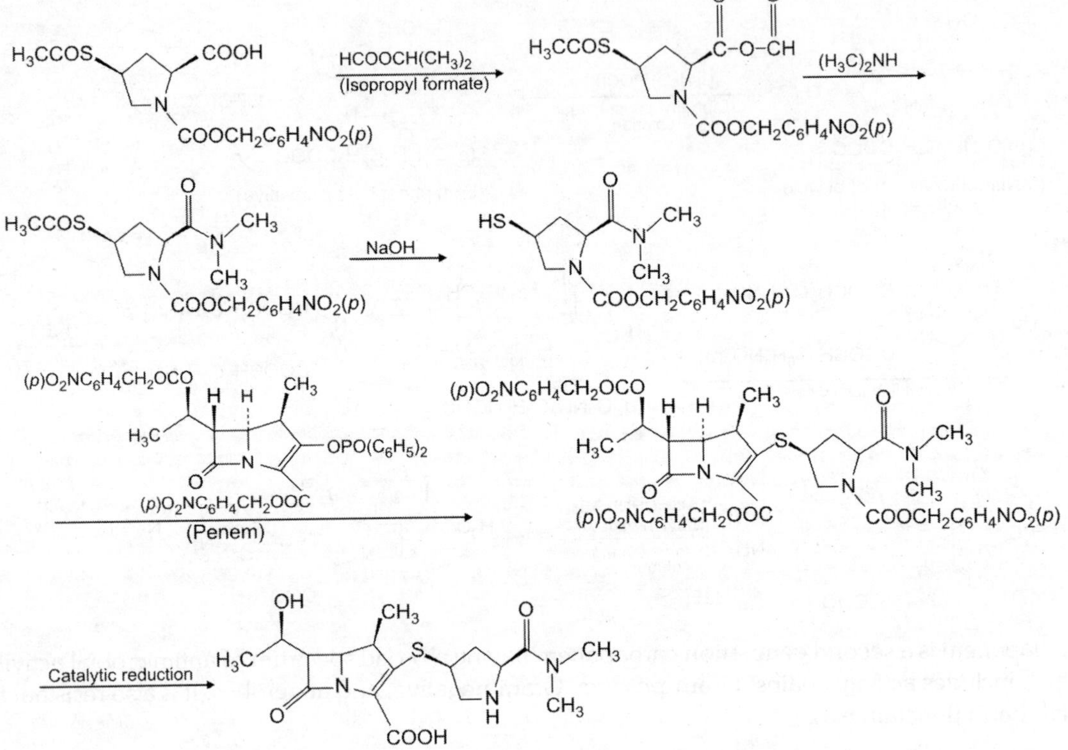

It is a second generation carbapenem and possesses the same activity as biapenem (38).

Ertapenem

(4R,5S,6S)-3-[[3S,5S)-5-[[(3-Carboxyphenyl)amino]carbonyl]-3-pyrrolidinyl]thio]-6-[(1R)-1-hydroxyethyl]-4-methyl-7-oxo-1-azabicyclo[3.2.0]hept-2-ene-2-carboxylic acid

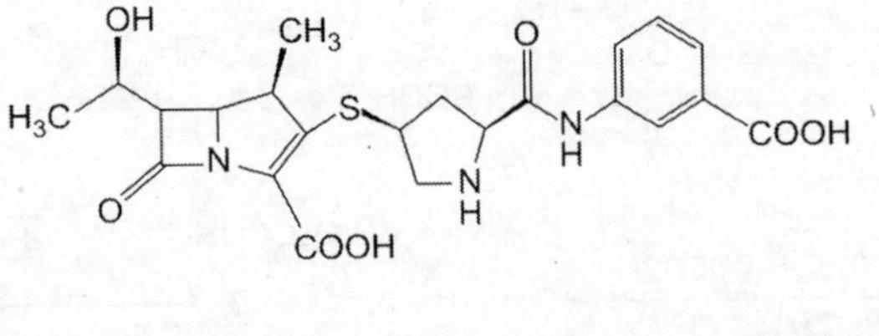

Synthesis

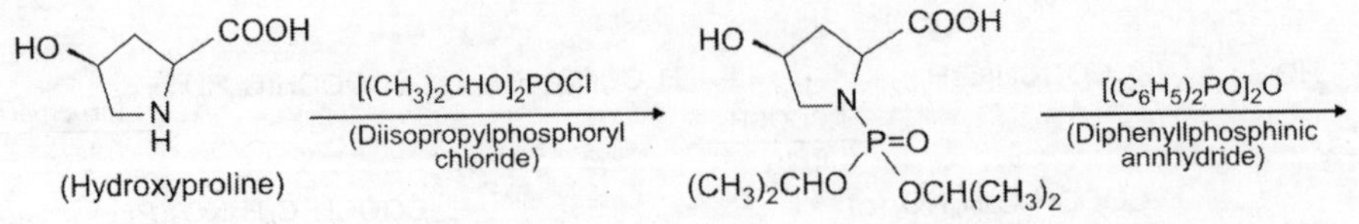

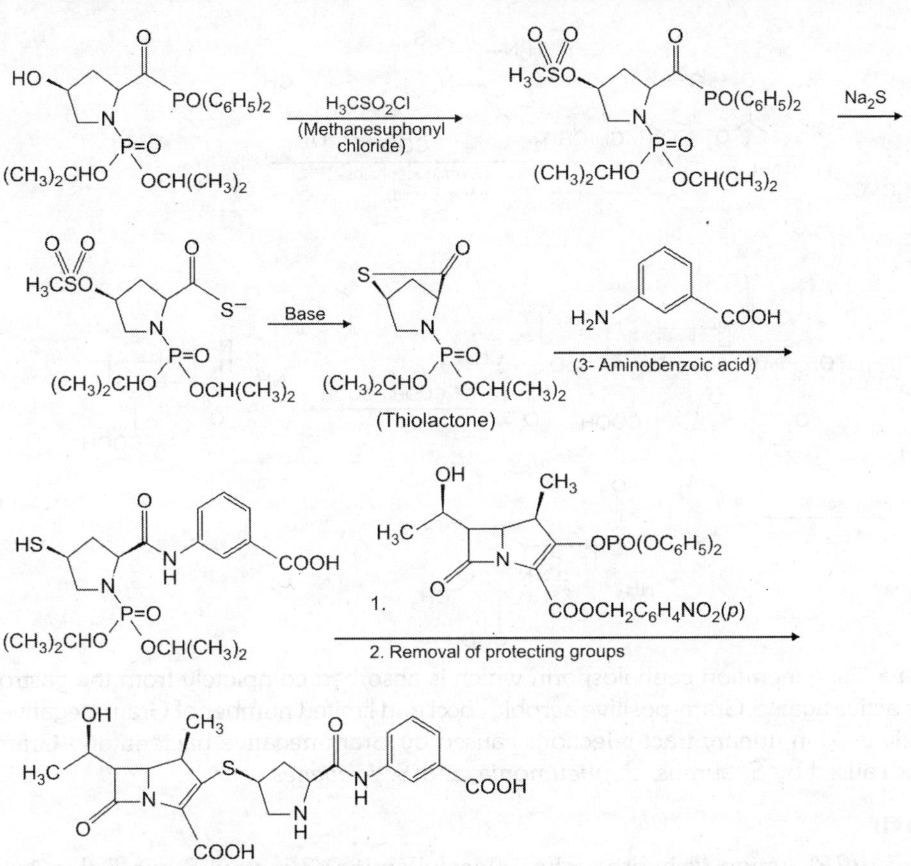

It is a second generation carbapenem and possesses the same activity as biapenem (38).

CEPHALOSPORINS : FIRST GENERATION
Cephalexin

(6R,7R)-7-[[(2R)-Aminophenylacetyl]amino]-3-methyl-8-oxo-5-thia-1-azabicyclo[4. 2. 0]oct-2-ene-2-carboxylic acid

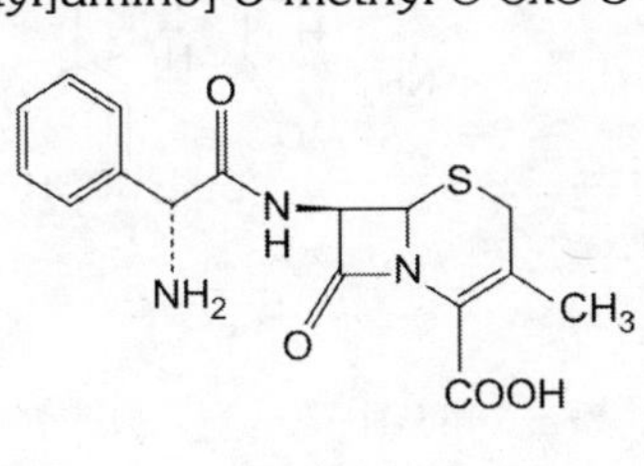

Synthesis

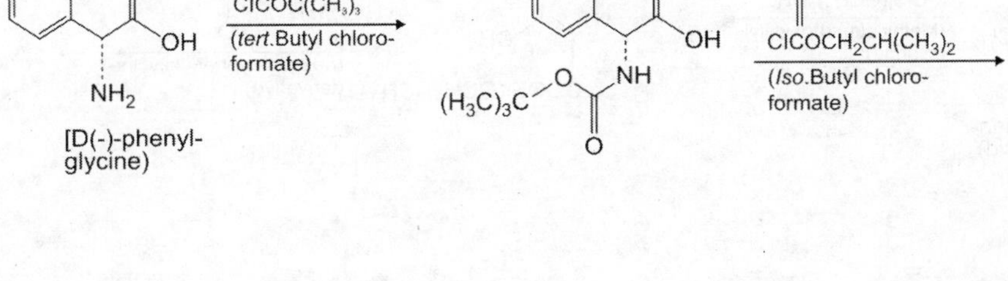

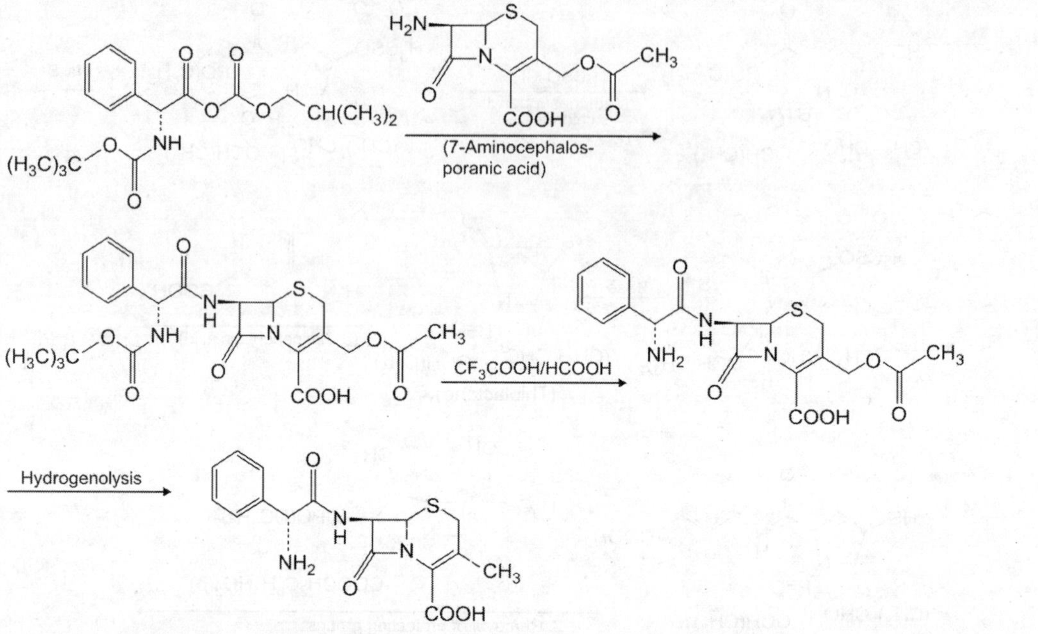

This is a first generation cephalosporin which is absorbed completely from the gastrointestinal tract. It is active against Gram-positive aerobic cocci and limited number of Gram-negative bacteria. It is widely used in urinary tract infections caused by Gram-negative bacteria and Gram-positive infections caused by *S. aureus*, *S. pneumonia*, and *S. pyogenes*.

Cefadroxil

(6*R*,7*R*)-7-[[(2*R*)-Amino-(4-hydroxyphenyl)acetyl]amino]-3-methyl-8-oxo-5-thia-1-azabicylo-[4.2.0]oct-2-ene-2-carboxylic acid

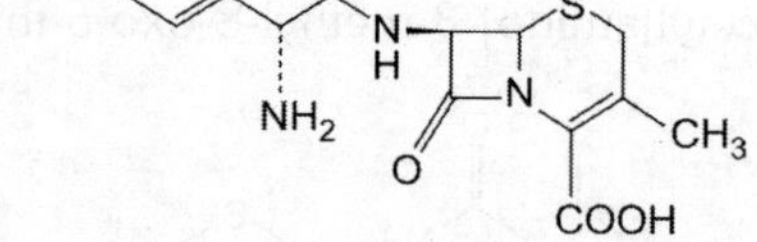

Synthesis

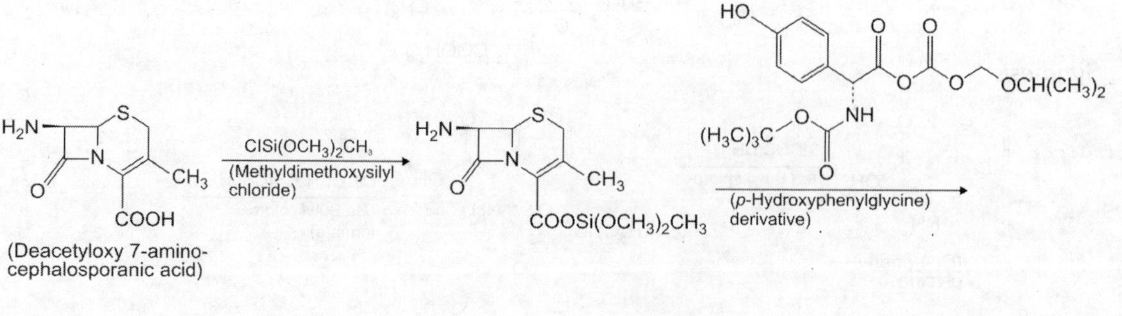

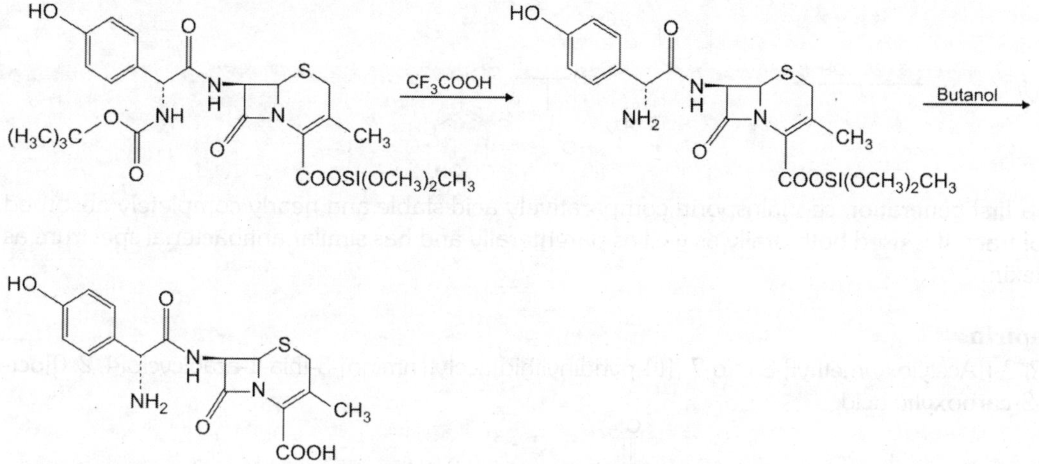

It is a first generation cephalosporin with a side chain similar to that of amoxicillin (17). It is given orally and has a prolonged duration of action which permits once-a-day dosing. The antibacterial spectrum is similar to that of cephalexin.

Cephradine

(6R,7R)-7-[[(2R)-Amino-1, 4-cyclohexadien-1-ylacetyl] amino]-3-methyl-8-oxo-5-thia-1-azabicylo-[4. 2. 0]oct-2-ene-2-carboxylic acid

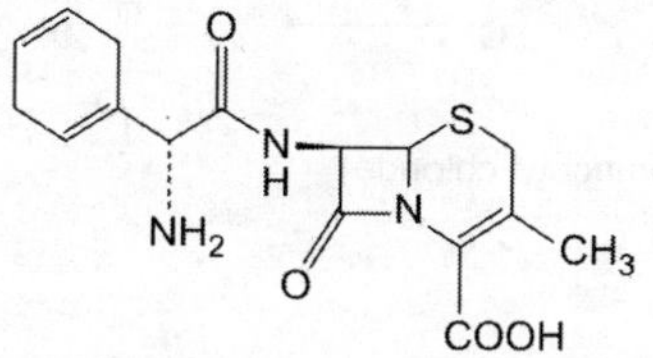

Synthesis

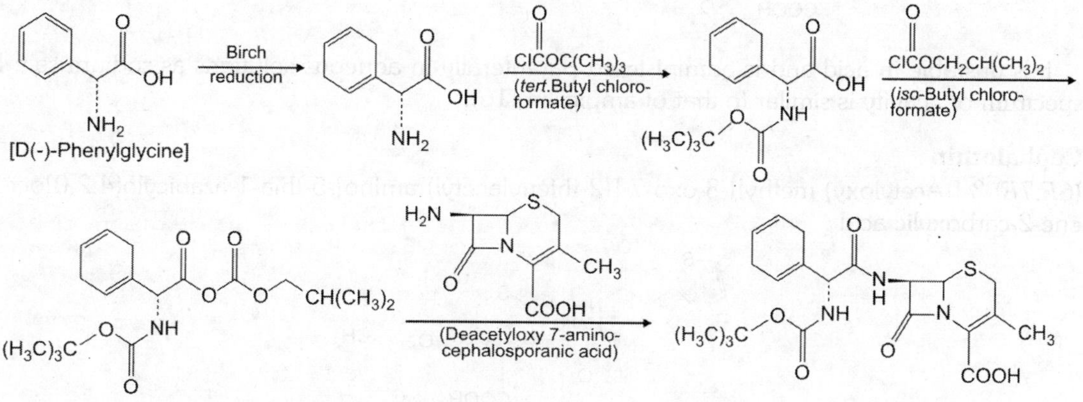

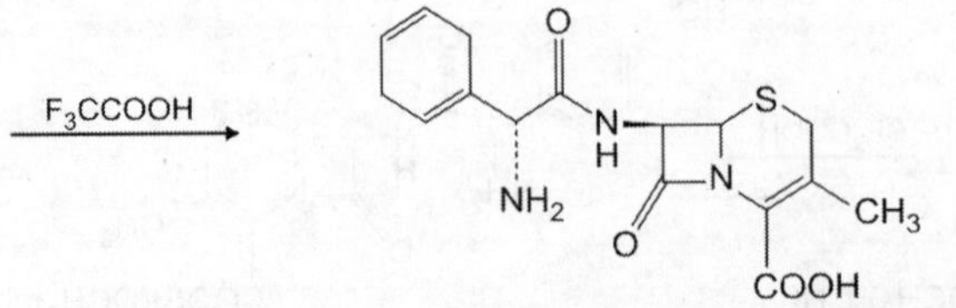

It is a first generation cephalosporin comparatively acid stable and nearly completely absorbed from GI tract. It is used both orally as well as parenterally and has similar antibacterial spectrum as cephalexin.

Cephapirin

(6*R*,7*R*)-3-[(Acetyloxy)methyl]-8-oxo-7-[[(4-pyridinylthio)acetyl] amino]-5-thia-1-azabicyclo[4. 2. 0]oct-2-ene-2-carboxylic acid.

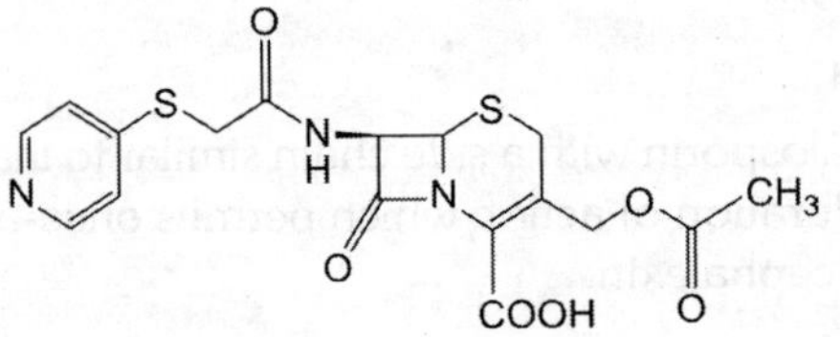

Synthesis

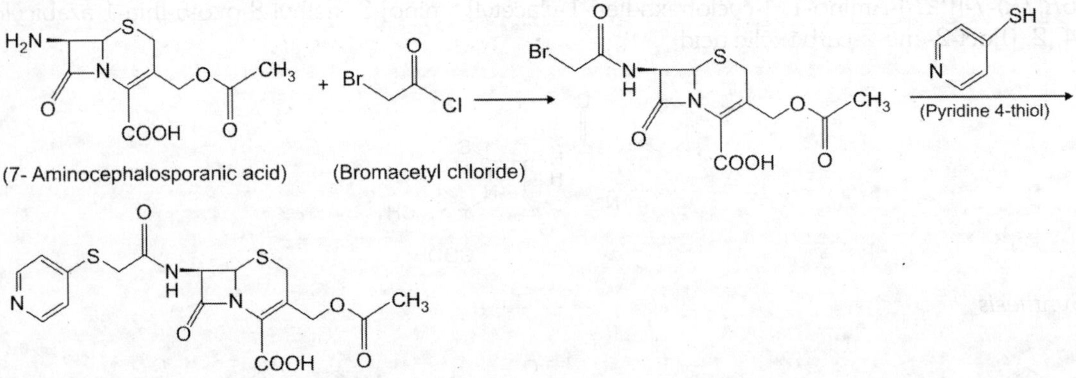

(7- Aminocephalosporanic acid)   (Bromacetyl chloride)

It is unstable in acid and is administered parenterally in aqueous solutions as sodium salt. Its spectrum of activity is similar to that of ampicillin (16).

Cephalothin

(6*R*,7*R*)-3-[(Acetyloxy) methyl]-8-oxo-7-[(2-thienylacetyl) amino]-5-thia-1-azabicylo[4.2.0]oct-2-ene-2-carboxylic acid

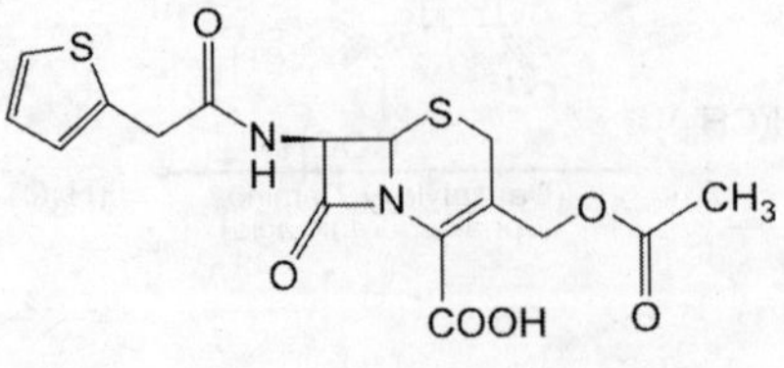

Synthesis

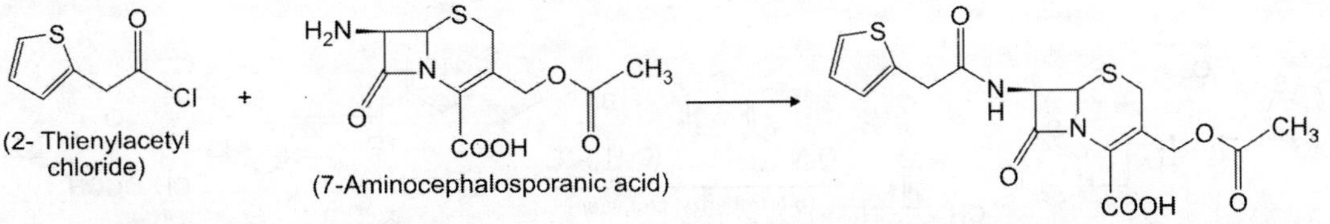

(2- Thienylacetyl chloride) + (7-Aminocephalosporanic acid) →

Like cephapirin it is unstable towards acid and is therefore adminstered parenterally as sodium salt. It has similar activity as cephapirin.

Cefazolin

(6*R*,7*R*)-3-[[(5-Methyl-1,3,4-thiadiazol-2-yl)thio]methyl]-8-oxo-7-[(1*H*-tetrazol-1-ylacetyl)amino]-5-thia-1-azabicylo[4. 2. 0]oct-2-ene-2-carboxylic acid

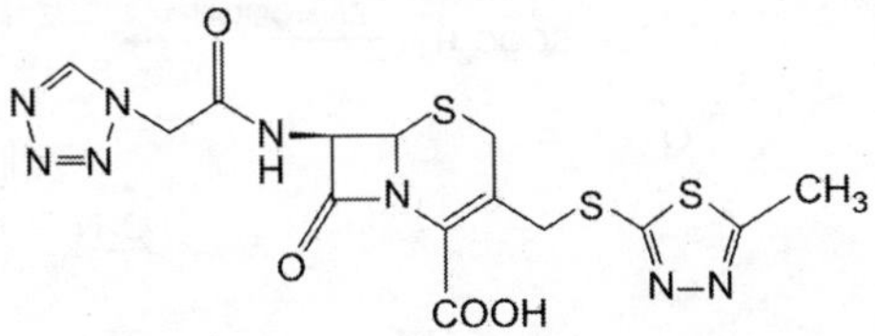

Synthesis

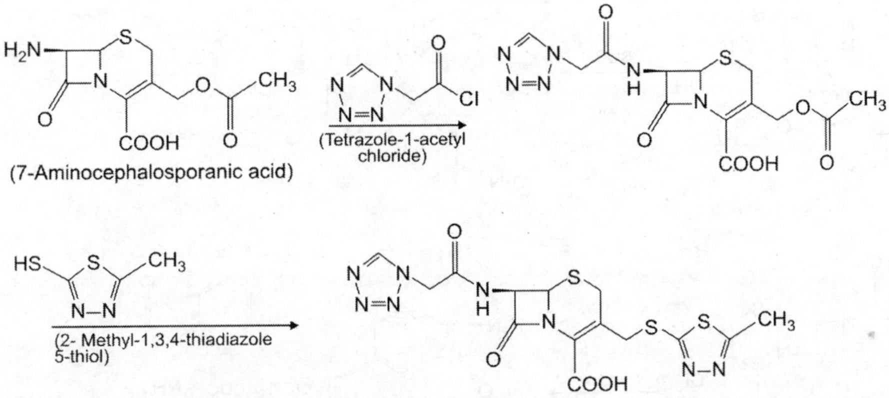

(7-Aminocephalosporanic acid) (Tetrazole-1-acetyl chloride)

(2- Methyl-1,3,4-thiadiazole 5-thiol)

It is administered parenterally as sodium salt. It has longer half-life because of slower renal clearance.

CEPHALOSPORINS : SECOND GENERATION

Cefaclor

(6*R*,7*R*)-7-[[(2*R*)-Aminophenylacetyl] amino]-3-chloro-8-oxo-5-thia-1-azabicylo[4. 2. 0]oct-2-ene-2-carboxylic acid

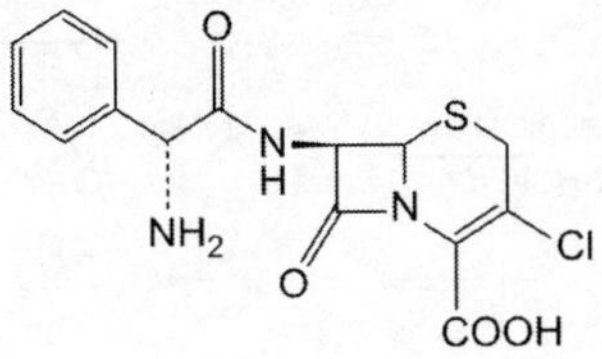

Synthesis

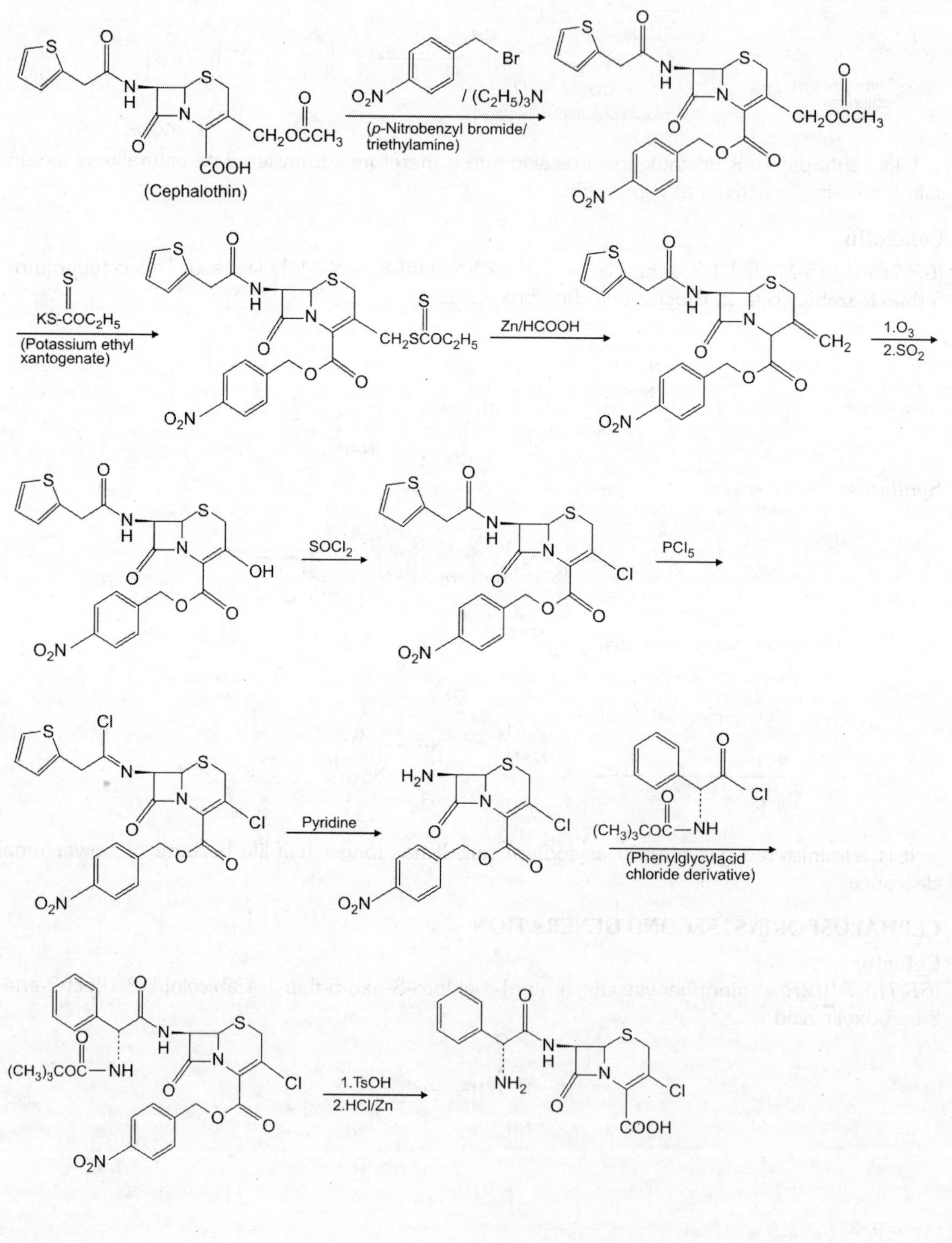

Br
O_2N
/ $(C_2H_5)_3N$
(*p*-Nitrobenzyl bromide/
triethylamine)
(Cephalothin)
COOH
CH_2OCCH_3
KS-COC$_2$H$_5$
(Potassium ethyl
xantogenate)
$CH_2SCOC_2H_5$
Zn/HCOOH
CH_2
1.O_3
2.SO_2
OH
$SOCl_2$
Cl
PCl_5
Pyridine
H_2N
$(CH_3)_3COC$—NH
(Phenylglycylacid
chloride derivative)
1.TsOH
2.HCl/Zn
NH_2

It is a second generation cephalosporin. Cefaclor is acid stable and can therefore be administered orally. The antibacterial spectrum is similar to cephalexin.

Cefprozil

(6*R*,7*R*)-7-[[(2*R*)-Amino(4-hydroxyphenyl) acetyl] amino]-8-oxo-3-(1-propenyl)-5-thia-1-azabicylo[4. 2. 0]oct-2-ene-2-carboxylic acid

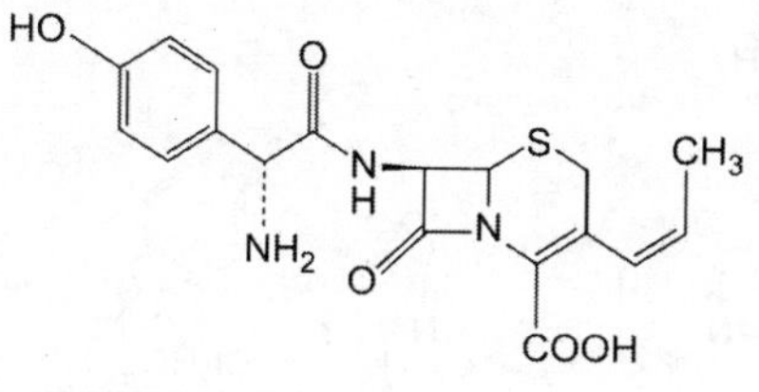

(Z) 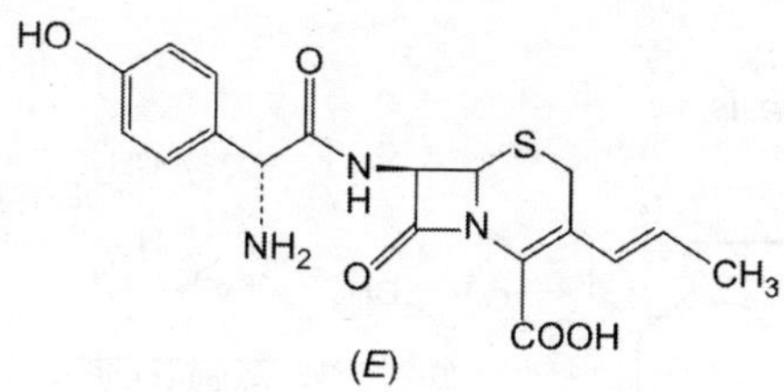   (E)

Synthesis

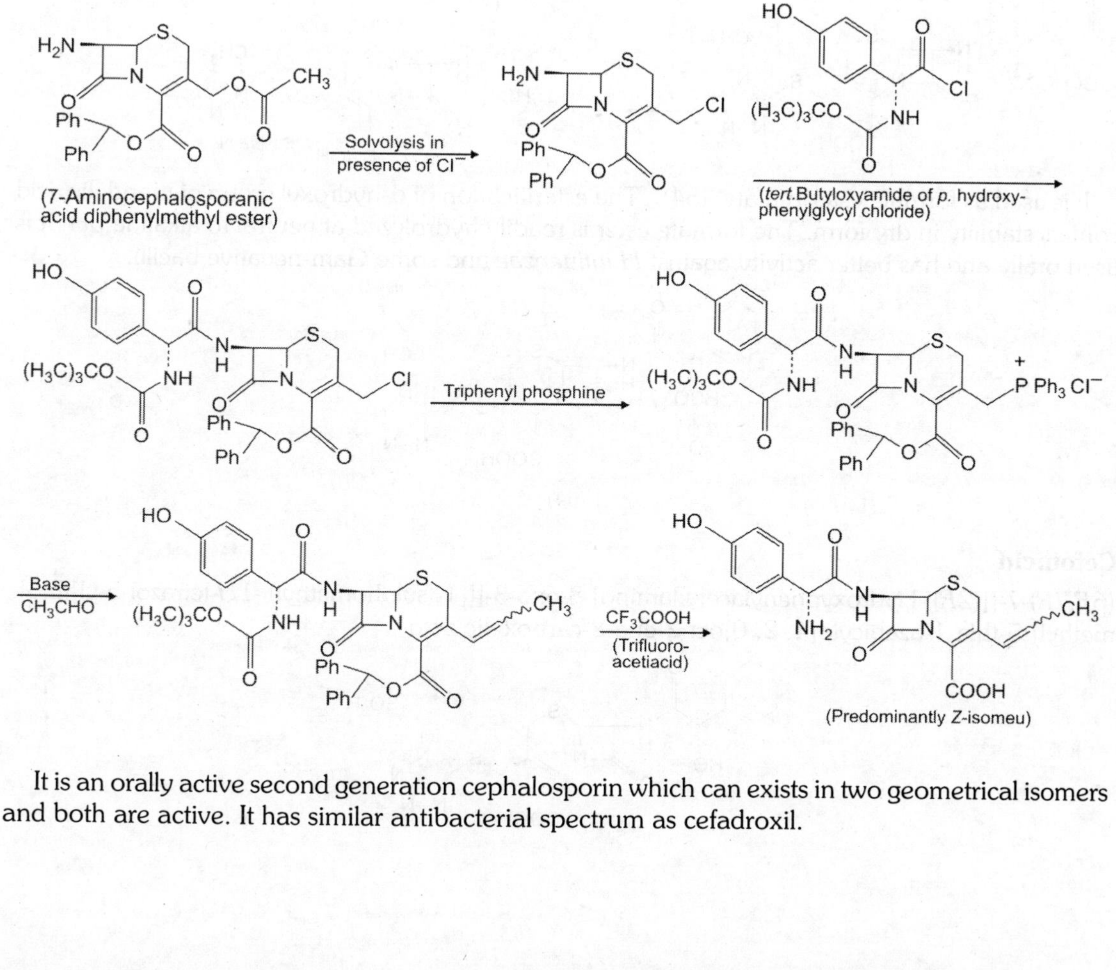

(7-Aminocephalosporanic acid diphenylmethyl ester)

(*tert*.Butyloxyamide of *p.* hydroxy-phenylglycyl chloride)

(Predominantly *Z*-isomeu)

It is an orally active second generation cephalosporin which can exists in two geometrical isomers and both are active. It has similar antibacterial spectrum as cefadroxil.

Cefamandole

(6R,7R)-7-[[(2R)-Hydroxyphenylacetyl] amino]-3-[[(1-methyl-1H-tetrazol-5-yl)thio]-methyl]-8-oxo-5-thia-1-azabicylo[4. 2. 0]oct-2-ene-2-carbcxylic acid

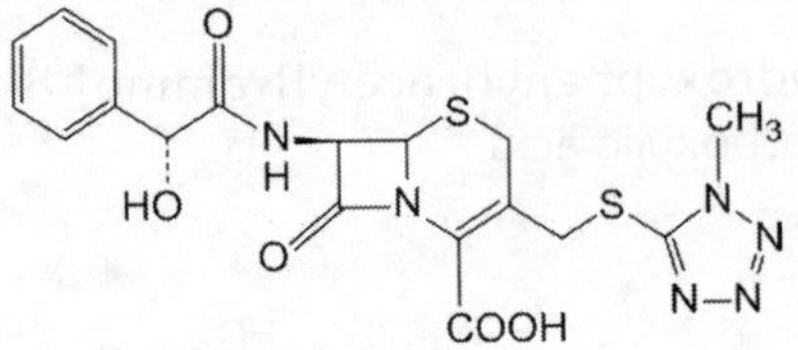

Synthesis

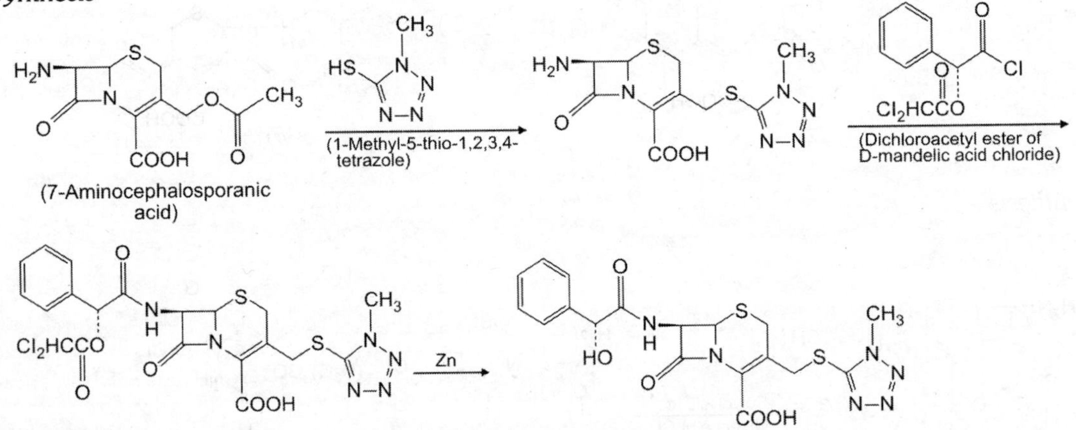

(7-Aminocephalosporanic acid)

(1-Methyl-5-thio-1,2,3,4-tetrazole)

(Dichloroacetyl ester of D-mandelic acid chloride)

It is used as formate ester [nafate, (54)]. The esterification of α-hydroxyl group of mandelic acid confers stability in dry form. The formate ester is readily hydrolyzed at neutral to alkaline pH. It is used orally and has better activity against *H.influenzae* and some Gam-negative bacilli.

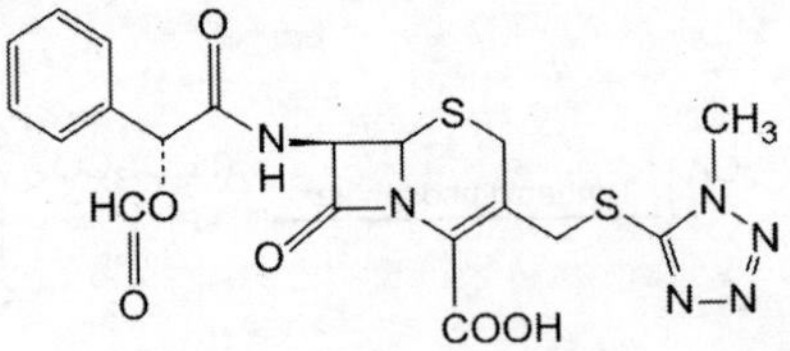

(54)

Cefonicid

(6R,7R)-7-[[(2R) -Hydroxyphenylacetyl]amino]-8-oxo-3-[[[1-(sulphomethyl) -1H-tetrazol-5-yl]thio]-methyl]-5-thia-1-azabicylo[4. 2. 0]oct-2-ene-2-carboxylic acid

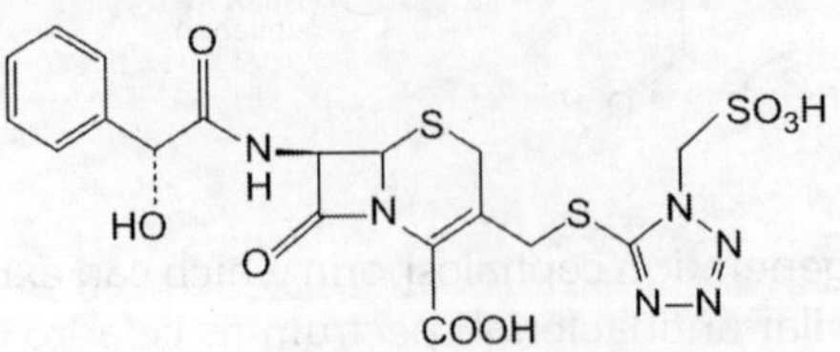

Synthesis

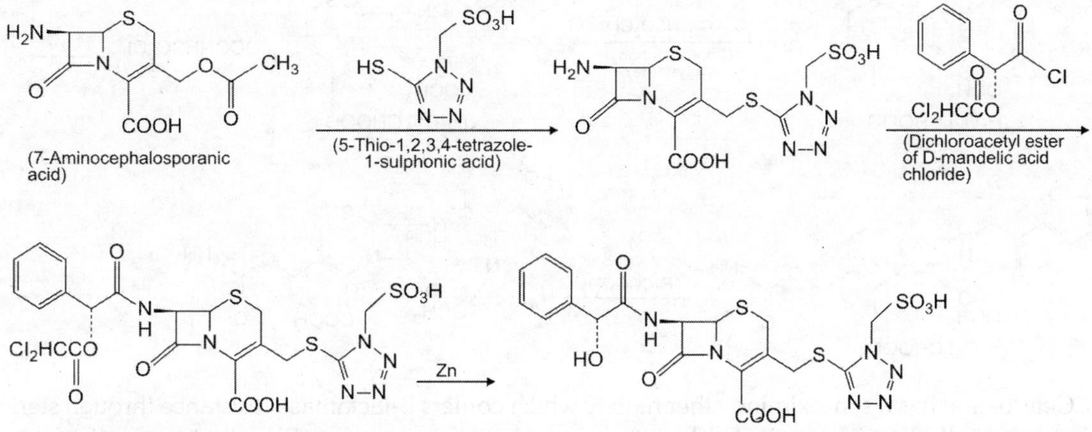

It is a second generation cephalosporin. It has a longer half-life than other members. It is used as a parenteral preparation as a disodium salt.

Cefuroxime

(6R,7R)-3-[[(Aminocarbonyl) oxy]methyl]-7-[[(2Z)-2-furanyl(methoxyimino)aceyl]amino]-8-oxo-5-thia-1-azabicyclo[4. 2. 0] oct-2-ene-2-carboxylic acid

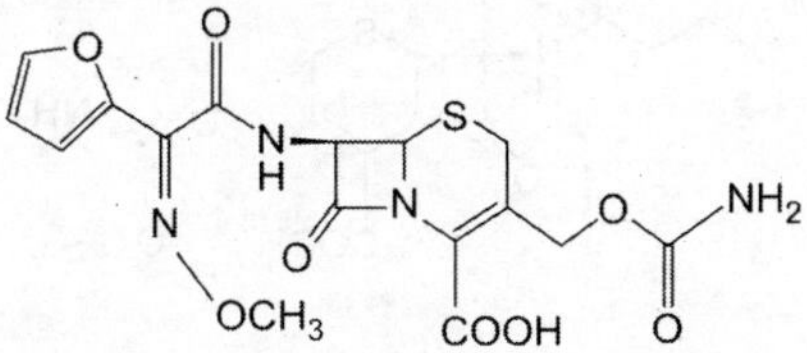

Synthesis

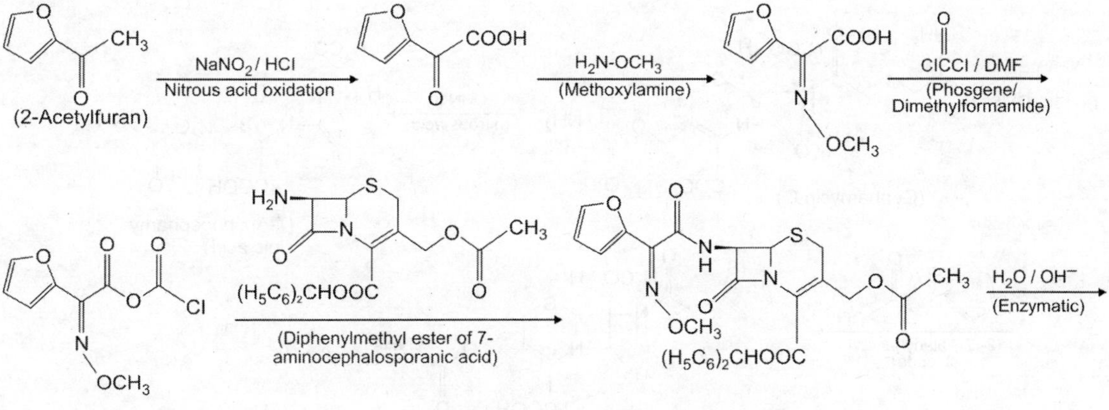

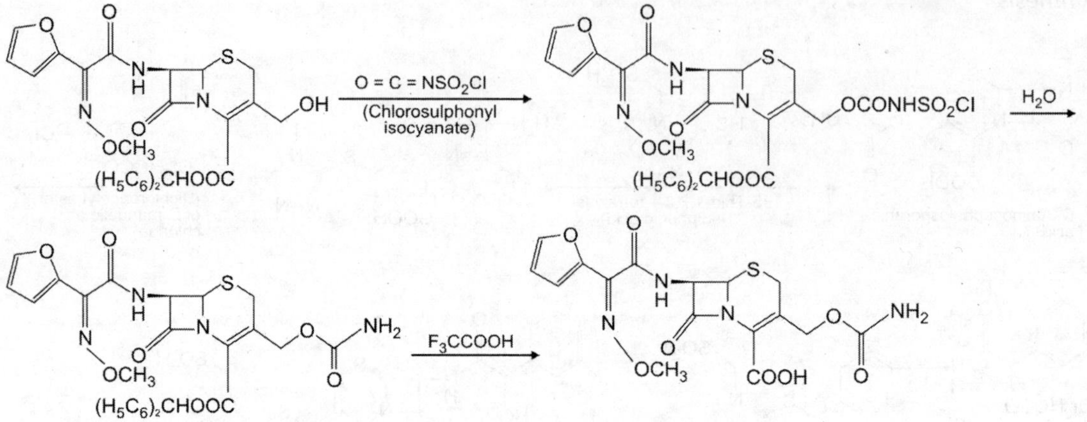

Cefuroxime has a syn-oximino ether moiety which confers β-lactamase resistance through steric hinderance. It is active against β-lactamase producing microorganisms that are resistant to cefamandole such as *E. coli, K. pneumonia, N. gonorrhoeae, H. influenzae*, and some Gram-negative microorganisms. It is administered orally.

Cefoxitin

(6R,7S)-3-[[(Aminocarbonyl)oxy]methyl]-7-methoxy-8-oxo-7-[(2-thienylacetyl)-amino]-5-thia-1-azabicyclo[4.2.0]oct-2-ene-2-carboxylic acid

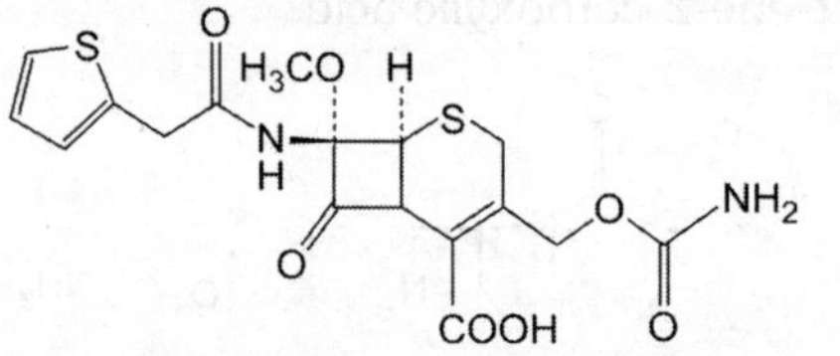

Synthesis

Route 1

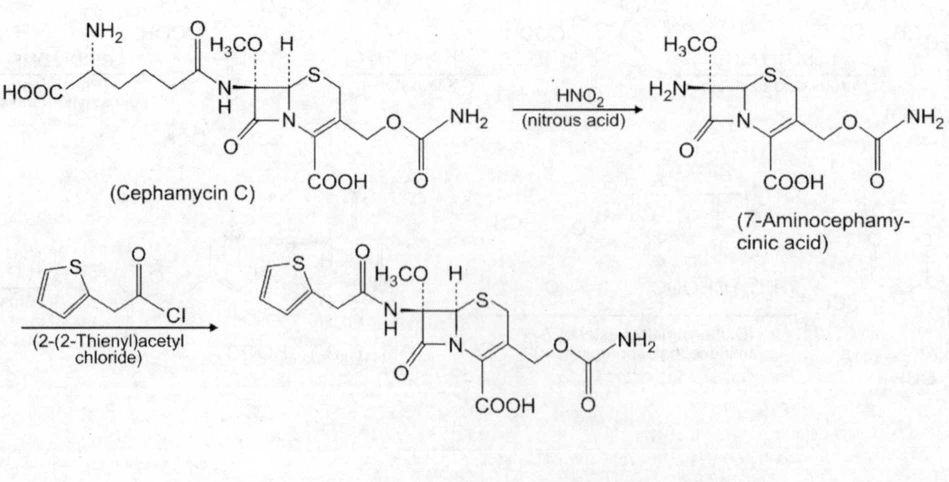

Route 2

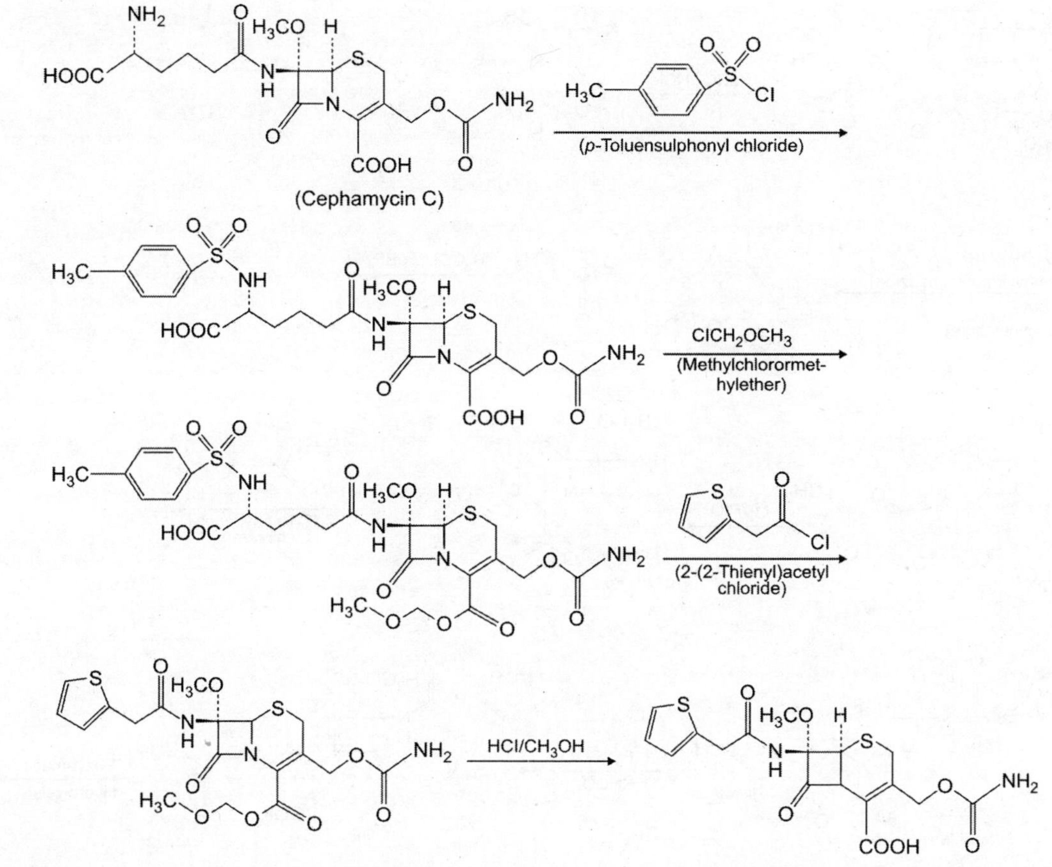

(Cephamycin C)

(p-Toluensulphonyl chloride)

ClCH₂OCH₃ — written as $ClCH_2OCH_3$
(Methylchlorormet-hylether)

(2-(2-Thienyl)acetyl chloride)

HCl/CH₃OH — HCl/CH_3OH

Route 3

(7-Aminocephalosporanic acid)

(p-Toluenesulphonyl chloride)

$(H_5C_6)_2C = N^+ = N$
(Diphenyldiazomethane)

Removal of tosyl Group

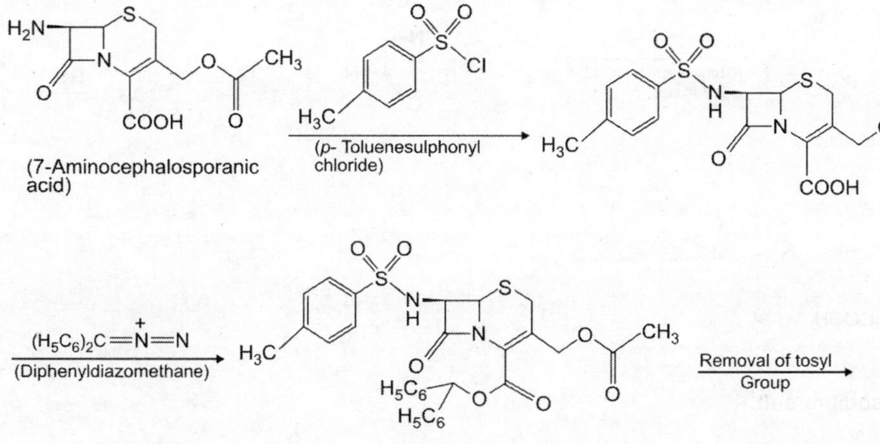

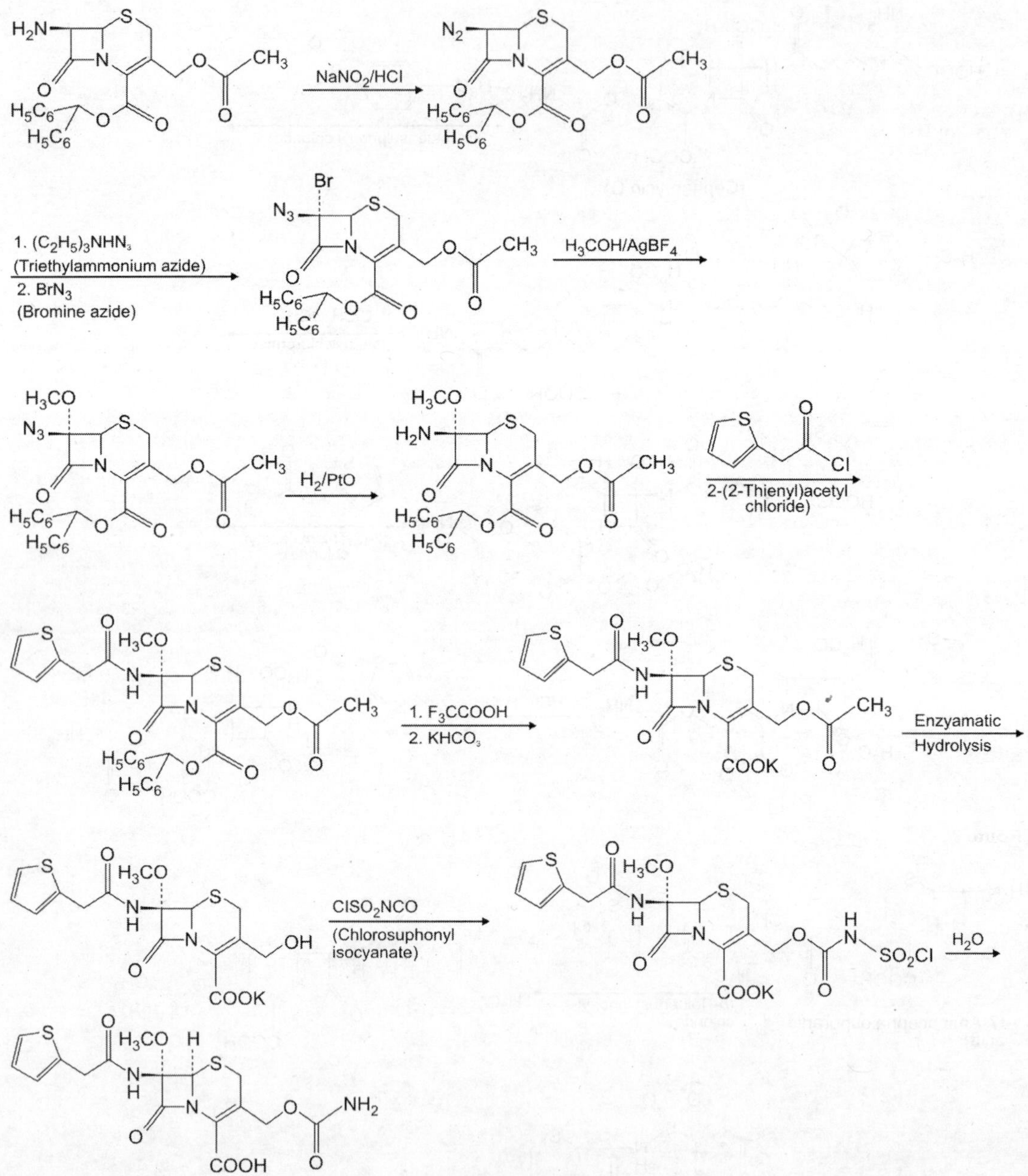

It is given orally as sodium salt.

Cefmetazole

(6R,7S)-7[[[(Cyanomethyl)thio]acetyl] amino]-7-methoxy-3-[[(1-methyl -1H-tetrazol-5-yl)thio]-methyl]-8-oxo-5-thia-1-azabicyclo[4.2.0]oct-2-ene-2-carboxylic acid

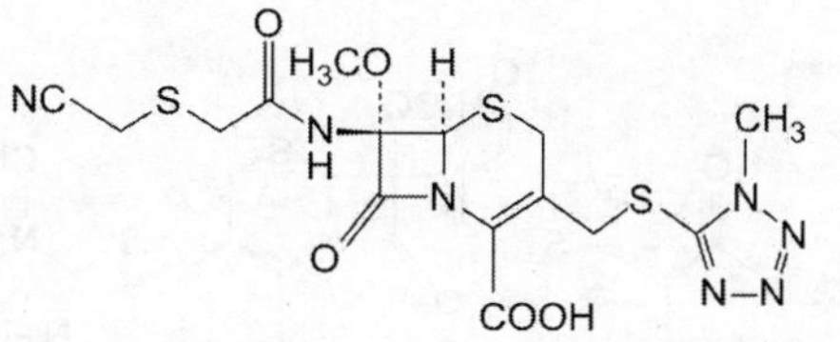

Synthesis

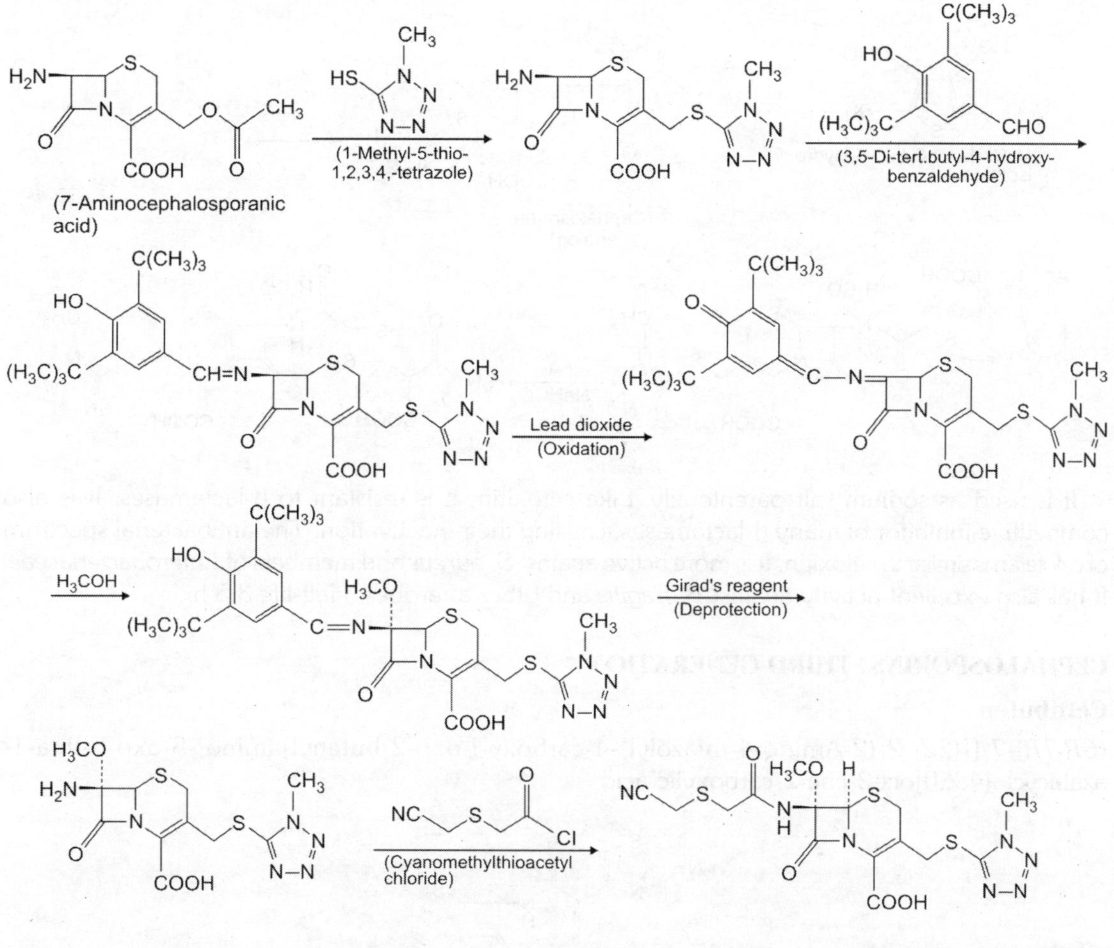

It is more active against members of *Enterobacteriaceae* family and β-lactamase producing strains and is administered as sodium salt parenterally.

Cefotetan

(6R,7S)-7-[[(4-(2-Amino-1-carboxy-2-oxoethylidene)-1, 3-dithietan-2-yl]carbonyl]-amino]-7-methoxy-3-[[(1-methyl-1H-tetrazol-5-yl)thio]methyl]-8-oxo-5-thia-1-azabicyclo[4. 2. 0]oct-2-ene-2-carboxylic acid

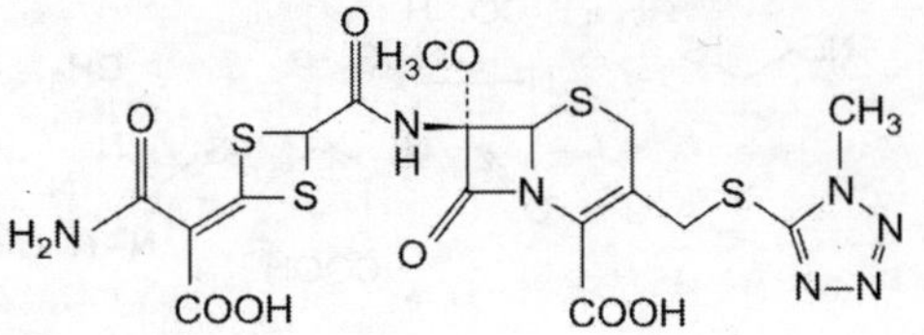

Synthesis

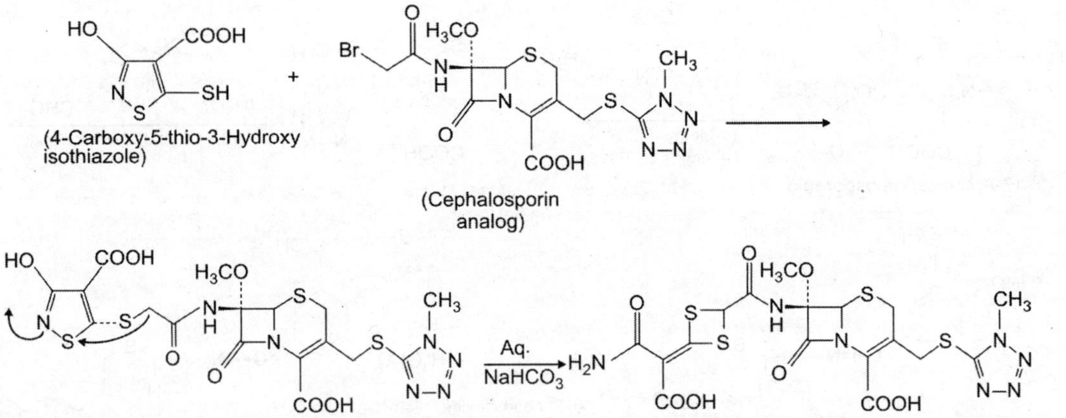

(4-Carboxy-5-thio-3-Hydroxy isothiazole)

(Cephalosporin analog)

It is used as sodium salt parenterally. Like cefoxitin, it is resistant to β-lactamases. It is also competitive inhibitor of many β-lactamases, causing their inactivation. The antibacterial spectrum of cefotetan is similar to cefoxitin. It is more active against *S. aureus* and members of *Enterobacteriaceae*. It has also excellent activity against *B. fragilis* and other anerobes. Half-life 3.5 hr.

CEPHALOSPORINS : THIRD GENERATION

Ceftibuten

(6R,7R)-7-[[(2Z)-2-(2-Amino-4-thiazolyl)-4-carboxy-l-oxo-2-butenyl]amino]-8-oxo-5-thia-1-azabicyclo[4.2.0]oct-2-ene-2-carboxylic acid

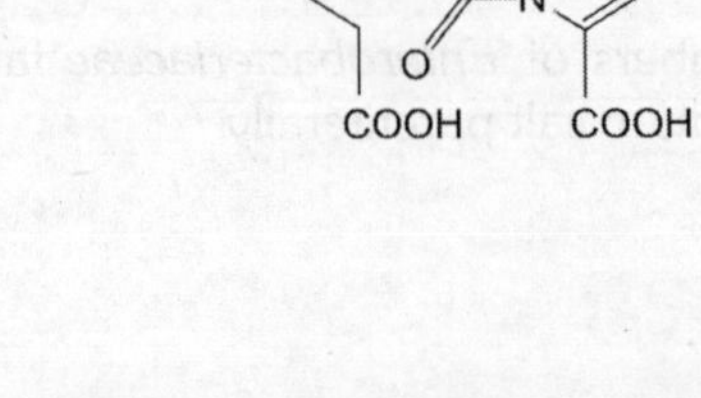

Synthesis

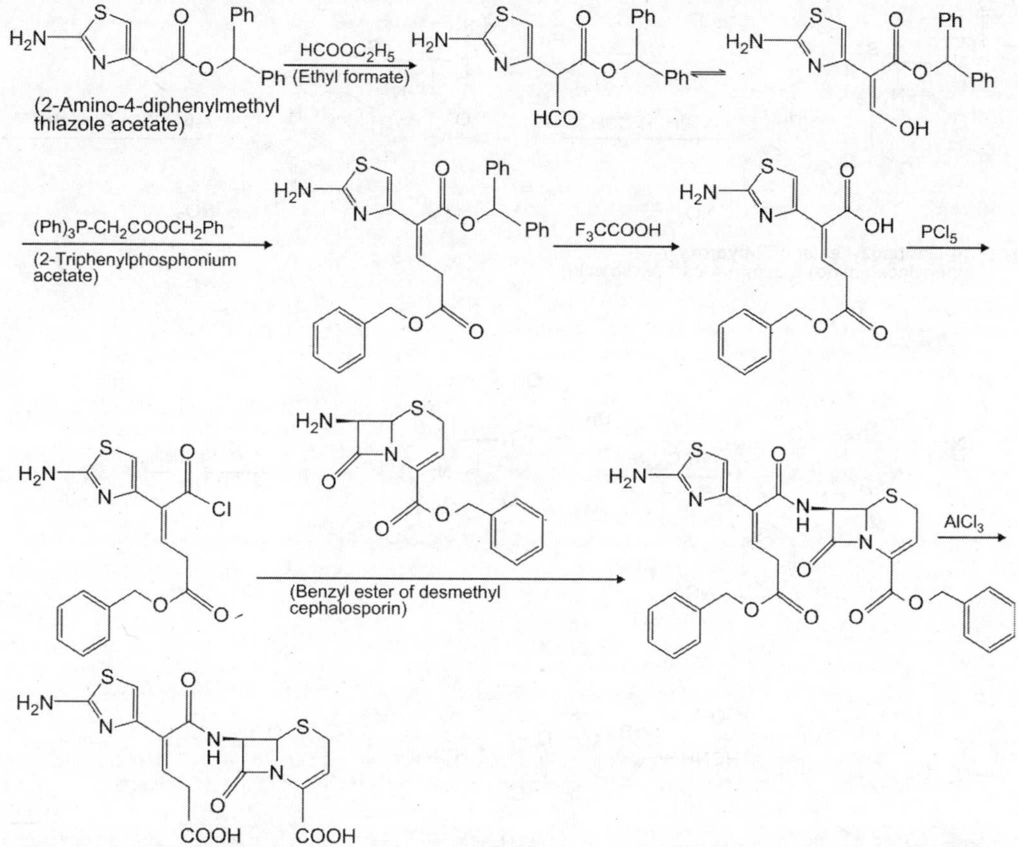

It is carbon analog of oximino-cephalosporin in which an oximino group has been replaced by methylene carbon. This replacement does not affect its activity particularly resistance to β-lactamases. It is orally active and is used for respiratory tract, urinary tract, and gynecological infections.

Ceftizoxime

(6R,7R)-7-[[[(2Z)-(2-Amino-4-thiazolyl)(methoxyimino) acetyl] amino]-8-oxo-5-thia-1-azabicyclo-[4.2.0]oct-2-ene-2-carboxylic acid

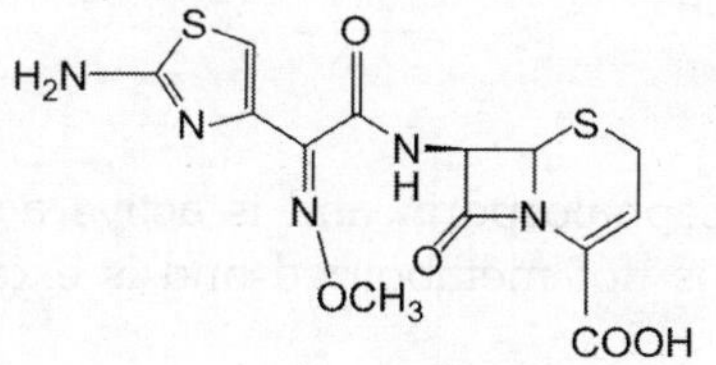

Synthesis

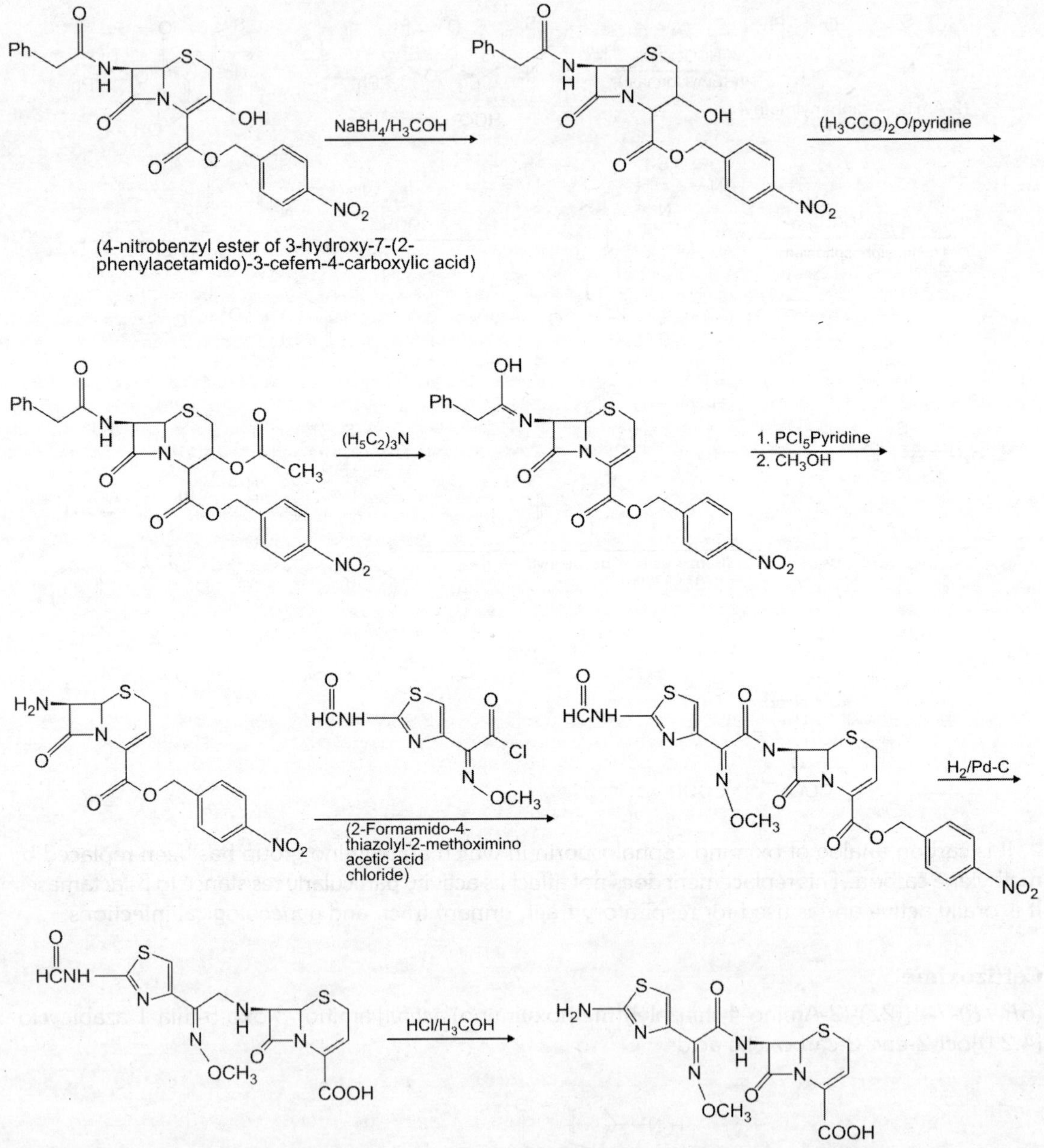

(4-nitrobenzyl ester of 3-hydroxy-7-(2-phenylacetamido)-3-cefem-4-carboxylic acid)

It is a β-lactamase resistant cephalosporin and is active against *Enterobacteria*, *E. coli*, *K. pneumoniae*, *aerogenes*, etc. It is not metabolized and is excreted as such. It is administered parenterally.

Cefotaxime

(6R,7R)-3-[(Acetyloxy) methyl]-7-[[(2Z)-2-amnio-4-thiazolyl)(methoxyimino)-acetyl]amino]-8-oxo-5-thia-1-azabicyclo[4. 2. 0.]oct-2-ene-2-carboxylic acid

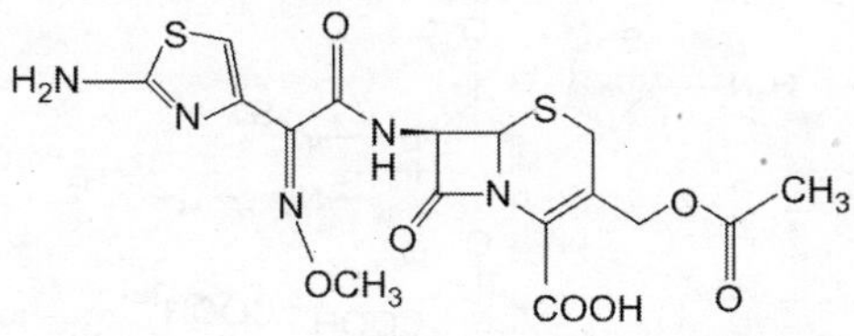

Synthesis

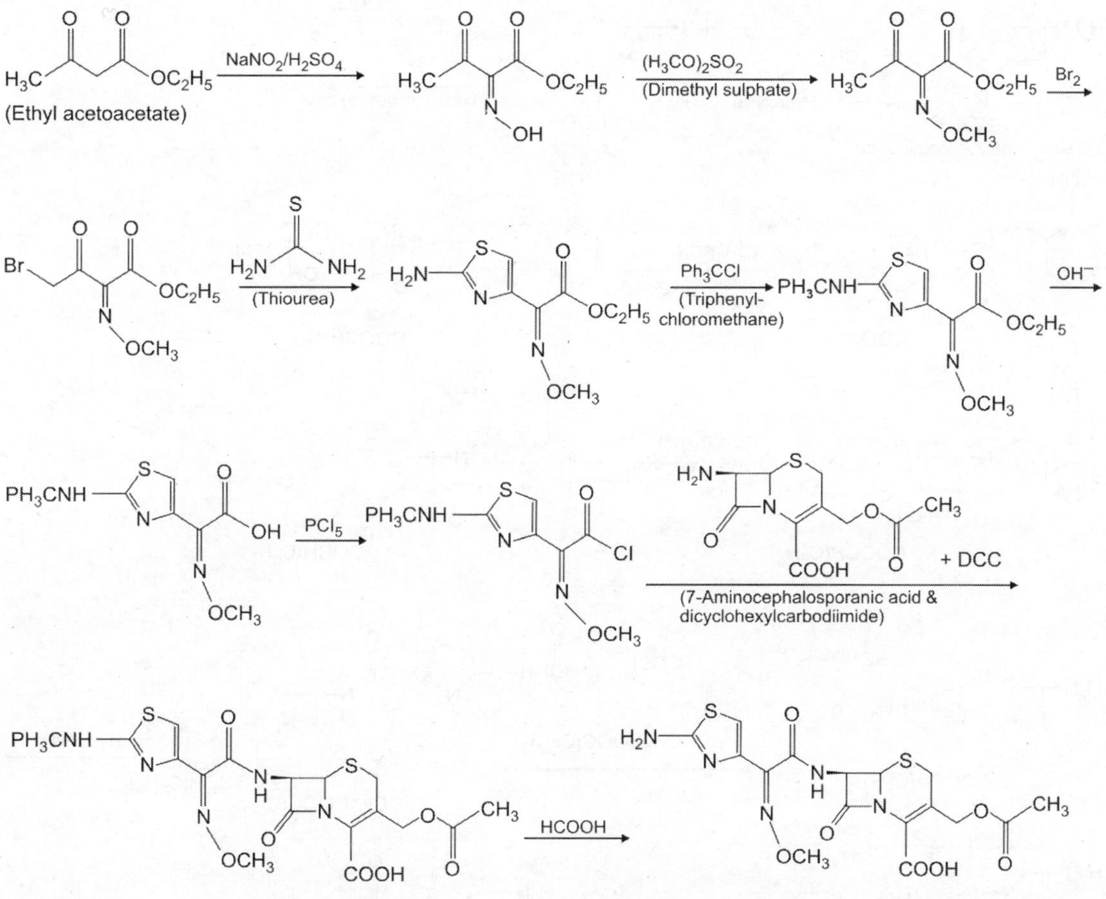

Cefotaxime has excellent Gram-positive and Gram-negative activity against both aerobic and anaerobic organisms. It is also active against β-lactamase producing microorganisms. The *syn*-isomer is more active than the *anti*-isomer. The greater potency of the *syn*-isomer is partly due to steric hinderance and partly due to greater affinity to PBP. It is adminstered parenterally.

Cefixime

(6R,7R)-7-[[(2Z)(2-Amino-4-thiazolyl)(carboxymethoxy) imino]acetyl]amino-3-ethenyl-8-oxo-5-thia-1-azabicyclo[4. 2. 0]oct-2-ene-2-carboxylic acid

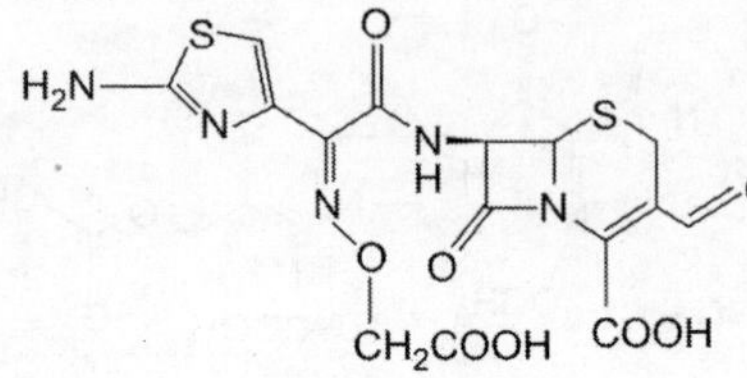

Synthesis

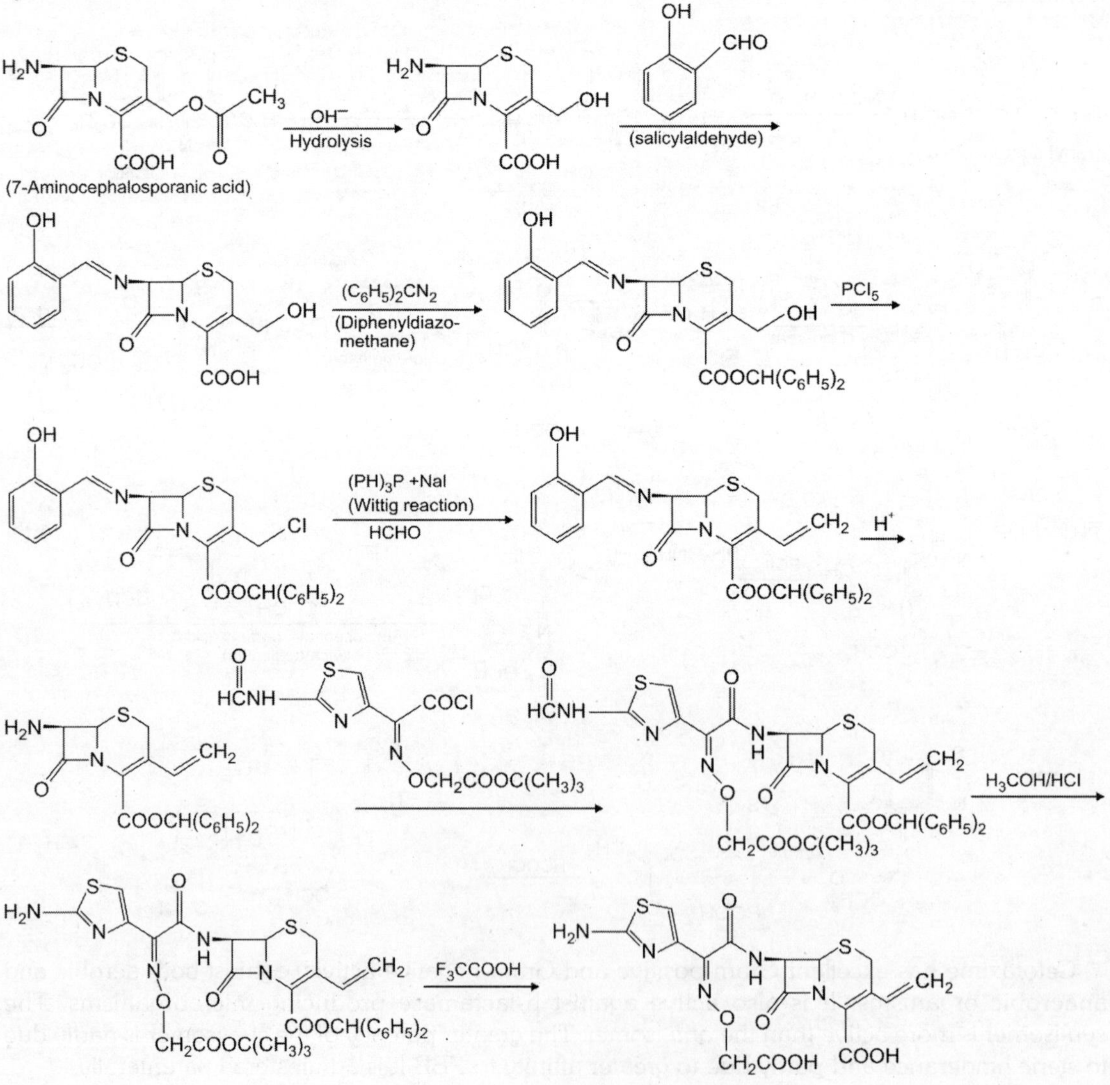

Cefixime is orally active third generation cephalosporin. It has good oral absorption (40-50%) and is a broad-spectrum cephalosporin that is resistant to β-lactamases. Effective against β-lactamase **producing microorganisms including** E. coli, Klebsiella species, Pseudomonas, Enterobacter, streptococci, gonococci, and influenzae. Half-life 3 to 4 hr.

Ceftazidime

1-[[(6R,7R)-7-[[(2Z)-(2-Amino-4-thiazolyl)][(1-carboxy-1-methylethoxy) imino] acetyl] amino]-2-carboxy-8-oxo-5-thia-1-azabicyclo[4. 2. 0]oct-2-en-3-yl]methylpyridium inner salt

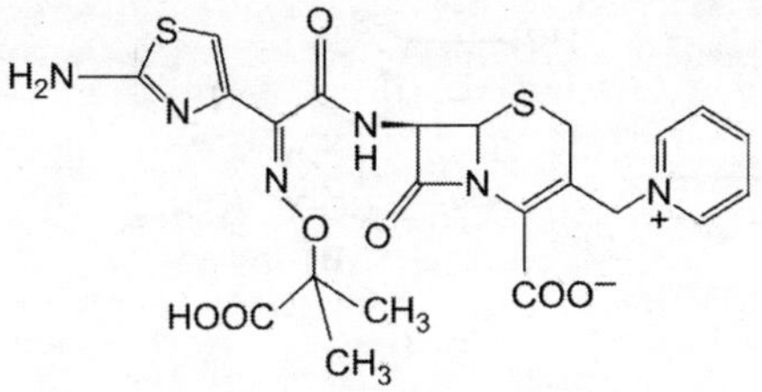

Synthesis

Step 1

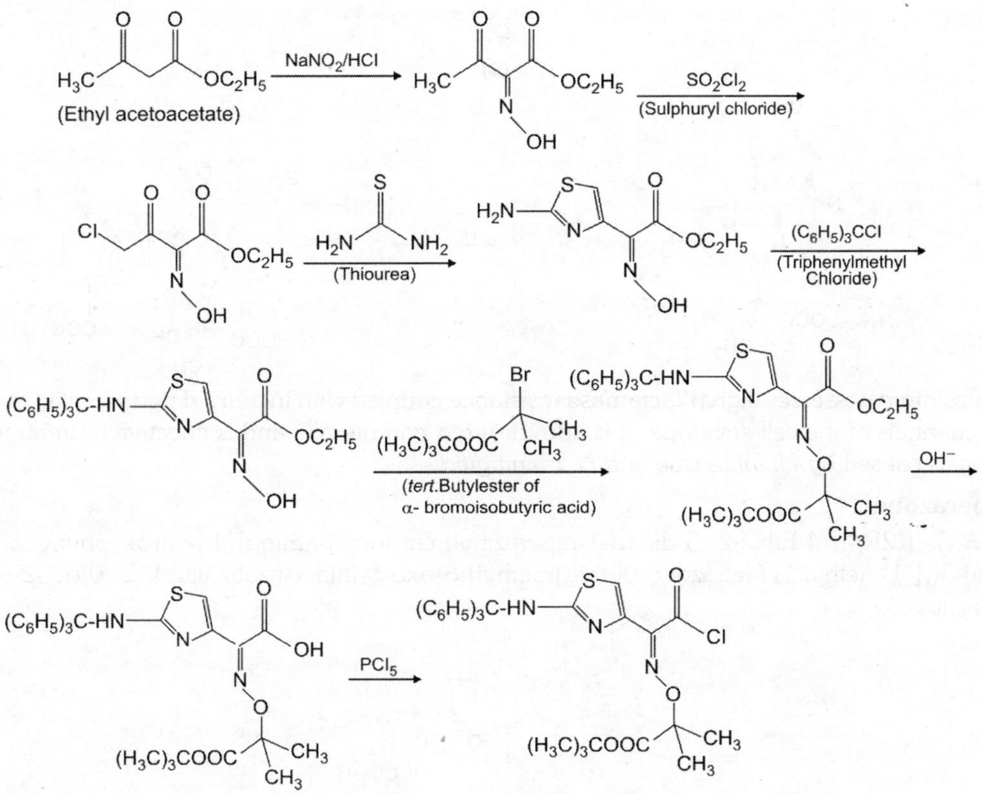

(A)

Step 2

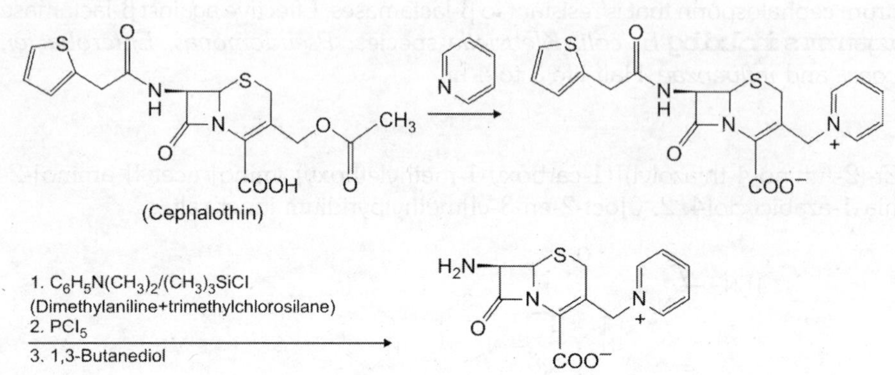

(Cephalothin)

1. $C_6H_5N(CH_3)_2/(CH_3)_3SiCl$
(Dimethylaniline+trimethylchlorosilane)
2. PCl_5
3. 1,3-Butanediol

Step 3

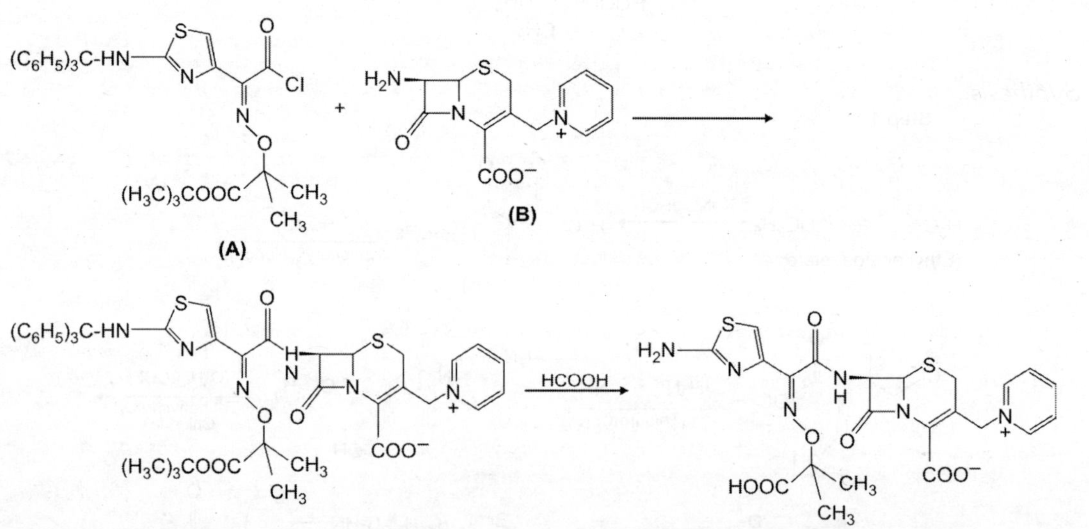

(B)

(A)

(B)

   Ceftazidime possesses high β-lactamase resistance coupled with increased permeability through porin channels of the cell envelope. It is administered parenterally and is effective in treatment of meningitis caused by *H. inluenzae* and *N. meningitidis.*

Cefoperazone

(6*R*,7*R*)-7-[[(2*R*)-[[(4-Ethyl-2, 3-dioxo-1-piperazinyl) carbonyl] amino](4-hydroxyphenyl)acetyl]-amino]-3-[[(1-methyl-1*H*-tetrazol-5-yl)thio]methyl]-8-oxo-5-thia-1-azabicylo[4. 2. 0]oct-2-ene-2-carboxylic acid

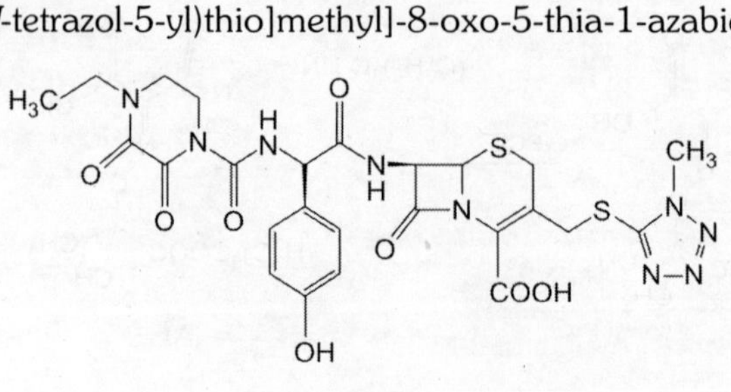

Synthesis

Step 1

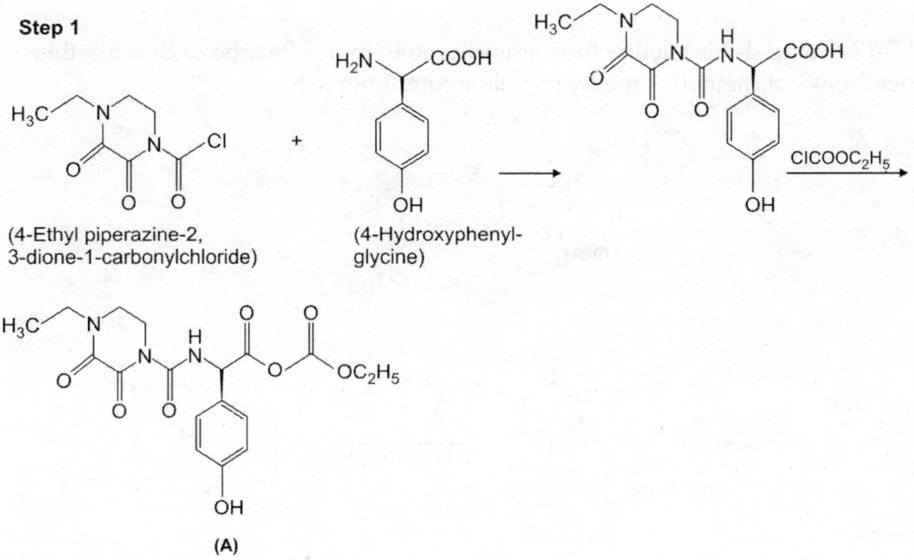

(4-Ethyl piperazine-2,
3-dione-1-carbonylchloride)

(4-Hydroxyphenyl-
glycine)

ClCOOC$_2$H$_5$

(A)

Step 2

(7-Aminocephalos-
poranic acid)

HCOCl
(Formylchloride)

HCl

(A)

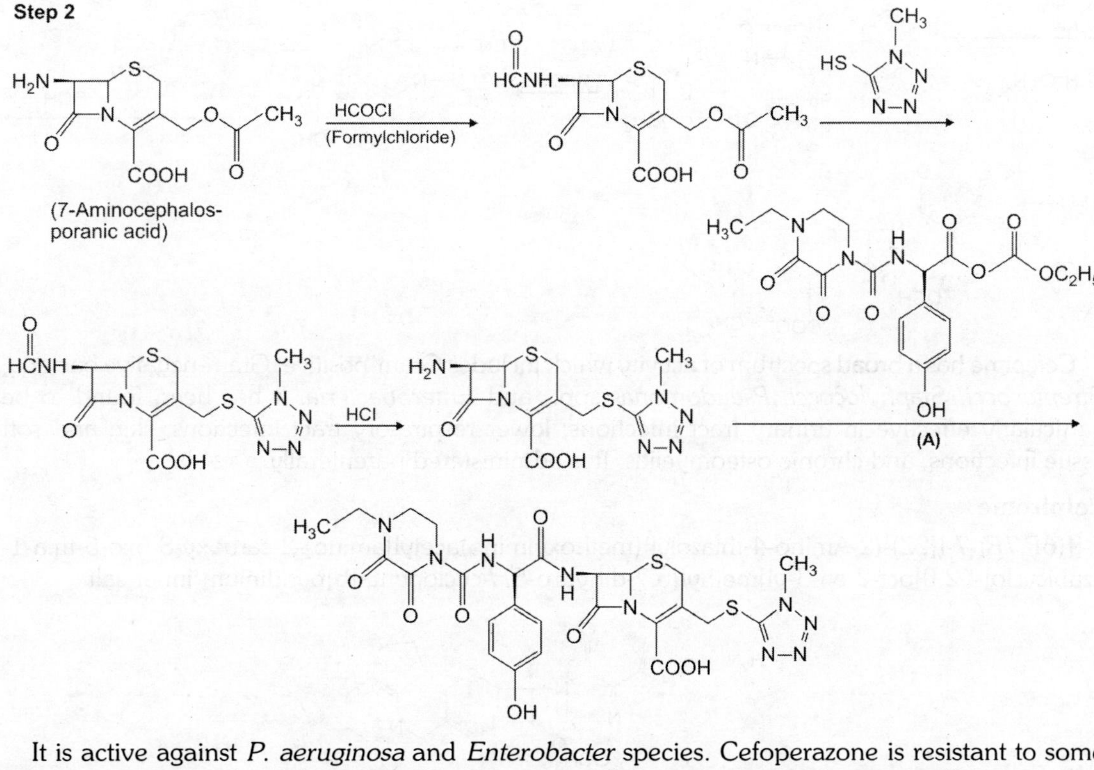

It is active against *P. aeruginosa* and *Enterobacter* species. Cefoperazone is resistant to some β-lactamases which hydrolyze penicillins but not to all. It is administered parenterally.

CEPHALOSPORINS : FOURTH GENERATION

Cefepime

1-[[[(6R,7R)-7-[[(2Z)-(2-Amino-4-thiazolyl)methoxyimino)acetyl]amino]-2-carboxy-8-oxo-5-thia-1-azabicyclo[4.2.0]oct-2-en-3-yl]methyl]-1-methylpyrrolidinium inner salt

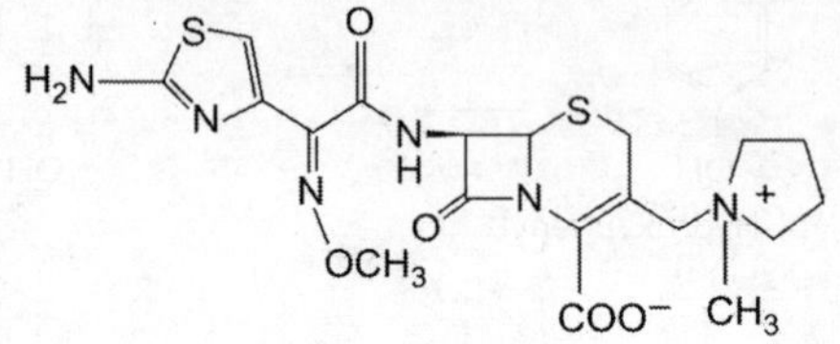

Synthesis

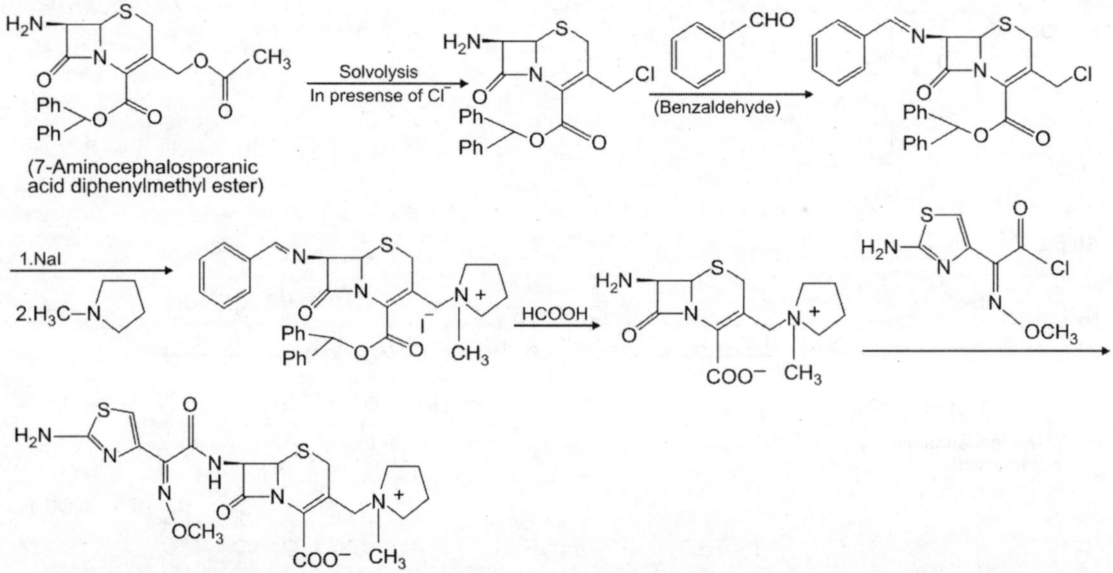

(7-Aminocephalosporanic acid diphenylmethyl ester)

Cefepime has a broad spectrum of activity which includes Gram-positive, Gram-negative bacteria, *Streptococci, Staphylococci, Pseudomonas* spp., and *Enterobacteria*. It has been found to be particularly effective in urinary tract infections, lower respiratory tract infections, skin and soft tissue infections, and chronic osteomyelitis. It is administered parenterally.

Cefpirome

1-[[[(6R,7R)-7-[[2Z)-(2-Amino-4-thiazolyl)(methoxyimino)acetyl]amino]-2-carboxy-8-oxo-5-thia-1-azabicyclo[4.2.0]oct-2-en-3-yl]methyl]6,7-dihydro-5H-cyclopenta[b]pyridinium inner salt

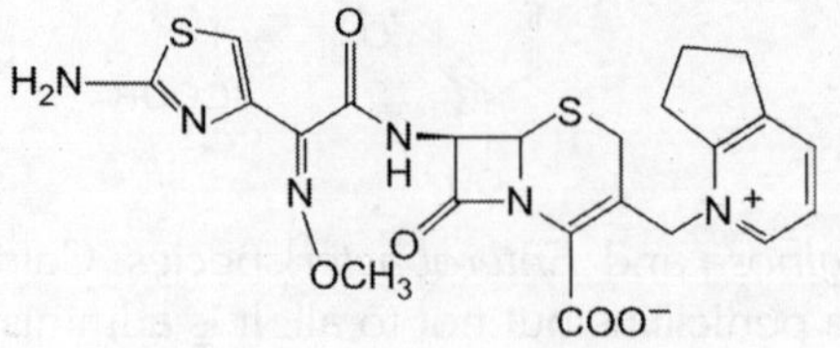

Synthesis

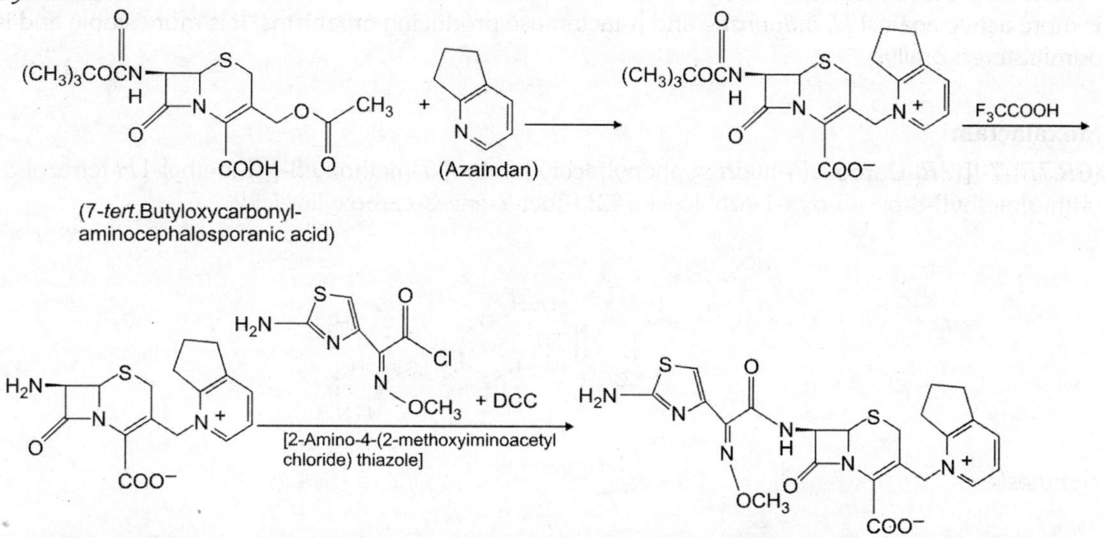
(CH3)3COCN
COOH
(Azaindan)
F3CCOOH
(7-tert.Butyloxycarbonyl-aminocephalosporanic acid)
+ DCC
[2-Amino-4-(2-methoxyiminoacetyl chloride) thiazole]
COO−

It has a broad spectrum of activity and is active against methicillin (12) resistant *Staphylococci*, penicillin resistant pneumococci, and β-lactamase producing strains of *E. coli*, *Enterobacter*, *Citrobacter*, and *Serratia* species. It is administered parenterally.

CARBACEPHEMS AND OXACEPHEMS

Loracarbef

(6*R*,7*S*)-7-[[(2*R*)-Aminophenylacetyl]amino]-3-chloro-8-oxo-1azabicyclo[4.2.0]oct-2-ene-2-carboxylic acid

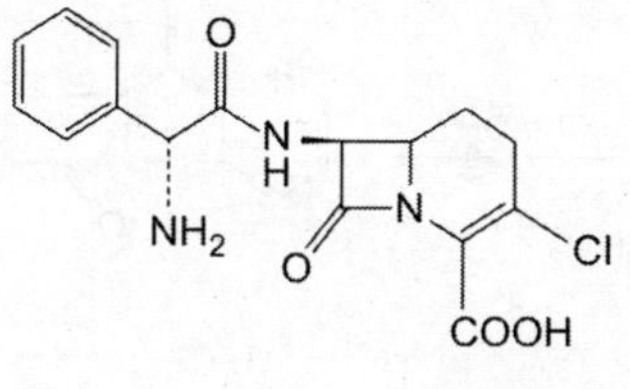

Synthesis

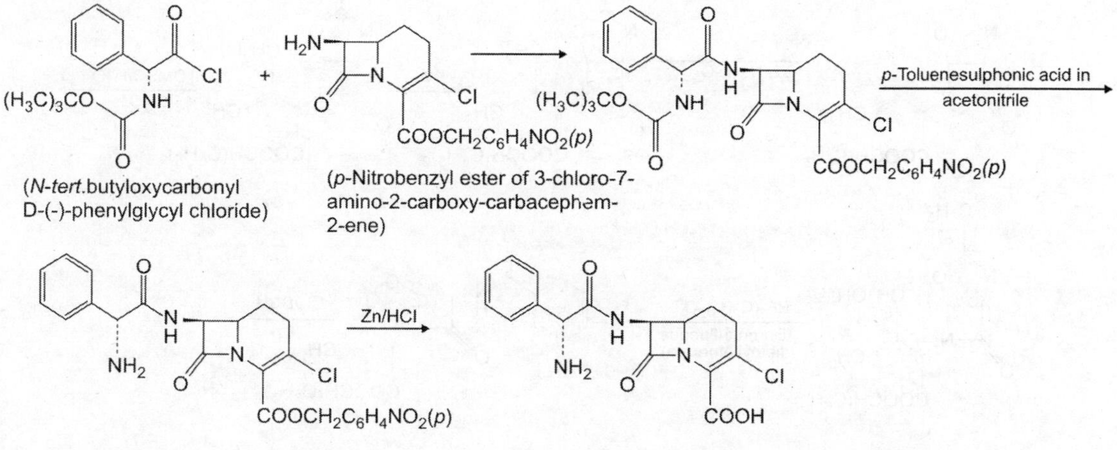
(N-tert.butyloxycarbonyl D-(-)-phenylglycyl chloride)
(p-Nitrobenzyl ester of 3-chloro-7-amino-2-carboxy-carbacephem-2-ene)
p-Toluenesulphonic acid in acetonitrile
COOCH2C6H4NO2(p)
Zn/HCl
COOH

Loracarbef is an isosteric analog of cefaclor and has similar antibacterial spectrum. However, it is more active against *H. influenzae* and β-lactamase producing organisms. It is more stable and is administered orally.

Moxalactam

(6R,7R)-7-[[(2R)-Carboxy(4-hydroxyphenyl)acetyl]amino]-7-methoxy-3-[[(I-methyl-1H-tetrazol-5-yl)thio]methyl]-8-oxo-5-oxa-1-azabicyclo[4.2.0]oct-2-ene-2-carboxylic acid

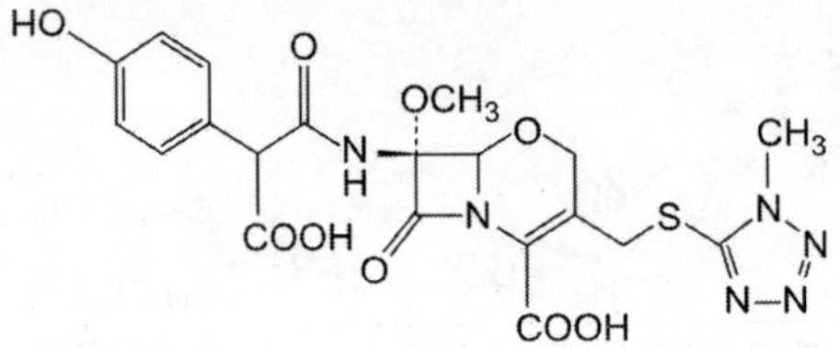

Synthesis

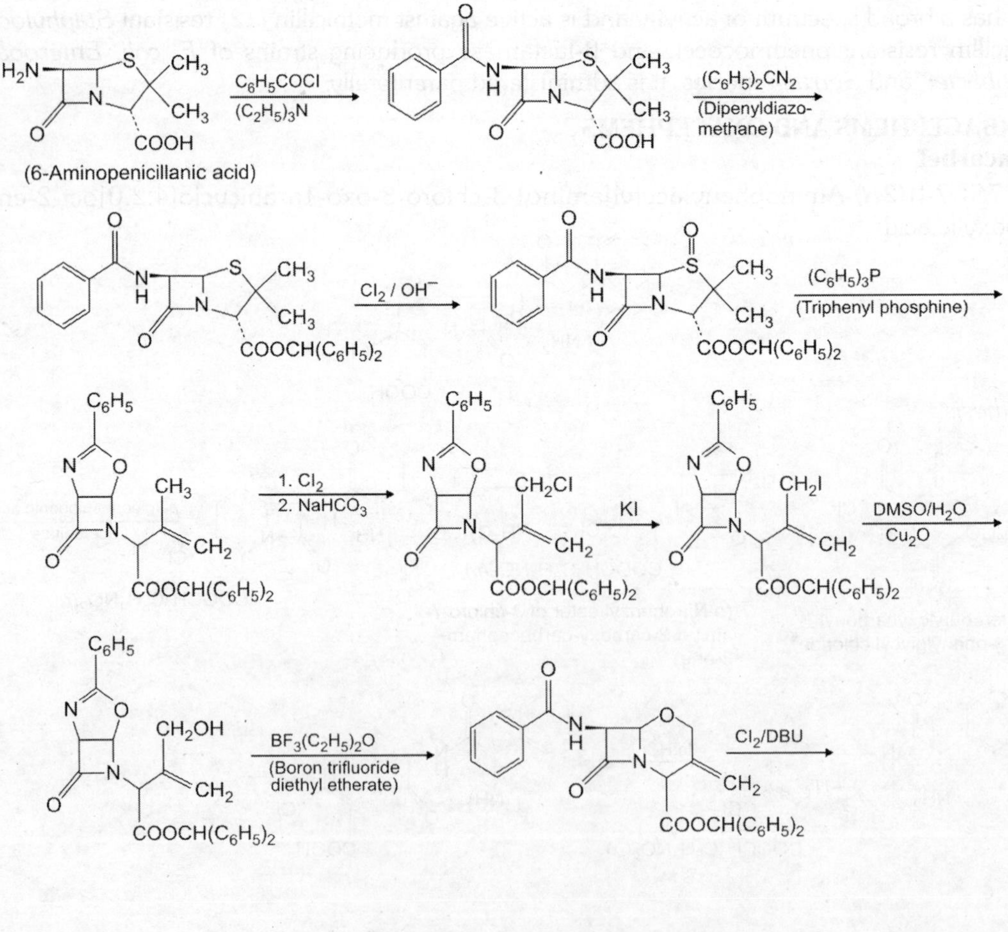

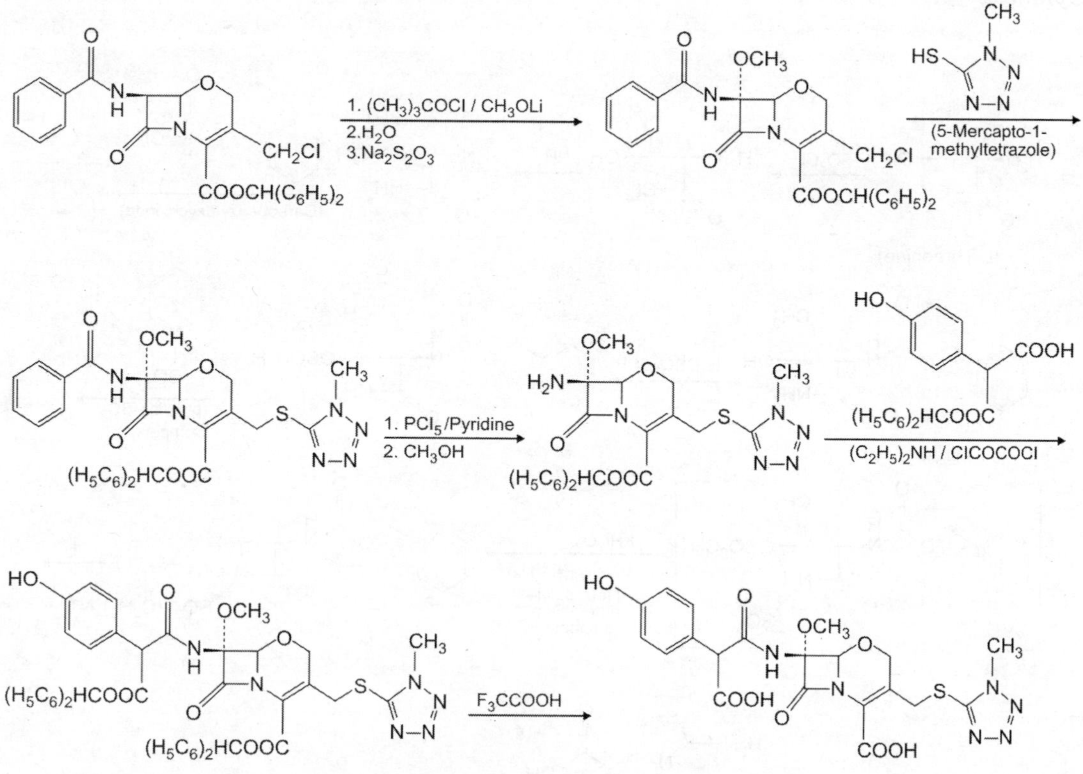

1. (CH₃)₃COCl / CH₃OLi
2.H₂O
3.Na₂S₂O₃

(5-Mercapto-1-methyltetrazole)

1. PCl₅/Pyridine
2. CH₃OH

(C₂H₅)₂NH / ClCOCOCl

F₃CCOOH

(DBU = 1,7-diazabicylo[4.5.0] undecene)

Moxalactam is active against many microorganisms which are resistant to various antibiotics such as penicillins (including semisynthetic penicillins), tetracyclines, cephalosporins, and aminoglycosides. It is also highly resistant to action of β-lactamase and penicillinase producing Gram-positive and Gram-negative microorganisms.

MONOBACTAMS
Aztreonam

[2S-[2α,3β(Z)]]-2-[[[1-(2-Amino-4-thiazolyl)-2-[(2-methyl-4-oxo-1-sulpho-3-azetidinyl)amino]-2-oxoethylidene]amino]oxy]-2-methylpropanoic acid

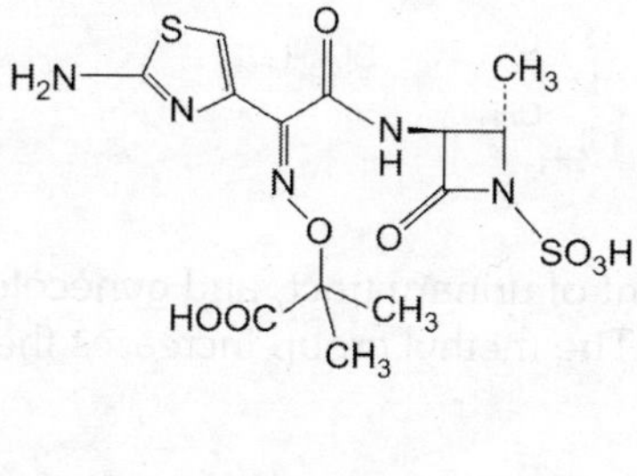

Synthesis

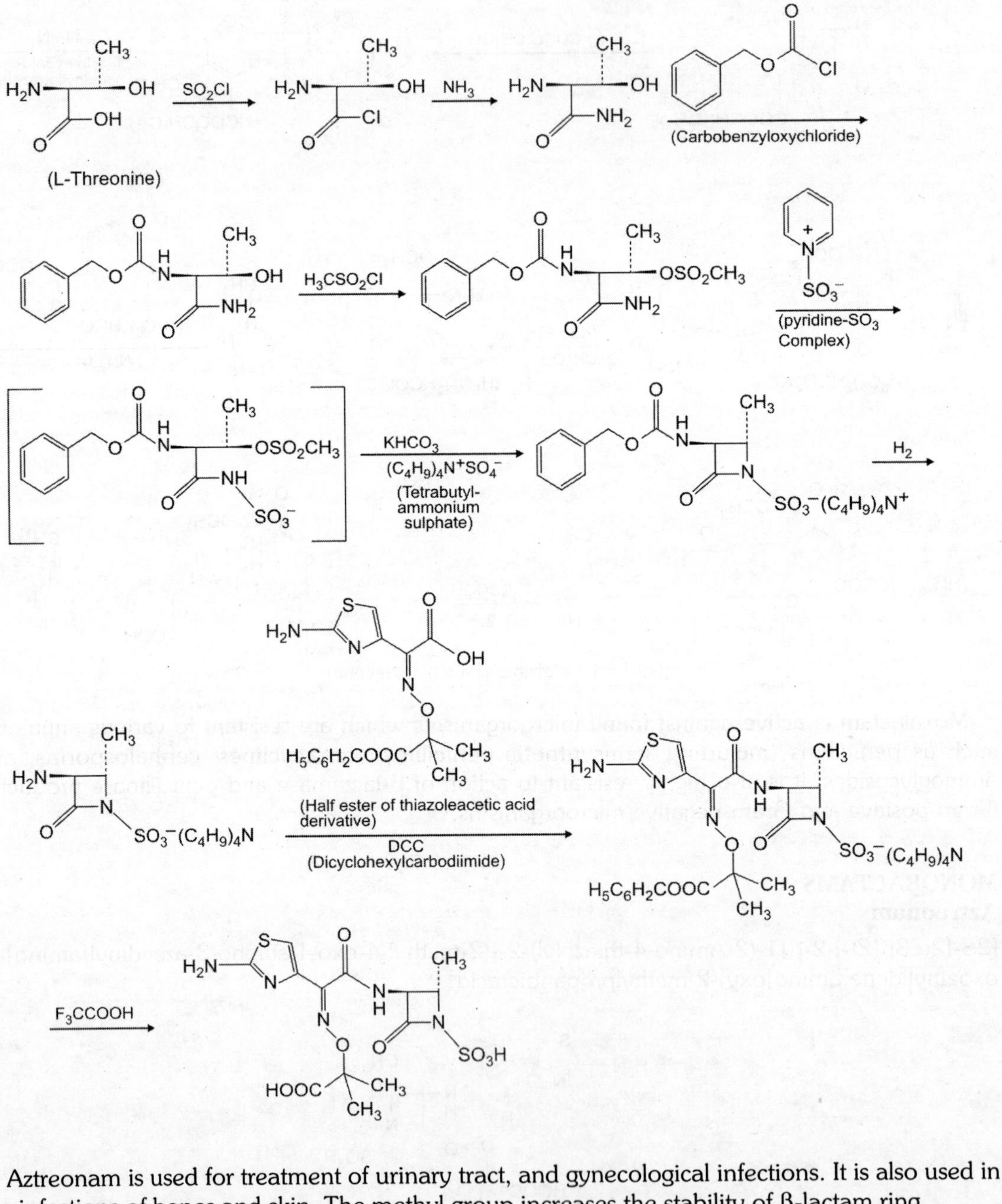

Aztreonam is used for treatment of urinary tract, and gynecological infections. It is also used in the infections of bones and skin. The methyl group increases the stability of β-lactam ring.

Tigemonam

[[(Z)-[1-(2-Amino-4-thiazolyl)-2-[[(3S)-2,2-dimethyl-4-oxo-1-(sulfooxy)-3-azetidinyl]amino]-2-oxoethylidene]amino]oxy]acetic acid

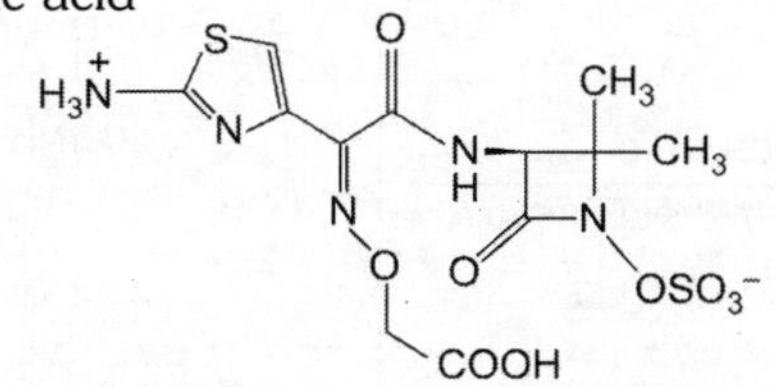

Synthesis

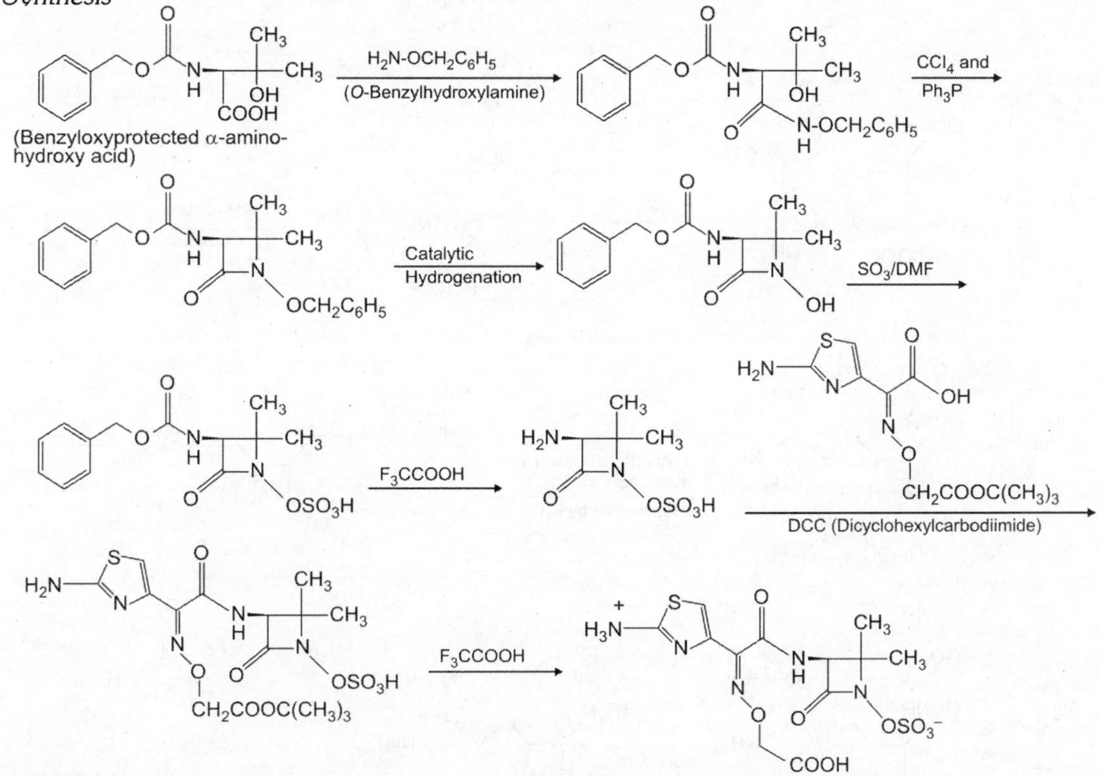

It has similar antibacterial spectrum as aztreonam (49). However, it is more active against *Enterobacter* species including *E. coli, Proteus, Serratia, Klebsiella,* and *Citrobacter.*

Carumonam

[[(Z)-[2-[[2S,3S)-2[[(Aminocarbonyl)oxy]methyl]-4-oxo-1-sulpho-3-azetidinyl]-amino]-1-(2-amino-4-thiazolyl)-2-oxoethylidene]amino]oxy]acetic acid

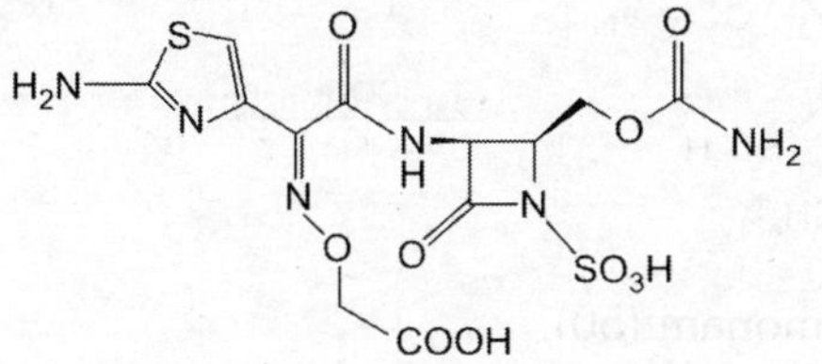

Synthesis

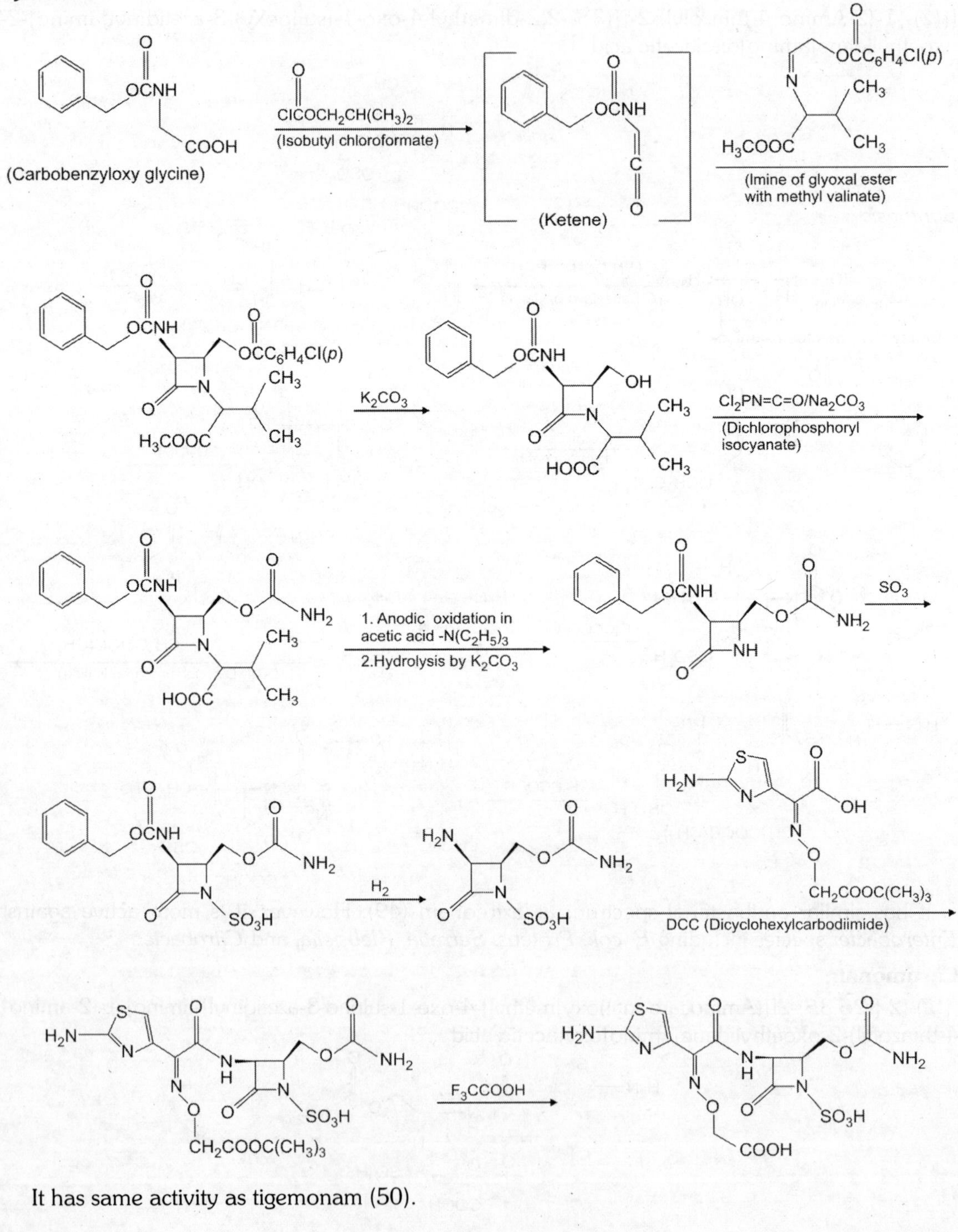

It has same activity as tigemonam (50).

PEPTIDE ANTIBIOTICS

SOME OF the bacterial species produce antibiotics which have been found to be cyclic peptides. In addition to natural amino acids, these cyclic peptides contain unnatural amino acids in D-configuration. Further in addition to the amino acids, these cyclic peptides may also contain a heterocyclic ring, fatty acids, or sugars, etc. Polypeptide antibiotics may be acidic, basic, or zwitterionic, depending on the number of free amino, carboxylic, or guanidino groups present in the molecule.

The peptide antibiotics are water soluble and highly lethal to susceptible microorganisms. They attach themselves to the bacterial cell wall/membrane and interfere with their semipermeability. This way the essential metabolites leak out and undesireable substances pass in. These antibiotics can be highly toxic to the host also.

The peptide antibiotics are used only for serious situations where there are few alternatives or for topical use. Microorganisms are rarely able to develop resistance to these agents. They are generally unstable so their solutions should be protected from heat, light, and extremes of pH.

INDIVIDUAL COMPOUNDS

Bacitracin

It is produced from a strain of *Bacillus subtilis*. It is a mixture of at least 9 bacitracins. The commercial product contains principally A (1) with smaller amounts of B, D, E, and F_1-F_3. Bacitracin is active against Gram-positive organisms. It inhibits mucopeptide cell wall synthesis.

(1)

Polymyxin

Polymyxin is produced by *B. polymyxia*. So far polymyxin B_1 (2), B_2 (3), D_1 (4), D_2 (5), and E_1 [colistin *A*, (6)] have been identified. Polymyxin B which is a mixture of polymyxin B_1 and B_2 is used as a sulphate salt. It is useful against Gram-negative microorganisms. Its main use is in topical applications against local infections in wounds and burns.

$$
\begin{array}{c}
\text{DAB} \rightarrow \text{D–X} \rightarrow \text{Y} \\[-2pt]
| \\[-2pt]
\gamma\text{-NH}_2 \\[-2pt]
\text{R} \rightarrow \text{DAB} \rightarrow \text{Thr} \rightarrow \text{Z} \rightarrow \text{DAB} \qquad \text{Thr} \leftarrow \text{DAB} \leftarrow \text{DAB} \\[-2pt]
| \qquad\qquad\qquad\qquad\qquad | \qquad\quad | \\[-2pt]
\gamma\text{-NH}_2 \qquad\qquad\qquad\qquad \gamma\text{-NH}_2 \ \gamma\text{-NH}_2
\end{array}
$$

	R	X	Y	Z
(2)	MOC	Phe	Leu	DAB
(3)	MHP	Phe	Leu	DAB
(4)	MOC	Leu	Thr	D-Ser
(5)	MHP	Leu	Thr	D-Ser
(6)	MOC	Leu	Leu	DAB

DAB=L-α,γ- Diaminobutryl
MHP=6-Methylheptanoyl
MOC=(+)-6-Methyloctanoyl

Teicoplanin

It is a mixture of five closely related peptide antibiotics namely A_2-1 (7), A_2-2 (8), A_2-3 (9), A_2-4 (10), and A_2-5 (11). These antibiotics are produced by *Actinoplanes teichomyceticus*. Teicoplanin

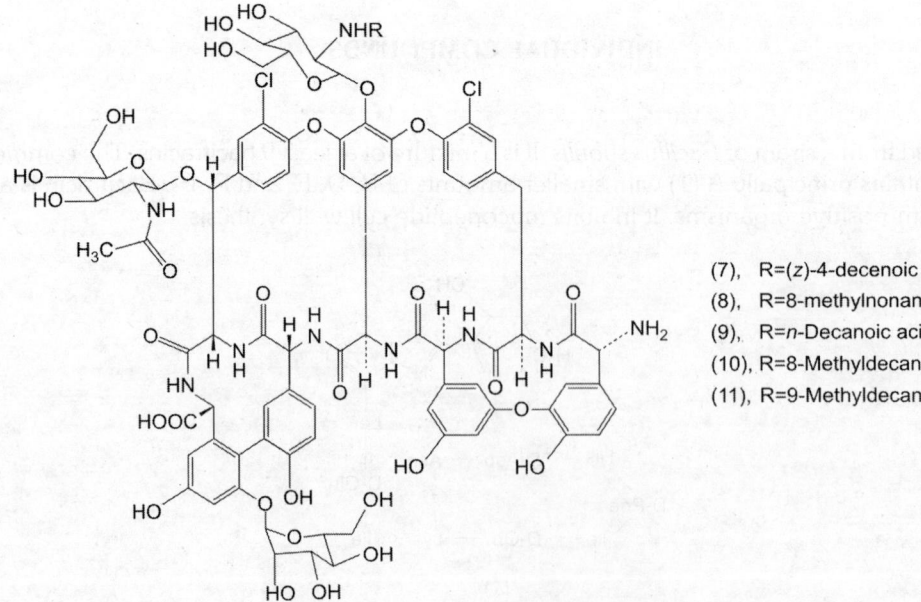

(7), R=(z)-4-decenoic acid
(8), R=8-methylnonanoic acid
(9), R=*n*-Decanoic acid
(10), R=8-Methyldecanoic acid
(11), R=9-Methyldecanoic acid

is active against Gram-positive organisms including *Staphylococci, Streptococci, Enterococci, Clostridium, Corynbacterium*, etc. It appears to impair the bacterial cell wall synthesis by complexing with D-ala-D-ala dipeptide of the peptidoglycan and preventing the cross-linking of the cell wall.

Vancomycin

It is a glycopeptide (12) obtained from *Streptomyces orientalis*. It is active against Gram-positive cocci particularly *Streptococci, Staphylococci*, and *Pneumococci*. It inhibits cell wall synthesis by preventing the synthesis of cell wall mucopeptide polymer.

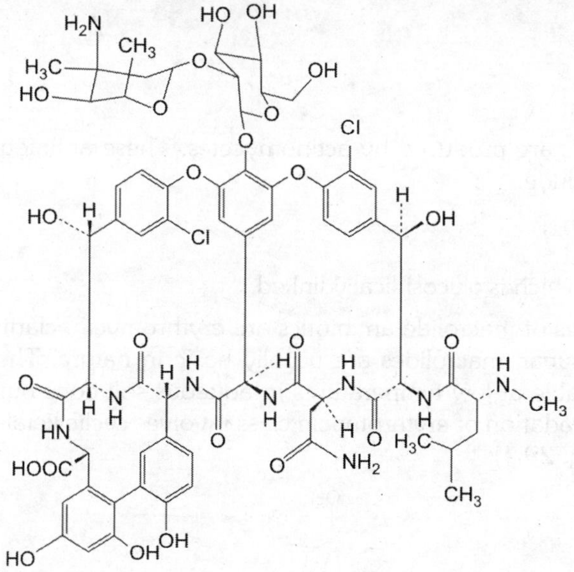

(12)

MACROLIDE ANTIBIOTICS

MACROLIDE ANTIBIOTICS are produced by actinomycetes. These antibiotics have three common features which include:

(a) a large lactone ring,
(b) a keto group, and
(c) an amino sugar which is glycosidically linked.

Some of the examples of macrolide antibiotics are erythromycin, clarithromycin, etc. Because of presence of amino sugar, macrolides are usually basic in nature. The free bases are slightly soluble in water and stable at low temperatures in aqueous solutions but get degraded in acids. The acid catalysed degradation of erythromycin class involves cyclic ketal formation which results in their inactivation (Fig. 29.1).

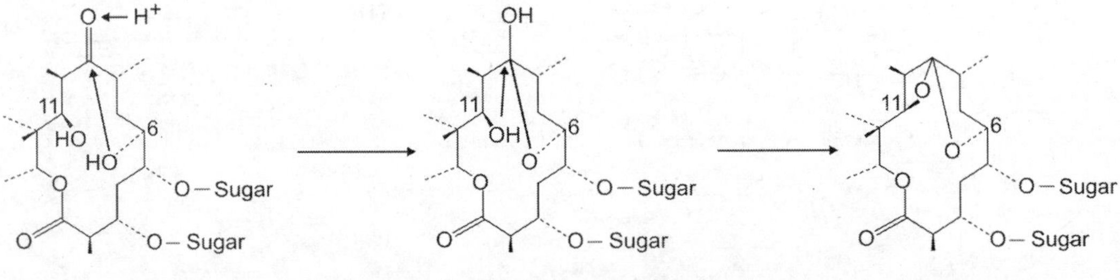

Fig. 29.1: Acid catalysed degradation of erythromycin class of antibiotics

Macrolide antibiotics are effective against Gram-positive bacteria, both cocci and bacilli, and Gram-negative cocci especially *Neisseria* species. Further they are active against penicillin resistant bacterial strains.

Mechanism of Action

The macrolides inhibit translocation of aminoacyl t-RNA following binding to 50S subparticle. As a result, the protein synthesis is blocked.

Resistance

Three mechanisms for the resistance to macrolides have been proposed and these include:

(a) decreased or poor binding of macrolide antibiotics,

(b) expulsion of the drug from the cell by some microorganisms, and

(c) lack of penetration of cell wall particularly in case of Gram-negative microorganisms.

INDIVIDUAL COMPOUNDS

Erythromycin

It is a mixture of erythromycin A(1), erythromycin B(2), and erythromycin C(3). The commercial preparation is mainly composed of erythromycin A(1). It is produced by fermentation using *Streptomyces erythraeus*.

	R	R'
(1)	OH	CH_3
(2)	H	CH_3
(3)	OH	H

Erythromycin Stearate

It is a stearic acid salt of erythromycin. It is acid labile and is film coated to protect it from acid degradation. In alkaline pH of the alimentary canal, it is hydrolysed to base erythromycin which is absorbed.

Erythromycin Ethylsuccinate

It is the ethyl succinate mixed ester involving the 2'-hydroxyl of desosamine. It is absorbed as such and slowly hydrolysed in the body.

Erythromycin Estolate

It is salt of 2'-propionate ester (desosamine) with lauryl sulphate. It is claimed to provide higher blood levels.

Clarithromycin

6-O-Methylerythromycin

It is obtained by methylation of 6-hydroxy group of erythromycin A(1). It is well absorbed following oral administration. It exhibits greater potency against *M. pneumoniae* and *H. influenzae*. It occurs as a white crystalline solid that is particularly insoluble in water and sparingly soluble in alcohol.

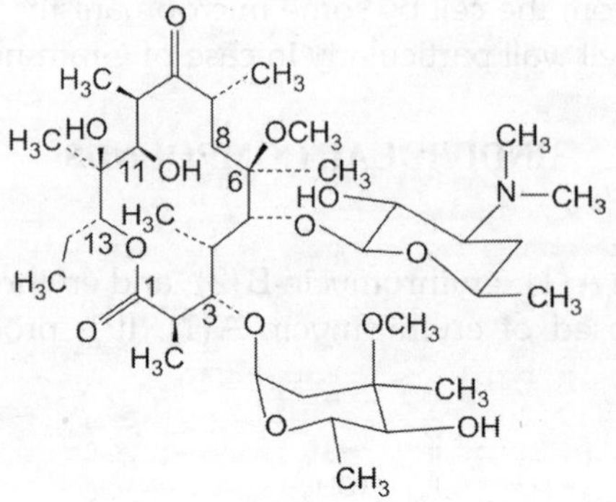

(4)

Troleandomycin and Oleandomycin

Troleandomycin (5) is the triacetyl derivative of oleandomycin (6). It is considered to have the same activity as erythromycin (1).Troleandomycin (5) is mainly used for upper respiratory tract infections caused by *S. pyogenes* and *S. pneumoniae*.

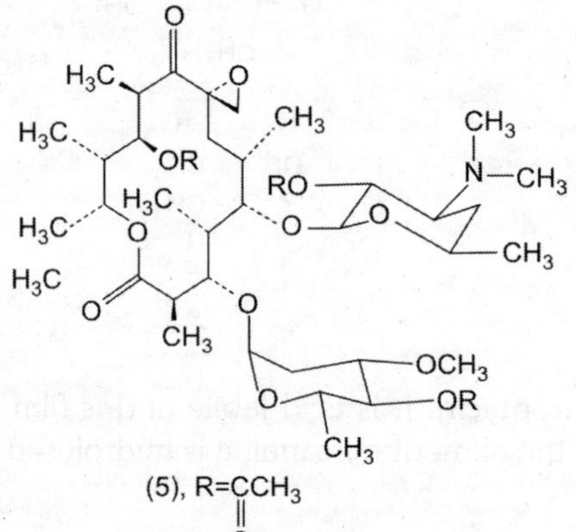

(5), R=CCH$_3$
         ‖
         O

(6), R=H

AMINOGLYCOSIDE ANTIBIOTICS

SOME of the aminoglycoside antibiotics include streptomycin, gentamicin, kanamycin, netilmicin, and spectinomycin. The various aminoglycoside antibiotics are all water soluble basic substances. They are not absorbed in significant amounts from gastrointestinal tract and they are given through parenteral routes. They do not cross blood-brain barrier and their plasma half-life is 2–3 hr. Elimination is through kidneys and about 50–60% of the dose is excreted unchanged within 24 hr. Since elimination is mostly through kidneys, if the renal function is impaired the drug may accumulate to toxic levels. The most important side effect of aminoglycoside antibiotics are damage to 8th cranial nerve and to kidneys.

Antibacterial Spectrum

The aminoglycoside antibiotics are effective against many aerobic Gram-negative and Gram-positive bacteria. The Gram–negative aerobes against which they are active include, *Proteus vulgaris, Pseudomonas aeruginosa, Escherichia coli, Acinetobacter sp., Citrobacter sp., Enterobacter sp., Klebsiella sp., Shigella sp., and Salmonella sp.* The Gram-positive aerobes against which they are active include *Staphyllococcus epidermis.*

Mechanism of Action

Aminoglycoside antibiotics are bactericidal. They inhibit protein biosynthesis by binding to 16S-ribosomal DNA portion of 30S-ribosomal subparticle. This results in impairment of proof-reading function of ribosomes. As a result there is mistranslation of RNA-template which results in wrong selection of amino acid and formation of what are known as non-sense proteins. Synthesis of these unnatural proteins results in upsetting of bacterial membrane function. Further, their presence destroys the semipermeability of the membrane resulting in increased permeation of aminoglycoside antibiotics which may result in complete inhibition of the protein synthesis. Although aminoglycoside antibiotics are highly polar, they are able to penetrate the bacterial cell wall by binding initially to lipopolysaccharides then diffusing into the cell in small amounts.

Resistance

Resistance to aminoglycoside antibiotics may arise from:

(a) production of enzymes (plasmid controlled) that inactivate the antibiotic by acylation, phosphorylation, or adenylation,

(b) prevention of drug access, and

(c) alteration of binding site on 30S so that drug does not bind.

INDIVIDUAL COMPOUNDS

Streptomycin and its Analogs

Streptomycin (1) is produced by *Streptomyces griseus*. It was introduced in 1943 for the treatment of tuberculosis. It is active against gram-positive and gram-negative bacteria. Streptomycin (1) is used as a valuable adjunct to other treatment modalities in tuberculosis. It is not absorbed when given orally and is administered through intramuscular route. The resistance to streptomycin (1) is due to *O*-acylation, *O*-phosphorylation, and *O*-adenylation of various functional groups.

The other analogs of streptomycin include dihydrostreptomycin (2) and hydroxystreptomycin (3).

(1), R = CHO, R' = CH$_3$

(2), R = CH$_2$OH, R' = CH$_3$

(3), R = CHO, R' = CH$_2$OH

It causes toxic effects on 8th cranial nerve resulting in loss of hearing.

Kanamycin

Kanamycin is a mixture of at least three components namely kanamycin A (4), kanamycin B (5), and kanamycin C (6) with kanamycin A predominating.

	R	R'
(4),	NH$_2$	OH
(5),	NH$_2$	NH$_2$
(6),	OH	NH$_2$

Kanamycin is usually used against intestinal infection (bacillary dysentery) and systemic infections arising from Gram-negative bacilli (*Klebsiella, Proteus, Enterobacter*) that have developed resistance to other antibiotics. Kanamycin is absorbed poorly when given orally so preferred route is intramuscular.

Amikacin

Amikacin (7) is a semisynthetic derivative of kanamycin A (4) and is obtained by the acylation of 1-amino group of desoxystreptamine by L-γ-amino-α-hydroxybutyric acid. This acylation prevents adenylation and phosphorylation of the amino sugar resulting in increased potency and enhanced spectrum of activity of amikacin (7). It is used for treatment of infections caused by *Mycobacterium tuberculosis* and severe infections caused by *Pseudomonas aeruginosa*. The L-isomer is more active than D-isomer.

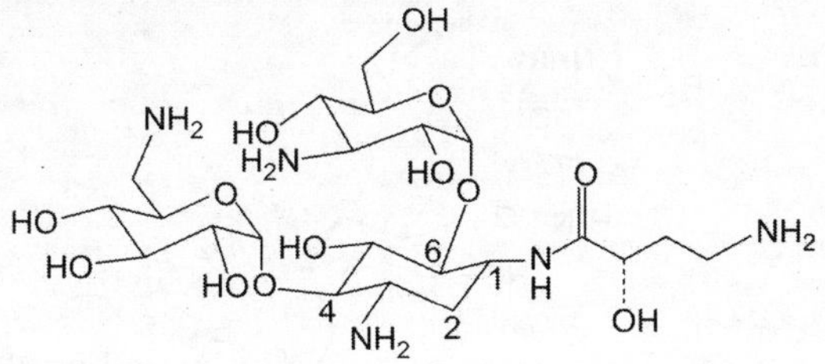

(7)

Paromomycin

Paromomycin consists of two fractions namely paromomycin I (8) and paromomycin II (9). It has broad-spectrum antibacterial activity and is used for the treatment of gastrointestinal infections caused by *Salmonella* and *Shigella* species. It is mainly used for the treatment of intestinal amoebiasis.

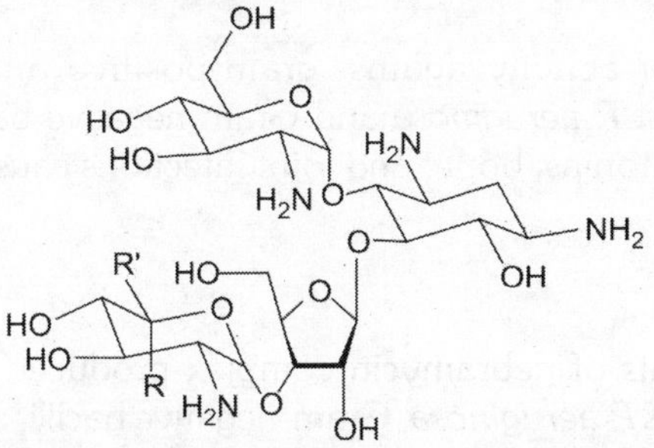

	R	R'
(8),	CH_2NH_2	H
(9),	H	CH_2NH_2

Neomycin

Neomycin is a mixture of three components namely neomycin A, neomycin B, and neomycin C with neomycin B (10) predominating. It is obtained by fermentation process using *Streptomyces fradiae*.

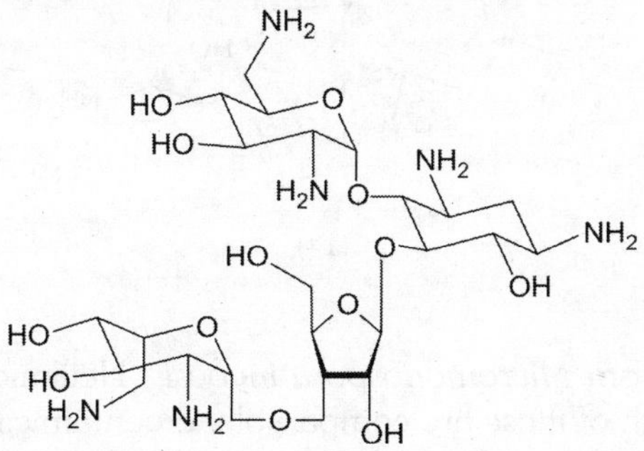

(10)

It is used in *E. coli* infections. Neomycin is considered as one of the useful antibiotics for gastrointestinal and dermatological infections. It has a broad-spectrum of activity against a variety of organisms and low incidence of hypersensitivity. Further, development of resistance is also rare.

Gentamicin

Commercially, it is obtained using *Micromonospora purpurea*. Gentamicin is a mixture of gentamicin C_1 (11), gentamicin C_2 (12), and gentamicin C_{1a} (13).

(11), R = R' = CH_3
(12), R = CH_3, R' = H
(13), R = R' = H

Gentamicin has a broad-spectrum of activity against gram-positive and gram-negative microorganisms. It has high activity against *P. aeruginosa* and Gram-negative bacilli. It is used for urinary tract infections, burns, some pneumonias, bone, and joint infections caused by susceptible Gram-positive bacteria.

Tobramycin

Tobramycin (14) is one of the components of nebramycin complex produced by *Streptomyces tenebrarius*. It is used against most strains of *P. aeruginosa*, Gram-negative bacilli, and *staphylococci*.

(14)

Sisomicin and Netilmicin

Sisomicin (15) is obtained from *Micromonospora inyoesis*. Netilmicin (16), is the semisynthetic analog of sisomicin (15). Both of these are comparable to gentamicin in activity against strains of *Enterobacter*, *P. aeruginosa*, and *S. aureus*. Netilmicin (16) is also active against many strains which are resistant to gentamicin. This is attributed to resistance to inactivation of netilmicin by the enzymes which adenylate or phosphorylate gentamicin and sisomicin (15). This perhaps is due to introduction of ethyl group in sisomicin (15) which results in lower affinity of netilmicin (16) to these inactivating enzymes.

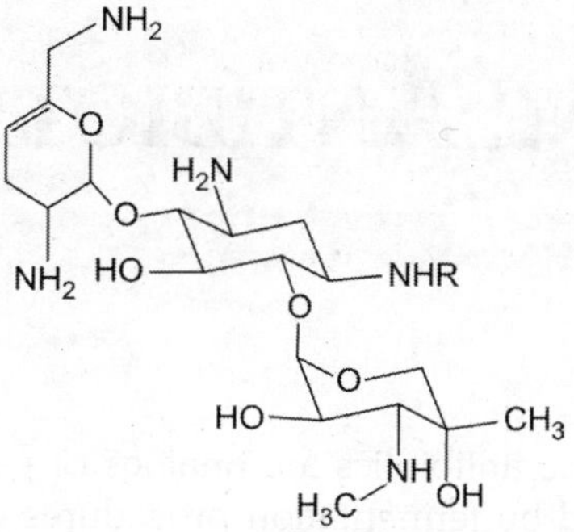

(15), R=H;   (16), R=C_2H_5

Spectinomycin

Spectinomycin (17) is produced by *Streptomyces spectabilis*. It is an aminocyclitol antibiotic which is a broad-spectrum antibiotic and active against gram-positive and gram-negative bacteria. It exerts bacteriostatic action and is inferior to other aminoglycoside antibiotics.

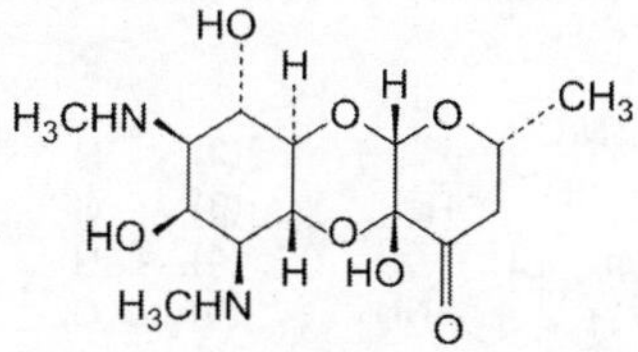

(17)

TETRACYCLINE ANTIBIOTICS

THE BROAD-SPECTRUM tetracycline antibiotics are analogs of partially reduced naphthacene (1). These antibiotics are obtaind by fermentation procedures using *Streptomyces* species or by chemical transformations of natural products. Some of these constitute tetracycline (2), chlortetracycline (3), oxytetracycline (4), demeclocycline (5), doxycycline (6), minocycline (7), sancycline (8), methacycline (9), meclocycline (10), and rolitetracycline (11).

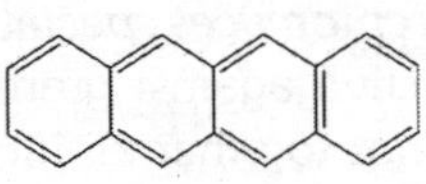

(1)

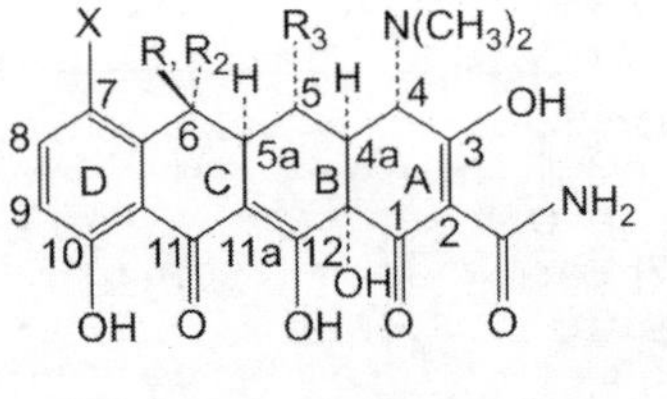

	X	R_1	R_2	R_3
(2)	H	OH	CH_3	H
(3)	Cl	OH	CH_3	H
(4)	H	OH	CH_3	OH
(5)	Cl	OH	H	H
(6)	H	H	CH_3	OH
(7)	$N(CH_3)_2$	H	H	H
(8)	H	H	H	H

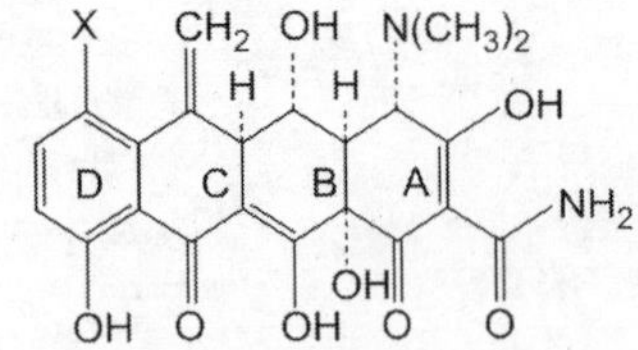

(9), X=H;   (10), X=Cl

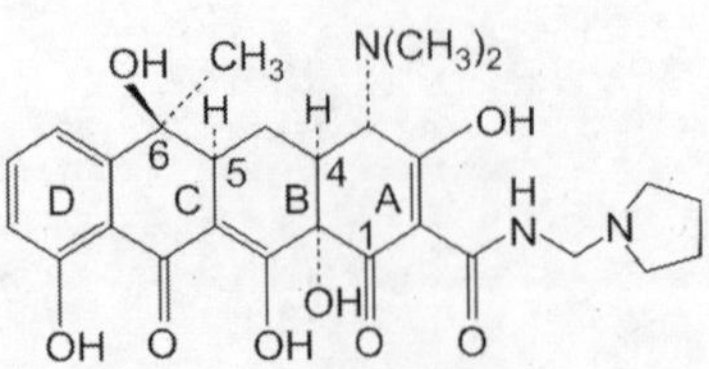

(11)

800

The carbon atoms 4, 4a, 5, 5a, 6, and 12a are potentially chiral depending upon the substitution. Thus, oxytetracycline (4) and doxycycline (6), each having 5α-hydroxyl have six asymmetric carbon atoms, while others possess only five asymmetric carbon atoms.

Tetracyclines are amphoteric in nature with three pKa values and these are:

(*a*) pKa_1 of 2.8—3.3 due to conjugated trione system (C_1 to C_3),
(*b*) pKa_2 of 7.2—7.8 due to phenolic-enone system (C_{10}-C_{12}),
(*c*) pKa_3 of 9.1—9.7 due to diethylamino group (C_4).

Tetracyclines undergo epimerization at C_4 in solutions of intermediate pH range. These isomers are called epi-tetracyclines. Under acidic conditions an equilibrium is established. The 4-epi-tetracyclines possess much less activity than the natural tetracyclines. Tetracyclines with *tert*-hydroxyl at postion 6 undergo dehydration with strong acids and bases, involving α-hydrogen at 5a position. This results in shift of double bond between 11a and 12 (12) to 11-11a (13) to form a stable naphthalene system. These anhydro-products (12) and (13) are inactive.

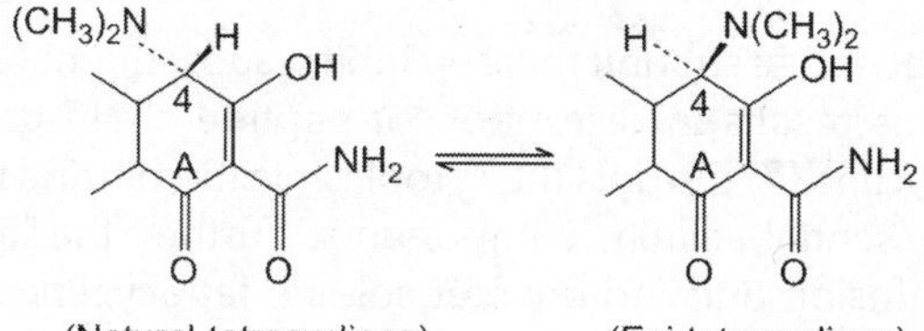

(Natural-tetracyclines)　　　(Epi-tetracyclines)

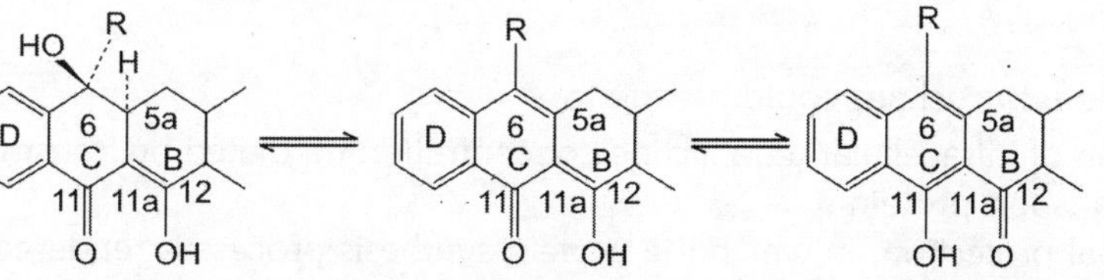

(12)　　　　　　　　(13)

Tetracyclines form stable chelates with metals including calcium, magnesium, aluminium, and iron. Such chelates are insoluble. This results in impaired absorption of tetracyclines in presence of milk, calcium, magnesium, aluminium, and antacids. Tetracyclines have affinity for calcium. This affinity results in deposition of tetracyclines in newly formed bones and teeth.

Structure-activity Relationship

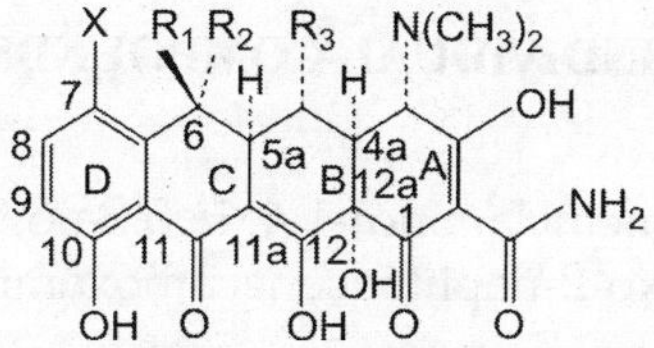

(*a*) For activity, derivatives with less than four rings are inactive.
(*b*) Any drastic change in the substitution at carbons 1, 2, 3, 4, 10, 11, 11a and 12 results in loss of activity.
(*c*) Substituents in ring A can be modified slightly. For good activity, the substituents at carbon 1, 2, 3 must be intact.

(d) Replacement of amide function at C-2 reduces or abolishes the activity.

(e) Aminoalkylation of amide nitrogen [rolitetracycline, (11)] results in more water soluble derivatives.

(f) The dimethylamino group at C-4 should have α-orientation, the 4-epi-analogs are much less active.

(g) A *cis* A/B ring fusion with α-OH at 12a is essential for activity.

(h) The enolizable β-diketone moiety of C_{11}-C_{11a}-C_{12} seems to be essential.

(i) Substituents at carbons 5, 5a, 6, 7, 8 and 9 can be changed or modified resulting in retention and sometimes improvement in activity.

(j) Hydroxyl group at carbon 5 leads to better antimicrobial activity, examples, oxytetracycline (4) and doxycycline (6).

(k) Electron withdrawing groups at carbon 7 (chloro) and strong electron donating groups (dimethylamino) at carbon 7 enhance the activity, examples, chlortetracycline (3), demeclocycline (5), and minocycline (7).

Mechanism of Action

Tetracyclines bind to 30S ribosomal subunit thereby inhibit subsequent binding of aminoacyltransfer RNA to the ribosomes. This results in disruption of peptide chain growth. The more lipophilic tetracyclines such as minocycline (7) disrupts the cytoplasmic membrane function resulting in leakage of nucleotides and other essential cellular components. Further, the lipophilic tetracyclines enter bacterial cell by passive diffusion and more water soluble tetracyclines enter through water-lined protein porin routes.

Resistance

The resistance to tetracyclines could be due to:

1. Reduction of intracellular tetracycline concentration mediated by transmembrane-spanning active transport protein.

2. Ribosomal protection, in which the protein synthesis process is rendered resistant to action of tetracycline.

Spectrum of Activity

Tetracyclines have broadest spectrum of activity. They are active against whole range of Gram-positive, Gram-negative, spirochetes, mycoplasma, rickettesia, and chlamydiae.

Because of incomplete absorption, their effetiveness against natural bacterial flora of intestines may result in superinfection caused by *Candida albicans*.

INDIVIDUAL COMPOUNDS

Tetracycline

[4S-(4α,4aα,5aα,6β,12aα)]-4-(Dimethylamino)-1,4,4a,5,5a,6,11,12a-octahydro-3, 6, 10, 12, 12a-pentahydroxy-6-methyl-1, 11-dioxo-2-naphthacenecarboxamide

Synthesis

(Chlortetracycline)

Commercially, it is obtained by controlled hydrogenolysis of chlortetracycline (3) in which process the 7-chloro group is removed. It is also obtained by fermentation process utilizing *Streptomyces aureofaciens*.

It is stable in acid solutions with a pH above 2. It is more stable than chlortetracycline (3) in alkaline solution but like other tetracyclines, they lose potency.

Tetracycline gives higher plasma concentration than oxytetracycline (4) or chlortetracycline (3). It is also found in in higher concentration in spinal fluid than other tetracyclines. Food and milk lower the blood levels.

Chlortetracycline Hydrochloride

[4S-(4α,4aα,5aα,6β,12aα)]-7-Chloro-4-dimethylamino-1,4,4a,5,5a,6,11,12a-octahydro-3, 6, 10, 12, 12a-pentahydroxy-6-methyl-1,11-dioxo-2-naphthacenecarboxamide hydrochloride

It is obtained by fermentation using *Streptomyces aureofaciens*. It is used as hydrochloride salt. Oral and parenteral forms of chlortetracycline are not now used because of poor bioavailability. It is mainly used in form of ointment for topical application and also as ophthalmic solution.

Oxytetracycline Hydrochloride

[4S-(4α,4aα,5α,5aα,6β,12aα)]-4(Dimethylamino)-1,4,4a,5,5a,6,11,12a-octahydro-3,5,6,10, 12,12a-hexahydroxy-6-methyl-1, 11-dioxo-2-naphthacenecarboxamide hydrochloride

Both base and hydrochloride are absorbed rapidly. However, the free base is less bitter than the hydrochloride salt. So free base is preferred for oral use. It is also used as intramuscular and intravenous injection. It is obtained by fermentation using *Streptomyces rimosus*.

Demeclocycline

[4S-(4α,4aα,5aα,6β,12aα)]-7-Chloro-4-(dimethylamino)-1,4,4a,5,5a,6,11,12a-octahydro-3,6,
10,12,12a-pentahydroxy-1,11-dioxo-2-naphthacenecarboxamide

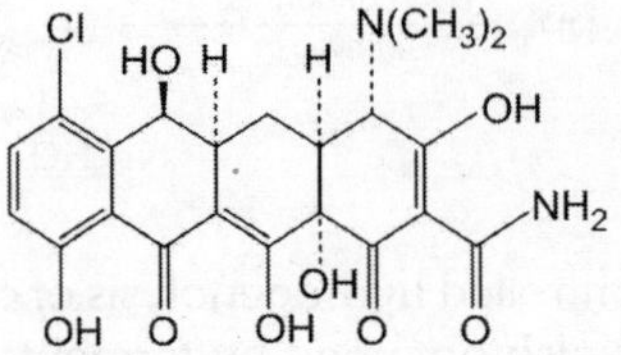

It has been isolated from mutant strains of *S. aureofaciens*. It differs from chlortetracycline (3) in absence of methyl group at C-6.

It has antibiotic spectrum like that of other tetracyclines. Further, it shows slower rate of elimination, as a result it is more effective.

Doxycycline Hydrate

[4S-(4α,4aα,5aα,5aα,6α,12aα)]-4-(Dimethylamino)-1,4,4a,5,5a, 6,11,12a-octahydro-3,5,10,12,
12a-pentahydroxy-6-methyl-1,11-dioxo-2-naphthacenecarboxamide hydrate

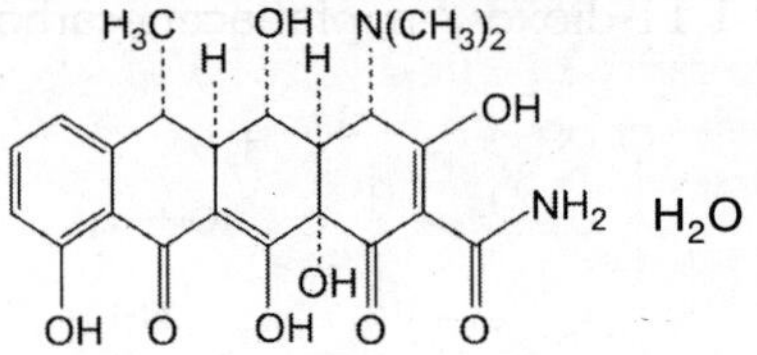

Synthesis

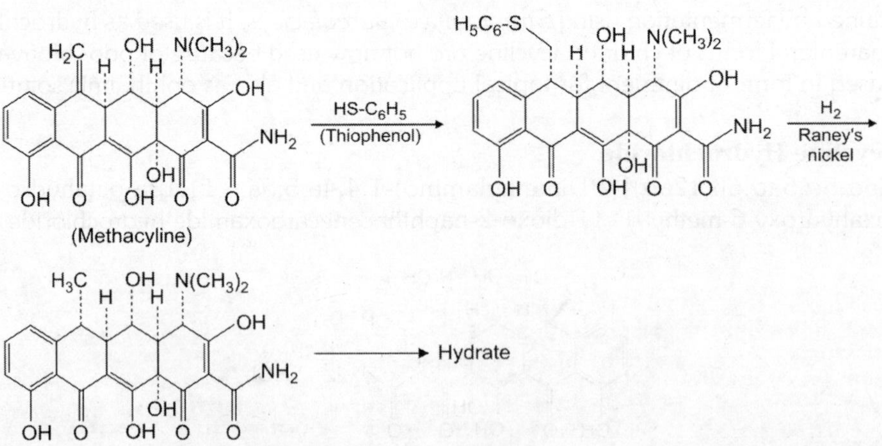

It is 6β-dehydroxyoxytetracycline. The absence of hydroxyl group gives the stability to the molecule. The 6α-methyl analog has better and more activity than the 6β-methyl analog.

It does not accumulate in patients with impaired renal function.

Minocycline

[4S-(4α,4aα,5aα,12aα)]-4,7-Bis(Dimethylamino)-1,4,4a,5,5a,6,11,12a-octahydro-3,10,12,12a-tetrahydroxy-1,11-dioxo-2-naphthacenecarboxamide

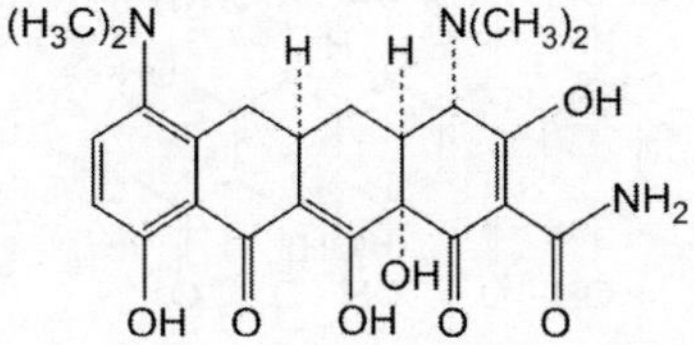

Synthesis

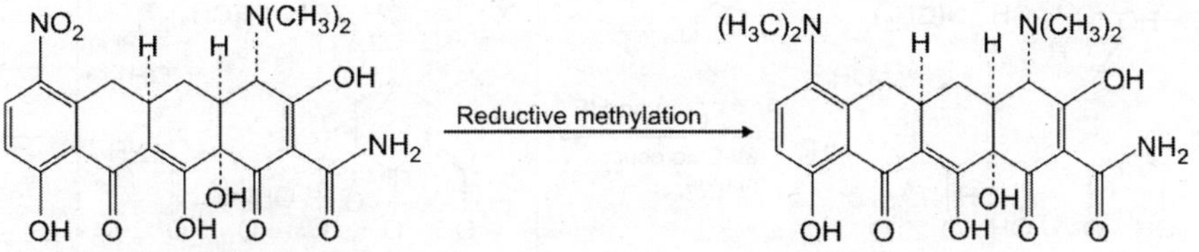

(7-Nitro-6-demethyl-
6-deoxy tetracycline)

It is the most potent tetracycline currently in use. Like doxycycline (6) it also lacks 6-hydroxyl group and is stable towards acids. It is well absorbed when given orally to give high plasma levels. Further, it has long serum half-life and slow urinary excretion. It is effective against resistant strains of *Staphylococci*. It has been recommended for chronic bronchitis and other respiratory tract infections. It is also used in urinary tract infections.

Methacycline

[4S-(4α,4aα,5α,5aα,12aα)]-4-Dimethylamino-1,4,4a,5,5a,6,11,12a-octahydro-3,5,10,12,12a-pentahydroxy-6-methylene-1,11-dioxo-2-naphthacenecarboxamide

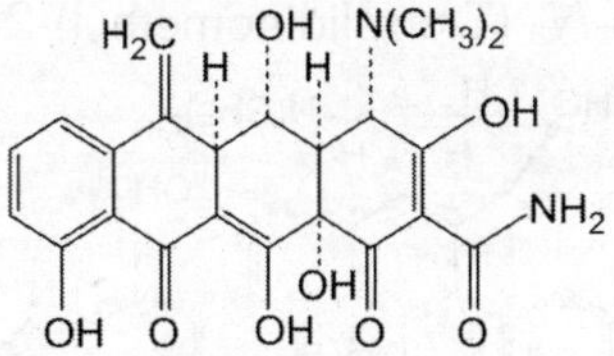

Synthesis

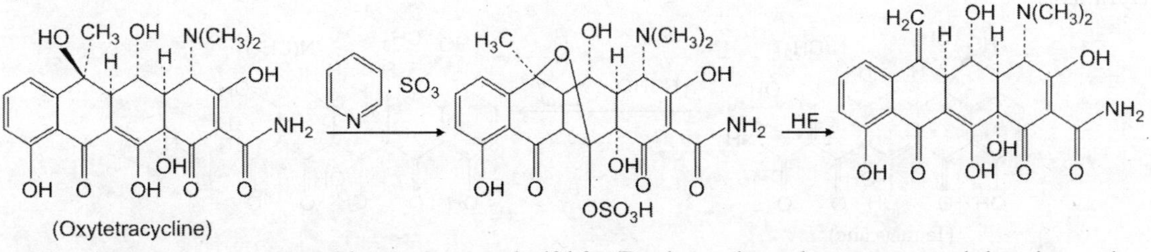

(Oxytetracycline)

It has greater potency and longer serum half-life. Further it has also greater stability than other tetracyclines. It is used as hydrochloride salt.

Meclocycline

4S-(4α,4aα,5α,5aα,12aα)]-7-Chloro-4-(dimethylamino)-1,4,4a,5,5a,6,11,12a-octahydro-3,5,10,12,12a-pentahydroxy-6-methylene-1,11-dioxo-2-naphthacenecarboxamide

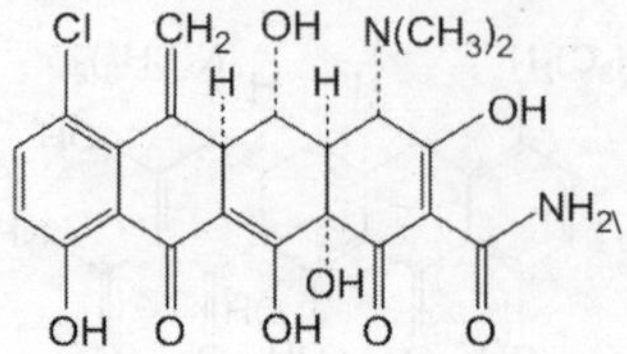

Synthesis

(Oxytetracycline)

(N-Chlorosucci-nimide)

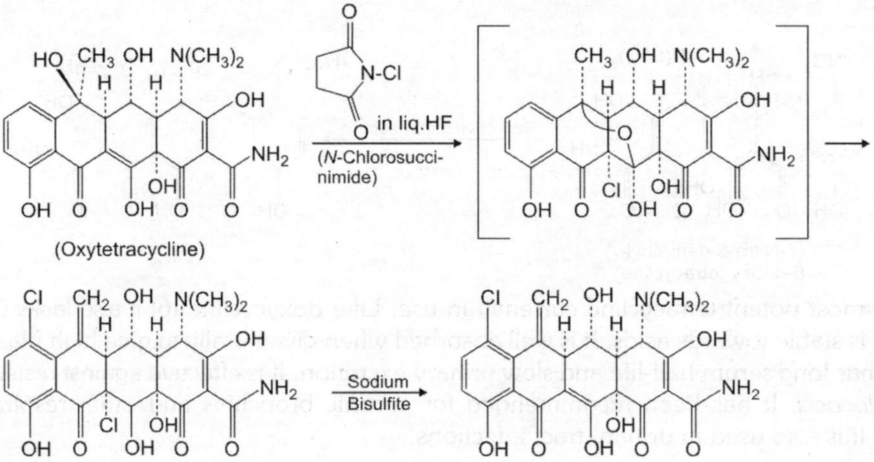

It is a semisynthetic tetracycline obtained from oxytetracycline (4). It is much more active in vitro.

Rolitetracycline

4S-(4α,4aα,5aα,6β,12aα)]-4-(Dimethylamino)-1,4,4a,5,5a,6,11,12a-octahydro-3,6,10,12,12a-pentahydroxy-6-methyl-1,11-dioxo-N- (1-prrolidinomethyl)-2-naphthacenecarboxamide

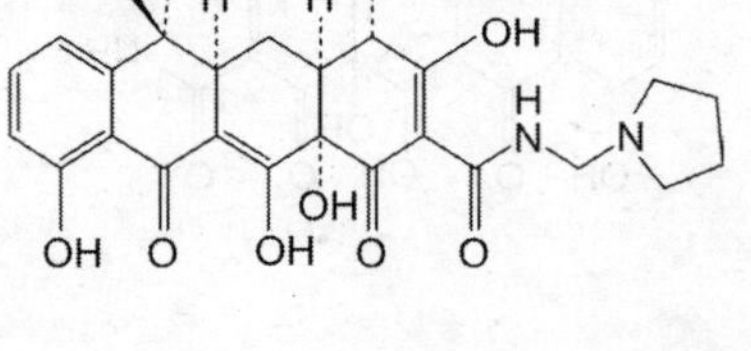

Synthesis

(Tetracycline)

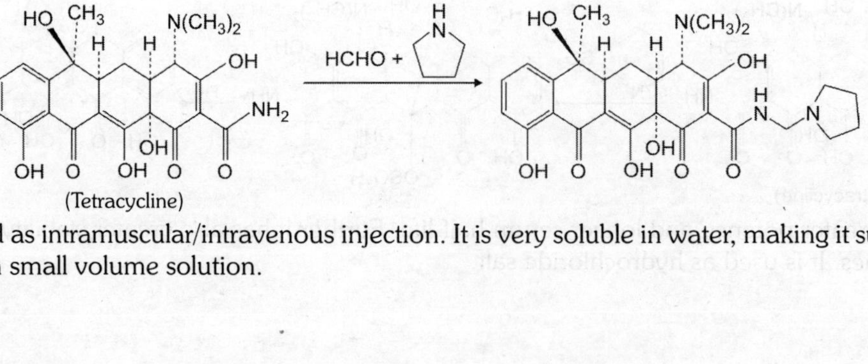

It is used as intramuscular/intravenous injection. It is very soluble in water, making it suitable for injection in small volume solution.

MISCELLANEOUS ANTIBIOTICS

CHLORAMPHENICOL

CHLORAMPHENICOL (1) was originally produced by fermentation using *Streptomyces venezuelae*. However, it is now produced completely by synthesis.

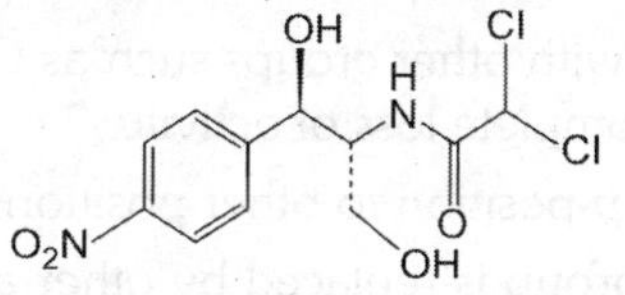

(1)

Chloramphenicol (1) is a white crystalline compound. It is highly soluble in alcohol and polar solvents. It has two asymmetric carbon atoms and can exist in four isomers, D-and L-*erythro* isomers (2a) and (2b), respectively and D-and L-*threo* isomers (3a) and (3b), respectively. The biological activity resides almost exclusively in the D(-)-*threo* (3a). The other isomers namely D-and L-*erythro* [(2a) and (2b), respectively] and L-*threo* isomer (3b) are inactive.

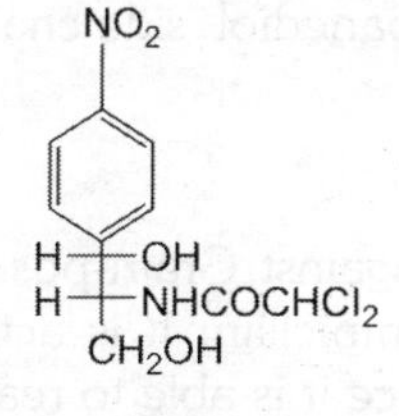

(2a)

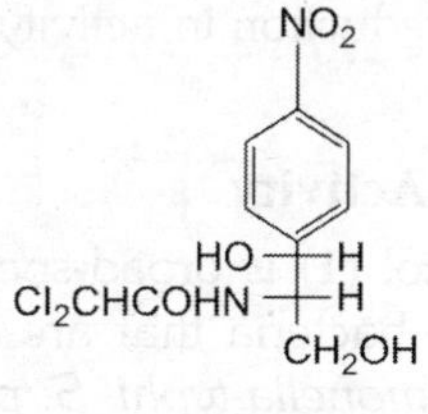

(2b)

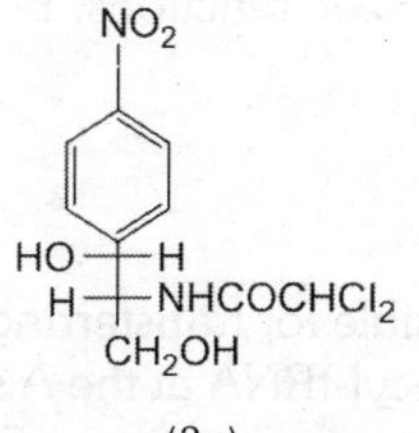

(3a)

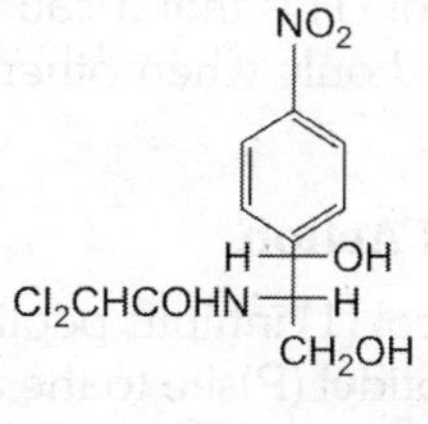

(3b)

807

Chloramphenicol (1) is bitter in taste. However, its palmitate ester (4) is tasteless and is used for oral pediatric formulations. The palmitate ester (4) is a prodrug of chloramphenicol (1) and is readily hydrolyzed after absorption to chloramphenicol (1). The sodium succinate ester (5) is water soluble and is used for parenteral formulations.

(1), R = H

(4), R = $C(CH_2)_{14}CH_3$; (5), R = CCH_2CH_2COONa

Structure-activity Relationships

Studies on structure-activity relationship have shown that:

1. Replacement of nitro group with other groups such as CN, $CONH_2$, SO_2NHR, NH_2, Br, Cl, F, I, etc. results in some or complete loss of activity.

2. Shifting of nitro group from *p*-position to other positions results in loss of activity.

3. Compounds where phenyl group is replaced by other aromatic rings such as naphthalene. alicyclic rings, heterocyclic rings like pyridyl, were less potent than chloramphenicol (1) itself.

4. Of the four isomers, only the D(-)-*threo* (3a) isomer is antibacterially active.

5. The primary alcoholic group also seems to be essential for the activity. Its removal or substitution by other groups like alkyl, etc. results in loss of activity.

6. Replacement of dichloroacetyl group with other acyl groups such as dibromoacetyl also results in loss of activity.

7. Similar reduction in activity is also observed when the propanediol side chain is extended.

Antibacterial Activity

Chloramphenicol (1) is broad-spectrum antibiotic and is active against Gram-positive as well as Gram-negative bacteria that are resistant to penicillin G and ampicillin. It is active against *H. influenzae*, *Salmonella typhi*, *S. pneumoniae*, and *B. fragilis*. Since it is able to reach the CNS in therapeutic concentration it has been found useful in meningitis. One of the serious toxic effects of chloramphenicol (1) is that it causes blood dyscrasias and other toxic reactions. Because of this it is recommended only when other antibiotics fail.

Mechanism of Action

Chloramphenicol (1) inhibits peptidyltransferase which is responsible for transferring peptide chain attached to peptidyl (P)site to the amino acid attached to aminoacyl-tRNA at the A site, this results in inhibition of protein synthesis.

INDIVIDUAL COMPOUNDS

Chloramphenicol

D-(-)-*threo*-*N*-Dichloroacetyl-1-*p*-nitrophenyl-2-amino-1,3-propanediol

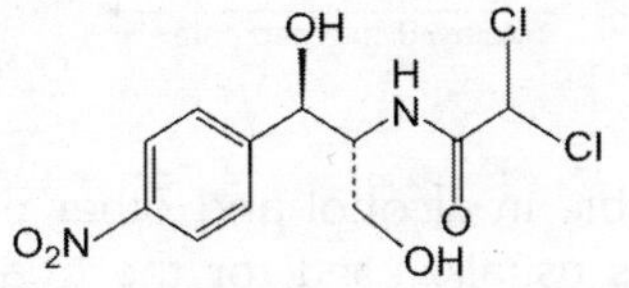

Synthesis

Route 1

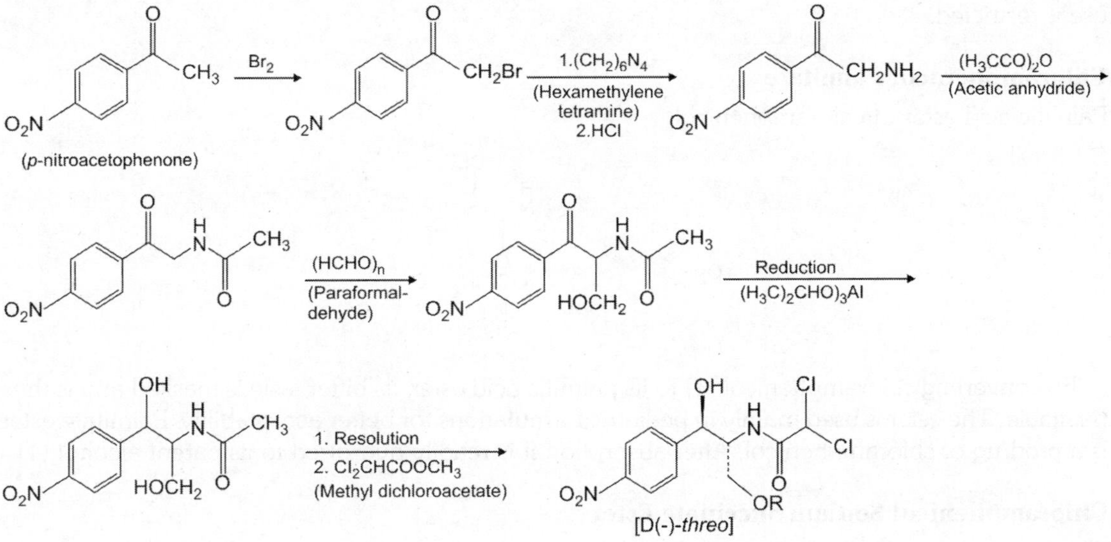

Route 2

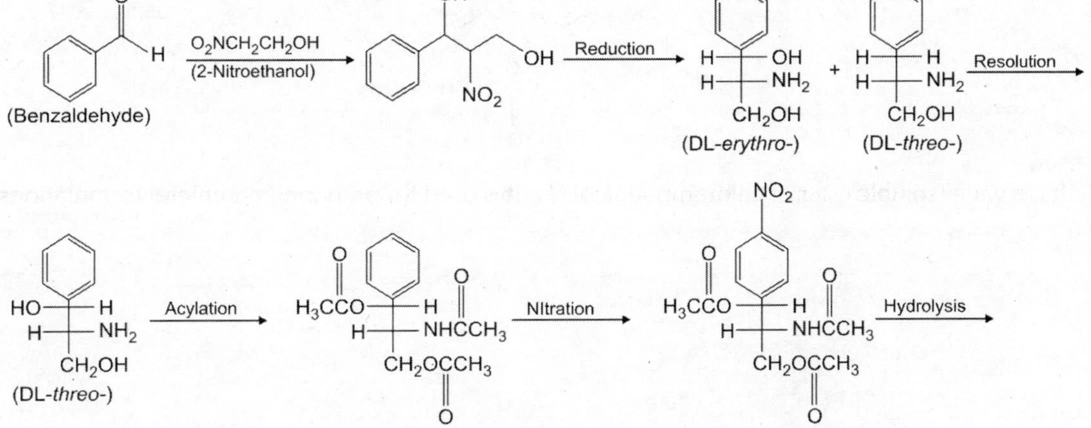

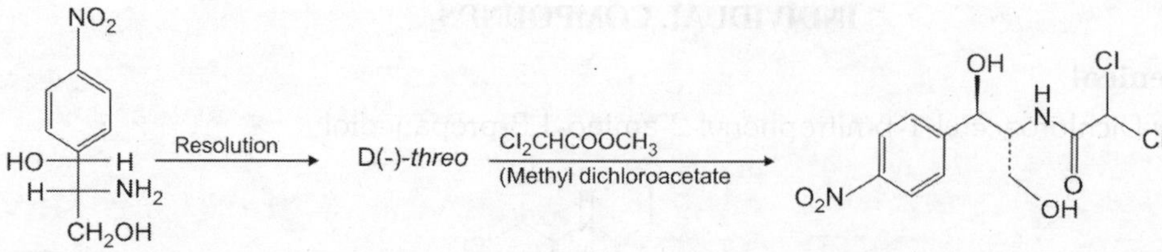

Chloramphenicol is highly soluble in alcohol and other polar solvents but is slightly soluble in water. It has a bitter taste. It is usually used for the treatment of serious infections due to Gram-positive and Gram-negative bacteria and also for the treatment of meningitis because it can penetrate central nervous system. Since it causes blood dyscrasias and other toxic side reactions its use is restricted.

Chloramphenicol Palmitate

Palmitic acid ester of chloramphenicol

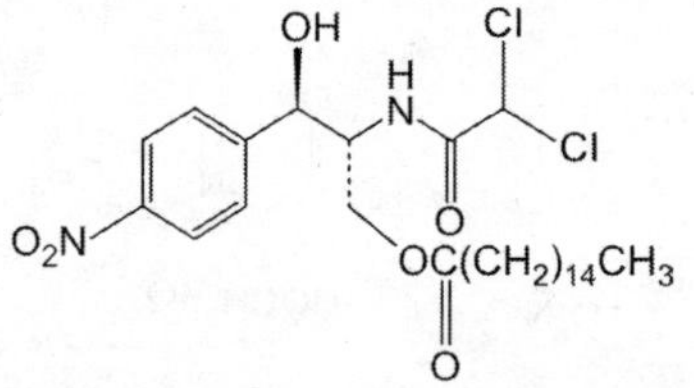

By converting chloramphenicol (1) to its palmitic acid ester, its bitter taste is masked and is thus palatable. The ester is used mainly in pediatric formulations for better acceptability. Palmitate ester is a prodrug of chloramphenicol. After absorption it is readily hydrolsed to its parent alcohol (1).

Chloramphenicol Sodium Succinate Ester

Chloramphenicol monosuccinate sodium salt

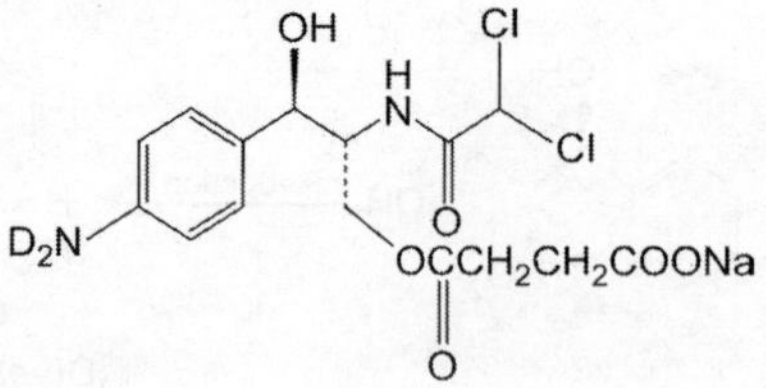

It is a water soluble ester of chloramphenicol (1). It is used for preparing parenteral formulations.

CHAPTER
33

CHEMOTHERAPY OF ACID-FAST INFECTIONS

THE AEROBIC BACILLI, belonging to genus *Mycobacterium,* is acid-fast bacilli because its cell wall has a high content of lipid, making it hydrophobic and thus resistant to decolorization by acid after staining. The pathogenic forms of acid-fast bacilli are various tubercle bacilli, the bacilli of human and rat leprosy, the bacilli which produce chronic enteritis in cattle, and the vole bacilli which causes disease in field mice.

Mycobacterium tuberculosis is the most important pathogenic form of mycobacterium. It is the causative organism of tuberculosis in humans (human type), cattle (bovine type), and birds (avian type). The other disease, the leprosy, is caused by *Mycobacterium leprae.*

Compared to other common infections, mycobacterial infections are protracted. Common infections are acute and induce a sharp defensive reactions on the part of the host and they last for short duration. The mycobacterial infections, on the other hand, are slow, and a long-drawn process. They are chronic in character and they take much longer time to get eradicated as compared to common infections.

TUBERCULOSIS

Tuberculosis, caused by *Mycobacterium tuberculosis*, has been known from the earliest recorded history. It is transmitted via respiratory route. It primarily affects lungs (pulmonary form), but it can affect other tissues or organs (extrapulmonary tuberculosis) also. Thus, in addition to pulmonary tuberculosis, there are tuberculosis meningitis, tuberculosis enteritis, tuberculosis laryngitis, tuberculosis osteomyelitis, and host of others.

In pulmonary tuberculosis, after the organisms gain entry into the alveoli, they are ingested by pulmonary macrophages. This results in stimulation of surrounding fibroblasts to enclose the infection site leading to the formation of tubercles. The infection, which is thus contained, may lie dormant for years and may reappear later either through reactivation or through another invasion. In tuberculosis there is extensive tissue destruction and as the disease advances, the live, virulent bacilli become isolated in cavities and debris of necrotic tissue. The tubercle formation and the tissue debris allow the chemotherapeutic agents to reach the bacilli in sub-lethal doses. This leads to emergence of resistant strains. Sometime there may be cross-resistance to other drugs also. Multidrug-resistant tuberculosis (MDR-TB) has assumed alarming proportion. It is estimated that MDR-TB may have fatality rate of more than 50%.

The AIDS patients have been found to develop infections caused by *Mycobacterium avium* and *Mycobacterium intracellulare*. These two organisms are difficult to distinguish and are considered complex, thus the acronym *Mycobacterium avium-intracellulare* (MAC).

In case of non-AIDS patients, lungs are usually involved but in case of AIDS patients, the infection can involve bone marrow, lymph nodes, liver or even blood.

CHEMOTHERAPY

Considering the nature of the disease, an effective tuberculostat should be such that it is able to penetrate the tubercle and enter the phagocytes, within which the parasites are growing, in sufficient concentration. It should be highly toxic to the parasite and of course least toxic to the host. Further since the drug has to be used for long time it should be slow in producing resistant strains.

Almost all substances used for other diseases have been tried against tuberculosis and this includes oils, inorganic compounds, gold salts, etc. However, none of them is used nowadays.

Calmette developed a vaccine from a virulent strain of bovine tubercle bacilli which was attenuated by prolonged culture outside the body. This attenuated strain is known as Bacillus Calmette-Guerin or BCG vaccine. The vaccine has been administered to millions of humans in the hope of producing prophylaxis. However, there is no evidence that the vaccine produces resistance in human beings, at the same time it is considered to be of some benefit.

SYNTHETIC ANTITUBERCULAR DRUGS

The observation that sulphanilamide (1) had weak activity against tubercle bacilli led to testing of various sulphonamides for their activity. However, they were effective at toxic levels only. Structure-activity relationship studies led to synthesis of dapsone [4, 4'-diaminodiphenylsulphone, DDS, (2)], which was effective against leprosy. It was not effective against tuberculosis because of its high toxicity.

(1)   (2)

p-Aminosalicylic Acid and its Derivatives

Some salts of benzoates and salicylates have been found to increase the oxygen uptake by tubercle bacilli. These observations led to investigation of these salts in the hope of finding compounds from benzoates and salicylates which would decrease the oxygen uptake by tubercle bacilli. This study led to discovery of p-aminosalicylic acid (3) commonly called PAS, which was found to be an effective tuberculostat.

(3)

Antitubercular-activity of p-Aminosalicylic acid (3)

p-Aminosalicylic acid (3) is absorbed well and rapidly from gastrointestinal tract. It is also excreted rapidly, mainly via urine, about half appearing as the *N*-acetyl derivative (4), and a large fraction as glycyl derivative (5).

(4)   (5)

The drug is relatively non-toxic, though common side effect, with usual 12 g/day dose, is gastrointestinal irritation which can be sufficiently severe to discontinue the treatment. *p*-Aminosalicylic acid (3) produces resistant strains but the emergence of resistant strains is markedly delayed when *p*-aminosalicylic acid (3) is given along with streptomycin or isoniazid (isonicotinic acid hydrazide). The utility of *p*-aminosalicylic acid (3) is based on this characteristic rather than its activity which is 1/10th of dapsone (2) or 1/50th of streptomycin. It also increases the serum concentration of isoniazid when given along with it. *p*-Aminosalicylic acid (3) is active against growing bacilli, its effect is reversed by *p*-aminobenzoic acid.

Thiosemicarbazones

While testing various sulphonamides, thiosemicarbazone of *p*-acetamidobenzaldehyde [thiacetazone (6)], an intermediate in synthesis of sulphathiadiazole (7), was found to possess antitubercular activity. Its activity was comparable to that of streptomycin and was half as active as isoniazid. However, the drug is not well tolerated in man as well as in animals. It produces considerable gastrointestinal disorders and is not clinically used now. The drug has been reinvestigated as a substitute for *p*-aminosalicylic acid (3) in oral regimen with isoniazid. It is claimed that this combination of thiacetazone (6) with isoniazid suppresses the emergence of resistant strains.

(6)   (7)

Nicotinic Acid and other Heteroecycle Derivatives

Based on the report by Chorine that nicotinamide (8) had weak antitubercular activity, structure-activity relationship studies were carried out on nicotinamide (8). This led to finding of in vivo antitubercular activity in thioisonicotinamide (9). It was found to be active against isoniazid resistant and susceptible organisms. Further, increased potency without any increase in toxicity was observed in 2-alkyl derivatives. The most potent among them was the 2-ethylthioisonicotinamide known as ethionamide (10). Ethionamide (10) has about 1/10th the activity and 1/5th the toxicity of that of isoniazid and is about 4-times as active as streptomycin. Ethionamide (10) when given alone results in rapid emergence of resistant strains. Prothionamide (11), a 2-*n*-propyl analog, has similar activity as ethionamide (10) but has limited clinical use.

(8)   (9)   (10)

(11)   (12)

The investigations of other heterocyclic rings led to the discovery of pyrazinamide (12). It is about 2-times as active as *p*-aminosalicylic acid (3) and 7-times as active as nicotinamide (8).

Pyrazinamide (12) is active against both streptomycin and isoniazid resistant strains. However, when used alone, resistant strains develop very fast. Further, it has severe hepatotoxicity. It is usually reserved in treatment of chronic tuberculosis which is resistant to major drugs.

Hydrazides

During 1950's, three groups of investigators reported independently and simultaneously the exceptional antitubercular activity of isoniazid [INH, (13)].

Structure-activity relationship in isoniazid (13)

(13)   (13a)

1. Substitution of pyridine ring by benzene, piperidine, or thiazole nucleus results in loss of activity with the exception of 2-thiazole carboxyhydrazide which is said to be active.
2. Substitution of alkylidene, cycloalkylidene, and arylalkylene groups for H^2 and H^3 (13a) has little effect on the activity. This may be because they are hydrolyzed to isoniazid (13) itself.
3. Substitution of an alkyl, cycloalkyl, or aralkyl group for H^2 (13a) generally results in highly active derivatives, but aryl substitution is detrimental.
4. The position 4 in pyridine ring is the position of choice for acid hydrazide group.
5. Acylation with carbonyl compounds diminishes and acylation with arylsulphonyl groups seems to abolish the activity.
6. Substitution of H^1 and H^2 (13a) by alkyl groups diminishes the activity.

7. Compounds substituted with alkyl groups for H^1, H^2 and H^3 (13a) were either weakly active or inactive.

8. Substitution of alkyl group for both H^2 and H^3 (13a) gives highly active compounds but the activity decreases with the increase in size of the substituent.

9. Substitution of H^1 (13a) by an alkyl group is detrimental for the activity.

Isoniazid (13) is highly effective drug in small doses. It has been shown to be non-toxic and well tolerated. However, CNS stimulation, peripheral neuritis, and gastric intolerance have been reported. It can penetrate the dense fibrous tissues surrounding the tubercle in high concentration. It can also enter and inhibit tubercle bacilli growing within phagocytic cells. One of the disadvantage of isoniazid (13) treatment is that it gives rise to isoniazid-resistant strains readily. However, the emergence of such strains can markedly be delayed by using combination of isoniazid (13) with streptomycin or *p*-aminosalicylic acid (3).

Diamines

During random screening, *N*, *N*-diisopropyl ethylenediamine (14) was found specifically antimycobacterial. Extensive modification of the molecule led to the synthesis of 2,2'-(ethylenediimino)di-1-butanol or ethambutol (15). Out of the two isomers, the (+)-isomer was found to be more active.

(14)   (15)

Clinically, ethambutol (15) alone is effective against acute and chronic pulmonary tuberculosis and also against renal and vesicular diseases. Further ethambutol (15) in combination with isoniazid (13) and streptomycin has been found to be a better combination. Ethambutol (15) with ethionamide (10) has been found to be highly effective in treatment of tuberculosis resistant to streptomycin, isoniazid (13), and *p*-aminosalicylic acid (3). Ethambutol (15) is well tolerated and relatively free from toxicity.

ANTIBIOTICS

Streptomycin

In addition to being active against a variety of bacteria, streptomycin (16) also inhibits *Mycobacterium tuberculosis*. It is an aminoglycoside antibiotic isolated from the fermentation broth of *Streptomyces species*. Streptomycin (16) was infact the first substance to be used against tuberculosis in humans. The minimum dose required is 4 mg/kg per day subcutaneously. Continued use of streptomycin (16) is associated with damage of eighth cranial nerve which results in deafness and vertigo. These toxic effects are lessened by use of combination therapy.

To overcome the toxicity, various modifications in structure have been made and include.

1. Reduction of formyl group of the streptose to CH_2OH in streptomycin (16) yields dihydrostreptomycin (17), which had similar activity as that of streptomycin (16) but caused delayed deafness.

2. Oxidation of formyl group of streptose in streptomycin (16) to COOH group led to loss of activity. Similar loss of activity followed when the formyl group was treated with reagents like hydroxylamine, semicarbazone, and phenylhydrazine.

3. Acetylation of *N*-methylamino group in *N*-methy-L-glucosamine portion of streptomycin (16) and dihydrostreptomycin (17) caused some reduction of activity.

4. Hydroxystreptomycin (18) [CH_3 group of streptose in (16) is converted to CH_2OH] has similar activity as that of streptomycin (16).

5. Derivatives of guanidine functions were less active and more toxic. Hydrolysis of guanidine to amino groups abolishes the activity.

6. Streptidine, streptose, and N-methylglucosamine are individually inactive.

7. Substitution of methyl group in methylamino group of glucosamine by hydrogen or higher alkyl group results in reduction in activity.

Streptomycin (16) is absorbed poorly when given orally, but is absorbed rapidly from subcutaneous or intramuscular sites. It is excreted unchanged in urine in about 12 hr. Resistance to streptomycin (16) emerges rapidly but when used with other drugs, the development of resistance is suppressed. It inhibits protein synthesis by binding to 30S ribosomal site thus disrupting the protein synthesis and formation of abnormal proteins.

Rifamycins

These are a group of chemically related antibiotics obtained by fermentation from cultures of *Streptomyces mediterrani*. They contain a macrocyclic ring bridged across two adjacent positions of an aromatic nucleus. The rifamycins and their semisynthetic analogs possess a broad-spectrum of activity. They are most active against Gram-positive bacteria and *M. tuberculosis*. Some of the rifamycins include rifamycin B (19), rifamycin S (20), rifamycin X (21), rifamycin SV (22), and rifampin (23).

Rifampin (23) is the most active agent presently in use in clinical practice. It is a derivative of rifamycin SV (22) which is lacking a substituent at position 3. Rifampin (23) inhibits DNA-dependent RNA polymerase (DDRP) and is highly active against rapidly dividing intra- and extracellular bacilli.

Rifabutin (24), another antibiotic belonging to this class is used for disseminated MAC in AIDS patients. It has higher activity than rifamycins against MAC organisms.

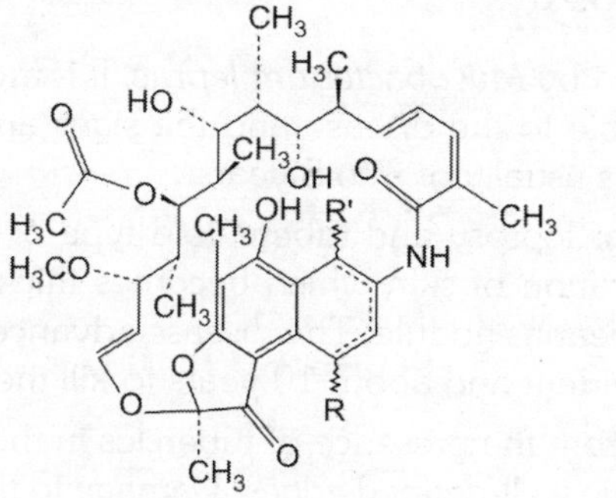

	R	R'
(19),	OCH_2COOH	OH
(20),	$= O$	$= O$
(21),	$\overset{+}{=}N\overset{-}{=}N$	$= O$

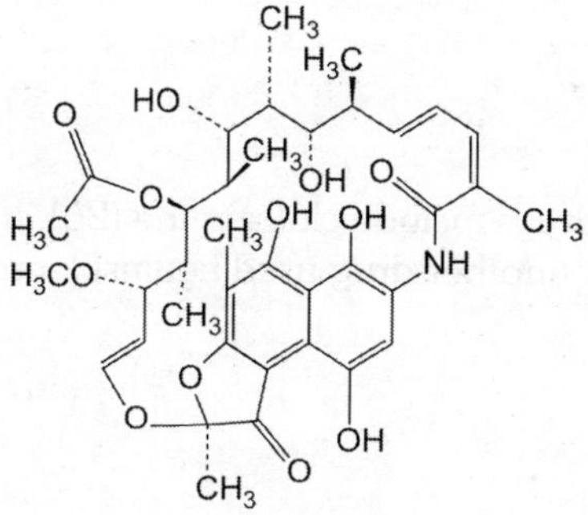

(22)

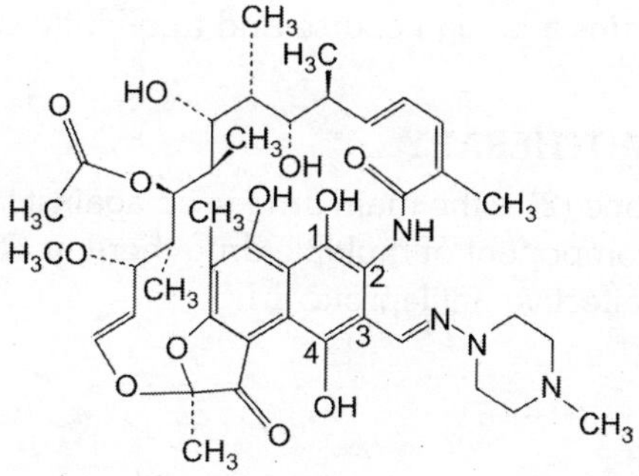

(23)

Cycloserine (25), an antibiotic, has been isolated from the fermentation tanks of three different *Streptomyces* species, namely, *S. orchidaceus*, *S. garyphalus*, and *S. lavendulus*. It exhibits antibiotic activity in vitro against a wide spectrum of Gram-positive and Gram-negative organisms but is weakly active against tuberculosis. Further, it shows frequent toxic reactions. As a result it is not used against tuberculosis. It is, however, given in combination with isoniazid (13).

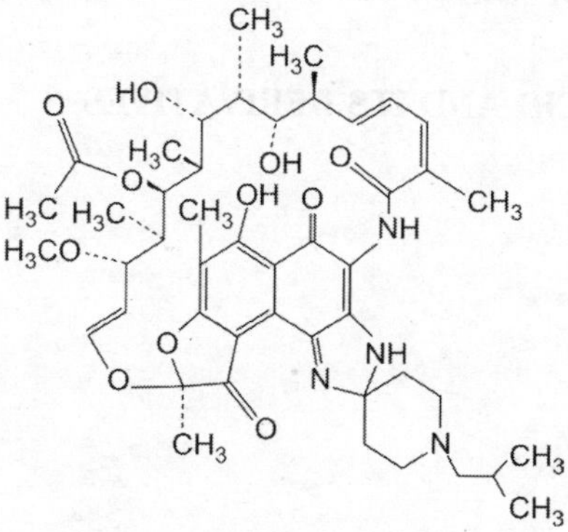

(24)

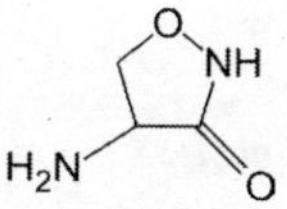

(25)

LEPROSY

Another mycobacterium disease, leprosy, is caused by *Mycobacterium leprae*. It is more prevalent in tropical countries. Chlidren are more susceptible to the disease and the signs and symptoms appear much later in life. The incubation period is usually of 3 to 5 years.

Leprosy is of two types, lepromatus or nodular leprosy and tuberculoid type of leprosy. The lepromatus type is characterized by diffuse infiltration of skin which becomes thickened, glossy and corrugated. The localized infiltration may appear as nodule. The disease advances slowly and it takes more than 5 years to become clinically evident and about 10 years to kill the patient.

The tuberculoid type of leprosy gets its name from the presence of tubercles in the lesions. It is characterized by erythematous macules which have well-defined edges. Damage to the peripheral nerves is the serious feature of this type of leprosy. The disease goes through long period of remission followed by acute phases during which additional nerve damage takes place. The tuberculoid form runs a benign course and frequently cures itself.

CHEMOTHERAPY

Dapsone (2) is the main drug used against leprosy. Other drugs include clofazimine (26). It is used as a component of multiple drug therapy. Rifampin (23) is another drug used against leprosy and is an effective antileprotic drug.

(26)

INDIVIDUAL COMPOUNDS

ANTITUBERCULAR DRUGS : p-AMINOSALICYLIC ACID AND ITS DERIVATIVES

p-Aminosalicylic Acid

4-Amino-2-hydroxybenzoic acid

Synthesis

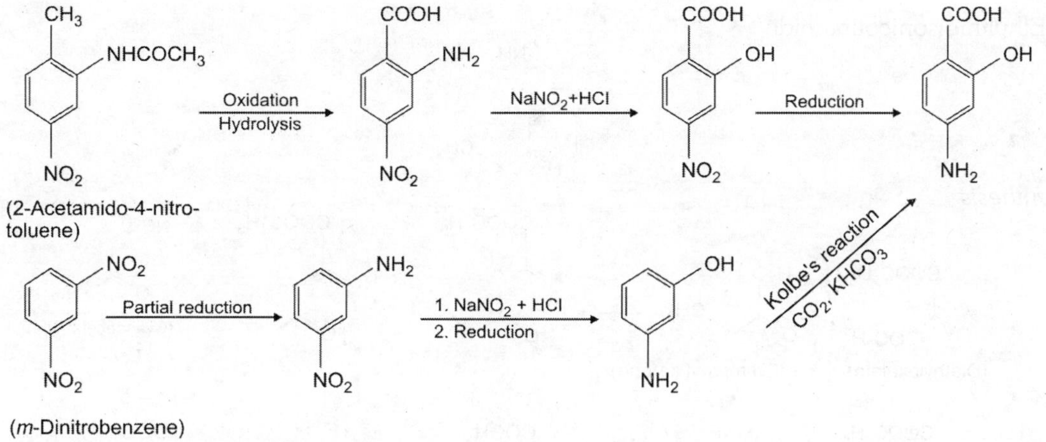

(2-Acetamido-4-nitro-
toluene)

(*m*-Dinitrobenzene)

p-Aminosalicylic acid or PAS is slightly soluble in water (about 0.1%). Its salts such as sodium PAS and calcium PAS are more soluble.

p-Aminosalicylic acid was once a popular antitubercular drug, however, since its use is associated with rapid development of resistant strains and severe side effects, its use is now restricted. It is used in cases where there is intolerance to other drugs. Its mechanism of action is thought to involve interference in incorporation of PABA into folic acid.

ANTITUBERCULAR DRUGS : THIOSEMICARBAZONES

Thiacetazone

p-Acetamidobenzaldehyde thiosemicarbazone

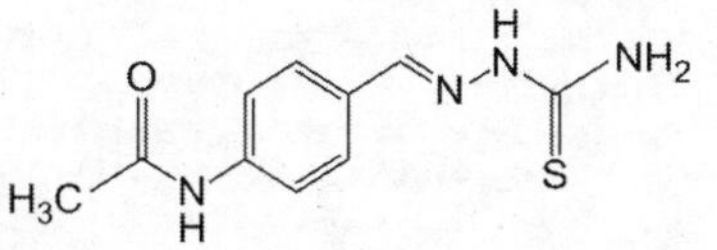

Synthesis

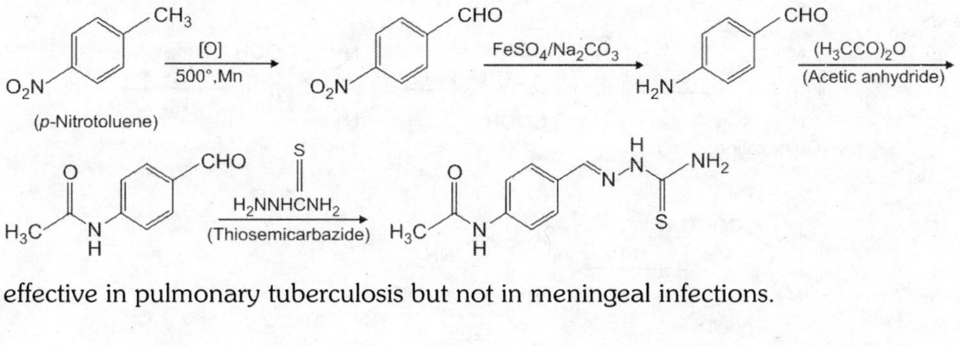

(*p*-Nitrotoluene)

(Thiosemicarbazide)

It is effective in pulmonary tuberculosis but not in meningeal infections.

ANTITUBERCULAR DRUGS : NICOTINIC ACID AND OTHER HETERDCYCLE DERIVATIVES

Ethionamide

2-Ethylthioisonicotinamide

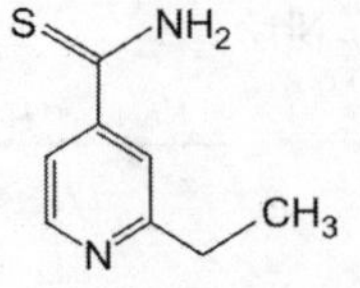

Synthesis

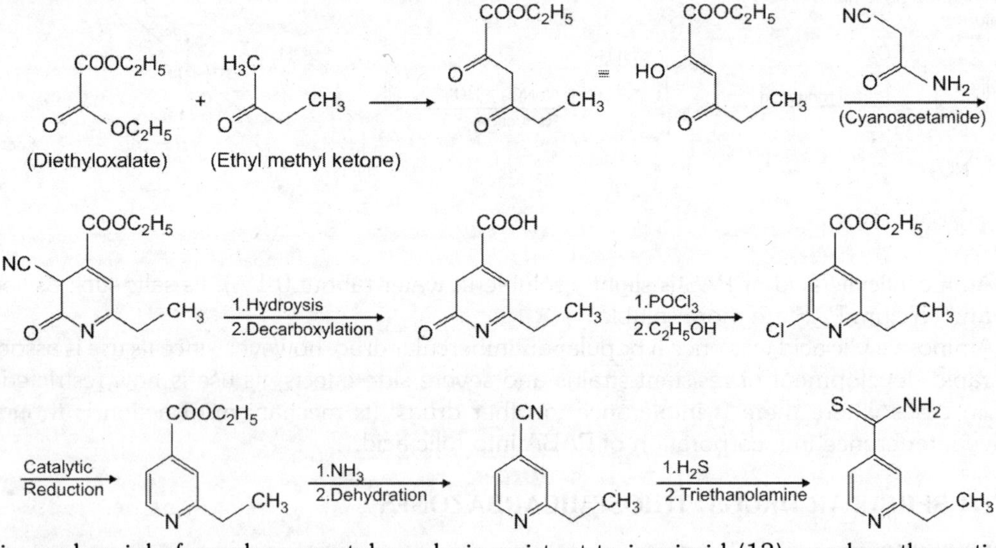

It is used mainly for pulmonary tuberculosis resistant to isoniazid (13) or when the patient is intolerant to other drugs. It acts by inhibiting the incorporation of cysteine and methionine in proteins.

Pyrazinamide

Pyrazinecarboxamide

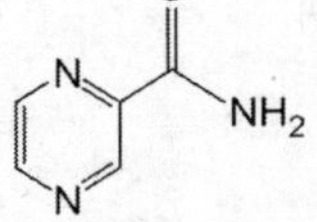

Synthesis

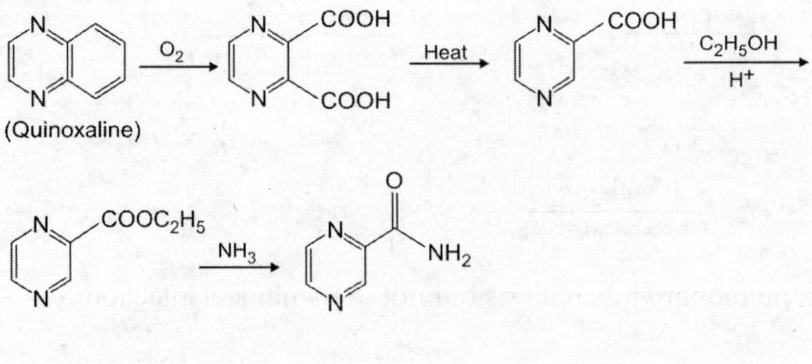

It is a white crystalline powder that is sparingly soluble in water. Although its structure resembles that of isoniazid (13) and ethionamide (10) but its mechanism of action is different. The active species of pyrazinamide is pyrazinoic acid (27) which is formed by the action of pyrazinamidase on pyrazinamide. The pyrazinoic acid (27) so produced lowers the pH of the immediate surroundings and the *Mycobacterium* is not able to grow. The organisms that produce pyrazinamidase are thus susceptible to pyrazinamide while as resistant strains do not produce this enzyme. Further metabolism of pyrazinoic acid (27) results in 5-hudroxypyrazinoic acid.

ANTITUBERCULAR DRUGS : HYDRAZIDES

Isoniazid

4-Pyridinecarboxylic acid hydrazide

Synthesis

Isoniazid is a colourless crystalline solid. It is remarkably effective against mycobacterium. It is bactericidal against replicating microorganisms and bacteriostatic against non-replicating organisms. Mycobacterium is reported to lose its acid fastness after treatment with isoniazid. This suggests that isoniazid interferes with cell wall development. The mechanism of action of isoniazid is inhibition of the synthesis of mycolic acids which are high molecular weight β-hydroxy fatty acids and important components of cell wall. For inhibition of synthesis of mycolic acid, it is necessary that isoniazid gets first activated. This bioactivation is carried out by mycobacterial catalase-peroxidase enzyme complex, which results in active species which attack the enzyme required for the mycolic acid synthesis. Resistance to isoniazid has been attributed to loss of catalase-peroxidase activity by the mycobacterium.

Isoniazid is a safe drug, incidence of toxic effects are minimal. The principal toxic effects include peripheral neuritis, gastrointestinal disturbances, mainly constipation and loss of appetite and hepatotoxicity. The peripheral neuritis is overcome by administration of vitamin B_6.

Isoniazid is completely absorbed after its administration and is well distributed in all the parts of the body. The principal metabolites include N-acetylisoniazid (29), isonicotinic acid (30), acetylhydrazide (31), and diacetylhydrazide (32).

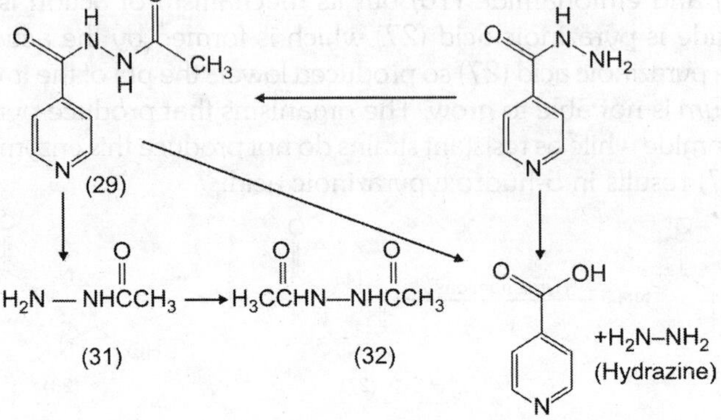

O=C(NH-NH-CH3)... (29)

H2N—NHCCH3 → H3CCHN—NHCCH3
(31)   (32)

(30)

+H2N—NH2
(Hydrazine)

ANTITUBERCULAR DRUGS : DIAMINES

Ethambutol

(+)–2, 2'-(ethylenediimino)di-1-butanol

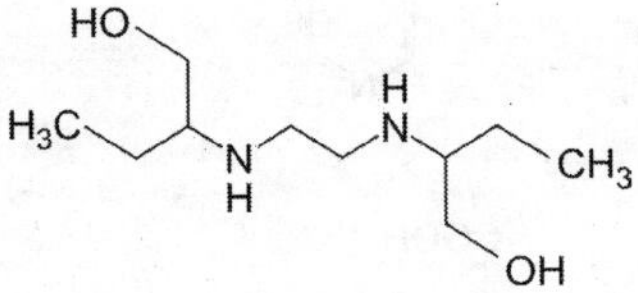

Synthesis

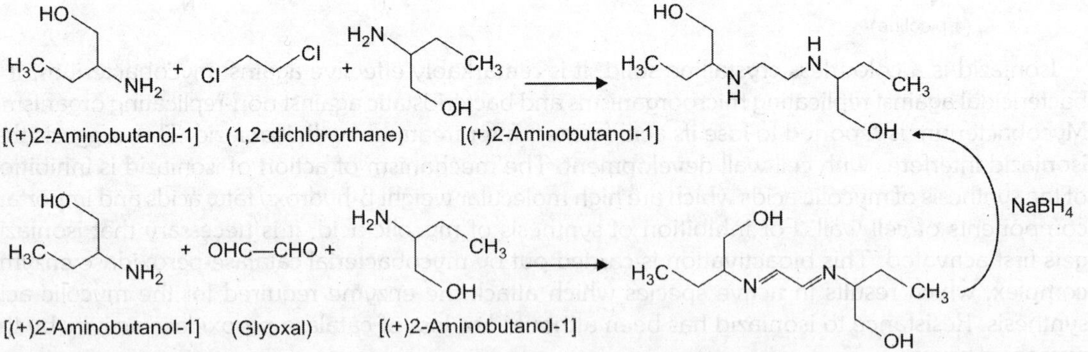

[(+)2-Aminobutanol-1]   (1,2-dichlororthane)   [(+)2-Aminobutanol-1]

[(+)2-Aminobutanol-1]   (Glyoxal)   [(+)2-Aminobutanol-1]

NaBH4

Exists in three forms the (+), (–) and the *meso*-form. It is stereospecific in its action. The toxicities of (+)-, (–)-, and *meso*-isomers are equal but they vary considerably in their activities. The (+)-isomer is about 200-500-times more active than (–)-isomer and 16-times more active than the *meso*-isomer. Its mechanism of action is unknown. The proposed mechanism of its action involves inhibition of transfer of mycolic acid into mycobacterial cell wall thus interfering with the cell wall synthesis.

Ethambutol is mostly excreted unchanged (about 85%), rest of it is excreted as (33) and (34).

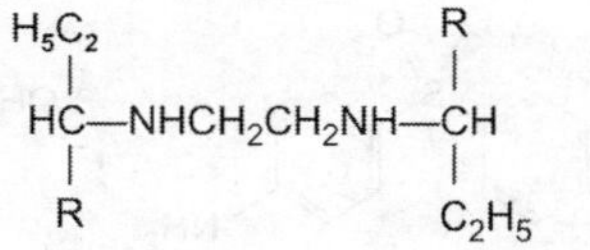

$$H_5C_2$$
$$|$$
$$HC-NHCH_2CH_2NH-CH$$

(33), R=CHO   (34), R=COOH

ANTILEPROTIC DRUGS

Dapsone

4,4'-Sulphonylbisbenzeneamine

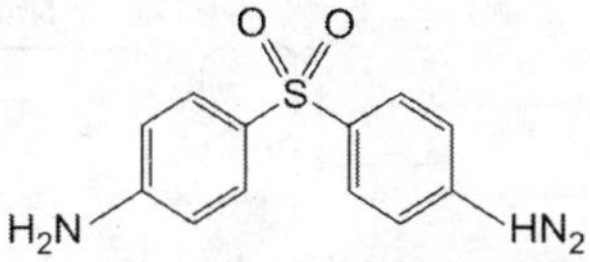

Synthesis

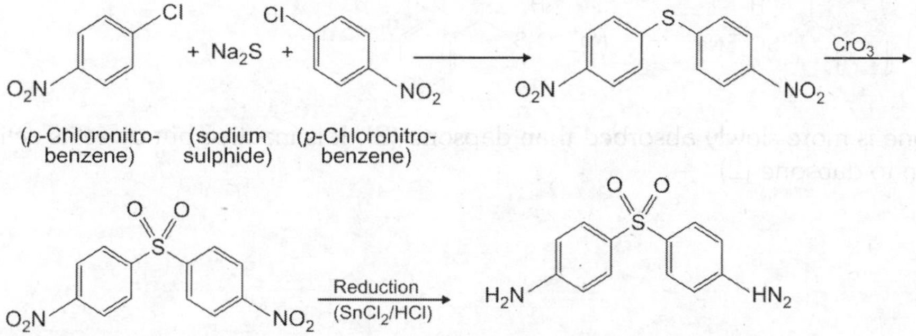

Dapsone is nearly insoluble in water and is very weakly basic. It causes GI irritation. Despite the lack of solubility, it is efficiently absorbed from GI tract.

It acts in similar manner as sulphonamides through competitive inhibition of PABA, thus inhibiting the synthesis of dihydrofolic acid.

Solapsone

Di(γ-phenylpropylamino)-4,4'-diphenylsulphone α,α',γ,γ'-sodium tetrasulphonate

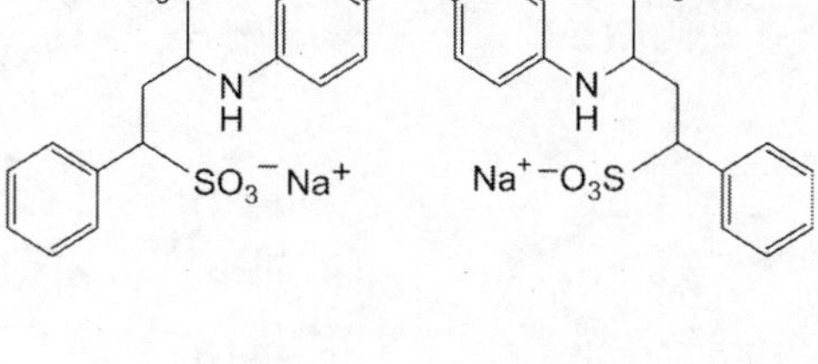

Synthesis

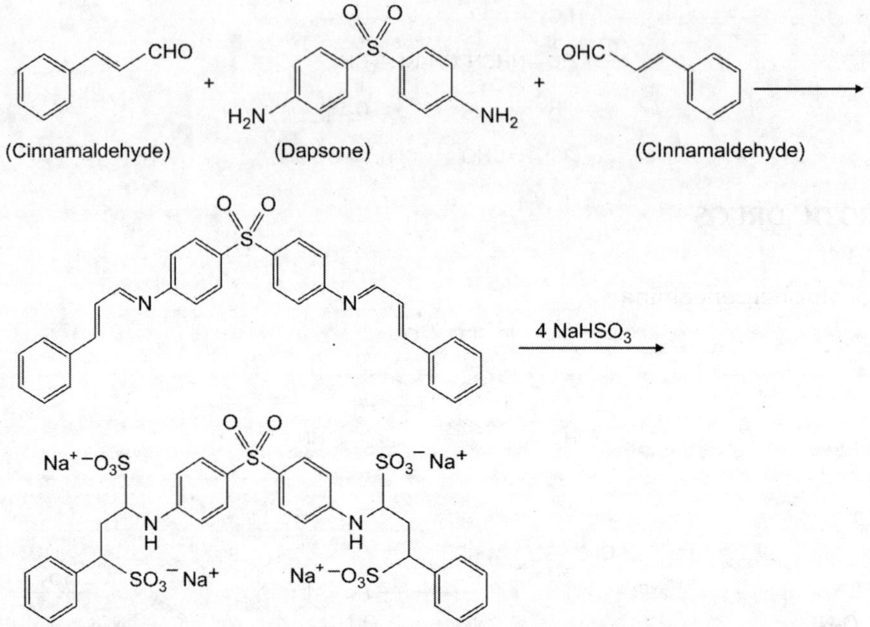

(Cinnamaldehyde)   (Dapsone)   (CInnamaldehyde)

4 NaHSO$_3$

Solapsone is more slowly absorbed than dapsone (2). It is inactive but owes its activity due to metabolism to dapsone (2).

CHAPTER

34

ANTIFUNGAL AGENTS

FUNGI is a general term and it includes yeasts, molds, rusts, and mushrooms. Fungi are heterotrophic (saprophytic, parasitic, symbiotic, or hyperparasitic) spore bearing organisms. They differ from algae by lack of photosynthetic ability and from protozoa by lack of motility and possession of well-defined cell wall made up of chitin. Fungi reproduce both asexually as well as sexually. In the asexual reproduction, spores are formed without involving the fusion of nuclei or sex cells. In sexual reproduction, there is formation and fusion of two types of sex cells or gametes.

Some of the diseases caused by fungi in humans are given in Table 34.1.

Table. 34.1: Fungal diseases in humans.

	Disease	*Causative organism*
1.	Athelete's foot, ring worm of skin, hair, nails	Dermatophytes (*Trichophyton sp., Microsporum sp., Epidermophyton sp.*)
2.	Candidiasis of skin, nails, mucous membrane	*Candida albicans*
3.	Aspergillosis	*Aspergillus sp.*
4.	Blastomycosis	*Blastomyces brasiliensis, Blastomyces dermatidis*
5.	Chromoblastomycosis	*Cladosporium sp.*
6.	Candiasis	*Candida albicans*
7.	Coccidioidomycosis	*Coccidioides sp.*
8.	Cryptococcosis	*Cryptococcus neoformans*
9.	Histoplasmosis	*Histoplasma capsulatum*
10.	Mucromycosis	*Mucor sp., Rhizopus sp.*
11.	Protothecosis	*Protheca sp.*
12.	Rhinosporidiosis	*Rhinospordium sp.*
13.	Sporotrichosis	*Sporotricosis sp.*

ANTIFUNGAL AGENTS

ANTIBIOTICS
Griseofulvin
Griseofulvin (1) is an antifungal antibiotic produced by *Penicillium griseofulvum*. It has been used systemically for infections caused by *Trichophyton, Microsporum* and *Epidermophyton species*.

It possesses very low toxicity and acts as a mitotic spindle poison. In vitro, it rapidly arrests cell division in metaphase. It has a selective toxicity towards fungi which is because it concentrates in tissues which are rich in keratin, a site where the dermatophytes establish the infection.

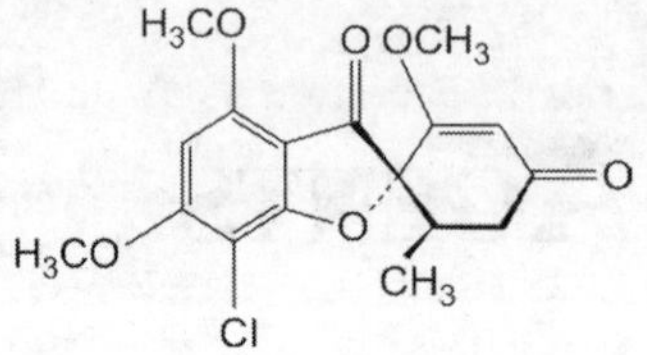

(1)

Polyene Antibiotics

The polyene antibiotics useful as antifungal agents include amphotericin B (2), nystatin A_1 (3), and natamycin (4). The polyene antibiotics contain a large lactone ring with 4 to 7 unsubstituted conjugated double bonds. The double bonds are in all-*trans* configuration. Polyenes are water insoluble and unstable because of high unsaturation. They have high affinity for sterol containing membranes. This results in alteration in permeability of cell and they lose essential organic and inorganic cell constituents. Further, among the sterols containing membranes also, polyenes have high affinity for the ergosterol containing membranes than those containing cholesterol. This gives selectivity towards fungi which contain such membrane.

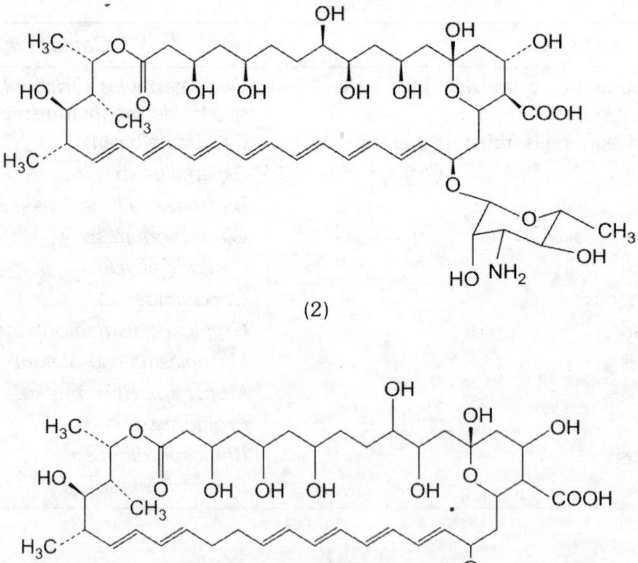

(2)

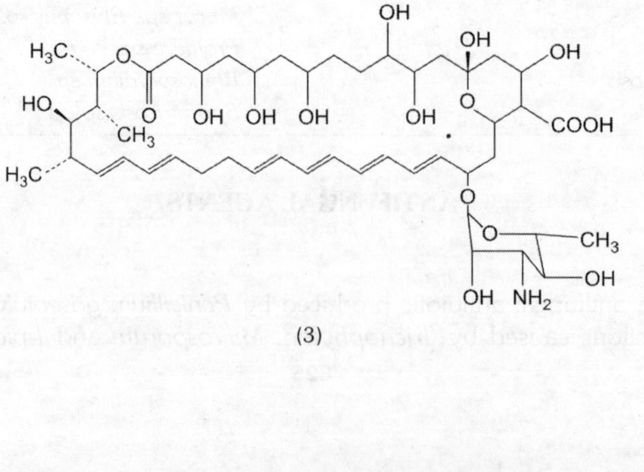

(3)

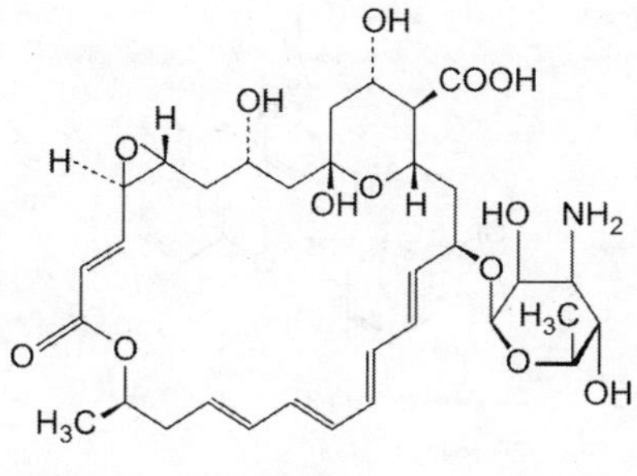

(4)

Amphotericin B (2) is administered intravenously or intrathecally as a colloidal dispersion in aqueous sodium deoxycholate solution in patients with systemic mycoses.

Nystatin is a mixture of nystatin A_1, A_2 and A_3. Nystatin A_1 (3) which is the major component is employed as a cutaneous, vaginal, or oral preparation in non-systemic candidiasis. Natamycin (4) is used as 5% suspension applied topically for the treatment of infections of eye.

AZOLES

These constitute the imidazole and triazole analogs. The clinically useful imidazole analogs include oxiconazole (5), lanoconazole (6), omoconazole (7), ketoconazole (8), chlormidazole (9), butoconazole (10), clotrimazole (11), flutrimazole (12), croconazole (13), neticonazole (14), miconazole (15), econazole (16), sulconazole (17), fenticonazole (18), isoconazole (19), sertaconazole (20), and tioconazole (21). Among the triazoles, fluconazole (22), voriconazole (23), itraconazole (24), saperconazole (25), and terconazole (26) are some of the important drugs.

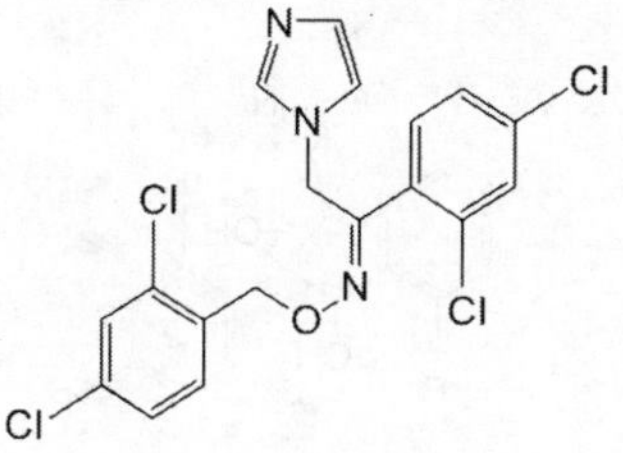

(5)

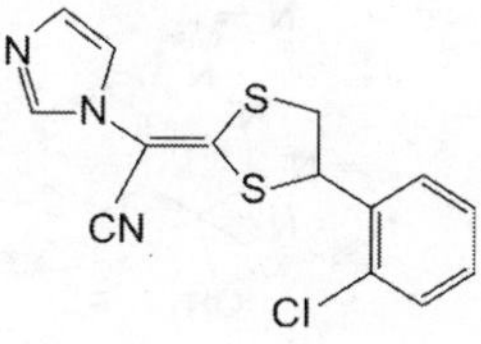

(6)

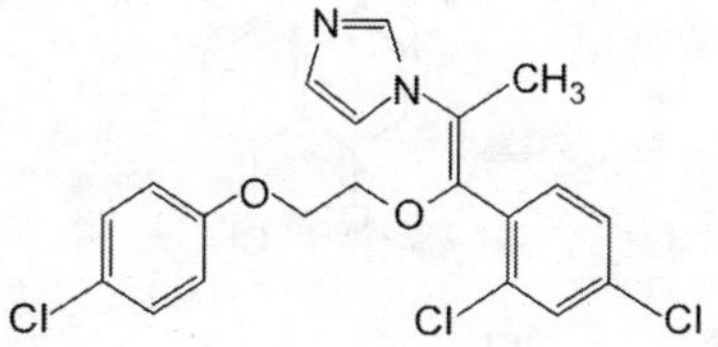

(7)

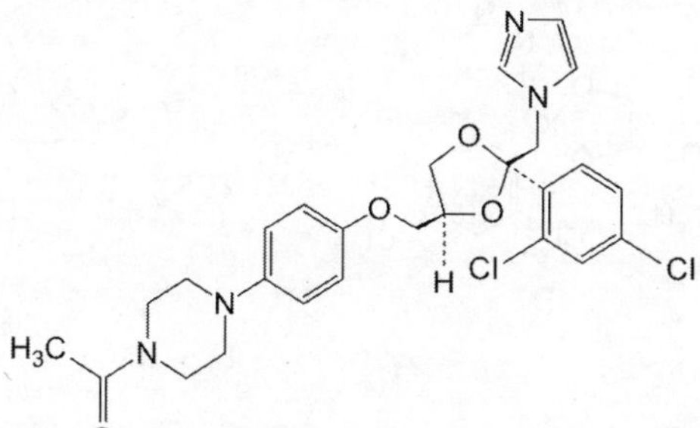

(8)

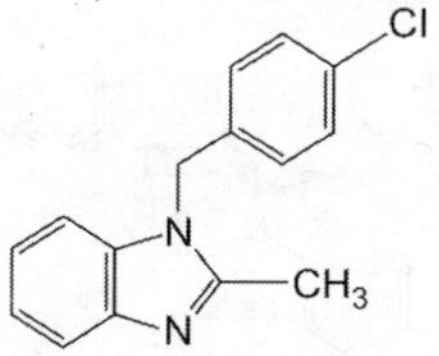

(9)

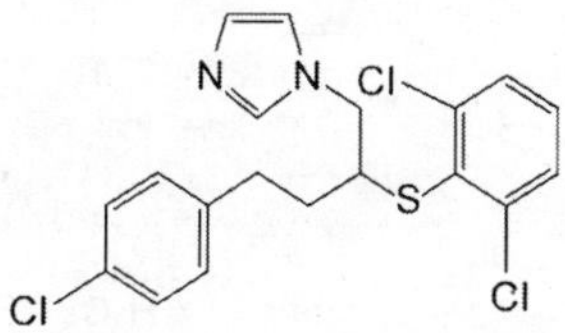

(10)

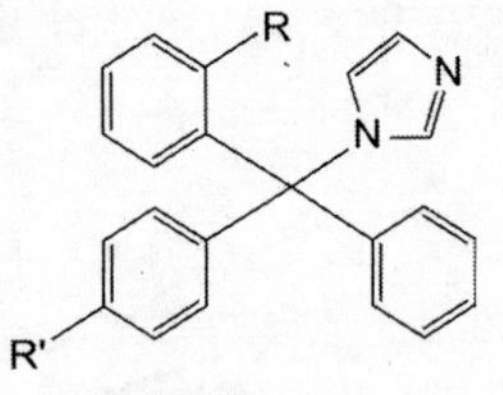

(11), R = Cl; R' = H
(12), R = R' = F

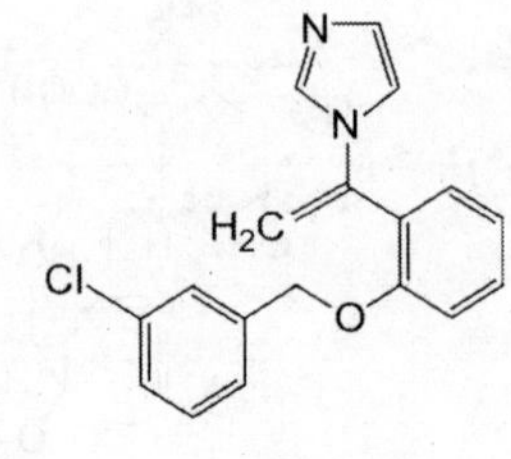

(13)

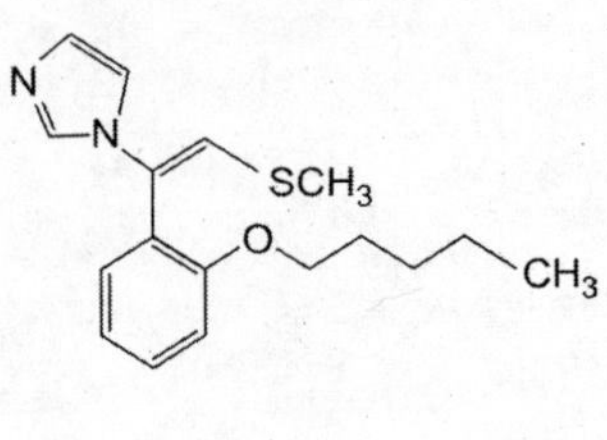

(14)

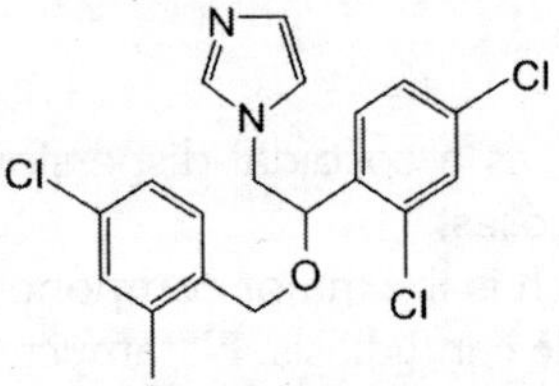

(15)

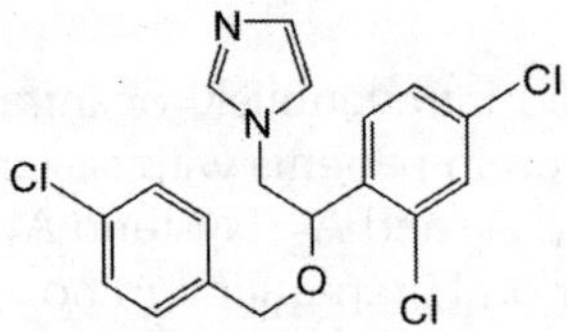

(16)

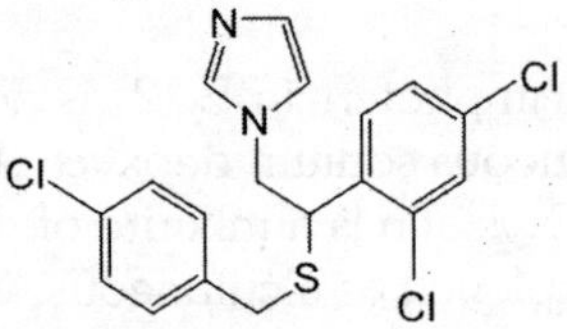

(17)

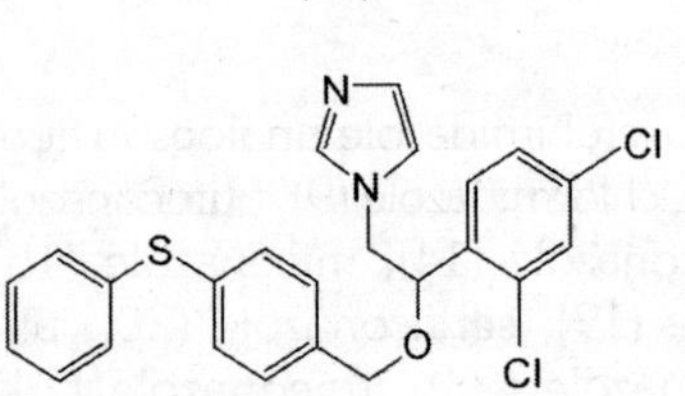

(18)

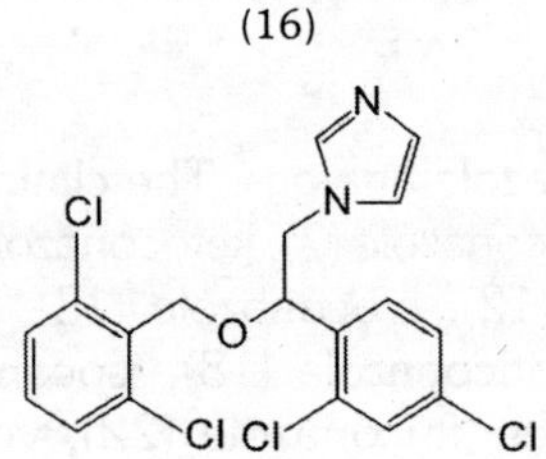

(19)

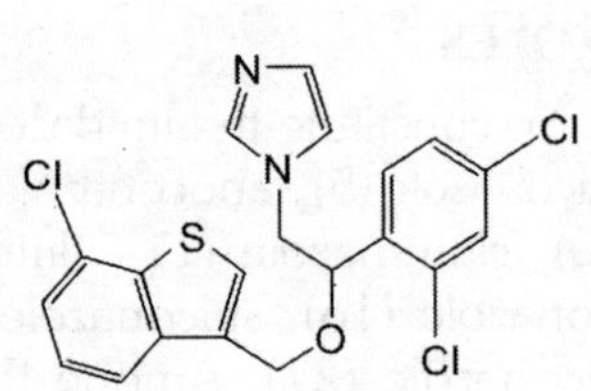

(20)

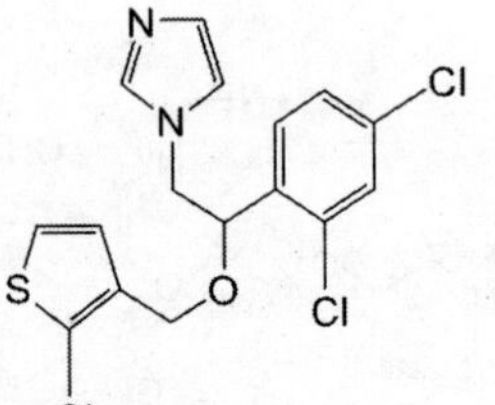

(21)

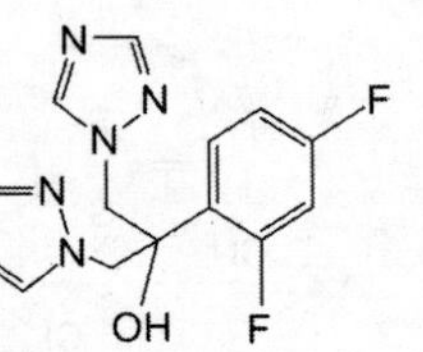

(22)

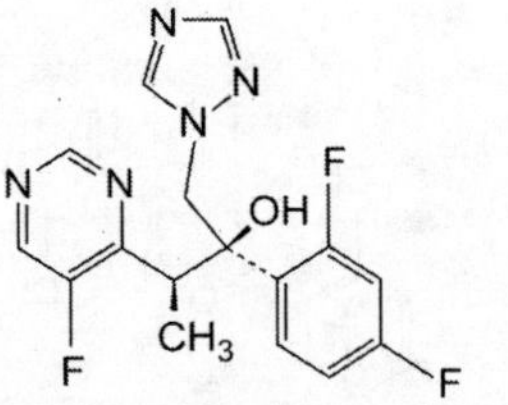

(23)

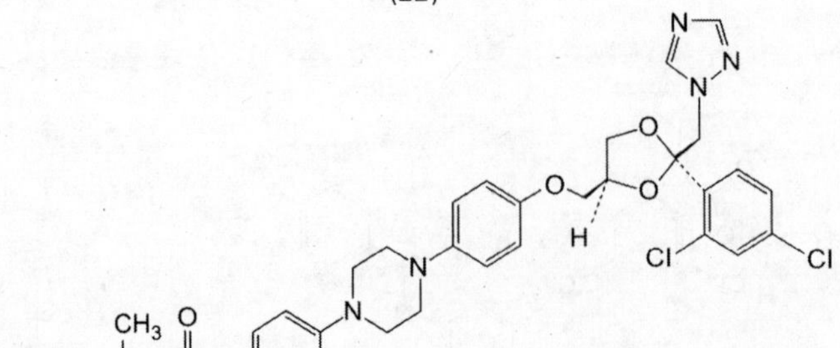

(24)

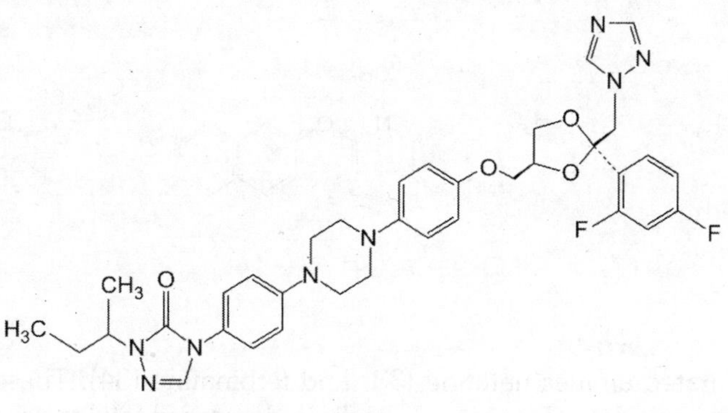

(25)

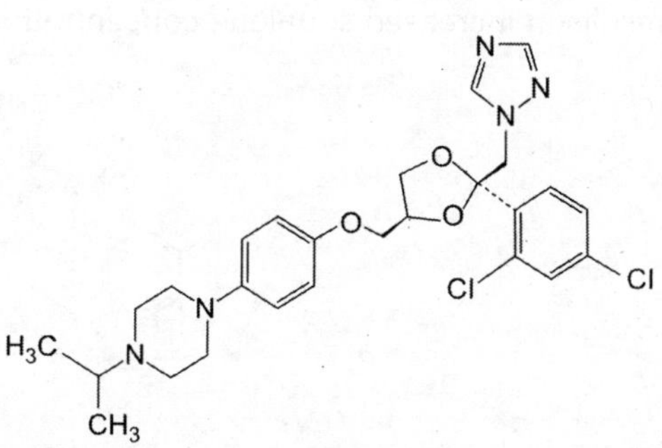

(26)

Azoles act by inhibition of 14α-demethylase heme, which is required for oxidation and finally for removal of 14α-methyl group in the ergosterol biosynthesis. This results in inhibition of ergosterol biosynthesis. The proposed mechanism involves formation of a bond between basic nitrogen of azoles with heme iron of the 14α-demethylase heme. This results in inability of the enzyme to carry out the oxidation.

PHENOLS

Phenols have been used for the treatment of superficial mycoses. Some of the compounds belonging to this class include salicylanilide (27), 3,5-dibromosalicylaldehyde (28), ethyl vanillate (29), pyrogallol triacetate (30), tolnaftate (31), and haloprogin (32). Haloprogin (32), an iodinated acetylenic compound is used as a topical application.

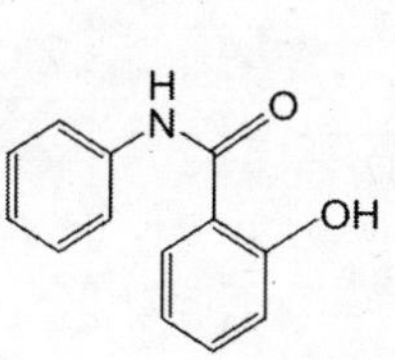

(27)

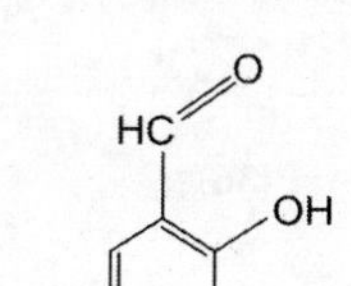

(28)

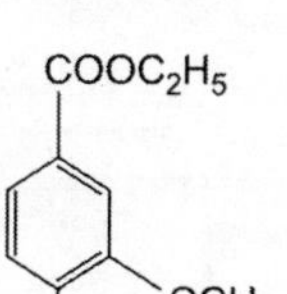

(29)

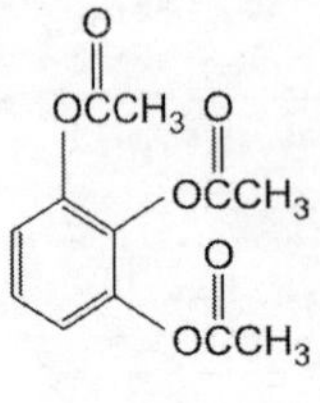

(30) 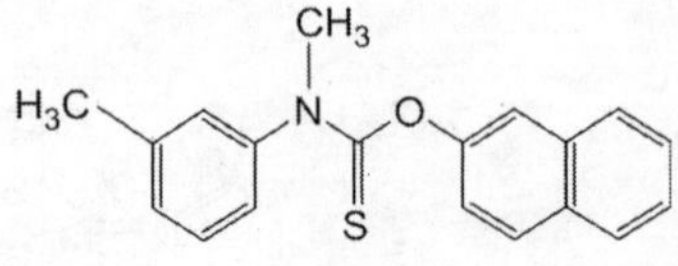   (31) 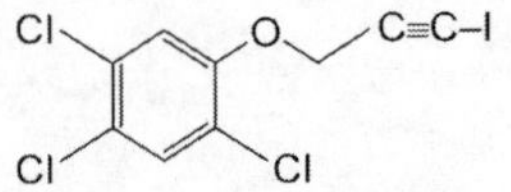   (32)

AMINES

These include unsaturated amines naftifine (33) and terbinafine (34). These compounds act by inhibition of squalene epoxidase. This in turn results in decreased total sterol content of fungal cell membrane which affects the functioning of membrane embedded transport proteins. The inhibition of squalene epoxidase also results in increased squalene concentration which itself is toxic.

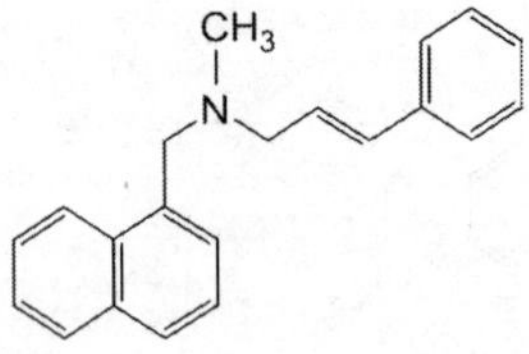

(33) 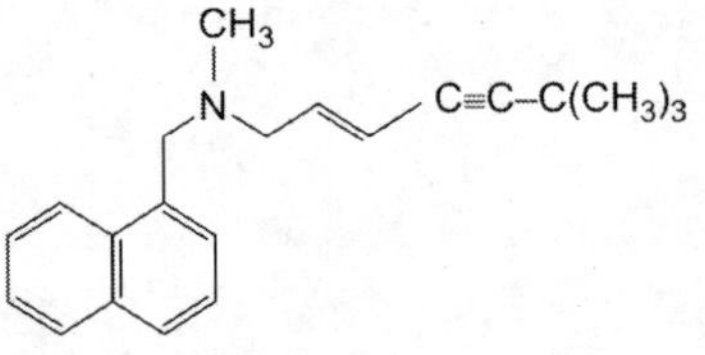   (34)

MISCELLANEOUS COMPOUNDS

Flucytosine (35) is a powerful antifungal agent used in treatment of systemic fungal infections caused by *Cryptococcus neoformans* and *Candida sp.* Flucytosine (35) is actually a prodrug and is inactive. It is oxidized by fungal deaminase to fluorouracil (36) and then converted to 5-fluorodeoxyuridine monophosphate (37). 5-Fluorodeoxyuridine monophosphate (37) is an inhibitor of thymidylate synthase, an enzyme involved in the biosyntheses of RNA and proteins.

Among the metal salts, zinc undecylenate (38) has been used as an application.

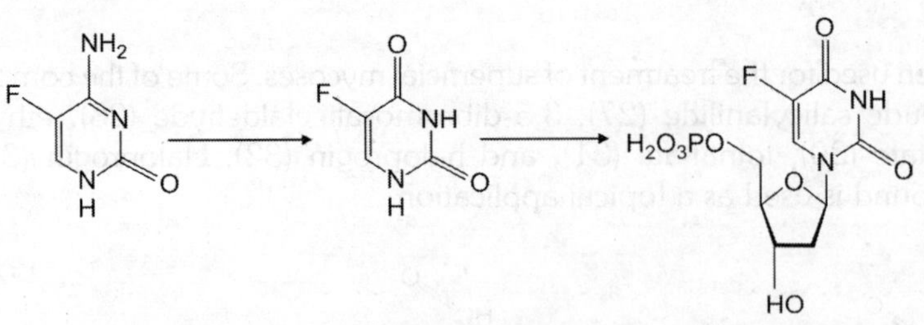

(35)   (36)   (37)

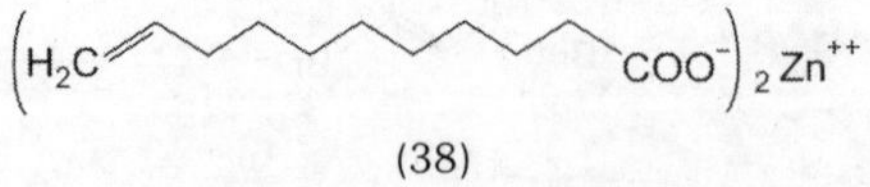

(38)

INDIVIDUAL COMPOUNDS

AZOLES : IMIDAZOLES

Oxiconazole

(Z)-1-(2, 4-Dichlorophenyl)-2-(1H-imidazol-1-yl)ethanone O-[(2, 4-dichlorophenyl) methyl] oxime

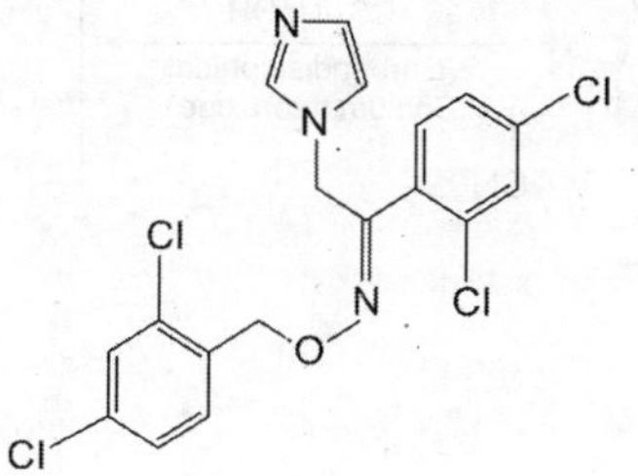

Synthesis

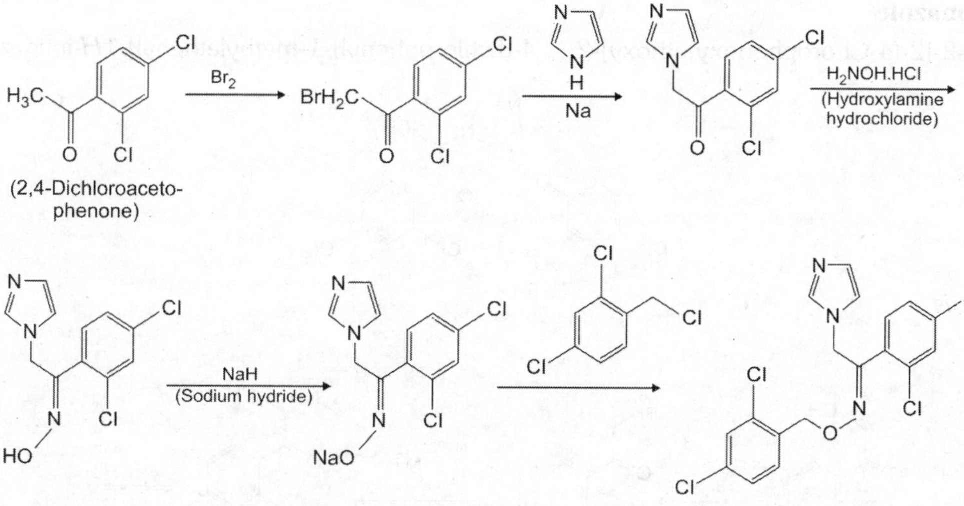

(2,4-Dichloroaceto-
phenone)

It is a broad-spectrum antifungal agent and used in cream and lotion form.

Lanoconazole

(E)–(±)-α-[4-(2-Chlorophenyl)-1,3-dithiolan-2-ylidene]-1H-imidazole-1-acetonitrile

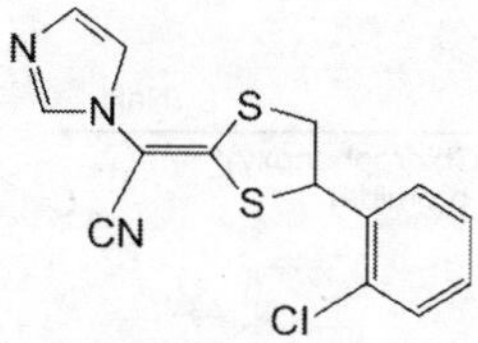

Synthesis

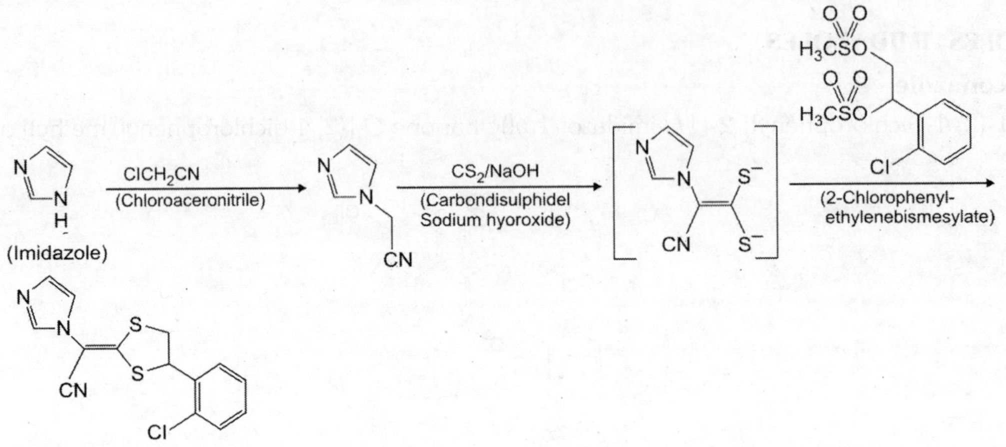

It is a broad spectrum antifungal agent.

Omoconazole

1-[(1Z)-2-[2-(4-Chorophenoxy)ethoxy]-2-(2,4-dichlorophenyl)-1-methylethenyl]-1H-imidazole

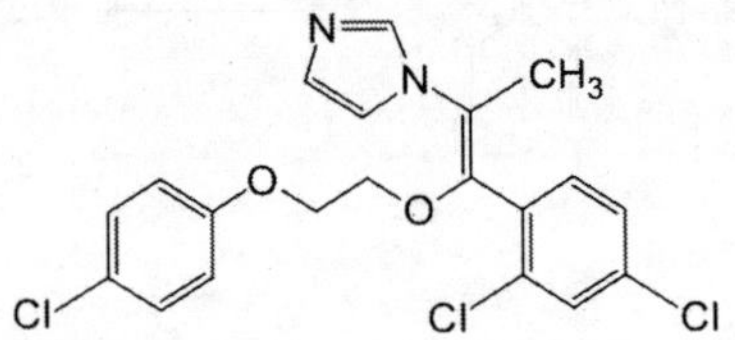

Synthesis

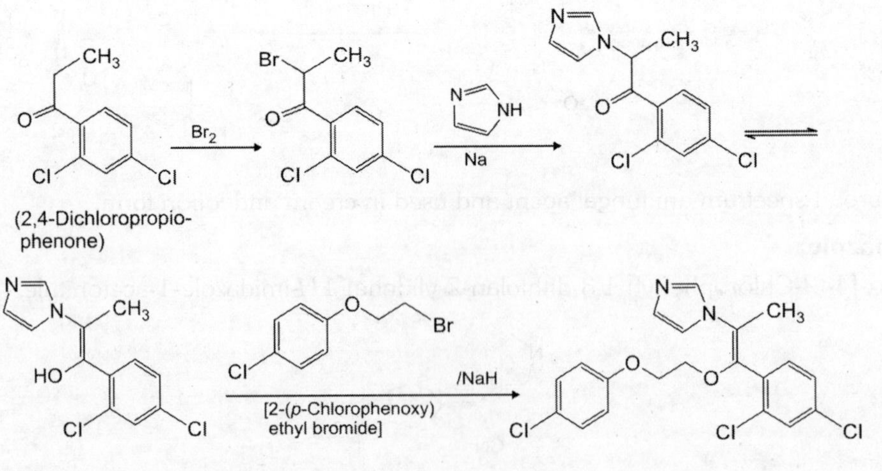

Same activity as lanoconazole (6).

Ketoconazole

cis-1-Acetyl-4-[4-[[2-(2,4-dichlorophenyl)-2-(1H-imidazol-1-ylmethyl)-1, 3-dioxolan-4-yl]methoxy]-phenyl] piperazine

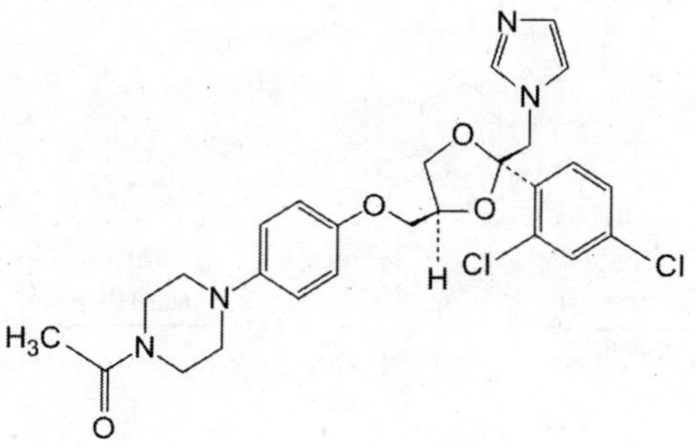

Synthesis

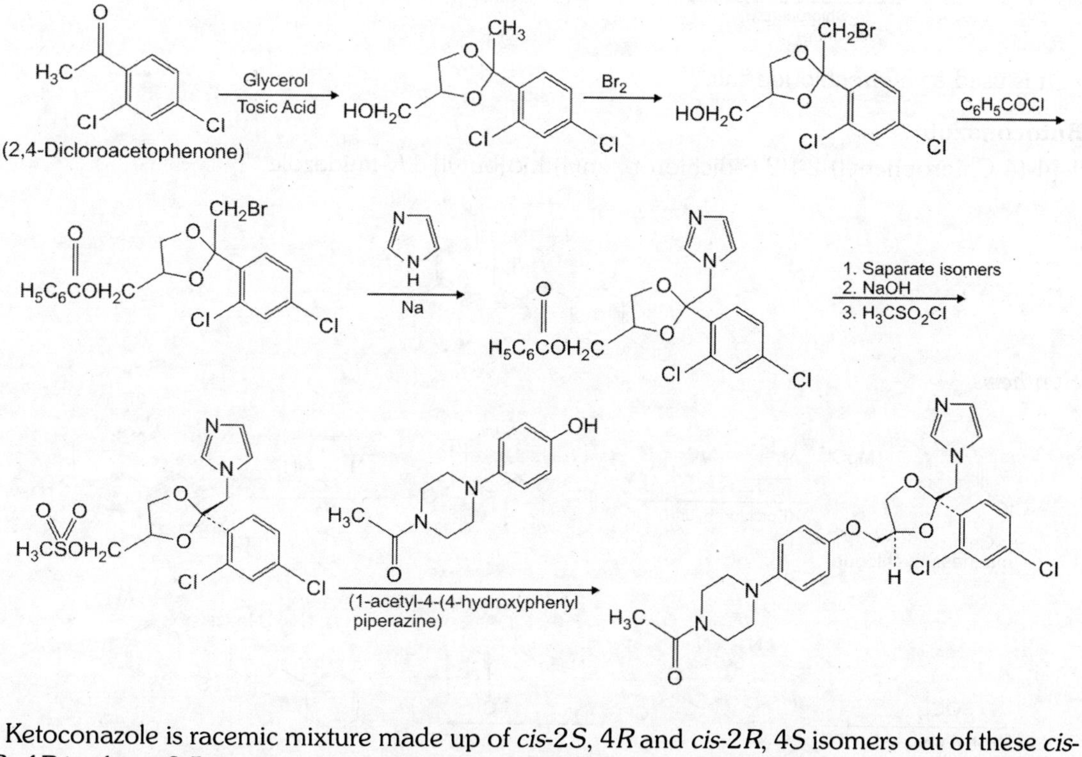

Ketoconazole is racemic mixture made up of *cis-2S, 4R* and *cis-2R, 4S* isomers out of these *cis-2S, 4R* is about 2.5 times more active than *cis-2R, 4S* isomer. The *trans*-isomers are much less active. It is used for systemic fungal infections of candidiasis, coccidioidomycosis, blastomycosis, histoplasmosis, and chromomycosis.

Chlormidazole

1-[(4-Chlorophenyl)methyl]-2-methyl-1*H*-benzimidazole

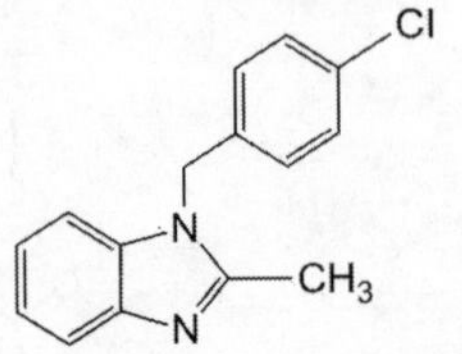

Synthesis

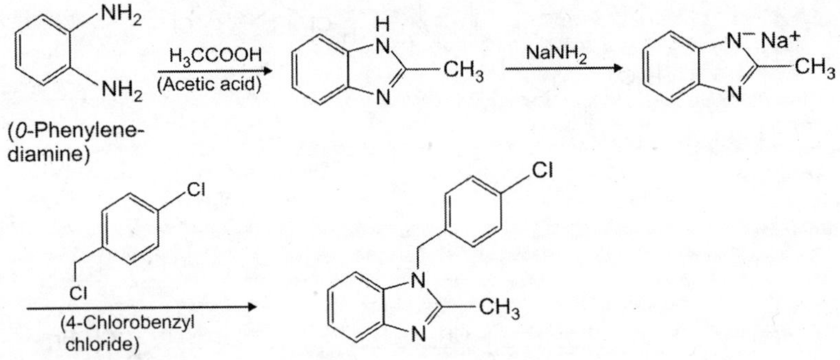

It is used as hydrochloride salt.

Butoconazole

1-[4-(4-Chlorophenyl)-2-[(2,6-dichlorophenyl)thio]butyl]-1*H*-imidazole

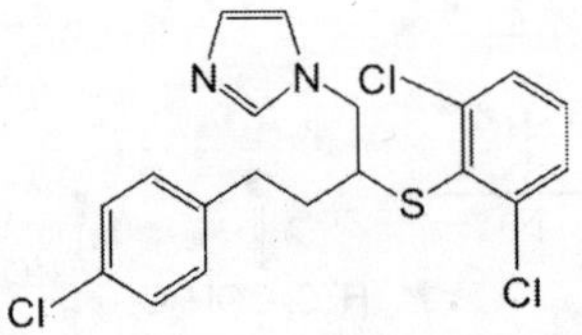

Synthesis

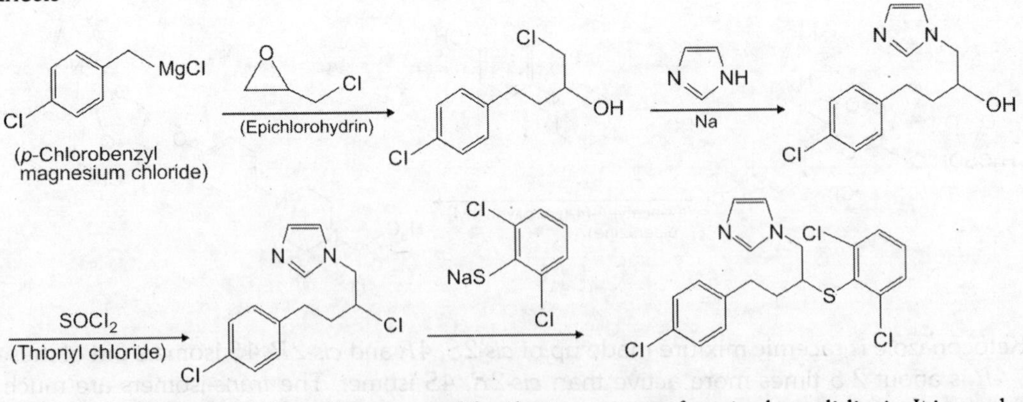

It is a broad-spectrum antifungal agent used for the treatment of vaginal candidiasis. It is marketed as cream of nitrate salt.

Clotrimazole

1-[(2-Chlorophenyl)-diphenylmethyl]-1*H*-imidazole

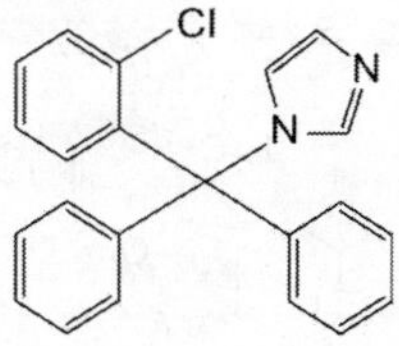

Synthesis

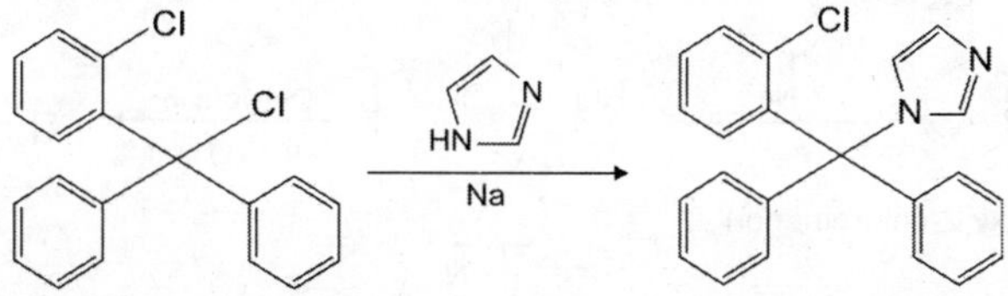

(2-Chlorophenyldiphenyl
methyl chloride)

It is a broad-spectrum antifungal agent and is used systemically as well as a topical application. When used orally it causes gastrointestinal disturbances. It is used in tinea infections.

Flutrimazole

1-[(2-Fluorophenyl)-(4-fluorophenyl)phenylmethyl]-1*H*-imidazole

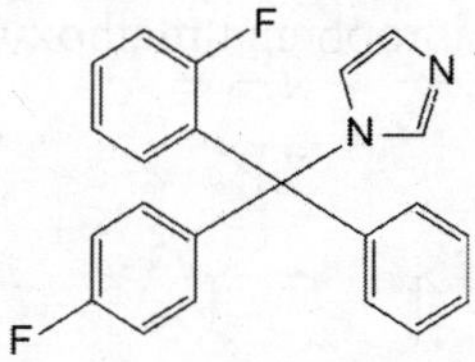

Synthesis

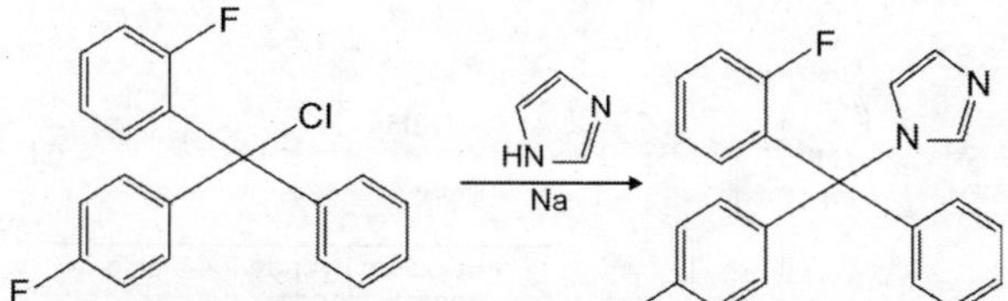

(2-Fluorophenyl-4-
fluorophenylphenyl
methylchloride)

It is used topically.

Croconazole

1-[1-[2-[(3-Chlorophenyl)methoxy]phenyl]ethenyl]-1*H*-imidazole

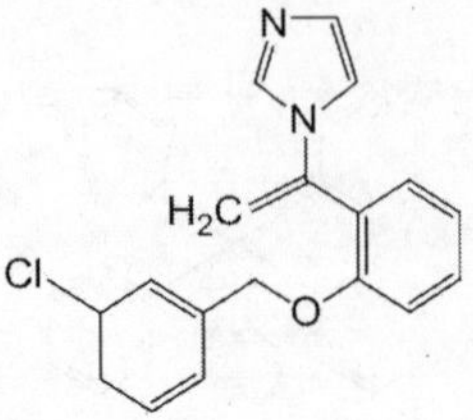

Synthesis

(2-*m*-Phenoxy-2-chlorethenol)

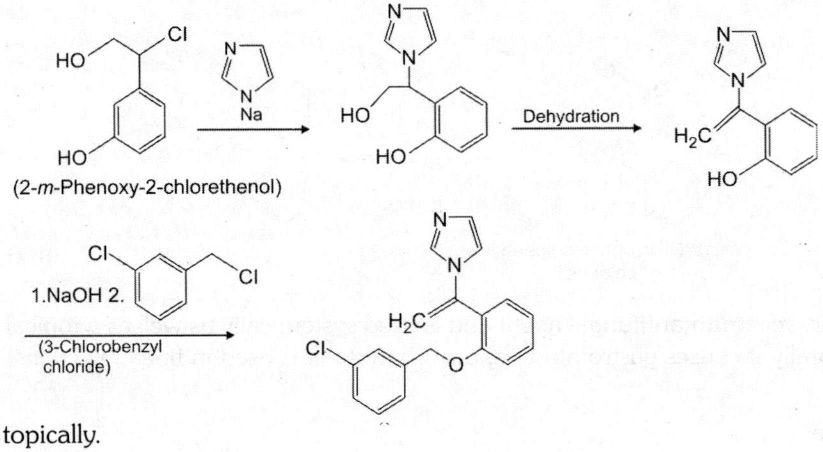

It is used topically.

Miconazole

1-[2-(2,4-Dichlorophenyl)-2-[(2,4-dichlorophenyl)methoxy]ethyl]-1*H*-imidazole

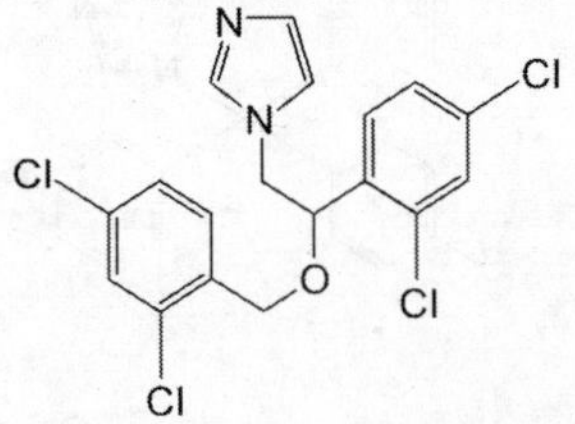

Synthesis

(Intermediate from oxiconazole)

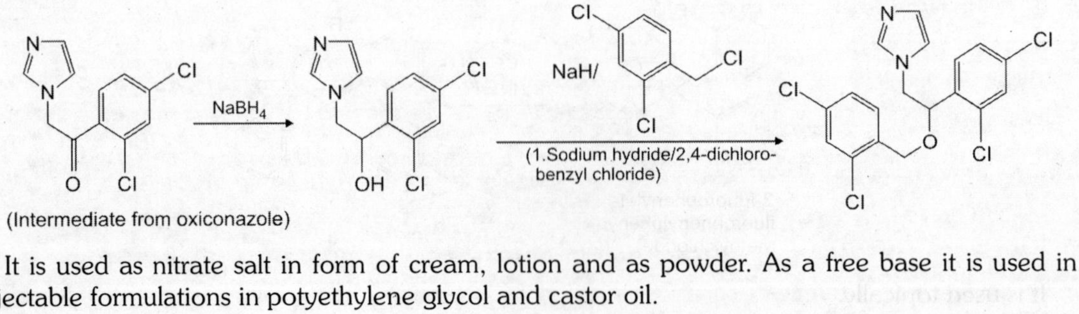

It is used as nitrate salt in form of cream, lotion and as powder. As a free base it is used in injectable formulations in potyethylene glycol and castor oil.

Econazole

1-[2-[(4-Chlorophenyl)-methoxy]-2-(2,4-dichlorophenyl)ethyl]-1*H*-imidazole

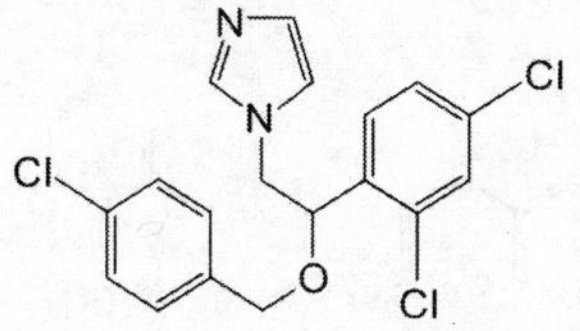

Synthesis

(Intermediate from miconazole)

1. NaH/

(Sodium hydride/4-Chlorobenzyl chloride)

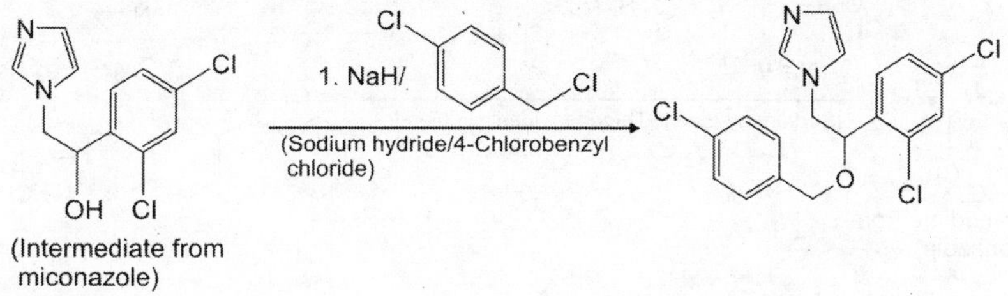

It is used topically.

Sulconazole

1-[2-[[(4-Chlorophenyl)methyl)thio]-2-(2,4-dichlorophenyl)ethyl]-1*H*-imidazole

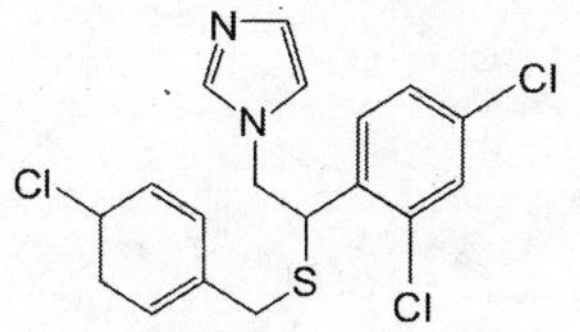

Synthesis

(Intermediate from miconazole)

SOCl₂

(4-Chlorobenzylthiol)

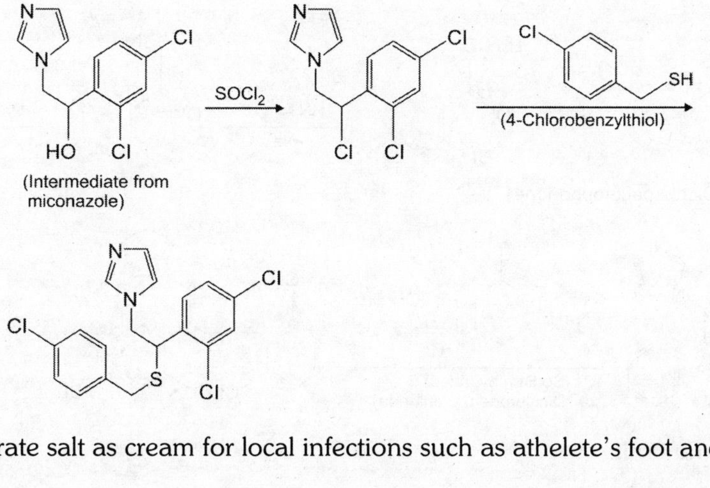

It is used as nitrate salt as cream for local infections such as athelete's foot and ringworm.

Fenticonazole

1-[2-(2,4-Dichlorphenyl)-2-[[4-phenylthio) phenyl] methoxy] ethyl]-1*H*-imidazole

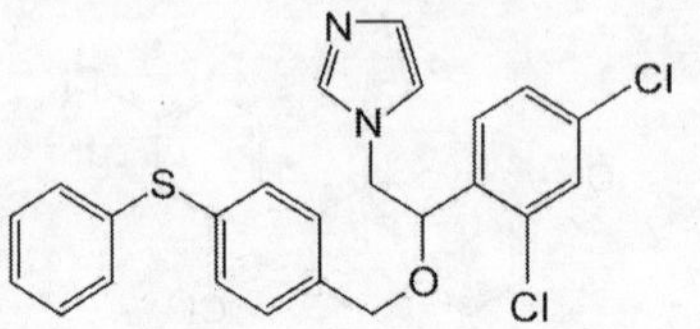

Synthesis

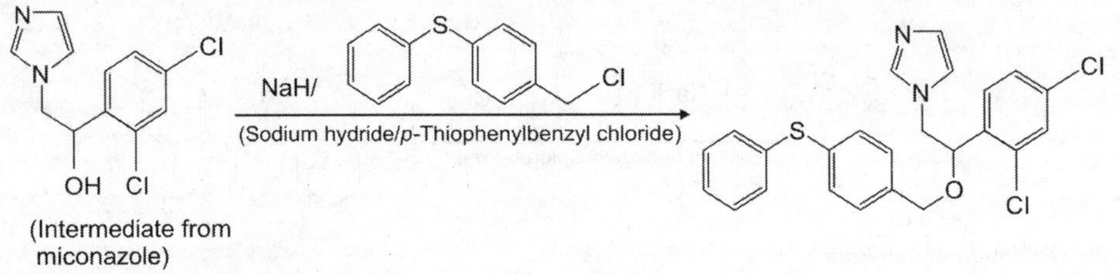
NaH/
(Sodium hydride/p-Thiophenylbenzyl chloride)
(Intermediate from miconazole)

It is used topically as solution or in form of ointment.

Isoconazole

1-[2-(2, 4-Dichlorophenyl)-2-[(2, 6-dichlorophenyl) methoxy] ethyl]-1*H*-imidazole

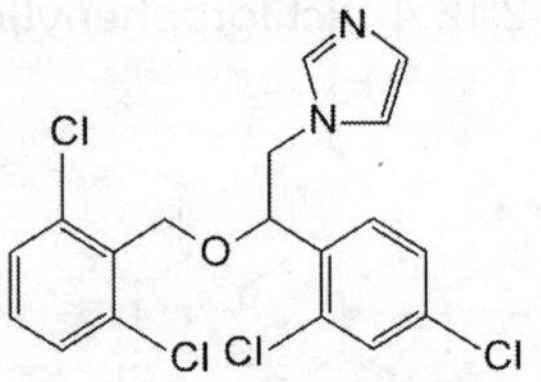

Synthesis

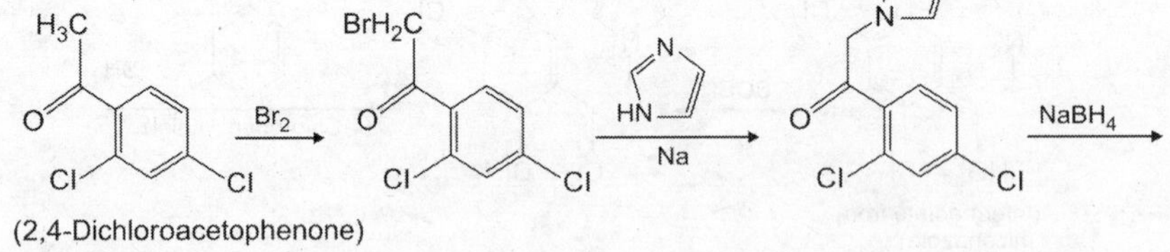
Br2
Na
NaBH4
(2,4-Dichloroacetophenone)

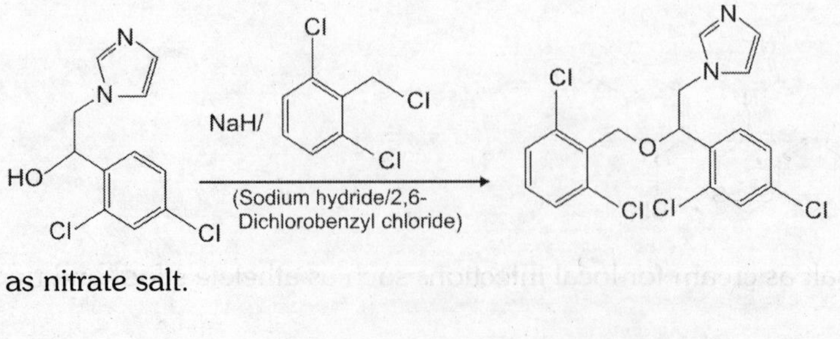
NaH/
(Sodium hydride/2,6-Dichlorobenzyl chloride)

It is used as nitrate salt.

Sertaconazole

1-[2-[7-Chlorobenzo[b]thien-3-yl)methoxy]-2-(2,4-dichlorophenyl)ethyl]-1*H*-imidazole

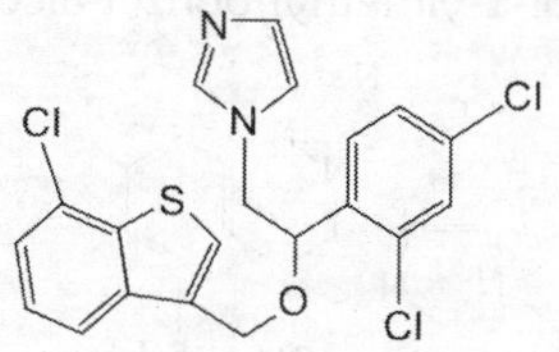

Synthesis

(Intermediate from miconazole)

NaH/ (Sodium hydride/7-Chloro-3-chloromethyl benzothiophene)

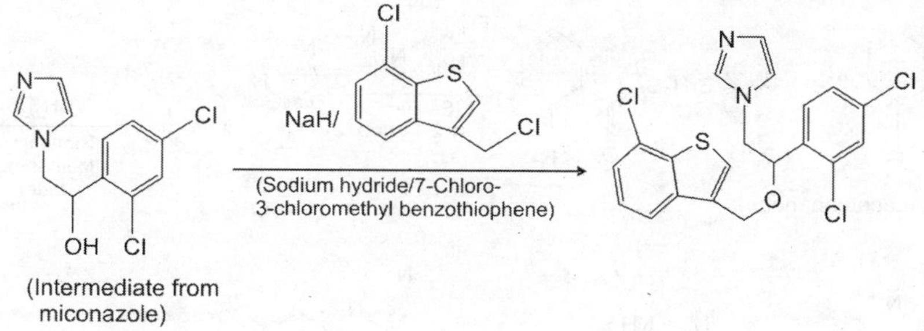

It is used as nitrate salt.

Tioconazole

1-[2-[(2-Chloro-3-thienyl)methoxy]-2-(2, 4-dichlorophenyl)ethyl]-1*H*-imidazole

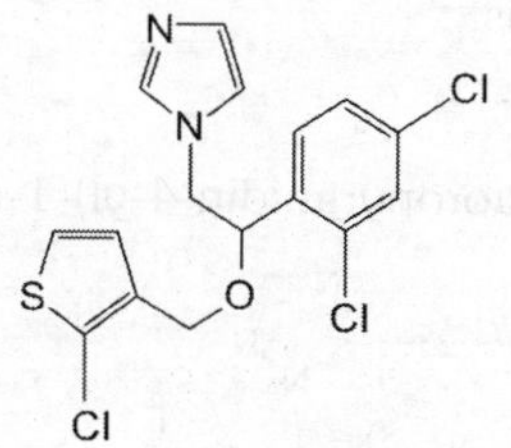

Synthesis

(Intermediate from miconazole)

NaH/ (Sodium hydride/2-Chloro-3-chloromethylthiophene)

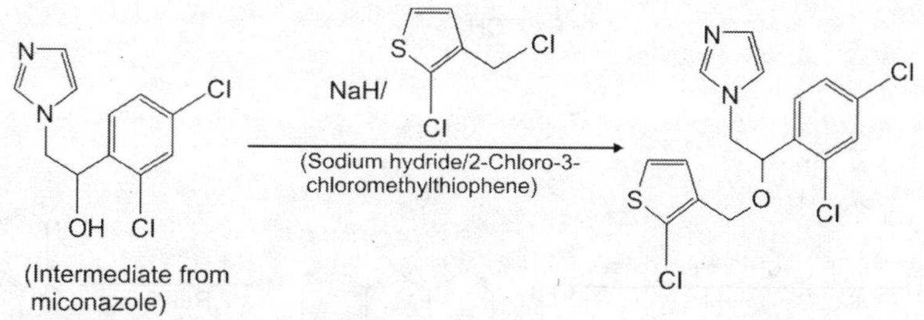

It is used for infections in vagina as vaginal ointment.

AZOLES : TRIAZOLES

Fluconazole

2, 4-Difluoro-α,α-bis(1H-1,2,4-triazol-1-ylmethyl)benzyl alcohol

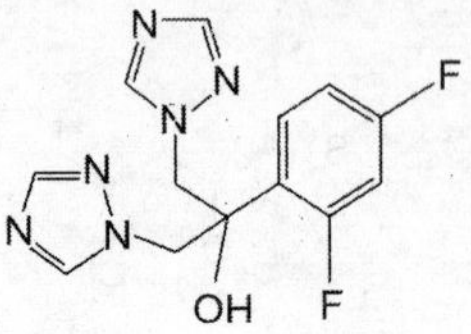

Synthesis

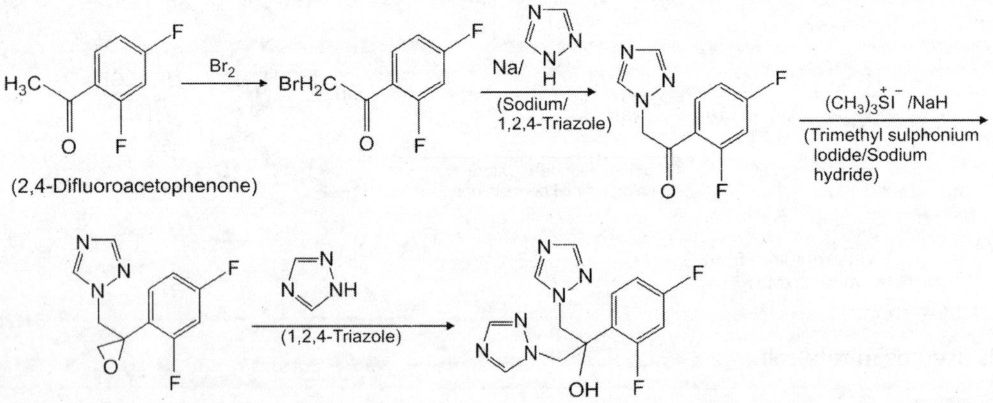

(2,4-Difluoroacetophenone)

(Sodium/
1,2,4-Triazole)

$(CH_3)_3\overset{+}{S}\overset{-}{I}$ /NaH

(Trimethyl sulphonium
Iodide/Sodium
hydride)

(1,2,4-Triazole)

Fluconazole is absorbed well and has a long half-life ranging from 27 to 34 hr. It is used in various dosage forms including tablets, or as oral suspension and is recommended for disseminated deep organ candidiasis.

Voriconazole

2R,3S-2-(2,4-Difluorophenyl)-3-(5-fluoropyrimidin-4-yl)-1-(1H-1,2,4-triazol-1-yl)butan-2-ol

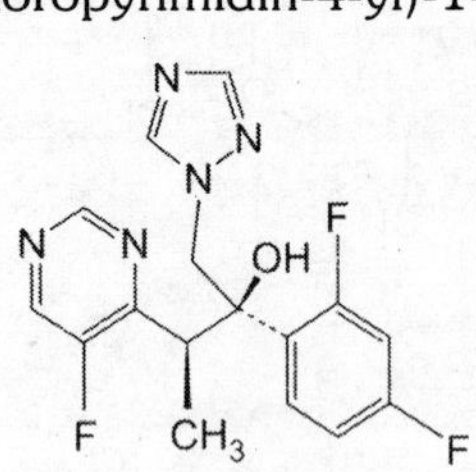

Synthesis

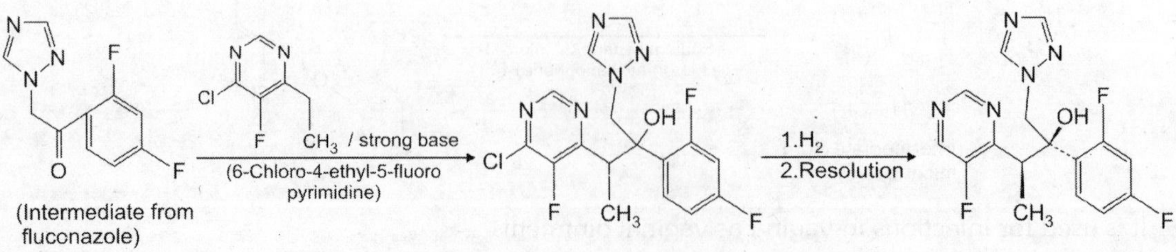

(Intermediate from
fluconazole)

$F \quad CH_3$ / strong base

(6-Chloro-4-ethyl-5-fluoro
pyrimidine)

1.H_2
2.Resolution

It is a potent antifungal agent and is active against a variety of fungi including clinically important pathogens.

Saperconazole

4-[4-[4-[4-[[2-(2,4-Difluorophenyl)-2-(1*H*-1,2,4-triazol-1-ylmethyl)-1,3-dioxalan-4-yl]methoxy]-phenyl]1-piperazinyl]phenyl]-2,4-dihydro-2-(1-methylpropyl)-3*H*-1,2,4-triazol-3-one

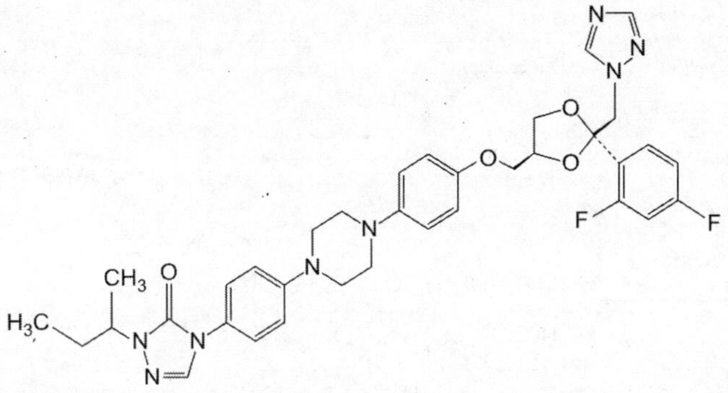

Synthesis

Step 1

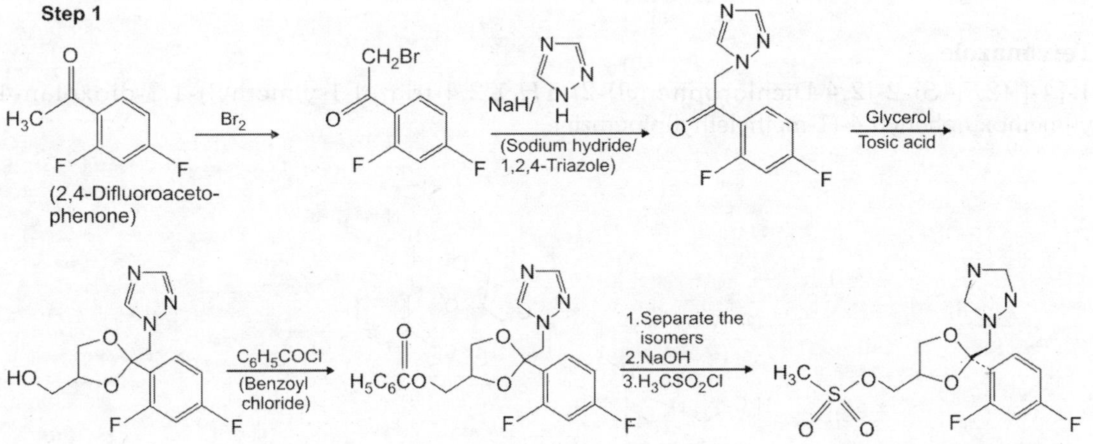

(2,4-Difluoroaceto-phenone)

NaH/ (Sodium hydride/ 1,2,4-Triazole)

Glycerol Tosic acid

C₆H₅COCl (Benzoyl chloride)

1. Separate the isomers
2. NaOH
3. H₃CSO₂Cl

(A)

Step 2

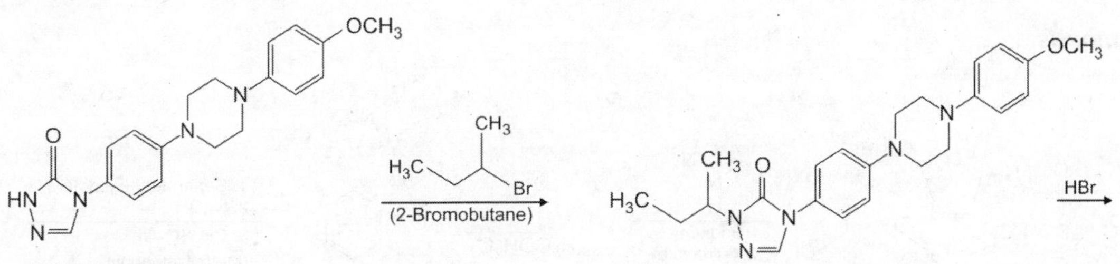

(Triazolone analog)

(2-Bromobutane)

HBr

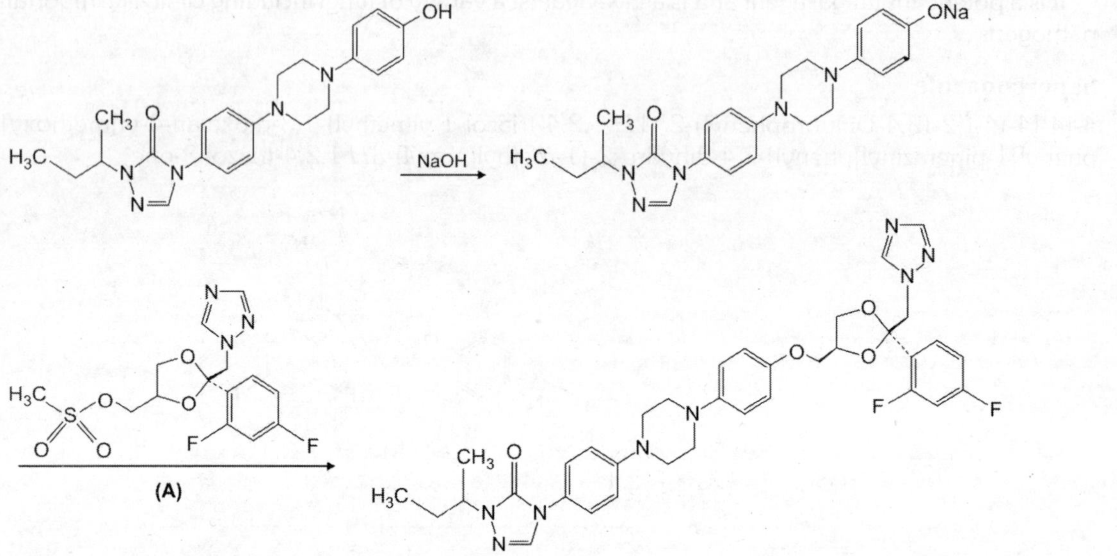

Activity similar as in case of voriconazole (23).

Terconazole

1-[4-[[(2R,4S)-2-(2,4-Dichlorophenyl)-2-(1H-1,2,4-triazol-1-ylmethyl)-1,3-dioxolan-4-yl]methoxy]phenyl]-4-(1-methylethyl)piperazine

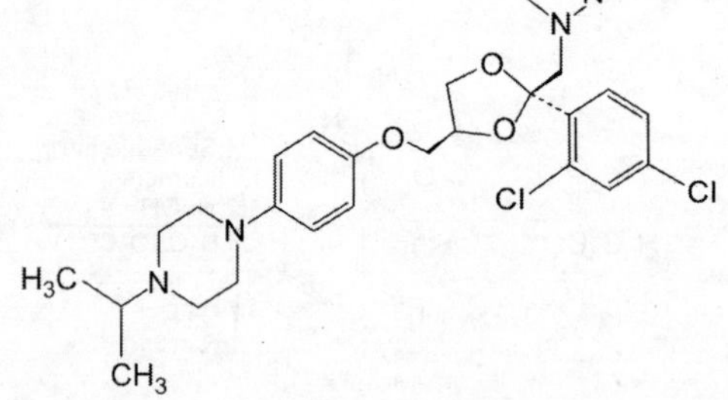

Synthesis

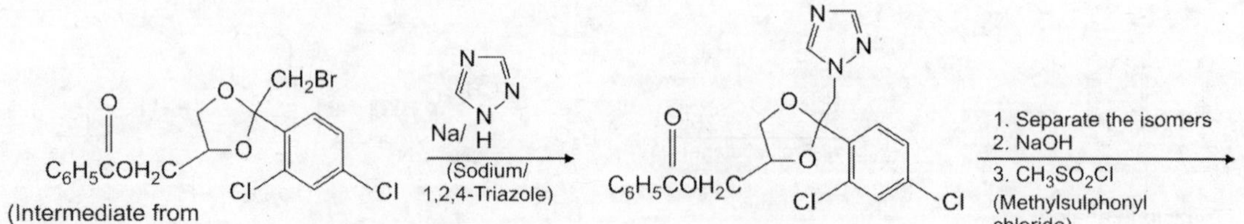

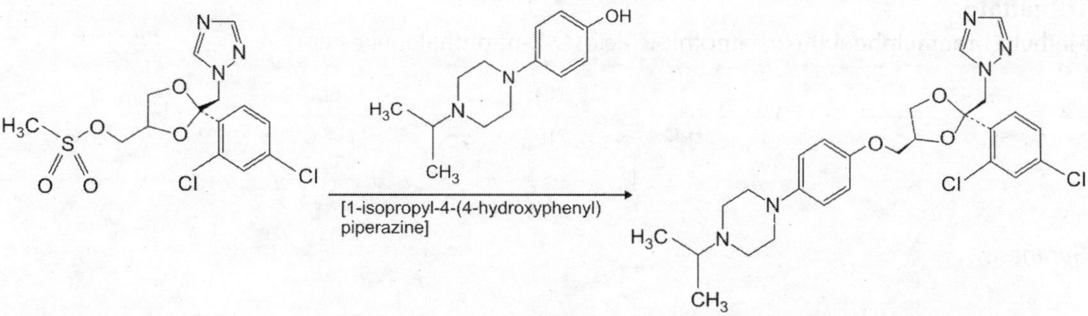

It is exclusively used for vaginal infections caused by *C.albicans* and other *Candida* species.

PHENOLS

Salicylanilide

2-Hydroxy-*N*-phenylbenzamide

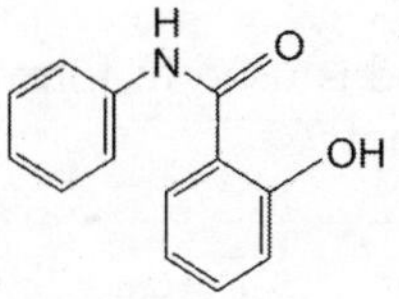

Synthesis

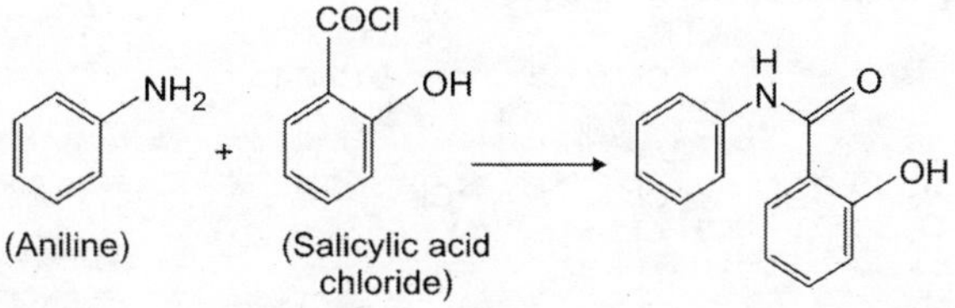

(Aniline)   (Salicylic acid chloride)

It is used topically

Pyrogallol triacetate

1,2,3-Trihydroxybenzene acetate

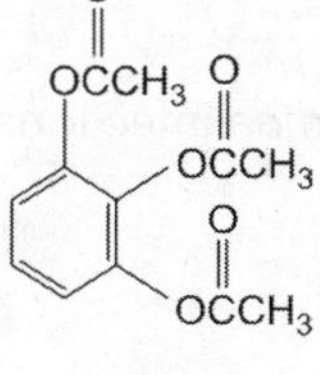

Synthesis

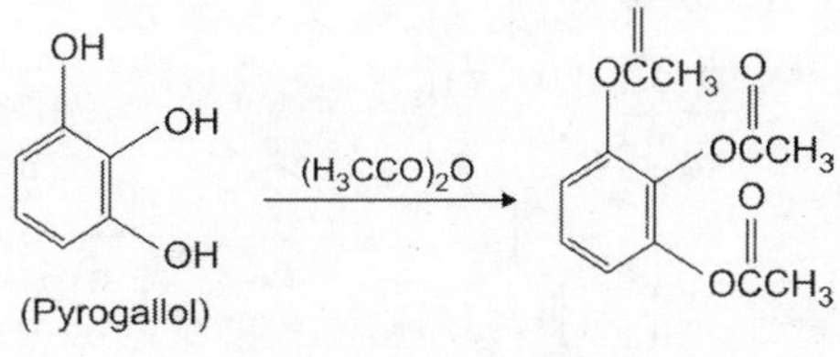

(Pyrogallol)

It is used topically

Tolnaftate

Methyl (3-methylphenyl)-carbamothioic acid *O*-2-naphthalenyl ester

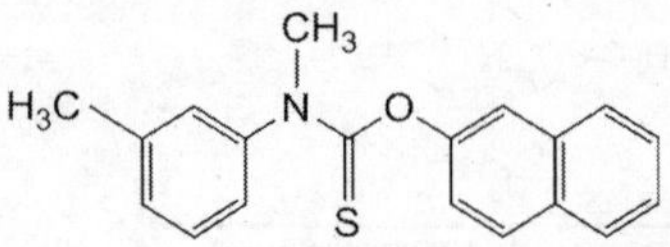

Synthesis

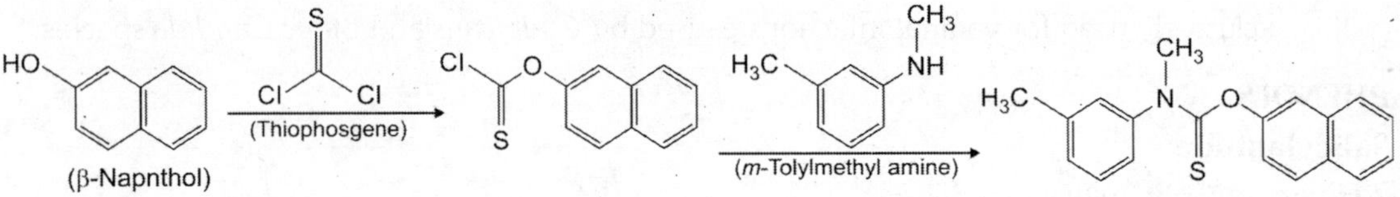

It is active against dermatophytes and is used in form of creams, powders, aerosols, gels, and solutions for ringworm and athelete's foot.

Haloprogin

3-Iodo-2-propynyl 2,4,5-trichlorophenyl ether

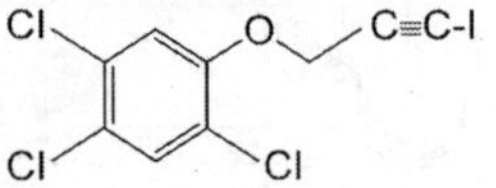

Synthesis

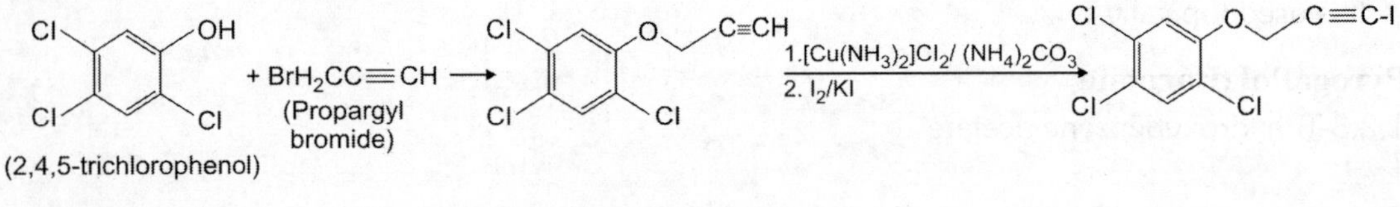

It is used topically for superficial *Candida* infections.

AMINES

Naftifine

(*E*)-*N*-Cinnamyl-*N*-methyl-1-naphthalenemethylamine

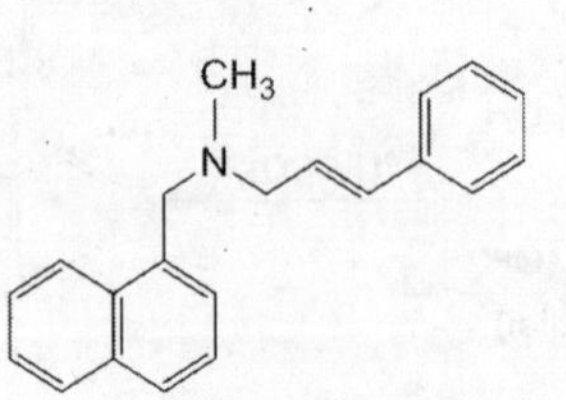

Synthesis

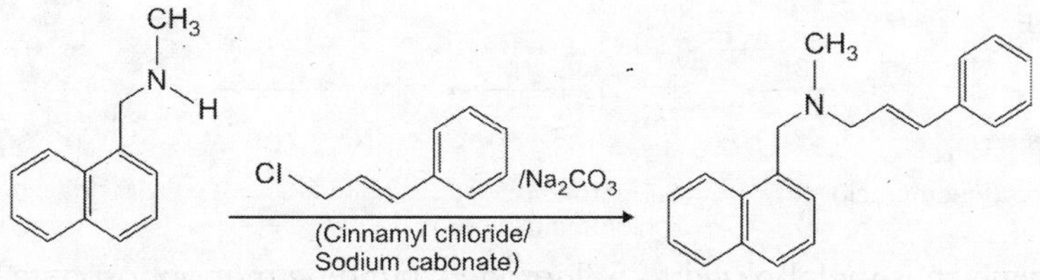

It is used as gel and cream as a topical application for the treatment of ringworm and athelete's foot.

Terbinafine

N-[(2*E*)-6, 6-Dimethyl-2-hepten-4ynyl]-*N*-methyl-1-naphthalenemethanamine

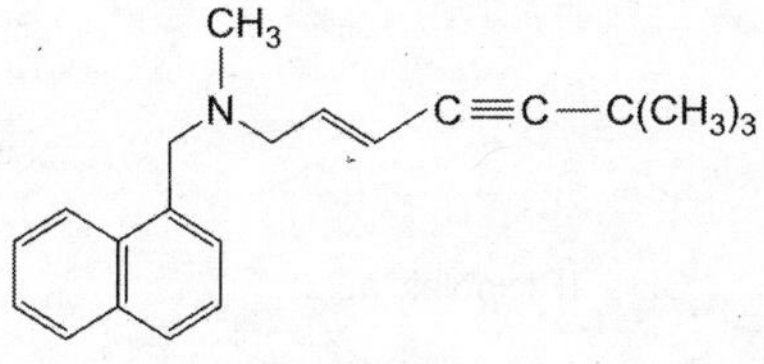

Synthesis

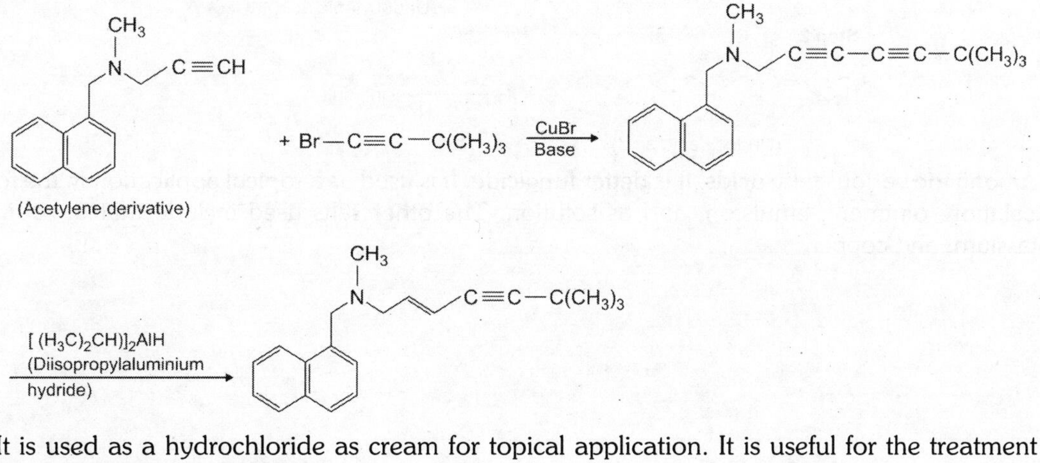

It is used as a hydrochloride as cream for topical application. It is useful for the treatment of ringworm infection of nails.

MISCELLANEOUS COMPOUNDS
Flucytosine

4-Amino-5-fluoro-2(1*H*)-pyrimidinone

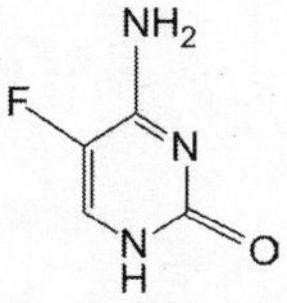

Synthesis

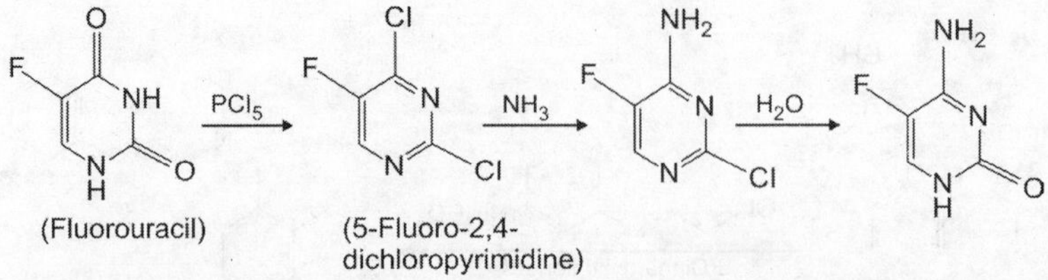

(Fluorouracil)   (5-Fluoro-2,4-dichloropyrimidine)

It is a prodrug which is metabolized to 5-fluorodeoxyuridine monophosphate (37), a powerful inhibitor of thymidylate synthase. It is used for treatment of systemic fungal infections.

Zinc Undecylenate
10-Undecenoic acid zinc salt

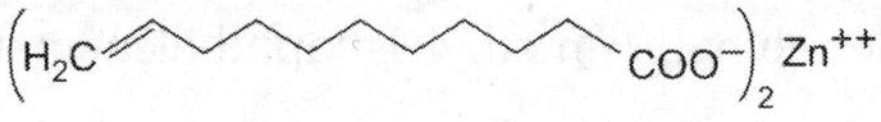

Synthesis

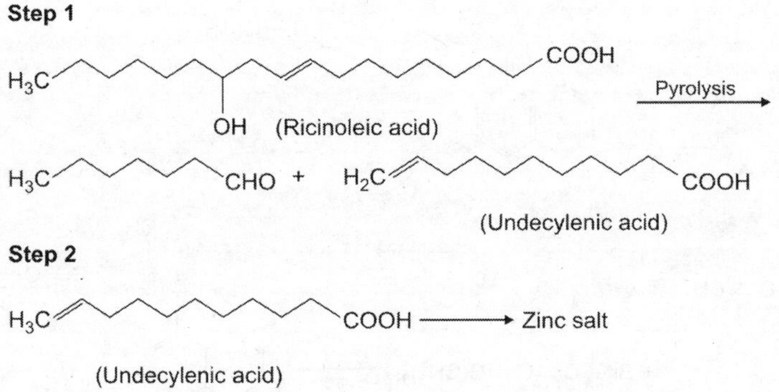

Step 1

OH   (Ricinoleic acid)

(Undecylenic acid)

Step 2

(Undecylenic acid)

Among the various fatty acids, it is better fungicide. It is used as a topical application in the form of solution, ointment, emulsion, and as solution. The other salts used include that of sodium, potassium, and copper.

ANTIVIRAL AGENTS

V IRUSES are smallest microorganism varying in size from 0.02-0.40 μm. They consist essentially of nucleic acids, either ribonucleic acid (RNA) or deoxyribonucleic acid (DNA), enclosed in a protein coat called nucleocapsid (Fig. 35.1). In some viruses, there is a lipoprotein envelope, which may contain antigenic viral glycoprotein as well as phospholipids. These may be aquired when the virus nucleocapsid buds through the nuclear membrane or the plasma membrane of the host cell. Certain viruses also contain enzymes that initiate their replication in the host cell. The whole infective particle is known as virion. In different types of virus, the genome may be double or single stranded.

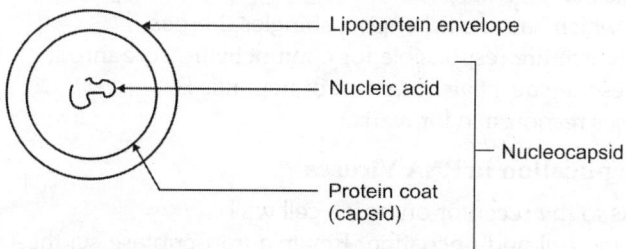

Fig. 35.1: Components of virus particle (virion).

Viruses are filterable through porcelain filters and can be seen and identified by electron microscope. Viruses are causative organisms of a wide variety of infections in both animals and humans. The type of disease and symptoms depend upon the group and species of viruses.

Viruses are classified according to nucleic acid of which they are made-up of, the DNA and RNA virus.

The protein coats of the nucleocapsid, the presence or absence of envelope, play an important role in the initial stages of viral infection. The reactive site on the capsid or the envelope become attached to the receptor sites on the host cell. The penetration, uncoating, and release of the virions depend on the structural coat proteins. It is this process which is susceptible to the action of antiviral drugs. The study of the properties of viral coat proteins plays an important role in the development of effective antiviral agents.

VIRUS LIFE HISTORY

Viruses are intracellular parasites with no metabolic machinery of their own. In order to replicate, they have to attach to and enter the living host cell, plant, animal, or bacteria, and use its metabolic processes.

The binding sites on the virus are polypeptides on the envelope or capsid. The receptor on the host cell, to which the virus attaches, are the cytokines, neurotransmitters or hormones, ion channels, integral membrane glycoproteins, etc. After entering the host cell, it removes its coat. Once in host cell, the nucleic acid of virus then uses the host cell's machinery for synthesizing the nucleic acids and proteins and manufacture of new virion particles.

Virus replication requires DNA or RNA synthesis of viral proteins and glycosylation. The various steps involved in two types of viruses are as follows.

Steps involved in Replication in DNA Viruses

1. Attachment of virus to cell wall of host cell.
2. Penetration of cell wall by pinocytosis.
3. Uncoating of virus and transfer of viral DNA to the nucleus of host's cell.
4. Early transcription into mRNA.
5. Early translation of viral mRNA into enzymes for viral DNA synthesis.
6. Synthesis of viral DNA and late transcription of viral mRNA.
7. Late translation of mRNA into viral structural proteins.
8. Assembly of virus particles into nucleus.
9. Budding from nucleus and release of virions.

Examples of DNA viruses and the diseases they cause include:

(a) Pox viruses which cause smallpox.
(b) Herpes viruses which cause chickenpox, shingles, herpes.
(c) Adeno viruses which are responsible for conjunctivitis, sore throat.
(d) Hepadna viruses the causative organism of hepatitis B.
(e) Papilloma viruses responsible for warts.

Steps involved in Replication in RNA Viruses

1. Binding of virus to the receptor on host's cell wall.
2. Penetration in the cell and uncoating. Reverse transcriptase synthesizes a double stranded DNA copy of viral RNA.
3. DNA copy enters host's nucleus and integrates with host's DNA forming provirus.
4. Transcription of provirus into genomic RNA and mRNA for translation into viral proteins.
5. The completed viruses are then released by budding and many replicate without killing host cell.

Examples of RNA viruses and the diseases they cause include:

(a) Rubella viruses responsible for German measles.
(b) Rhabdo viruses responsible for rabies.
(c) Picorna viruses the causative organisms for poliomyelitis, meningitis, cold.
(d) Arena viruses responsible for meningitis, lassa fever.
(e) Arbo viruses which is responsible for yellow fever, anthropod borne encephalitis.
(f) Retroviruses responsible for AIDS, T-cell leukemia.

Virus can infect all living cells. As indicated earlier they are parasitic and multiply at the expense of host's metabolic system. Virus may start its infectious cycle immediately or remain dormant in the cellular site of the host for long periods until something triggers them to reproduce. Once they are active, they may produce cytotoxic effects or cause numerous diseases in animals or humans.

The major routes of transmission of viral infections in humans are through respiratory tract, gastrointestinal tract, genital tract, skin, urine, blood, and placenta. Viral infections may occur through air, water, food, milk, or, environmental sources.

Whether the host survives the effects of viral infection depends on the immune response of host and also on the severity of infection. Immune response is obtained by production of B lymphocytes derived from bone marrow and T lymphocytes derived from thymus with the help of macrophages. Specific immune response to viral diseases depends on antibodies formed by humoral (B cells), local (secretory IgA system), and cell mediated (T cells) immunities.

APPROACHES FOR PREVENTION OF VIRAL INFECTIONS

Immunization

Prevention of viral infection by conferring artificially acquired active immunity with vaccines is the main approach for preventing most of the viral diseases. Safe and highly effective vaccines are available for prevention of polio, rubella, measles, mumps, influenza, yellow fever, encephalitis, rabbies, smallpox, and hepatitis B. However, attempts to develop vaccines for prevention of infection with herpes virus, Epstein-Barr virus, cytomegalovirus (CMV), respiratory syncytial virus (RSV), and human immunodeficiency virus (HIV) have so far proved to be futile.

An effective vaccine against a chronic viral disease such as aquired immunodeficiency syndrome (AIDS) should have the following characteristics:

1. It should be sufficiently antigenic to induce an effective antibody response even in very young patients.
2. It should not cause disease that is designed to prevent or cause some other toxic manifestations.
3. It should produce a lasting immunity.

As it seems these conditions are difficult to meet for the viruses that cause acute infections and chronic cases become still more complicated.

As compared to bacterial infections, the development of drugs against viral infections has been slow because:

1. Viruses are difficult to grow in synthetic cultures as compared to bacteria. The most commonly used cell cultures in virology are derived from primates (humans and monkeys) and rodents (hamsters and mice).
2. Since biochemically virus is simple, there are fewer targets for chemotherapeutic agents.

One of the approaches to viral infections is chemoprophylaxis, an approach where chemical agents act by interfering with a step in early infectivity. Some of the most successful chemoprophylactics are those that interfere with penetration of virus into host cell. However, there are also other approaches and these include:

1. Inhibition and interference of virus attachment to host cell receptor, virus penetration, and uncoating.
2. Inhibition of virus-associated enzymes such as DNA polymerase and others.
3. Inhibition of transcription processes.
4. Interference with virus regulatory processes.
5. Interference with glucosylation, phosphorylation, sulfation, etc.
6. Interference with assembly of viral proteins.
7. Interference with release of virus from cell surface membrane.

ANTIVIRAL AGENTS

AGENTS INHIBITING VIRUS ATTACHMENT PENETRATION AND EARLY VIRAL REPLICATION

These include admantane analogs, amantadine (1) hydrochloride, rimantadine (2) hydrochloride, and interferons. Amantadine (1) inhibits penetration of RNA virus particles into host cell. It also inhibits early stages of viral replication blocking the uncoating of viral genome and transfer of nucleic acid into the host cell. Rimantadine (2) is more effective and has less side effects. It interferes with virus uncoating by inhibiting the release of specific protein. It may also act by inhibiting reverse transcriptase or the synthesis of virus specific RNA and does not affect absorption and penetration.

(1)   (2)

The interferons (IFN) are a family of inducible proteins synthesized by mammalian cells and now produced by recombinant DNA technology. There are at least three types of interferons, namely α-, β-, and γ-interferons, constituting a family of hormones involved in cell growth and regulation and modulation of immune reaction. IFNγ termed 'immune interferon' is produced by T lymphocytes as part of immunological response to both viral and non-viral antigens which include bacteria and their products, ricketisae, protozoa, fungal polysaccharides and a range of polymeric materials, and other cytokines. IFNα and IFNβ are produced by B and T lymphocytes, macrophages, and fibroblasts in response to the presence of viruses and cytokines. Interferons act partly by augmenting host's immune response.

IFNα possesses a broad-spectrum of activity. It acts on virus infected cells by binding to the specific cell surface receptors. It inhibits the transcription and translation of mRNA into viral nucleic acid and protein. Interferons may also act by blocking synthesis of a cleaving enzyme required for viral release.

Interferon α-2a is used for hepatitis B infections and AIDS related Kaposi sarcoma. Interferon α-2b is used for hepatitis C.

NEURAMINIDASE INHIBITORS

Hemaglutinin and neuraminidase are the enzymes present in the lipid envelope of influenza virus. Hemaglutinin is necessary for binding of the virus to the receptors of target cell. This binding takes place through glycoprotein of the virus. Bound to this glycoprotein is sialic acid (3) through a glycosidal bond (4) on the terminal sugar of the glycoprotein. Before the glycoprotein gets attached to the receptor on the cell, it has to be activated. This activation takes place after the sialic acid (3) is cleaved by neuraminidase. Inhibition of neuraminidase, thus results in prevention of viral attachment to the target cell receptors as well as the pathogenicity. Neuraminidase also prevents viral inactivation by respiratory mucous. Some of the neuraminidase inhibitors include 2-deoxy-2, 3-dehydro-N-acetylaminoneuraminic acid [DANA, (5)], zanamivir (6), and oseltamivir (7). DANA (5) is neuraminidase inhibitor but it lacks specificity for the viral neuraminidase. Zanamivir (6) which has a guanidine group at position 4 is an effective drug against influenza virus A and B. Oseltamivir (7) has also been found to be effective against influenza virus A and B. Oseltamivir (7) is a prodrug the active form of which is the free acid (8).

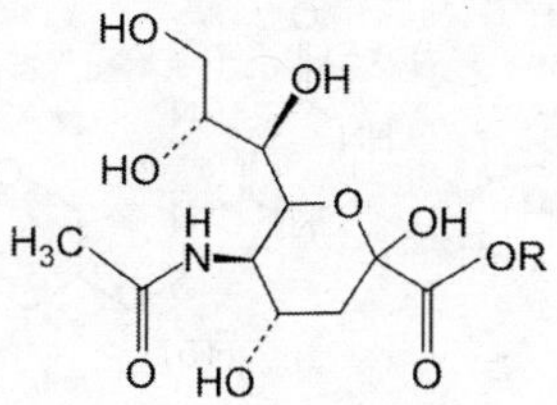

(3), R=H
(4), R=sugar-protein
    (Glycoprotein)

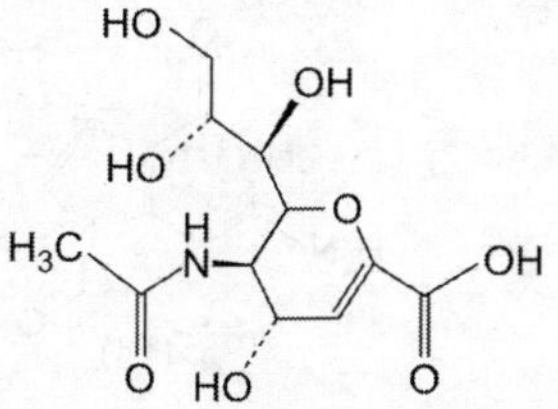

(5)

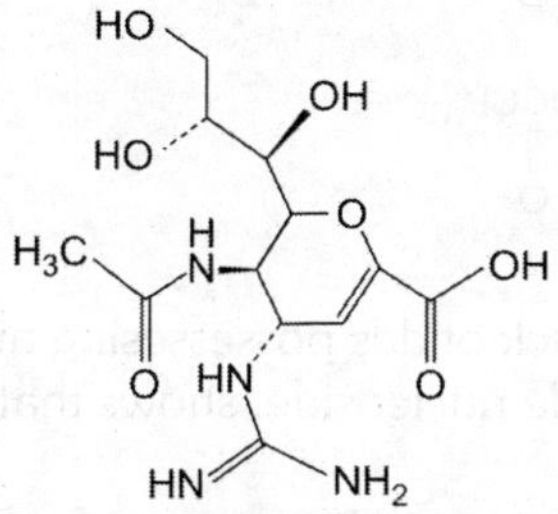

(6)

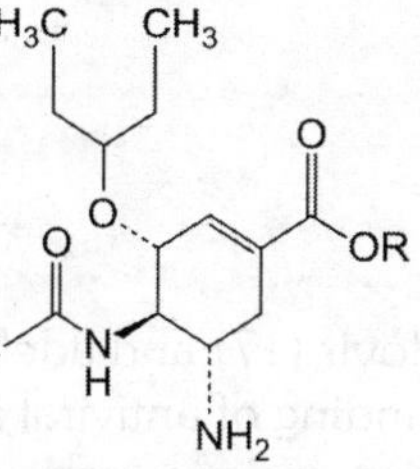

(7), R=C₂H₅
(8), R=H

DNA POLYMERASE INHIBITORS

These include pyrimidine and purine nucleosides like idoxuridine (9), trifluridine (10), and vidarabine (11).

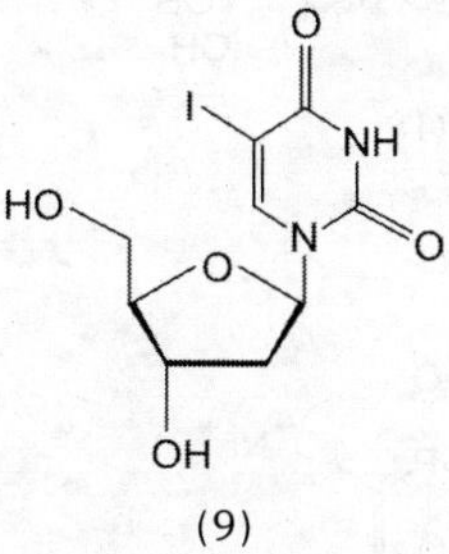

(9) 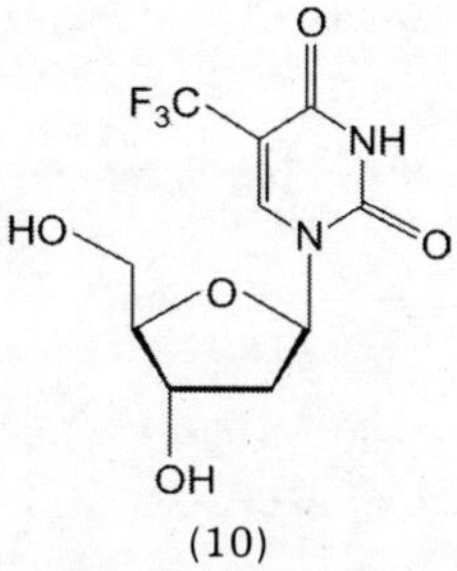   (10) 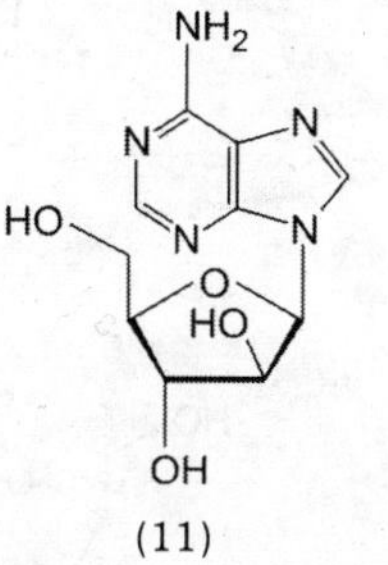   (11)

Replacement of sugar moiety of pyrimidine and purine nucleosides by open chain compounds containing a hydroxyl or hydroxymethyl group has led to another class of antiviral compounds. Some of these compounds which have been successfully used in clinical practice include acyclovir (12), valacyclovir (13), ganciclovir (14), penciclovir (15), and famciclovir (16).

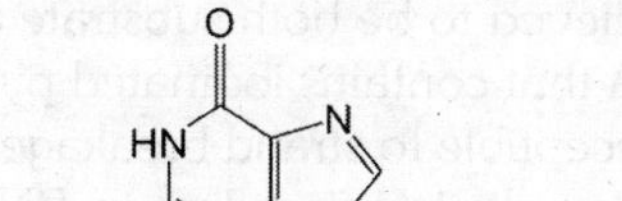

(12) 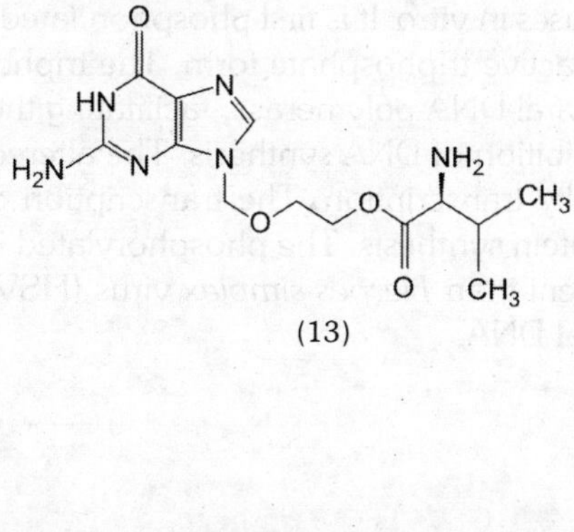   (13)

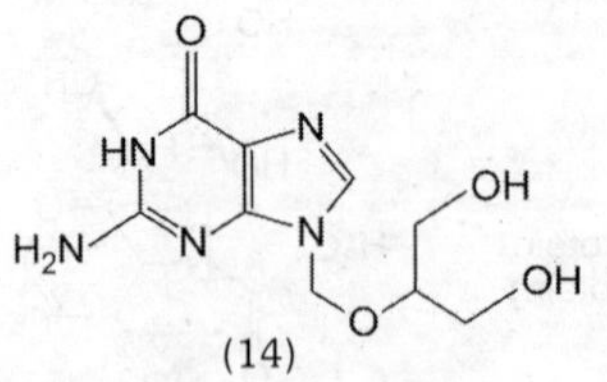

(14)

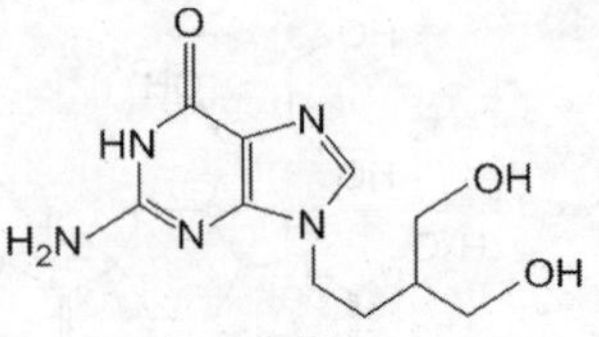

(15)

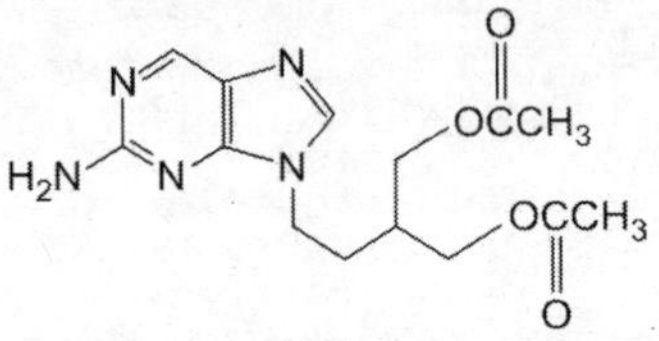

(16)

Cidofovir (17) and adefovir (18) represent the acyclonucleotides possessesing antiviral activity.

The finding of antiviral activity in ribavirin (19), a triazole nucleoside, shows that the pyrmidine and purine moieties are not indispensable.

Foscarnet sodium (20) represents the non-nucleoside compound possessesing antiviral activity.

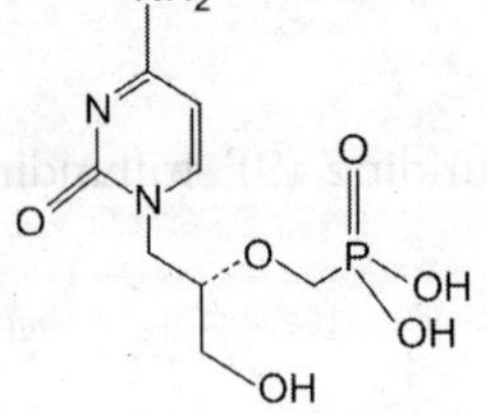

(17)

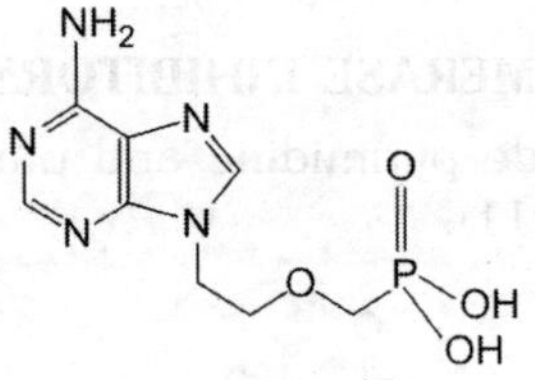

(18)

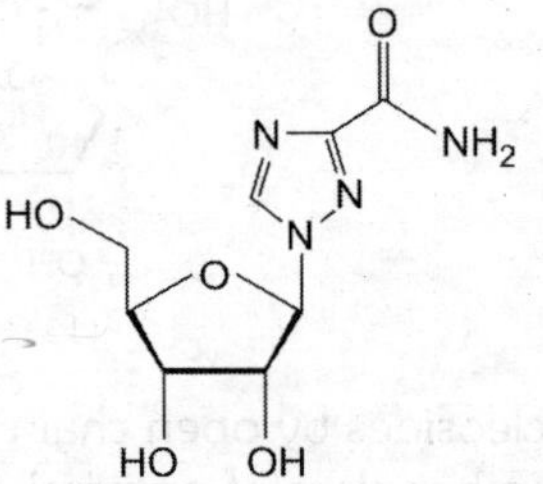

(19)

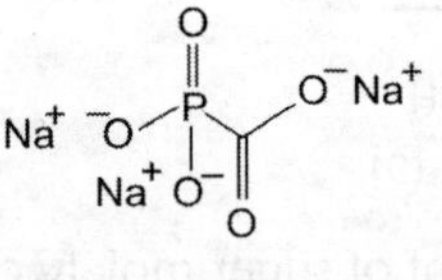

(20)

Idoxuridine (9) is an iodinated analog of uridine. It inhibits replication of a number of DNA viruses in vitro. It is first phosphorylated by the host cell virus encoded enzyme thymidine kinase to an active triphosphate form. The triphosphate form is believed to be both substrate and inhibitor of viral DNA polymerase, facilitating the synthesis of DNA that contains iodinated pyrimidine and inhibition of DNA synthesis. The altered DNA is more susceptible to strand breakage and leads to faulty transcription. The transcription of iodinated DNA results in miscoding in RNA and faulty protein synthesis. The phosphorylated idoxuridine (9) inhibits cellular DNA polymerase to a lesser extent than *Herpes simplex* virus (HSV) DNA polymerase which is necessary for the synthesis of viral DNA.

Trifluridine (10) is similar to idoxuridine (9) and contains trifluoromethyl group instead of iodine at position 5 of uridine. It has similar activity as that of idoxuridine (9). Trifluridine (10) monophosphate is irreversible inhibitor of thymidylate synthetase. The triphosphate analog inhibits the incorporation of thymidine triphosphate into DNA by DNA polymerase. Further incorporation of trifluridine (10) into cellular DNA results in a fragile poorly functioning DNA.

Vidarabine (11) inhibits viral DNA synthesis. After getting phosphorylated, the triphosphate analog competes with deoxyadenosine triphosphate for viral DNA polymerase. It is also incorporated into cellular and viral DNA where it acts as a chain terminator. The triphosphate analog of vidarabine (11) also inhibits enzymes that are involved in methylation of uridine to thymidine.

As indicated earlier, acyclovir (12) is a non-sugar analog of guanine. It is highly active against *Hepes simplex* virus type 1 and less active against type 2. It is first converted to monophosphate by thymidine kinase. It has more affinity (>200 times) to viral thymidine kinase than the mammalian kinase. Thus, it shows some selectivity towards viral thymidine kinase. After being converted to triphosphate analog, it competes with endogenous deoxyguanosine triphosphate for the DNA polymerase and inhibits the enzyme. It is also incorporated into viral DNA during DNA synthesis. Since acyclovir (12) lacks 3′-OH group of sugars, therefore, it terminates further elongation of DNA chain.

Valacyclovir (13) is a prodrug of acyclovir (12). It is hydrolyzed to acyclovir (12) after oral administration.

Ganciclovir (14) is an analog of acyclovir (12) with an additional hydroxyl group on the side chain. After administration, it is converted to monophosphate and then to triphosphate. The monophosphate reaches the infected cells 10-times faster than the uninfected cells. The triphosphate inhibits selectively the viral DNA polymerase. The triphosphate analog is also incorporated into viral DNA which results in strand breakage and cessation of chain elongation.

Penciclovir (15) is structurally related to acyclovir (12). Its metabolite acts by inhibiting the viral DNA polymerase.

Famciclovir (16) is 6-deoxy diacylated analog of penciclovir (15). It is inactive and is infact a prodrug of penciclovir (15).

Cidofovir (17) possesses broad-spectrum of activity against several DNA viruses. After getting absorbed, it is additionally phosphorylated by the host cell enzymes to its active metabolite, cidofovir diphosphate. The diphosphate is a competitive inhibitor of viral DNA polymerase and also gets incorporated into viral DNA strand where it causes chain termination.

Adefovir (18), an adenosine analog used for Hepatitis B, is activated through phosphorylation by adenylate kinase to its diphosphate. The diphosphate inhibits hepatitis B virus DNA polymerase. It is also incorporated into viral DNA which leads to DNA chain termination.

Ribavirin (19), a triazole analog, is activated through conversion to triphosphate by adenosine kinase. The triphosphate inhibits viral specific RNA polymerase resulting in disruption of mRNA and nucleic acid synthesis.

Foscarnet (20) is phosphorylated analog of formic acid. It acts by inhibiting DNA polymerase without requiring any activation.

NUCLEOSIDE REVERSE TRANSCRIPTASE INHIBITORS (NRTIs)

In the replication of HIV-1, reverse transcription takes place. During this, genomic RNA from virus is converted to cDNA–RNA complex then into double stranded DNA ready for integration into the host chromosomes. The enzyme that catalyzes this is known as reverse transcriptase (RT).

Reverse transcriptase operates at two steps:

(*i*) Creation of cDNA-RNA complex,

(*ii*) RNA chain is digested away by RNase-H while reverse transcriptase creates the double stranded unintegrated DNA.

The synthesis of viral DNA under the direction of reverse transcriptase (RT) requires purines and pyrimidine nucleotides. Accordingly, a variety of chemically modified nucleosides have been investigated. Two such modifications include:

(*a*) Replacement of 3'- hydroxyl group by 3'- azido group.

(*b*) Removal of 3'-hydroxy group of deoxynucleosides resulting in dideoxynucleosides, examples include dideoxyadenosine, dideoxycytidine, and dideoxythymidine.

All of these compounds have similar mechanism of action which leads to chain – terminating blockade due to lack of 3'- hydroxyl group needed for DNA propagation.

Some of the compounds in this class include the pyrimidine and purine nucleosides zidovudine (21), zalcitabine (22), stavudine (23), didanosine (24), and dideoxyadenosine (25). Pyrimidine analogs with thiosugars include lamivudine (26) and emtricitabine (27). The other analogs include tenofovir (28) and abacavir (29).

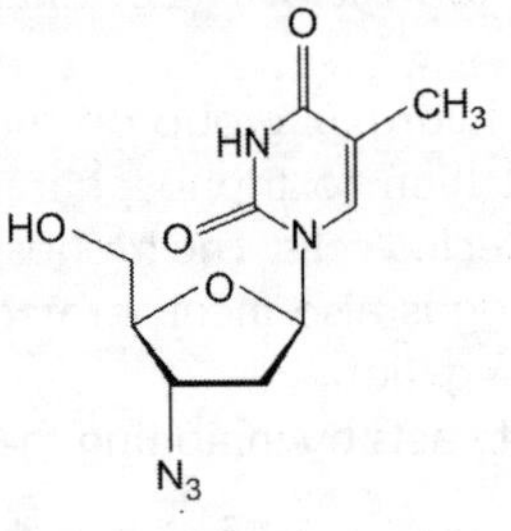

(21) 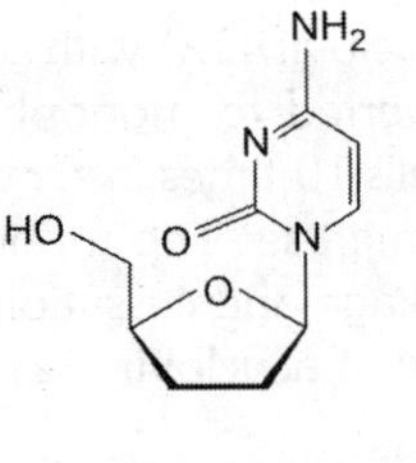   (22) 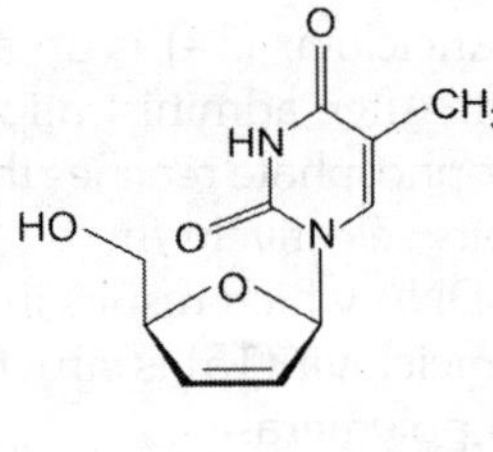   (23)

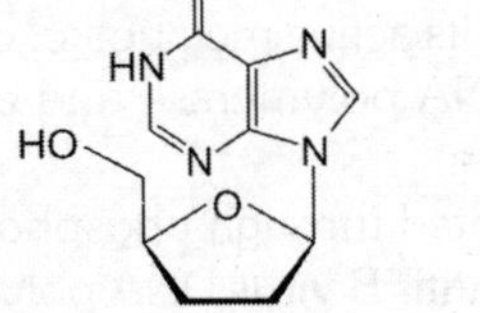

(24) 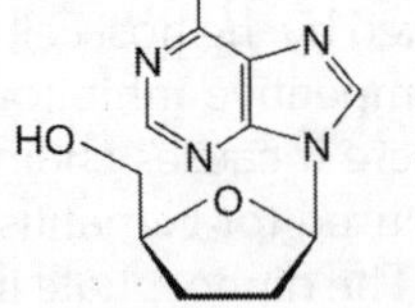   (25) 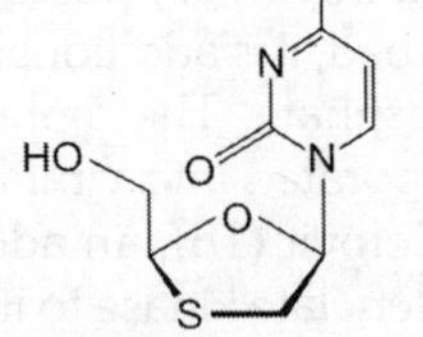   (26)

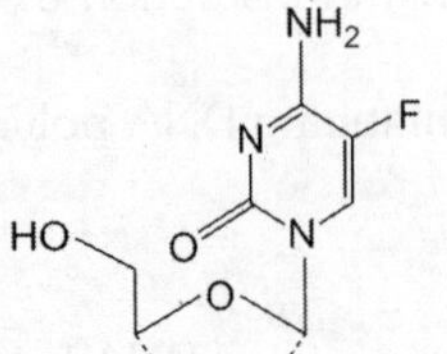

(27) 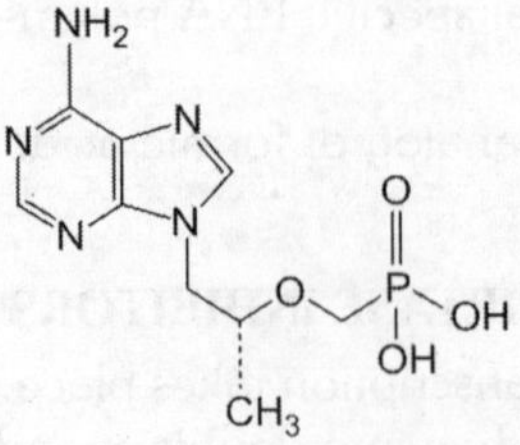   (28) 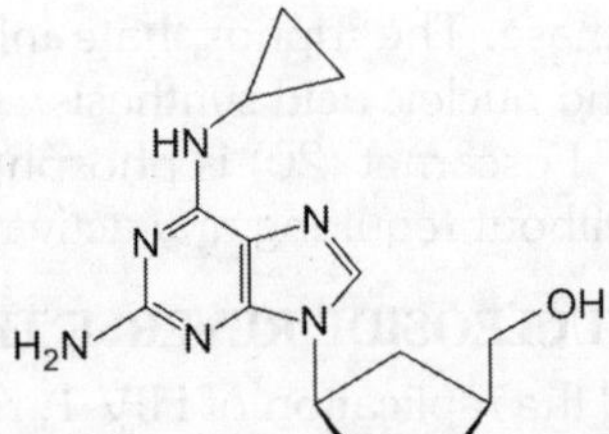   (29)

Zidovudine (21) is converted to 5'- mono-, di- and tri-phosphate by thymidine kinase. These phosphates are then incorporated into proviral DNA because RT uses zidovudine (21) triphosphate as a substrate. This process results in termination of DNA chain elongation step owing to presence of azido group in zidovudine (21). The multiplication of the HIV is halted by selective inhibition of RT and thus viral DNA-polymerase.

Zalcitabine (22) is transported across the membrane by carrier-facilitated diffusion. After monophosphorylation by deoxycytidine kinase, it is further metabolized to dideoxycytidine-5'-triphosphate (ddCTP) by cellular kinases. The triphosphate inhibits RT by competitive inhibition with deoxycytidine phosphate (dCTP). ddCTP causes termination of the elongation of viral DNA chain.

Stavudine (23) is activated through triphosphorylation at 5'-position. The triphosphate analog competitively inhibits the incorporation of thymidine triphosphate (TTP) into retroviral DNA by RT. It also causes termination of viral DNA elongation through its incorporation into DNA.

Didanosine (24) is activated to dideoxyadenosine triphosphate (ddATP). This compound causes chain termination because of absence of 3'-hydroxyl group.

Dideoxyadenosine (25) ia an adenosine analog. It acts as inhibitor of RT after getting phosphorylated to triphosphate.

Lamivudine (26) is a sulphur analog of dideoxycytidine. It is converted to 5'-triphosphate, which is the active form. The triphosphate competes with normal substrate for incorporation into viral DNA by inhibiting HIV reverse transcriptase. Emtricitabine (27) has similar mechanism of action as zalcitabine (22). Out of the two enantiomers the (–)-enantiomer is more active than (+)-enantiomer. The active form of emtricitabine (27) is the triphosphate which after incorporation into the viral DNA leads to termination of DNA elongation.

Tenofovir (28), is used for HIV. It is used as its prodrug, disoproxil ester (30). After absorption the ester disoproxil (30) is hydrolyzed to tenofovir (28), which is analogous to adefovir (18). The active form of tenofovir (28) is the diphosphate, which inhibits HIV reverse transcriptase. Further, incorporation of tenofovir (28) diphosphate into viral DNA results in premature termination of DNA chain and inhibition of DNA polymerase.

(30)

Abacavir (29) is used along with other nucleoside drugs for the tratment of HIV and AIDS. It passes blood-brain barrier efficiently. After absoption it is metabolized by phosphorylation to mono, di, and triposphates.

NONNUCEOSIDE REVERSE TRANSCRIPTASE INHIBITORS (NNRTIs)

These compounds have been developed recently and do not require bioactivation. However, resistance to these develops rapidly. Nonnucleoside reverse transcriptase inhibitors (NNRTIs) are highly potent and they inhibit HIV-1 at nanomolar concentrations. They do not inhibit the RT of

HIV-2 and simian immunodeficiency virus (SIV). They have high therapeutic indices and do not affect mammalian DNA polymerases. When given together, the nucleoside reverse transcriptase inhibitors (NRTIs) and NNRTIs exhibit synergistic effect on HIV, since they act by different mechanisms on RT. No cross-resistance has been observed between NRTIs and NNRTIs. However cross-resistance has been observed within NNRTIs.

Some of the clinically useful NNRTIs include nevirapine (31), delavirdine (32), and efavirenz (33).

(31)   (32)   (33)

Nevirapine (31) acts by binding directly to RT and thus blocking RNA and DNA dependent polymerase activity by causing disruption of the catalytic site of the enzyme. The HIV-2 and DNA polymerases are not inhibited by nevirapine (31).

Delavirdine (32) is a powerful NNRTI and is specific to HIV-1. It directly inhibits RT and DNA directed DNA polymerase activity of HIV-1 thereby causing the chain termination.

Efavirenz (33) is the latest NNRTI. It is a potent inhibitor of wild type as well as resistant mutant of HIV-1.

HIV-PROTEASE INHIBITORS

The HIV-protease is an enzyme that is essential for viral growth. It is responsible for the post-translation modification of core proteins which have been identified as p7, p9, p17 and p24 and play a role in the infectivity of the virus.

In HIV, the mRNA transcribed from provirus is translated into two biochemically inert polyproteins. A virus specific protease then converts polyproteins into various structural and functional proteins by cleavage at appropriate positions. Since the protease does not occur in the host, it is a good target for chemotherapeutic intervention. The HIV-specific protease inhibitors bind to the site where cleavage occurs and their use in combination with reverse transcriptase inhibitors gives good results. The active site of the HIV-protease has a triad Asp-Thr-Gly. This site is blocked by the HIV- protease inhibitors. Some of these inhibitors include saqinavir (34), ritonavir (35), indinavir (36), nelfinavir (37), amprenavir (38), lopinavir (39), atazanavir (40), fosamprenavir (41), and tipranavir (42).

(34)

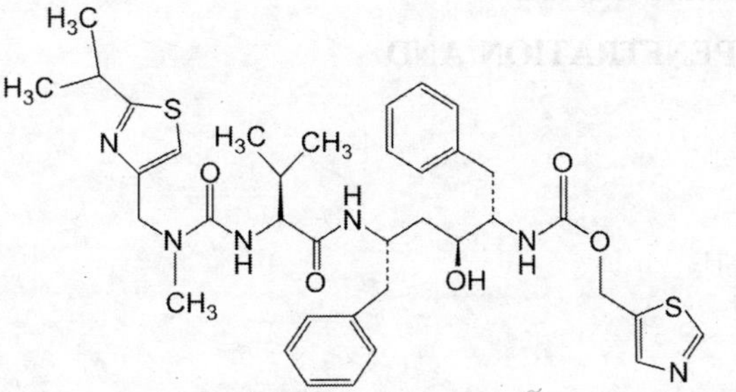

(35)

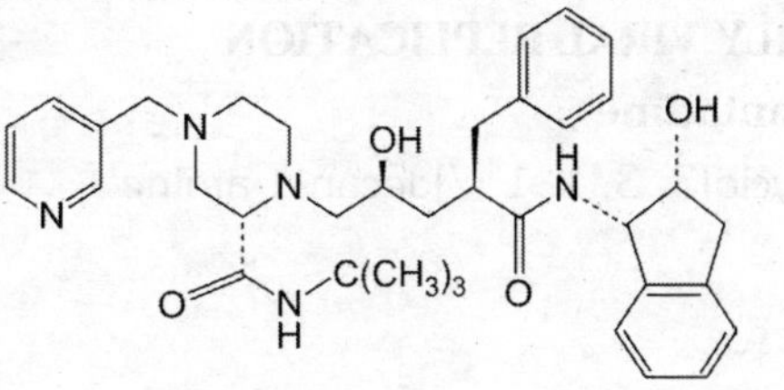

(36)

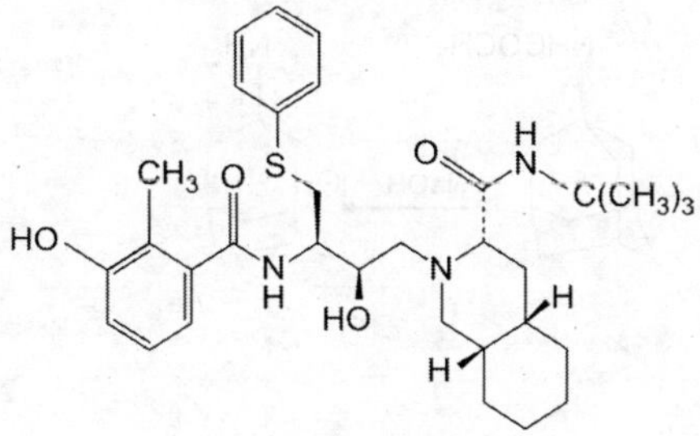

(37)

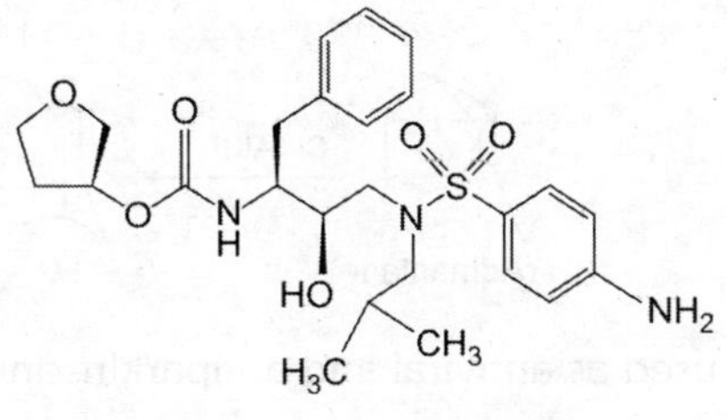

(38)

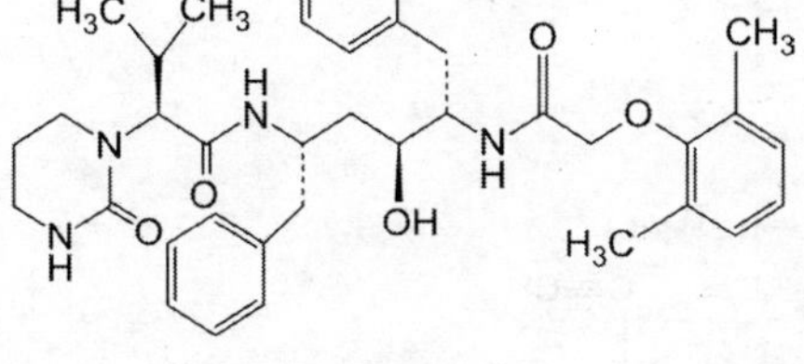

(39)

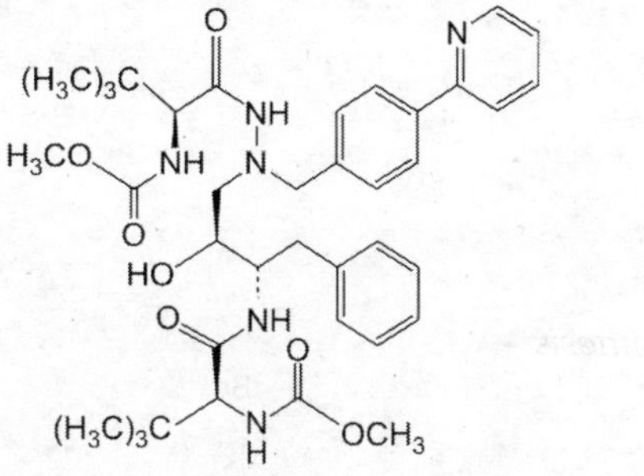

(40)

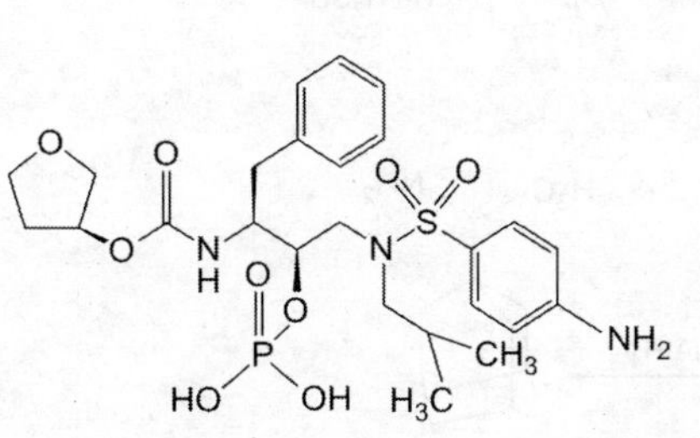

(41)

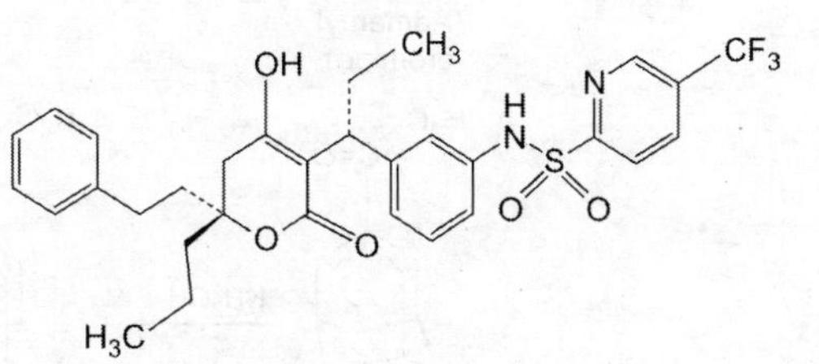

(42)

INDIVIDUAL COMPOUNDS

AGENTS INHIBITING VIRUS ATTACHMENT PENETRATION AND EARLY VIRAL REPLICATION

Amantadine

Tricyclo[3. 3. 1. $1^{3, 7}$]decan-1-amine

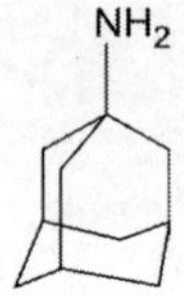

Synthesis

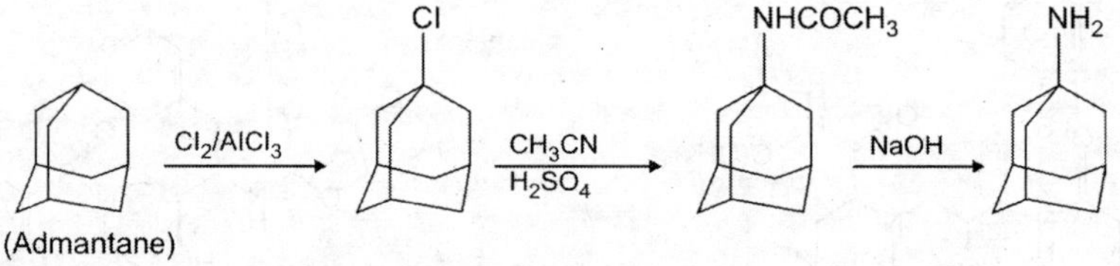

It is used as antiviral and antiparkinsonian drug.

Rimantadine

α-Methyltricyclo[3. 3. 1. $1^{3, 7}$]decane-1-methanamine

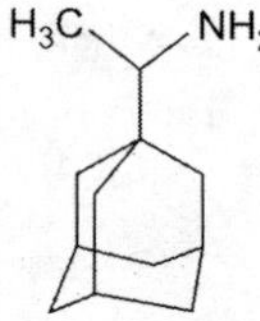

Synthesis

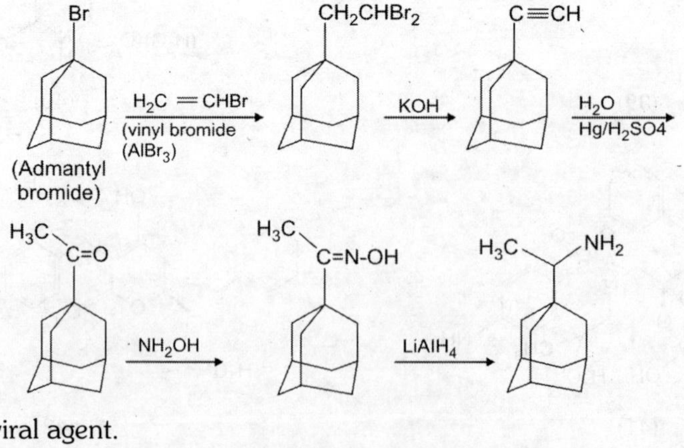

It is used as antiviral agent.

NEURAMINIDASE INHIBITORS
Zanamivir
4-Guanidino-2,4-dideoxy-2,3-dehydro-*N*-acetylneuraminic acid

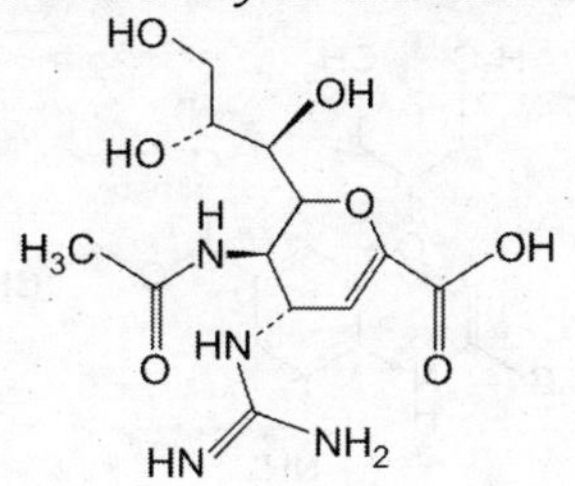

Synthesis

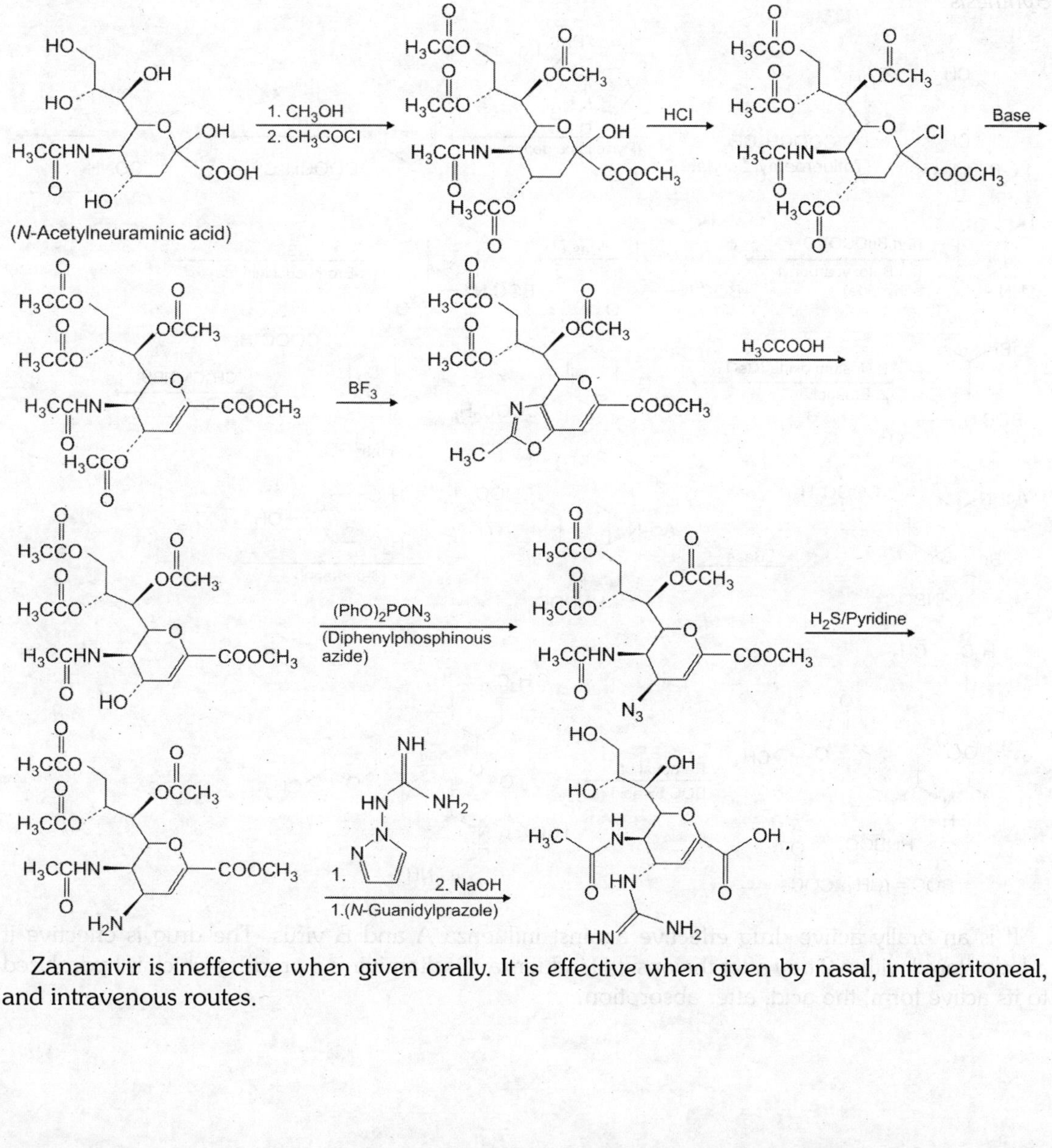

Zanamivir is ineffective when given orally. It is effective when given by nasal, intraperitoneal, and intravenous routes.

Oseltamivir

(3R,4R,5S)-4-(Acetylamino)-5-amino-3-(1-ethylpropoxy)-1-cyclohexene-1-carboxylic acid ethyl ester.

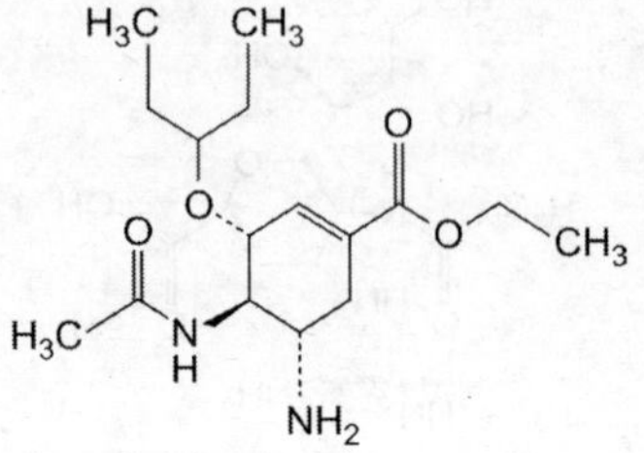

Synthesis

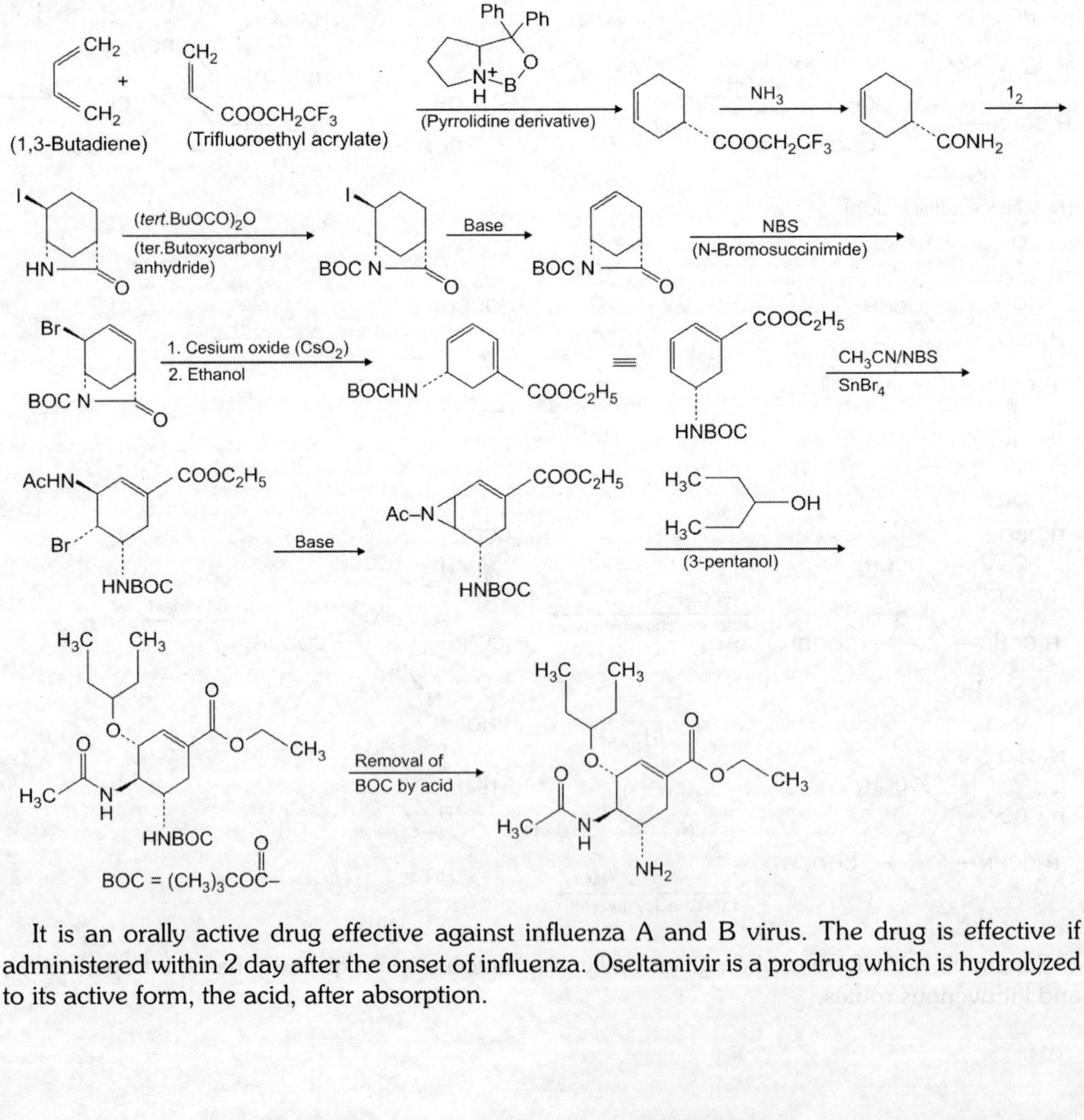

BOC = $(CH_3)_3CO\overset{O}{\overset{\|}{C}}$–

It is an orally active drug effective against influenza A and B virus. The drug is effective if administered within 2 day after the onset of influenza. Oseltamivir is a prodrug which is hydrolyzed to its active form, the acid, after absorption.

DNA POLYMERASE INHIBITORS

Idoxuridine

2'-Deoxy-5-iodouridine

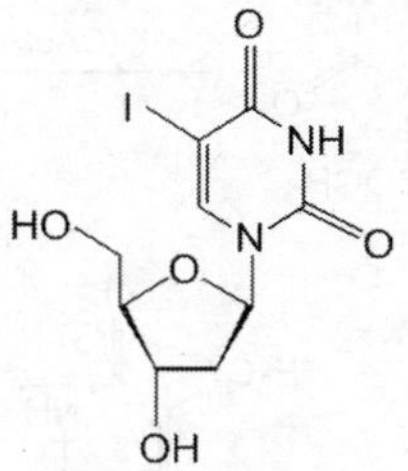

Synthesis

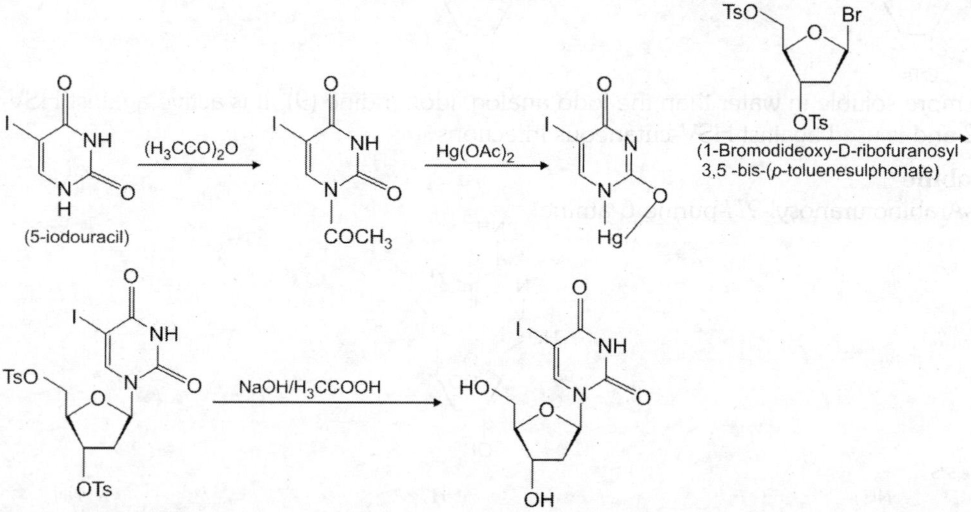
$(H_3CCO)_2O$
$Hg(OAc)_2$
(1-Bromodideoxy-D-ribofuranosyl 3,5 -bis-(*p*-toluenesulphonate)
(5-iodouracil)
$NaOH/H_3CCOOH$

It is used as opthalamic drops and ointment for the treatment of HSV-keratoconjunctivits which causes blindness. It has also been used in the HSV infections of mouth and nose in DMSO solution. The common toxicity associated with it includes pain, burning, hypersensitivity, and edema. Systemic administration leads to bone marrow toxicities.

Trifluridine

α,α,α-Trifluorothymidine

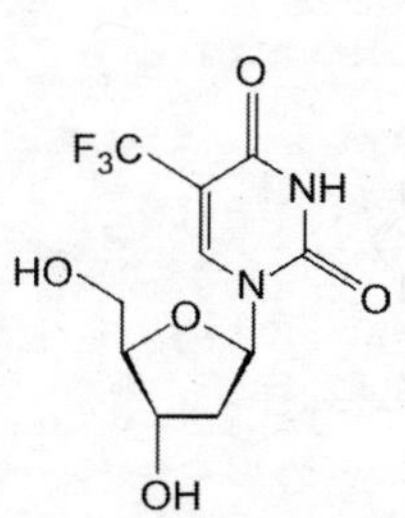

Synthesis

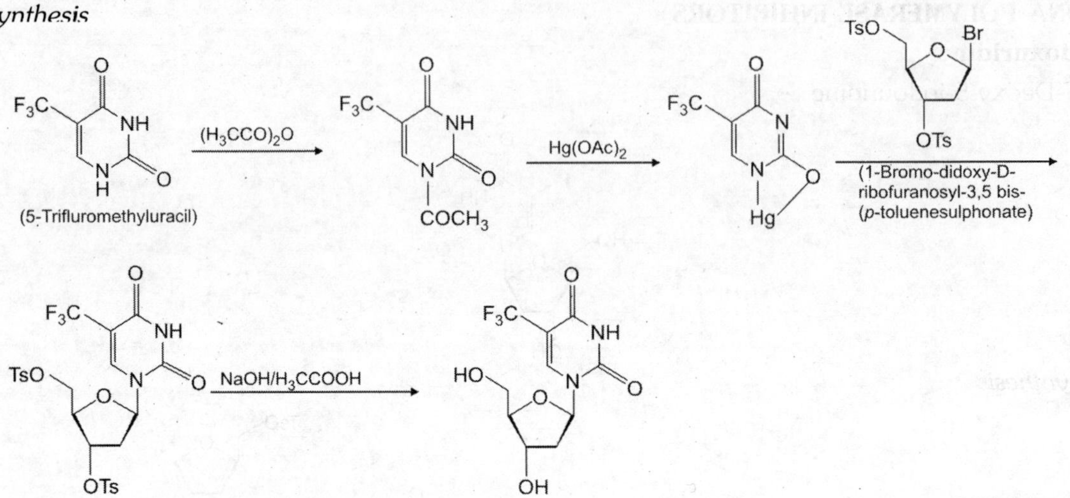
(H3CCO)2O
Hg(OAc)2
(1-Bromo-didoxy-D-ribofuranosyl-3,5 bis-(p-toluenesulphonate)
(5-Trifluromethyluracil)
NaOH/H3CCOOH

It is more soluble in water than the iodo analog, idoxuridine (9). It is active against HSV-1 and HSV-2 and is used against HSV-cutaneous infections.

Vidarabine

9-β-D-Arabinofuranosyl-9*H*-purine-6-amine

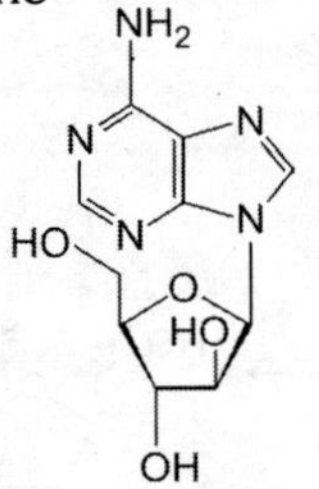

Synthesis

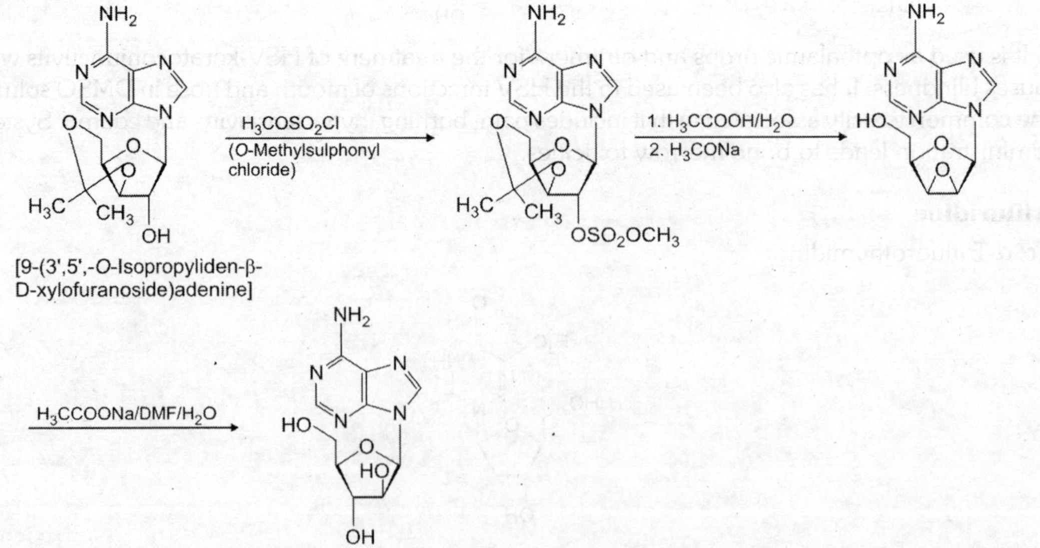
H3COSO2Cl
(O-Methylsulphonyl chloride)
1. H3CCOOH/H2O
2. H3CONa
[9-(3',5',-O-Isopropyliden-β-D-xylofuranoside)adenine]
H3CCOONa/DMF/H2O

It is mainly used in human HSV-1 and HSV-2 encephalitis infections. It has poor solubility so it has to be administered by constant flow intravenous infusion. It has largely been replaced by acyclovir (12).

Acyclovir

2-Amino-1,9-dihydro-9-[(2-hydroxyethoxy)methyl]-6*H*-purin-6-one

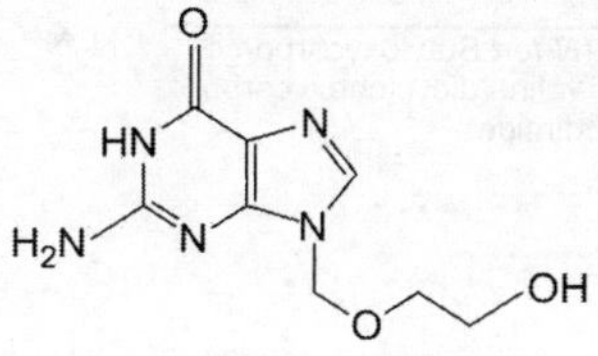

Synthesis

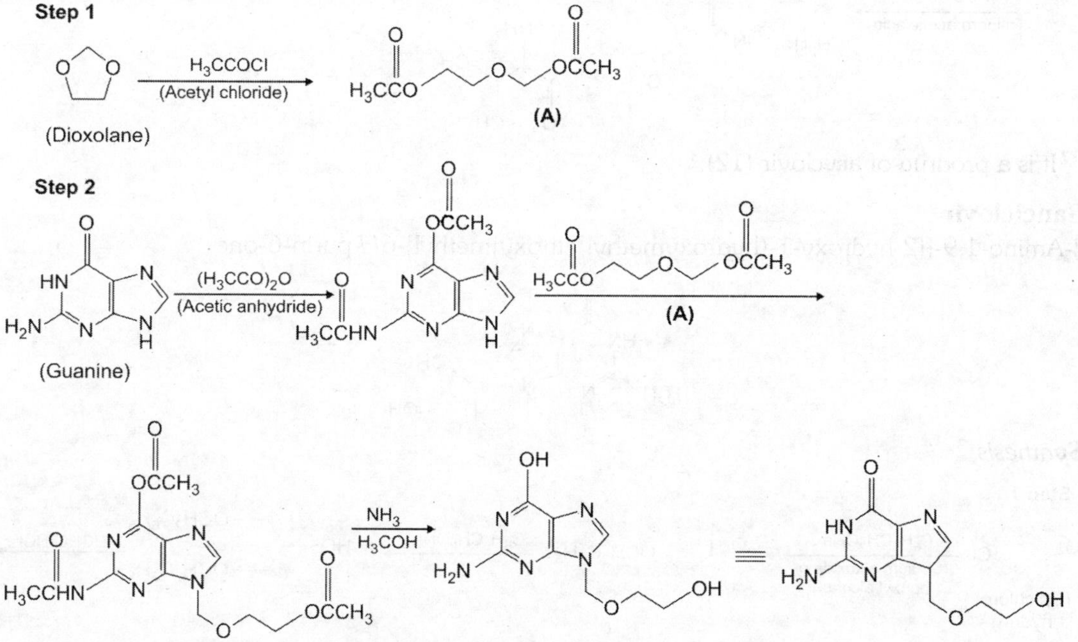

Step 1

(Dioxolane)

Step 2

(Guanine)

It is active against several DNA viruses including HSV-1 and HSV-2. It is also active against chickenpox caused by *varicella-zoster virus* (VZV).

Valacyclovir

L-Valine 2-[(2-amino-1,6-dihydro-6-oxo-9*H*-purin-9-yl)methoxy]ethyl ester

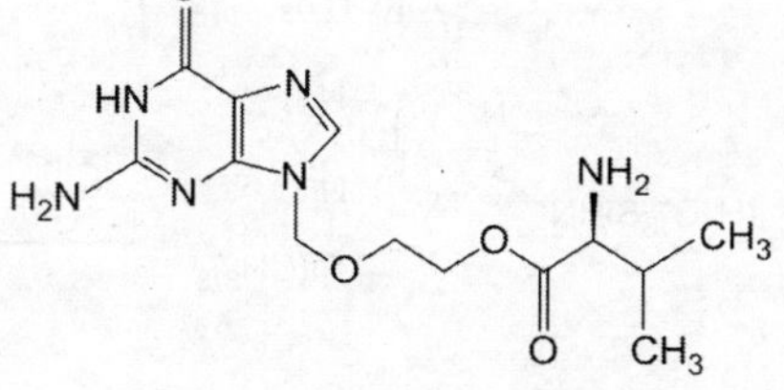

Synthesis

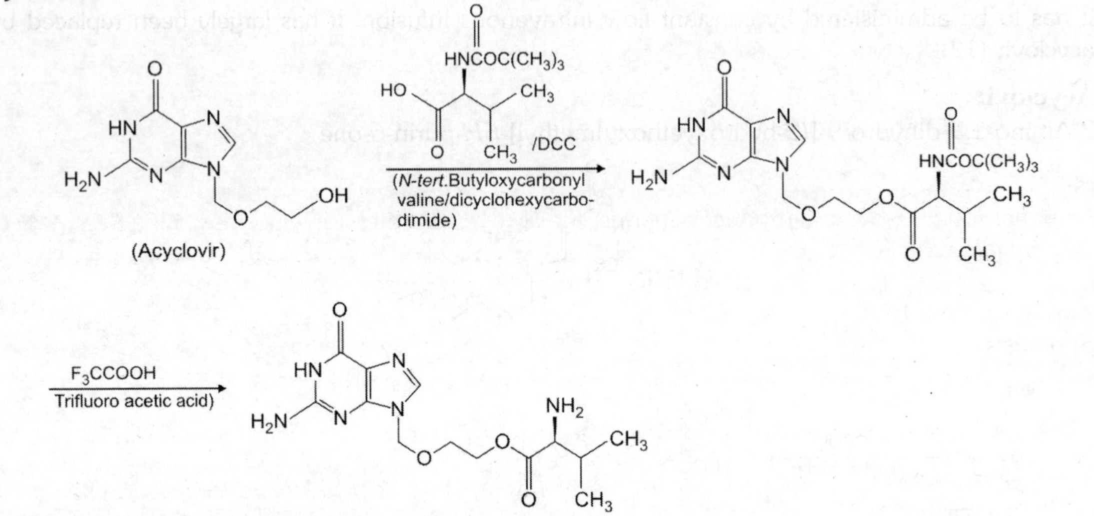

It is a prodrug of acyclovir (12).

Ganciclovir

2-Amino-1,9-[[2-hydroxy-1-(hydroxymethyl)ethoxy]methyl]-6*H*-purin-6-one

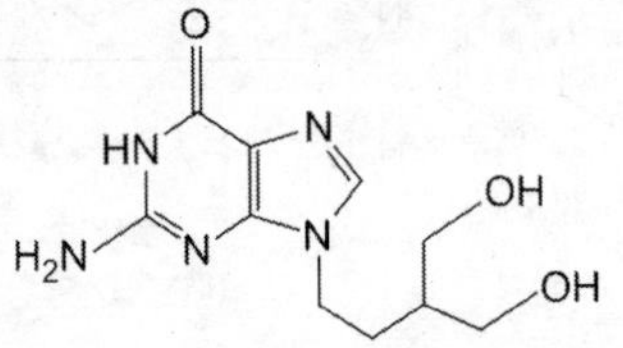

Synthesis

Step 1

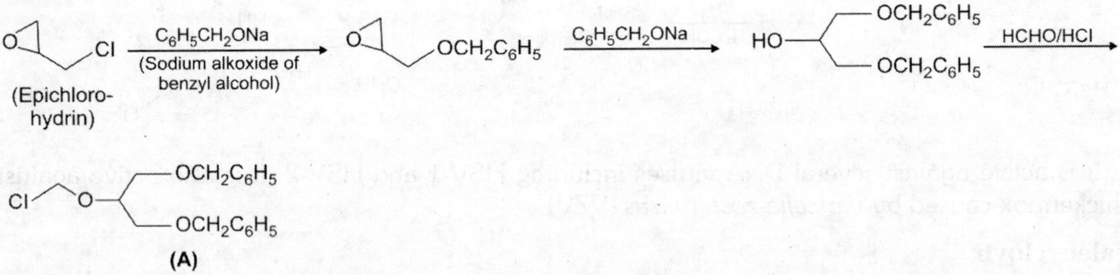

Step 2

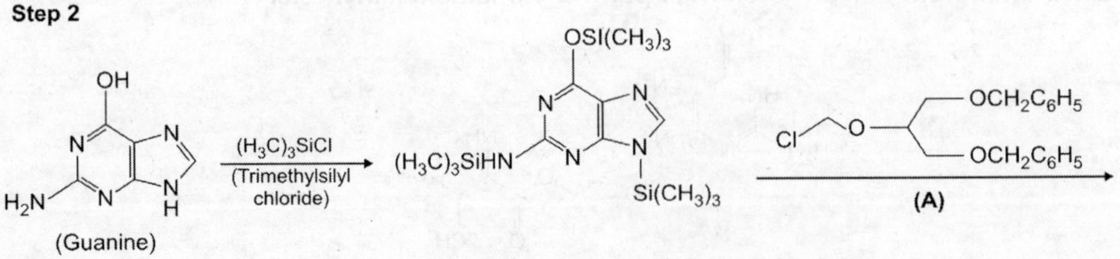

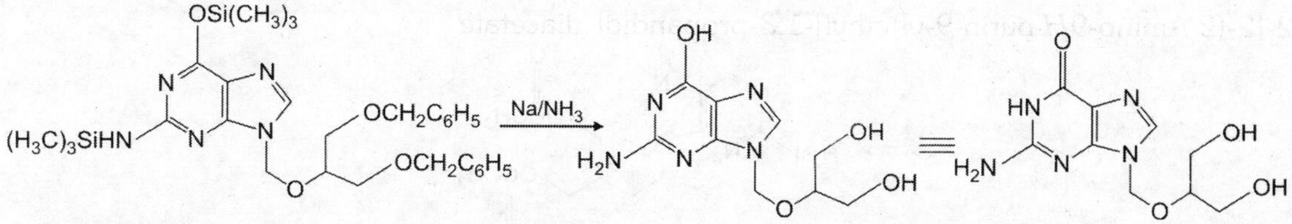

Ganciclovir is toxic and produces anemia due to myelosuppression. It is used in the treatment of *cytomegalo virus* (CMV).

Penciclovir

2-Amino-1,9-dihydro-9-[4-hydroxy-3-(hydroxymethyl)butyl-6*H*-purin-6-one

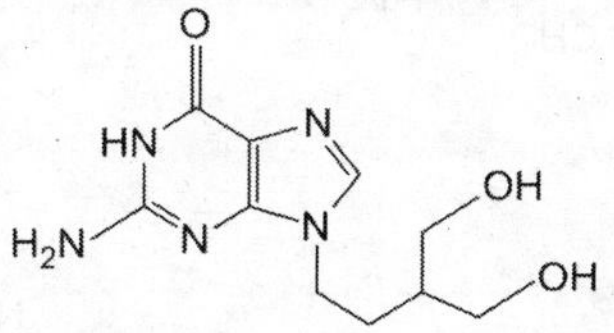

Synthesis

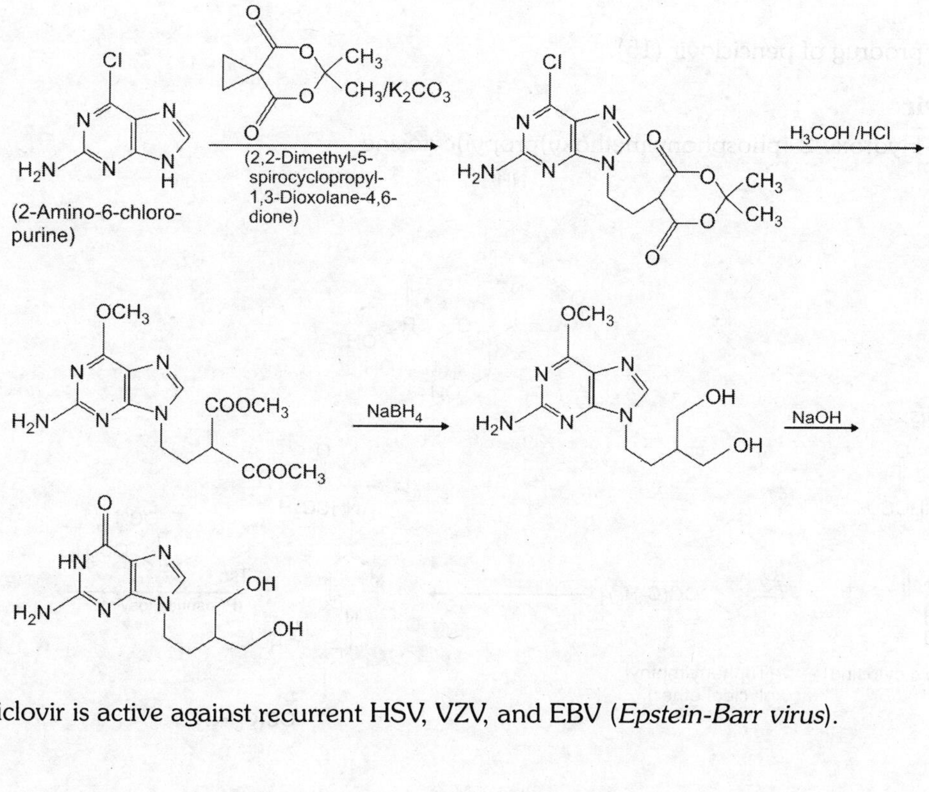

Penciclovir is active against recurrent HSV, VZV, and EBV (*Epstein-Barr virus*).

Famciclovir

2-[2-(2-Amino-9*H*-purin-9-yl)ethyl]-1,3-propandiol diacetate

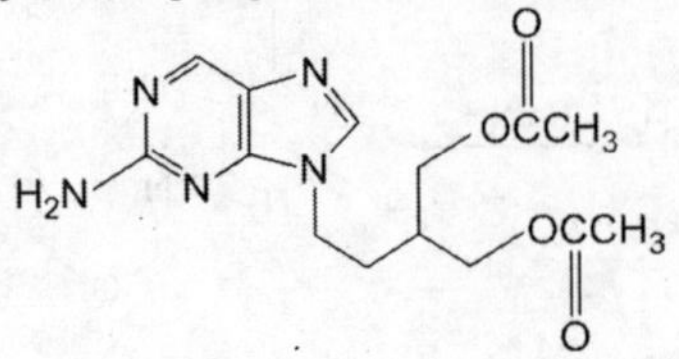

Synthesis

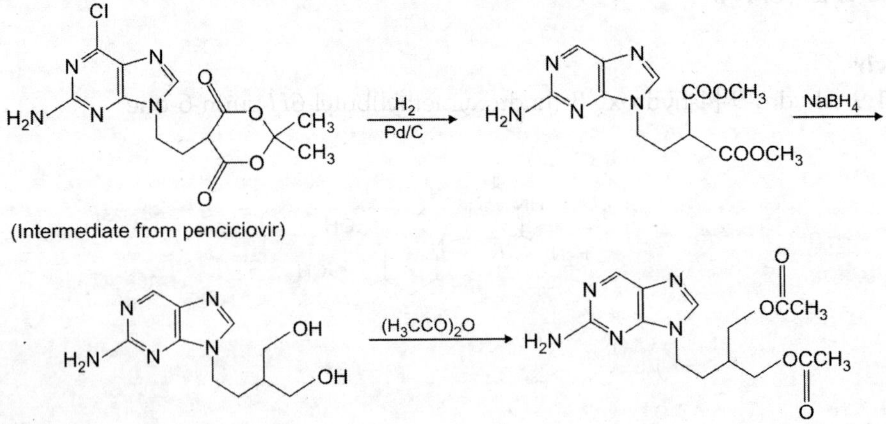

(Intermediate from penciciovir)

It is a prodrug of penciclovir (15).

Cidofovir

(*S*)-1-[3-Hydroxy-2-(phosphonylmethoxy)propyl)cytosine

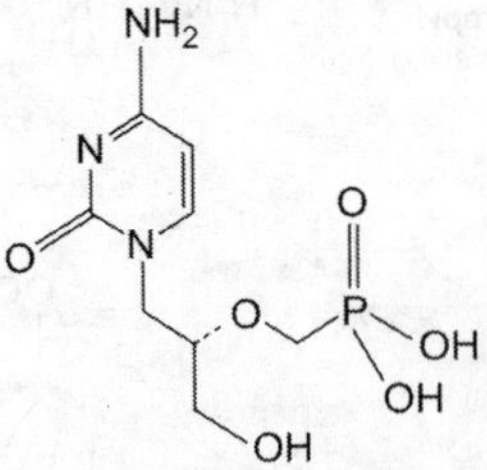

Synthesis

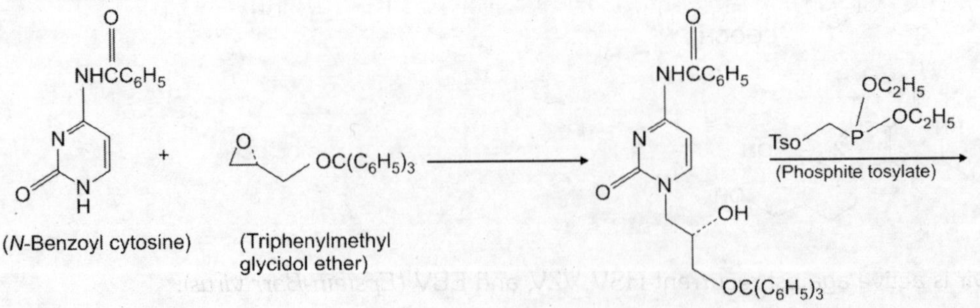

(*N*-Benzoyl cytosine)   (Triphenylmethyl glycidol ether)

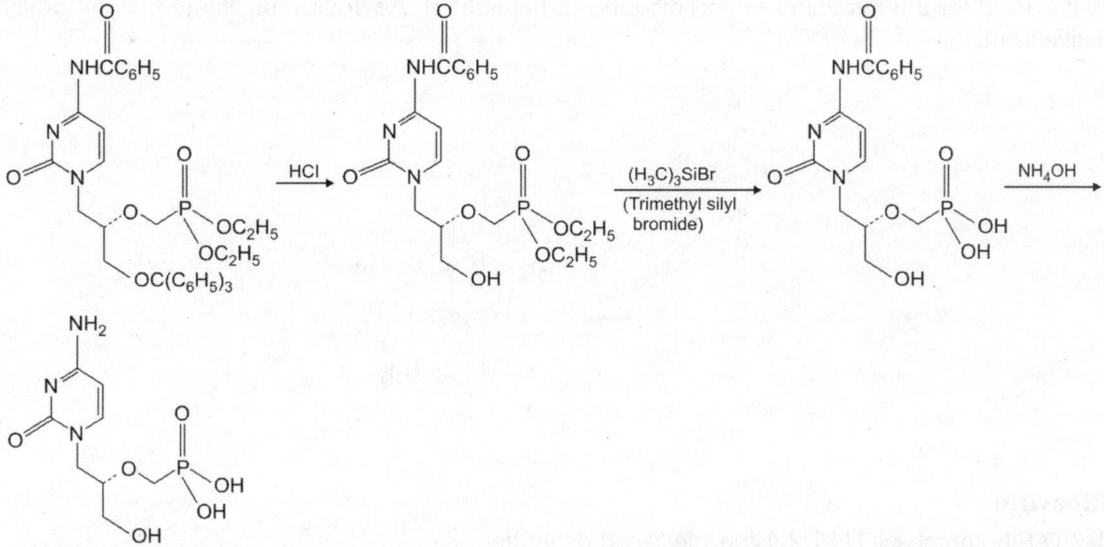

Its active form is the diphosphate, obtained by phosphorylation of phosphonate by cellular kinases. The diphosphate acts as antimetabolite to deoxycytosine triphosphate. It is competitive inhibitor of viral DNA polymerase and is incorporated in viral DNA strand which leads to termination of DNA Chain.

Adefovir

9-(2-Phosphonylmethoxyethyl)adenine

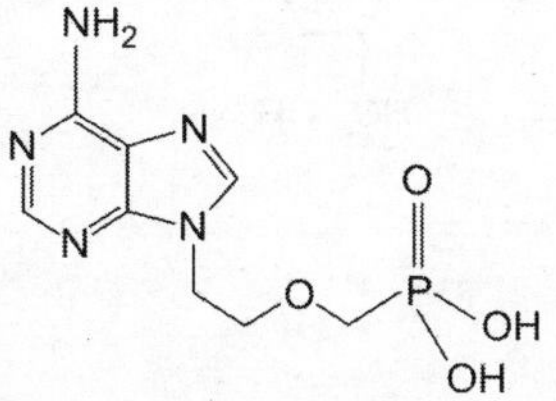

Synthesis

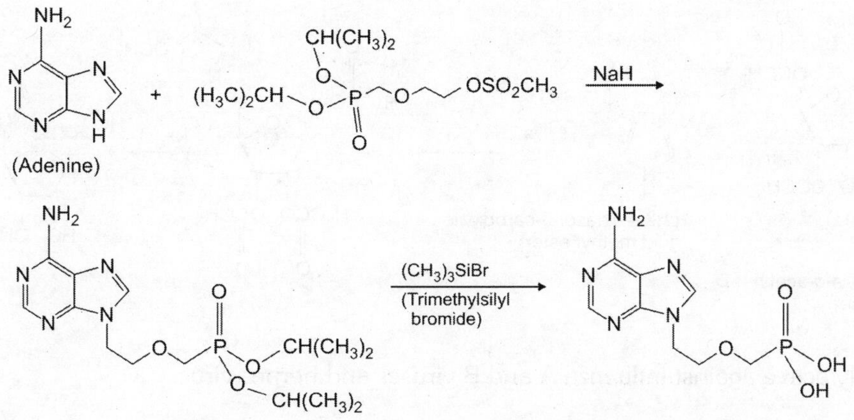

It is used for the treatment of chronic form of hepatitis B. Adefovir dipivoxil (43) is the orally active from.

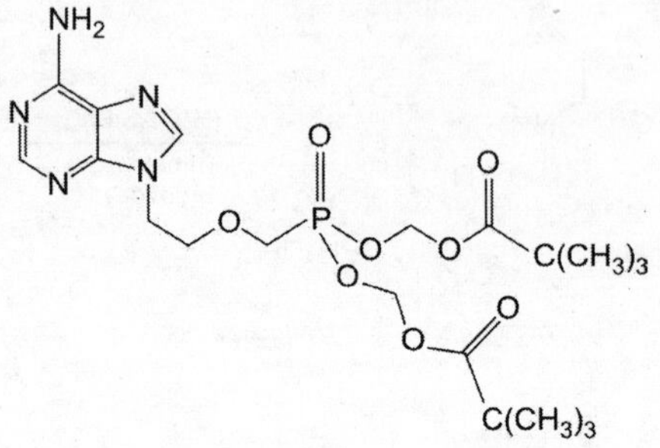

(43)

Ribavirin

1-β-D-Ribofuranosyl-1H-1,2,4-triazole-3-carboxamide

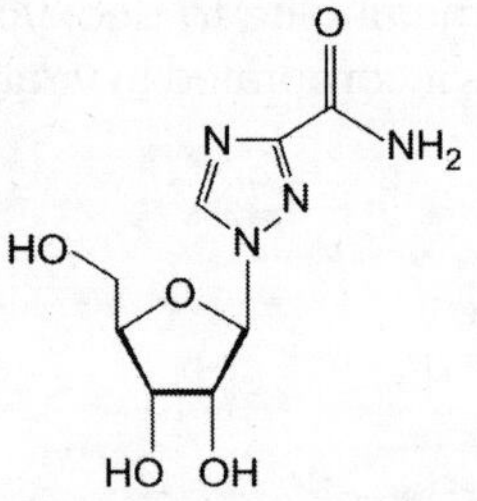

Synthesis

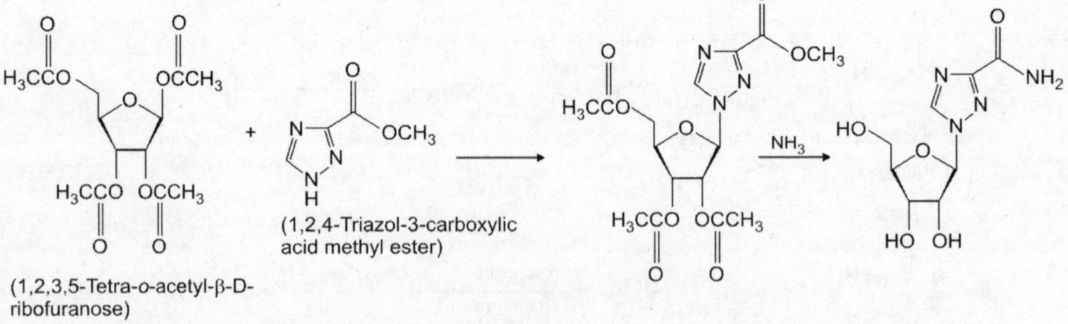

(1,2,3,5-Tetra-o-acetyl-β-D-ribofuranose)

(1,2,4-Triazol-3-carboxylic acid methyl ester)

It is highly active against influenza A and B viruses and herpes virus.

NUCLEOSIDE REVERSE TRANSCRIPTASE INHIBITORS (NRTIs)

Zidovudine

3'-Azido-3'-deoxythymidine

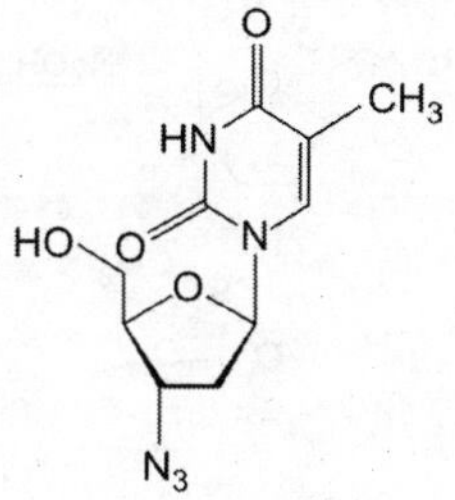

Synthesis

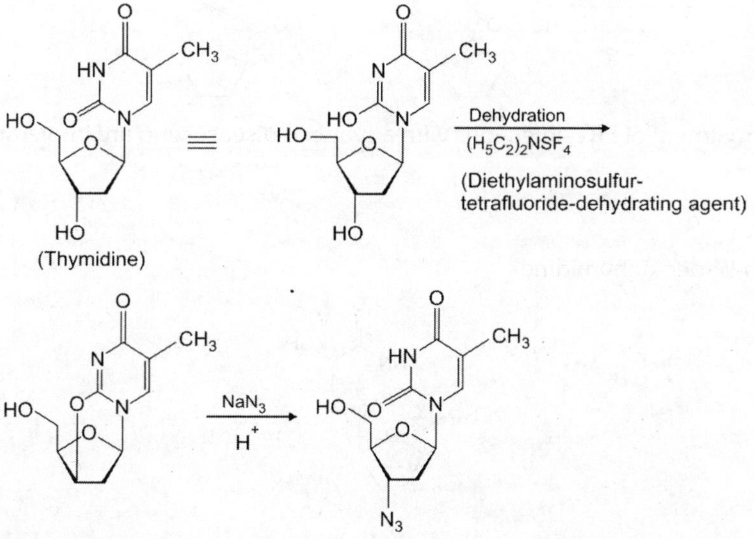

It is commonly known as AZT. It is effective against HIV-1, HIV-2, and HTLV-1 (Human T-cell lymphotropic vitus –1).

Zalcitabine

2', 3'-Dideoxycytidine

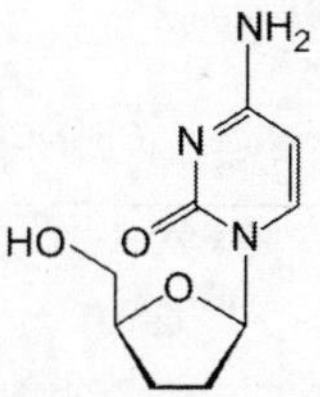

Synthesis

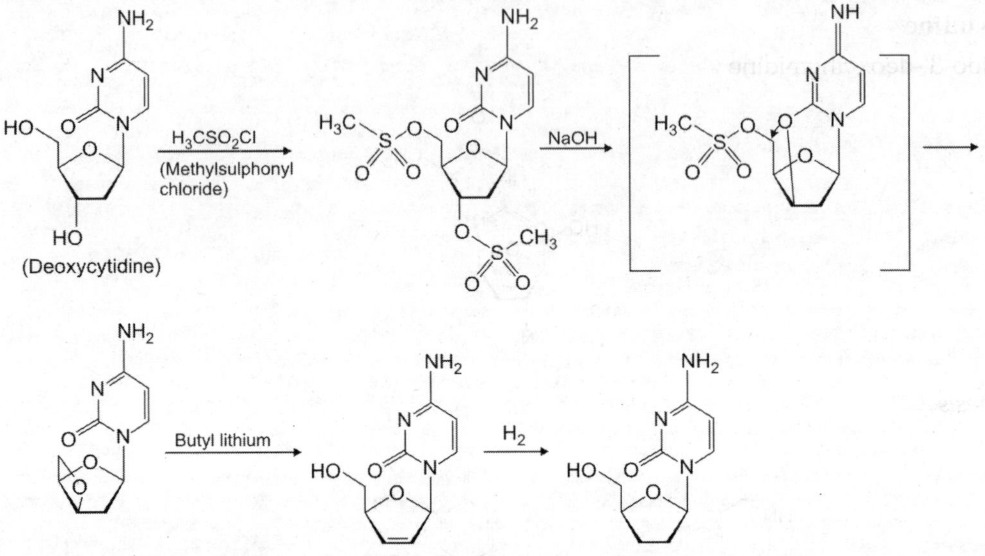

NH$_2$ ... HO (Deoxycytidine) → H$_3$CSO$_2$Cl (Methylsulphonyl chloride) → ... NaOH → ...

NH$_2$ ... → Butyl lithium → HO ... → H$_2$ → HO ...

Used for the treatment of HIV-infections with advanced disease who are intolerant to zidovudine (21).

Stavudine

2′, 3′-Didehydro-3′-deoxythymidine

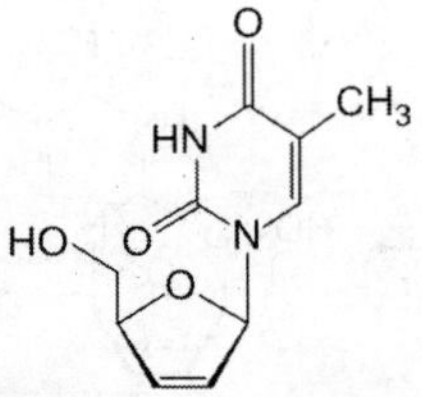

Synthesis

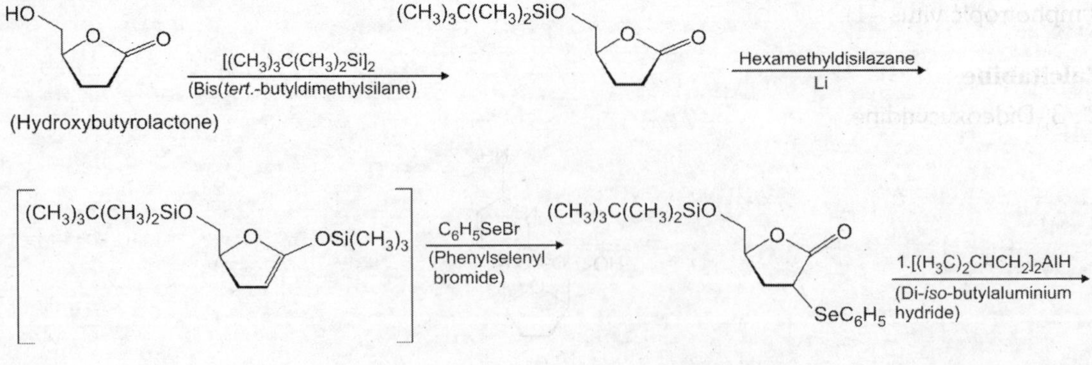

HO ... (Hydroxybutyrolactone) → [(CH$_3$)$_3$C(CH$_3$)$_2$Si]$_2$ (Bis(*tert.*-butyldimethylsilane)) → (CH$_3$)$_3$C(CH$_3$)$_2$SiO ... → Hexamethyldisilazane, Li →

(CH$_3$)$_3$C(CH$_3$)$_2$SiO ... OSi(CH$_3$)$_3$ → C$_6$H$_5$SeBr (Phenylselenyl bromide) → (CH$_3$)$_3$C(CH$_3$)$_2$SiO ... SeC$_6$H$_5$ → 1.[(H$_3$C)$_2$CHCH$_2$]$_2$AlH (Di-*iso*-butylaluminium hydride)

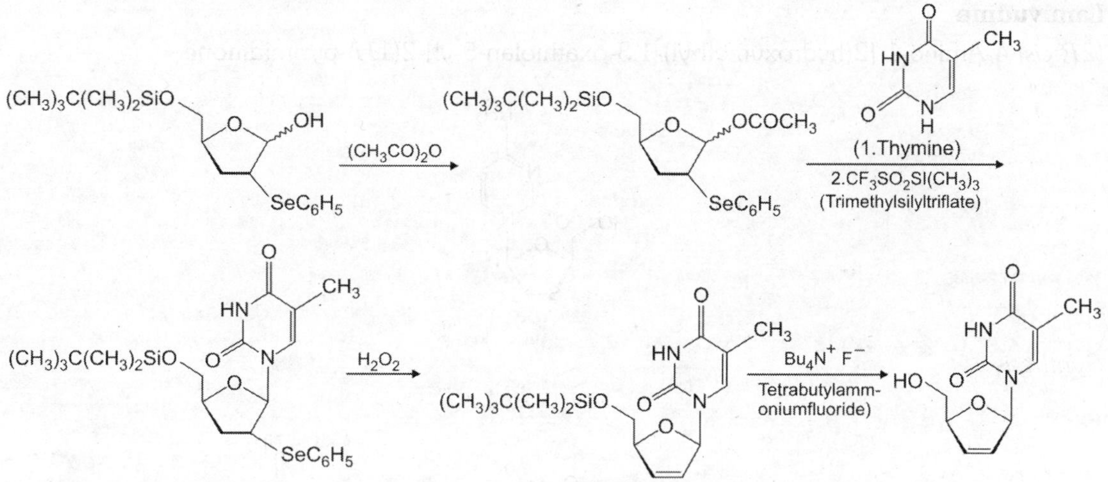

Stavudine is recommended for patients with advanced HIV infections.

Didanosine

2′, 3′-Dideoxyinosine

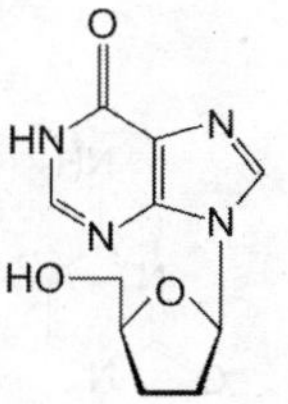

Synthesis

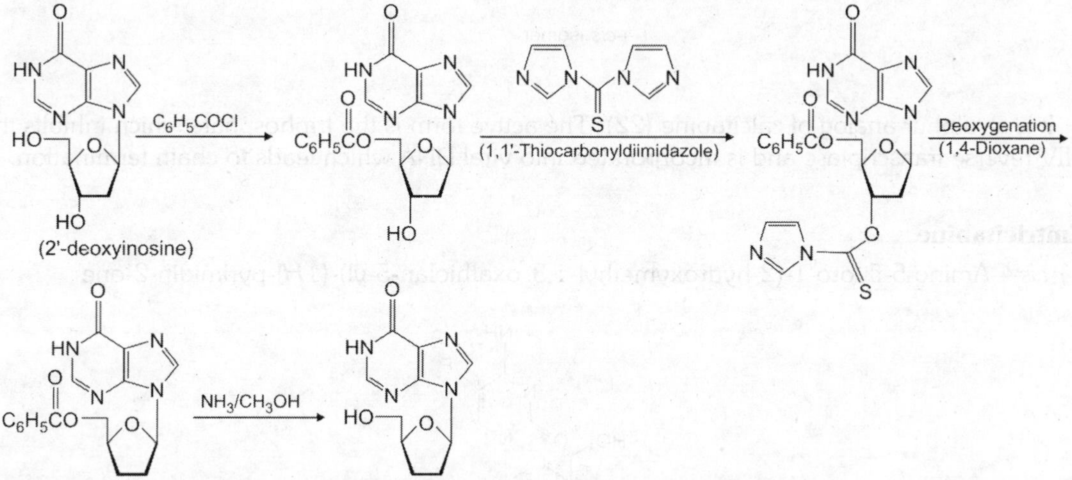

Didanosine is given in advanced HIV infection to patients who are intolerant to zidovudine (21).

Lamivudine

(2*R*-cis)-4-Amino-1-[2(hydroxymethyl)-1,3-oxathiolan-5-yl]-2(1*H*)-pyrimidinone

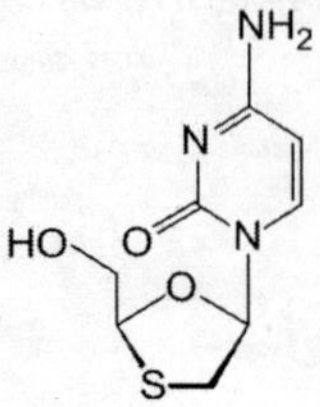

Synthesis

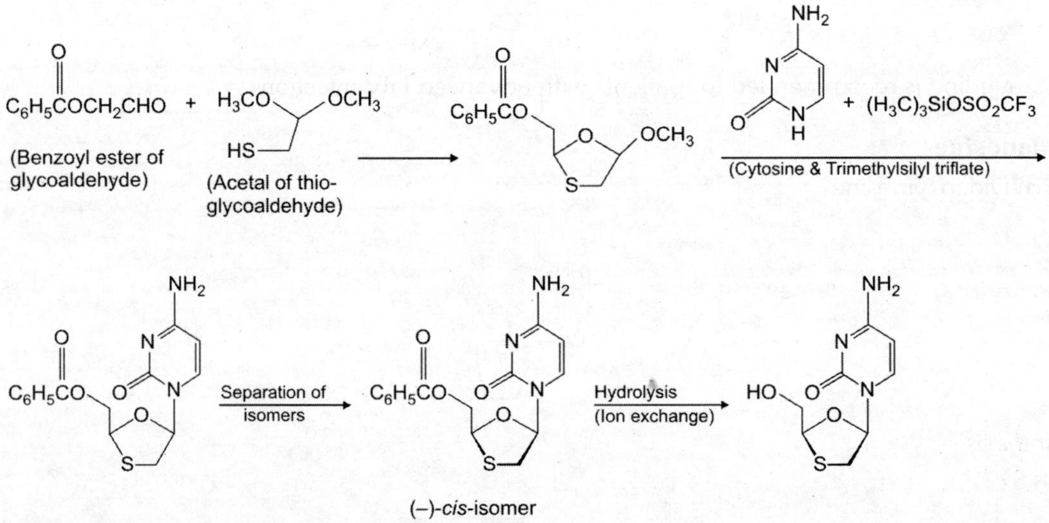

(−)-*cis*-isomer

It is a sulphur analog of zalcitabine (22). The active form is the triphosphate which inhibits the HIV reverse transcriptase and is incorporated into viral DNA which leads to chain termination.

Emtricitabine

(-)-*cis*-4-Amino-5-fluoro-1-(2-hydroxymethyl-1,3 oxathiolan-5-yl)-(1*H*)-pyrimidin-2-one

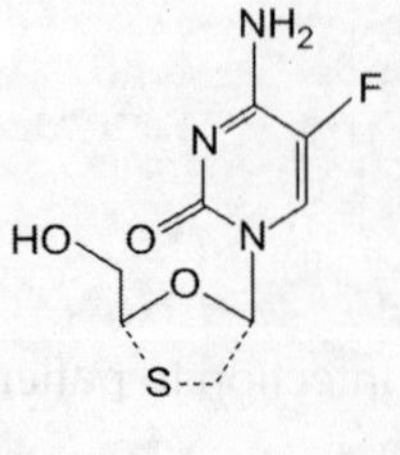

Synthesis

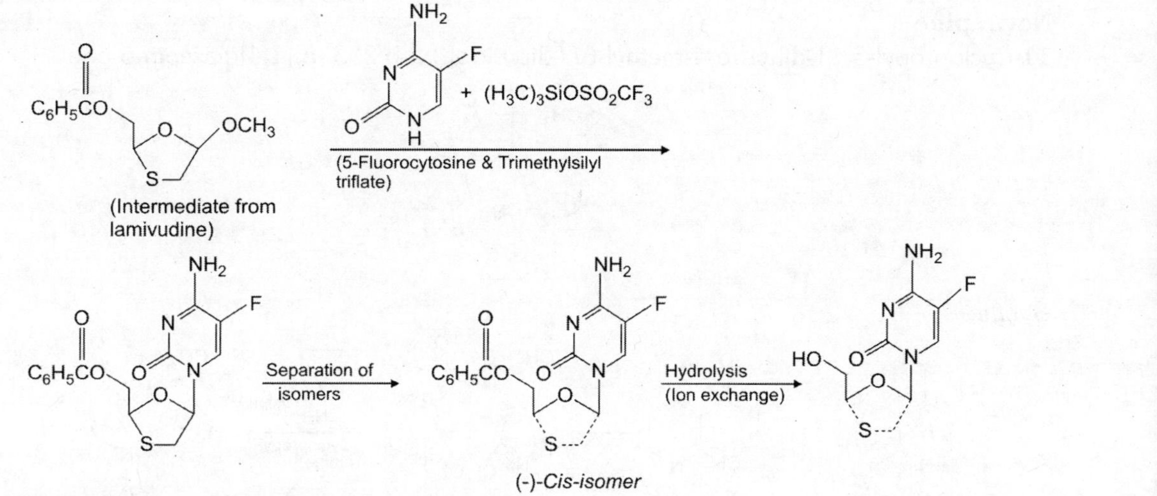

(Intermediate from lamivudine)

(5-Fluorocytosine & Trimethylsilyl triflate)

(-)-*Cis-isomer*

Separation of isomers

Hydrolysis (Ion exchange)

It is an orally active reverse transcriptase inhibitor.

Tenofovir

(*R*)-9-(2-Phosphonomethoxypropyl)adenine

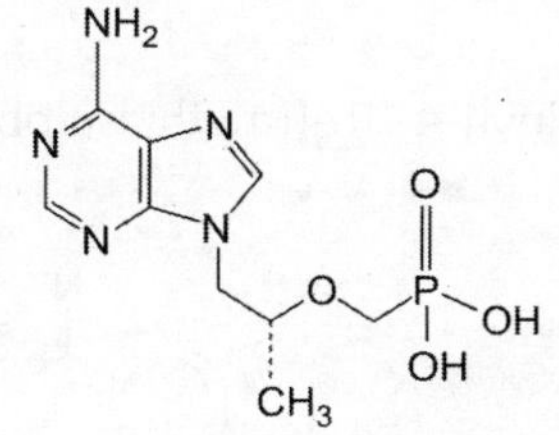

Synthesis

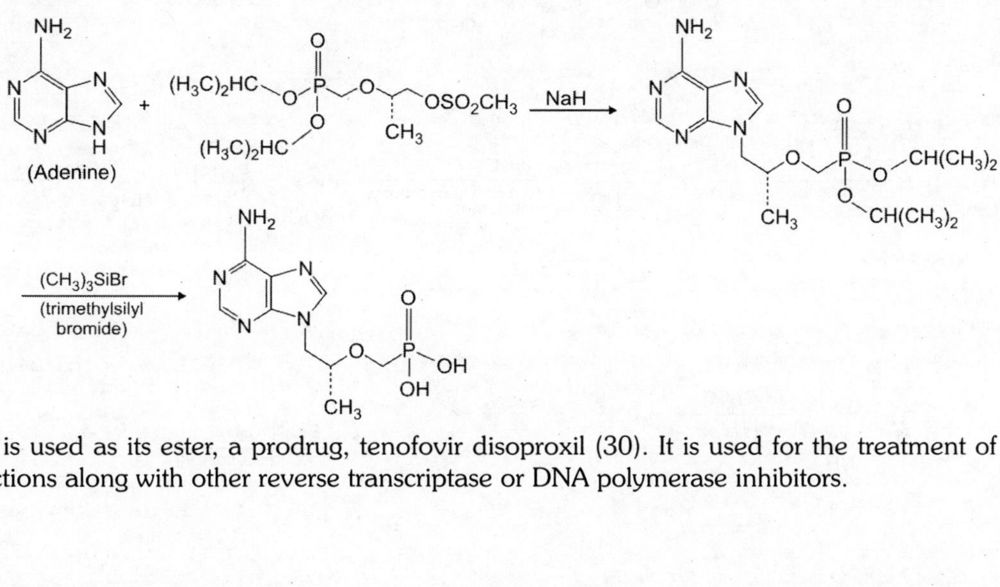

(Adenine)

NaH

(CH₃)₃SiBr
(trimethylsilyl bromide)

It is used as its ester, a prodrug, tenofovir disoproxil (30). It is used for the treatment of HIV infections along with other reverse transcriptase or DNA polymerase inhibitors.

NONNUCLEOSIDE REVERSE TRANSCRIPTASE INHIBITORS (NNRTIs)
Nevirapine
11-Cyclopropyl-5,11-dihydro-4-methyl-6H-dipyrido[3,2-b:2',3'-e][1,4]diazepin-6-one

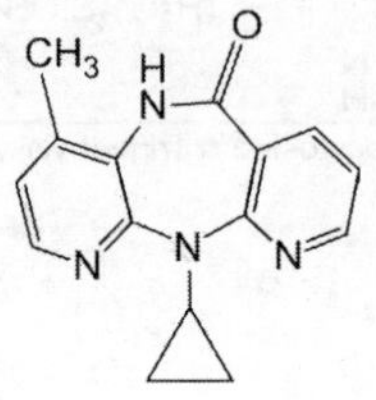

Synthesis

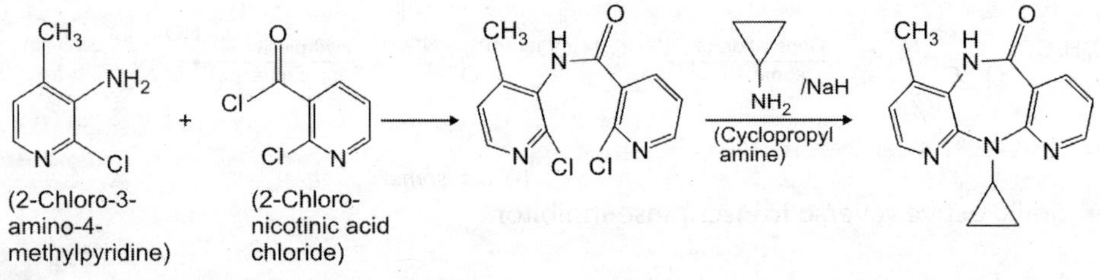

(2-Chloro-3-amino-4-methylpyridine) + (2-Chloro-nicotinic acid chloride)

Nevirapine is used along with other nucleoside inhibitors for HIV-1.

Delavirdine
1-[3-[(1-Methylethyl)amino]-2-pyridinyl]-4-[[5-[(methylsulphonyl)amino]-1H-indol-2yl]carbonyl]piperazine

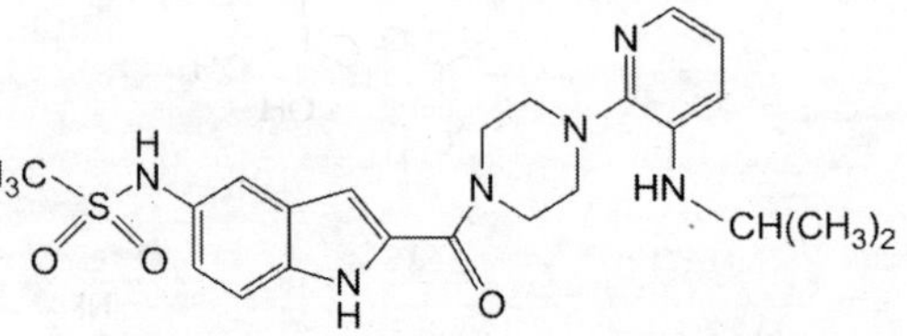

Synthesis

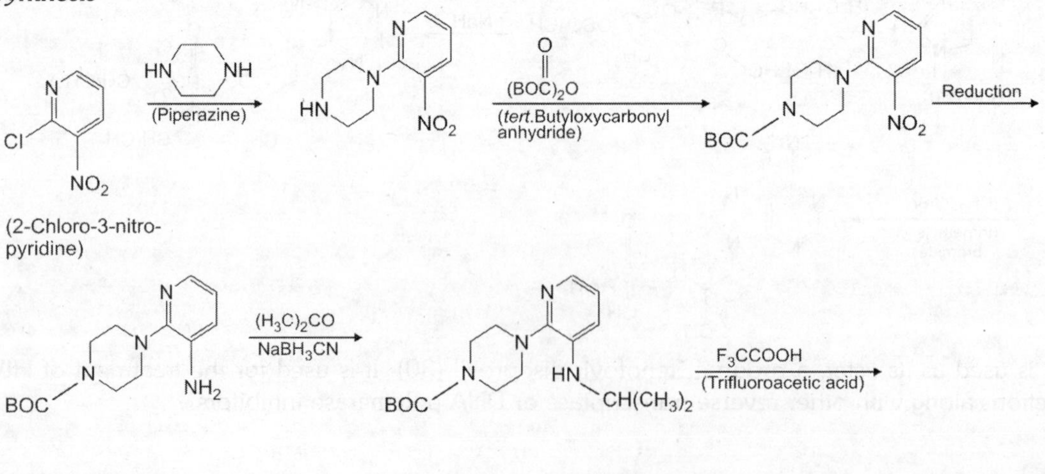

(2-Chloro-3-nitro-pyridine)

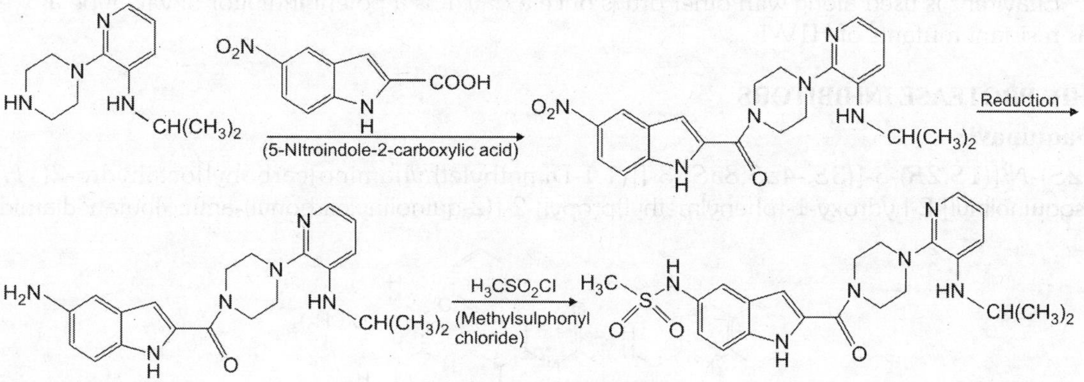

Efavirenz

(4S)-6-Chloro-4-(cyclopropylethynyl)-1,4-dihydro-4-(trifluoromethyl)-2H-3,1-benzoxazin-2-one

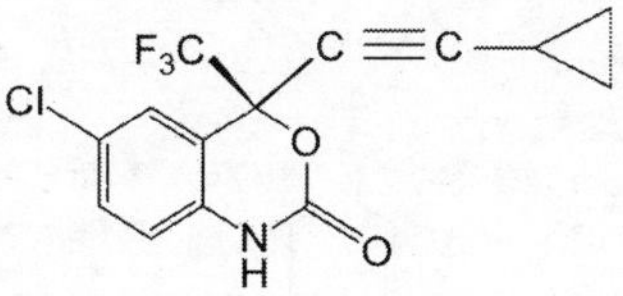

Synthesis

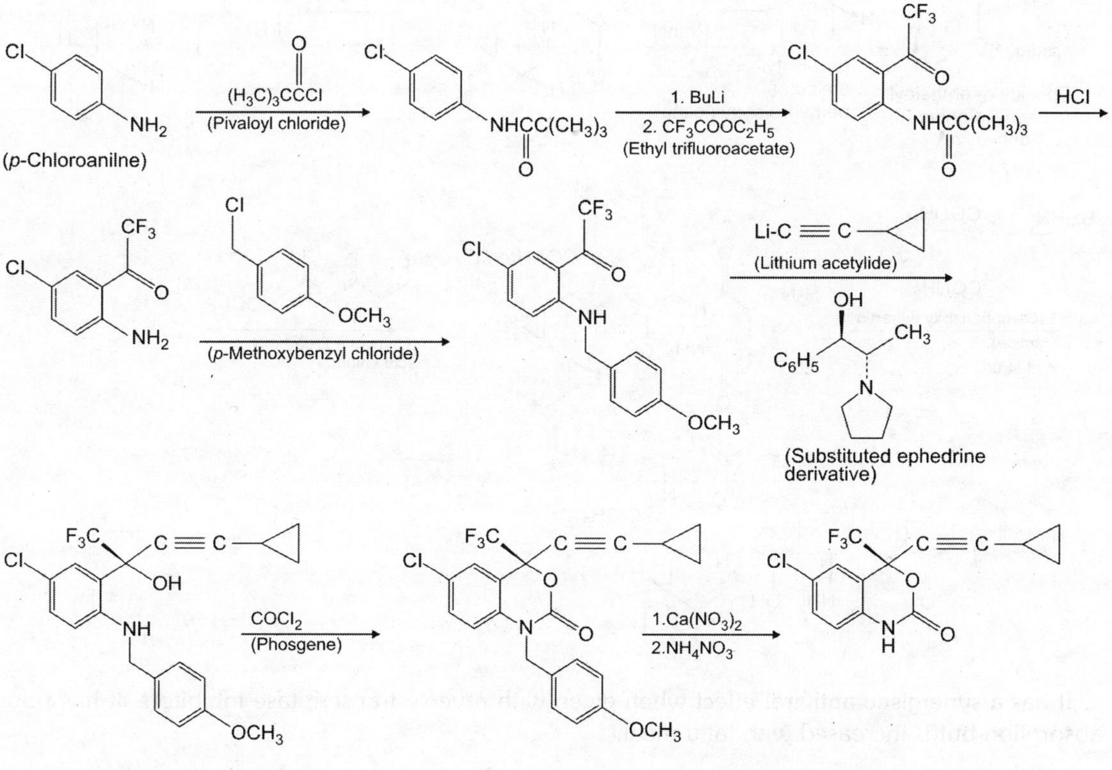

Effavirenz is used along with other drugs once a day. It is a potent inhibitor of wild type as well as resistant mutants of H1V-1.

HIV PROTEASE INHIBITORS

Saquinavir

(2S)-N^1[(1S,2R)-3-[(3S,-4aS,8aS)-3-[[(1,1-Dimethylethyl)amino]carbonyl]octahydro-2(1H)-isoquinolinyl]-2-hydroxy-1-(phenylmethyl)propyl]-2-[(2-quinolinylcarbonyl)-amino]butanediamide

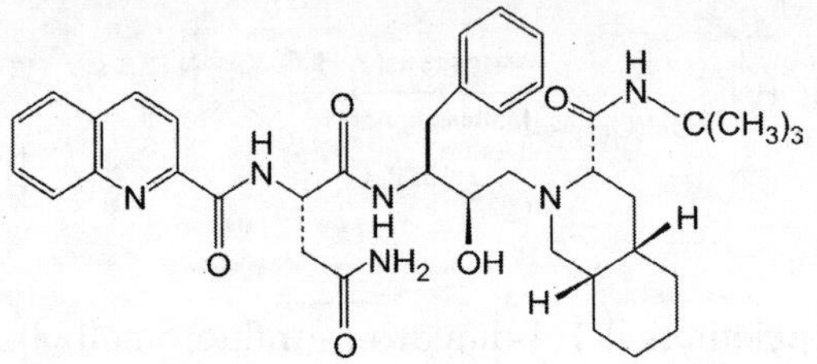

Synthesis

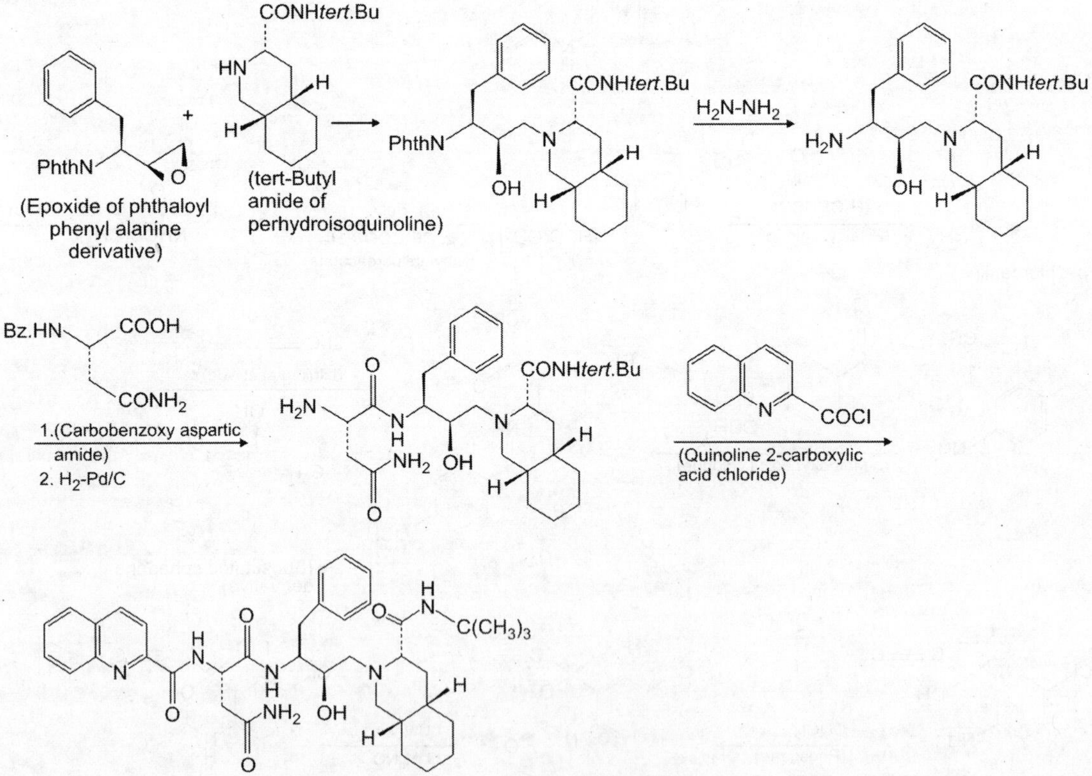

It has a synergistic antiviral *effect* when given with *reverse* transcriptase inhibitors. It has poor absorption but is increased with fatty meal.

Ritonavir

(2*S*,3*S*,5*S*)-5-[*N*-[*N*-[[*N*-Methyl-*N*-[(2-isopropyl-4-thiazolyl)methyl]amino]carbonyl]valinyl]amino]-2-[*N*-[(5-thiazolyl)methoxycarbonyl]amino]1,6-diphenyl-3-hydroxyhexane

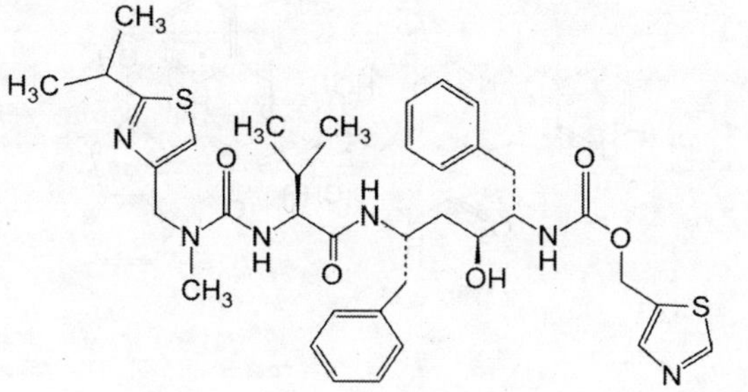

Synthesis

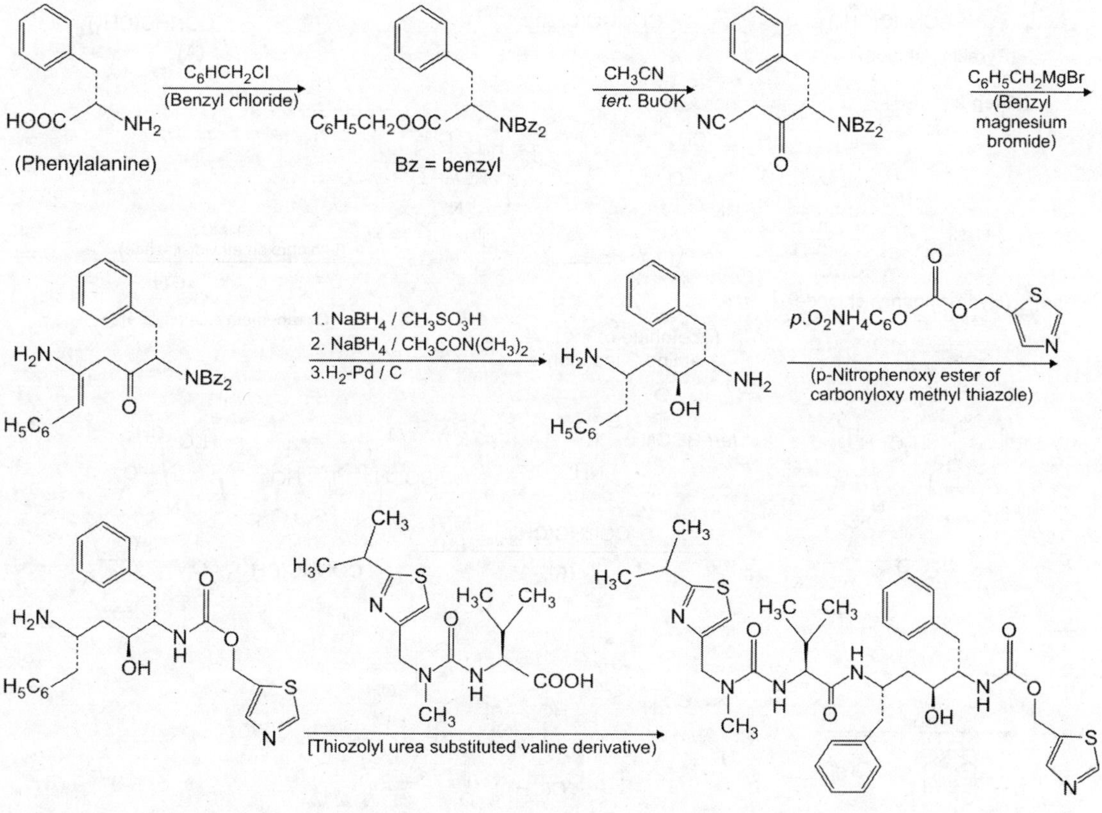

Ritonavir is peptidomimetic inhibitor of both HIV –1 and HIV –2 protease.

Indinavir

2,3,5-Trideoxy-*N*-[(1*S*,2*R*)-2,3-dihydro-2-hydroxy-1*H*-inden-1-yl]-5-[(2*S*)-2-[[(1,1-dimethylethyl)- amino]carbonyl]-4-(3-pyridinylmethyl)-1-piperazinyl]-2-(phenylmethyl)-D-*erythro*-pentonamide.

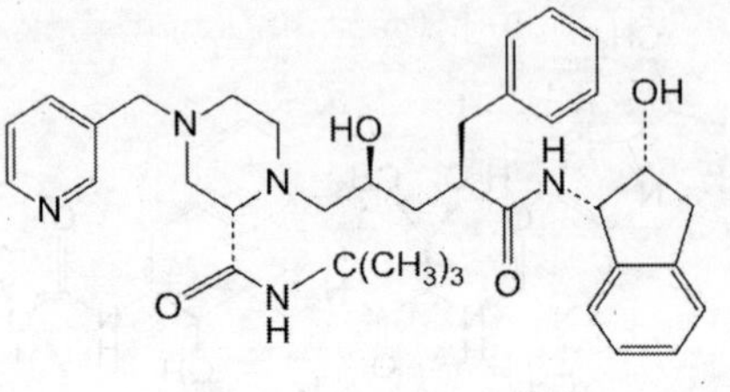

Synthesis

Step 1

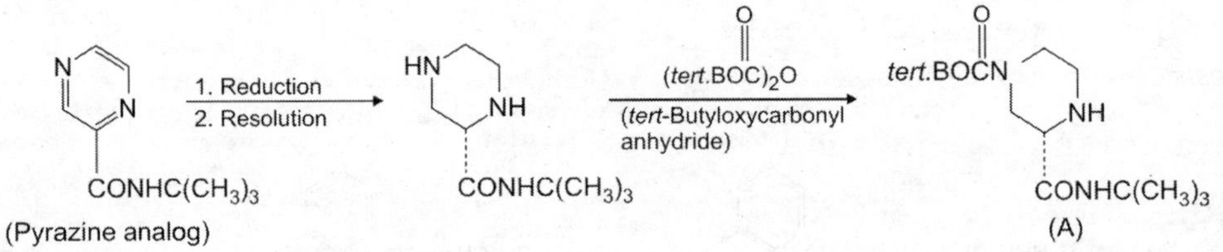

Step 2

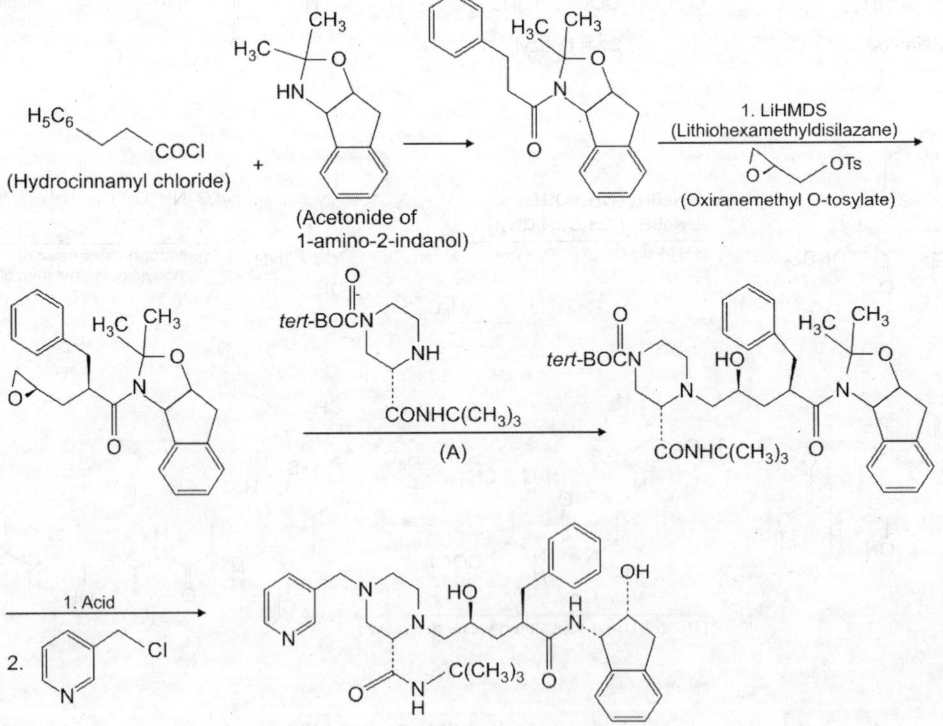

It is administered along with a high fat diet to get higher serum concentrations.

Nelfinavir

(3S,4aS,8aS)-N-(1,1-Dimethylethyl)decahydro-2-[(2R,3R)-2-hydroxy-3-[(3-hydroxy-2-methylbenzoyl)amino]-4-(phenylthio)butyl]-3-isoquinolinecarboxamide

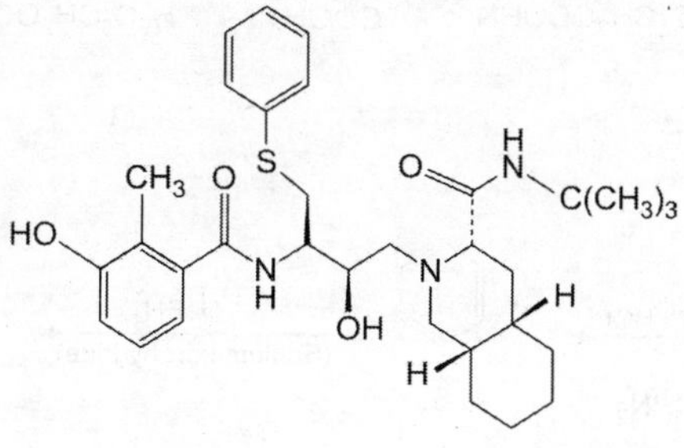

Synthesis

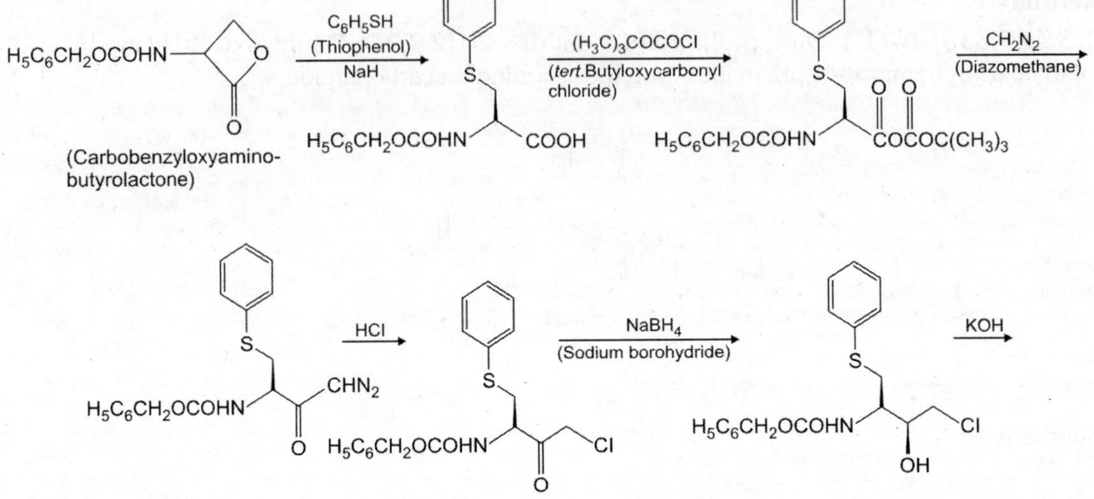

$H_5C_6CH_2OCOHN$

(Carbobenzyloxyamino-
butyrolactone)

C_6H_5SH
(Thiophenol)
NaH

$H_5C_6CH_2OCOHN$ COOH

$(H_3C)_3COCOCl$
(tert.Butyloxycarbonyl
chloride)

$H_5C_6CH_2OCOHN$ $COCOC(CH_3)_3$

CH_2N_2
(Diazomethane)

$H_5C_6CH_2OCOHN$ CHN_2

HCl

$H_5C_6CH_2OCOHN$ Cl

$NaBH_4$
(Sodium borohydride)

$H_5C_6CH_2OCOHN$ Cl   OH

KOH

Step 1

$H_5C_6CH_2OCOHN$

HN

$C(CH_3)_3$

(perhydroisiquinoline
2-tert.butylamide

$H_5C_6CH_2OCOHN$ OH $C(CH_3)_3$

HBr

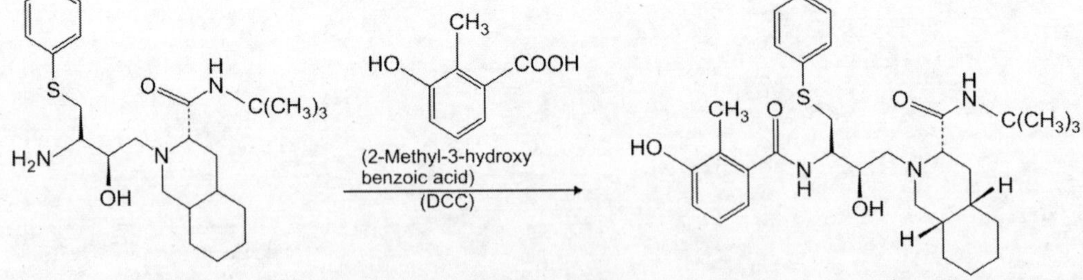

H_2N OH $C(CH_3)_3$

CH_3
HO   COOH

(2-Methyl-3-hydroxy
benzoic acid)
(DCC)

CH_3 HO   OH $C(CH_3)_3$

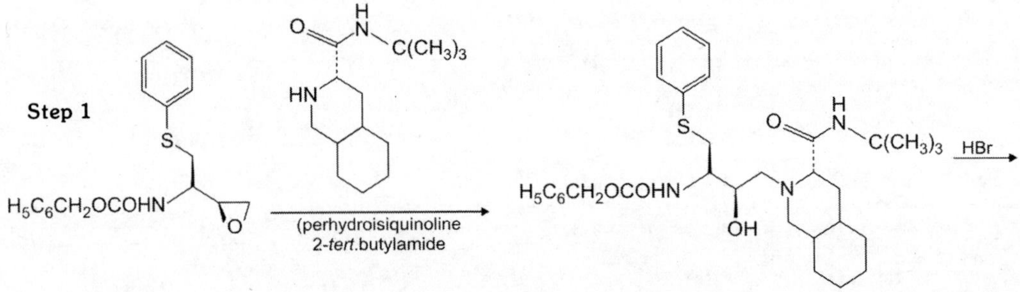

It is used as a mesylate. It is effective against HIV –1, HIV –2 wild type and zidovudine (21) resistant strains.

Amprenavir

[(1S,2R)-3-[[(4-Aminophenyl)sulphonyl](2-methylpropyl)amino]-2-hydroxy-1-(phenylmethyl)propyl]carbamic acid (3*S*)-tetrahydro-3-furanyl ester

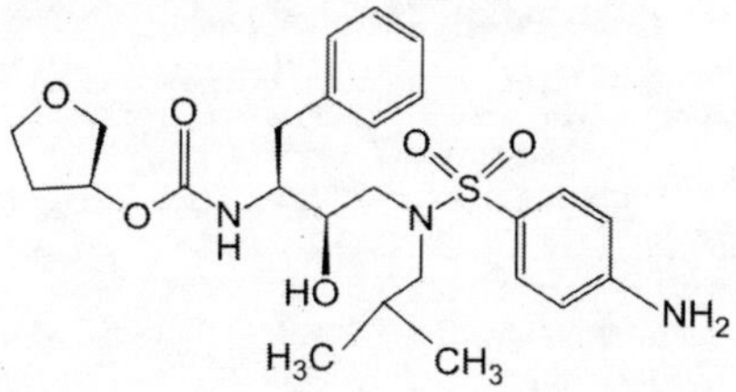

Synthesis

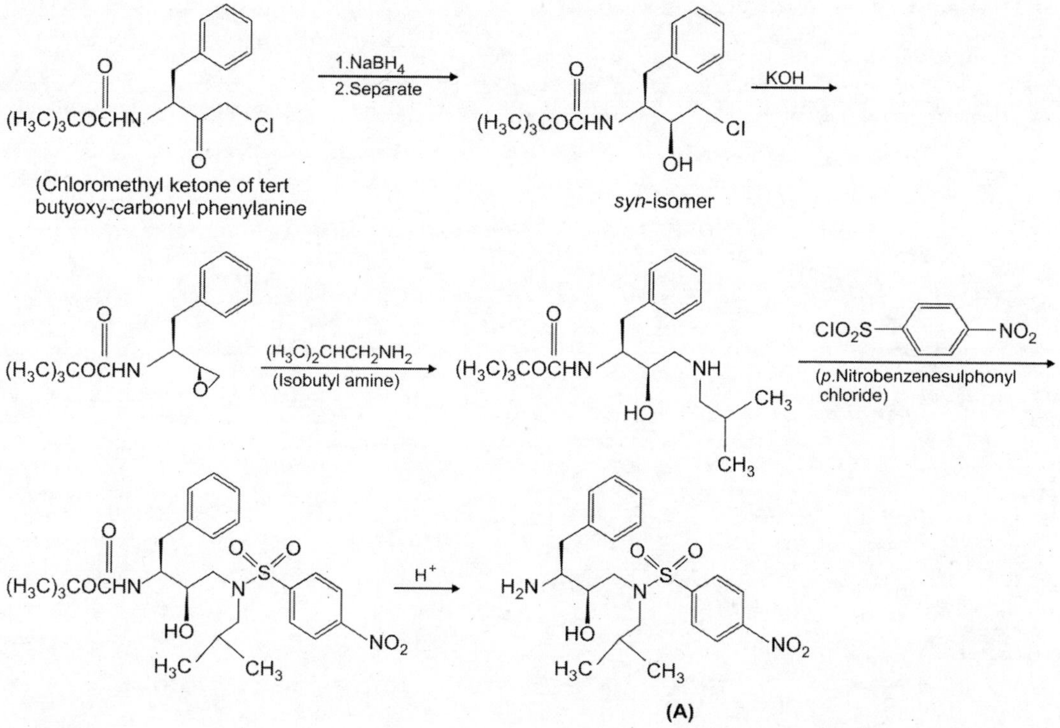
1.NaBH4
2.Separate
KOH
(Chloromethyl ketone of tert butyoxy-carbonyl phenylanine
syn-isomer
(H3C)2CHCH2NH2
(Isobutyl amine)
ClO2S-⟨⟩-NO2
(p.Nitrobenzenesulphonyl chloride)
H+
(A)

Step 2

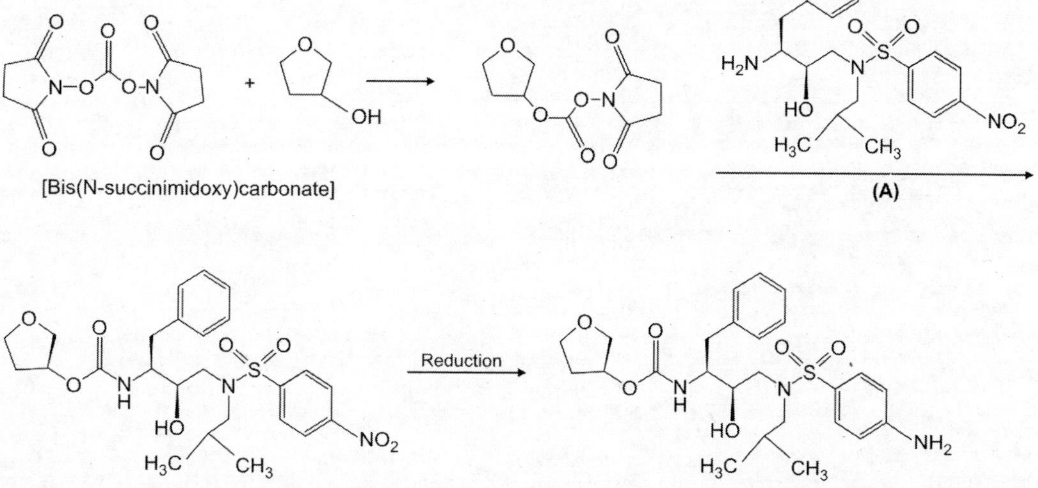
[Bis(N-succinimidoxy)carbonate]
(A)
Reduction

Section X

Chemotherapy—Drugs Used in Cancer

CHAPTER 36

ANTICANCER AGENTS

THE MEDICAL TERM for cancer is neoplasm. Neoplasm means "relatively autonomous growth of tissue", building up to form a solid mass or tumor. Tumors can be benign or malignant and the word cancer is associated with malignant tumor. Like cancer, benign tumors are caused by abnormal growth but they do not metastasize. Benign tumors are rarely life-threatening, grow within a well-defined capsule which limits their size and maintain characteristics of cell of origin and are thus usually differentiated.

Malignant tumors are life-threatening, invade surrounding tissues and spread to different areas of body by breaking away from tumor and traveling to different organs through blood. The transplanted cells grow into new tumors. This process is known as metastasis.

The different type of cancers fall into four groups, i.e. carcinomas, sarcomas, gliomas, and lymphomas which include leukemias and myelomas. Carcinomas arise from epithelial tissues which includes skin and most of soft organ. Cancers of bones, cartilage and muscles are known as sarcomas. Cancers of brain and nervous system are termed as gliomas while lymphomas arise from lymphatic system. Leukemias are characterized by uncontrolled growth of white blood cells. The myelomas arise from bone marrow.

Malignant tumor formation could be through:

1. Mutation.
2. Addition of new genetic material such as addition and integration of viral genetic material into cell's gene as a result of infection by tumor producing viruses.
3. Viruses.
4. Chemicals, such as polycyclic aromatic hydrocarbons, benzo[a]pyrene (1), pyrene (2), etc. inhaled through smoking, exposure to asbestos particles, compounds of beryllium, cadmium, chromium, nickel, lead, and amines.

(1)

(2)

Cancer is very difficult to treat, the present day therapy can at the most increase the lifespan of a cancer patient but not radically cure the patient unless treated at early stage.

There are basically four approaches to cancer treatment and these include, surgery, radiation therapy, immunological approach, and chemotherapy.

Surgical approach is used when the tumor is in early stage of development and the surgeon has the confidence of removing the entire tumor without affecting the vital organs. Surgery is also used in combination with other approaches such as chemotherapy.

Radiation therapy involves destruction of cancerous tissues by Ionizing, thermal, or photodynamic radiation. It is not painful and there are few side effects. Radiation therapy requires that the tumor is localized so that radiation does not affect other vital organs.

The immunological approach uses immune system, especially T cell and B cell lymphocytes to eradicate the cancerous cells. Currently highly purified interferons, especially interferon – 2 is used for this purpose.

The chemotherapeutic approach is complimentary to radiation and surgical approaches. It is used to reduce the size of the tumor before the surgery or sensitize the tumor to radiation therapy. Chemotherapy is not effective in case of large tumors because they cannot reach the inside of the tumor in sufficient concentration to destroy them. This is because the inner of the tumor is not profused well by blood. Further, the anticancer agents lack selectivity towards cancer cells, as a result most of the chemotherapeutic agents are highly toxic and they kill both normal as well as malignant cells.

The various classes of chemotherapeutic agents used against cancers are:

1. Alkylating agents.   2. DNA Cross-linking agents-Organoplatinum complexes.
3. Antimetabolites.   4. Antibiotics.
5. Plant products.   6. Hormones and antihormones.
7. Inhibitors of protein kinase.   8. Miscellaneous compounds.

ALKYLATING AGENTS

These are the agents which alkylate the nucleophilic sites of the biomolecules, as a result they are not able to carry out the normal functions. The various classes of alkylating agents together with the compounds used in clinical practice are discussed below.

Nitrogen Mustards

Although mustard gas (3) has some antileukemic properties but it could not be used in clinical practice because of its low solubility in water and vesicant properties. Attention was next focused on nitrogen mustards (4). Nitrogen mustards (4) had certain advantages and these included their ease of handling since their salts were solids and water soluble. The nitrogen mustards (4) owe their antitumor activity due to their ability to cyclize to a highly reactive ethylenimmonium ions (5) at physiological pH. The immonium ions (5) then alkylates the biomolecules to yield (6). The process then gets repeated with another β-chloroethyl residue.

Some of the nitrogen mustards used in clinical practice include mechlorethamine [mustine or HN2,(9)] used in Hodgkin's disease and novembichin (10), claimed to be less toxic than mechlorethamine (9) and possessesing comparable activity against leukemia and Hodgkin's disease.

(9)   (10)

Structure-activity relationship studies have shown that the reactivity of nitrogen mustards could be reduced by making nitrogen less nucleophilic. This would result in less toxic and more seiective nitrogen mustards. One way to achieve this is to replace electron releasing alkyl group by electron withdrawing group such as phenyl group, example, chlorambucil (11). Chlorambucil (11) has been found to be less toxic and it can be administered orally.

(11)   (12)

Nitrogen mustards of important naturally occuring compounds have also been prepared and found to possess clinically useful antineoplastic activity and include nitrogen mustards of phenylalanine, 6-methyluracil and estradiol. The nitrogen mustard of L-phenylalanine commonly known as melphalan [L-sarcolysin, (12)], is more active than the D-isomer, indicating that the L-isomer is preferentially transported into cells by L-amino acid transporter. It is used in ovarian carcinoma and multiple myeloma. 5-Bis(β-chloroethyl)amino-6-methyluracil [dopan, (13)], the nitrogen mustard of 6-methyluracil, is active against Hodgkin's disease. Estramustine (14a), a C_3-N,N-bis(2-chloroethyl) carbamic acid ester of estradiol, has been found to be useful in prostate cancer. Its antineoplastic activity has been attributed to inhibition of mitosis and not as an alkylator of DNA, as was thought earlier. It binds to microtubule associated proteins to promote microtubule disassembly. Its 17-disodiumphosphate ester (14b) is also used.

(13)

(14a), R = H
(14b), R = PO$_3$Na$_2$

Among the nitrogen mustards of organophosphorus compunds, two compunds, namely, cyclophosphamide (15) and ifosfamide (16) are the clinically useful compounds.

(15)   (16)

Cyclophosphamide (15) is not itself active, it requires bioactivation to phosphoramide mustard (17) (Fig. 36.1), which is responsible for alkylationn of DNA. Cyclophosphamide (15) has been found to be useful in leukemia and myeloma.

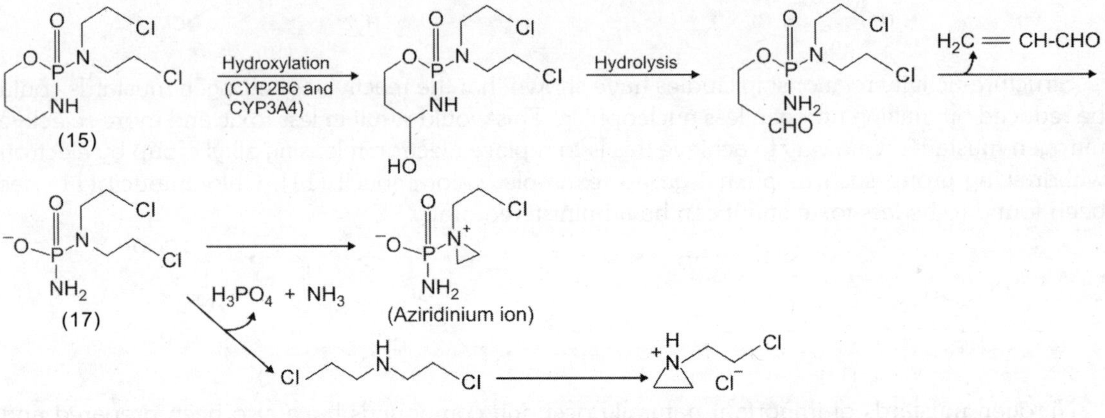

Fig. 36.1: Bioactivation of cyclophsphamide (15).

Ifosfamide (16) is an analog of cyclophosphamide (15) in which the two β-chloroethyl residues are on two different nitrogen atoms rather than on the same nitrogen. Like cyclophosphamide (15), it also requires bioactivation to phosphoramide mustard (18) (Fig. 36.2). It is used for testicular carcinoma.

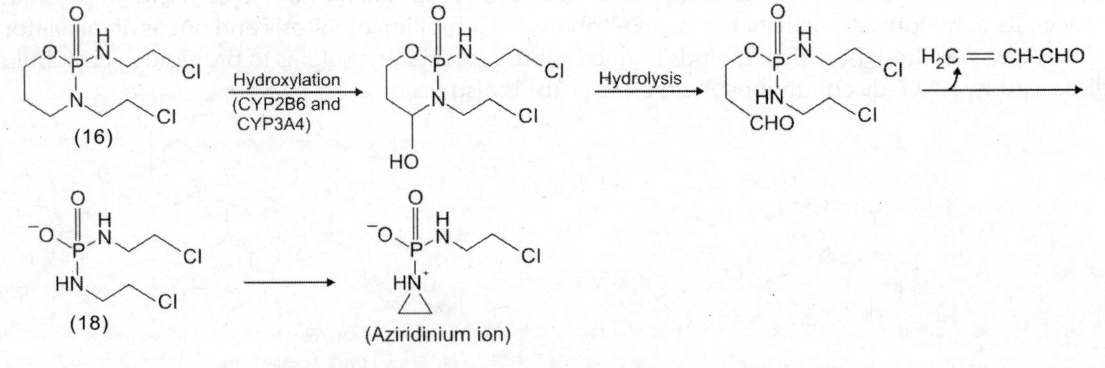

Fig. 36.2: Bioactivation of ifosfamide (16).

Nitrogen Mustard N-Oxides

Nitrogen mustard N-oxides (19) have better therapeutic index because of lower toxicity as compared to nitrogen mustards (4). The nitrogen mustard N-oxides (19) act in the same manner as the nitrogen mustards (4), giving initially a highly reactive oximmonium ion which acts as an alkylating agent. The only nitrogen mustard N-oxide which has received clinical acceptance is mechlorethamine oxide [HN2-oxide, (20)].

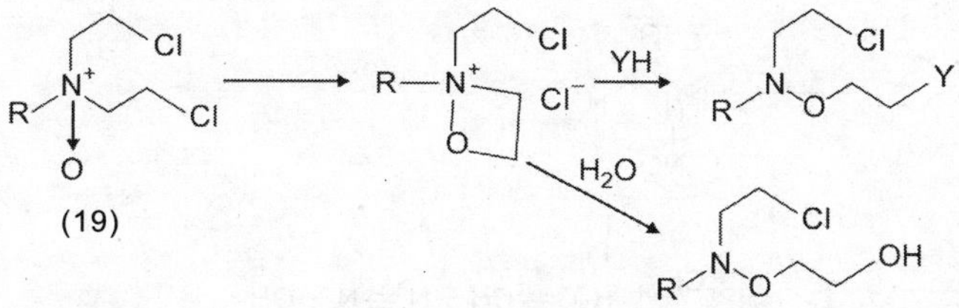

(19)

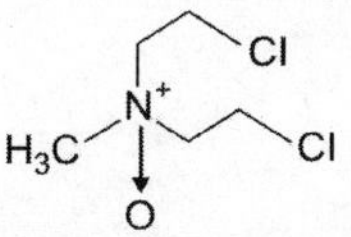

(20)

Ethylenimines

Ethylenimines constitute another class of alkylating agents. Some of these include triethylen-emelamine [TEM, (21)]. It is as toxic as mechlorethamine (9) and is used in leukemia and ovarian cancer. Triethylenephosphoramide [TEPA, (22)] and thiotepa [TSPA, (23)] are the other ethylenimines which are used in carcinoma of breast, bladder, and ovaries.

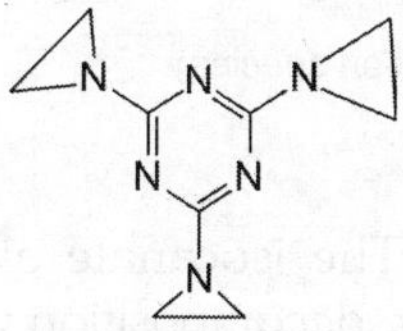

(21)

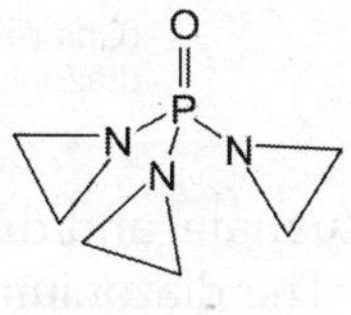

(22)

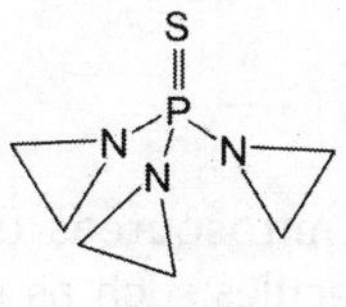

(23)

Methanesulphonates

Alkylenebismethanesulphonate esters (24) have shown sufficient antineoplastic activity. The most important among them is busulfan [myleran, (24), $n = 4$]. It is used in chronic myelocytic leukemia.

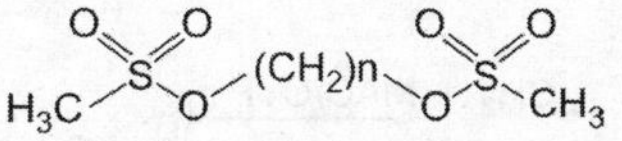

(24)

Nitrosoureas

The nitrosoureas is another class of compounds which produce an alkylating species and include nitrosomethylurea (25), carmustine (26), and lomustine (27).

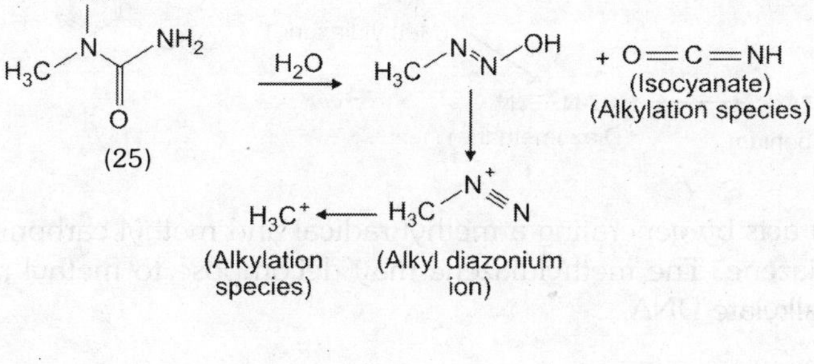

(25)

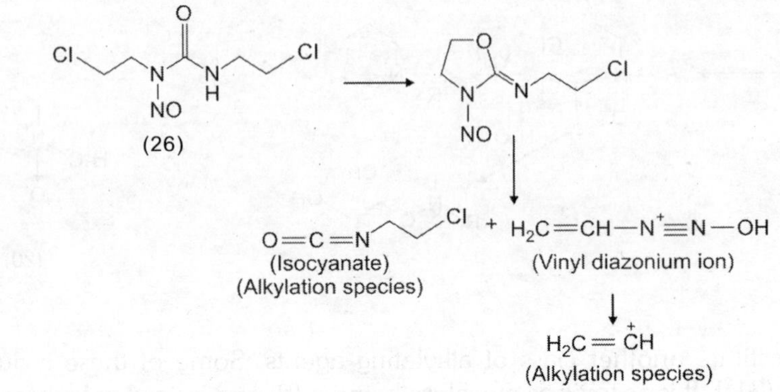

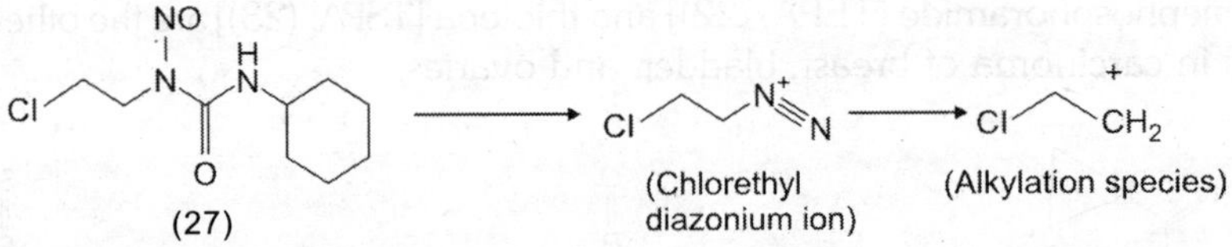

The nitrosoureas decompose to isocyanate and/diazonium ions. The isocanate alkylates biomolecules such as proteins and RNA. The diazonium ion, on further, decomposition yields a carbonium ion which alkylates the DNA.

Miscellaneous Alkylating Agents

This class of antineoplastics agents include substances which are having different structures at the same time act by of alkylating the biomolecules. Some of these include procarbazine (28), dacarbazine (29), altretamine (30), and temozolomide (31).

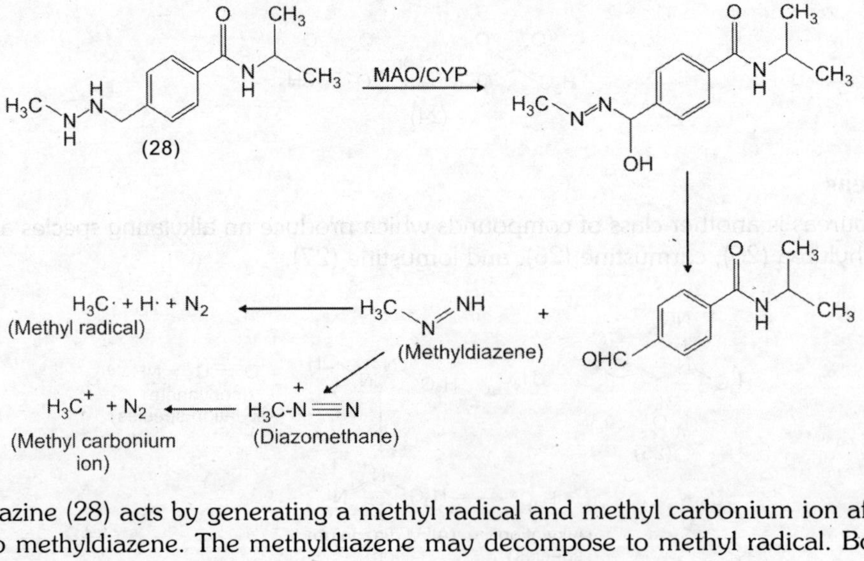

Procarbazine (28) acts by generating a methyl radical and methyl carbonium ion after getting oxidized to methyldiazene. The methyldiazene may decompose to methyl radical. Both radical and carbonium ion alkylate DNA.

Dacarbazine (29), an imidazole derivative, is thought to alkylate the DNA molecule through methyl carbonium ion which is generated after it is metabolized to methyl diazonium ion.

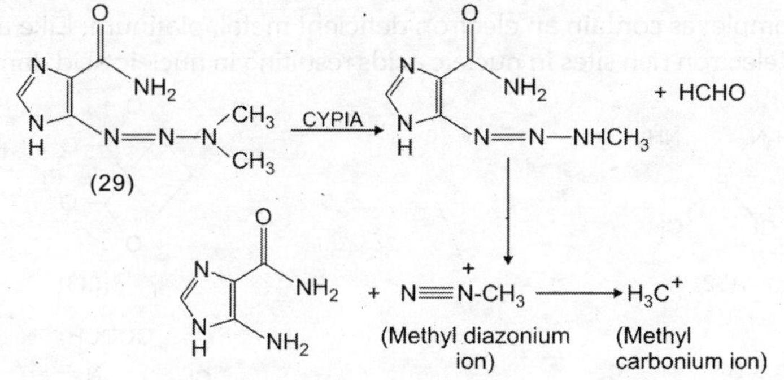

Altretamine (30), a hexamethylmelamin, acts through iminium ion. The iminium ion is generated by oxidation of methyl to hydroxymethyl group and subsequent dehydration.

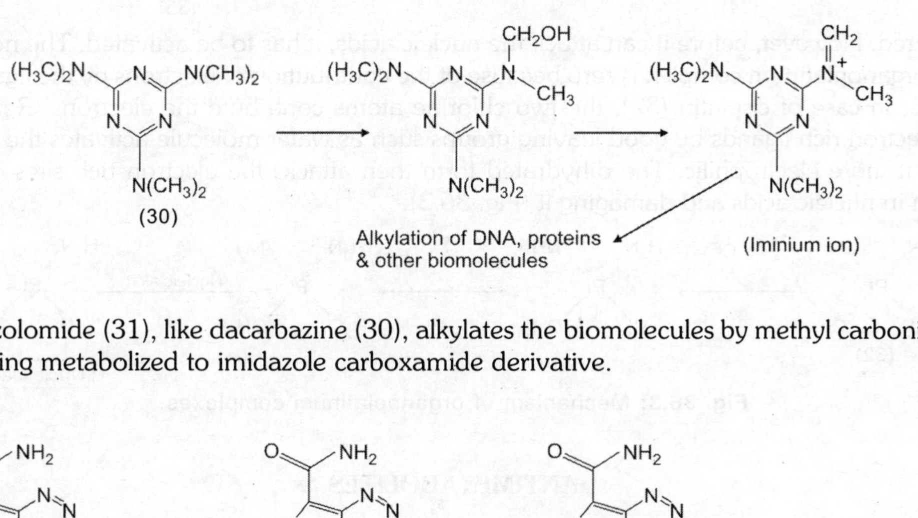

Temozolomide (31), like dacarbazine (30), alkylates the biomolecules by methyl carbonium ion after getting metabolized to imidazole carboxamide derivative.

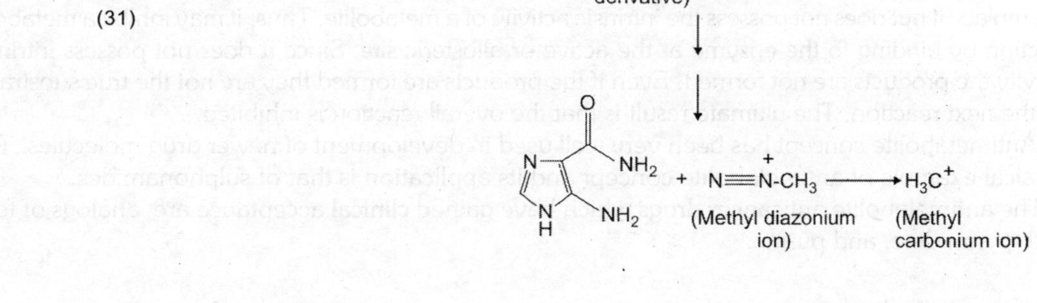

DNA CROSS LINKING AGENTS – ORGANOPLATIUM COMPLEXES

These include cisplatin (32), carboplatin (33), oxaliplatin (34), and satraplatin (35). The organoplatinum complexes contain an electron deficient metal, platinum. Like alkylating agents, it can also attack the electron rich sites in nucleic acids resulting in nucleic acid damage which cannot

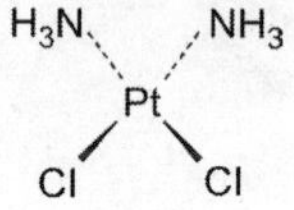

(32) 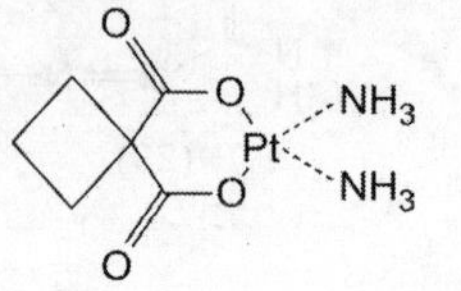   (33)

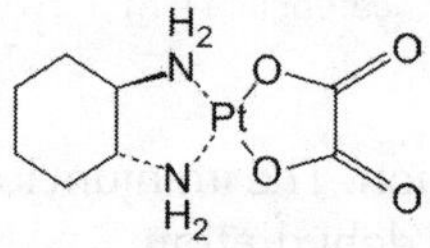

(34) 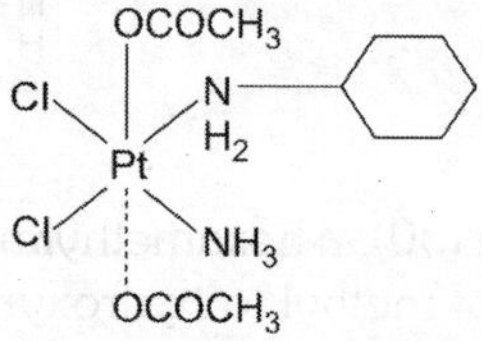   (35)

be repaired. However, before it can attack the nucleic acids, it has to be activated. The net charge on the organoplatinum complex is zero because of the contribution of electrons by the ligands. For example, in case of cisplatin (32), the two chlorine atoms contribute the electrons. Removal of these electron rich ligands by good leaving groups such as water molecule activates the complex making it more electrophilic. The dihydrated form then attacks the electron rich sites of amino nitrogen in nucleic acids and damaging it (Fig. 36.3).

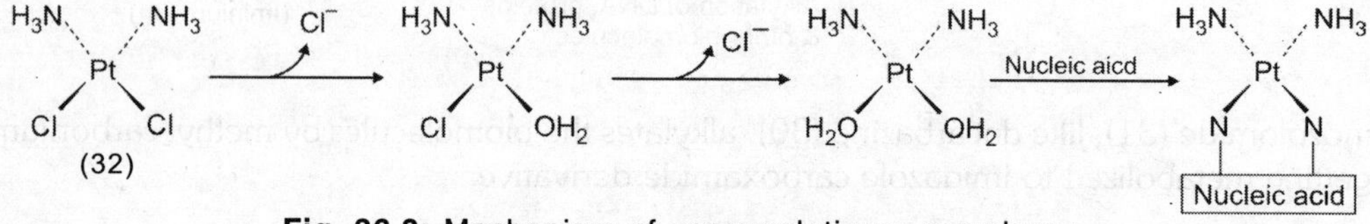

Fig. 36.3: Mechanism of organoplatinum complexes.

ANTIMETABOLITES

A metabolite is a substance involved in the biochemical process leading to the formation and maintenance of living cell. Antimetabolites are substances which interfere with the normal biological functions or synthesis of a metabolite. An antimetabolite closely resembles a metabolite and thus, can replace it but does not possess the intrinsic activity of a metabolite. Thus, it may inhibit a metabolic reaction by binding to the enzyme at the active or allosteric site. Since it does not possess intrinsic activity the products are not formed. Even if the products are formed they are not the true substrates for the next reaction. The ultimate result is that the overall reaction is inhibited.

Antimetabolite concept has been very well used in development of newer drug molecules. The classical example of antimetabolite concept and its application is that of sulphonamides.

The antimetabolite anticancer drugs which have gained clinical acceptance are analogs of folic acid, pyrimidine, and purine.

Folic Acid Analogs

Folic acid (36), as 5, 6, 7, 8-tetrahydrofolic acid (37), is involved in one carbon metabolism required for syntheses of purines and pyrimidines, and then in the syntheses of nucleic acids (see Sulphonamides and Quinolones). Methorexate (38) is a powerful inhibitor of dihydrofoliate reductase. It is also an inhibitor of glycine amide ribonucleotide transformylase, a key enzyme in synthesis of purines. Inhibition of dihydrofoliate reductase results in lower concentration of tetrahydrofoliate so one carbon transfer does not take place, this results in inhibition of DNA synthesis. Alternately, inhibition of dihydrofoliate reductase results in increased concentrations of 7,8-dihydrofoliate in the cells this in turn results in feedback inhibition of thymidylate synthase.

Replacement of pyrazine ring by pyrrole ring and NH by CH_2 at position 10 in folic acid (36) results in another antifoliate, pemetrexed (39). It inhibits various enzymes. which include dihydrofoliate reductase, glycine amide ribonucleotide transformylase, and thymidylate synthase.

(36)

(37)

(38)

(39)

Pyrimidine Analogs

The pyrimidine analogs used as anticancer agents include fluorouracil (40), tetetrahydrofuran analog of fluorouracil (40), tegafur (41). The pyrimidine ncleosides, include floxuridine (42), capecitabine (43), cytarabine (44), gemcitabine (45), azacitidine (46), and decitabine (47).

(40)

(41)

(42)

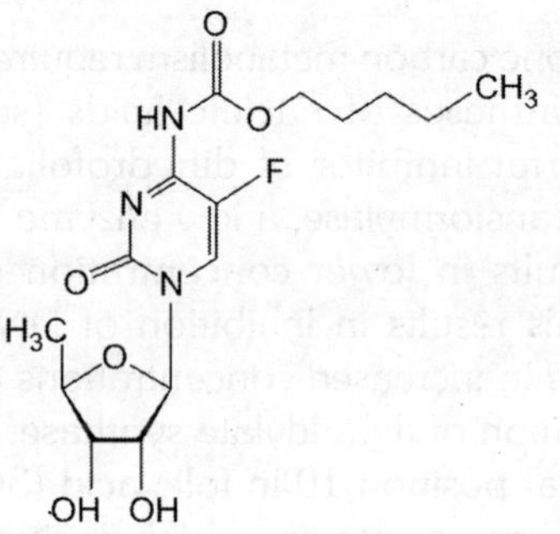

(43)

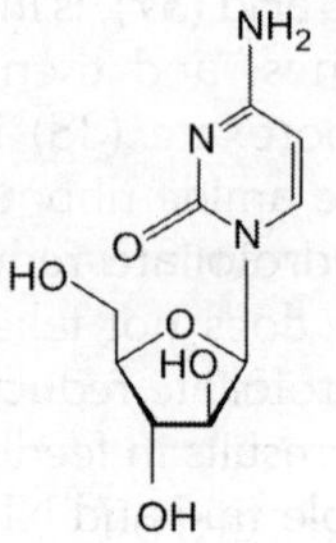

(44)

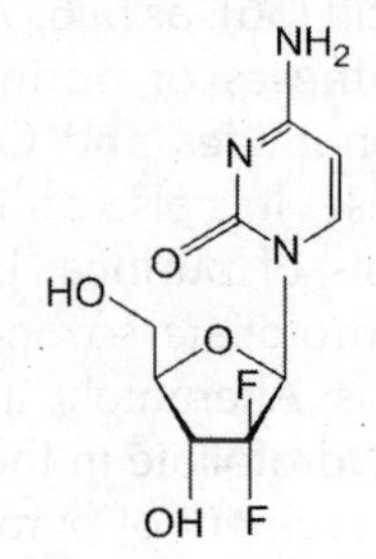

(45)

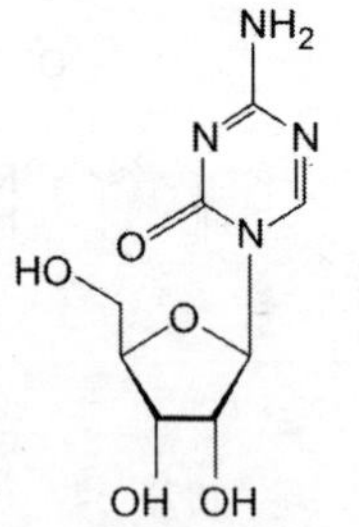

(46)

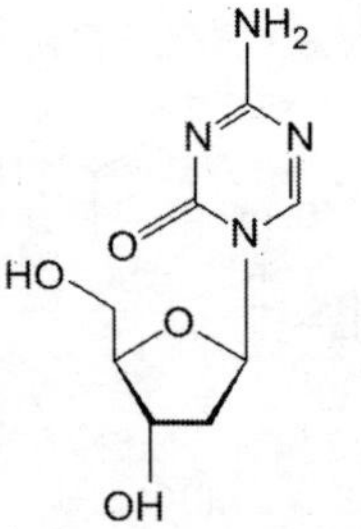

(47)

Fluorouracil (40) is an inhibitor of thymidylate synthase, an enzyme responsible for conversion of 2'-deoxyuridylic acid (48) to 2'-deoxythymidylic acid (49). Fluorouracil (40) is first of all activated to 5-fluoro-2'-deoxyuridine monophosphate (50) which then binds to thymidylate synthase and inhibits it. As a result, 2'-deoxyuridylic acid is not converted to (49) and the cell dies.

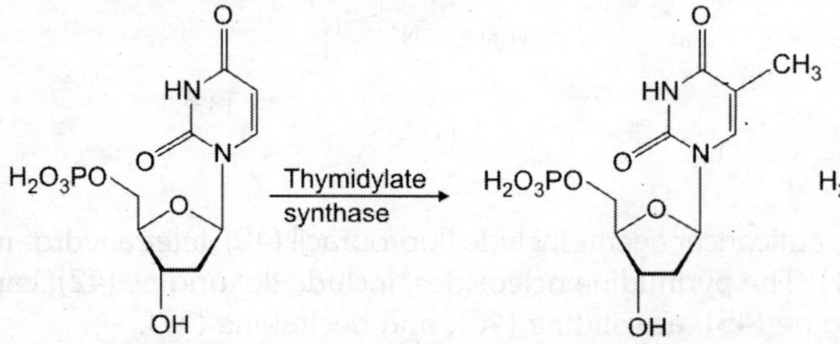

(48)

(49)

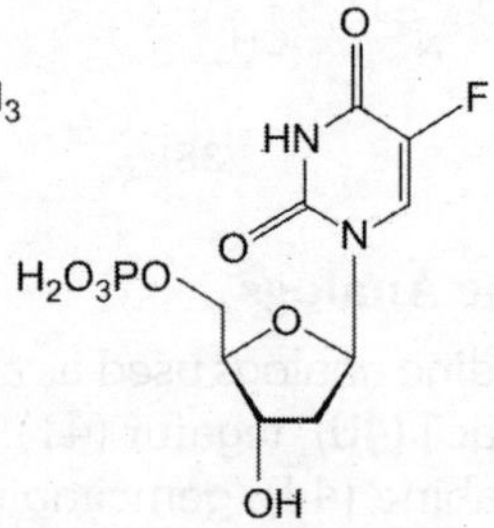

(50)

The tetrahydrfuran analog, tegafur (41), is first converted to fluorouracil (40) which then inhibits thymidylate synthase.

Floxuridine (42), the 2'-deoxyribonucleoside of fluorouracil, is first converted to 5-fluoro-2'-deoxyuridine monophosphate (50), the active metabolite of fluorouracil.

Capecitabine (43), a carbamylated analog, is a prodrug. It is converted to active form, 5'-deoxy-5-fluorocytidine (51), by carboxyesterase. It also inhibits thymidylate synthase after getting metabolized to fluorouracil (40) which is then converted to active form 5-fluoro-2'-deoxyuridine monophosphate (50).

Cytarabine (44) and gemcitabine (45) act by interfering with DNA synthesis by inhibiting both DNA polymerase and reductase after getting mon-,di-, and triphosphorylated.

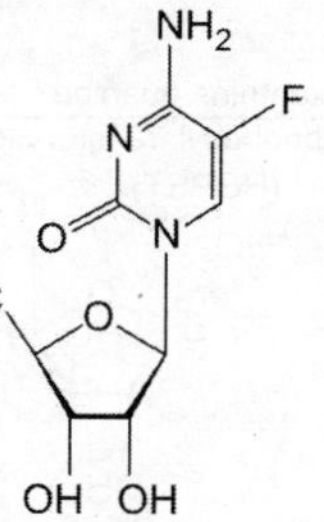

(51)

Azacitidine (46) and decitabine (47) act by demethylating the DNA residues on genes responsible for differentiation and growth, a mechanism which is opposite to that of DNA alkylators like nitrogen mustards and other alkylators, discussed earlier.

Purine Analogs

Clinically useful purine and purine nucleosides as anticancer agents include mercaptopurine (52), thioguanine (53), vidarabine (54), cladribine (55), clofarabine (56), and fludarabine (57).

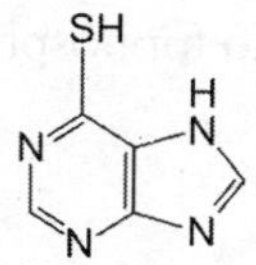

(52) 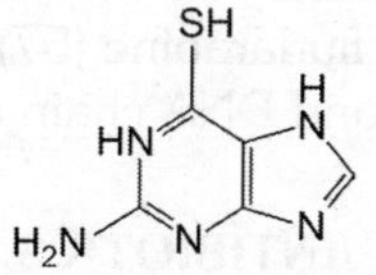 (53) 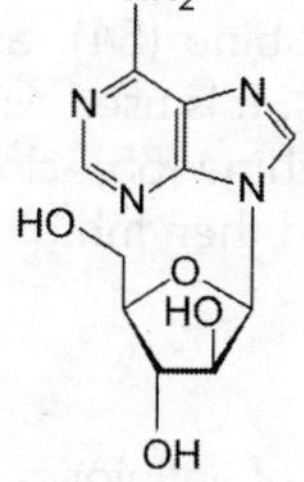 (54)

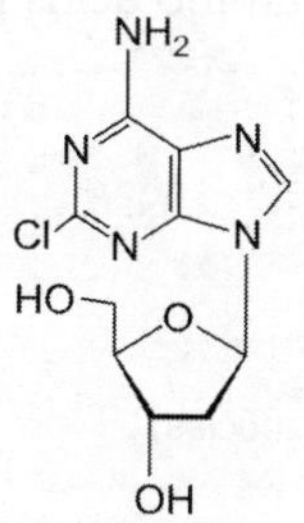

(55) 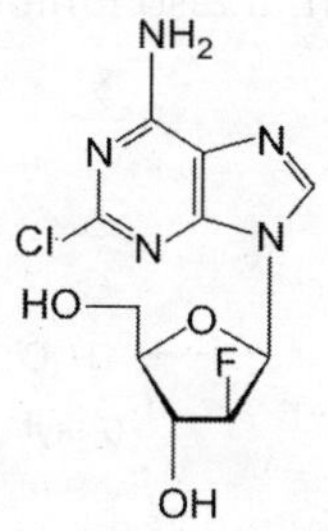 (56) 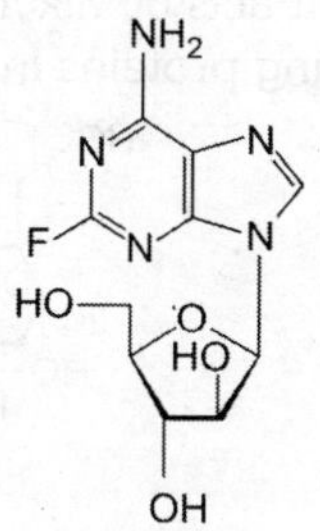 (57)

Both mercaptopurine [thiol isoster of hypoxanthine, (52)] and thioguanine [thiol isostere of guanine, (53)] after getting activated to corresponding ribonucleotides [(52a) and (53a), respectively) inhibit purine synthesis involving conversion of 5-phosphoribosylpyrophosphate into 5-phosphoribosylamine. In addition they also inhibit chain elongation as diphosphate and triphosphate.

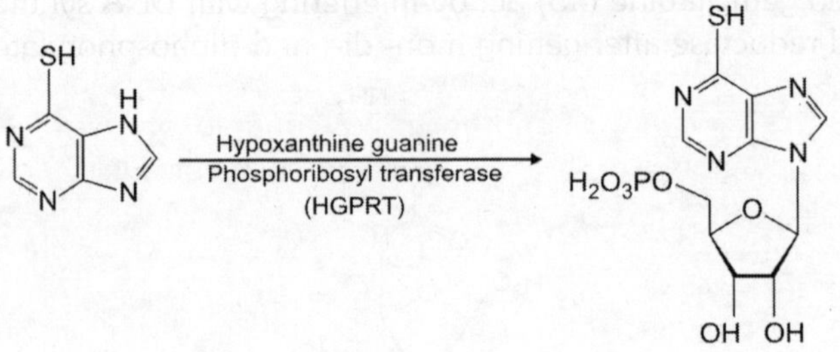

(52)   (52a)

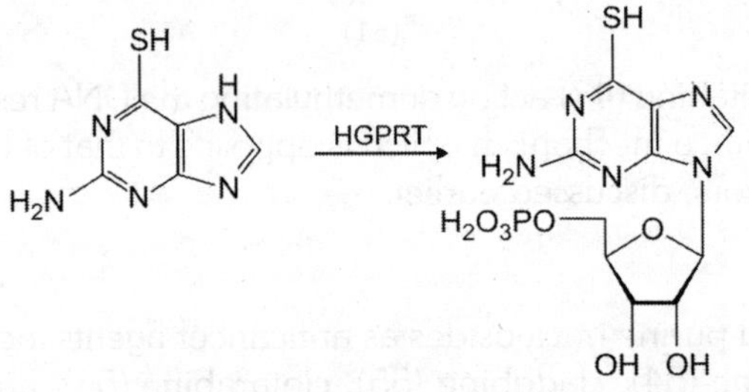

(53)   (53a)

Vidarabine (54), as mono-, di-, and triphosphate acts by inhibiting the early steps in DNA synthesis. It is used as a antiviral agent rather as an anticancer agent.

Cladribine (55), clofarabine (56), and fludarabine (57) get activated first to triphosphate nucleotide and then inhibit DNA polymerase and DNA chain elongation.

ANTIBIOTICS

Number of antibiotics have found clinical use in cancer.

Streptozocin (58), an antibiotic produced by *Streptomyces achromogenes* contains a nitrosourea moiety. It acts by alkylating the DNA chain. It also inhibits the synthesis of amino acids necessary for making proteins in cancer cells.

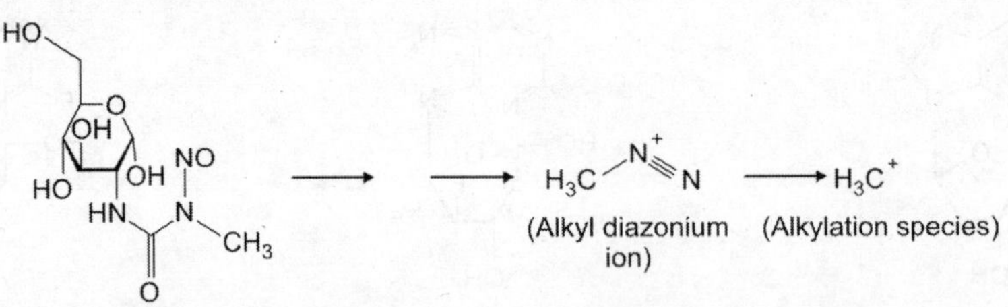

(58)   (Alkyl diazonium   (Alkylation species)
                   ion)

Dactinomycin (59) obtained from fermentation tanks of *Streptomyces parvulus* belongs to actinomycetes group. It intercalates the double helical structure of DNA leading to unwinding of the helical structure resulting in inhibition of nucleic acid synthesis.

Daunorubicin (60) and doxorubicin (61) belong to anthracyclin class of antibiotics. Daunorubicin (60) is obtained from *Steptomyces peucetius* and doxorubicin (61) from *Streptomyces peucetius* var. *caesius*. While daunorubicin (60) has been found to be active against acute leukemias, doxorubicin (61) is a broad-spectrum anticancer antibiotic. It is presently the most widely used anticancer antibiotic. Another anthracycline, idarubicin (62) is 4-demethoxy analog of daunorubicin (60). Idarubicin (62) is less toxic than daunorubicin (60) and doxorubicin (61). The mechanism of their action is similar to dactinomycin (59), i.e. they intercalate the DNA molecule and thus inhibit the nucleic acid synthesis.

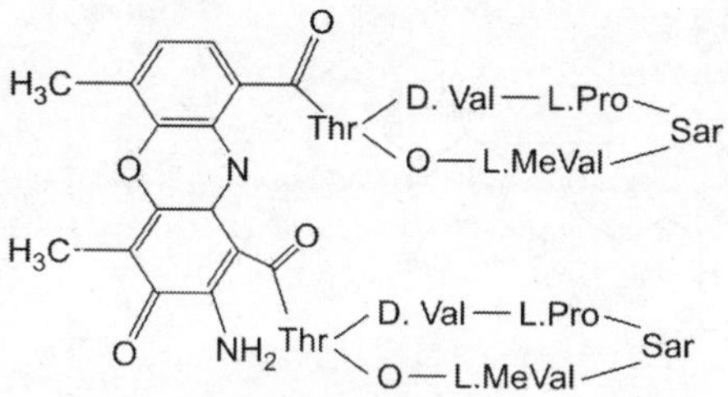

(59)

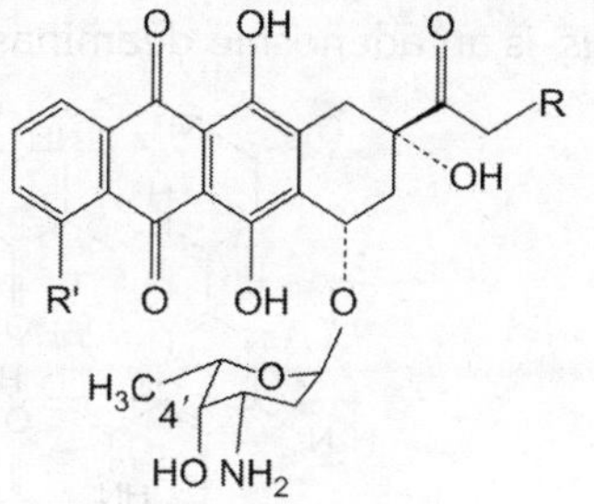

(60), R = H, R' = OCH$_3$
(61), R = OH, R' = OCH$_3$
(62), R = R' = H

Analogs of doxorubicin (61) have been prepared and include its 4'-epimer, epirubicin (63), pirarubicin (64), and valrubicin (65). Some of these are being used in clinical practice.

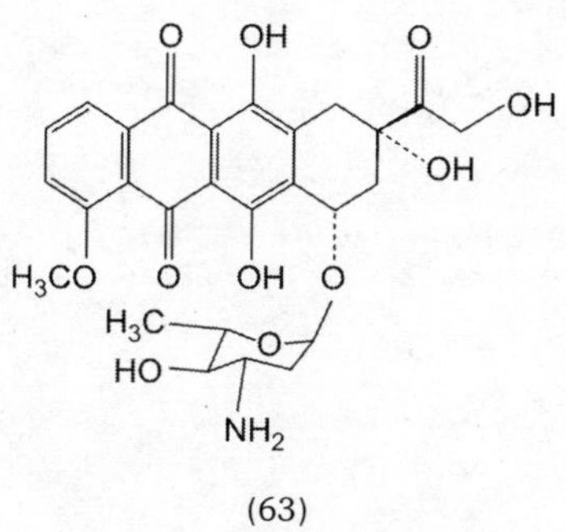

(63)

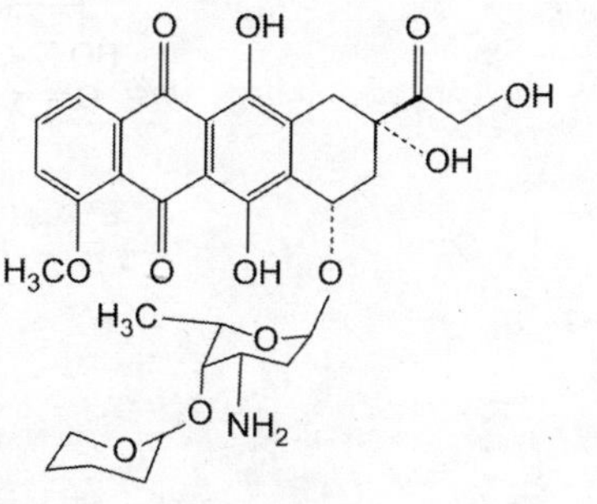

(64)

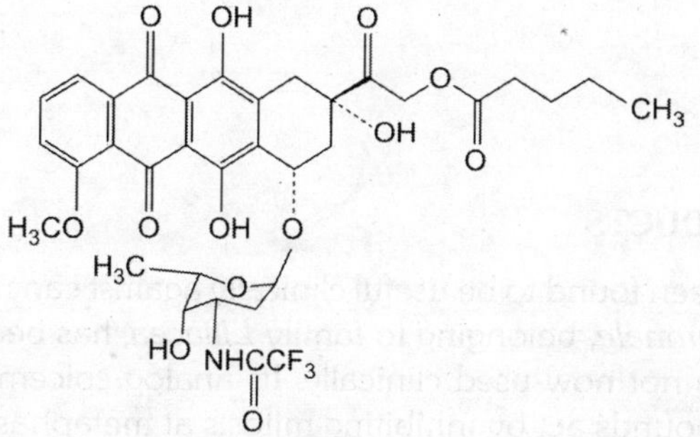

(65)

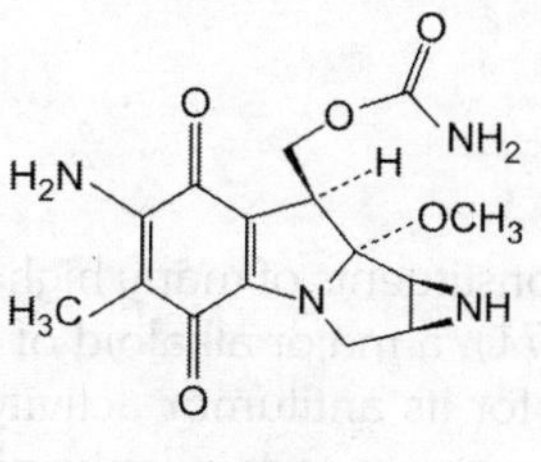

(66)

Mitomycin C (66) is an antibiotic isolated from *Streptomyces caespitosus*. It acts by alkylation. Mitomycin C (66) contains number of functional groups which could be responsible for its action and these include quinone moiety, the aziridine moiety, and the carbamate moiety. It seems all the three functional groups are involved in the alkylation of DNA.

Bleomycin, the derivative of bleomycinic acid (67), is a mixture of bleomycin A_2 (68) and bleomycin B_2 (69). It has been isolated from *Streptomyces verticillus*. Naturally occurring bleomycin contains copper which is removed during processing. The copper free bleomycin is active and it is believed that it acts through chelation of ferrous iron (Fe^{2+}). Pentostatin (70) obtained from *Streptomyces antibioticus*, is an adenosine deaminase inhibitor.

(67), R=OH
(68), R=HN(CH$_2$)$_3$S(CH$_3$)$_2$
(69), R=HN(CH$_2$)$_4$NHCNH$_2$

(70)

PLANT PRODUCTS

The active constituents of many higher plants have been found to be useful clinically against cancer Colchicine (71), a major alkaloid of *Colchicum autumnale*, belonging to family *Liliacea*, has been long known for its antitumor activity. However, it is not now used clinically. Its analog colcemid (72) is active against certain leukemias. These compounds act by inhibiting mitosis at metaphase.

The most important antitumor agents from plants are the vinca alkaloids obtained from *Catharanthus rosa*, family *Apocynacea*. Of the various alkaloids, vincristine (73), vinblastine (74), and the semi-synthetic alkaloid vinorelbine (75) have shown very good activity.

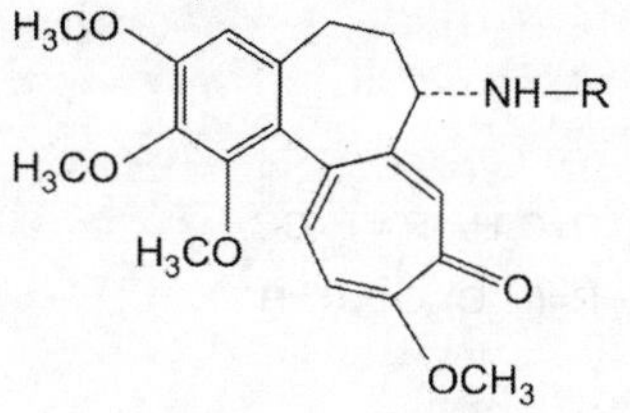

(71), R = $\overset{\overset{O}{\|}}{CCH_3}$;   (72), R = CH_3

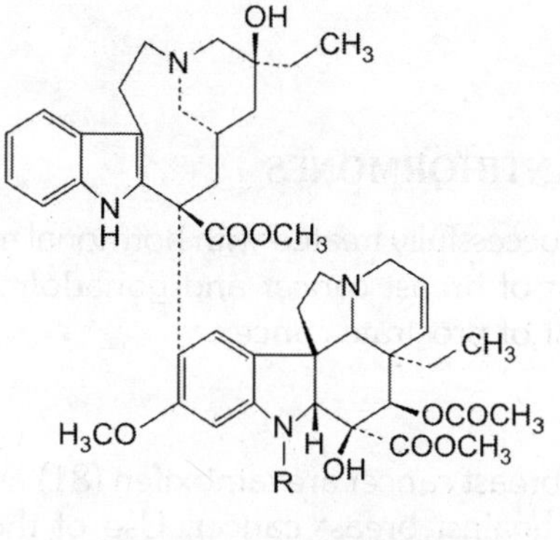

(73), R=CHO
(74), R=CH₃

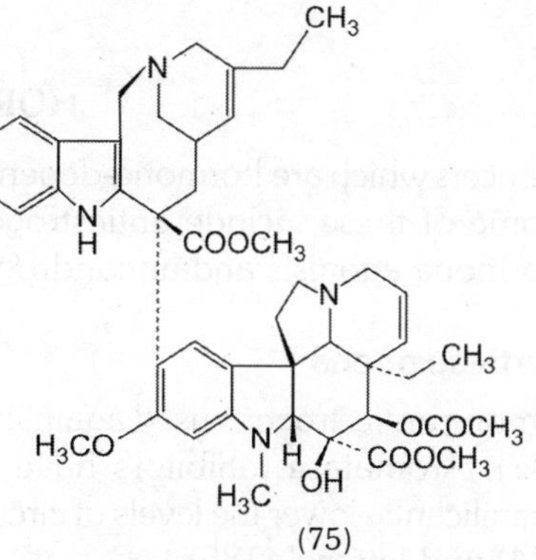

(75)

Vinca alkaloids cause mitotic arrest by promoting dissolution of microtubules in cells. Vinblastine (74) causes inhibition of mitosis. These compounds are used against different types of tumors.

Podophyllotoxin, (76) a constituent of the resin of *Podophyllum peltatum*, family *Berberidaceae*, has shown antineoplastic activity. It acts by destroying the structural organization of mitotic apparatus. It is highly toxic. Analogs such as etoposide (77) and teniposide (78) have been found to be promising.

One of the most important plant product used against cancer is paclitaxel (79) obtained from *Taxus brevifolia*, family *Taxaceae*. Paclitaxel (79) acts as a spindle poison and thereby inhibits mitosis. However, unlike vinca alkaloids it does not cause depolymerization. Docetaxel (80), another taxoid, is used against metastatic breast cancer and nonsmall cell lung cancer.

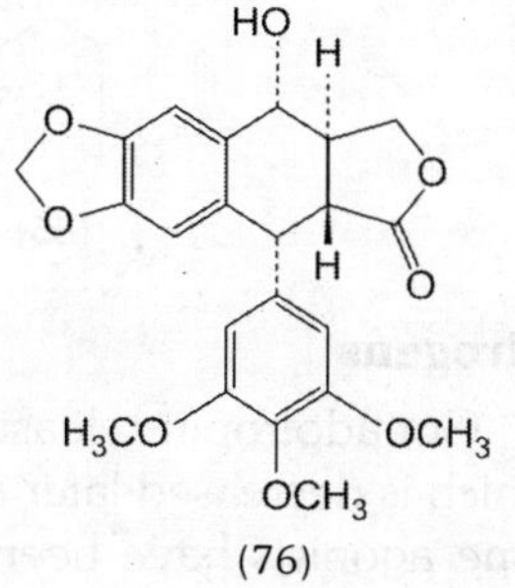

(76)

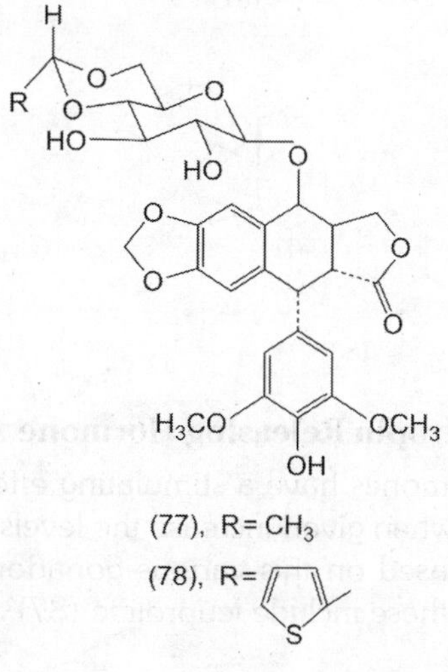

(77), R= CH₃

(78), R=

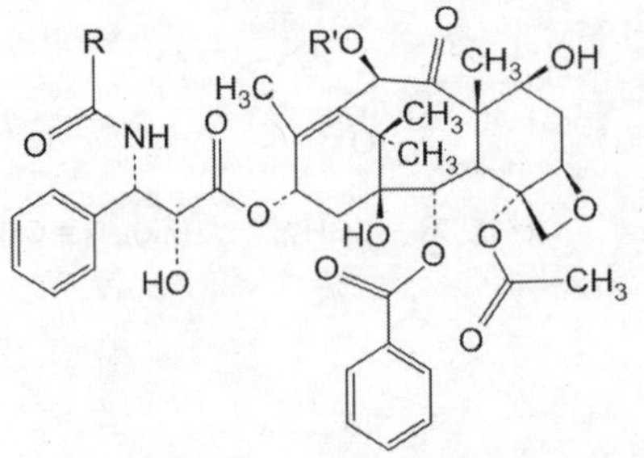

(79), R=C₆H₅; R'= H₃CC
(79), $R=C_6H_5$; $R'=H_3C\overset{O}{\overset{\|}{C}}$
(80), $R=(H_3C)_3CO$; $R'=H$

HORMONES AND ANTIHORMONES

Cancers which are hormone-dependent have been successfully treated with hormonal manipulations. Some of these include antiestrogens for treatment of breast cancer and gonadotropin releasing hormone agonists and antiandrogens for treatment of prostrate cancer.

Antiestrogens

Among antiestrogens used against estrogen related breast cancer are tamoxifen (81) and toremifene (82). Aromatase inhibitors have also been used against breast cancer. Use of these inhibitors siginifically lower the levels of circulating estradiol (83). Two of these compounds include anastrozole (84) and letrozole (85).

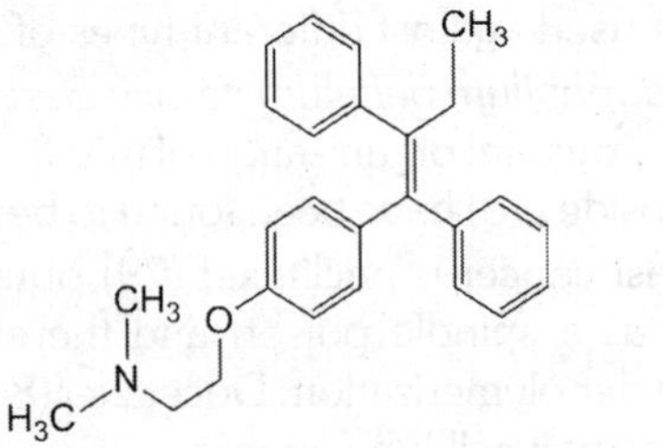

(81)

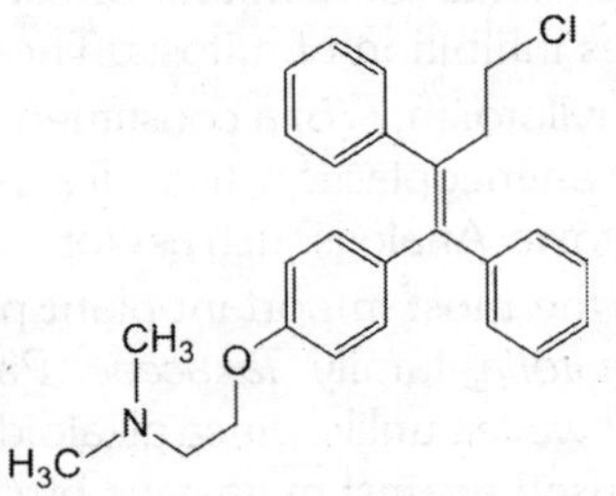

(82)

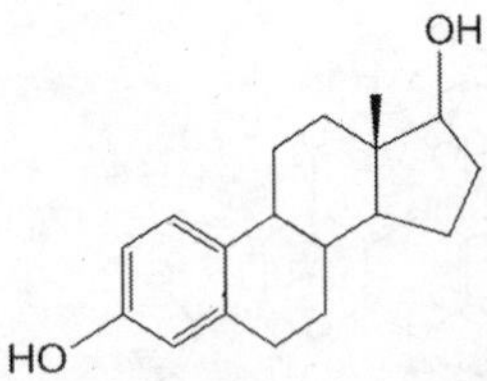

(83)

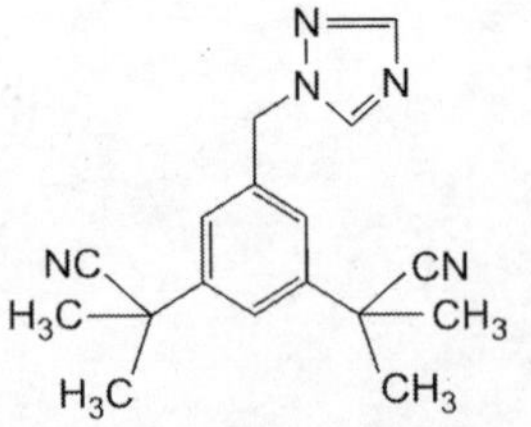

(84)

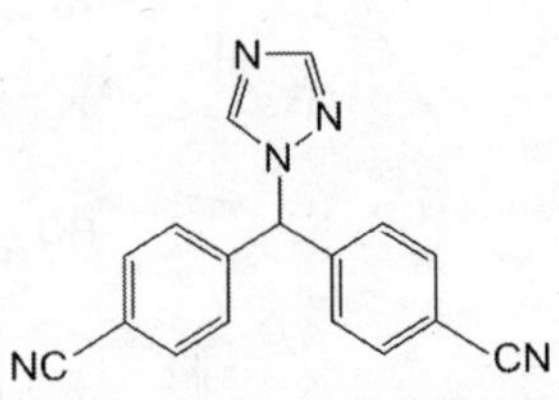

(85)

Gonadotropin Releasing Hormone Agonists and Antiandrogens

Male hormones have a stimulating effect on prostate cancers. Gonadotropin releasing hormone agonists when given increase the levels of testosterone (86) which is decreased later after about 4 weeks. Based on this various gonadotropin releasing hormone agonists have been developed. Some of these include leuprolide (87) and goserelin (88).

(86)

5-oxoPro-His-Trp-Ser-Tyr-D-Leu-Leu-Arg-Pro-NHC$_2$H$_5$

(87)

5-oxoPro-His-Trp-Ser-Tyr-D-Ser(*t*-Bu)-Leu-Arg-Pro-NHNHCONH$_2$

(88)

Another approach to the treatment of prostate cancer is use of antiandrogens. Some of these include flutamide (89), bicalutamide (90), and nilutamide (91). All of these are non-steroidal. They act by inhibiting androgen receptor translocation to the nucleus in the target tissue. Prostate cancer has also been treated with gonadotropin releasing hormone antagonists. One of such antagonist is abarelix, a peptide. It bears some resemblance to gonadotropin releasing hormone.

(89)   (90)   (91)

INHIBITORS OF PROTEIN KINASES

Protein kinases are involved in normal signaling pathways. They interact with extracellular ligands such as growth factors and hormones and then transmit signals across the cell membrane to the cytoplasm and nucleus. The signal transduction mediated by protein kinases involve phosphorylation of hydroxyl groups of serine, tyrosine, and/or threonine residues of protein substrate through transfer of phosphoryl group of ATP by protein kinase in presence of Mg^{++}. The protein phosphatase removes the phosphate group from the phosphoprotein. Two types of protein kinases are known and these include protein tyrosine kinases (PTKs) and serine/threonine kinases (STKs).

Protein tyrosine kinases have been further subdivided into receptor tyrosine kinases (RTKs) and non-receptor tyrosine kinases (NRTKs). Receptor tyrosine kinases (RTKs) also known as growth factor receptor kinases are transmembrane cell surface proteins. The extracellular domain of receptor tyrosine kinases (RTKs) act as receptor for a particular hormone/growth factor and the intracellular domain functions as kinase. The receptor tyrosine kinases (RTKs) get activated by binding of hormone/growth factor to the receptor in the extracellular domain, leading to oligomerization and phosphorylation/activation of intracellular domain. The activated intracellular domain then activates the downstream signalling protein, the non-receptor tyrosine kinases (NRTKs).

Receptor tyrosine kinases (RTKs) include receptors of insulin (IRK), growth factors such as epidermal growth factor (EGF), basic fibroblast growth factor (bFGF), and nervegrowth factor (NGF).

The non-receptor tyrosine kinases (NRTKs) include members of Src family, Fak, Jak, Abl, and Zap 70.

Overexpression and enhanced protein kinase activity can lead to carcinogenesis and many human cancers. As a result of these studies, inhibitors of protein kinases have been developed and these include imatinib (92), dasatinib (93), erlotinib (94), gefitinib (95), lapatinib (96), sorafenib (97), and sunitinib (98). Most of these are used in combination with other drugs.

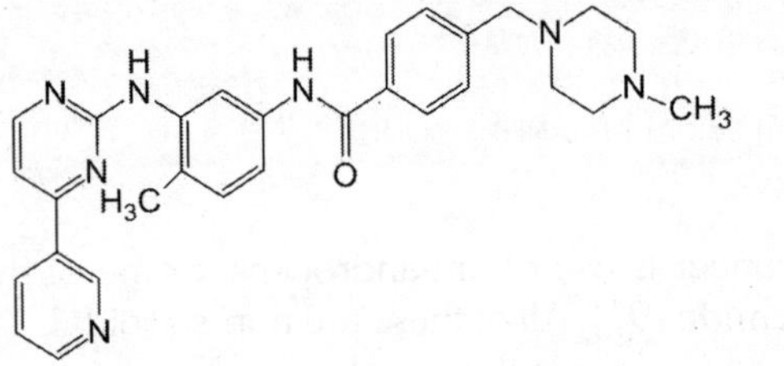

(92)

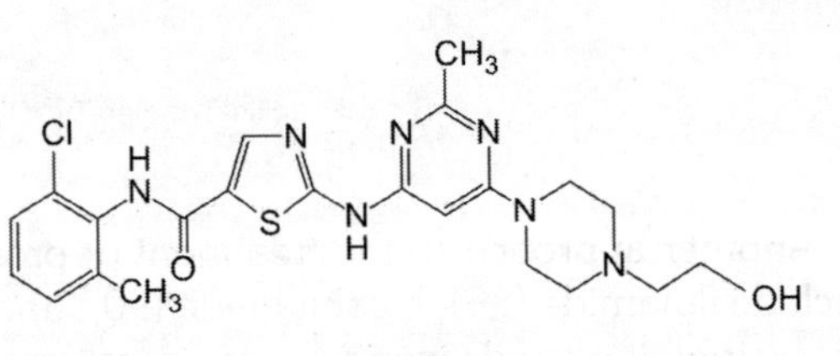

(93)

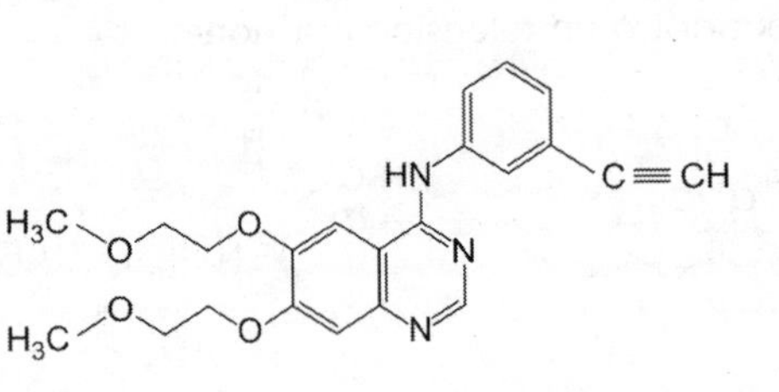

(94)

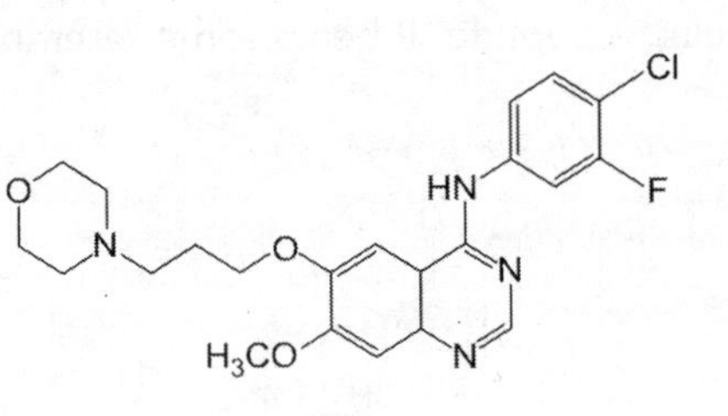

(95)

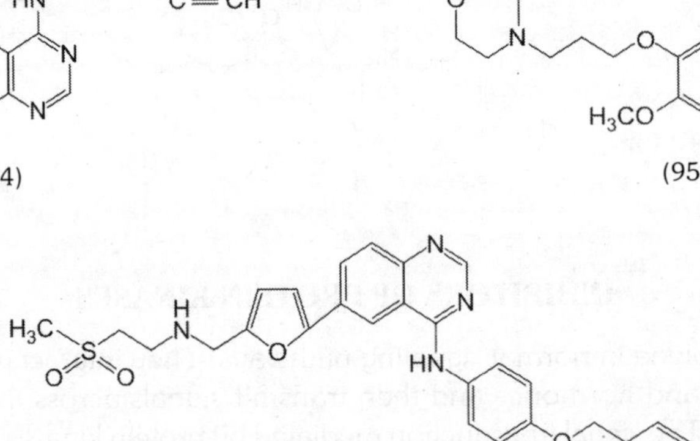

(96)

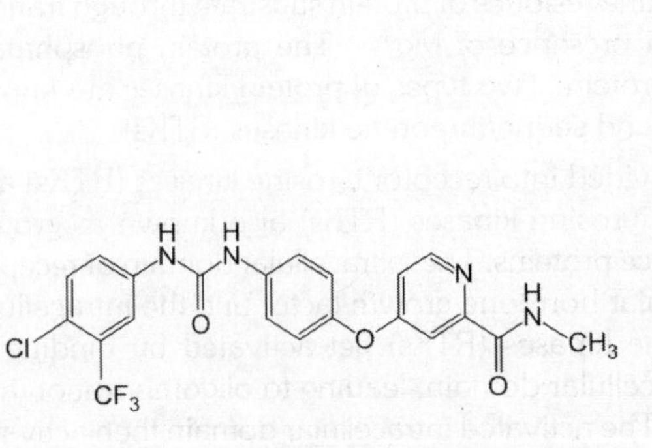

(97)

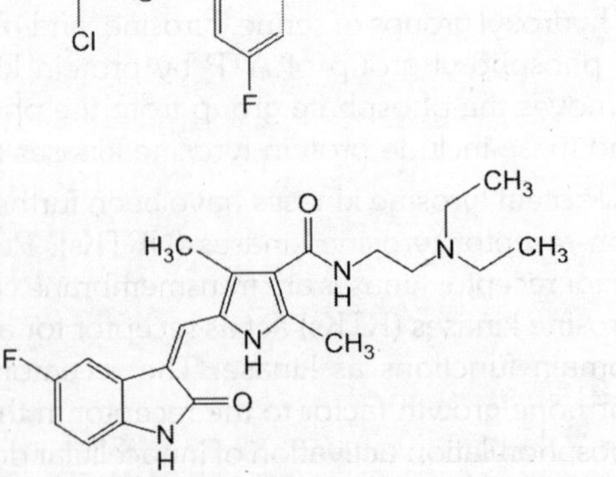

(98)

MISCELLANEOUS COMPOUNDS

This constitutes a group of compounds with different types of structures. Ribonucleotide diphosphate reductase, required for the DNA synthesis, is inhibited by hydroxyurea (99) through chelation of its cofactor Fe^{2+}. Mitotane (100) is used in adrenal cortex carcinoma. Its half-life is 18–159 days suggesting that most of the drug is stored in tissues.

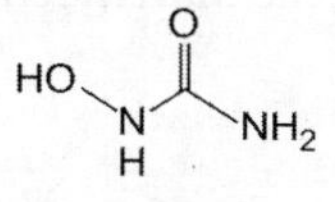

(99) 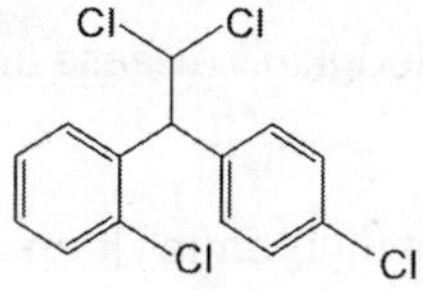   (100)

Tretinoin (101) is all *trans*-retinoic acid and a normal metabolite of vitamin A_1 (102). It is used against leukemia. Alitretinoin (103), a 9-*cis*-retinoic acid analog inhibits Kaposi sarcoma cells. It acts by activating retinoid receptors which express genes that are responsible for cell growth differentiation and apoptosis.

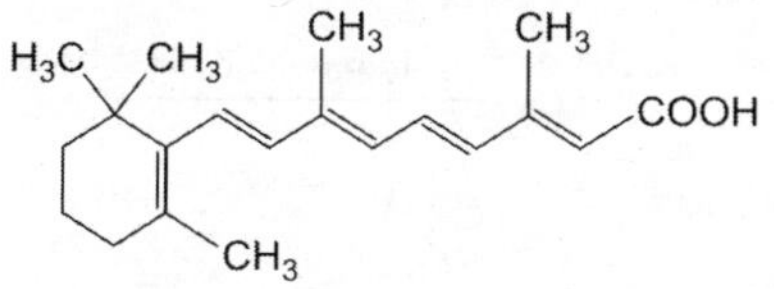

(101) 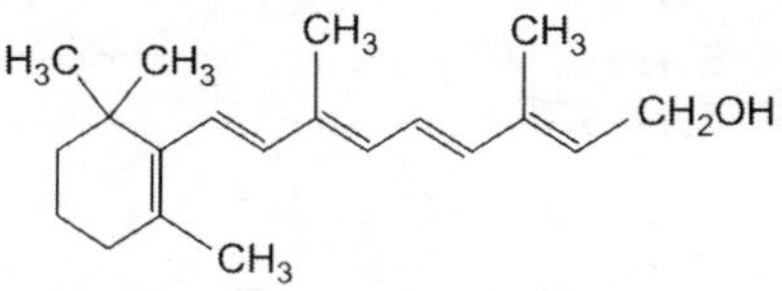   (102) 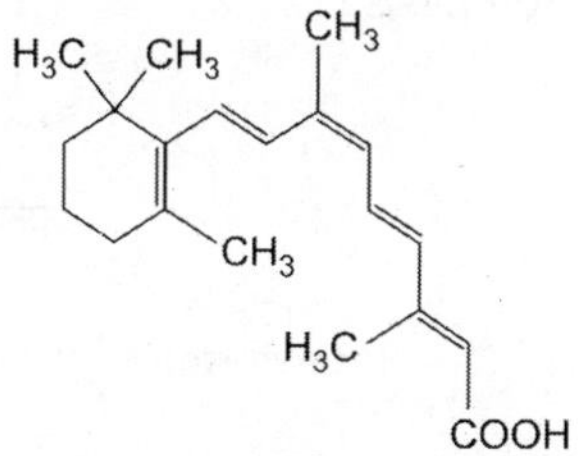   (103)

INDIVIDUAL COMPOUNDS

ALKYLATING AGENTS : NITROGEN MUSTARDS

Mechlorethamine

N-Methyl-2,2'-dichlorodiethylamine

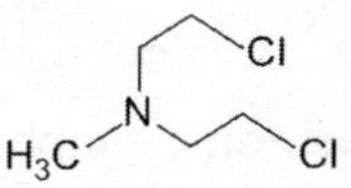

Synthesis

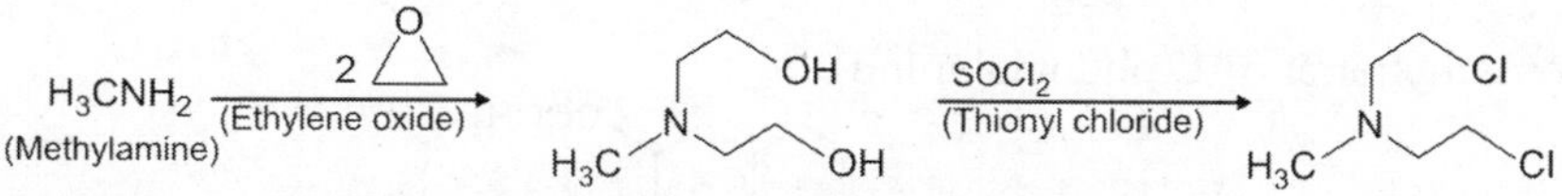

It is effective against Hodgkin's disease. Toxic effects include depression of bone marrow.

Novembichin

2-Chloro-*N*,*N*-bis(2-chloroethyl)prpanamine

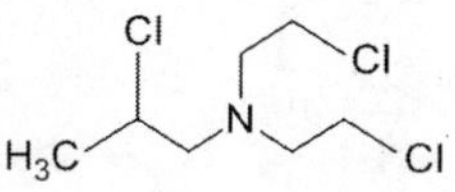

Synthesis

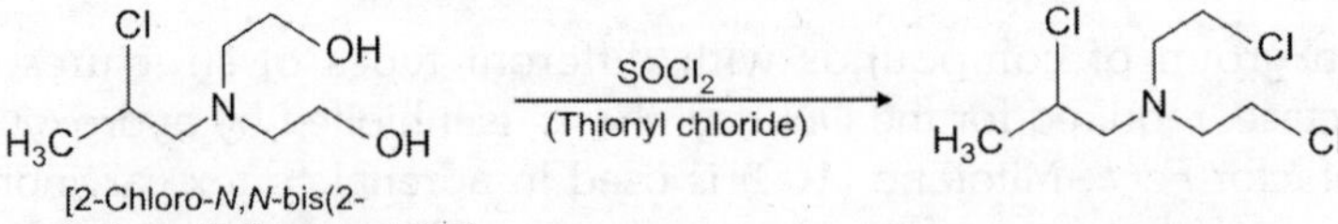

[2-Chloro-*N*,*N*-bis(2-hydroxyethyl) propanamine]

It is used in Hodgkin's disease and in certain leukemias. It is less toxic than mechlorethamine (9).

Chlorambucil

4-[Bis (2-chloroethyl) amino]benzenebutanoic acid

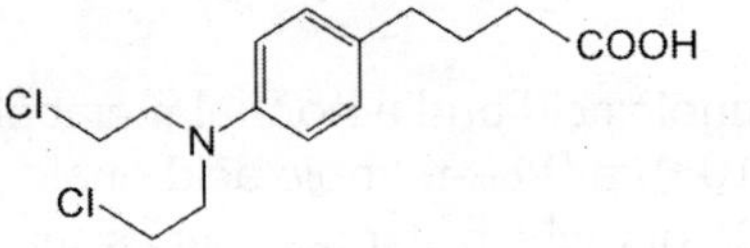

Synthesis

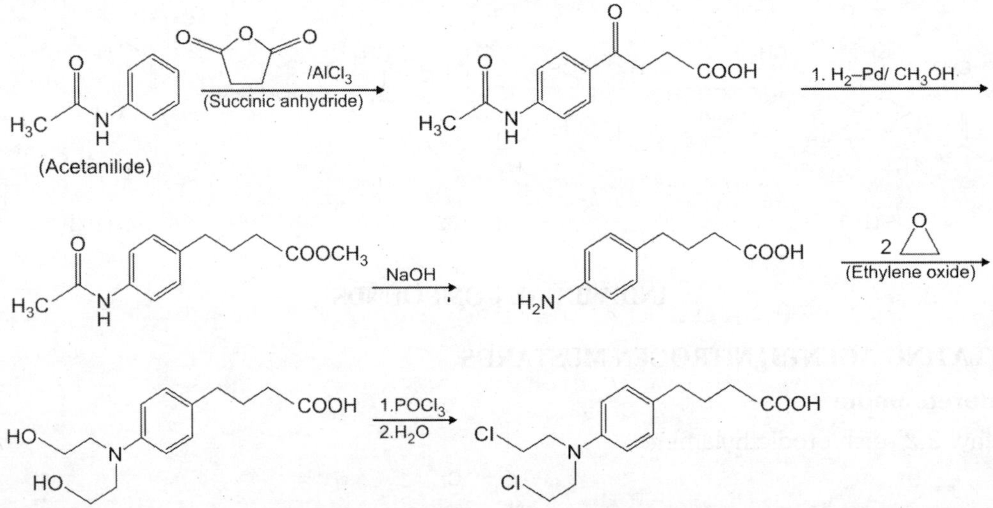

It is adminstered orally and is used for chronic lymphatic anemia and for multiple myelomas.

Melphalan

4-[Bis (2-chloroethyl)amino]-L-phenylalanine

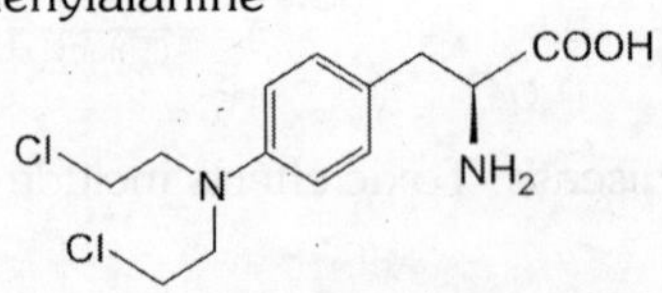

Synthesis

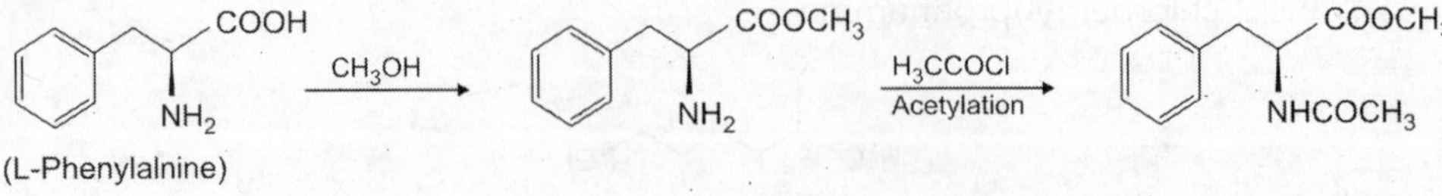

(L-Phenylalnine)

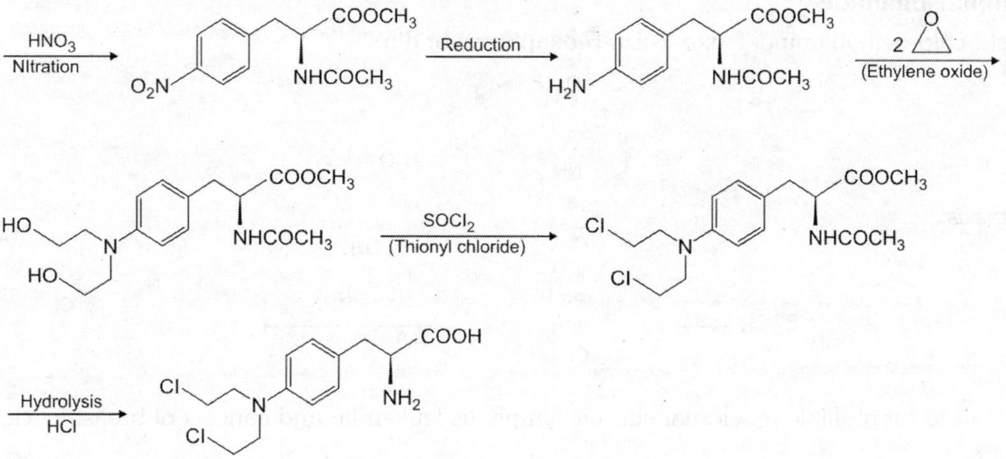

It is used both intravenously as well as orally for the treatment of multiple myeloma, cancers of breast, neck, and ovaries.

Estramustine

Estradiol 3-bis(2-chloroethyl)carbamate

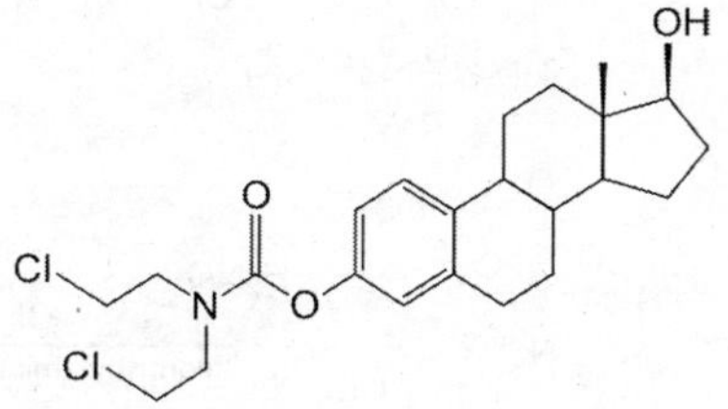

Synthesis

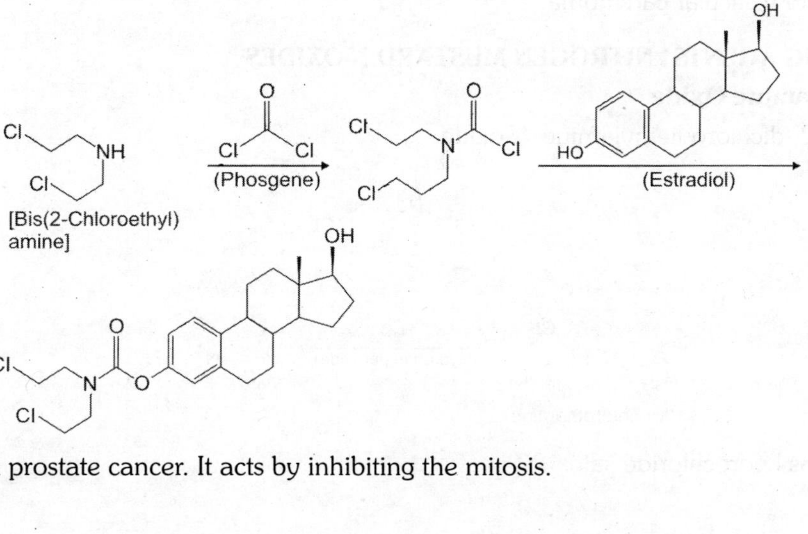

It is used in prostate cancer. It acts by inhibiting the mitosis.

Cyclophosphamide

1-Bis(2-chloroethyl)amino-1-oxo-2-aza-5-oxaphosphoridin

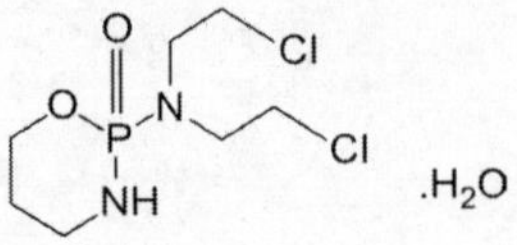

Synthesis

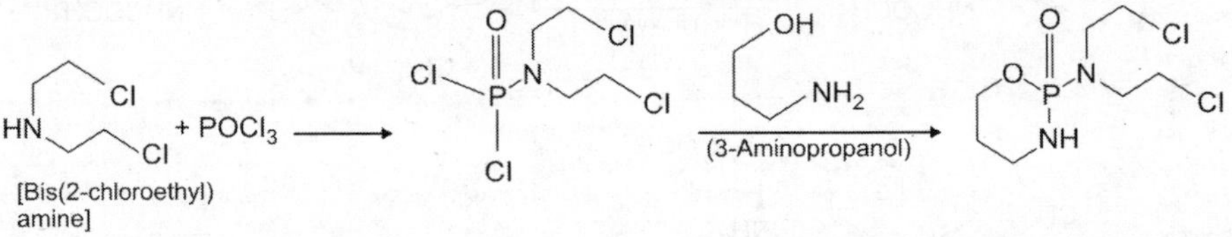

[Bis(2-chloroethyl)
amine]

It is used for multiple myeloma, chronic lymphatic leukemia, and cancers of breast, neck, and ovaries.

Ifosfamide

3-(2-Chloroethyl)-2-[(2-chloroethyl)amino]tetrahydro-2H-1,3,2-oxazaphosphorin-2-oxide

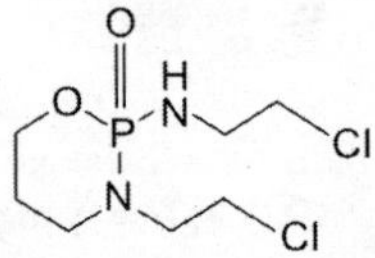

Synthesis

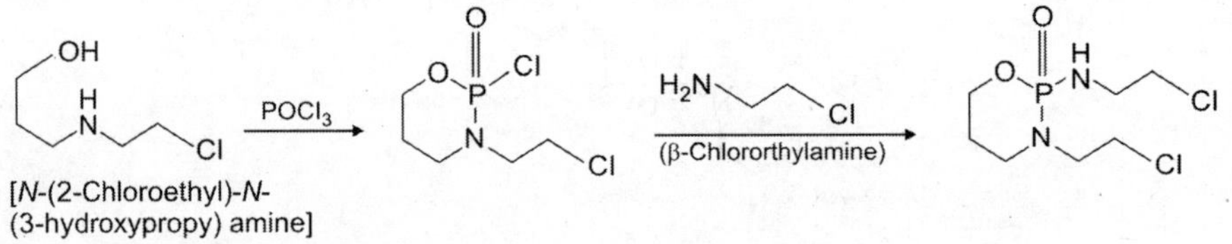

[N-(2-Chloroethyl)-N-
(3-hydroxypropy) amine]

It is used for testicular carcinoma.

ALKYLATING AGENTS : NITROGEN MUSTARD N-OXIDES

Mechlorethamine Oxide

N-Methyl-2-2'-dichlorodiethylamine N-oxide

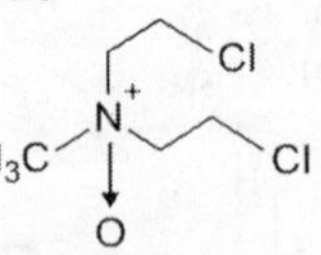

Synthesis

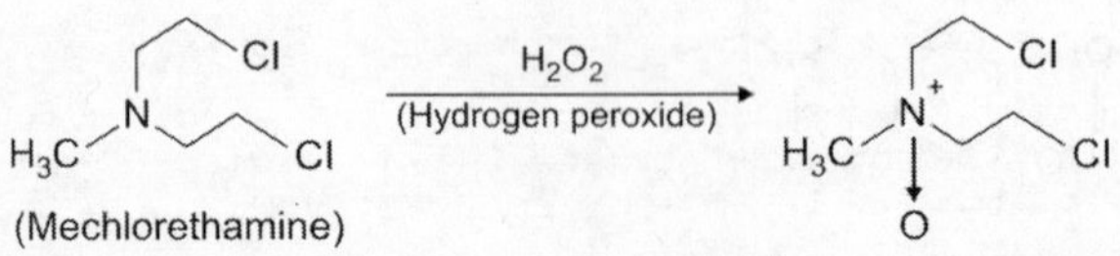

(Mechlorethamine)

It is used as hydrochloride salt.

ALKYLATING AGENTS : ETHYLENIMINES
Thiotepa
Tris(1-aziridinyl)phosphine sulphide

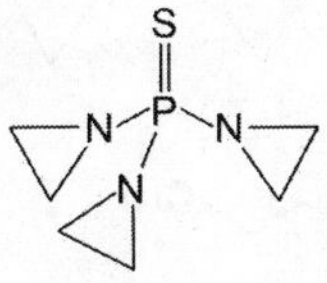

Synthesis

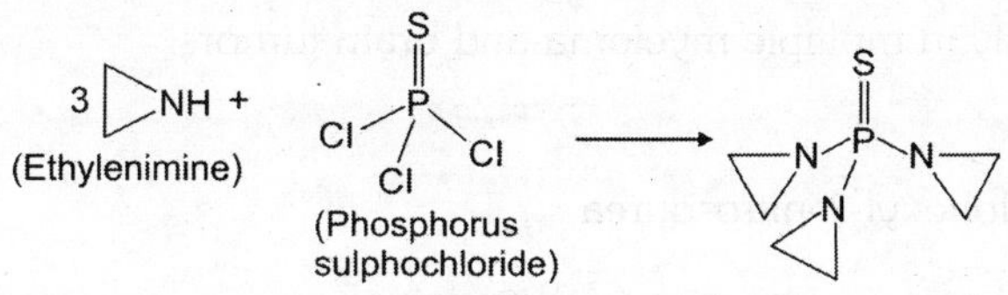

It is used against a wide variety of tumors. It has been particularly useful in breast, ovarian, bronchogenic carcinoma, and malignant lymphomas. It is highly toxic to bone marrow.

ALKYLATING AGENT : METHANESULPHONATES
Busulfan
1, 4-Butanediol dimethanesulphonate ester

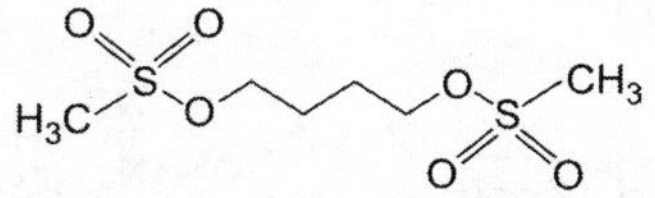

Synthesis

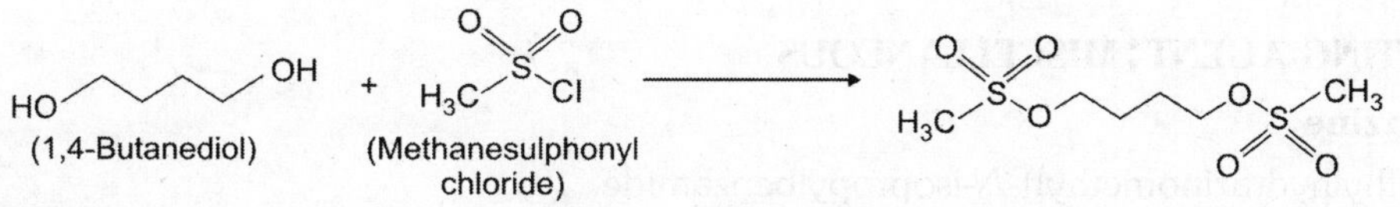

It is a bifunctional alkylating agent. It alkylates N^7 of guanine, thiol groups of glutathione, and cysteine. It is used in chronic granulocytic leukemia.

ALKYLATING AGENT : NITROSOUREAS
Carmustine
N,N-Bis(2-chloroethyl)-*N*-nitrosourea

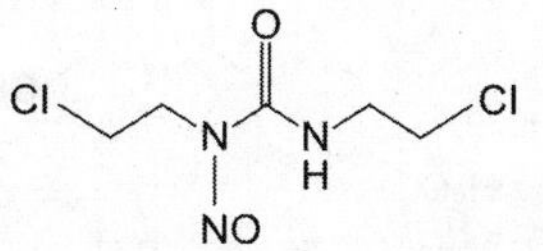

Synthesis

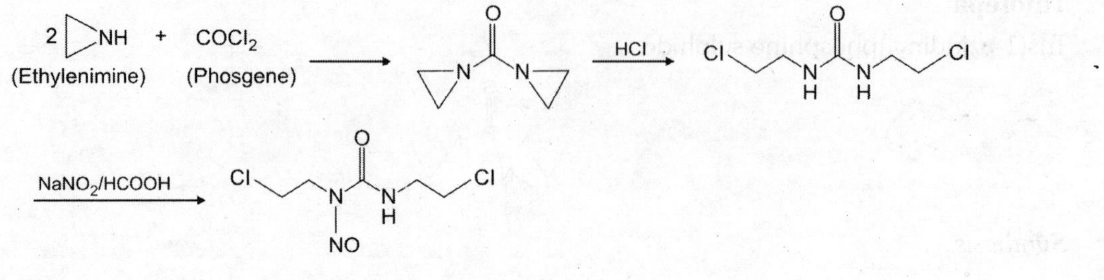

It is used intravenously in multiple myeloma and brain tumors.

Lomustine

1-(2-Chloroethyl)-3-cyclohexyl-1-nitrosourea

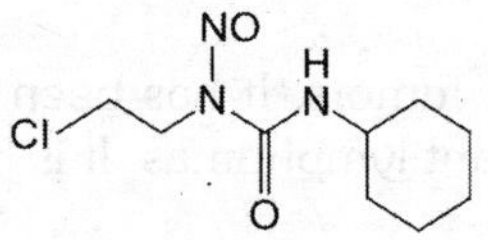

Synthesis

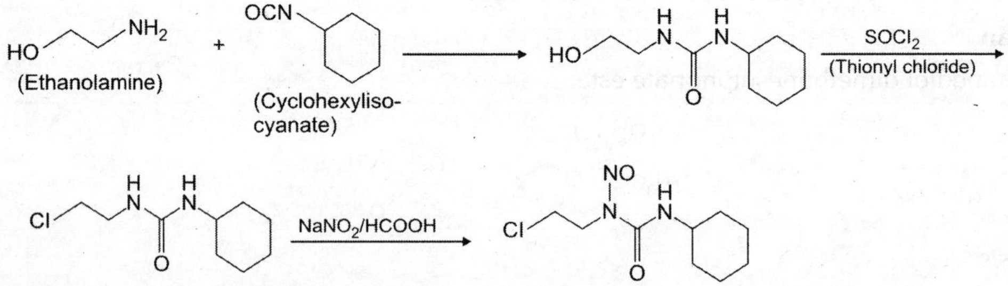

ALKYLATING AGENT : MISCELLANEOUS

Procarbazine

p-(N^1-Methylhydrazinomethyl)-*N*-isopropylbenzamide

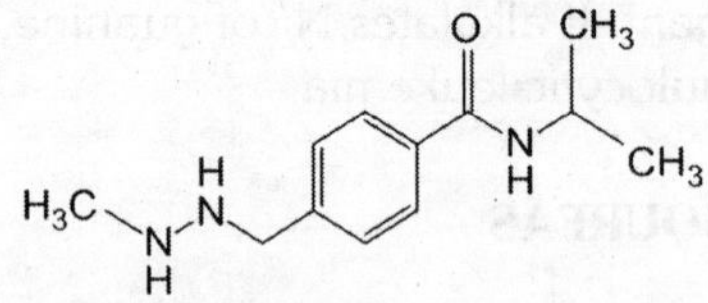

Synthesis

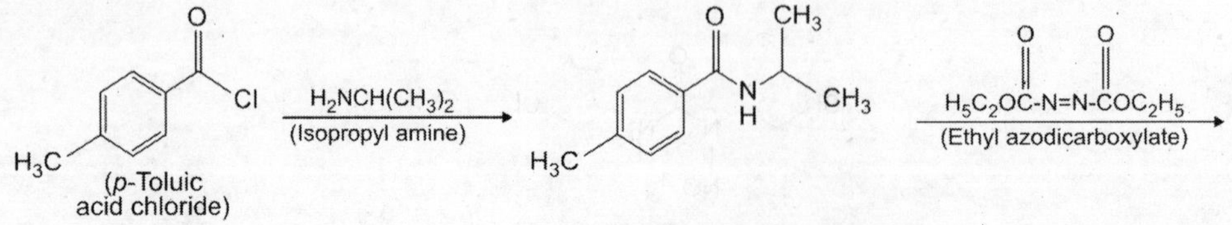

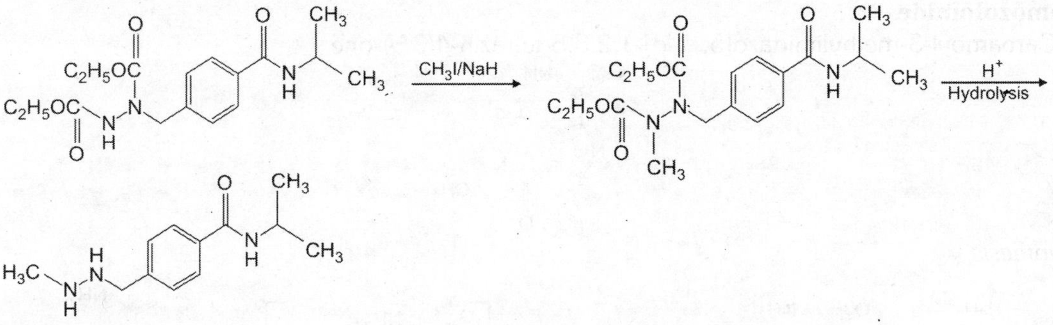

Procarbazine is used for the treatment of Hodgkin's disease and brain cancer.

Dacarbazine

5-(3,3-Dimethyl-1-triazenyl)-1H-imidazole-4-carboxamide

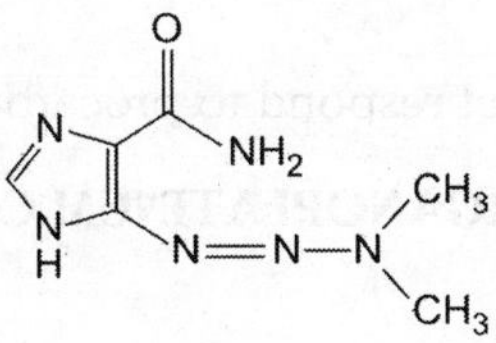

Synthesis

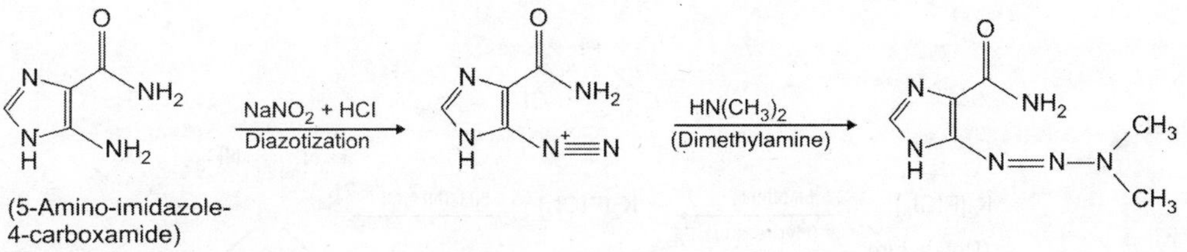

(5-Amino-imidazole-4-carboxamide)

It is indicated in metastatic malignant melanoma. Some of the side effects observed include anorexia, nausea and vomiting.

Altretamine

2,4,6-Tris(dimethylamino)-s-triazine

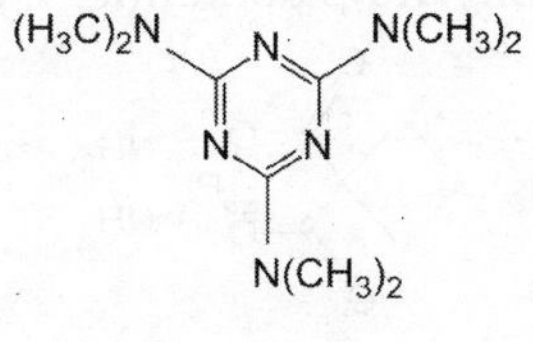

Synthesis

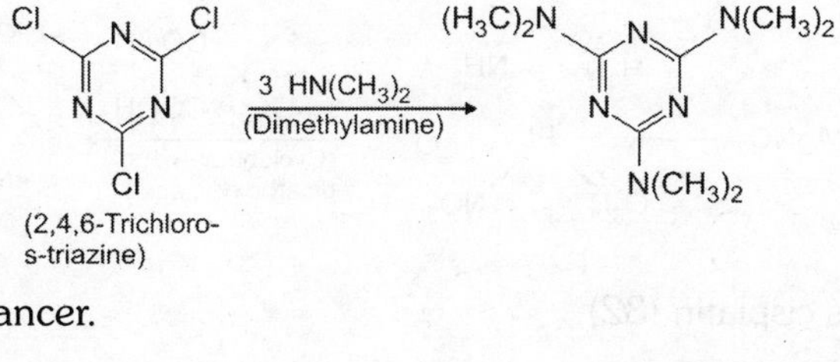

(2,4,6-Trichloro-s-triazine)

It is used in ovarian cancer.

Temozolomide

8-Carbamoyl-3-methylimidazo[5, 1-d]-1,2,3,5-tetrazin-4(3H)-one

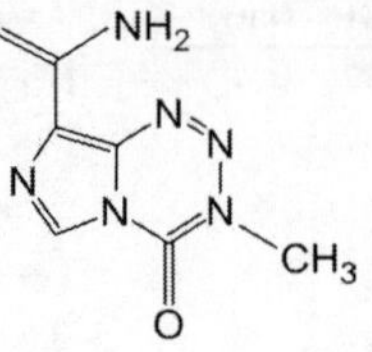

Synthesis

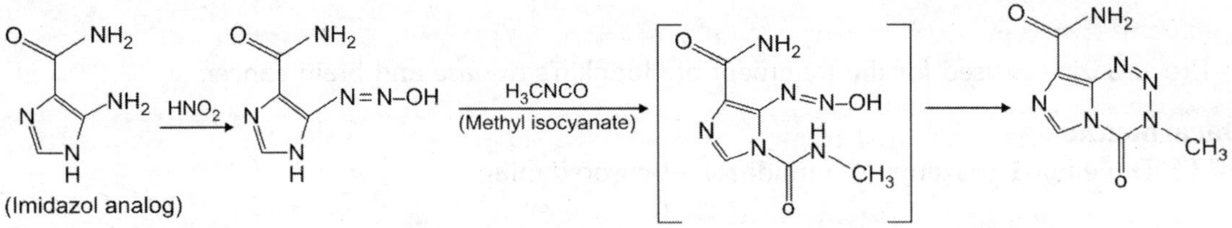

It is used for the patients who do not respond to procarbazine (28) or nitrosoureas.

DNA CROSS-LINKING AGENTS : ORGANOPLATINUM COMPLEXES

Cisplatin

cis-Diamminedichloroplatinum

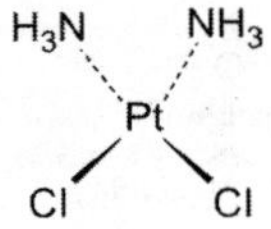

Synthesis

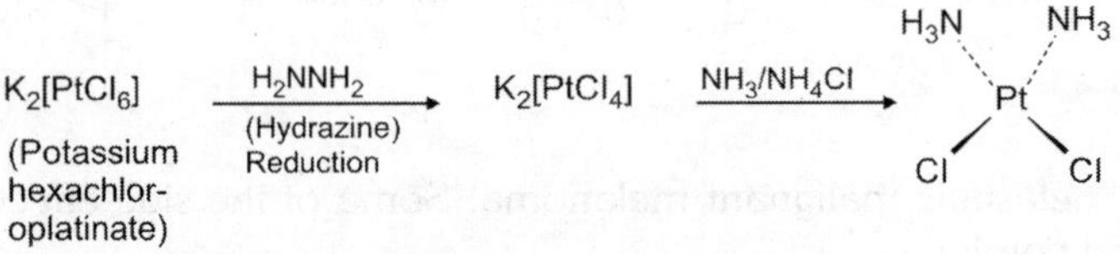

It is used in case of cancinomas of testicles, ovaries, spleen, etc.

Carboplatin

cis-Diammine(1,1-cyclobutanedicarboxylato)platinum(II)

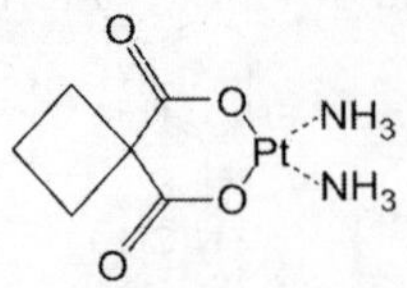

Synthesis

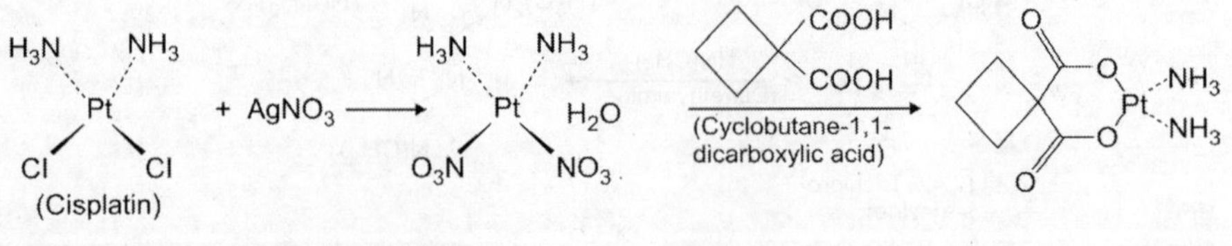

It has similar activity as cisplatin (32).

ANTIMETABOLITES : FOLIC ACD ANALOGS

Methotrexate

N-[4-[[(2,4-Diamino-6-pteridinyl)methyl]methylamino]benzoyl]-L-glutamic acid

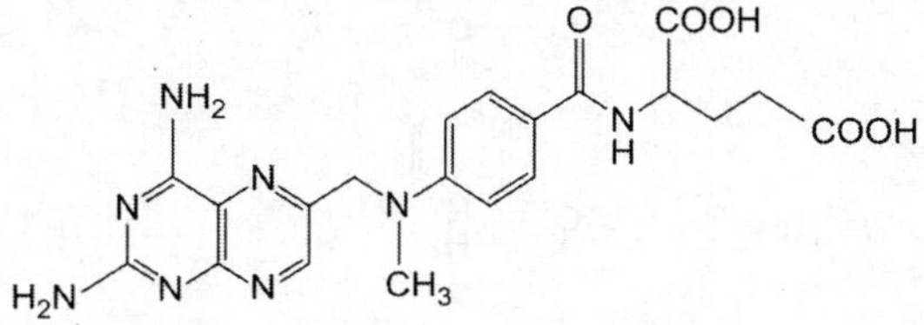

Synthesis

Step 1

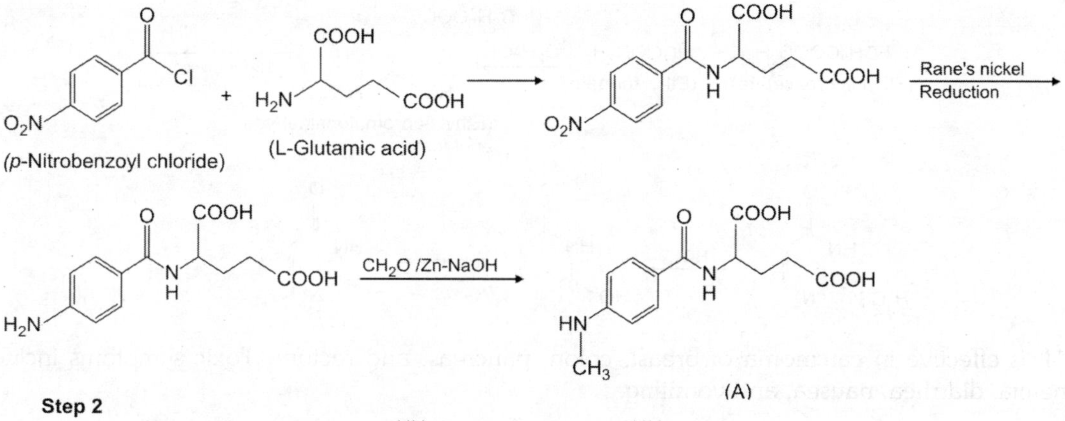
(p-Nitrobenzoyl chloride)
(L-Glutamic acid)
Rane's nickel
Reduction
CH2O /Zn-NaOH
(A)

Step 2

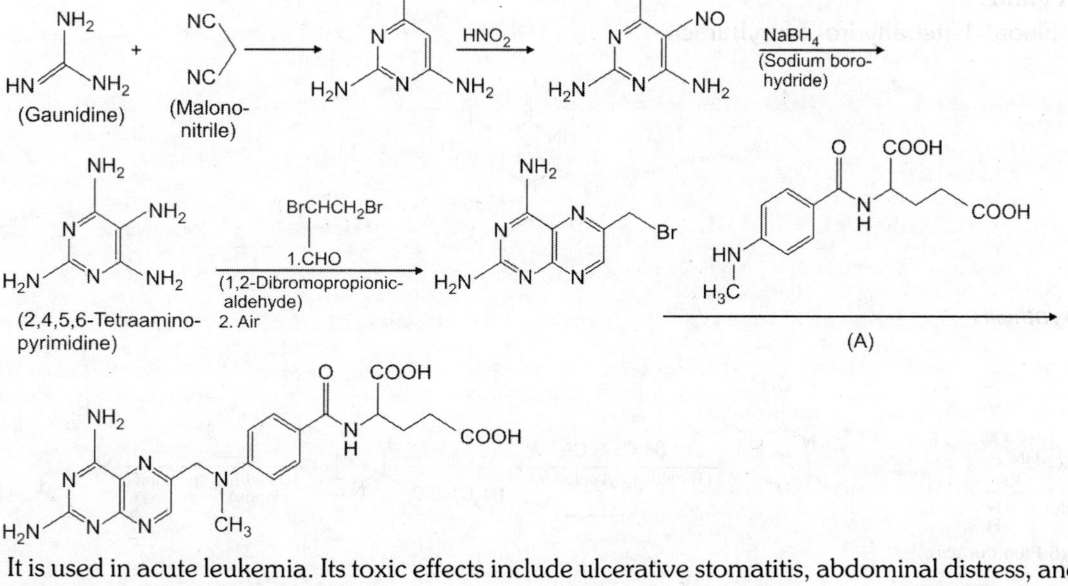
(Gaunidine)
(Malono-
nitrile)
HNO2
NaBH4
(Sodium boro-
hydride)
BrCHCH2Br
1.CHO
(1,2-Dibromopropionic-
aldehyde)
2. Air
(2,4,5,6-Tetraamino-
pyrimidine)
(A)

It is used in acute leukemia. Its toxic effects include ulcerative stomatitis, abdominal distress, and decrease of leukocytes (leukopenia).

ANTIMETABOLITES : PYRIMIDINE ANALOGS

Fluorouracil

2,4-Dioxo-5-fluoropyrimidine

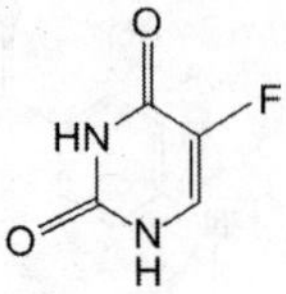

Synthesis

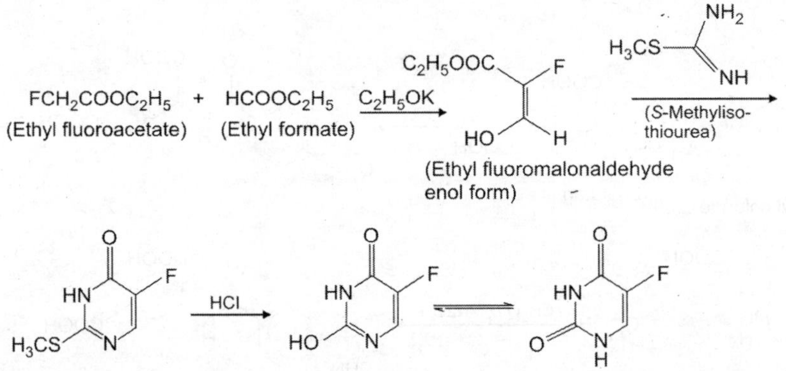

It is effective in carcinoma of breast, colon, pancreas, and rectum. Toxic symptoms include anemia, diarrhea, nausea, and vomiting.

Tegafur

5-Fluoro-1-(tetrahydro-2-furyl)uracil

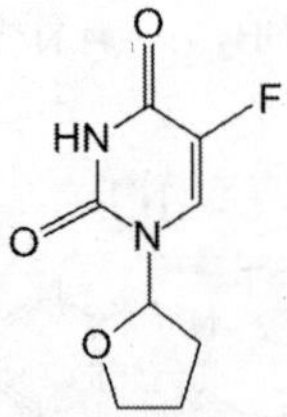

Synthesis

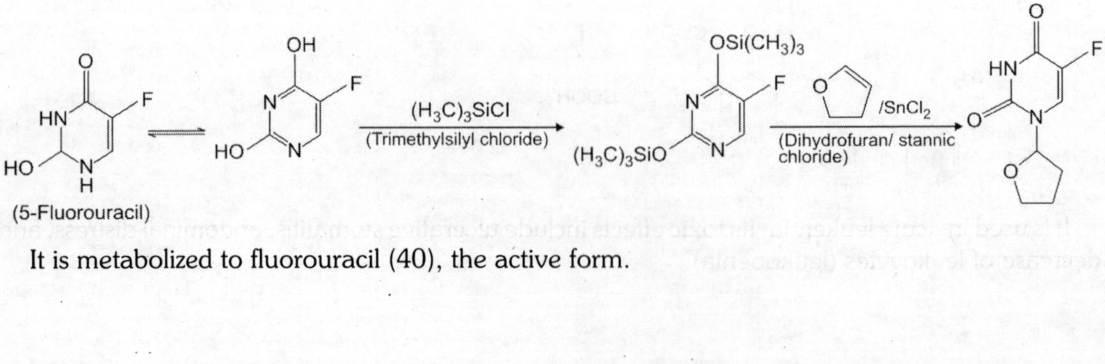

It is metabolized to fluorouracil (40), the active form.

Floxuridine

2'-Deoxy-5-fluorouridine

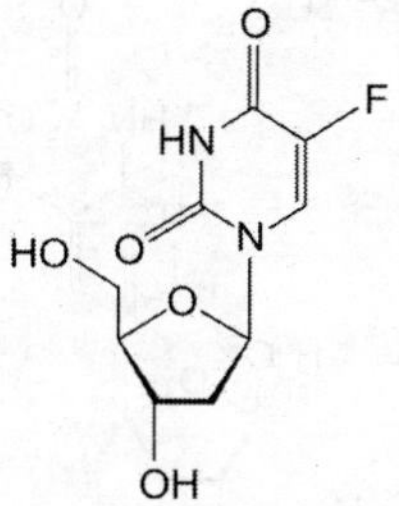

Synthesis

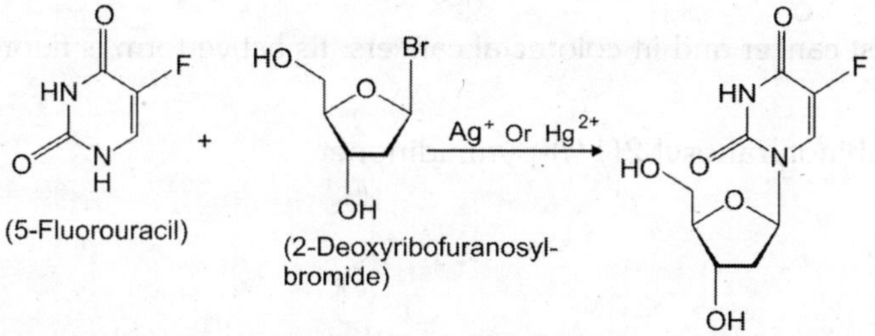
(5-Fluorouracil)
(2-Deoxyribofuranosyl-bromide)
Ag+ Or Hg2+

It is used for the liver cancer.

Capecitabine

5'-Deoxy-5-fluoro-*N*-[(pentyloxy)carbonyl]cytidine

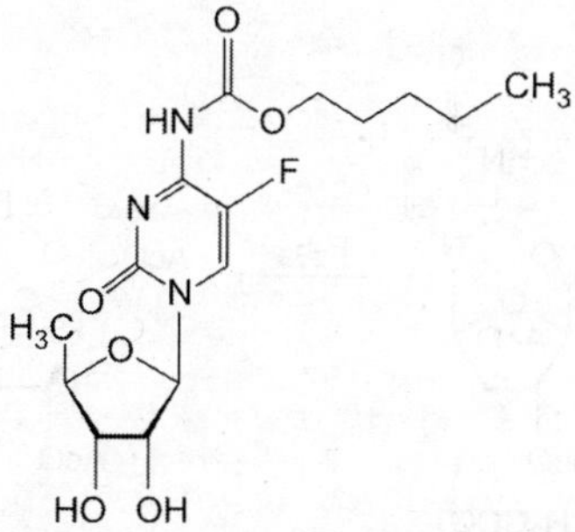

Synthesis

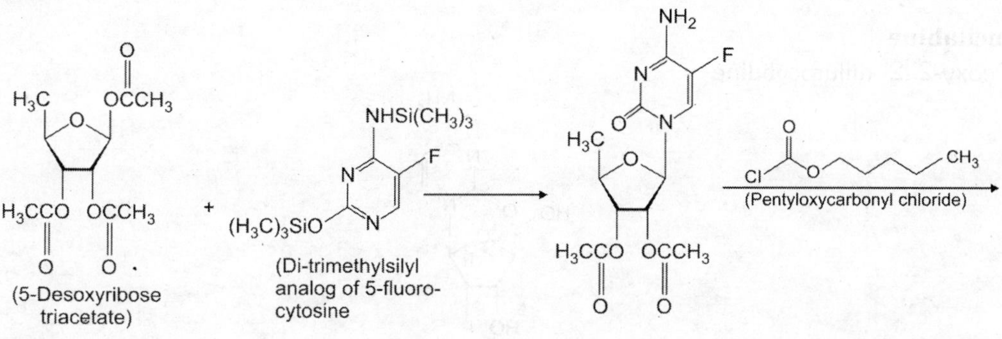
(5-Desoxyribose triacetate)
(Di-trimethylsilyl analog of 5-fluoro-cytosine)
(Pentyloxycarbonyl chloride)

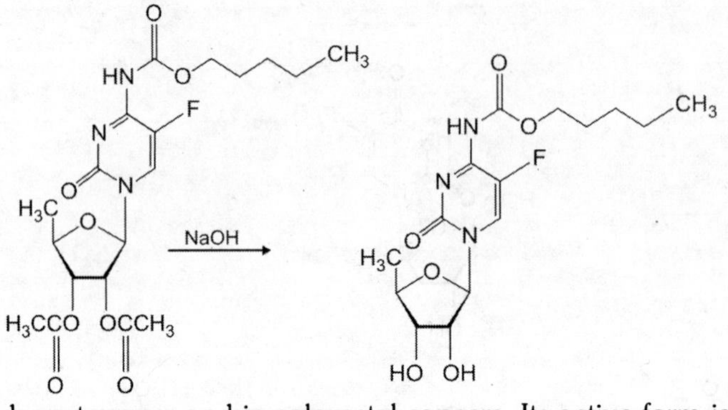

It is used in breast cancer and in colorectal cancers. Its active form is fluorouracil (40).

Cytarabine

4-Amino-1-β-D-arabinofuranosyl-2(1*H*)-pyrimidinone

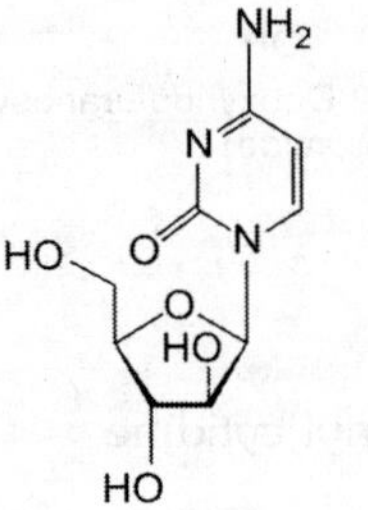

Synthesis

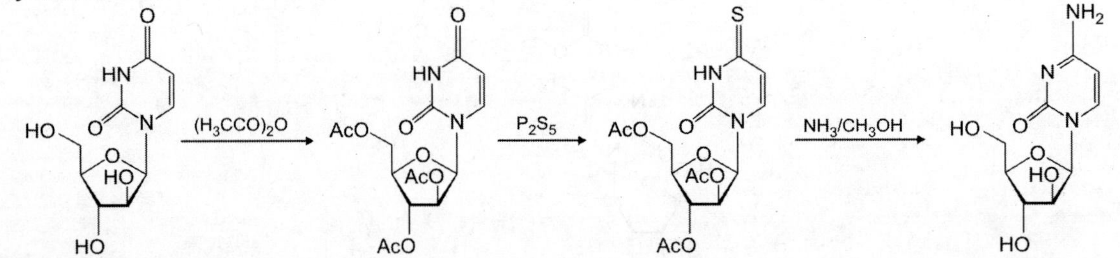

(1-β-D-Arabinofuranosyluracil)   (Ac = H₃CCO)

It is effective against leukemia.

Gemcitabine

2'-Deoxy-2',2'-diflurocytidine

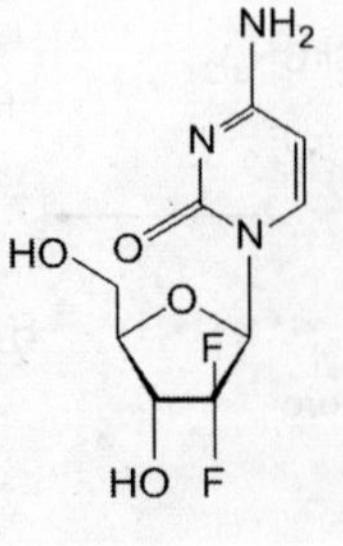

Synthesis

Step 1

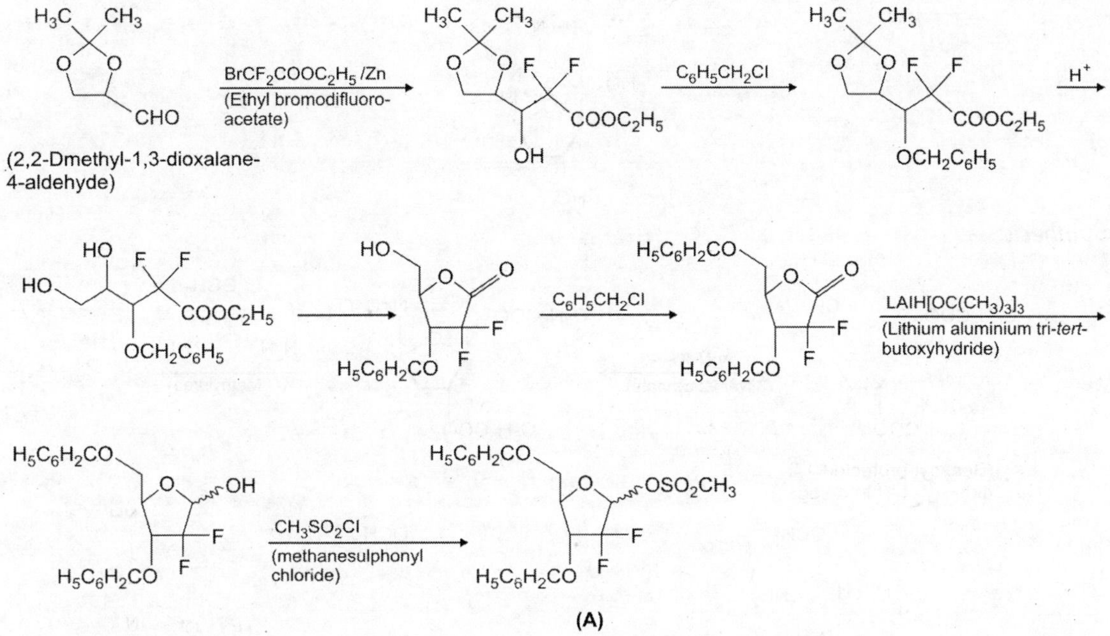

Step 2

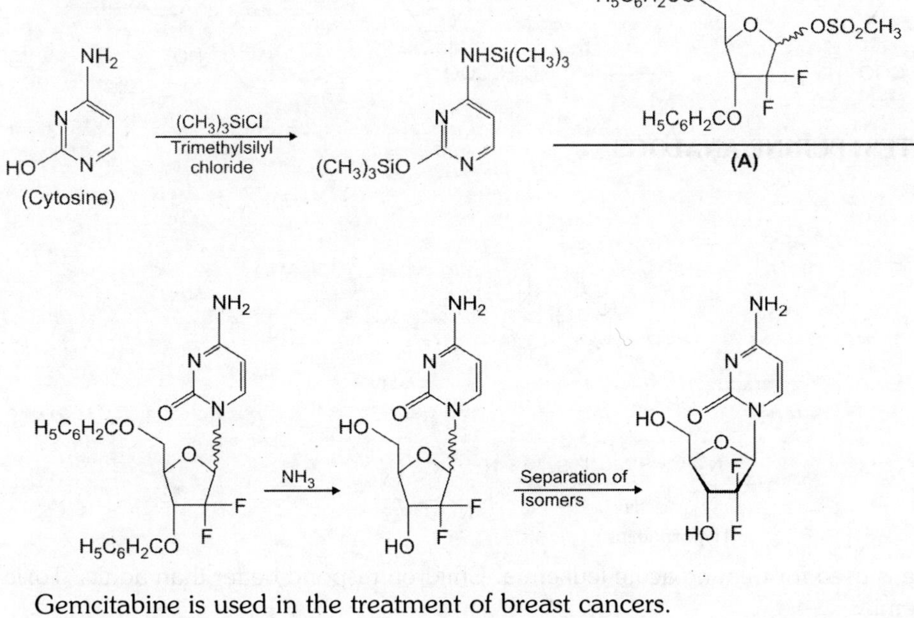

Gemcitabine is used in the treatment of breast cancers.

Decitabine

4-Amino-1-(2-deoxy-β-*erythro*-pentofuranosyl)-1,3,5-triazin-2(1*H*)-one

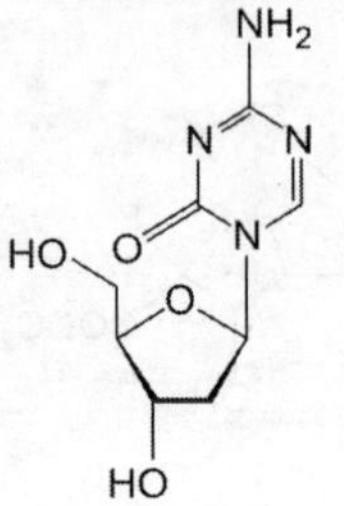

Synthesis

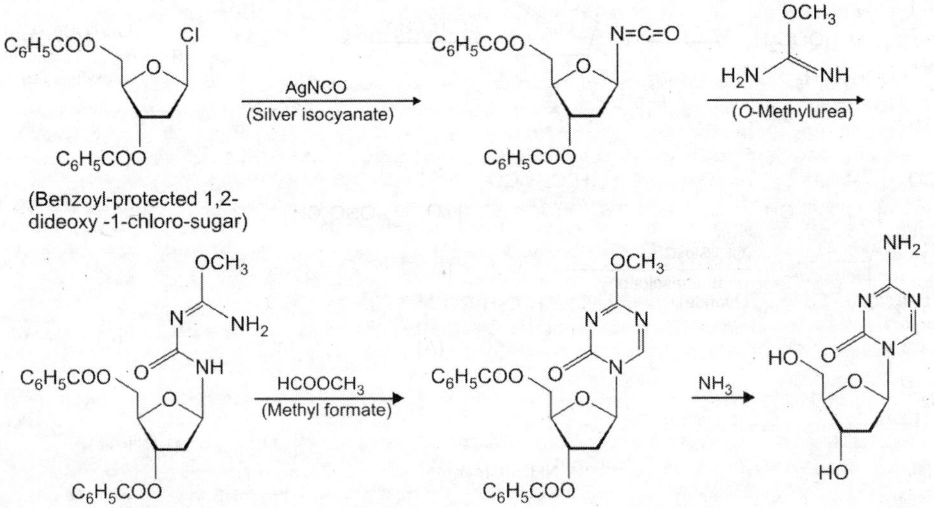

ANTIMETABOLITES : PURINE ANALOGS

Mercaptopurine

Purine-6-thiol

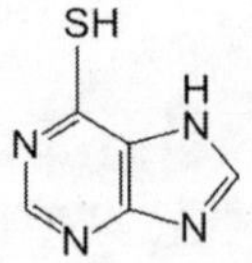

Synthesis

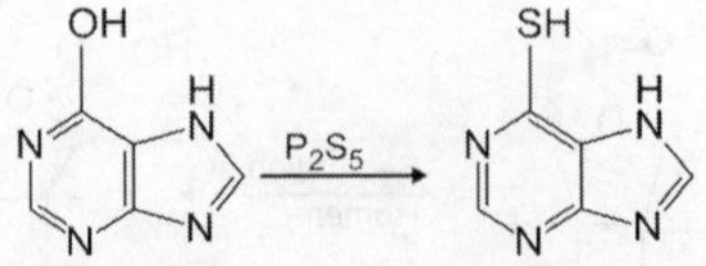

(Hypoxanthine)

Mercaptopurine is used for treating acute leukemia. Children respond better than adults. Toxic effect includes anemia.

Thioguanine
2-Aminopurine-6-thiol

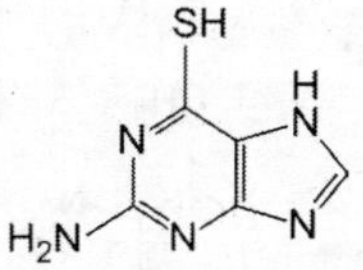

Synthesis

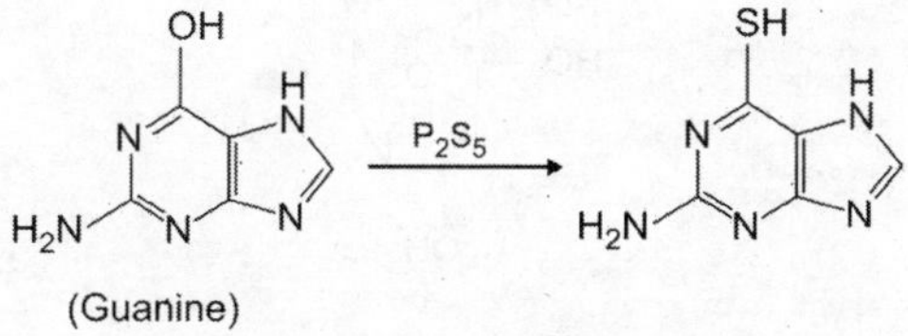

It is used in acute leukemia. Chief toxic effect is delayed bone marrow depression resulting in leukopenia and thrombocytopenia and eventual bleeding.

Vidarabine
See **ANTIVIRAL AGENTS**

Cladribine
2-Chloro-2′-deoxyadenosine

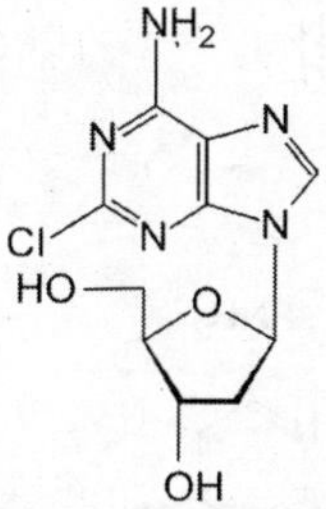

Synthesis

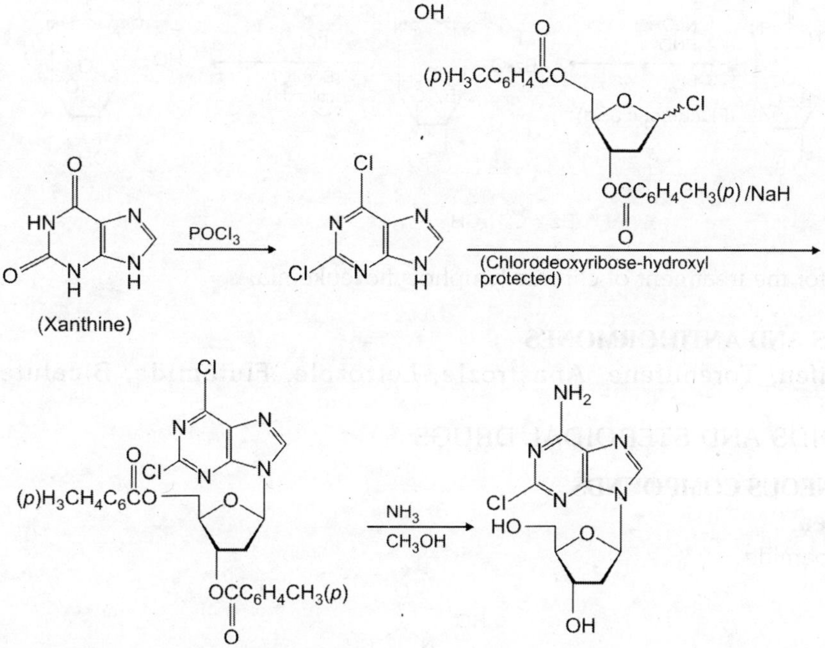

It is used for chronic lymphocytic leukemia.

Fludarabine
9-β-D-Arabinofuranosyl-2-fluoroadenine

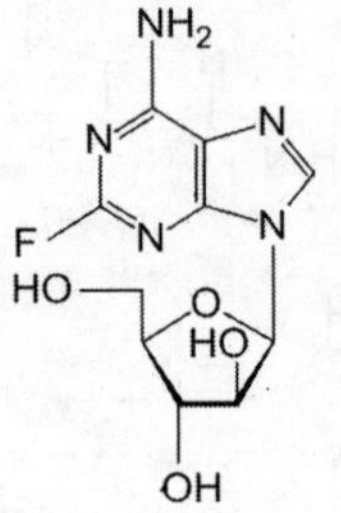

Synthesis

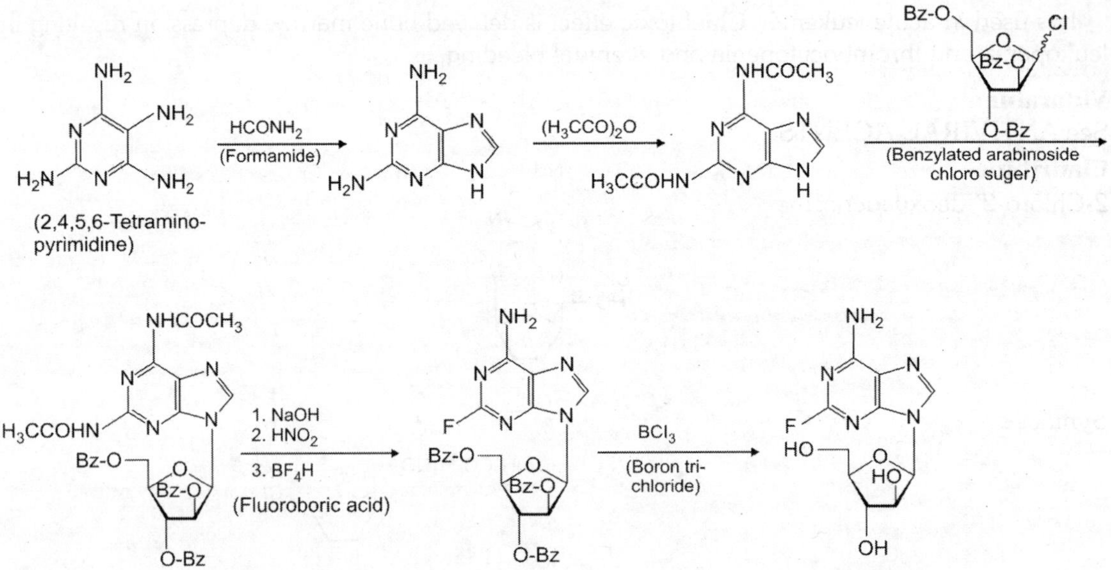

(2,4,5,6-Tetramino-pyrimidine)

Bz = C₆H₅CH₂

It is used for the treatment of chronic lymphocytic leukemia.

HORMONES AND ANTIHORMONES
For **Tamoxifen, Toremifene, Anastrozle, Letrozole, Flutamide, Bicalutamide, and Nilutamide**
See **STEROIDS AND STEROIDAL DRUGS**

MISCELLANEOUS COMPOUNDS
Hydroxyurea
Hydroxycarbamide

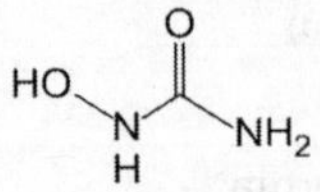

Synthesis

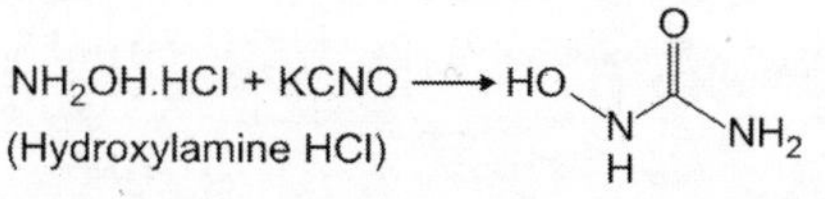

$$NH_2OH.HCl + KCNO \longrightarrow$$

(Hydroxylamine HCl)

Active against malanoma, leukemia, and ovarian carcinoma. Main toxicity against bone marrow.

Mitotane

2-(2-Chlorophenyl)-2-(4-chlorophenyl)-1,1-dichloroethane

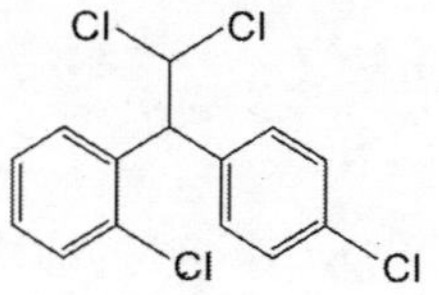

Synthesis

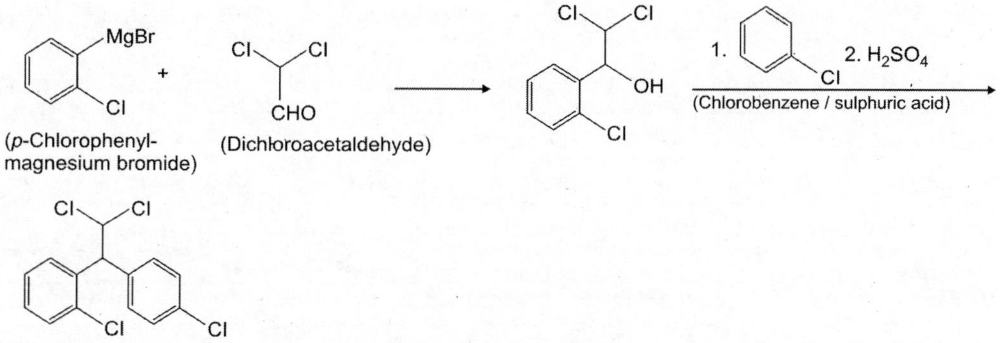

(*p*-Chlorophenyl-
magnesium bromide) (Dichloroacetaldehyde) (Chlorobenzene / sulphuric acid)

It is used for non-operable metastatic prostate carcinomas.

Section XI
Diagnostic Agents

DIAGNOSTIC AGENTS

DIAGNOSTIC AGENTS are used to detect the impaired function of the body organ or to recognize the abnormalities in the tissue structure. They are broadly classified into two categories

1. Clinical diagnostic agents used to determine the normal and pathological constituents in urine, blood, feces, and other body fluids/excrements. This also includes serological solutions and tissue staining dyes necessary for microscopic examination.

2. The second group includes:

    (a) Radiopaques, and

    (b) Compounds for testing functional capacity of various organs.

It is the second class of compounds that will be discussed here.

RADIOPAQUE SUBSTANCES

Any substance which when administered to a patient improves the visualization of an organ or tissue is called a contrast agent. A contrast agent can be negative or positive. A negative agent renders the structure of a tissue more translucent. Any substance that increases the radiopacity is a positive contrast agent. The substances in diagnostic radiology are positive contrast agents.

Some of the procedures used in diagnostic roentgenography include:

(a) Angiography,	for examination of blood vessels,
(b) Aortography,	for examination of aorta,
(c) Bronchography,	for examination of bronchial tree,
(d) Cholecystography,	for examination of gallbladder,
(e) Hepatography,	for examination of liver,
(f) Hysterosalpinography,	for examination of uterus and fallopian tube,
(g) Lymphangiography,	for examination of lymphatic duct,
(h) Myelography ,	for examination of subarachnoid space of spinal cord,
(i) Sialography,	for examination of salivary glands,
(j) Urography,	for examination of urinary tract, and
(k) Pyelography,	for examination of pelvis and ureter.

Radiopaque diagnostic agents can be inorganic as well as organic compounds. The inorganic compounds include barium sulphate, thorium oxide, and bismuth oxide. Out of these only barium sulphate is used and the other two, thorium oxide and bismuth oxide, are not used because of their acute and chronic toxicity. Barium sulphate is used as a suspension and is administered orally or by retrograde enema for the radiological examination of gastrointestinal tract.

Among the organic radiopaques, iodine compounds are usually more useful. They are more opaque and are used mostly in X-ray studies.

The characteristics of a radiopaque substances are:

1. It should have an adequate radiopacity which requires an iodine content of 50% or more.
2. The solution should be capable of selective concentration in certain structures such as gall-bladder, kidney, etc.
3. The substance should have high solubility. Solubility in the range of 40% and above is desirable.
4. The substance should be stable under the conditions of use, i.e. resist the change in vivo as well as during the storage.
5. The substance should have low toxicity with minimum of pharmacodynamic activity.

Organic compounds are used by two methods. The systemic and retrograde procedures. In the systemic procedure, the agent is administered orally or by intravenous method. The patient is given a preliminary test to determine individual's sensitivity. After this the patient is given a cathartic on the night before the administration of diagnostic agent. Food and liquids, which cause the blurring of the pictures, are withheld for 18 hr.

In the retrograde procedure, the diagnostic agent is introduced by the mechanical method. Iodinated compounds may be introduced into the urethra, bladder, vagina, lower bowel, ulcer area, or varicose tissue.

INDIVIDUAL COMPOUNDS

RADIOPAQUES : AGENTS USED FOR EXAMINATION OF GASTROINTESTINAL TRACT

Barium Sulphate

$$BaSO_4$$

It is an agent of choice for gastrointestinal roentgenography, and is administered orally or through rectal route as an aqueous suspension.

RADIOPAQUES : AGENTS USED FOR ANGIOGRAPHY AND UROGRAPHY

Diatrizoate Sodium

Sodium 3,5-bis(acetylamino)-2,4,6-triiodobenzoate

Synthesis

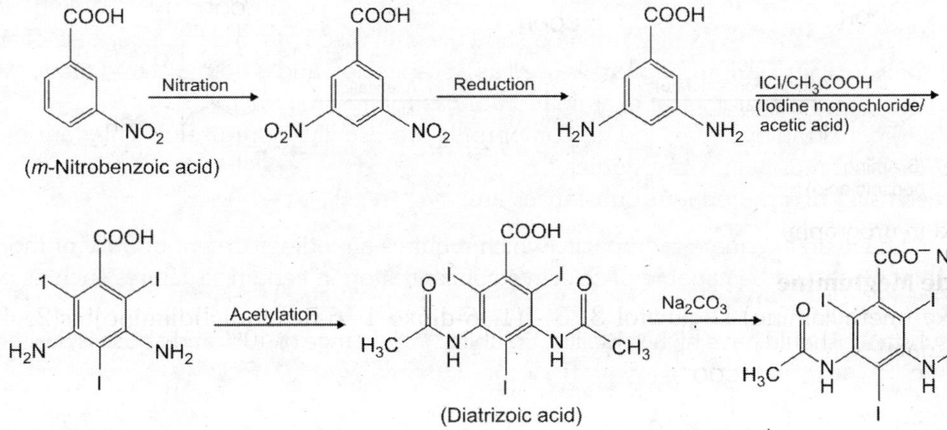

(*m*-Nitrobenzoic acid)

(Diatrizoic acid)

It is used in urography.

Diatrizoate Meglumine

1-Deoxy-1-(methylamino)-D-glucitol 3,5-bis(acetylamino)-2,4,6-triiodobenzoate

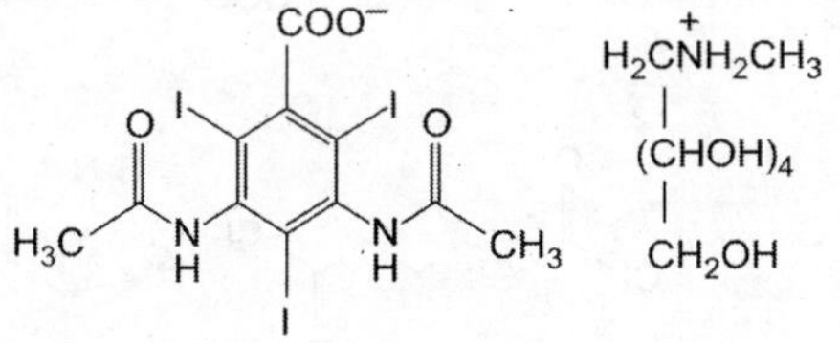

Synthesis

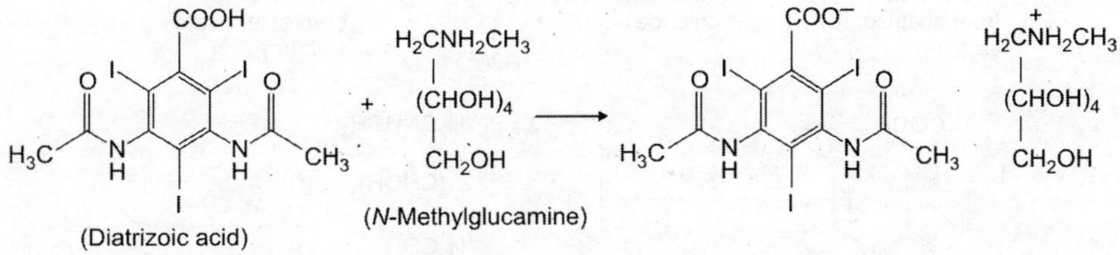

(Diatrizoic acid)   (*N*-Methylglucamine)

It is used for angiography and urography.

Acetrizoate Sodium

Sodium 3-(acetylamino)-2,4,6-triiodobenzoate

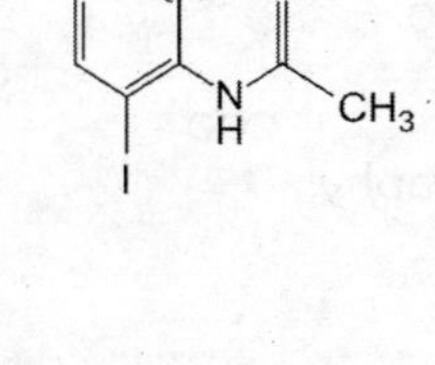

Synthesis

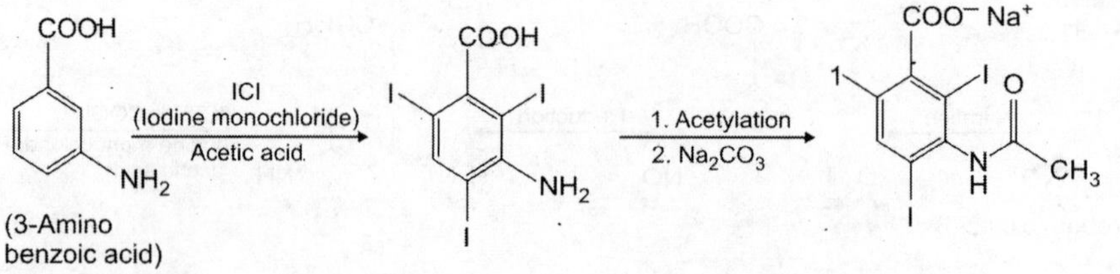

It is used in urography

Iodipamide Meglumine

Bis-1-deoxy-(methylamino)-D-glucitol 3, 3´-[(1, 6-dioxo-1, 6-hexandiyl)diimino]bis[2, 4, 6-triiodobenzoate]

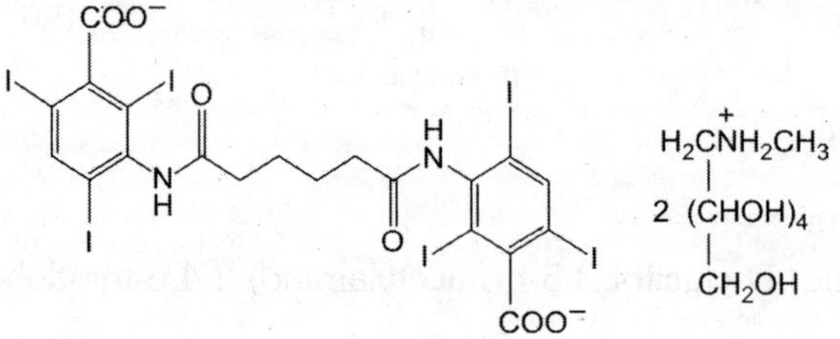

Synthesis

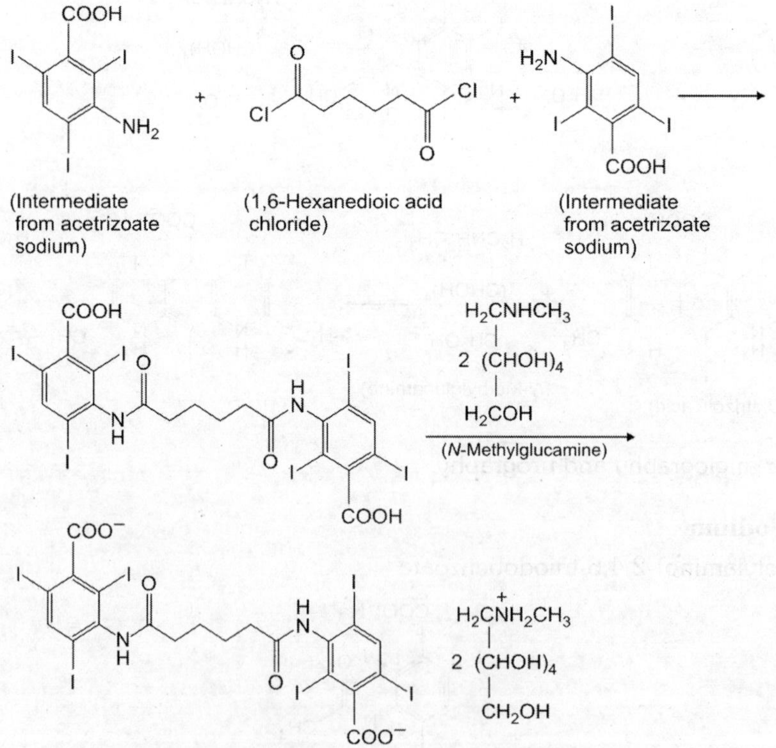

(Intermediate from acetrizoate sodium)

(1,6-Hexanedioic acid chloride)

(Intermediate from acetrizoate sodium)

(*N*-Methylglucamine)

It is used in angiography and urography.

Iothalamate Sodium

Sodium 3-(acetylamino)-2,4,6-triiodo-5-[(methylamino)carbonyl]benzoate

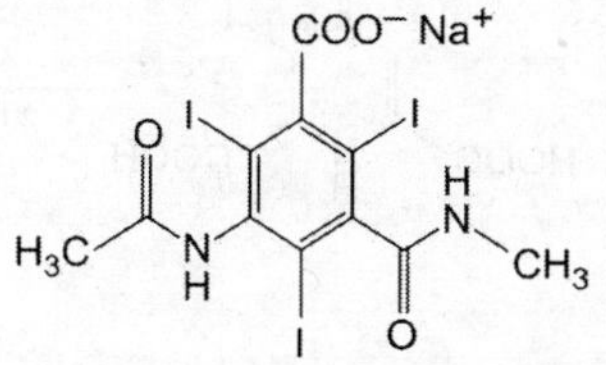

Synthesis

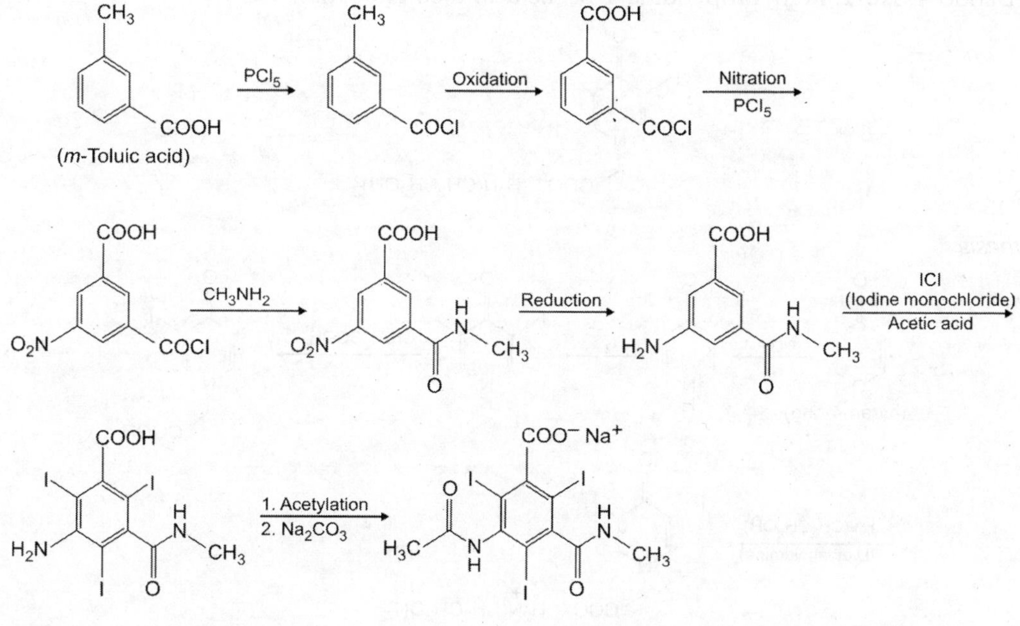

It is used in angiography.

Sodium Iodomethamate

1, 4-Dihydro-3, 5-diiodo-1-methyl-4-oxo-2, 6-pyridinedicarboxylic acid disodium salt

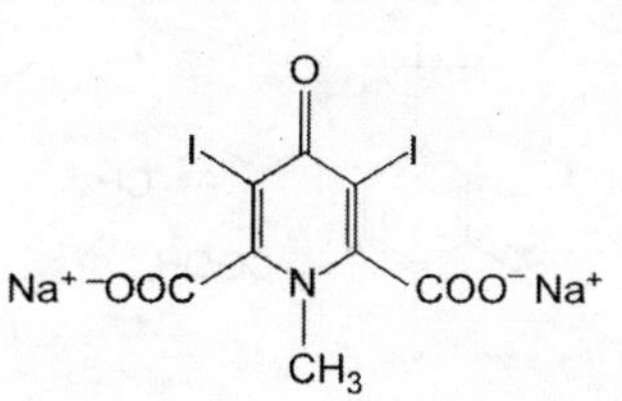

Synthesis

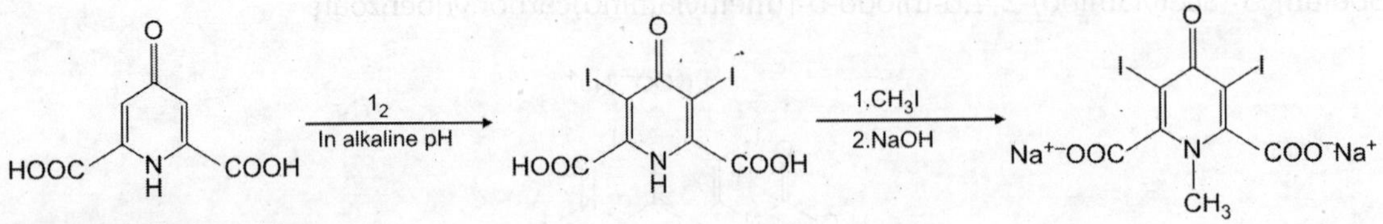

(4-Oxo-1,4-dihydropyridine
2,6-dicarboxylic acid)

It is used in urography.

Iodopyracet

3, 5-Diiodo-4-oxo-1,4-dihydropyridine-1-acetic acid diethanolamine salt

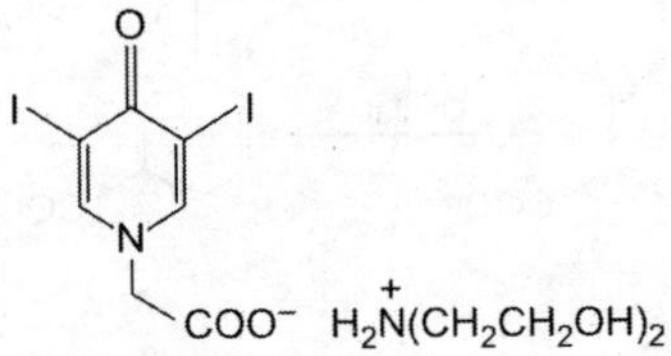

Synthesis

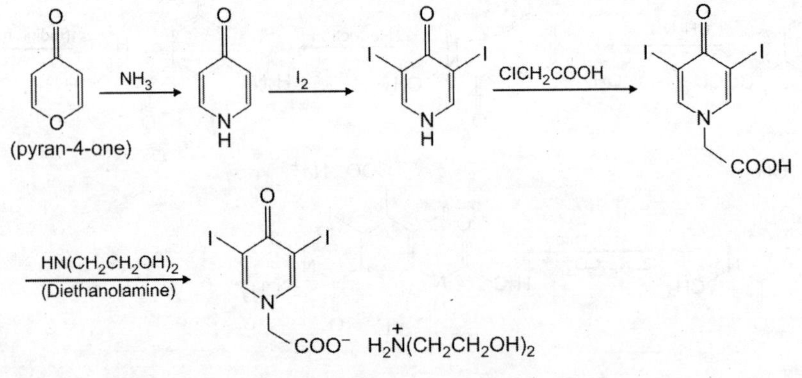

(pyran-4-one)

It is used in and angiography and urography.

RADIOPAQUES : AGENTS USED FOR CHOLECYSTOGRAPHY
Iopanoic Acid

3-(3-Amino-2,4,6-triiodophenyl)-2-ethylpropionic acid

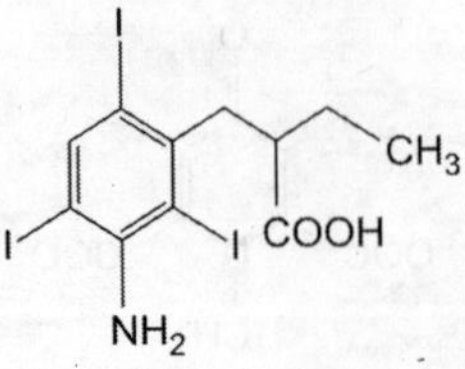

Synthesis

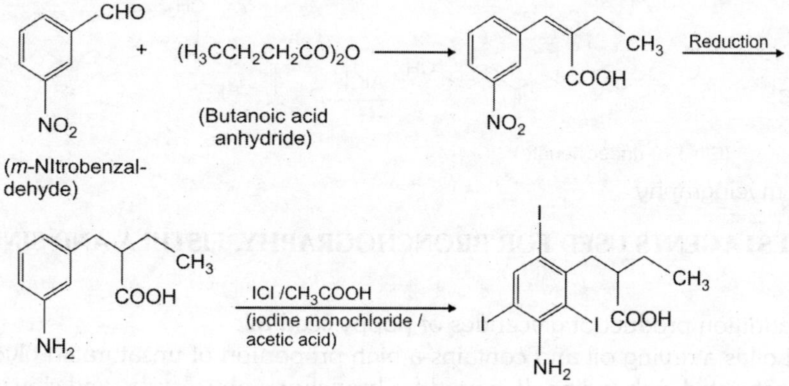

It is used for cholecystography.

Iodophthalein Sodium

Tetraiodophenolpthalein sodium

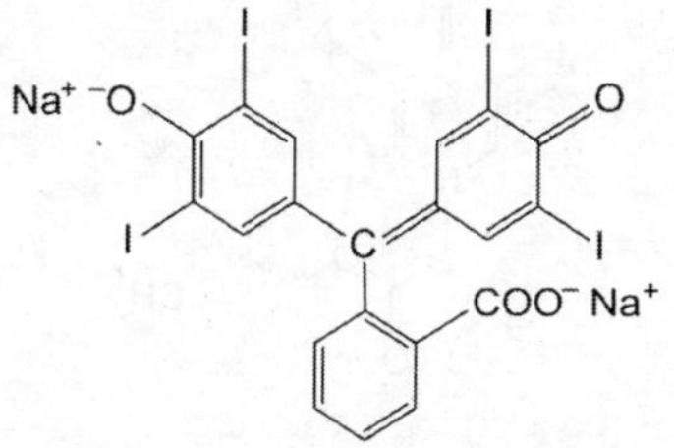

Synthesis

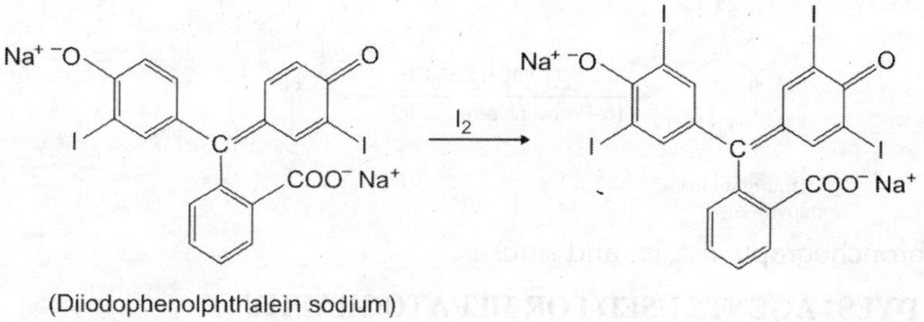

(Diiodophenolphthalein sodium)

It is used for cholecystography.

RADIOPAQUES : AGENTS USED FOR MYELOGRAPHY

Iophendylate

Ethyl 10-(p-iodophenyl) undecylate

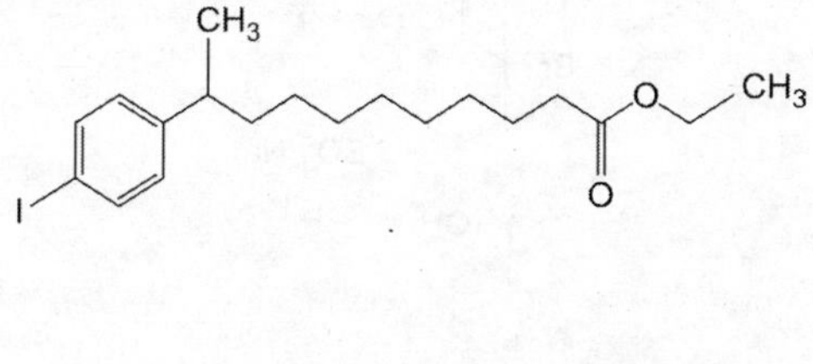

Synthesis

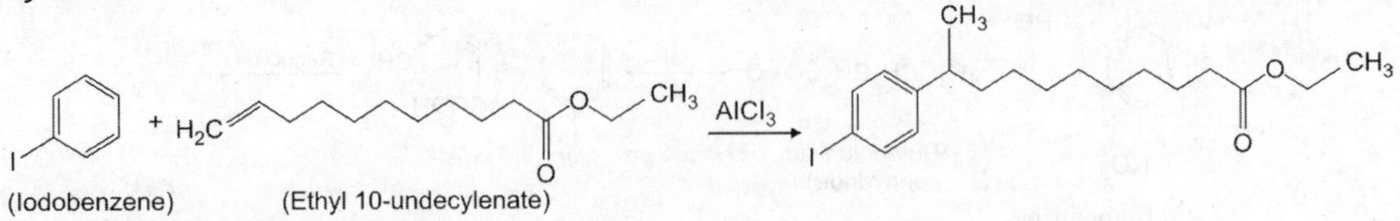

(Iodobenzene)
(Ethyl 10-undecylenate)
AlCl3

It is used in myelography.

RADIOPAQUES: AGENTS USED FOR BRONCHOGRAPHY, FISTULA AND SINUSES

Iodized Oil

Sterile iodine addition product of glycerides of poppy seed oil.

Poppy seed oil is a drying oil and contains a high proportion of unsaturated glycerides. These glycerides are saturated with iodine. It is used for bronchography, fistula, and sinuses.

Propyliodone

3,5-Diodo-4-pyridone-1-acetic acid propyl ester

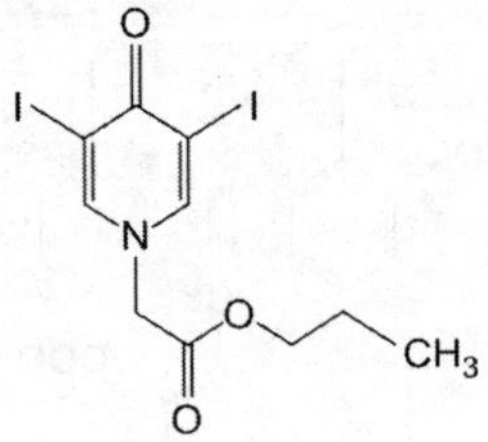

Synthesis

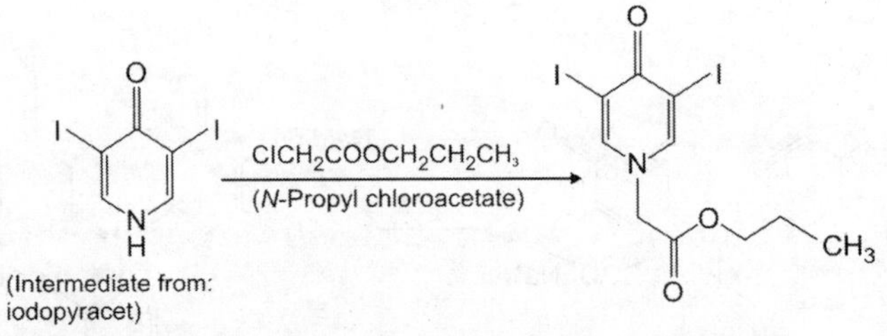

ClCH2COOCH2CH2CH3
(N-Propyl chloroacetate)
(Intermediate from: iodopyracet)

It is used in bronchograpy, fistula, and sinuses.

DIAGNOSTIC DYES: AGENTS USED FOR HEPATOGRAPHY

Sulphobromophthalein Sodium

Disodium phenoltetrabromophthalein sulphonate

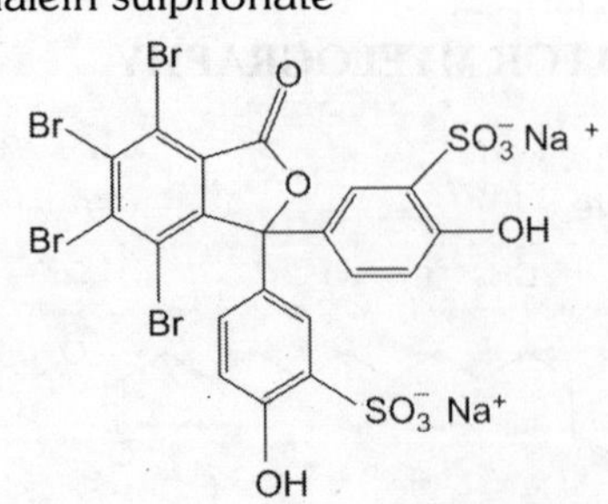

Synthesis

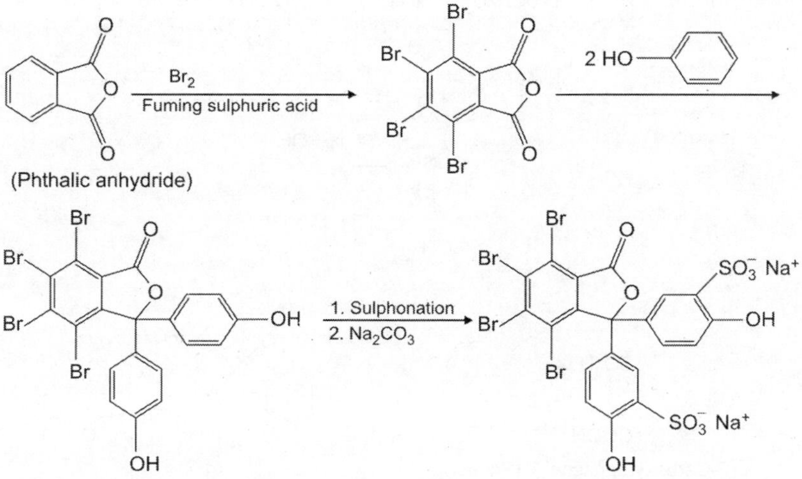

It is used for determining the liver function.

DIAGNOSTIC DYES : AGENTS USED FOR KIDNEY FUNCTION

Indigo Carmine

2-(1,3-Dihydro-3-oxo-5-sulpho-2H-indol-2-ylidene)-2, 3-dihydro-3-oxo-1H-indol-5-sulphonic acid disodium salt

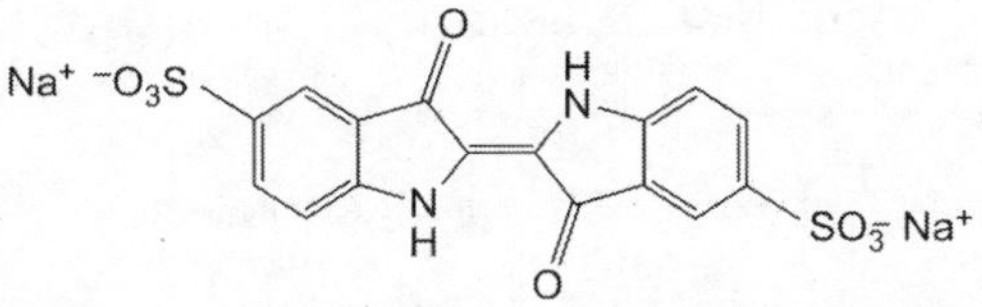

Synthesis

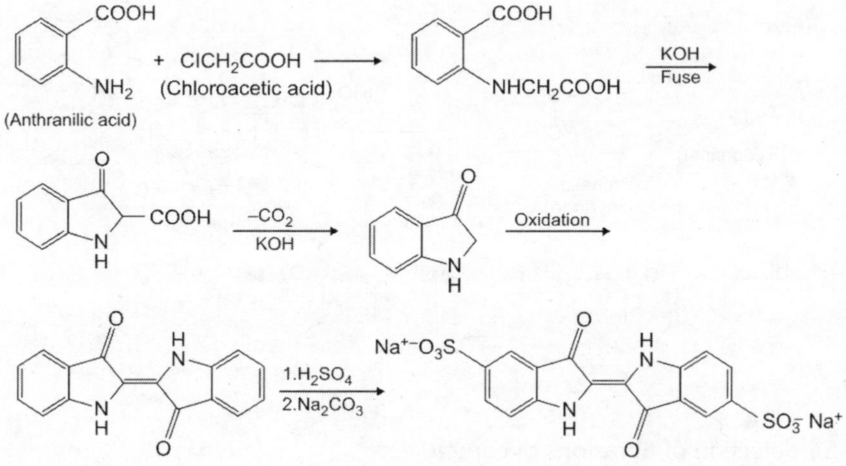

Phenolsulphonphthalein

3, 3-Bis(4-hydroxyphenyl)-3*H*-2, 1-benzoxathiole 1, 1-dioxide

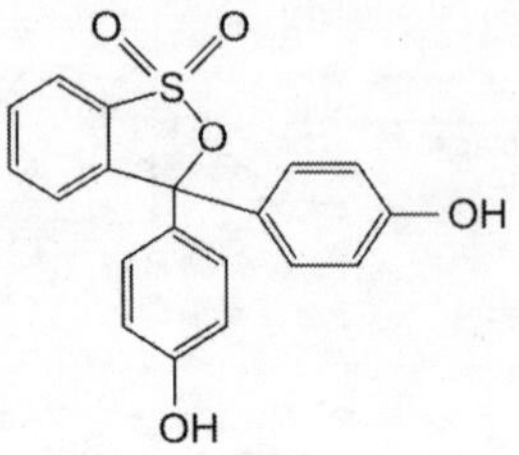

Synthesis

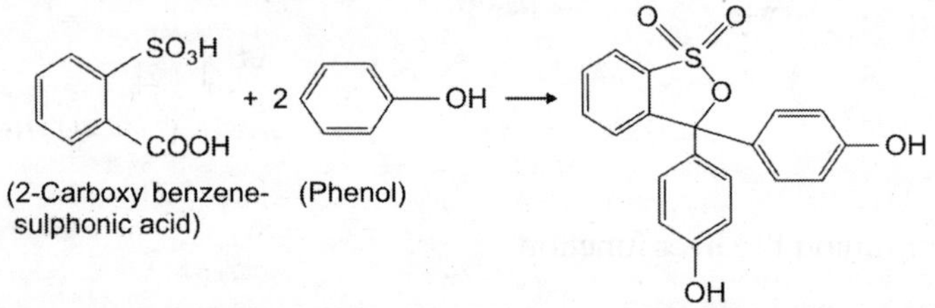

(2-Carboxy benzene-
sulphonic acid)   (Phenol)

DIAGNOSTIC DYES : MISCELLANEOUS

Fluorescein Sodium

Sodium 2-(6-sodiooxy-3-oxoxanthene-9-ylbenzoate)

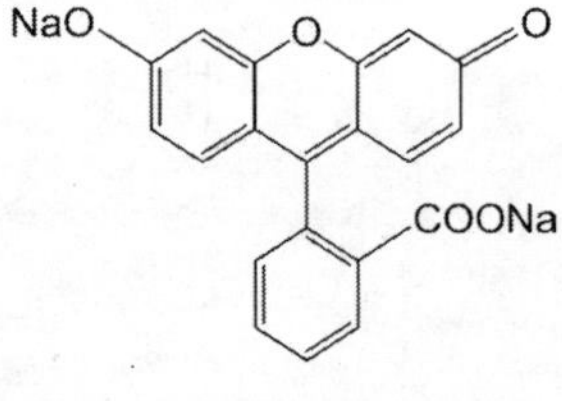

Synthesis

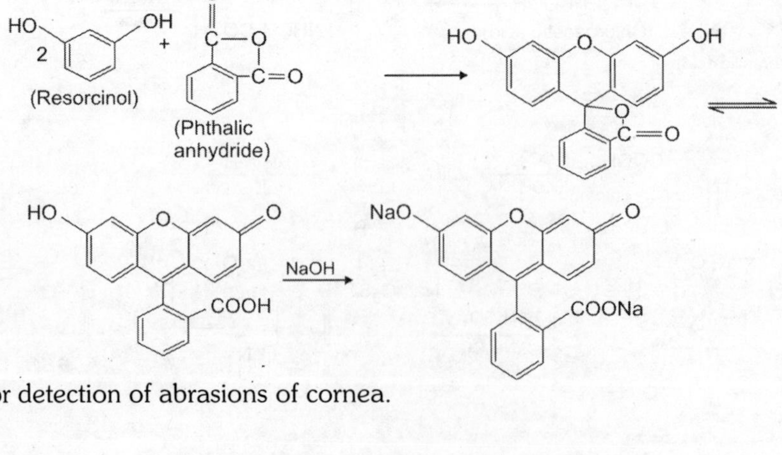

(Resorcinol)

(Phthalic
anhydride)

It is used for detection of abrasions of cornea.

Evans Blue

6,6′-[(3,3′-Dimethyl-[1,1′-biphenyl]-4,4′-diyl)bis(azo)]bis[4-amino-5-hydroxy-1,3-naphthalenedisulphonic acid] tetrasodium salt

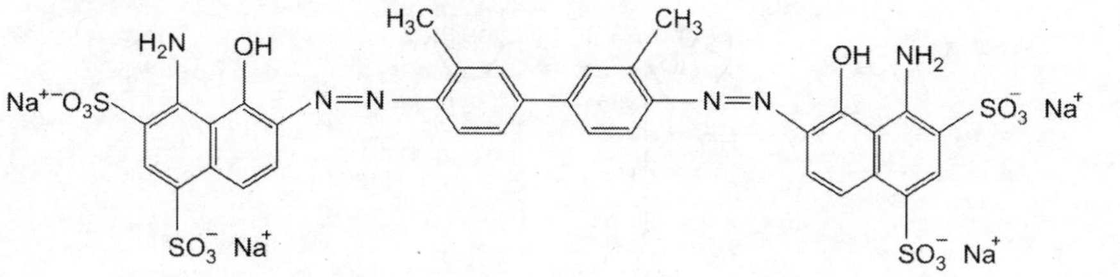

Synthesis

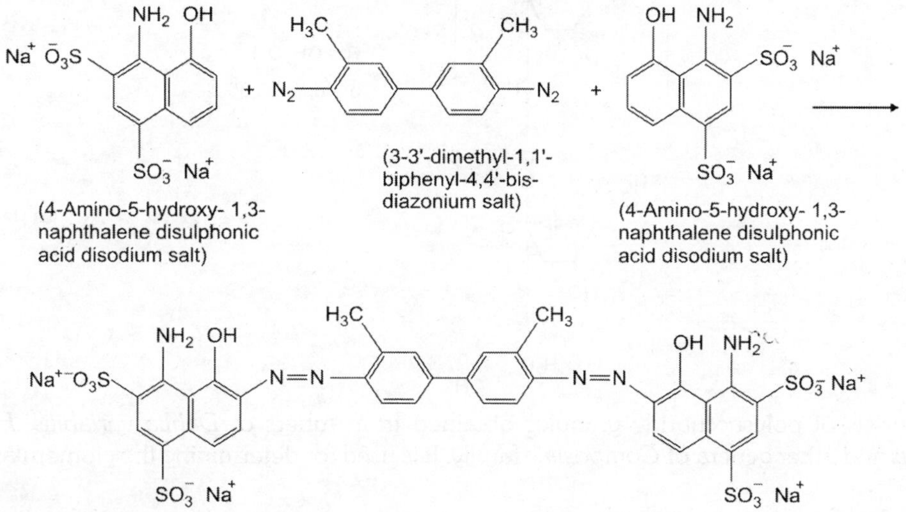

(4-Amino-5-hydroxy- 1,3-naphthalene disulphonic acid disodium salt)

(3-3′-dimethyl-1,1′-biphenyl-4,4′-bis-diazonium salt)

(4-Amino-5-hydroxy- 1,3-naphthalene disulphonic acid disodium salt)

It is used for determination of blood volume.

DIAGNOSTIC AGENTS : MISCELLANEOUS
Histamine

1*H*-Imidazole-4-ethanamine

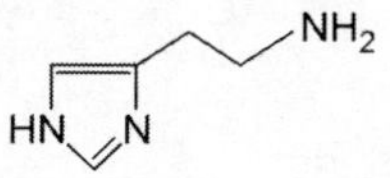

Synthesis

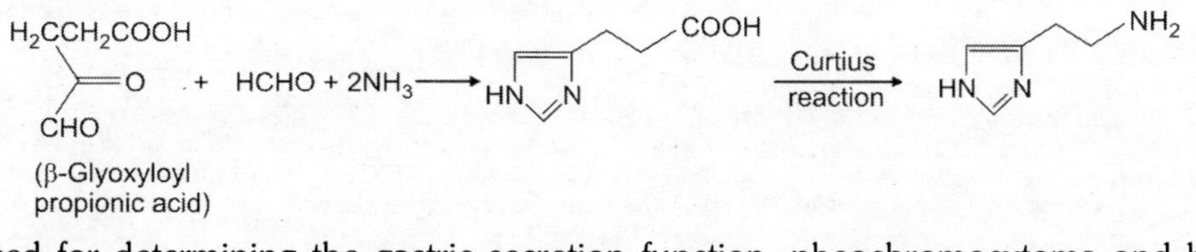

(β-Glyoxyloyl propionic acid)

It is used for determining the gastric secretion function, pheochromocytoma and bronchial hyperreactivity.

Inulin
Polysaccharide

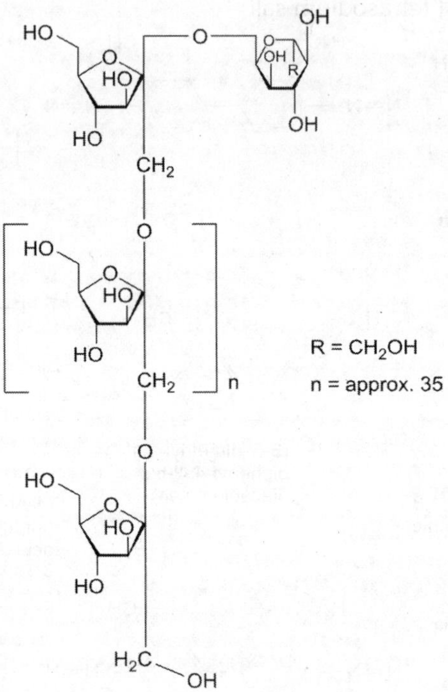

R = CH$_2$OH
n = approx. 35

It consists of polysaccharide granules obtained from tubers of *Dahlia variabilis, Helianthus tuberosus* and other genera of *Compositae* family. It is used for determining the glomerular filtration rate.

Section XII

Vitamins

VITAMINS

VITAMINS are organic substaces that are essential for the growth of humans and other vertebrates. Since the animals cannot synthesize their own requirement of vitamins, they have to be supplied from outside.

Vitamins constitute a group of compounds which have diverse structures. However, they have number of common properties which justifies their being grouped together. Thus,

(a) they are required in small quantities,

(b) they possess specificity of function,

(c) lack of these substances results in disease and each vitamin is related to a particular disease.

In the early stages, as they were discovered, they were identified by the alphabets A, B, C, D, etc. They have been also identified by the disease to which they are related, thus vitamin B_1 is also called aneurin – anti-neuritic, vitamin C is also known as antiscorbutic i.e., scurvy preventing and so on.

The word 'Vitamin' has come from "Vitamine" coined by Funk in 1912. According to him these substances were essential for life, so the word "Vita" and since such substances known at that time were containing nitrogen so the word 'amine". However since many of these substances are not basic in nature or do not contain nitrogen, the letter "e" has been dropped and the term "Vitamin" is used for such substances now.

Based on solubility, vitamins have been classified as fat soluble and water soluble vitamins. Fat soluble vitamins include vitamin A, D, E, and K. The water soluble vitamins are vitamin B group and vitamin C.

FAT SOLUBLE VITAMINS

VITAMIN A

Vitamin A constitute compounds possessing activity like that of retinol and include vitamin A_1 or retinol (1); vitamin A aldehyde or retinal (2); all-*trans*-retinoic acid (3); 11(4)-*cis*-retinal (4); 13(2)-*cis*-vitamin A or neovitamin A(5); all-*trans*-3(3′)-dehydroretinol (6); all-*trans*-3(3′)-dehydroretinal (7); 11(4)-*cis*-3(3′)-dehydroretinal (8).

(3)

(4)

(5)

(6)

(7)

(8)

Sources

The dietary sources include liver, milk, butter, cheese, eggs, fiesh liver oils, 11(4)-*cis*-3(3')-dehydroretinal (8) as careotenoids from fruits and vegetables. Purified vitamin A_1(1) is obtained by different methods and include:

(a) Saponification of fish liver oil and extraction of vitamin A_1 from non-saponifiable portion by a suitable solvent.

(b) By molecular distillation of non-saponifiable matter from which other substances such as sterols have been removed by freezing.

(c) Molecular distillation of fish liver oil. By this method free vitamin and its esters such as palmitate and myristate are obtained.

Pure crystalline vitamin A_1(1) is obtained in yellow plates or crystals, mp 62-64°C. It is unstable in light and oxygen and is preserved by excluding light and air in presence of an antioxidant.

Deficiency Diseases

Vitamin A is essential for growth, for the development and maintenance of epithelial tissues. It is also essential for vision particularly in dim light. Prolonged deficiency of Vitamin A may result in xerophthalmia, starting with night blindness leading to complete blindness. Vitamin A also enhances the function of immune system and thus protect against various infectious diseases and malignancies.

Vitamin A_1(1)

(all-*E*)-3,7-Dimethyl-9-(2',6',6'-trimethyl-1'-cyclohexen-1'-yl)-2,4,6,8-nonatetraen-1-ol; Retinol: all *trans*-retinol.

(1)

Solvated crystals from methanol, mp 62-64°C. Distills at 120-125°C at 0.005 mm pressure.

Structure

1. Molecular formula $C_{20}H_{30}O$
2. It forms esters with acids, indicating that oxygen function must be alcoholic. Further, the oxidation of vitamin A_1 results in an aldehyde indicating that the alcoholic group must be a primary alcohol.

3. Catalytic reduction of vitamin A_1 results in a compound having molecular formula $C_{20}H_{40}O$. This suggests that there must be five double bonds.

4. Ozonolysis produces one molecule of geronic acid (9) per molecule of vitamin A_1, indicating that there must be present one β-ionone (10) nucleus.

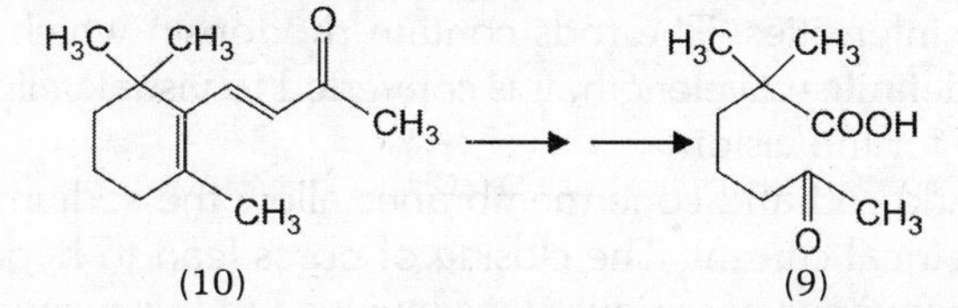

(10) → → (9)

5. Oxidation with permanganate produces two molecules of acetic acid. This indicates presence of $(-\overset{\text{O}}{\overset{\|}{C}}-CH_3)$ groups which has been further confirmed by chromic acid oxidation (Kuhn-Roth oxidation).

6. The above facts suggest that vitamin A_1 is half of the β-carotene (11) structure.

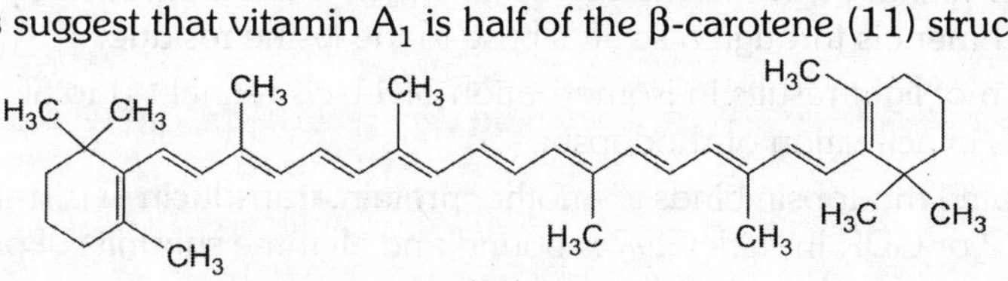

(11)

7. Further decahydrovitamin A_1 was synthesized from β-ionone. This was found to be identical with the compound obtained by reducing vitamin A_1.

8. The structure was further established by synthesis by Van Dorp et al (Fig. 38.1)

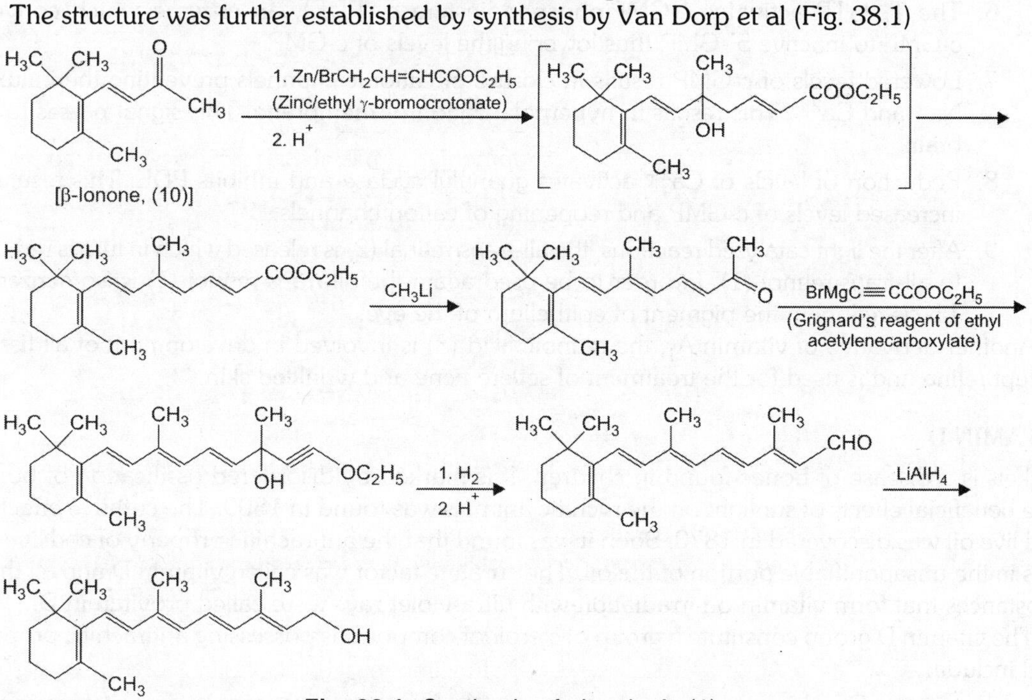

[β-Ionone, (10)]

1. Zn/BrCH$_2$CH=CHCOOC$_2$H$_5$ (Zinc/ethyl γ-bromocrotonate)
2. H$^+$

CH$_3$Li

BrMgC≡CCOOC$_2$H$_5$ (Grignard's reagent of ethyl acetylenecarboxylate)

1. H$_2$
2. H$^+$

LiAlH$_4$

Fig. 38.1: Synthesis of vitamin A_1 (1).

Biochemical Role

Vitamin A_1 [retinol, (1)] acts as a hormone and as a visual pigment of vertebrate eye. The vitamin A_1 derivative, retinal (2) is involved in response of rods and cone cells of the eye to the light. Rods are concerned with colorless vision at low intensities of light and the cones are concerned with color vision at high light intensities. The rods contain rhodopsin which is photosensitive. When acted upon by light of a definite wavelength, it is converted to visual yellow and initiate a series of chemical steps necessary for the vision.

In the resting state (dark) rod and cone membranes allow the sodium ions to enter freely and thus exhibit a steady electrical current. The closing of pores lead to hyperpolarzation resulting in neuronal response. The sequence of various steps involved in this response are as follows:

1. The all-*trans*-vitamin A_1 (1) isomerizes to 11-*cis*-retinol which then is oxidized to 11-*cis*-retinal (4).

2. The 11-*cis*-retinal (4) is attached to opsin which is the protein component of rhodopsin. This attachment is through a schiff's base to the lysine residue.

3. Absorption of light results in isomerization of 11-*cis*-retinal (4) to all-*trans*-retinal (2) and this results in activation of rhodopsin.

4. The activated rhodopsin binds to another protein, transducin (T). Transducin (T) can bind either GTP or GDP. In dark GDP is bound and all three subunits of protein T_α, T_β, and T_γ remain together and no signal is sent.

5. After excitation of rhodopsin and its binding to transducin (T), GDP is replaced by GTP and it dissociates in T_α-GTP and $T_{\beta\gamma}$.

6. The T_α-GTP activates c-GMP-phosphodiesterase (PDE), an enzyme which converts c-GMP to inactive 5'-GMP, thus lowering the levels of c-GMP.

7. Lowered levels of c-GMP results in closure of cationic channels preventing the influx of Na^+ and Ca^{2+}. This results in hyperpolarization of membrane. This signal passes to the brain.

8. Reduction of levels of Ca^{2+} activates guanylyl cyclase and inhibits PDE. This results in increased levels of c-GMP and reopening of cation channels.

9. After the light catalyzed reactions, the all-*trans*-retinal (2) is released which in turn is reduced to all-*trans*-retinol (1). In order to be used again the all-*trans*-retinol (1) is isomerized to 11-*cis*-retinol in the pigment of epithelium of the eye.

Another derivative of vitamin A_1, the retinoic acid (3) is involved in development of all tissues except retina and is used for the treatment of severe acne and wrinkled skin.

VITAMIN D

Rickets is a disease of bones found in children. It is marked by disordered ossification of bones. The beneficial effects of sunlight on the rachitic animals was found in 1800. The curative effects of cod live oil was discovered in 1870. Soon it was found that the antirachitic property of cod liver oil was in the unsaponifiable portion of the oil. The curative factor was called vitamin D and all those substances that form vitamin on irradiation with ultra-violet rays were called provitamin D.

The vitamin D group constitute a group of steroidal compounds possessing antirachitic property and include:

1. Vitamin D_1 which is a molecular compound of one molecule of calciferol and lumisterol.

2. Vitamin D_2 which is calciferol or ergocalciferol.
3. Vitamin D_3 or cholcalciferol.
4. Vitamin D_4 or 22, 23-dihydro-5,6-*cis*-ergocalciferol.

Sources

Occurs in fish liver oil. Animals are capable of producing their own requirement of vitamin D.

Deficiency Diseases

Deficiency of vitamin D results in rickets in children marked by disordered ossification of the bones.

Vitamin D_2(12)

$(3\beta,5Z,7E,22E)$-9,10-Secoergosta-5,7,10(19),22-tetraen-3-ol; Calciferol; Ergocalcifrol

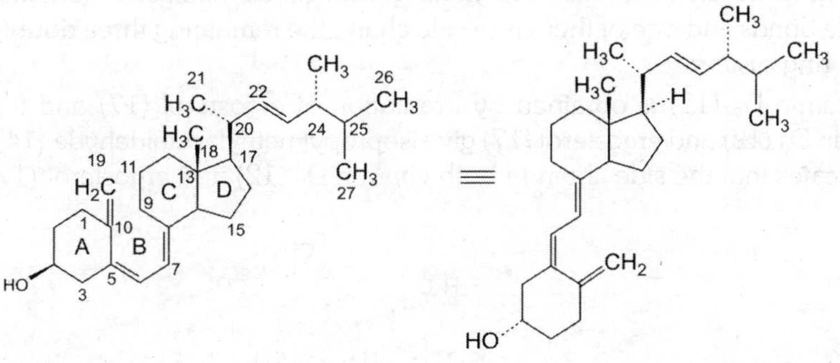

(12)

Prisms from acetone, mp 115-118, $[\alpha]_D^{25} + 85.6°$ (c = 3 in acetone).

Structure

Molecular formula $C_{28}H_{44}O$.

1. If forms esters with acids, so a hydroxyl group must be present in the molecule. The hydroxyl group was found to be secondary because on oxidation vitamin D_2 (12) gave a ketone.

2. Vitamin D_2 (12) on hydrogenation absorbs 4 molecules of hydrogens resulting in octa-hydrogenated molecule with molecular formula, $C_{28}H_{52}O$. This indicates that there are four double bonds present in the molecule and this corresponds to general formula C_nH_{2n-4}. The molecule, therefore, is tricyclic. Further, distillation of vitamin D_2 (12) with selenium does not give Diel's hydrocarbon (13) indicating that it does not contain 4 rings.

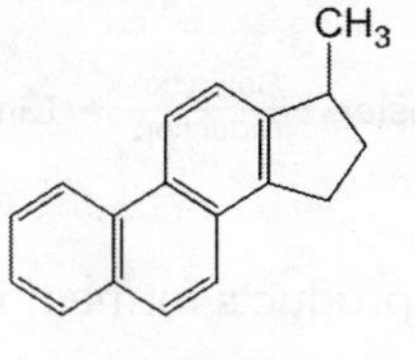

(13)

3. Ozonolysis of vitamin D_2 (12) gives isopropylmethylacetaldehyde (14), a keto acid (15), and formaldehyde (16).

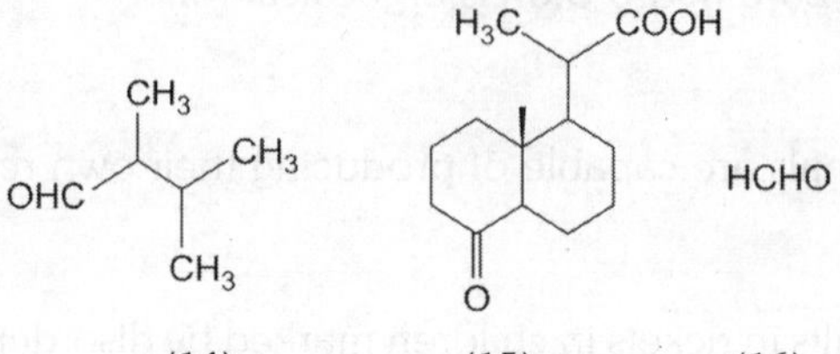

(14) (15) (16)

4. Formation of isopropylmethylacetaldehyde (14) and keto acid (15) indicate that there must be one double bond in side chain and formation of formaldehyde (16) indicates that there must be an exocyclic methylene group. Since molecule contains a total of four double bonds and one of them is in side chain, the remaining three double bonds must be in the ring system.

5. As vitamin D_2 (12) is obtained by irradiation of ergosterol (17) and further since both vitamin D_2 (12) and ergosterol (17) give isopropylmethylacetaldehyde (14) on ozonization, it indicates that the side chain in both vitamin D_2 (12) and ergosterol (17) are similar.

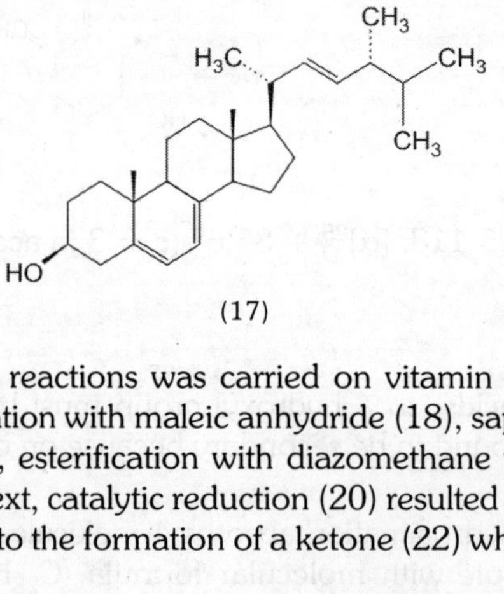

(17)

6. A set of the following reactions was carried on vitamin D_2 (12) acetate. The reactions involved adduct formation with maleic anhydride (18), saponification and formation of a dicarboxylic acid (19), esterification with diazomethane which resulted in formation of dimethyl ester (20). Next, catalytic reduction (20) resulted in dihydro compound (21) and finally ozonization led to the formation of a ketone (22) which had a molecular formula of $C_{19}H_{34}O$.

Vitamin D_2(12) acetate $\xrightarrow{\text{Maleic anhydride}}$ Maleic anhydride adduct of vitamin D_2 $\xrightarrow{\text{Saponification}}$

(18)

Dicarboxylic acid $\xrightarrow{CH_2N_2}$ Dimethyl ester $\xrightarrow[\text{reduction}]{\text{Catalytic}}$ Dihydro-compound $\xrightarrow{O_3}$ Ketone, $(C_{19}H_{34}O)$

(19) (20) (21) (22)

7. From these reactions and the products formed, the following can be concluded:

   (a) During the reduction it is the double bond which is getting reduced.

(b) The parent hydrocarbon of the ketone (22), $C_{19}H_{34}O$ must be $C_{19}H_{36}$. It must be containing two rings.

(c) The high number of hydrogens in the ketone (22) suggests that it contains a side chain and an angular methyl group.

(d) Based on the above, the two rings and the side chain must be corresponding to ring C and D of and the side chain at C_{17} of ergosterol (17).

(e) The formation of ketone also suggests that the ring C must be linked to ring B through a double bond. Based on the above, the ketone (22) must be having the following structure:

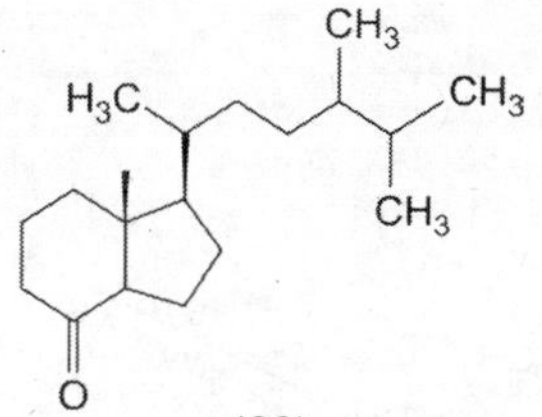

(22)

8. The dicarboxylic and (19) on dehydrogenation yielded naphthalene (23) and β-naphthoic acid (24) and the diester (20) on selenium dehydrogenation yielded 2,3-dimethyl naphthalene (25). Both of these reactions indicate that the adduct (18) formed between vitamin

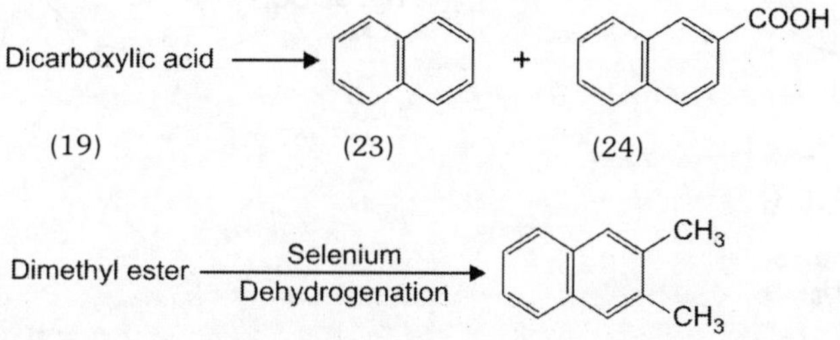

Dicarboxylic acid $\longrightarrow$

(19)   (23)   (24)

Dimethyl ester $\xrightarrow[\text{Dehydrogenation}]{\text{Selenium}}$

(20)   (25)

D (12) acetate and maleic anhydride must be involving exocyclic methylene group on the ring A. Based on this the structure of vitamin D_2 could be (12). The various reactions described above are explained in Fig. 38.2

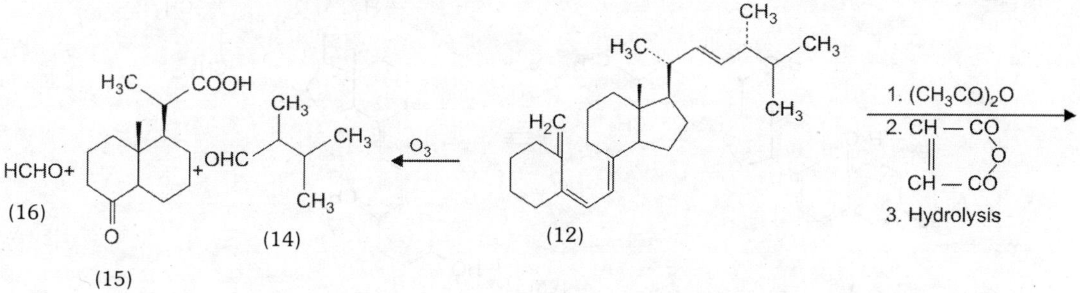

HCHO+

(16)

(15)

(14)

(12)

1. $(CH_3CO)_2O$
2. CH—CO
3. Hydrolysis

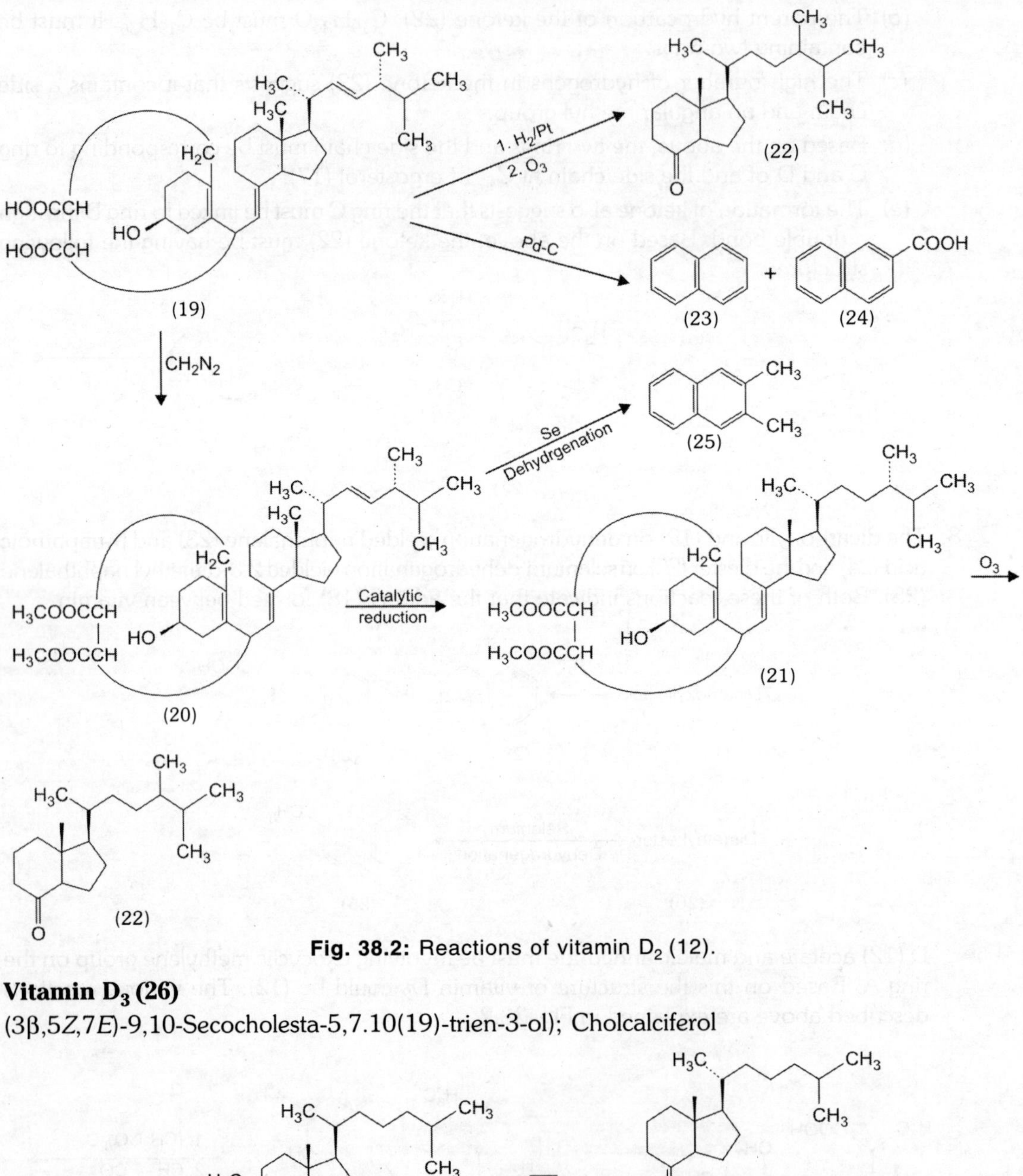

Fig. 38.2: Reactions of vitamin D₂ (12).

Vitamin D₃ (26)

(3β,5Z,7E)-9,10-Secocholesta-5,7.10(19)-trien-3-ol); Cholcalciferol

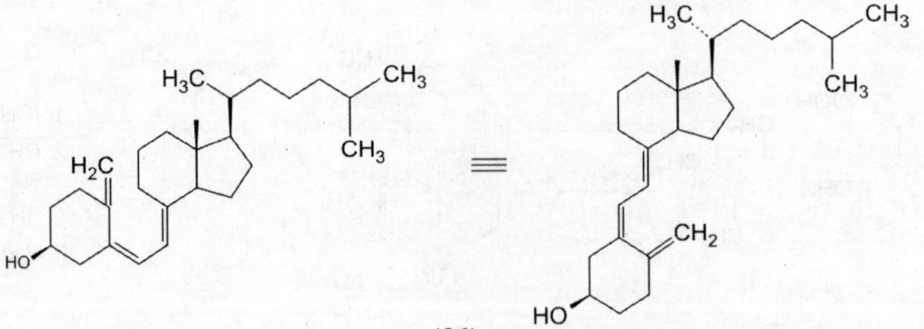

(26)

Cholesterol (27) when subjected to following set of reactions gave 7-dehydrocholesterol (28)

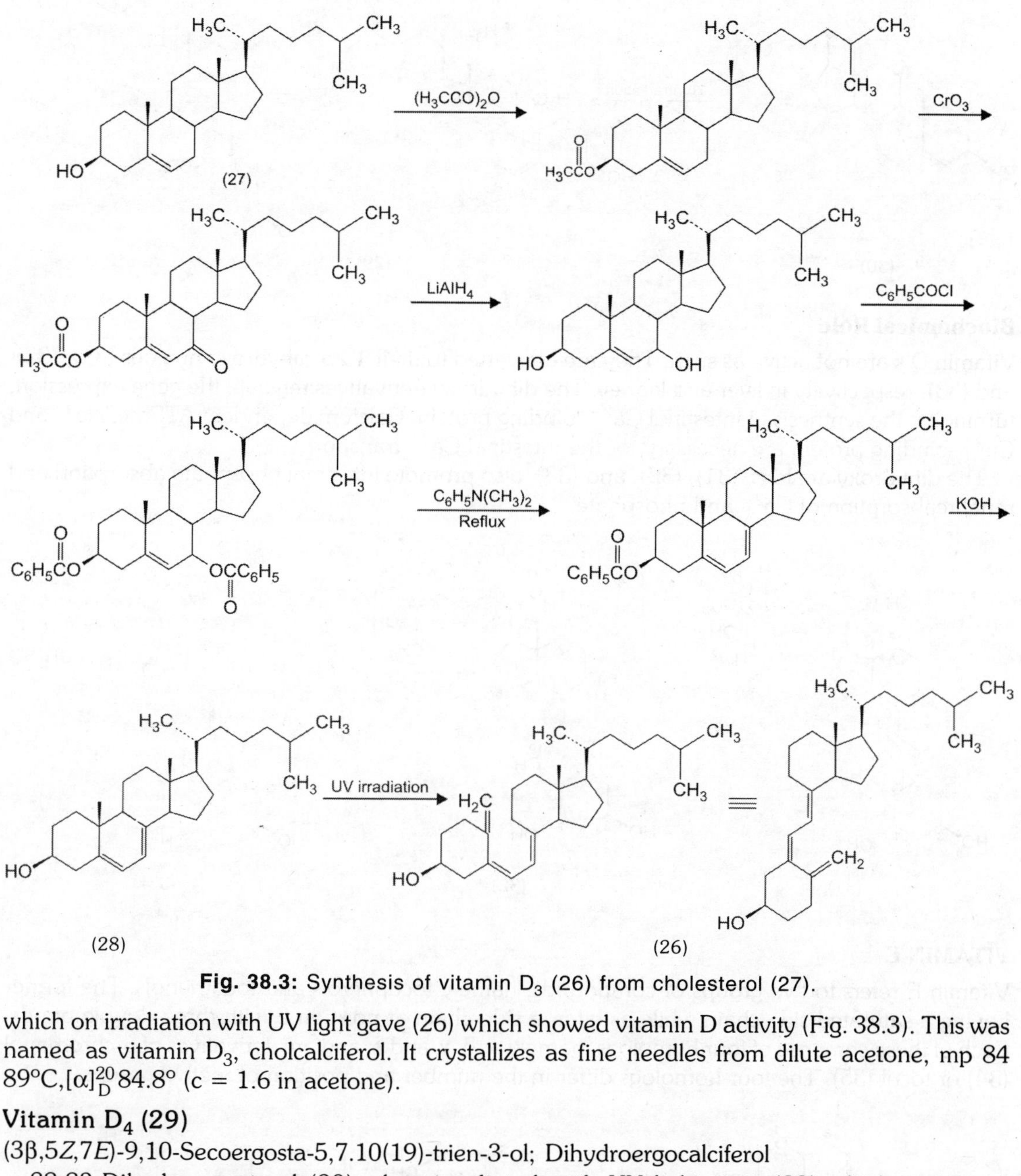

Fig. 38.3: Synthesis of vitamin D_3 (26) from cholesterol (27).

which on irradiation with UV light gave (26) which showed vitamin D activity (Fig. 38.3). This was named as vitamin D_3, cholcalciferol. It crystallizes as fine needles from dilute acetone, mp 84 89°C, $[\alpha]_D^{20}$ 84.8° (c = 1.6 in acetone).

Vitamin D_4 (29)

(3β,5Z,7E)-9,10-Secoergosta-5,7.10(19)-trien-3-ol; Dihydroergocalciferol

22,23-Dihydroergosterol (30) when irradiated with UV light gave (29) which possessed vitamin D activity. It was named as vitamin D_4, dihydroergocalciferol. It crystallizes from acetone, mp 96-98°C, $[\alpha]_D^{18}$ + 89.3° (c = 0.47 in acetone).

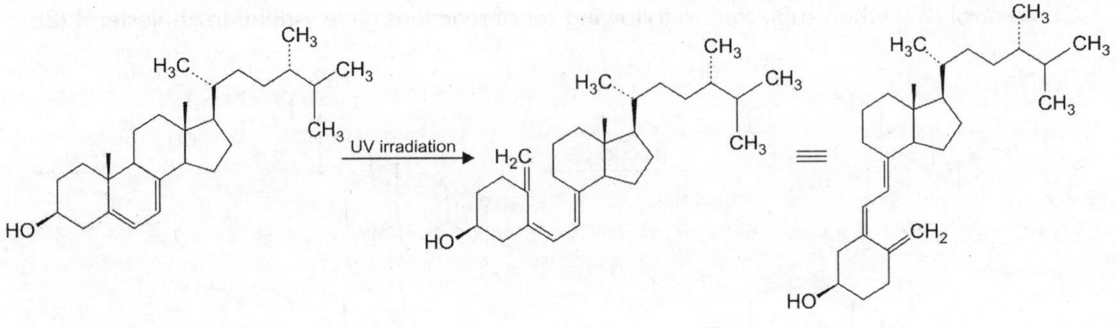

(30)   (29)

Biochemical Role

Vitamin D's are not active as such. They are converted to their 1,25-dihydroxy analogs (31), (32), and (33), respectively in liver and kidney. The dihydroxy derivatives regulate the gene expression, turning on the synthesis of intestinal Ca^{2+}-binding protein. Calcium dependent ATPase, Na^+, and Ca^{2+}-binding protein are necessary for the intestinal Ca^{2+} transport.

The dihydroxy analogs, (31), (32), and (33), also promote intestinal phosphate absorption and renal reabsorption of Ca^{2+} and phosphate.

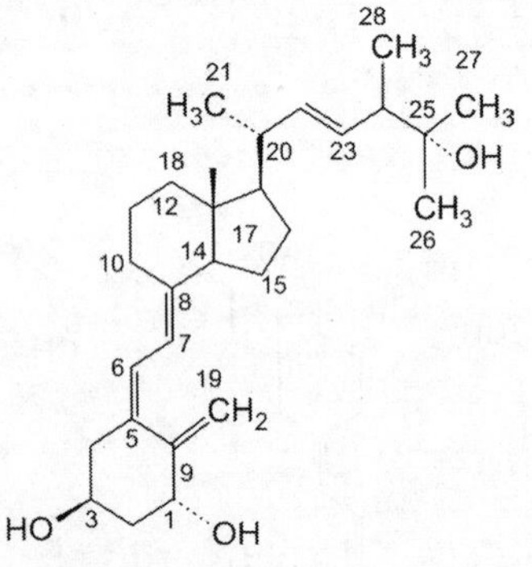

(31) 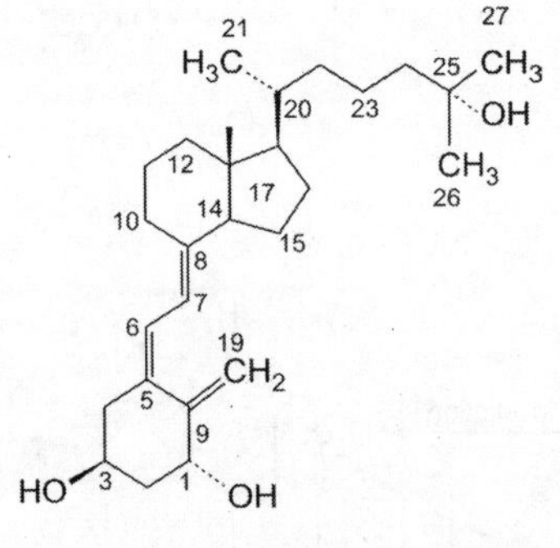   (32) 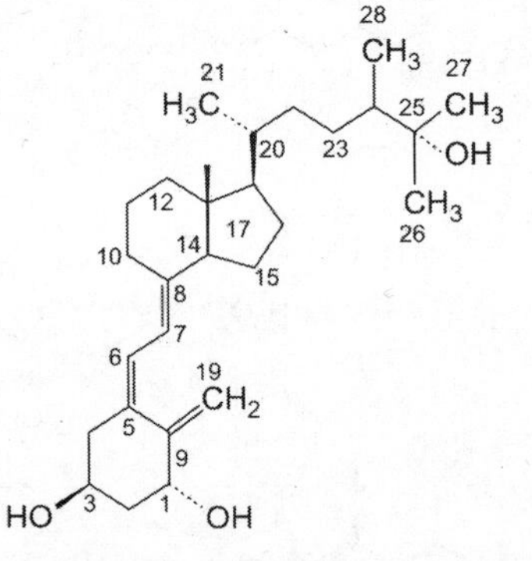   (33)

VITAMIN E

Vitamin E refers to two groups of compounds, namely tocopherols and tocotrienols. The former having a saturated side chain while as later, a side chain at position 2 with three double bonds. Each of these comprise of four homologs, namely α, β, γ, and δ, and are derivatives of 6-chromanol (34) or tocol (35). The four homologs differ in the number and position of methyl groups.

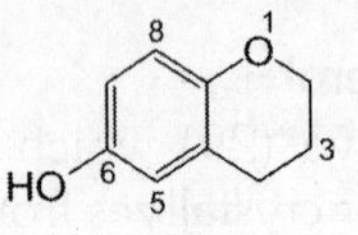

(34) 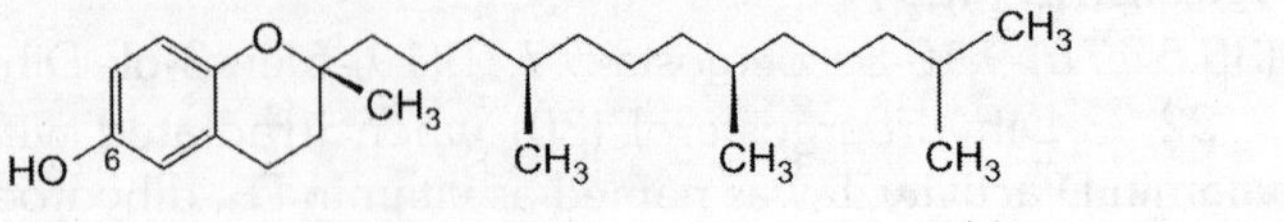   (35)

Tocopherols

These include, α-tocopherol [(+)-2,5,7,8-tetramethyl-2-(4', 8', 12'-trimethyltridecyl)-6-chromanol (36)]; β-tocopherol [(+)-2,5,8-trimethyl-2-(4',8',12'-trimethyltridecyl)-6-chromanol (37)]; γ-Tocopherol [(+)-2,7,8-trimethyl-2-(4', 8', 12'-trimethyltridecyl)-6-chromanol (38)]; and δ-Tocopherol [(+)-2,8-dimethyl-2-(4', 8', 12'-trimethyltridecyl)-6-chromanol (39)].

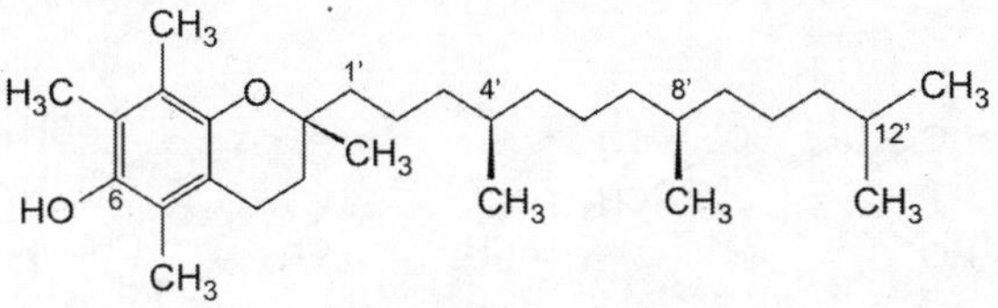

(36)

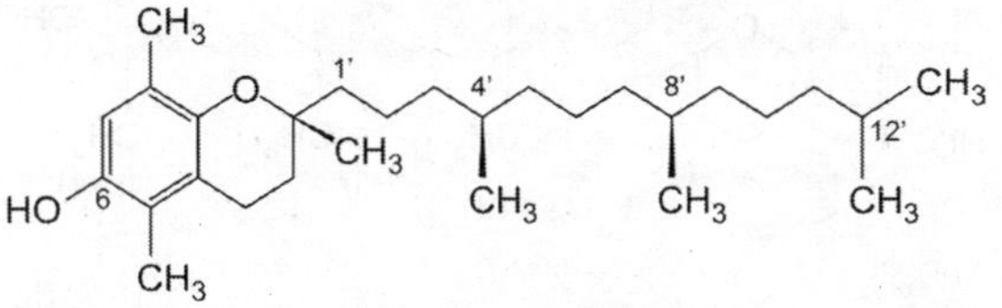

(37)

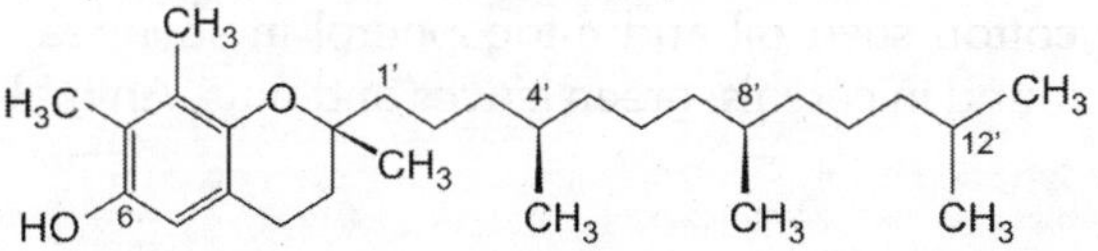

(38)

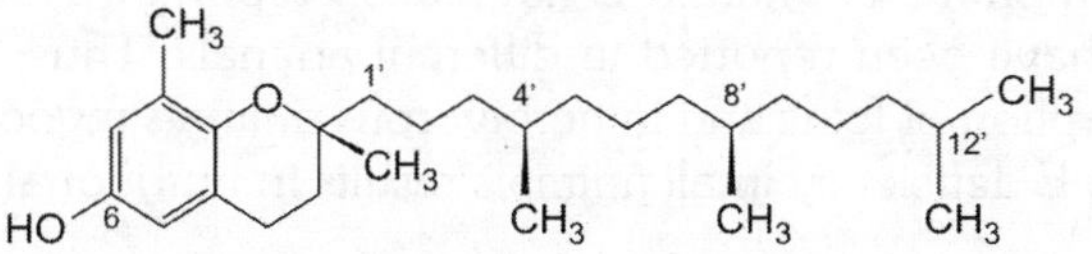

(39)

Trienols

α-Tocotrienol [(2R)-2,5,7,8-tetramethyl-2-(4',8',12'-trimethyl-3',7',11'-tridecatrienyl)-6-chromanol (40)]; β-tocotrienol [(2R)-2,5,8,-trimethyl-2-(4',8',12'-trimethyl-3',7',11'-tridcatrienyl)-6-chromanol (41)]; γ-Tocotrienol [(2R)-2,7,8-trimethyl-2-(4',8',12'-trimethyl-3',7',11'-tridecatrienyl)-6-chromanol (42)]; and δ-Tocotrienol [(2R)-2,8-dimethyl-2-(4',8',12'-trimethyl-3',7', 11'-tridecatrienyl)-6-chromanol (43)].

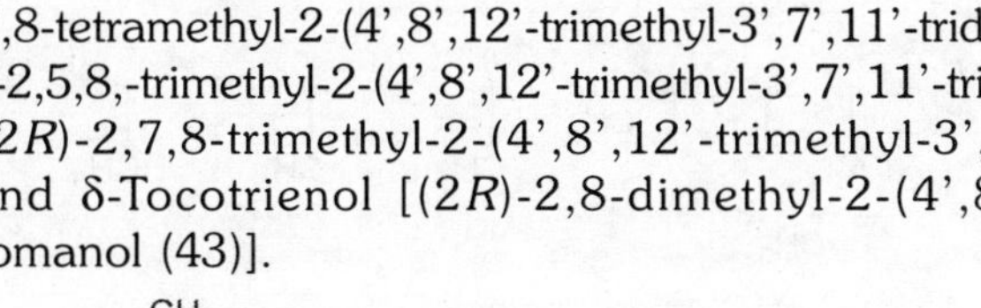

(40)

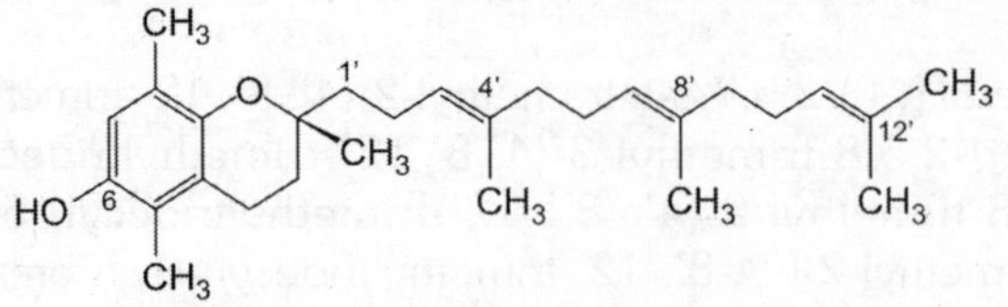

(41)

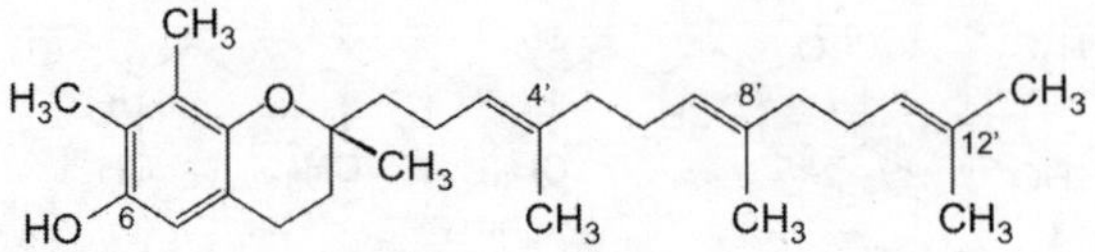

(42)

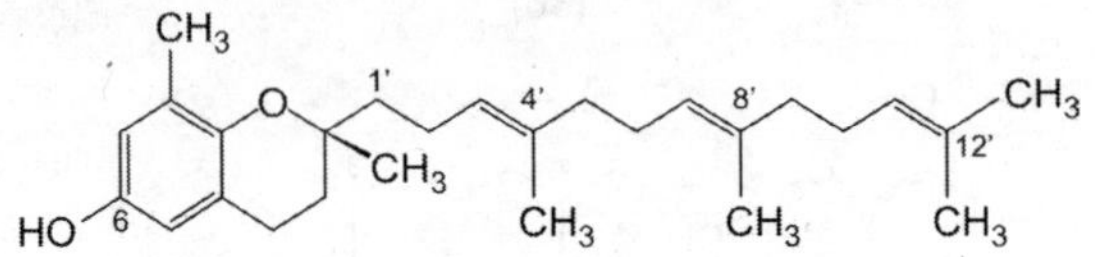

(43)

Sources

Tocopherols are found in free form in seed oils. α- and β-tocopherols are found in wheat germ oil. γ-tocopherol is found in cotton seed oil and δ-tocopherol in soyabean oil. In addition to these sources, vitamin E is also found in cereals, green leaves and nuts. Animals contain lower quantities of this vitamin.

Deficiency Diseases

No known deficiency symptoms of vitamin E have been reported. However, varying responses of vitamin E deficiency have been reported in different animals. Thus, in female rats, vitamin E deficiency results in resorption of fetus and in herbivorous animals myocardial degeneration takes place. In general vitamin E deficiency in all animals results in nutritional muscular dystrophy.

α-Tocopherol (36)

(+)-2,5,7,8-Tetramethyl-2-(4′,8′,12′-trimethyltridecyl)-6-chromanol

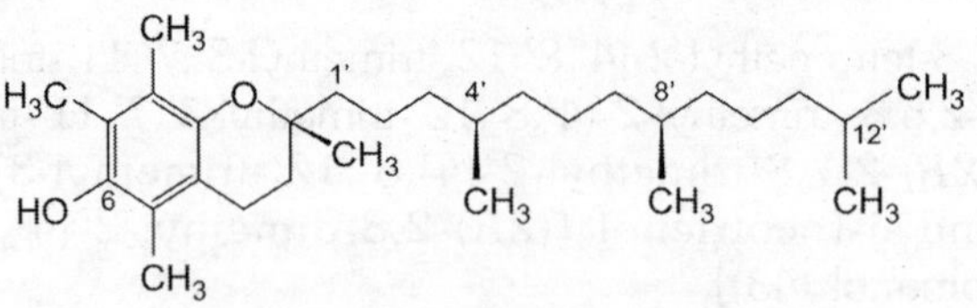

(36)

Structure

α-Tocopherol is a light yellow oil. It crystallizes as transparent needles, mp 2.5-3.5°, $[\alpha]^{25}_{546.1} + 0.32°$ (ethanol).

    1. Molecular formula $C_{29}H_{50}O_2$.

2. It forms monoesters and monoethers which indicates that it has one hydroxyl group. U.V. spectrum of α-tocopherol indicates that the hydroxyl group is phenolic in nature. The second oxygen was found to be a cyclic ether in nature.

3. Pyrolysis of α-tocopherol gives duroquinol (44), a known compound. Formation of duroquinol (44) confirms the presence of benzene nucleus in the molecule.

(44)

4. Oxidation with chromic acid under mild conditions converts α-tocopherol into dimethyl maleic anhydride (45), diacetyl (46), and an optically active lactone (47) with a molecular formula $C_{21}H_{40}O_2$.

(45)   (46)   (47)

5. The lactone (47) on hydrolysis yielded a hydroxy acid which readily lactonized indicating that hydroxyl and lactone were γ.

6. The hydroxyl group of the lactone (47) could neither be oxidized nor esterified. These observation indicated that the hydroxyl group was tertiary. Further when lactone (47) was hydrolyzed in presence of methyl alcohol, it gave a hydroxy ester which neither could be oxidized nor esterified confirming the tertiary nature of hydroxyl group.

(47)

7. α-Tocopherol (36) acetate on oxidation with chromic acid forms an acid (48) and a ketone (49). These compounds must be the oxidation products of lactone (47). Further, if one of the alkyl groups of the lactone (47) is methyl group then the formation of the acid (48) and the ketone (49) can be explained.

(47)   (48)

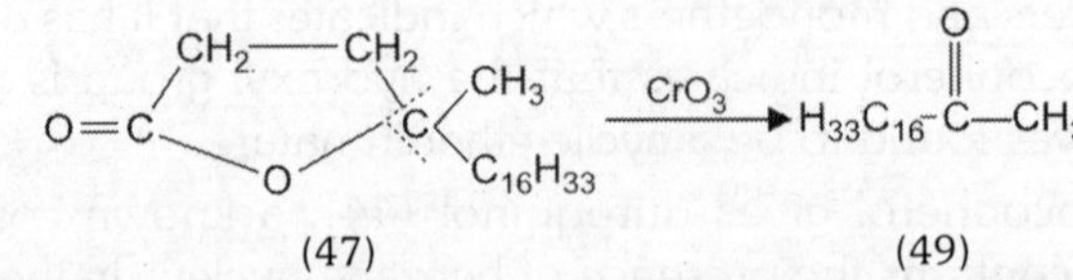

(47)　　　　　　　　　　　　　　　　　(49)

The Kuhn-Roth method of determining methyl group showed that acid (48) contained three methyl groups. Based on the observation that most of the naturally occurring compounds contain isoprene units, the acid was given the structure (48a) and the structure of corresponding γ-lactone could be (47a). Accordingly the α-tocopherol could be either chroman (50) or coumaran (51). U.V absorption spectra and subsequent synthesis of a-tocopherol indicated that it was having a chroman (50) structure. This was further confirmed by its synthesis (Fig. 38.4).

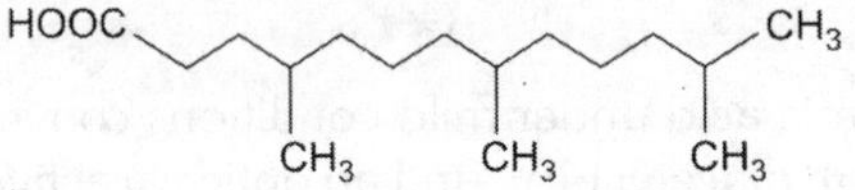

(48a)

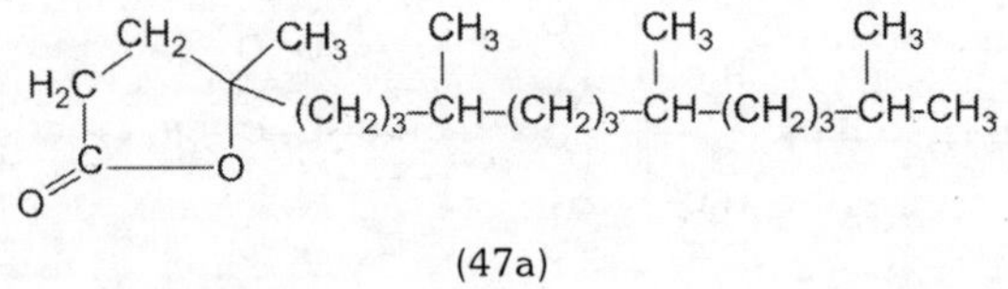

(47a)

(50)　　　　　　　　　　　　　　　　　(51)

Synthesis

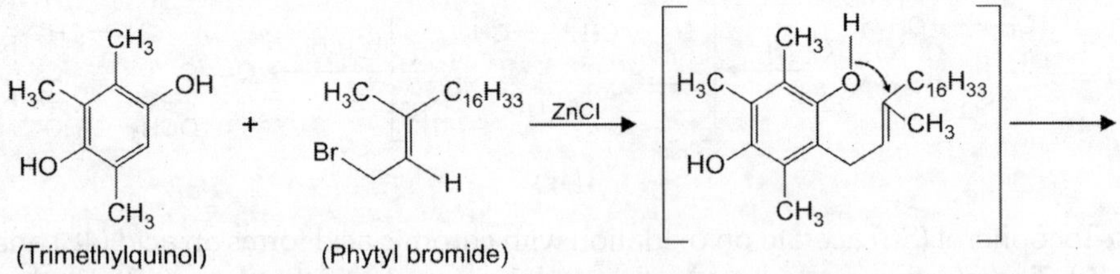

(Trimethylquinol)　　　　　(Phytyl bromide)

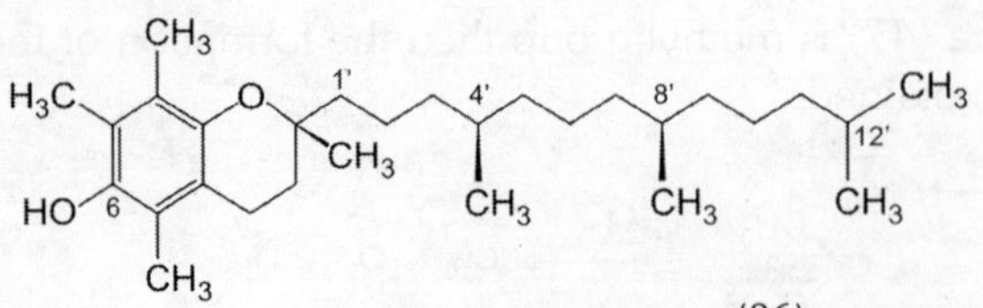

(36)

Fig. 38.4: Synthesis of α-tocopherol (36).

β-Tocopherol (37)

(+)-2,5,8-Trimethyl-2-(4',8',12'-trimethyltridecyl)-6-chromanol

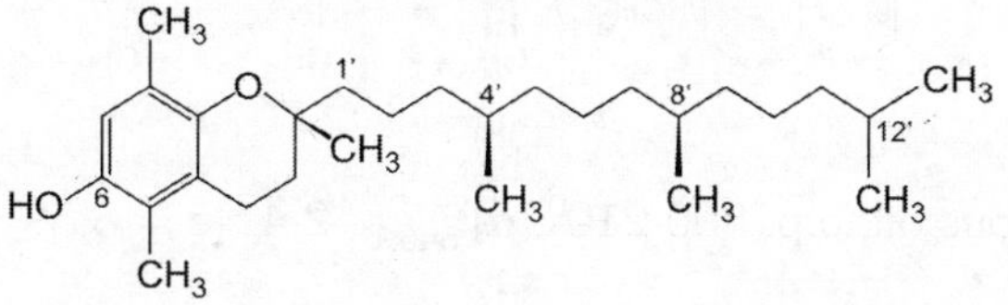

(37)

It is a pale yellow viscous oil, b.p. 200–210°, $[\alpha]_{546.1}^{25}$ +2.9° (c = 7.15 in ethanol).

Structure

1. Molecular formula $C_{28}H_{48}O_2$, which differs from α-tocopherol (36) by CH_2.
2. On pyrolysis β-tocopherol gives 2,3,5,-trimethylquinol (52) which differs from duroquinol (44) by CH_2.

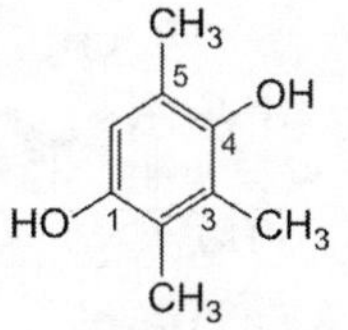

(52) 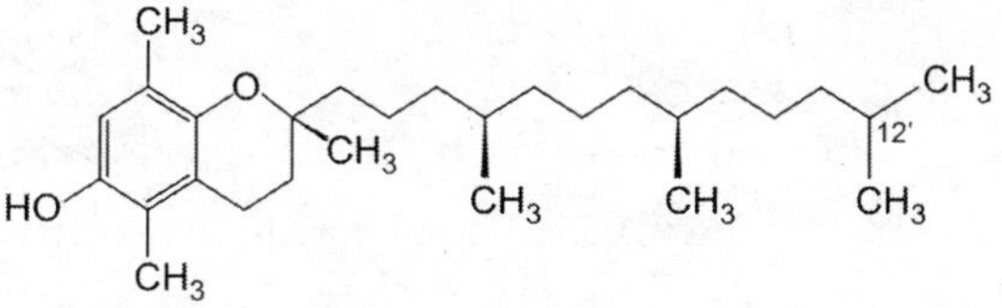   (37)

3. The tocopherols, thus, differ in benzenoid structure. Accordingly the β-tocopherol is (37), which is confirmed by synthesis (Fig. 38.5)

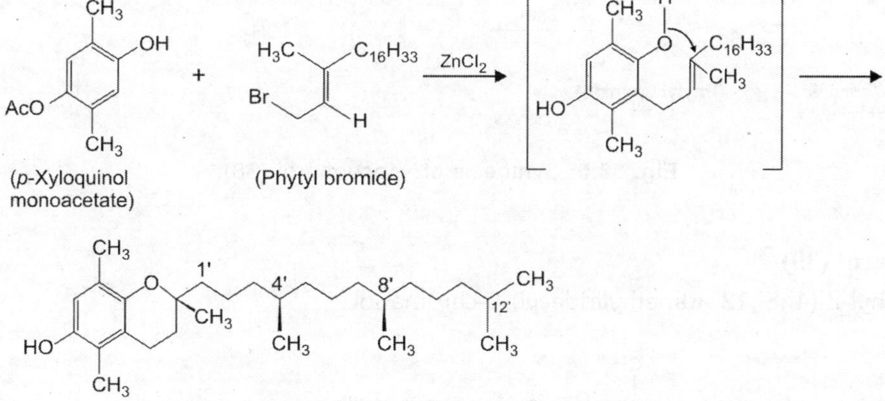

(37)

Fig. 38.5: Synthesis of β-tocopherol (37).

γ-Tocopherol (38)

(+)-2,7,8-trimethyl-2-(4',8',12'-trimethyltridecyl)-6-chromanol

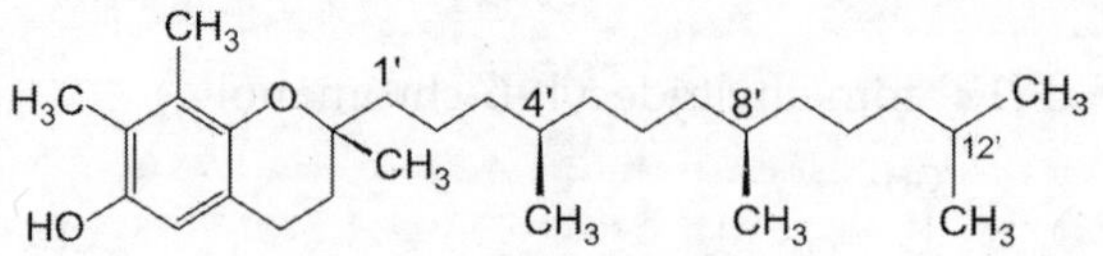

(38)

It is a pale yellow viscous oil, b.p. 200-210^0 $[\alpha]^{25}_{546.1}$ –2.4° (c = 8.59 in benzene).

Structure

1. Molecular formula $C_{28}H_{48}O_2$, which is the same as for β-tocopherol and therefore β- and γ-tocopherols must be isomers.

2. On pyrolysis γ-tocopherol yields 3,5,6,-trimethylquinol (53) which is isomeric with 2,3,5-trimethylquinol (52) confirming that β- and γ-tocopherols are isomers. Based on this the benzenoid ring in γ-tocopherol must be (54).

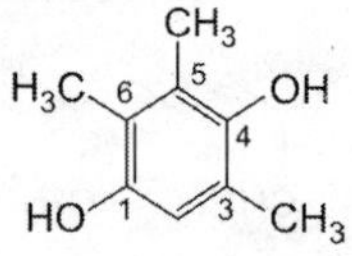

(53) 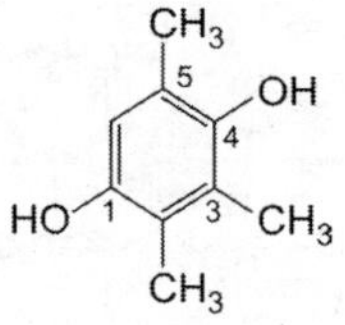   (52) 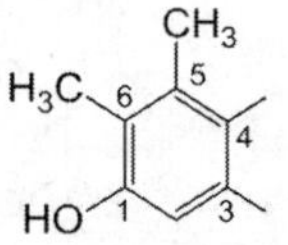   (54)

3. The structure was confirmed by the synthesis (Fig. 38.6).

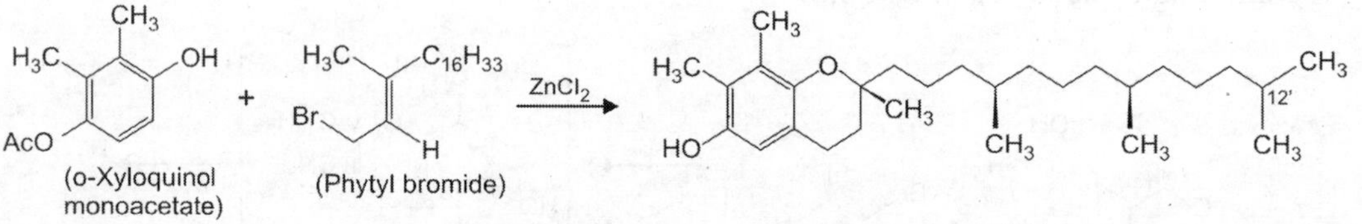

(o-Xyloquinol monoacetate)   (Phytyl bromide)   (38)

Fig. 38.6: Synthesis of γ-tocopherol (38).

δ-Tocopherol (39)

2,8-Dimethyl-2-(4',8',12'-trimethyltridecyl)-6-chromanol

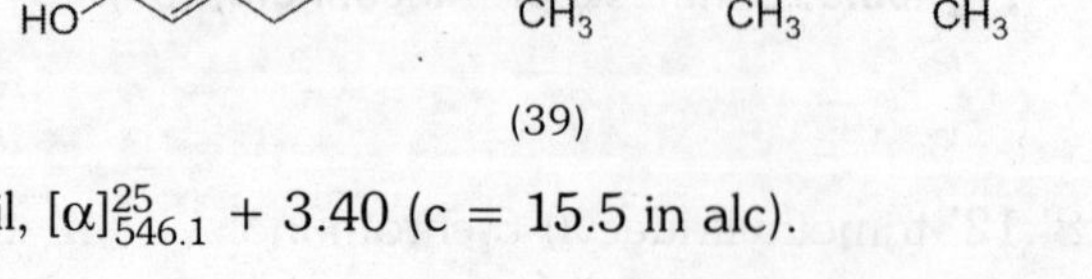

(39)

Pale yellow viscous oil, $[\alpha]^{25}_{546.1}$ + 3.40 (c = 15.5 in alc).

Structure

1. Molecular formula $C_{27}H_{46}O_2$.
2. The molecular formula of δ-tocopherol differs from β- and γ-tocopherols by CH_2.
3. On pyrolysis, δ-tocopherol yields 3,5-dimethylquinol (55) which differs from 3,5,6-trimethylquinol (55) by one methyl group indicating that the benzenoid portion of δ-tocopherol must be (56). Accordingly, δ-tocopherol must be (39). This was further confirmed by synthesis (Fig. 38.7).

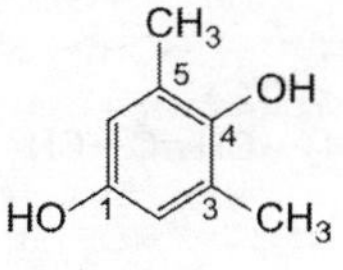

(55) 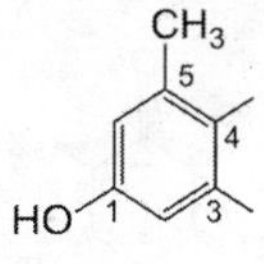   (56)

Synthesis

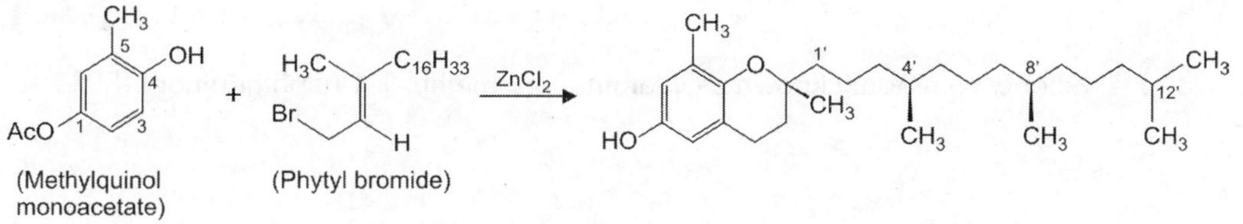

(Methylquinol monoacetate)   (Phytyl bromide)   (39)

Fig. 38.7: Synthesis of δ-tocopherol (39)

Biochemical Role

Tocopherols are lipophillic, as a result they associate with cell membranes, lipid deposits and lipoproteins in blood. The tocopherols react and destroy the most reactive forms of oxygen radicals and other free radicals thus preventing oxidative damage to membrane lipids which cause cell fragility. They also protect unsaturated fatty acids from oxidation. Vitamin E deficiency in humans is very rare, the principal symptom being presence of fragile erythrocytes.

VITAMIN K

Vitamin K is a general term used for naphthoquinone derivatives. These compounds have been classified into:

1. Phylloquinone [2-methyl-3-[(2'E,7'R,11'R)-3',7',11',15'-tetramethyl-2'-hexadecenyl]-1,4-naphthoquinone], commonly known as vitamin K_1 (57).

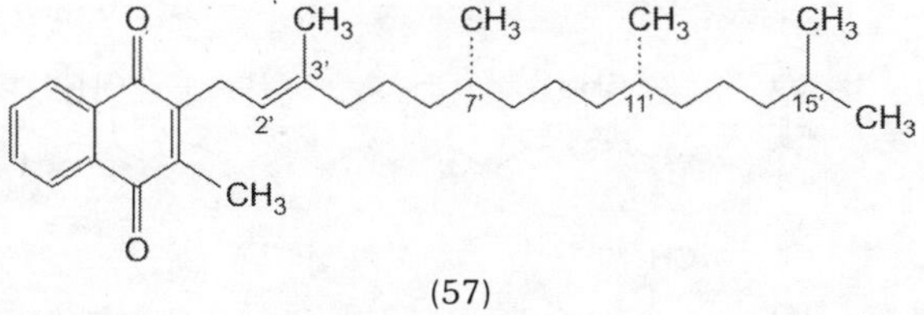

(57)

2. Menaquinones also known as vitamin K_2. They are 2-methyl-all *trans*-polyprenyl-1,4-naphthoquinones (58) and include:

(a) Menaquinone 4 or vitamin $K_{2(20)}$ [(all *E*)-2-methyl-3-(3',7',11',15'-tetramethyl-2',6'10'-14'-hexadecatetraenyl)-1,4-naphthalenedione (58a)].

(b) Menaquinone 6 or vitamin $K_{2(30)}$ [(all *E*)-2-methyl-3-(3',7',11',15',19',23',-hexamethyl-2',6',10',14',18',22'-tetracoshexaenyl)-1,4-naphthalenendione (58b)].

(c) Menaquinone 7 or vitamin $K_{2(35)}$ [(all *E*)-2-methyl-3-(3',7',11',15',19',23',27'-heptamethyl-2'.6',10',14',18',22',26'-octacosaheptaenyl)-1,4-naphthalenedione (58c)].

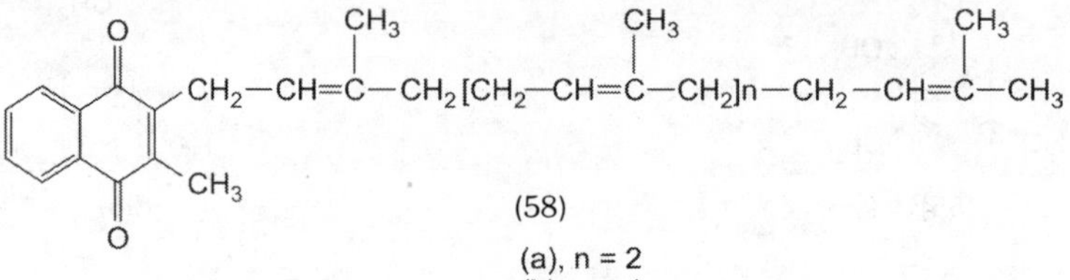

(58)

(a), n = 2
(b), n = 4
(c), n = 5

3. Menadione, commonly known as vitamin K_3 (2-methyl-1,4-naphthquinoe) (59).

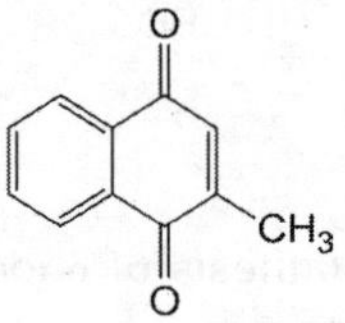

(59)

Sources

Vitamin K occur in all green leaves and vegetables, some of these include alfalfa, cabbage, cauliflower, spinach, etc.

Deficiency Diseases

Vitamin K helps in coagulation of blood. Its deficiency may result in increasing the clotting time and it is also possible that the blood may not clot at all resulting in death.

Vitamin K_1 (57)

2-Methyl-3-[(2'*E*,7'*R*,11'*R*)-3',7',11'15'-tetramethyl-2-hexadecenyl]-1,4-naphthoquinone; Phylloquione

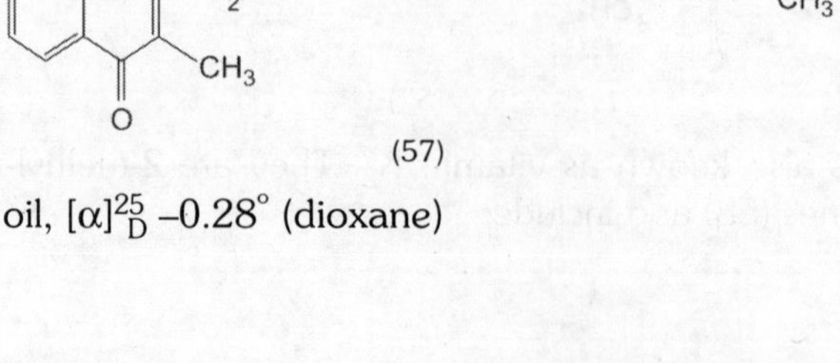

(57)

It is a yellow viscous oil, $[\alpha]_D^{25}$ –0.28° (dioxane)

Structure

1. Molecular formula $C_{31}H_{46}O_2$.
2. U.V. absorption spectra shows absorption maxima at 243, 249, 260, and 270 nm (ε 20,000). These bands are characteristics of 2,3-disubstituted 1,4-naphthoquinone. This indicates that vitamin K_1(57) is a 2,3-disubstituted naphthoquinone (60).

(60)

3. On catalytic hydrogenation, vitamin K_1(57) absorbs 4 moles of hydrogen yielding a substance with a molecular formula $C_{31}H_{54}O_2$. Since U.V absorption studies showed it to be analog of 1,4-naphthoquinone, 3 moles of hydrogen must have been used for reduction of naphthoquinone to naphthoquinol and the 4th molecule of hydrogen for the reduction of a double bond in side chain.
4. When vitamin K_1 (57) is oxidized with chromic acid, it gives phthalic acid, which must have been produced because of oxidation of quinone and side chain, indicating that there must be present a side chain in the naphthoquinone ring system.
5. Oxidation of vitamin K_1 (57) under controlled conditions, yields a compound having molecular formula $C_{13}H_{10}O_4$. Structural determination studies have shown it to be 2-methyl-1,4-naphthoquinone-3-acetic acid (61). These observations indicate that there is present a methyl group at position 2 and there is a side chain at position 3 which is oxidized to carboxylic acid.

(61)

6. Ozonolysis of diacetate of dihydrovitamin K_1 yielded diacetate of 2-methyl-1,4-naphthoquinol-3-acetic acid (62) and a ketone which was the same as obtained by oxidation of phytol (63). The ketone is accordingly (64).

(62)

(63)

(64)

Based on above the structure of vitamin K_1 must be (57).

Some of the reactions of vitamin K_1 (57) are given in Fig. 38.8 and synthesis in Fig. 38.9.

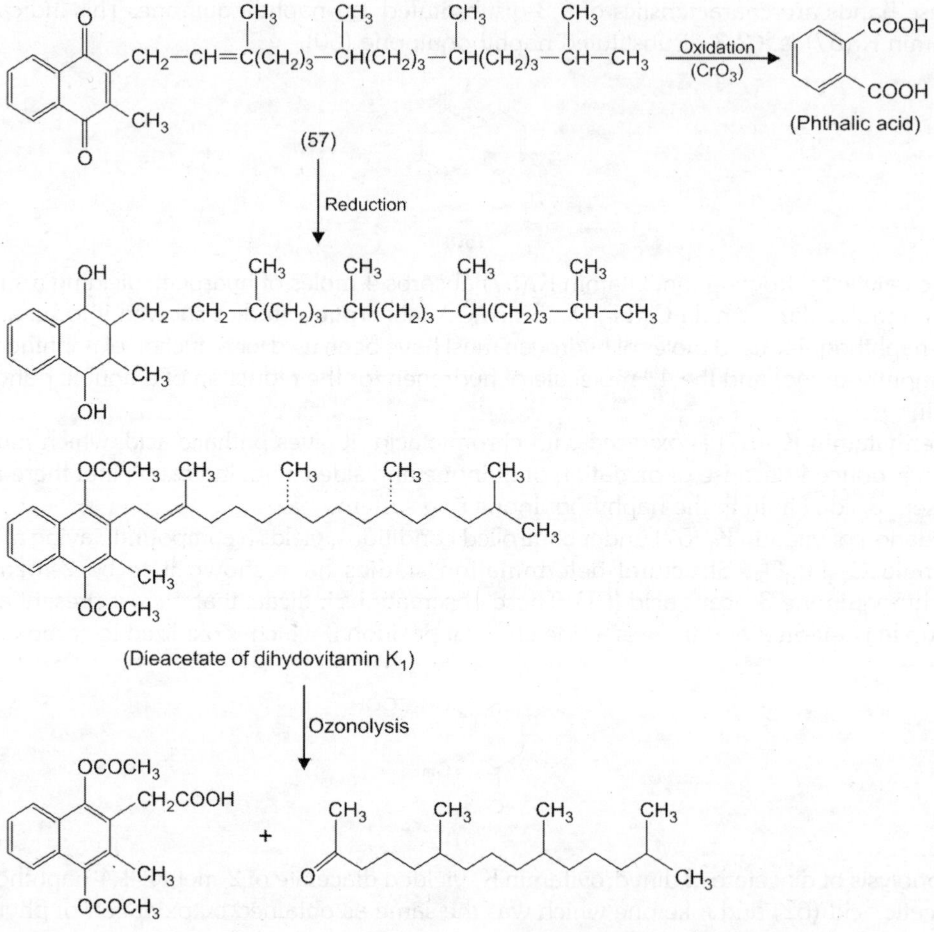

Fig. 38.8: Reactions of vitamin K_1 (57).

Synthesis

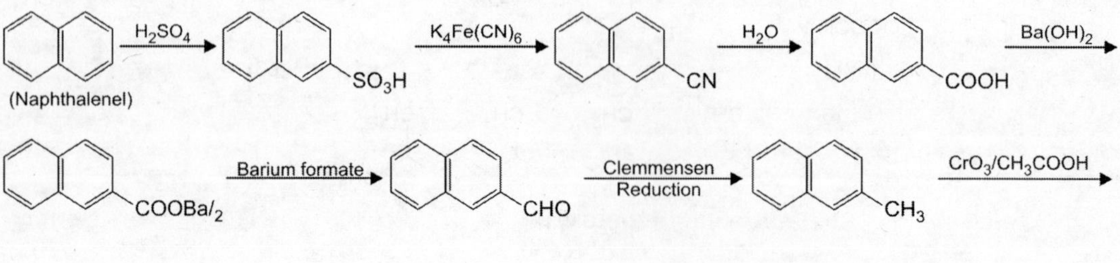

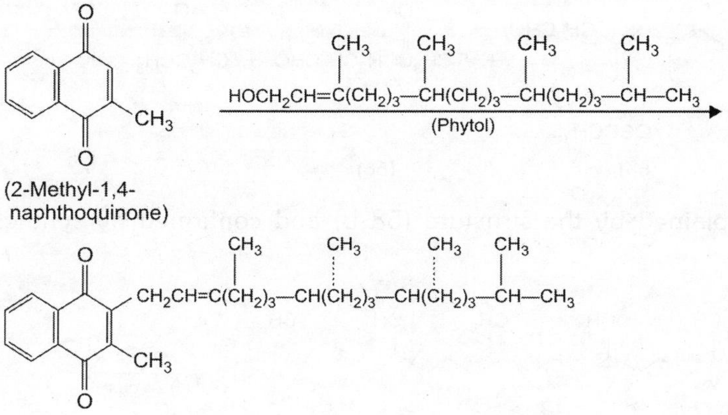

Fig. 38.9: Synthesis of vitamin K_1 (57).

Vitamin $K_{2(30)}$ (58b)

(all E)-2-Methyl-3-(3',7',11',15',19',23'-hexamethyl-2',6',10',14',18',22'-tetracoshexaenyl)-1,4-naphthalene dione; Menaquinone 6; 2-Difarnesyl-3-methyl-1,4-naphthoquinone

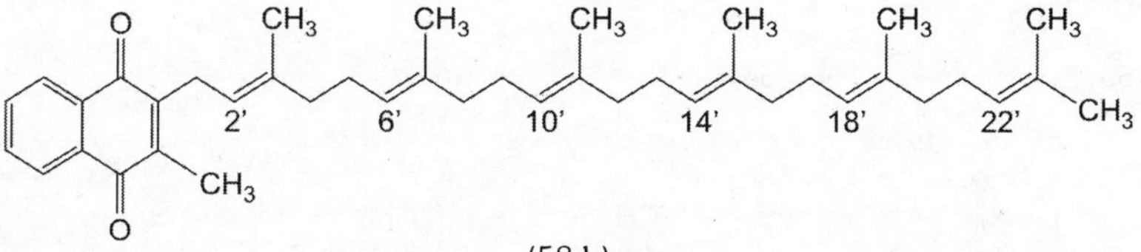

(58 b)

Yellow crystals mp 50° (acetone/alcohol) U.V max (petroleum ether, 243, 248, 261, 270, 325-328 nm) ($E^{1\%}_{1cm}$, 304, 320, 290, 292, 53).

Structure

1. Molecular formula $C_{41}H_{56}O$.
2. It shows ultraviolet spectrum similar to that of 1,4-napthoquinone indicating that like vitamin K_1 (57) it also contains 1,4-naphthoquinone system.
3. When reduced catalytically, it adds-up nine moles of hydrogen. Since 3 moles of hydrogen are used for reduction of 1,4-naphthoquinone, the other six moles of hydrogens must be used for reduction of six double bonds which must be present in the side chain. This was further confirmed by treating diacetyldihydro vitamin K_2 with bromine resulting in absorbtion of six bromine molecules.
4. Oxidation of vitamin $K_{2(30)}$ with permanganate gives phthalic acid, indicating that the benzene ring of 1,4-naphthoquinone is unsubstituted.
5. When a solution of vitamin $K_{2(30)}$ in acetic acid is treated with ozone and the product treated with zinc dust in ether, 1 mole of 1,4-diacetoxy-2-methylnaphthalene-3-acetaldehyde (65), 5 mole of laevulaldehyde (66) and one mole of acetone (67) are obtained.

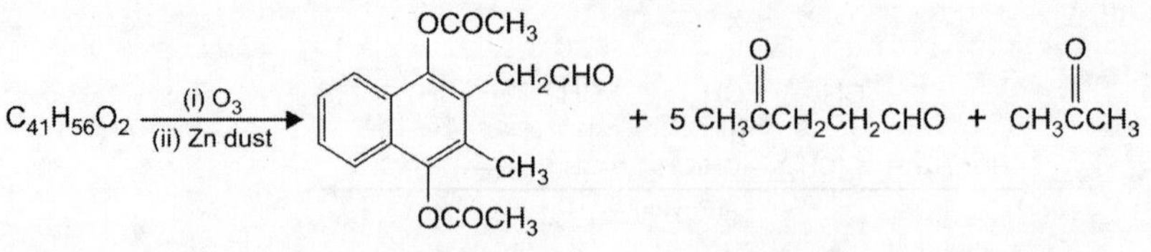
$C_{41}H_{56}O_2$
(i) O_3
(ii) Zn dust
$OCOCH_3$
CH_2CHO
CH_3
$OCOCH_3$
+ 5 $CH_3CCH_2CH_2CHO$ + CH_3CCH_3

(65) (66) (67)

6. These reactions can be explained by the structure (58 b) and confirmed by synthesis (Fig. 38.10)

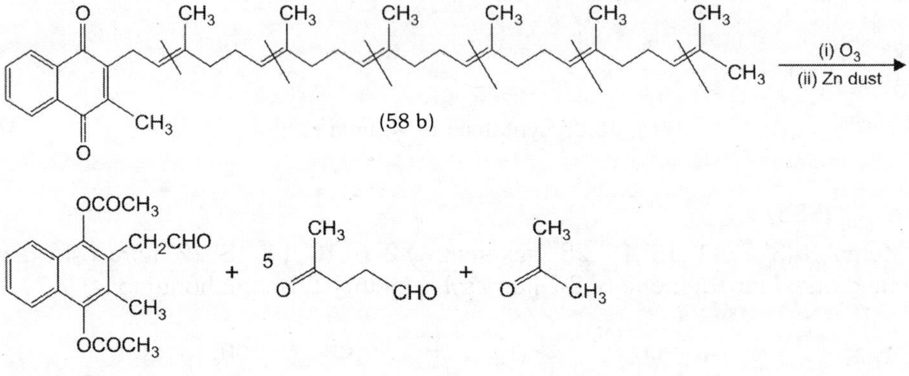
(58 b)
(i) O_3
(ii) Zn dust
$OCOCH_3$
CH_2CHO
CH_3
+ 5
CHO
+

(65) (66) (67)

Synthesis

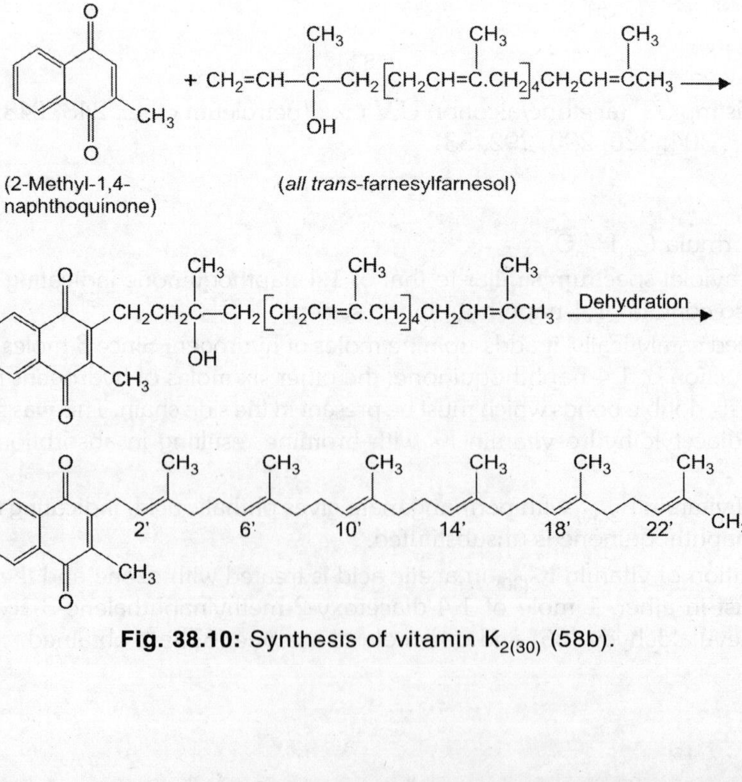
+ CH_2=CH—C—CH_2[CH_2CH=C.CH_2]$_4$$CH_2$CH=$CCH_3$
OH
(2-Methyl-1,4-naphthoquinone)
(all trans-farnesylfarnesol)
CH_2CH_2C—CH_2[CH_2CH=C.CH_2]$_4$$CH_2$CH=$CCH_3$
Dehydration
2'
6'
10'
14'
18'
22'

Fig. 38.10: Synthesis of vitamin $K_{2(30)}$ (58b).

Biochemical Role

The biochemical role of vitamin K is discussed under **Anticoagulants, Antiplatelet, and Thrombolytic Drugs.**

The water soluble vitamins include vitamin B group and ascorbic acid (vitamin C).

VITAMIN B GROUP

Vitamin B group constitutes, thiamine (vitamin B_1), riboflavin (vitamin B_2), nicotinic acid and nicotinamide (vitamin B_3), pantothenic acid (vitamin B_5), pyridoxine, pyridoxal, and pyridoxamine (vitamin B_6), biotin (vitamin B_7), Folic acid (vitamin B_9), and cyanocobalamin (vitamin B_{12}).

Thiamine (68)

3-[(4-Amino-2-methyl-5-pyrimidinyl)methyl]-5-(2-hydrxyethyl)-4-methylthiazolinium chloride; Vitamin B_1; Aneurin

(68)

Vitamin B_1 is commonly known as thiamine. It is obtained in crystalline form as a salt, thiamine chloride hydrochloride, mp 248° (dec.) and as mononitrate, mp 196-200° (dec).

Sources

The richest sources of thiamine are rice polishings, yeast, eggs, and liver. Green leafy vegetables, milk, fish, nuts, and legumes are also some of the sources of this vitamin.

Deficiency Diseases

Thiamine deficiency results in beriberi and the major organ affected are nervous system, cardiovascular system, and gastrointestinal tract.

Some of the compounds used in clinical practice include thiamine chloride hydrochloride and thiamine mononitrate.

Structure

1. The crystalline salt of thiamine, the thiamine chloride hydrochloride has the molecular formula $C_{12}H_{18}Cl_2N_4OS$.
2. The thiamine chloride hydrochloride on treatment with sodium sulphite yields compound (I) and compound (II) along with sodium chloride.

$$C_{12}H_{18}Cl_2N_4OS + Na_2SO_3 \longrightarrow C_6H_9NOS + C_6H_9N_3O_3S + 2NaCl$$

Compound I Compound II

Compound I

1. Molecular formula C_6H_9NOS.
2. The nitrogen was found to be tertiary because it does not react with nitrous acid.
3. The oxygen function was found to be alcoholic in nature. Further, the alcoholic function was found in the side chain, because the UV spectrum of the chloro derivative was the same as that of parent hydroxyl compound.
4. The sulphur atom was unreactive and did not give any reaction of a mercapto or sulphide group. These observation led to suggestion that compound I is a thiazole derivative.
5. Thiamine as well as compound I on oxidation with nitric acid gave an acid which was identified as 4-methylthiazole-5-carboxylic acid (69), having a molecular formula of $C_5H_5NO_2S$. A comparison of molecular formulas of compound I and (69) shows that this oxidation of compound has resulted in loss of one carbon atom. Based on this, compound I could be either (70) or (71). Both (70) and (71) account for the reactions shown by compound I. Since compound I was found to be optically inactive and (71) is asymmetric, so this can be excluded and structure of compound I must be (70). This was further confirmed by synthesis (Fig. 38.11).

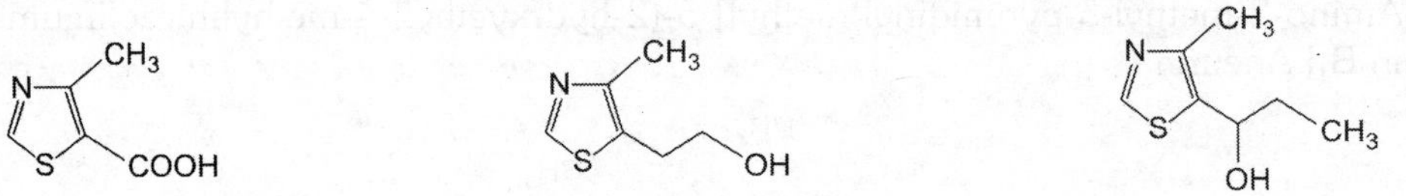

(69)   (70)   (71)

Synthesis

Step 1

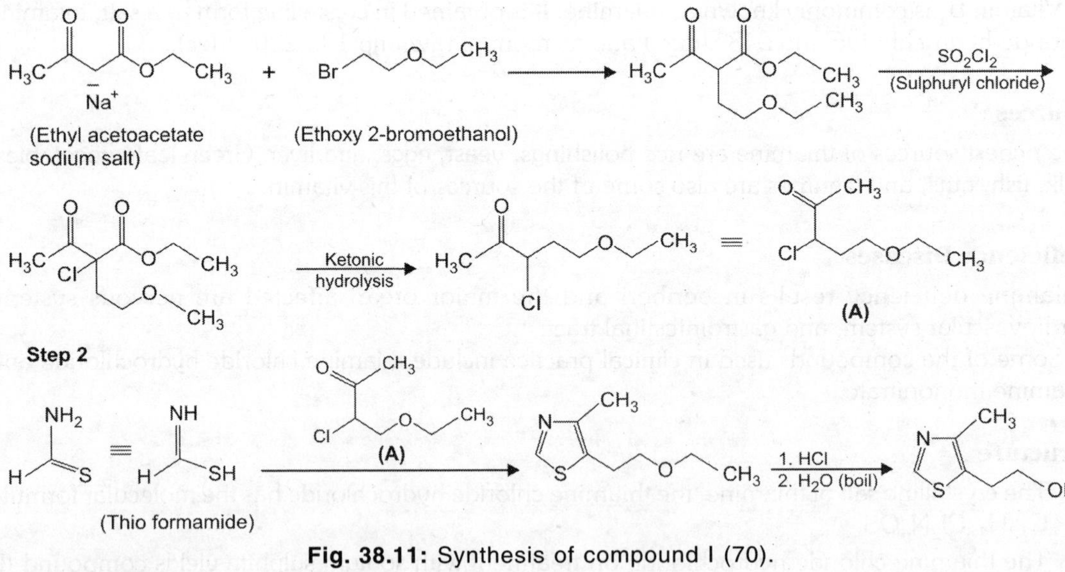

(Ethyl acetoacetate sodium salt)   (Ethoxy 2-bromoethanol)

Step 2

(Thio formamide)   (A)

Fig. 38.11: Synthesis of compound I (70).

Compound II

1. Molecular formula $C_6H_9N_3O_3S$.
2. When compound II is heated with water under pressure, it gives sulphuric acid indicating that sulphur must be present as sulphonic acid group.

3. Reduction of compound II with sodium in liquid ammonia gives aminodimethyl pyrimidine, which was found to be 2,5-dimethyl-4-aminopyrimidine (72). This was further confirmed by the synthesis of (72) (Fig. 38.12).

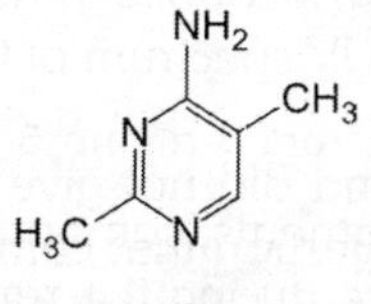

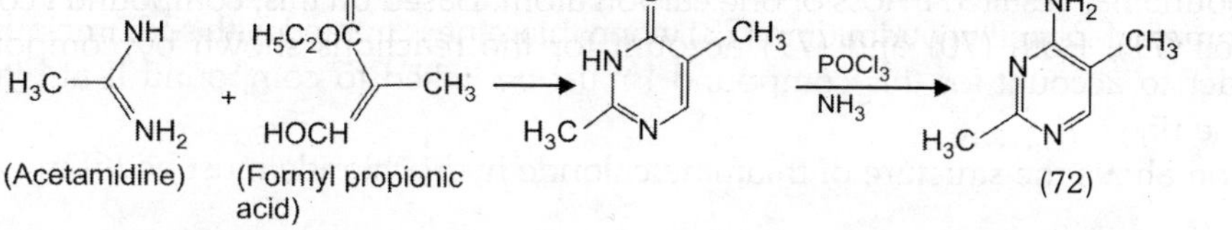

Fig. 38.12: Synthesis of 2,5-dimethyl-4-aminopyrimidine (72).

4. From the above it could be concluded that during the reduction of compound II by sodium in liquid ammonia, the sulphonic acid group is removed resulting in the formation of 2,5-dimethyl-4-aminopyrimidine. Thus, compound II is 2,5-dimethyl-4-aminopyimidine (72) with one hydrogen of 5-methyl group replaced by sulphonic acid group.

5. During the reduction of thiamine with sodium in liquid ammonia another compound was also isolated and it was identified as 4-amino-5-aminomethyl-2-methylpyrimidine (73). Its structure was further confirmed by its synthesis (Fig. 38.13).

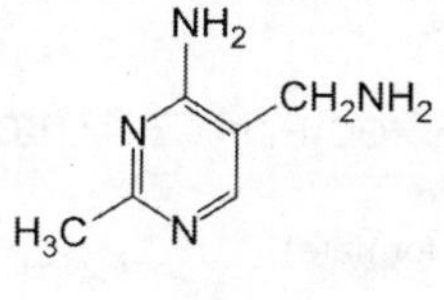

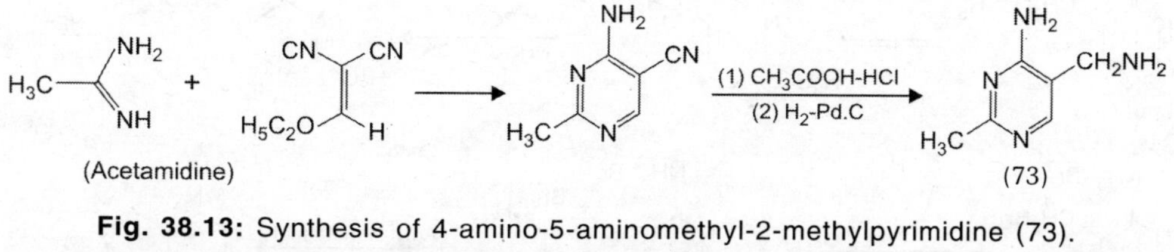

Fig. 38.13: Synthesis of 4-amino-5-aminomethyl-2-methylpyrimidine (73).

6. Thus, in 4-amino-5-methylamino-2-methylpyrimidine (73) there is an amino group instead of sulphonic acid group in compound II. Accordingly, it was concluded that sulphonic acid group in compound II must be linked to the methylene group at position 5. This was further confirmed by synthesis of compound II from (73) (Fig. 38.14).

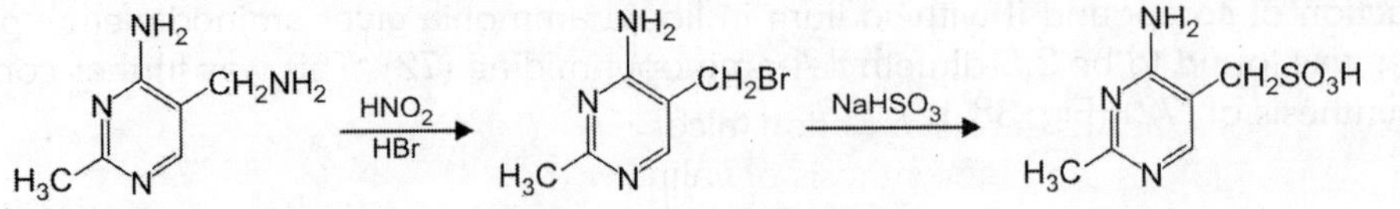

Fig. 38.14: Synthesis of compound II from 4-amino-5-methylamino-2-methylpyrimidine (73).

7. Next, the question is how the two fragments, compound I and compound II, are linked to each other in the parent compound. Since during the reaction of thiamine with sodium sulphite, sulphonic group is introduced into compound II, therefore, the point of attachment in compound II must be at CH$_2$ group at position 5 of the pyrimidine nucleus. Further, if compound II is linked to compound I through carbon, it is not possible to account for the formation of 4-amino-5-amniomethyl-2-methyl pyrimidine (73) when thiamine is treated with sodium/liquid ammonia. In order to account for this compound I must be linked to compound II at nitrogen of the thiazole ring.

Based on above the structure of thiamine chloride hydrochloride must be (68a)

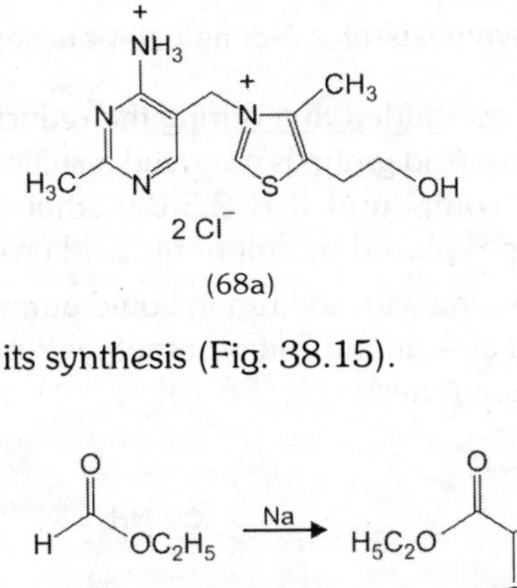

(68a)

This was further confirmed by its synthesis (Fig. 38.15).

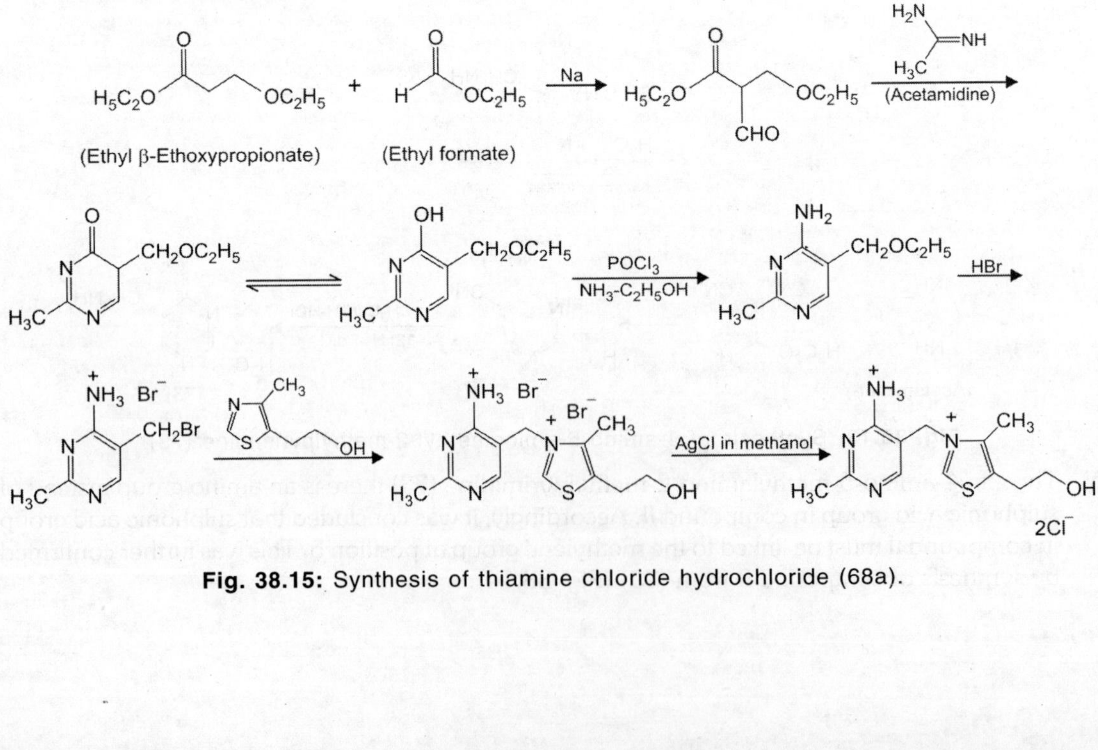

Fig. 38.15: Synthesis of thiamine chloride hydrochloride (68a).

Biochemical Role

Thiamine as thiamine pyrophosphate (74) is co-enzyme of many enzymes involved in various biochemical reactions such as decarboxylation (alcohol fermentation), synthesis of acyl CoA, carbon fixation in photosynthesis, and biosynthesis of valine and leucine as llustrated below (Fig. 38.16).

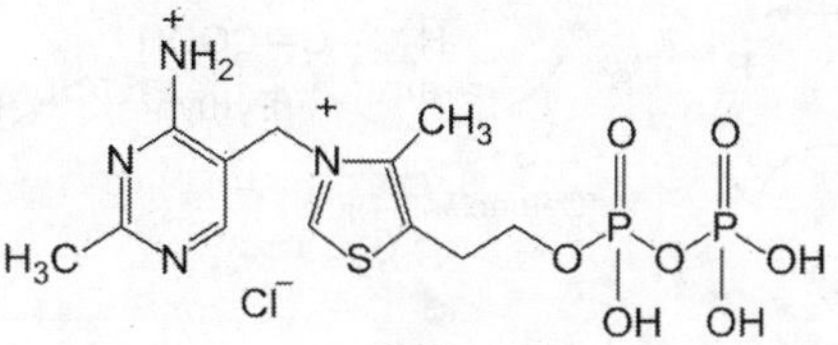

(74)

Alcohol fermentaion

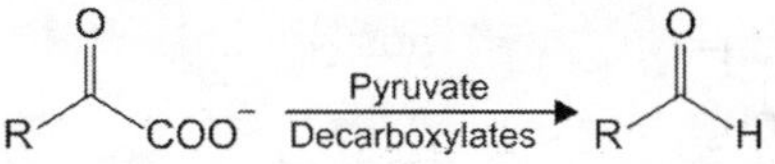

Synthesis of Acyl CoA

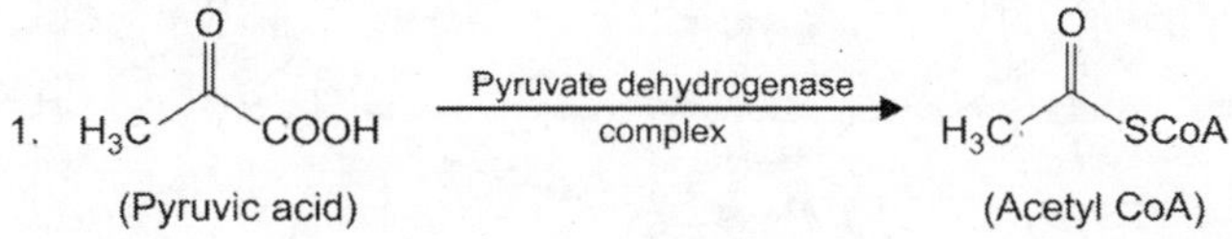

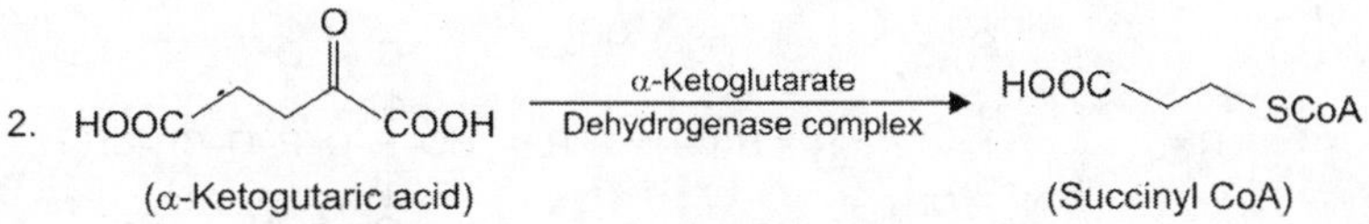

1. (Pyruvic acid) — Pyruvate dehydrogenase complex → (Acetyl CoA)

2. (α-Ketogutaric acid) — α-Ketoglutarate Dehydrogenase complex → (Succinyl CoA)

Photosynthesis

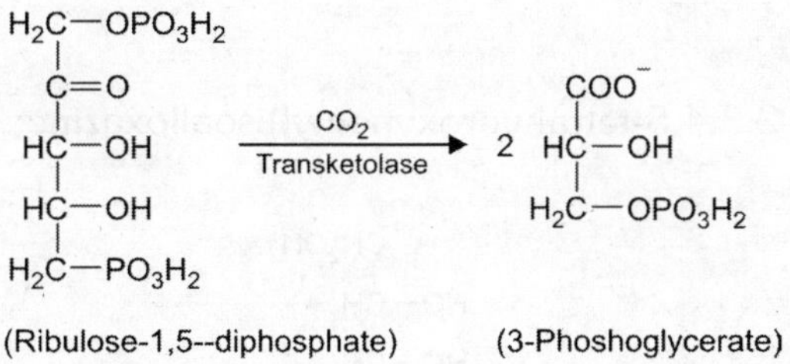

(Ribulose-1,5--diphosphate) — CO_2 Transketolase → 2 (3-Phoshoglycerate)

Synthesis of Valine and Leucine

Pyruvate — Acetoacetate Synthetase → (α-Acetolactate) → Valine / Leucine

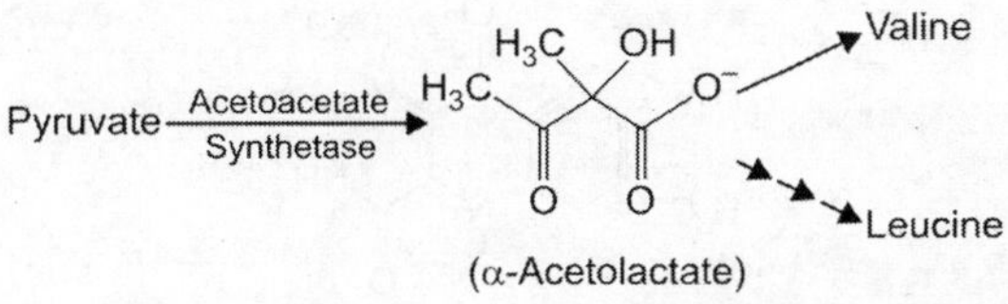

Fig. 38.16: Some of the thiamine pyrophosphate (74) dependent biochemical reactions.

The mechanism of pyruvate decarboxylation by thiamine pyrophosphate (74) is given below (Fig. 38.17).

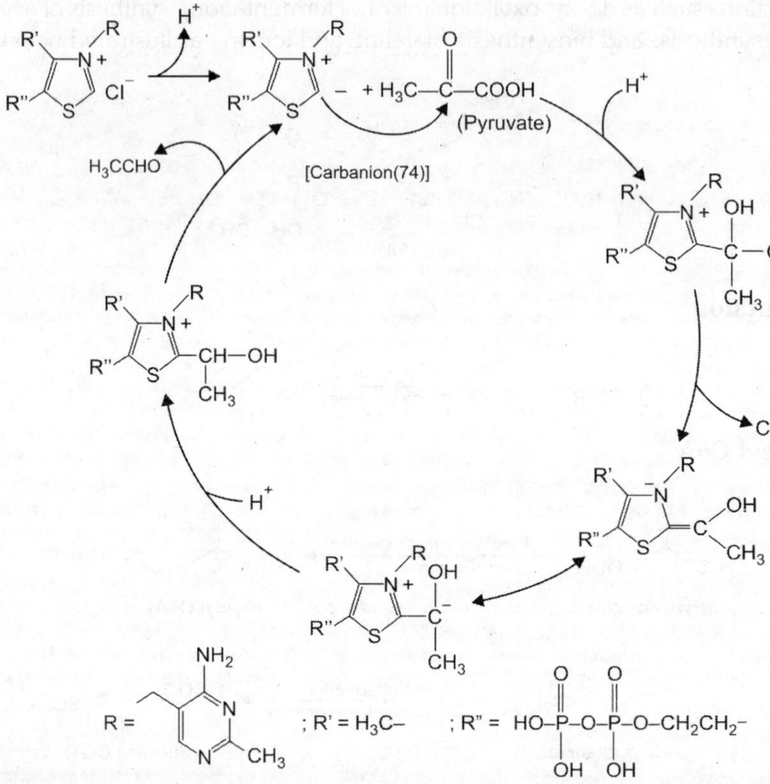

Fig. 38.17: Mechanism of pyruvate decarboxylation by thiamine pyrophosphate (74).

Riboflavin (75)

7,8-Dimethyl-10-(D-*ribo*-2,3,4,5-tetrahydroxypentyl)isoalloxazine; Vitamin B_2; Lactoflavin; Vitamin G

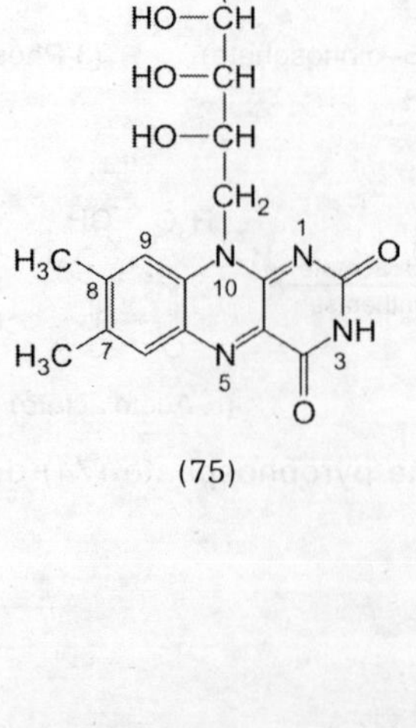

(75)

Riboflavin (75) crystallizes as orange-yellow needles from alcohol, mp 278-282°(dec.). Three different crystal forms having different solubilities in water have been isolated, $[\alpha]_D^{25}$ –112 to –120° (c = 50 mg/2ml 0.1N alcoholic NaOH diluted to 10 ml with water).

Sources

Riboflavin is found in eggs, milk, yeast green vegetables, and germinated seeds

Deficiency Diseases

Riboflavin deficiency causes ariboflavinosis. It is charecterzed by cheilosis – a disorder of lips, corneal and other changes in eye, and dermatitis seborrheia – an acute inflammatory form occurring on oily skin.

Structure

1. Molecular formula $C_{17}H_{20}N_4O_6$.
2. Silver salt of riboflavin on acetylation gives a tetraacetate, indicating the presence of four hydroxyl groups.
3. Oxidation of riboflavin with lead tetraacetate gives formaldehyde indicating the presence of a primary alcoholic group.
4. A solution of riboflavin in sodium hydroxide when exposed to light yields lumi-lactoflavin (76), molecular formula $C_{13}H_{12}N_4O_2$. The lumi-lactoflavin (76) on boiling with barium hydroxide yields one molecule of urea (77) and one molecule of barium salt of a β-keto. acid (78), the molecular formula of which was found to be $C_{12}H_{12}N_2O_3$.
5. The β-ketoacid (78) on treatment with acid loses one molecule of carbon dioxide and yields a compound with molecular formula $C_{11}H_{12}N_2O$ (79). Compound (79) was shown to be a lactam. Boiling of (79) with sodium hydroxide yields glyoxylic acid (80) and one molecule of a diamine $C_9H_{14}N_2$(81).

All these reactions are summarized in Fig. 38.18.

$$C_{17}H_{20}N_4O_6 \xrightarrow{\text{Light}} C_{13}H_{12}N_4O_2 \xrightarrow{\text{Ba(OH)}_2} H_2NCONH_2 + (C_{12}H_{12}N_2O_3)_2Ba$$

(75)   (76)   (77)   (78)

$$(C_{12}H_{12}N_2O_3)_2Ba \xrightarrow{\text{Acid}} C_{11}H_{12}N_2O \xrightarrow[\text{NaOH}]{\text{Boil with}} \begin{matrix} \text{CHO} \\ | \\ \text{COOH} \end{matrix} + C_9H_{14}N_2$$

(78)   (79)   (80)   (81)

Fig. 38.18: Reactions of riboflavin.

7. The diamine (81) was shown to be an analog of monomethyl-*o*-pheylenediamine (82) as it gave a blue preceipitate with ferric chloride. a characteristic of such compounds. The molecular formula of monomethyl-*o*-phenylendiamine (82) corresponds to $C_7H_{10}N_2$ which is two carbon and four hydrogens less than the diamine (81) obtained from lumi-lactoflavin (76). The structure of the diamine could then be either (81a) or (81b).

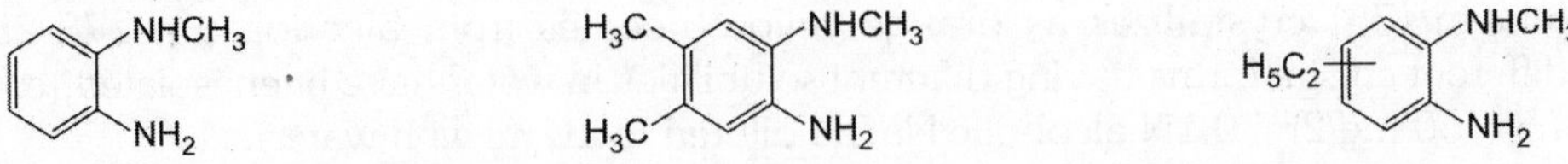

(82) (81a) (81b)

8. A comparision of (81a) obtained synthetically (Fig. 38.19) with (81) obtained from lumi-lactoflavin (76) showed that both were same. Accordingly (81) is *N*-methyl-4,5-diamino-*o*-xylene (81a).

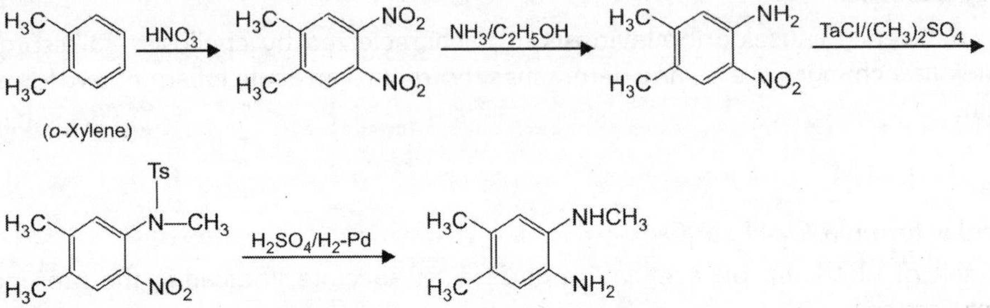

Fig. 38.19: Synthesis of N-methyl-4,5-diamino-o-xylene (81a).

9. Based on this, the structure of $C_{11}H_{12}N_2O$ which can readily produce glyoxylic acid (80) and the diamine (81a) is (79).

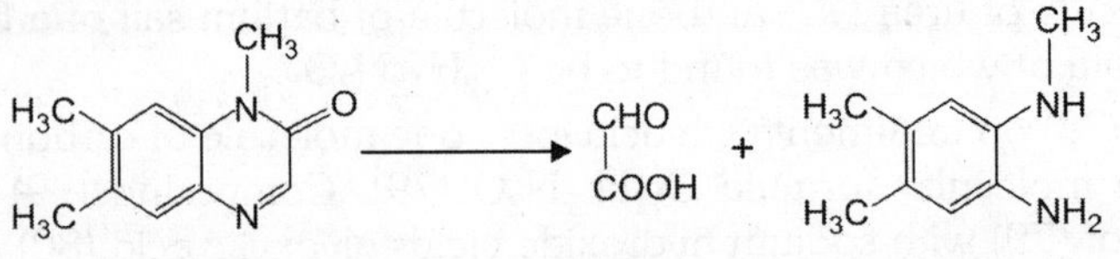

(79) (80) (81a)

Further, since lactam (79) is produced by decarboxylation of a β-ketoacid the structrue of β-ketoacid acid is (78).

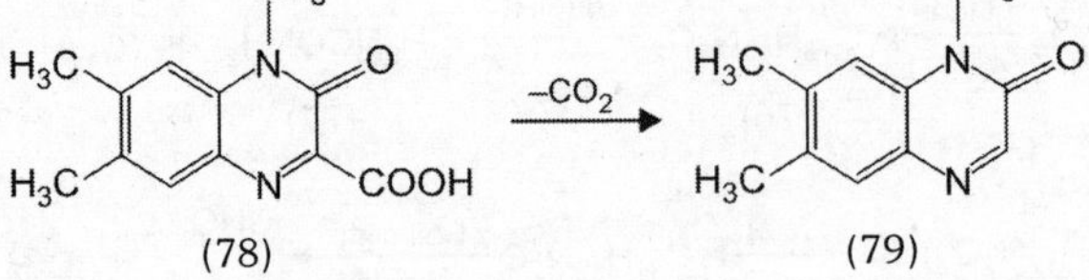

(78) (79)

10. The compound (78) along with urea is obtained from lumi-lactoflavin with barium hydroxide. Accordingly the structure of lumi-lactoflavin is (76).

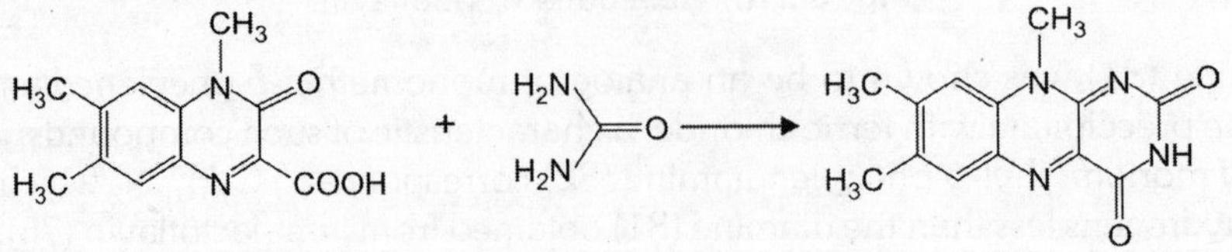

(78) (77) (76)

11. The structure of lumi-lactoflavin (76) was further confirmed by synthesizing it from *N*-methyl-4,5-diamino-*o*-xylene (81a) with alloxan (83)

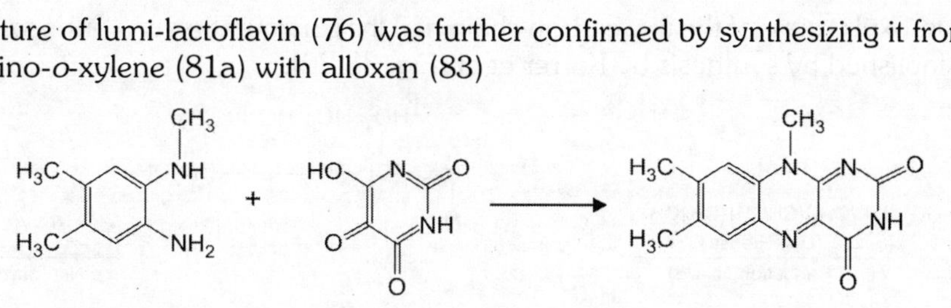

(81a) (83) (76)

Side Chain

1. Estimation of active hydrogen atoms by Zerewitnoff procedure shows that riboflavin contains five active hydrogen atoms. Out of these one must be on the nitrogen at position 3.
2. Since silver salt (84) of riboflavin forms tetraacetate (85) on acetylation, so there must be four hydroxyl groups' in the side chain.
3. Out of these four hydroxyl groups, one must be a primary alcoholic group because riboflavin on oxidation with lead tetraacetate gives one molecule of formaldehyde.
4. Further, the four hydroxyl groups must be attached to four carbons in a 1,2-glycol system, since riboflavin forms diisopropylidene derivative (86) on treatment with acetone.
5. All these observations indicate that there must be a five carbon chain attached to riboflavin and this can be accounted provided the riboflavin has the structure (75).

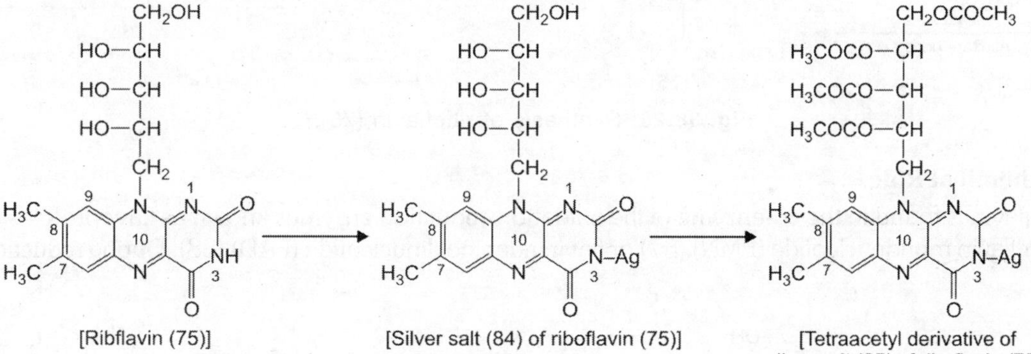

[Ribflavin (75)]

[Silver salt (84) of riboflavin (75)]

[Tetraacetyl derivative of silver salt (85) of riboflavin (75)]

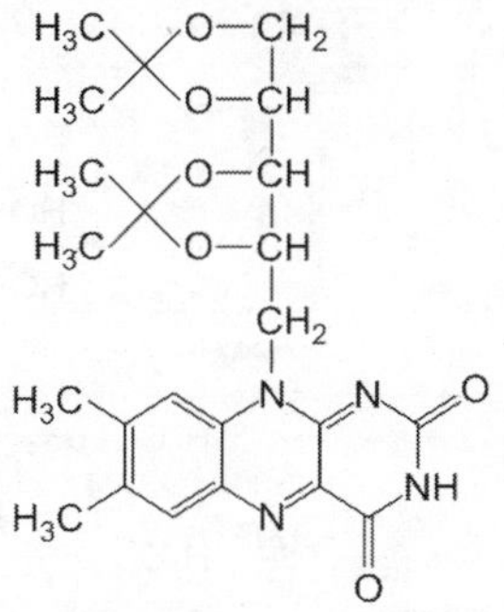

[Diisopropylidene derivative (86) of riboflavin (75)]

The four hydroxyl groups of the five carbon chain had the configuration of (-)-ribose. The structure was finally established by synthesis by Karrer et al (Fig. 38.20).

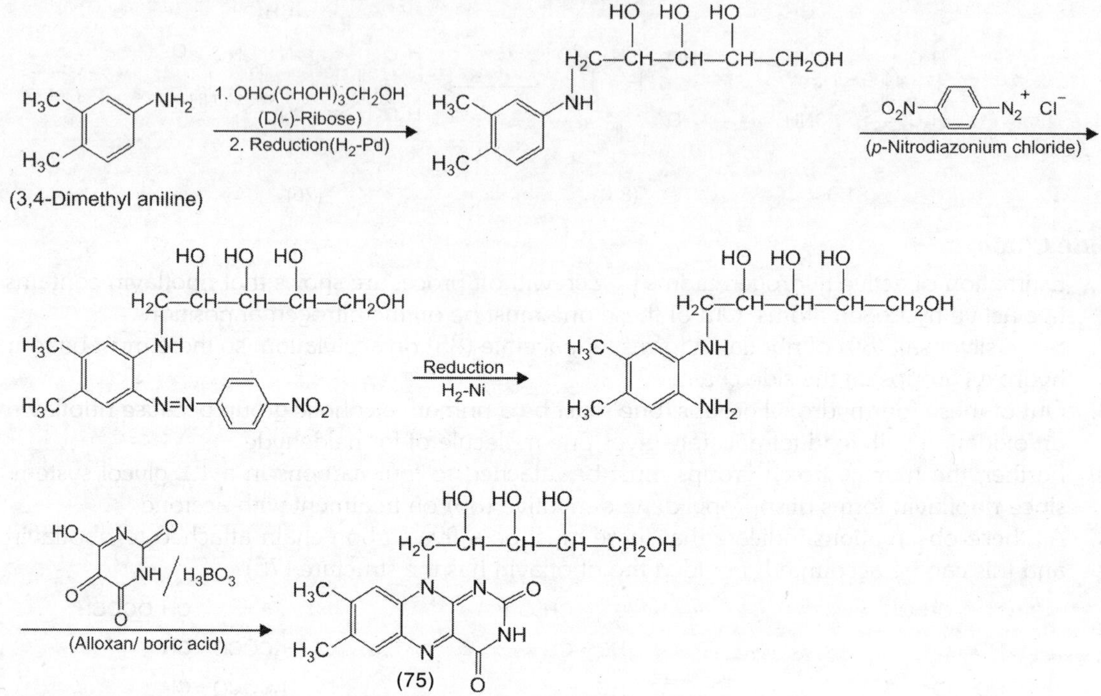

Fig. 38.20: Synthesis of riboflavin (75).

Biochemical Role

Riboflavin is found in the co-enzyme of the oxidation-reduction enzymes known as flavoproteins as either flavin mononucleotide (FMN) (87) or flavin adenine dinucleotide (FAD) (88). During reduction

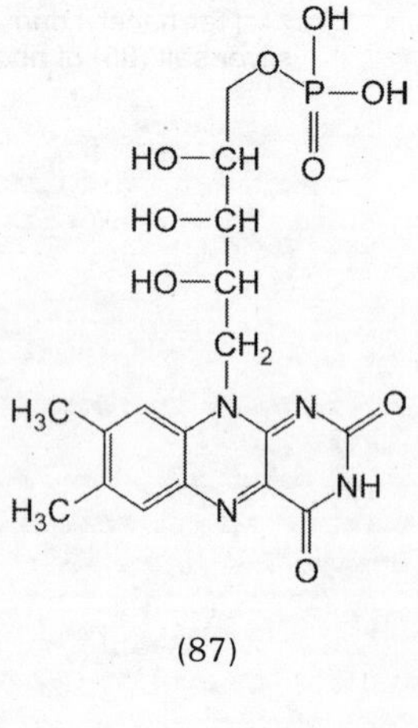

(87)

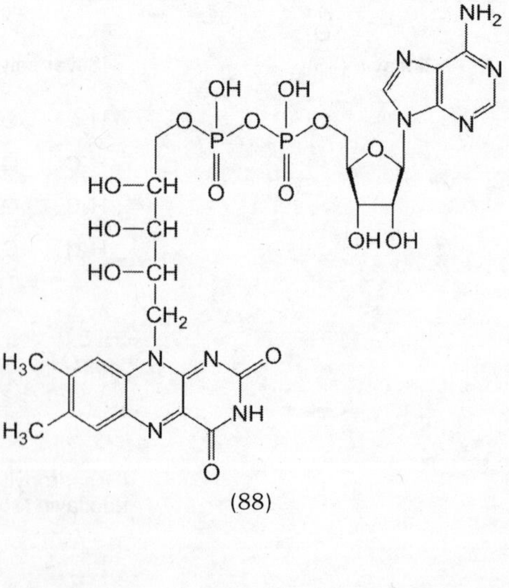

(88)

it is the isoalloxazine ring which undergoes reversible reduction accepting either one or two electrons in the form of one or two hydrogens (Fig. 38.21). The partially reduced forms, when only one electron is accepted, are FMNH$^+$ (89 a) and FADH$^+$ (89 b) and the fully reduced forms are FMNH$_2$ (90 a) and FADH$_2$ (90 b).

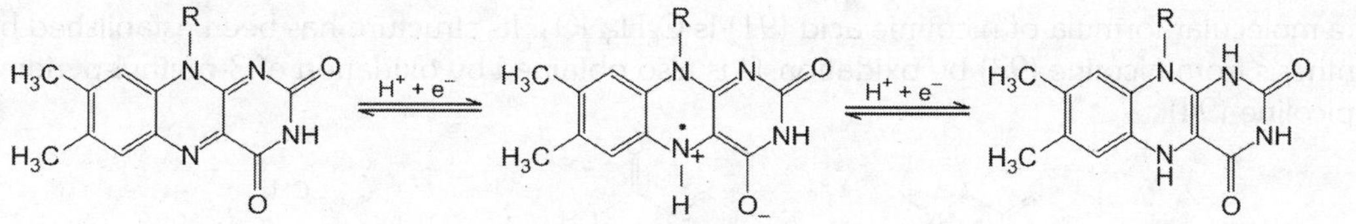

(a) FMN, R= H$_2$C.CH.CH.CH.CH$_2$OPO$_3$H$_2$; (b), FAD, R=H$_2$C.HC.HC.HC.H$_2$C

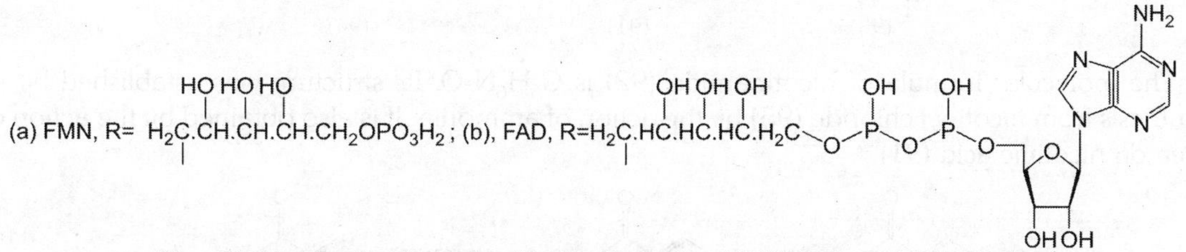

Fig. 38.21: Mechanism of oxidation involving FMN (87) and FAD (88).

Enzymes which use FMN (87) as co-enzyme include:

1. NADH dehydrogenase, and
2. Glycolate dehydrogenase

Enzymes which use FAD (88) as co-enzyme include:

1. Fatty acyl CoA dehydrogenase,
2. Dihydrolipoyl dehydrogenase,
3. Succinate dehydrogenase,
4. Glycerol-3-phosphate dehdrogenase, and
5. Thioredoxin dehydrogenase.

Nicotinic acid (91) and Nicotinamide (92)

Nicotinic acid [Pyridine 3-carboxylic acid, Niacin, (91)] and nicotinamide [Pyridine-3-carboxamide, Niacinamide, (92)] constitute vitamin B$_3$.

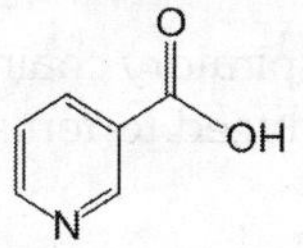

(91) 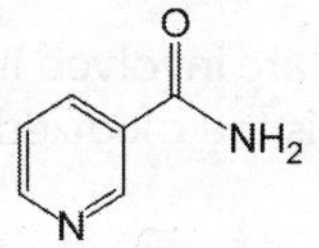   (92)

Nicotinic acid (91) crystallizes as needles from alcohol or water, mp 236.6°. Nicotinamide (92) crystallizes from benzene as needles, mp. 128-131°.

Sources

Nicotinic acid (91) is widely distributed in nature. Higher quantities are found in liver, fish, yeast, and cereal grains. Nicotinamide (92) occurs in wheat germ, yeast liver, barley, maize, and rice.

Deficiency Diseases

The deficiency of nicotinic acid (91) and nicotinamide (92) causes black tongue or pellagra.

Structure

The molecular formula of nicotinic acid (91) is $C_6H_5NO_2$. Its structure has been established by its synthesis from nicotine (93) by oxidation. It is also obtained by oxidation of 3-methyl-pyridine or β-picoline (94).

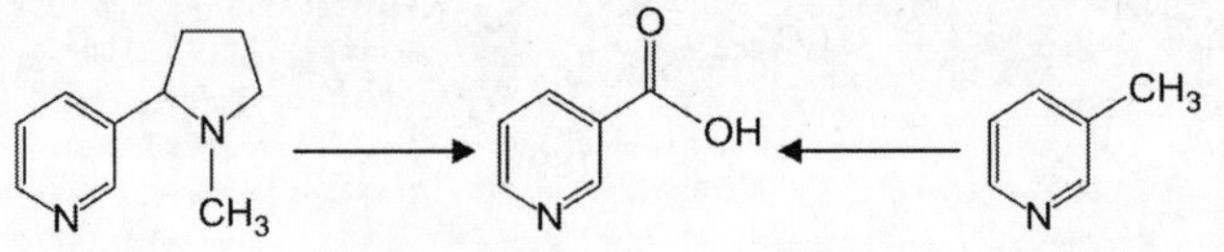

(93)   (91)   (94)

The molecular formula of nicotinamide (92) is $C_6H_6N_2O$. Its structure was established by its synthesis from nicotinyl chloride (95) by the action of ammonia. It is also obtained by the action of urea on nicotinic acid (91).

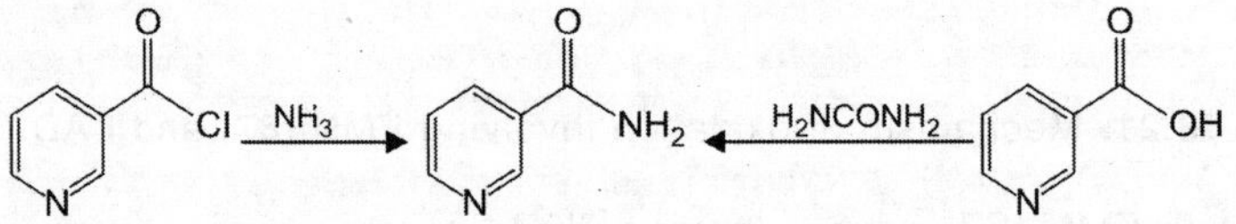

(95)   (92)   (91)

Biochemical Role

Nicotinamide (92) is a part of the co-enzyme I or NAD^+ (96) and co-enzyme II or $NADP^+$ (97).

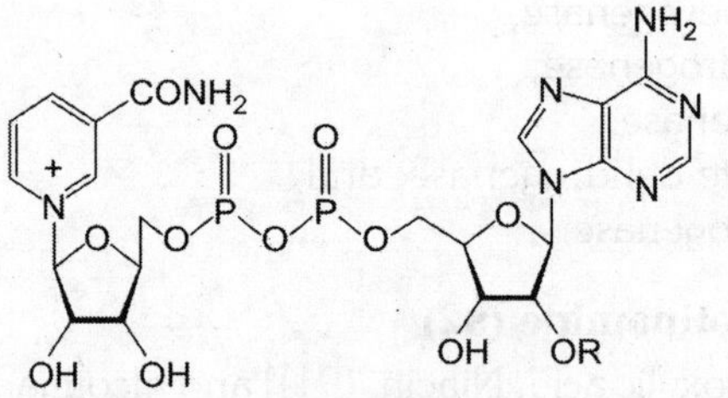

(96), R = H
(97), R = PO_3H_2

These enzymes are involved in oxidation-reduction reactions in respiratory chain. The quaternary form (98), which is the oxidized form, accepts hydrogens and is reduced to tertiary form (99).

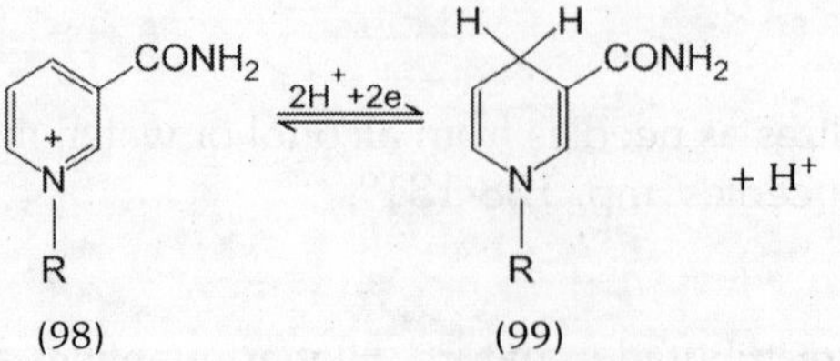

(98)   (99)

R represents the rest of molecule of NAD^+ and $NADP^+$

In many cells, the ratio of NAD$^+$ (oxidized form) to NADH (reduced form) is highly favouring the hydride transfer from substrate to NAD$^+$. On the other hand NADPH is generally present in greater amounts than NADP$^+$, favouring hydride transfer from NADPH to substrate.

When NAD$^+$ or NADP$^+$ is reduced, the hydride transfer could be to either side i.e. front side (100) or back side (101). Experimentally it has been found that an enzyme catalyzes only one type of transfer.

(100) (A side)   (101) (B side)

Accordingly, which face of NAD$^+$/NADP$^+$ is attacked depends upon the enzyme. Thus, yeast dehydrogenase and lactate dehydrogenase transfer a hydride onto (or remove ion from) A side of nicotinamide. So they are classified as type A dehydrogenases. Table 38.1 lists some of the enzymes and the corresponding coenzymes according to this classification. Some of the reactions catalyzed by NAD$^+$/NADP$^+$ linked dehdrogenases are listed in Fig. 38.22.

Table 38.1: Stereospecificity of nicotinamide dehydrogenases.

Enzyme	Co-enzyme	Stereochemical specificity of Nicotinamide ring (A or B)
Isocitrate dehydrogenase	NAD$^+$	A
α-Ketoglutarate dehydrogenase	NAD$^+$	B
Glucose 6-phosphate dehydrogenase	NADP$^+$	B
Malate dehydrogenase	NAD$^+$	A
Glutamate dehydrogenase	NAD$^+$/NADP$^+$	B
Glyceraldehyde 3-phosphate dehydrogenase	NAD$^+$	B
Lactate dehydrogenase	NAD$^+$	A
Alcohol dehydrogenase	NAD$^+$	A

NAD–linked Reactions

1. α-Ketoglutarate + CoA + NAD$^+$ $\rightleftharpoons$ Succinyl CoA + NADH + H$^+$
2. L-Malate + NAD$^+$ $\rightleftharpoons$ Oxaloacetate + NADH + H$^+$
3. Pruvate + CoA + NAD$^+$ $\rightleftharpoons$ Acetyl CoA + CO$_2$ + NADH + H$^+$
4. Glyceraldehyde 3-phosphate + Pi + NAD$^+$ $\rightleftharpoons$ 1,3-biphosphoglycerate + NADH + H$^+$
5. Lactate + NAD$^+$ $\rightleftharpoons$ Pyruvate + NADH + H$^+$
6. β-Hydroxyacyl CoA + NAD$^+$ $\rightleftharpoons$ β-Ketoacyl CoA + NADH + H$^+$

NADP–inked Reactions

1. Glucose 6-phosphate + NADP$^+$ $\rightleftharpoons$ 6-Phosphogluconate + NADPH + H$^+$

NAD–or NADP–linked Reactions

1. L-Glutamate + H$_2$O + NAD(P)$^+$ $\rightleftharpoons$ α-Ketoglutarate + NH$_4^+$ + NAD(P)H + H$^+$
2. Isocitrate + NAD(P)$^+$ $\rightleftharpoons$ α-Ketoglutarate + CO$_2$ + NAD(P)H$^+$ + H$^+$

Fig. 38.22: Some of the reactions catalyzed by NAD$^+$/NADP$^+$ linked dehydrogenases.

Pantothenic Acid (102)

D-(+)-*N*-(2,4-Dihydroxy-3,3-dimethylbutyryl)-β-alanine; Vitamin B$_5$; Chick-antidermatitis factor

(102)

Hygroscopic viscous oil which is unstable towards acids, bases and heat. $[\alpha]_D^{25}$ + 37.5.

Sources

It is widely distributed. The richest sources are egg yolk, liver, milk, vegetables, and fruits. It is also produced by green plants and moulds.

Deficiency Diseases

The deficiency symptoms of pantothenic acid are unknown in humans, this is because pantothenic acid is widely distributed vitamin. However, deficiency symptoms have been reported in chicks, rats, dogs, and swine. The deficiency in chicks results in dermatitis. In rats its deficiency results in retardation of growth, depigmentation of fur and spectacled eye condition. In dogs, the deficiency of pantothenic acid results in respiratory disturbances, degeneration of liver, and inflammation of digestive tract. In swine the deficiency symptoms include dermatitis and ulceration of digestive tract.

Structure

1. Molecular formula $C_9H_{17}NO_5$.
2. Reaction with diazomethane leads to the formation of a monomethyl ester indicating that pantothenic acid must be containing one carboxylic acid group.
3. It forms isopropylidene and benzylidene derivatives when treated with acetone and benzaldehyde, respectively. This indicates that it contains two hydroxyl groups which may have a 1,2 or 1,3 relationship. Since pantothenic acid does not react with periodic acid so the two hydroxyl groups may be at 1 and 3 positions.
4. Heating of pantothenic acid with dilute hydrochloric acid yielded two compounds, compound (A) and compound (B). Compound A which was a salt was found to be hydrochloride of β-alanine (103).

$$C_9H_{17}NO_5 \longrightarrow \underset{(A)}{C_3H_7NO_2} + \underset{(B)}{C_6H_{10}O_3}$$

$$\underset{(103)}{HOOCCH_2CH_2NH_2}$$

5. When treated with alkali, pantothenic acid forms β-alanine (103) and a salt of an acid which on acidification forms a lactone readily, indicating that the lactone must be a γ-lactone. The two groups, carboxyl and hydroxyl must be γ- to each other.
6. Compound B was shown to possess a *gem*-dimethyl group which was confirmed by formation of acetone when compound B was treated with barium permanganate.

7. Compound B also showed the presence of active hydrogen. As indicated earlier, pantothenic acid has been found to contain two hydroxyl groups, out of these one is accounted by the formation of γ-lactone. The second was shown to be α- to carbonyl group of lactone because sodium salt of lactone gave a canary yellow color with ferric chloride, a characteristic reaction of α-hydroxy acids. Based on this, the lactone must be having the structure (104) and compound B must (105) i.e. α, γ-dihydroxy-β–β-dimethyl butyric acid.

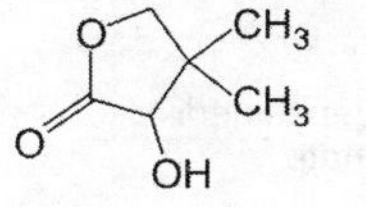

(104) 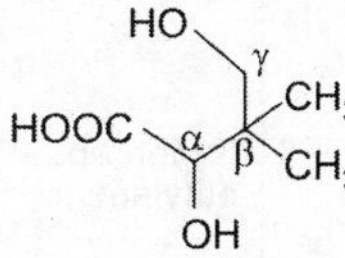   (105)

This was further confirmed by the synthesis of γ-lactone starting with Isobutyraldehyde (Fig. 38.23). The racemic mixture was resolved with quinine. The resolved (-)-form was found to be identical with the lactone (104) obtained from pantothenic acid.

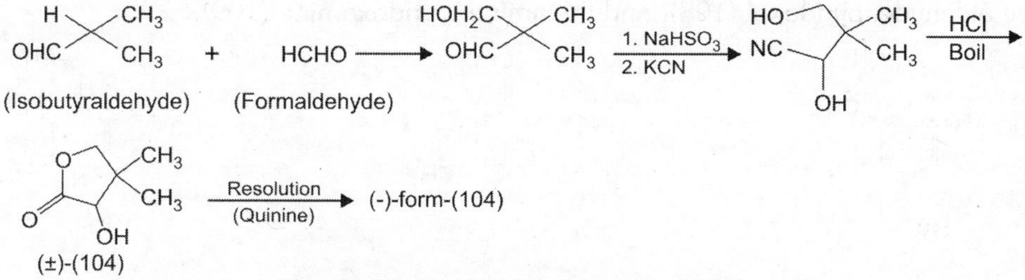

(Isobutyraldehyde)   (Formaldehyde)

(±)-(104)

Fig. 38.23: Synthesis of lactone (104).

8. Pantothenic acid does not contain a free amino group indicating that the amino group of β-alanine (103) must be present as an amide function. Thus, pantothenic acid is an amide and its structure must be (102). This was further confirmed by its synthesis (Fig. 38.24) by reacting lactone (104) with ethyl ester of β-alanine (103).

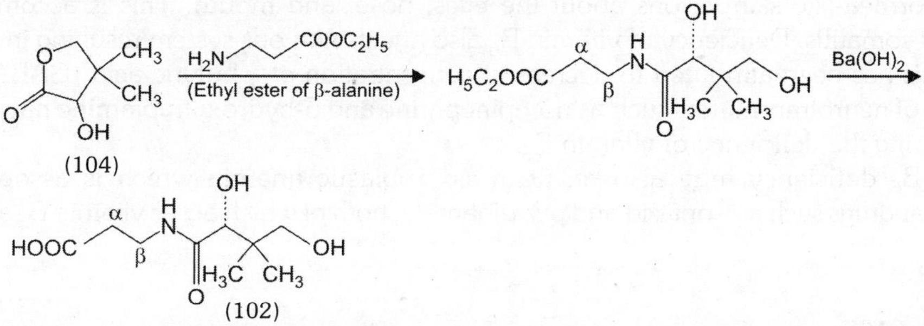

(104)

(Ethyl ester of β-alanine)

(102)

Fig. 38.24: Synthesis of pantothenic acid (102).

Biochemical Role

Pantothenic acid (102) is a component of Co-enzyme A (106) which is involved in activation of fatty acids before their β-oxidation. Co-enzyme A (106) is also involved in formation of acetyl Co A.

β-Mercapto-ethylamine | Pantothenic acid | 3-Phosphoadenosinedi-phosphate

(106)

Pyridoxine (107), Pyridoxal (108), and Pyridoxamine (109)

According to IUPAC, the term Vitamin B_6 is applied to all the three forms i.e the alcohol, pyridoxine (107), the aldehyde, pyridoxal (108), and the amine, pyridoxamine (109).

(107)   (108)   (109)

Sources

All the three forms of vitamin are found in abundance in seeds, cereals, wheat, and maize.

Deficiency Diseases

Since the vitamin B_6 is widely distributed, its deficiency is rare. Some of the deficiency symptoms include seborrhea-like skin lesions about the eyes, nose, and mouth. This is accompanied by glossitis and somatitis. Deficiency of vitamin B_6 also affects nervous system resulting in convulsive seizures. This has been attributed to decreased concentration of γ-butyric acid (GABA). Further, lower levels of neurotransmitters such as norepinephrine and 5-hydroxytryptamine have also been reported during the deficiency of vitamin B_6.

Vitamin B_6 deficiency may also result in sideroblastic anemia which is associated with antitubercular drugs such as isoniazid and pyrazinamide, both of which act as vitamin B_6 antagonists.

Structure

Pyridoxine (107)

3-Hydroxy-4,5-bis(hydroxymethyl)-2-methylpyridine

Hydrochloride as platelets from alcohol and acetone, mp. 160°.

1. Molecula formula $C_8H_{11}NO_3$.
2. It contains three active hydrogen atoms.

3. It is a weak base.

4. It showed the absence of methoxyl and methylamino groups.

5. Treatment of pyridoxine with diazomethane gave mono-methyl ether. The ether when treated with acetic anhydride gave a diacetyl derivative. These reactions indicate that the three oxygens must be present as three hydroxyl groups.

6. Pyridoxine gave positive test with ferric chloride indicating the presence of a phenolic group. This is further confirmed by the ready formation of mono-methyl ether with diazomethane. Further, the UV spectrum of pyridoxine was similar to 3-hydroxypyridine, indicating the presence of phenolic group at position 3. These results indicate that pyridoxine must be containing one phenolic group at position 3 and two alcoholic hydroxyl groups.

7. The mono-methyl ether of pyridoxine was unaffected by the action of lead tetraacetate indicating that the two hydroxyl groups were not on adjacent carbon atoms.

8. Careful oxidation of mono-methyl ether of pyridoxine with alkaline permanganate gave a product with molecular formula, $C_9H_7NO_7$, and possessed three carboxylic acid groups. This tricarboxylic acid gave blood-red color with ferrous sulphate, a characteristic reaction of pyridine 2-carboxylic acid. Thus, out of the three carboxylic acid groups in mono-methyl ether of tricarboxylic acid, one carboxylic group must be at position 2.

9. Oxidation of 3-methoxy analog of pyridoxine with alkaline permanganate gave carbon dioxide and an anhydride. The anhydride did not give any color reaction with ferrous sulphate. These observations led to the conclusion that the two carboxylic groups in anhydride must be present at the two adjacent carbon atoms and third carboxylic group produced during permanganate oxidation of 3-methoxy analog of pyridoxine, gets decarboxylated as carbon dioxide. Based on this the structure of 3-methoxy tricarboxylic acid could be either (110) or (111).

(110)   (111)

10. Since pyridoxine contains three oxygen atoms, out of which one is accounted by the phenolic group, the other two must be present as -CH_2OH. In addition to this there must be a methyl group which on oxidation gives third carboxylic group. Thus, pyridoxine could be (112) or (113).

(112)   (113)

11. Oxidation of pyridoxine 3-methyl ether with barium permanganate gave a dicarboxylic acid which did not give color reaction with ferrous sulphate, indicating that there is no carboxylic acid group at position 2. Accordingly the dicarboxylic acid could be either (114) or (115). Finally, Kuhn showed that the structure of methoxymethyl dicarboxylic acid was (114) by getting it from 4-methoxy-3-methylisoquinoline (116), a known compound by oxidation. The structure was further confirmed by synthesis of pyridoxine (107) from ethoxyacetylacetone (Fig. 38.25). The reactions of pyridoxine (107) are listed in Fig. 38.26.

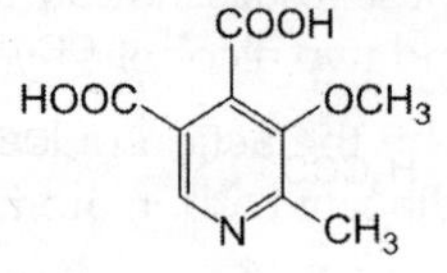

(114) 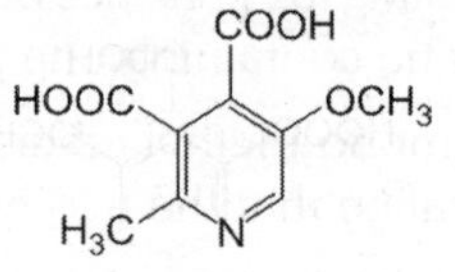   (115)

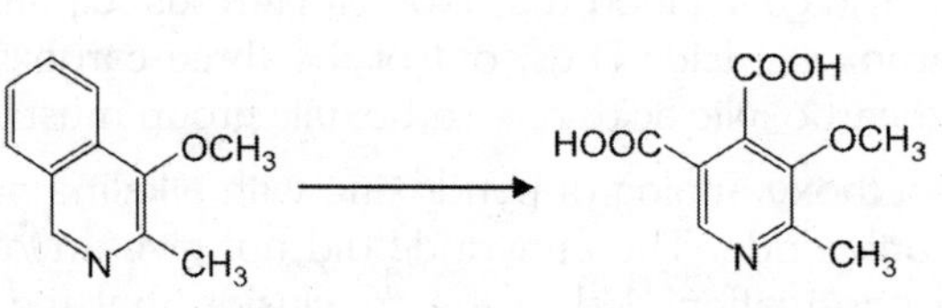

(116)   (114)

Synthesis

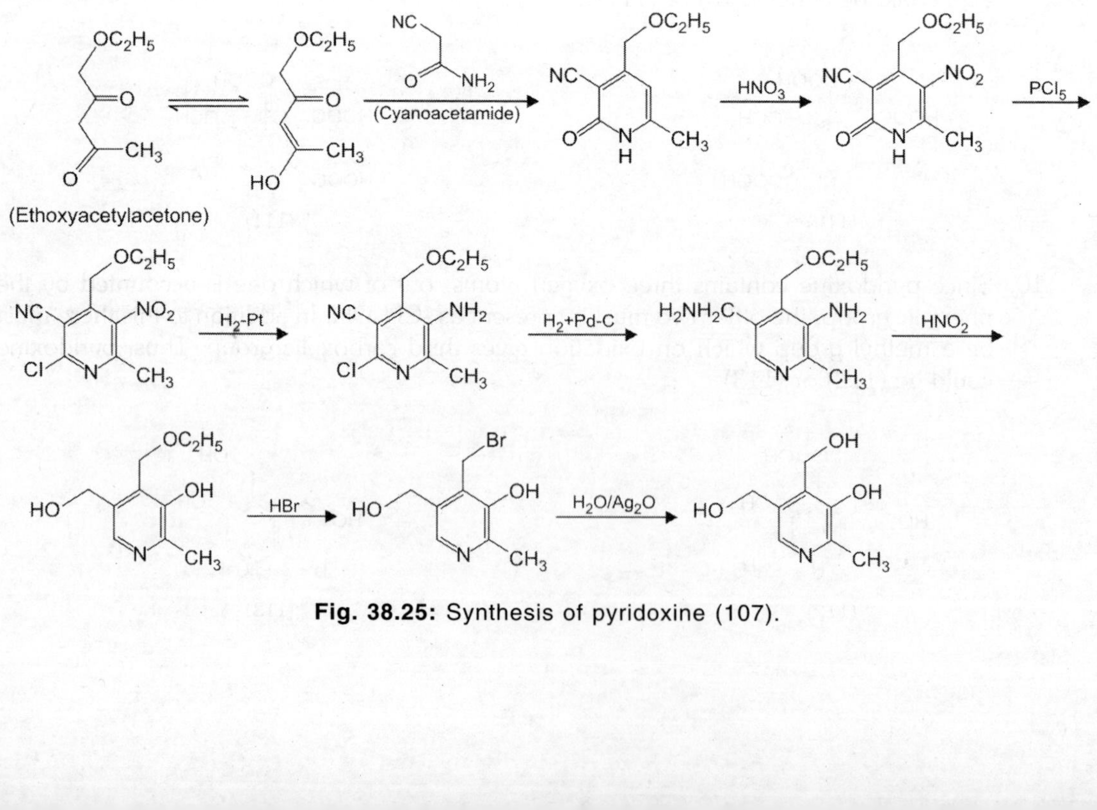

Fig. 38.25: Synthesis of pyridoxine (107).

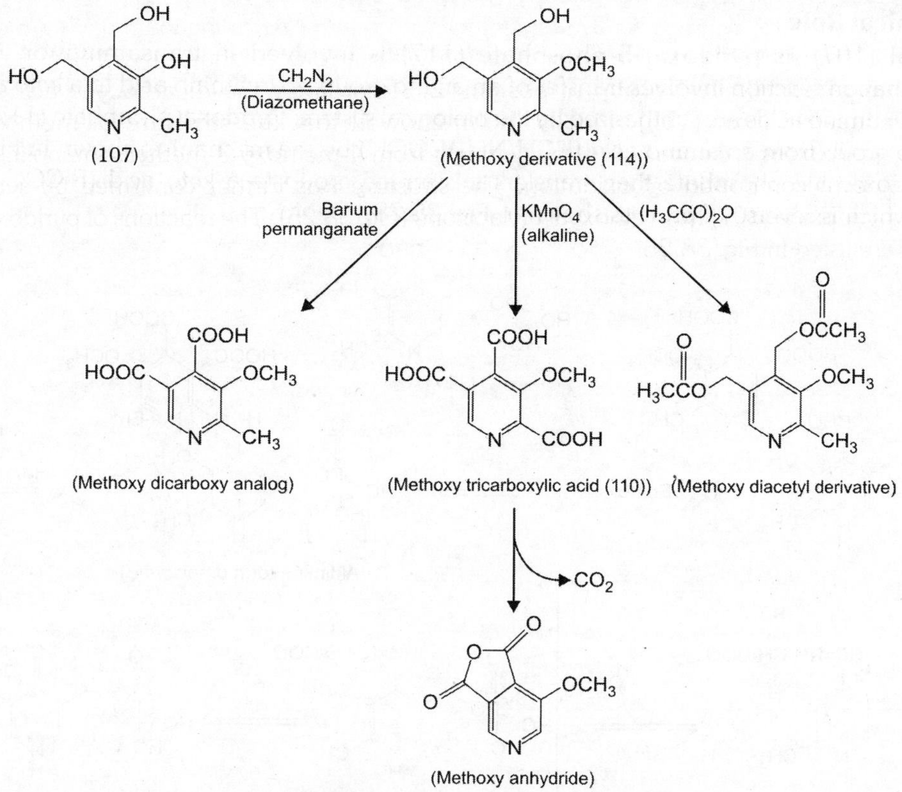

Fig. 38.26: Reactions of pyridoxine (107).

The structures of pyridoxal [5-hydroxymethyl-3-hydroxy-2-methyl-pyridine-4-aldehyde, (108)] and pyridoxamine [5-hydroxymethyl-3-hydroxy-4-aminomethyl-2-methylpyridine, (109)] were established by interconversion of pyridoxine (107), pyridoxal (108), and pyridoxamine (109) (Fig. 38.27).

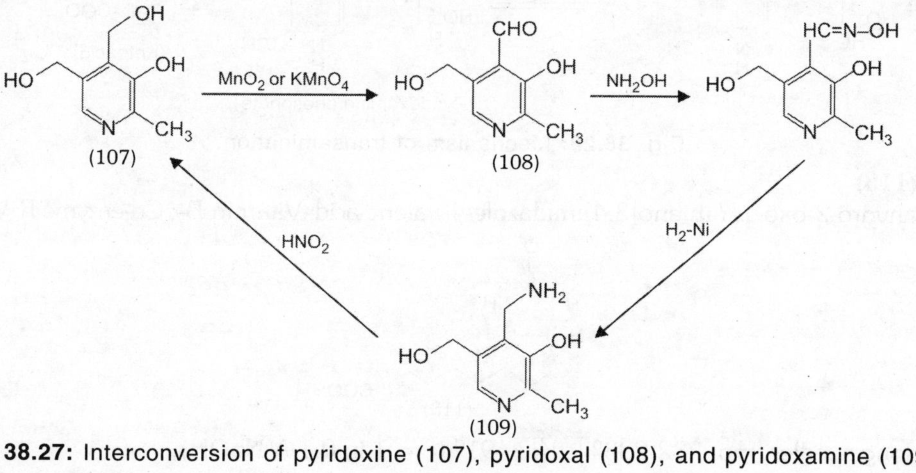

Fig. 38.27: Interconversion of pyridoxine (107), pyridoxal (108), and pyridoxamine (109).

Biochemical Role

Pyridoxal (107) as pyridoxal 5-phosphate (117) is involved in transamination reaction. Transamination reaction involves transfer of an amino group of an amino acid to a keto acid. This way newer amino acids are synthesized by the biological system. Pyridoxal phosphate (117) accepts an amino group from an amino acid ($RCH(NH_2)COOH$) by the mechanism shown in Fig. 38.28. The pyridoxamine phosphate then transfers this amino group to a keto acid ($R'COCOOH$) by process which is reverse of process shown in Fig. 38.28.

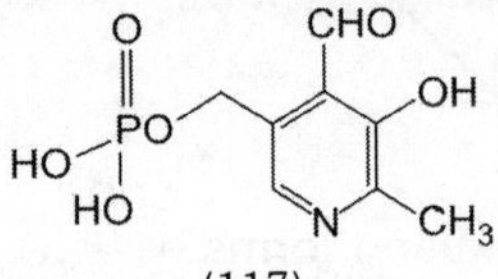

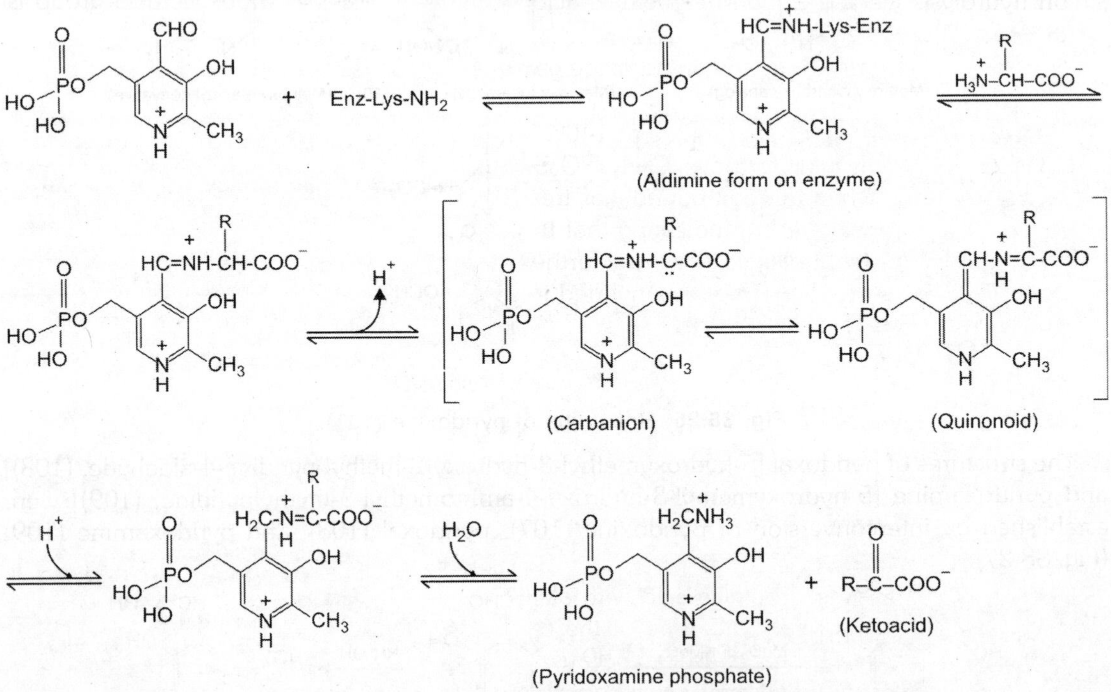

Fig. 38.28: Mechanism of transamination.

Biotin (118)

cis-Hexahydro-2-oxo-1H-thieno[3,4]imidazole-4-valeric acid; Vitamin B_7; Co-enzyme R; Vitamin H

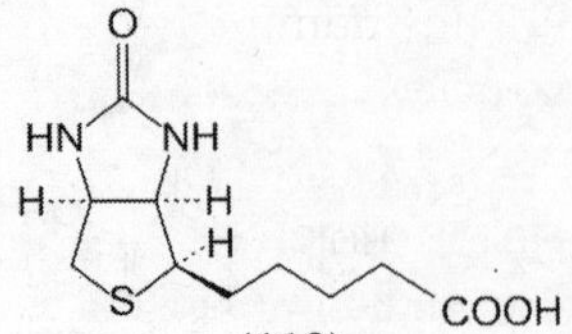

(118)

Fine long needles, mp. 232-233° $[\alpha]_D^{21} + 91°$ (c = 1 in 0.1 N NaOH).

Sources

The richest sources are liver, yeast, milk and eggs.

Deficiency Diseases

Include seborrheic dermatitis which is characterized by inflammation occurring in oily skin in areas having large sebaceous glands. Its deficiency also causes hyperesthesia – increased sensitivity to stimulus and glossites which is characterized by inflammation of tongue.

Structure

1. Molecular formula $C_{10}H_{16}N_2O_3S$.
2. It behaves as a saturated compound and forms an ester with methanol, $C_{11}H_{18}N_2O_3S$, which on hydrolysis yielded a mono carboxylic acid, indicating that one carboxylic acid group is present in the molecule.
3. Oxidation of biotin with hydrogen peroxide gave sulphur, indicating that sulphur was present as thioether.
4. When boiled with barium hydroxide at 140°, biotin yielded one molecule of carbon dioxide and an acid, molecular formula, $C_9H_{18}NO_2S$. This acid was found to contain two amino groups. Further, when this compound was treated with phenanthroquinone (119), it formed quinoxaline derivative (120) indicating that the two amino groups are present on adjascent carbon atoms of the molecule. This was further confirmed by treating the diaminocarboxylic acid with phosgene when it was reconverted to biotin.

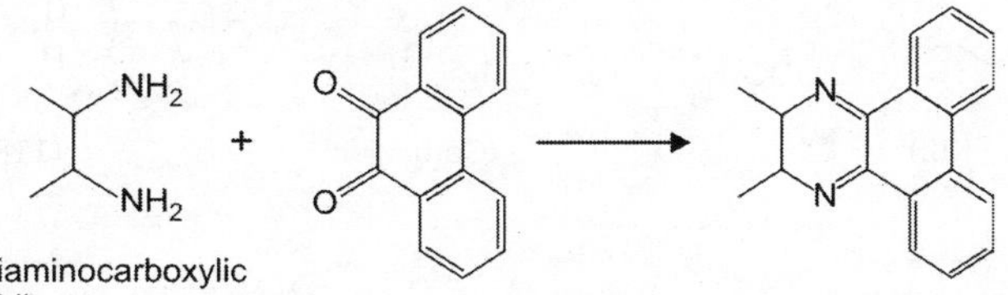

(Diaminocarboxylic acid)

(119) (120)

5. Oxidation of diaminocarboxylic acid with alkaline permanganate yielded adipic acid, a six carbon dicarboxylic acid. Since one of the carboxylic acid group is already present in the molecule the other must have resulted because of oxidation of the molecule. From this it could be concluded that in biotin there must be a chain containing a carboxylic acid group and the size of this chain must be -$(CH_2)_4COOH$, which can yield adipic acid on oxidation. This was further confirmed by converting the carboxylic acid group of biotin into amino group through the following set of reactions (Fig. 38.29). The amino analog of biotin (Fig. 38.29) on hydrolysis yielded a triamine (Fig. 38.29). The triamine, when subjected to oxidation by alkaline permanganate did not yield adipic acid.

$$\text{Biotin-COOH} \xrightarrow{CH_3OH/H^+} \text{Biotin-COOCH}_3 \xrightarrow{H_2N\text{-}NH_2} \text{Biotin-NHNH}_2 \longrightarrow \text{Biotin-}\overset{+}{N}_3$$

$$\text{Bion-NHCOOR} \xrightarrow{Ba(OH)_2} R\,(NH_2)_2\text{–}NH_2 \;\; \text{(Triamine)}$$

Fig. 38.29: Set of reactions showing conversion of biotin to triamine.

6. The diaminocarboxylic acid obtained by treatment of biotin with $Ba(OH)_2$ when subjected to exhaustive methylation reaction gave δ-(2-thienyl)-valeric acid (121), the structure of which was established by synthesis (Fig. 38.30).

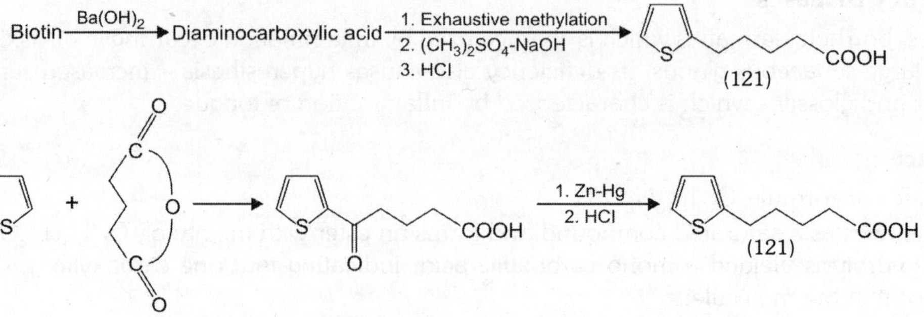

Fig. 38.30: Synthesis of δ-(2-thienyl) valeric acid (121).

7. Based on the above, sulphur must be present in a five membered ring and the structure of diaminocarboxylic acid must be (122). Further, since diaminocarboxylic acid (122) gives biotin on treatment with phosgene, the structure of biotin must be (118). This has been further confirmed by synthesis of biotin (118) (Fig. 38.31).

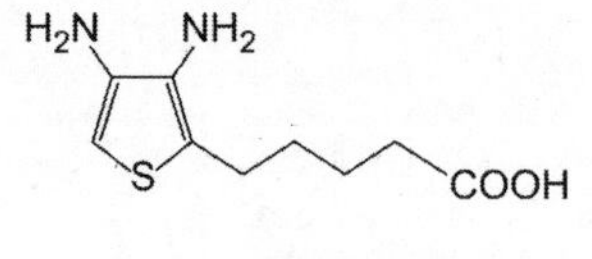

(122) 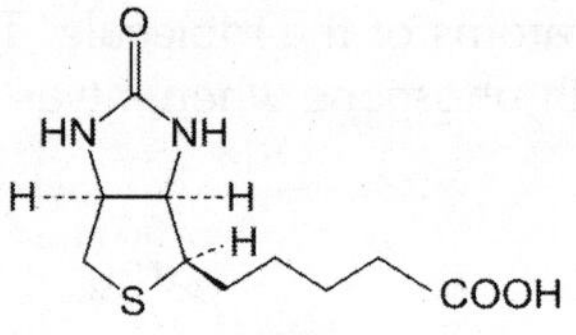   (118)

Synthesis

Step I

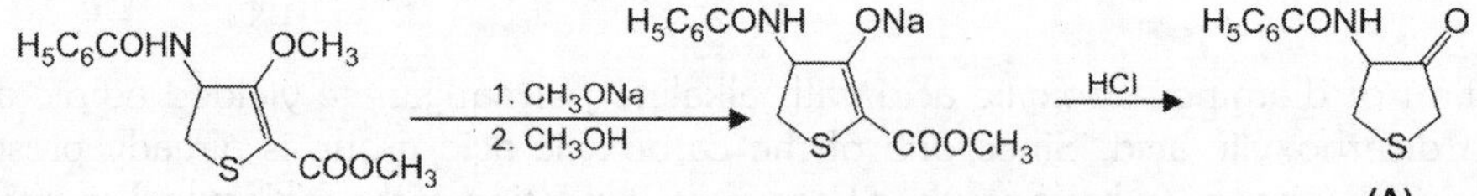

Step II

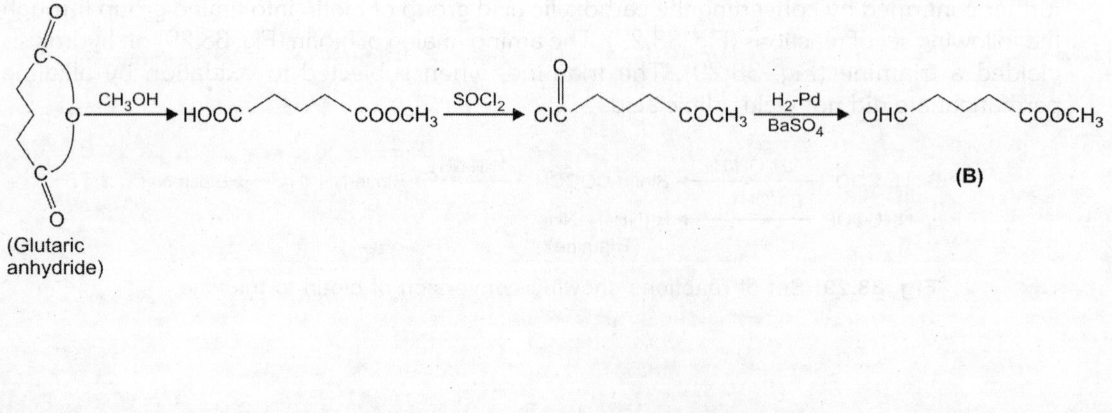

(Glutaric anhydride)

Step 3

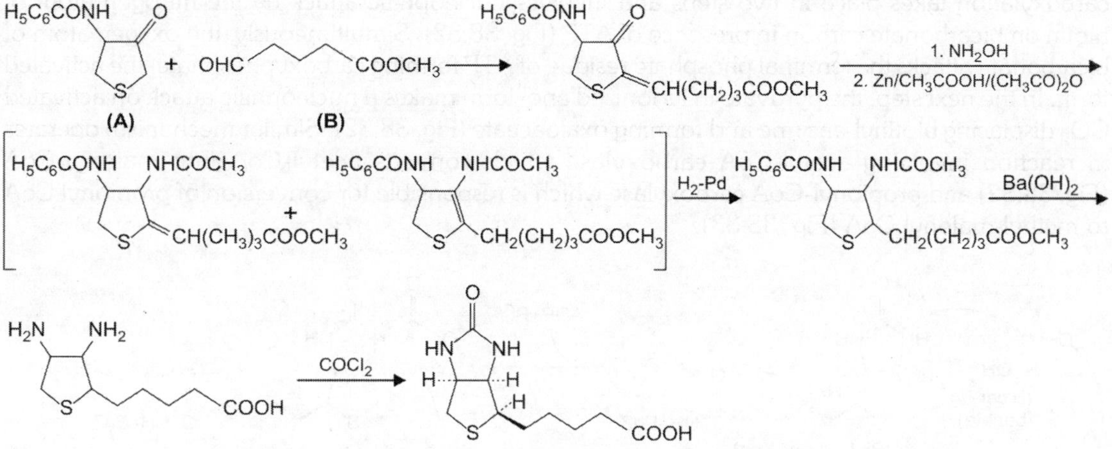

(118)

Fig. 38.31: Synthesis of biotin (118).

Biotin (118) has three asymmetric centres and these are 2,3, and 4. As a result there are eight isomers or four pairs of racemates possible and all of these are known. These incude (±)-biotin (118), (±)-epibiotin (123), (±)-allobiotin (124), and (±)-epiallobiotin (125). Of all the isomers (±)-biotin is biologically active.

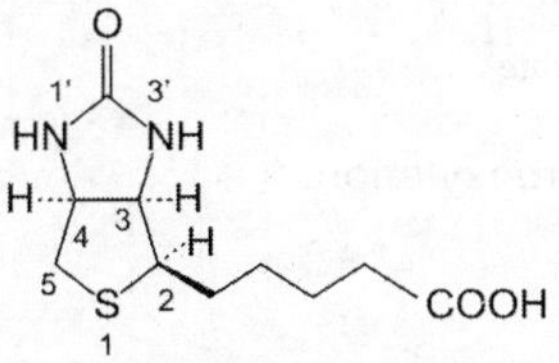

(118)

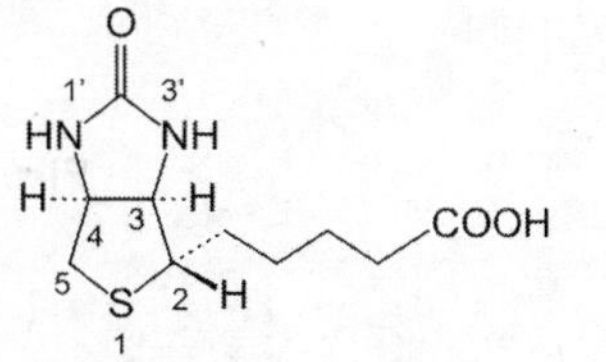

(123)

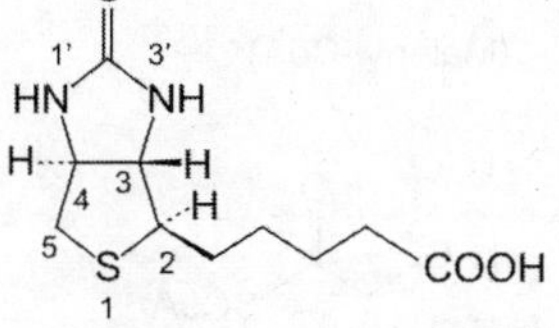

(124)

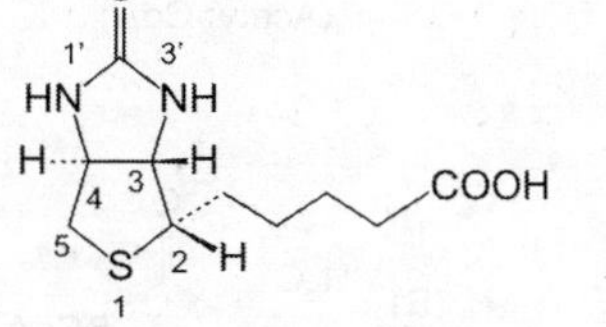

(125)

Biochemical Role

Biotin is involved in carboxylation reactions involving pyruvate carboxylase, propionyl carboxylase, and acetyl-CoA carboxylase.

In the carboxylation reaction biotin is attached to an enzyme through an amide linkage formed between carboxyl of the biotin and the ε-amino group of lysine residue of the enzyme. The carboxylation takes place in two steps and involves nucleophilic attack by the nitrogen atom of biotin on bicarbonate carbon in presence of ATP (Fig. 38.32). Simultaneously, the oxygen atom of bicarbonate attacks the terminal phosphate residue of ATP forming carboxyphosphate, the activated form. In the next step, the pyruvate in its ionized enol form makes a nucleophilic attack on activated CO_2 displacing biotinyl-enzyme and forming oxaloaceate (Fig. 38.32). Similar mechanism operates in reaction involving acetyl-CoA carboxylase which converts acetyl-CoA into malonyl-CoA (Fig. 38.32) and propionyl-CoA carboxylase which is responsible for conversion of propionyl CoA to methyl-malonyl CoA (Fig. 38.33).

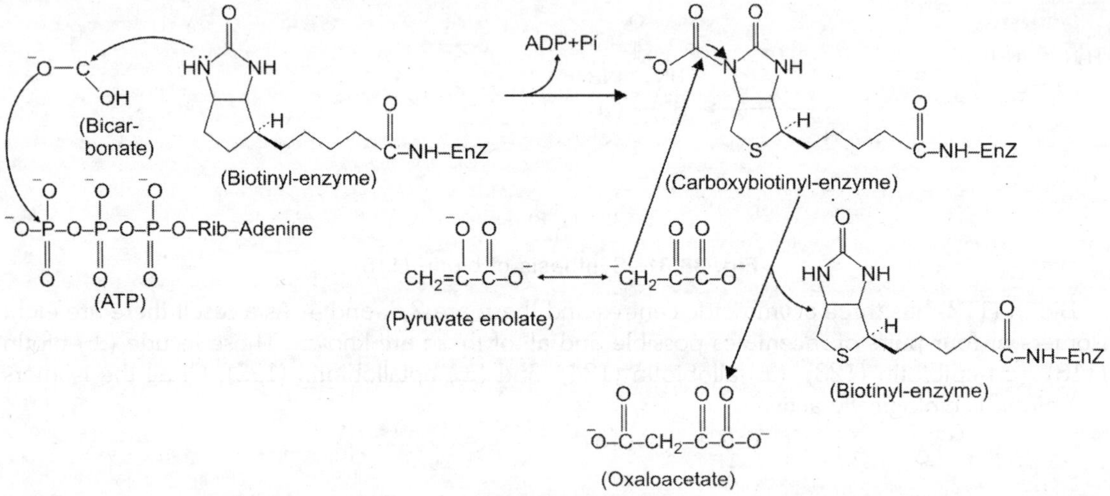

Fig. 38.32: Mechanism of carboxylation.

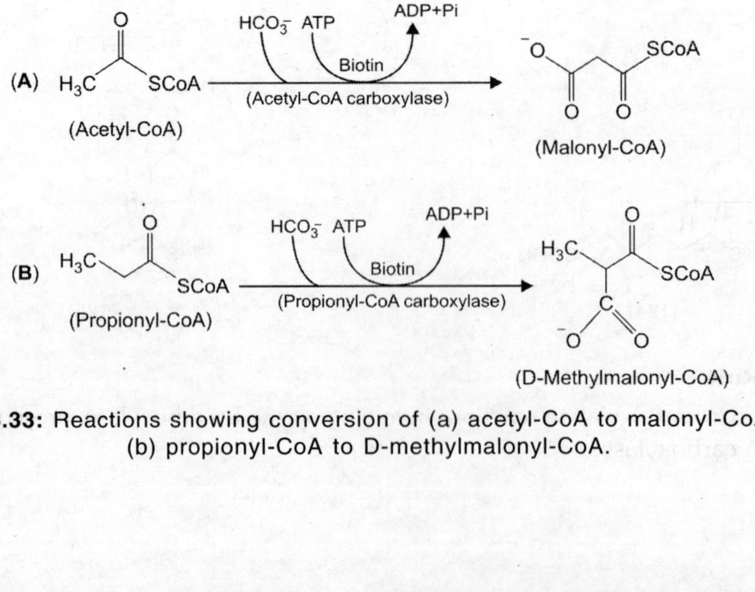

Fig. 38.33: Reactions showing conversion of (a) acetyl-CoA to malonyl-CoA and (b) propionyl-CoA to D-methylmalonyl-CoA.

Folic Acid (126)

N-[*p*[[2-Amino-4-hydroxy-6-pteridinyl)methyl]amino]benzoyl]glutamic acid; Liver *L.casei* factor; Pteroylglutamic acid; Vitamin B_9; Vitamin M

(126)

Thin platelets from hot water, darkens and chars from about 250°, $[\alpha]_D^{25} + 23°$ (c = 0.5 in 0.1*N* NaOH).

Sources

It is found in spinach leaves, present as free and combined with one or more additional L-(+)-glutamic acid molecule in liver, kidney, mushroom, yeast green leaves, and whey.

Deficiency Diseases

Folic acid deficiency leads to macrocytic anemia which is characterized by presence of abnormally large erythrocytes and decreased levels of blood platelets.

Structure

1. Folic acid or liver *Lactobacillus casei* factor, molecular formula $C_{19}H_{19}N_7O_6$, isolated from liver, has been found to be closely related to fermentation *L.casei* factor, molecular formula $C_{29}H_{33}N_9O_{12}$, isolated from fermentation residues.
2. Alkaline hydrolysis of the fermentation *L.casei* factor, in absence of oxygen, gave two molecules of D-glutamic acid (127) and DL-form of liver *L.casei* factor. However, alkaline hydrolysis in presence of air of the fermentation *L.casei* factor gave two compounds, namely compound (A) and (B).

(127)

3. ### Structure of Compound (A)

   (a) Molecular formula of compound (A) was found to be $C_7H_5N_5O_3$.
   (b) Compound (A) showed the presence of a carboxylic acid group, a hydroxyl group, and an amino group.
   (c) UV absorption spectrum of compound (A) showed it to be a pteridine derivative.
   (d) On treatment with chlorine water followed by hydrolysis, compound (A) yielded guanidine (128) as one of products, indicating that the amino group must be between the two nitrogens of pyrimidine ring of the pteridine moiety, that corresponds to position 2.

(128)   (129)   (130)

(*e*) Decarboxylation of the compound (A) gave a compound which was identical with 2-amino-4-hydroxypteridine (129), a known compound.

(*f*) The structure of compound (A) was established to be 2-amino-4-hydroxypteridine-6-carboxylic acid (130) by synthesis (Fig. 38.34).

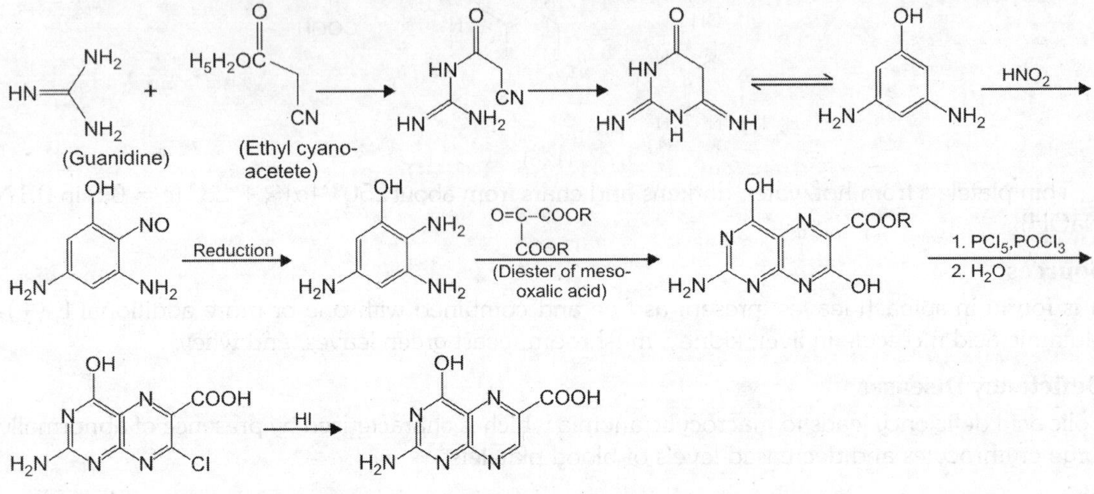

(130)

Fig. 38.34: Synthesis of compound (A) (130).

4. **Structure of compound (B)**

Compound B was found to be an aromatic amine containing free carboxylic acid groups. Hydrolysis of compound B yielded one molecule of *p*-aminobenzoic acid (131) and three molecules of glutamic acid (127) indicating that its structure is as given above.

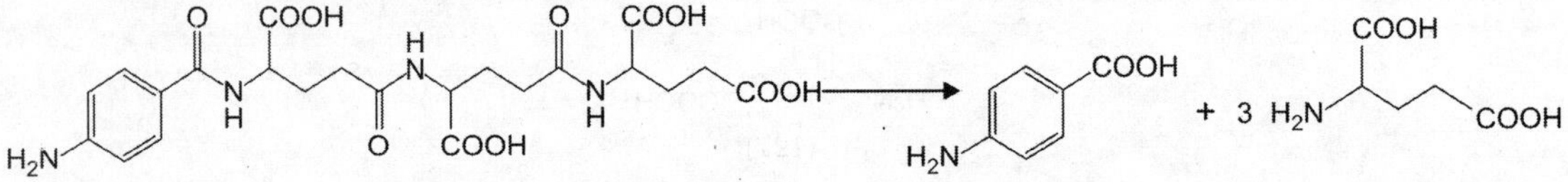

(Compound B) (131) (127)

5. Hydrolysis of fermentation of *L.Casei* factor with sulphurous acid gave an aldehyde (C) and an aromatic amine which on hydrolysis gave one molecule of *p*-aminobenzoic acid (131) and three molecules of glutamic acid (127), indicating that it was same as (B).
6. Compound (C), the aldehyde, when kept in dilute sodium hydroxide solution in absence of air gave compound (A) (130) and another compound (D). Compound (D) on vigorous hydrolysis gave 2-amino-5-methylpyrazine (132).

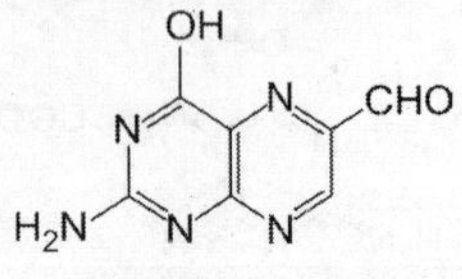

(Compound C)

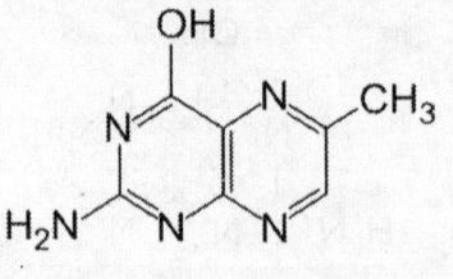

(Compound D)

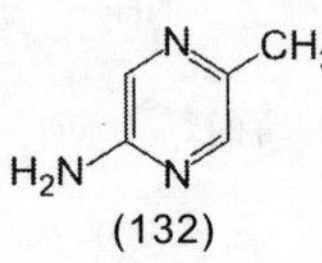

(132)

7. From the above it can be concluded that compound (D) is 2-amino-4-hydroxy-6-methyl-pteridine and compound (C) is 2-amino-4-hydroxypteridine-6-aldehyde.

8. The various product obtained after the hydrolysis of liver *L.casei* factor were 2-amino-4-hydroxypteridine-6-carboxylic acid (130), *p*-aminobenzoic acid (131), and glutamic acid (127) indicating that its structure must be (126). This was further confirmed by its synthesis (Fig. 38.35).

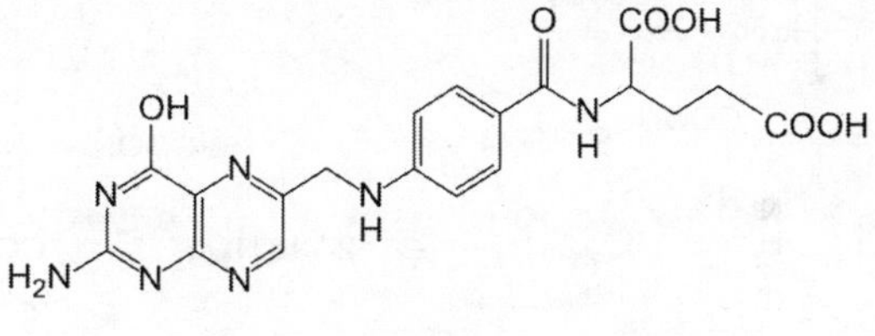

(126)

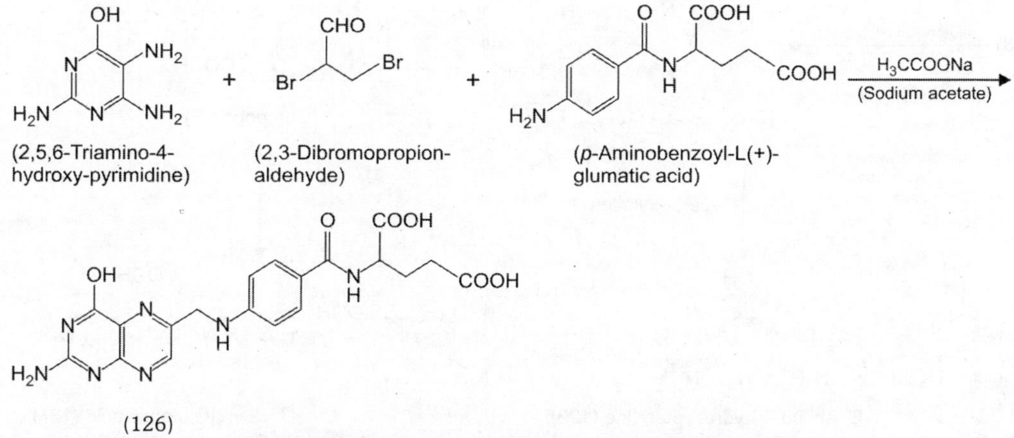

(2,5,6-Triamino-4-hydroxy-pyrimidine)

(2,3-Dibromopropion-aldehyde)

(*p*-Aminobenzoyl-L(+)-glumatic acid)

$H_3CCOONa$ (Sodium acetate)

(126)

Fig. 38.35: Synthesis of liver L.casei factor (126).

9. Since fermentation *L.casei* factor yields two glutamic acid (127) residues together with liver *L.casei* factor or folic acid (126), the structure of which has been established to be (126), the two glutamic acid (127) residues in fermentation factor must be joined to folic acid (126) by amide bonds. Accordingly, the structure of fermentation *L.casei* factor must be (133). The various reactions of fermentation *L.casei* (133) factor are summarized given in Fig. 38.36.

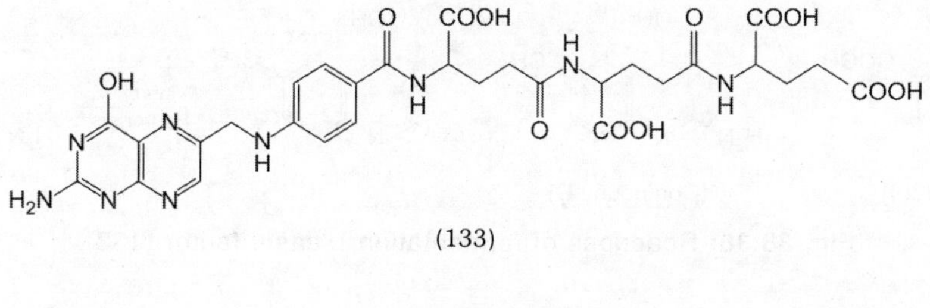

(133)

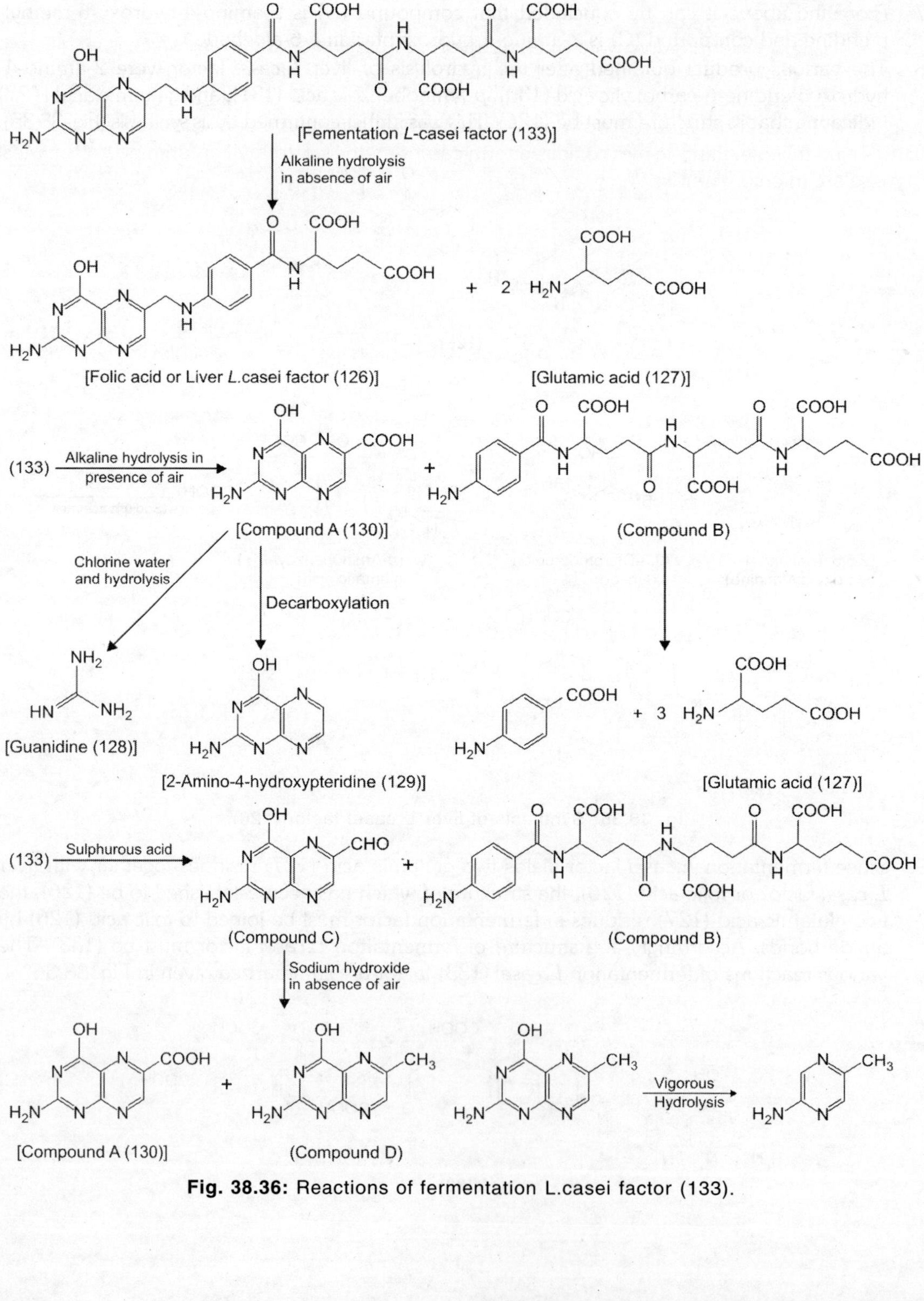

Fig. 38.36: Reactions of fermentation L.casei factor (133).

Biochemical Role

Folic acid (126), as tetrahydrofoliate (134), is involved in one carbon transfer which is involved in the synthesis of purines and pyrimidines required for the synthesis of nucleic acids. The one carbon group undergoing transfer in any of the three oxidation states is bonded to N^5 or N^{10} or both (Fig. 38.37). The most reduced from of co-factor carries a methyl group, a more oxidized form carries a methylene, and the most oxidized form carries methenyl, formyl, or forimino group. Most of these are interconvertible.

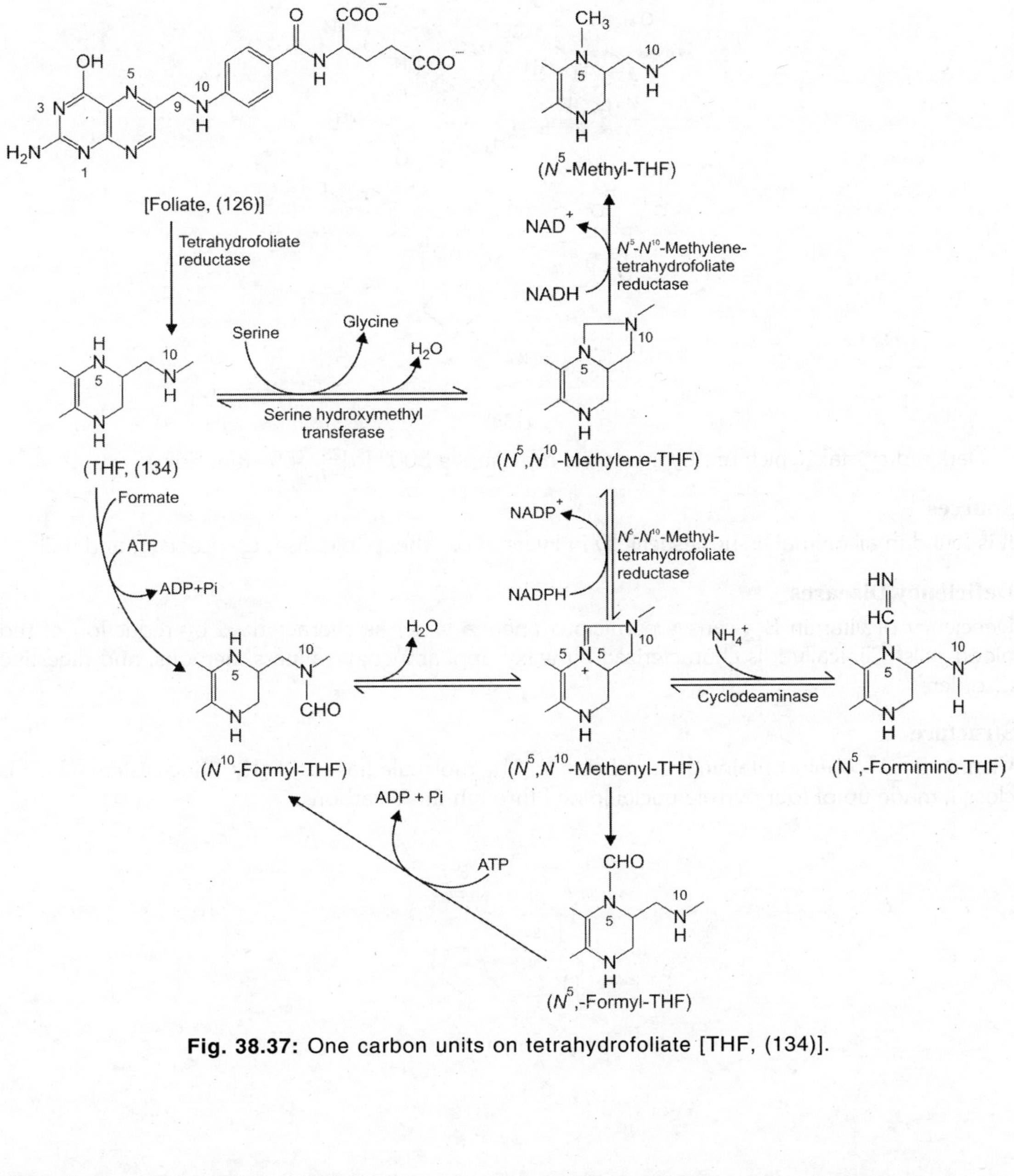

Fig. 38.37: One carbon units on tetrahydrofoliate [THF, (134)].

Cyanocobalamin (135)

5,6-Dimethylbenzimidazolylcyanocobamide; Vitamin B_{12}

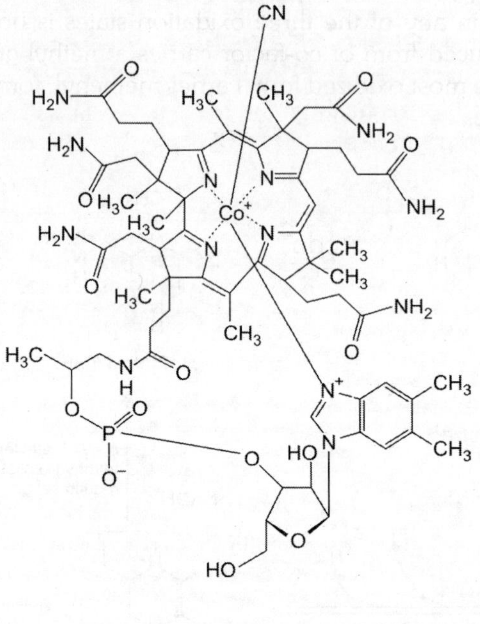

(135)

Dark red crystals which are hygroscopic, mp. Above 300° $[\alpha]^{23}_{656}$ -59° (aq. Soln).

Sources

It is found in all animal tissues especially in livers of ox, sheep, pig, fish, cheese, egg, and milk.

Deficiency Diseases

Deficiency of vitamin B_{12} causes pernicious anemia which is characterized by reduction of red blood cells. Clinically it is characterized by waxy appearance, weakness, nervous, and digestive disorders.

Structure

Vitamin B_{12} is cobalt containing red substance. The molecule has corin (136) ring system which is closed, made up of four pyrrole nuclei joined through three carbons.

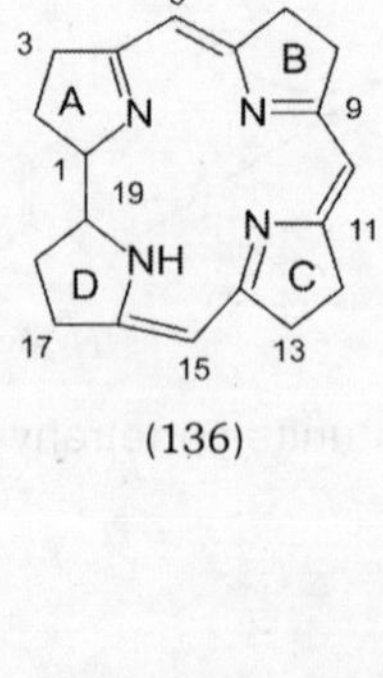

(136)

The four pyrrole rings are designated as A, B, C, and D. The numbering of the ring system is as shown in (136). The trivalent cobalt is held by co-ordinate bond with the three nitrogen of the pyrrole rings and nitrogen of benzimidazole and the cyanide ion.

The elemental analysis has given variable results and the most acceptable formula is $C_{63}H_{88}N_{14}O_{14}PCo$. It is optically active $[\alpha]^{23}_{656}$ -59 ± 9° (aq. Soln). It contains nine chiral centre namely, $C_1, C_2, C_3, C_7, C_8, C_{13}, C_{17}, C_{18},$ and C_{19}.

It is a polyacidic base and forms hexaperchlorate. Hydrolysis of vitamin B_{12} with hydrochloric acid produces D-1-aminopropan-2-ol (137), 5,6-dimethylbenzimimdazole (138), 1-α-D-ribofuranosyl-5,6-dimethylbenzimidazole (139), and its 3'-phosphate analog (140). Their structures have been established by UV spectrum and synthesis (Fig. 38.38).

D-1-Aminopropan-2-ol (137)

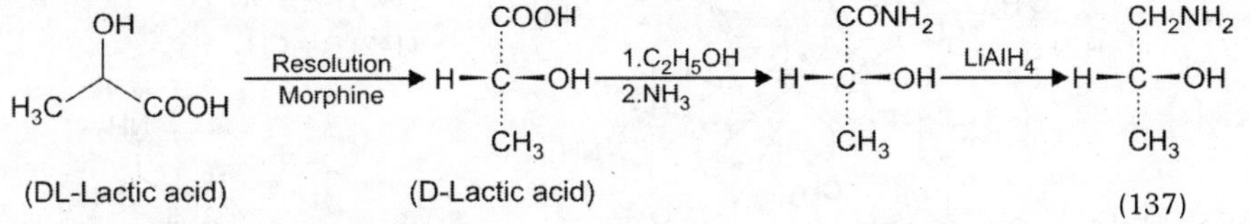

(DL-Lactic acid)   (D-Lactic acid)   (137)

5,6-Dimethylbenzimidazole (138)

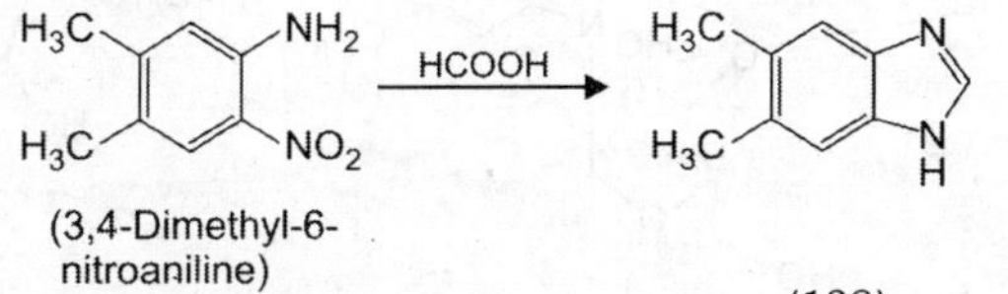

(3,4-Dimethyl-6-nitroaniline)   (138)

1-α-D-Ribofuranosyl-5,6-dimethylbenzimidazole (139)

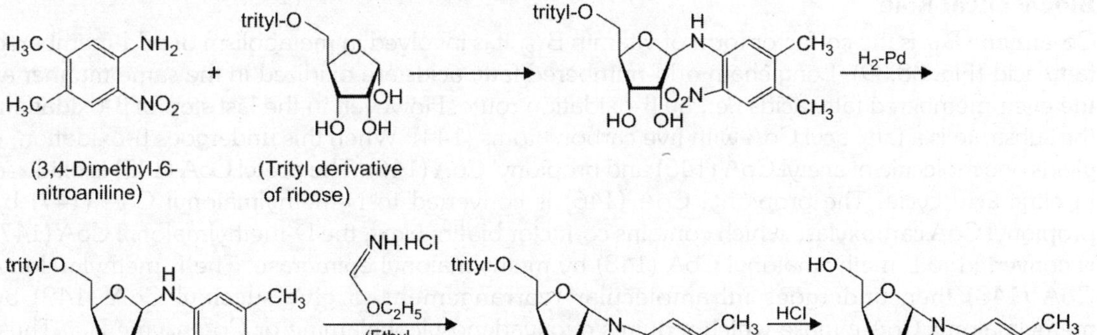

(3,4-Dimethyl-6-nitroaniline)   (Trityl derivative of ribose)

(Ethyl formamidinate)   (139)

Fig. 38.38: Synthesis of hydrolysis products of cyanocabalamin (135).

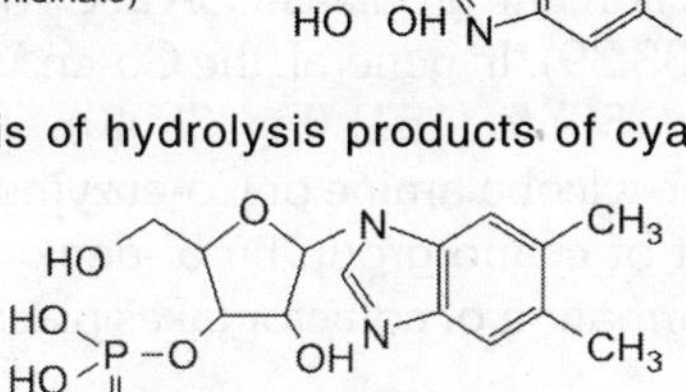

(140)

The vitamin contains six amido groups in the molecule. Alkaline hydrolysis gives a mixture of penta-and hexa-carboxylic acids and in both of them the nucleotide fragment is absent. The detailed x-ray analysis has established the structure of vitamin B_{12} as (135).

In addition to cyanocobalamine (135), the other forms of cabalamines include hydroxycobalamine (141), methylcobalamine (142), and 5'-deoxyadenosylcobalamine [Co-enzyme B_{12} (143)].

(135) R = –CN
(141) R = –OH
(142) R = CH3

(143) R =

Biochemical Role

Co-enzyme B_{12} is the co-factor form of vitamin B_{12}. It is involved in metabolism of odd-membered fatty acid (Fig. 38.39). Long chain odd-numbered fatty acids are oxidized in the same manner as the even-membered fatty acids i.e., by β-oxidation route. However, in the last step of β-oxidation, the substrate is a fatty acyl CoA with five carbon atoms (144). When this undergoes β-oxidation, it yields one molecule of acetyl CoA (145) and propionyl CoA (146). The acetyl CoA (145) is oxidized in citric acid cycle. The propionyl CoA (146) is converted to D-methylmalonyl CoA (147) by propionyl CoA carboxylase which contains co-factor biotin. Next, the D-methylmalonyl CoA (147) is converted to L-methylmalonyl CoA (148) by methylmalonyl epimerase. The L-methylmalonyl CoA (148) then undergoes intramolecular rearrangement to give succinyl CoA (149) by methylmalonyl CoA mutase which requires deoxyadenosylcobalamine or Co-enzyme B_{12}. Thus, in methylmalonyl CoA mutase reaction, the group -S-CoA at C_2 of the original propionate exchanges position with hydrogen at C_3(Fig. 38.39). In general, the Co-enzyme B_{12} (143) catalyzes the mutase reactions involving conversion of (150) to (151) (Fig. 38.40).

The formation of 5'-deoxyadenosylcobalamine or Co-enzyme B_{12} (143) from cyanocobalamine (135) takes place by replacement of cyano group by 5'-deoxyadenosyl group covalently bound through C-5' to the cobalt. This formation of cofactor takes place by cleavage of triphosphate from ATP (Fig. 38.41).

The mechanism of mutase reaction is given in (Fig. 38.42)

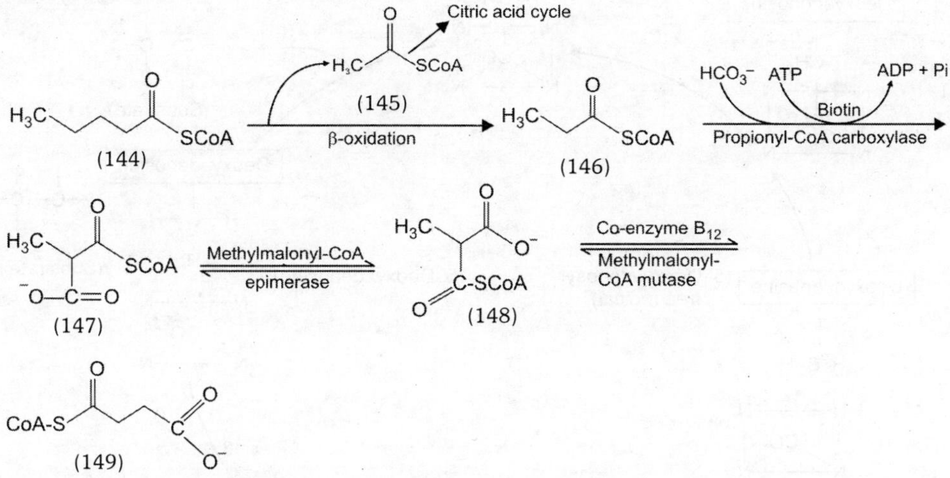

Fig. 38.39: β-Oxidation of odd-numbered fatty acids.

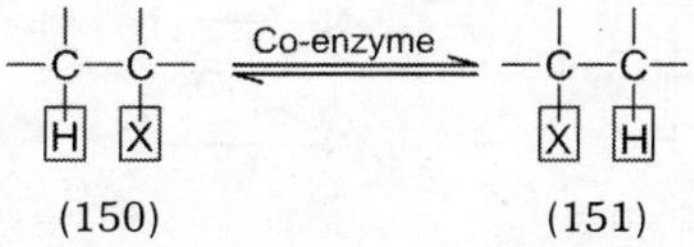

Fig. 38.40: Mutase reaction catalyzed by Co-enzyme B_{12} (143).

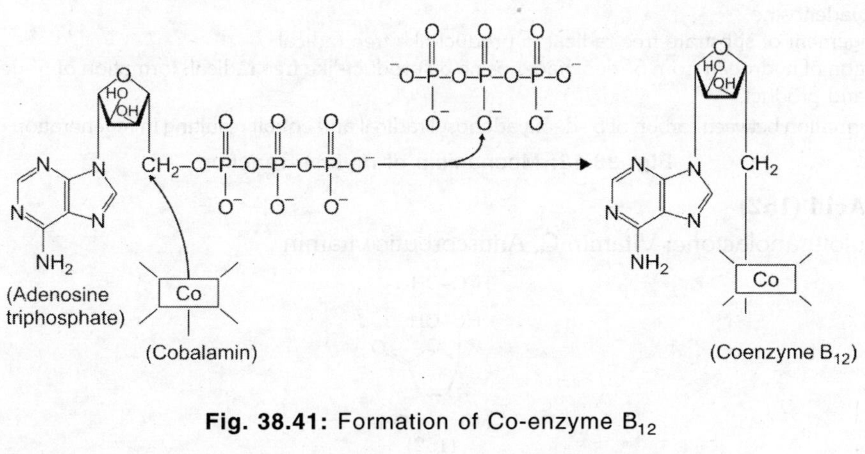

Fig. 38.41: Formation of Co-enzyme B_{12}

The mutase reaction takes place in 5 steps as shown in Fig. 38.42.

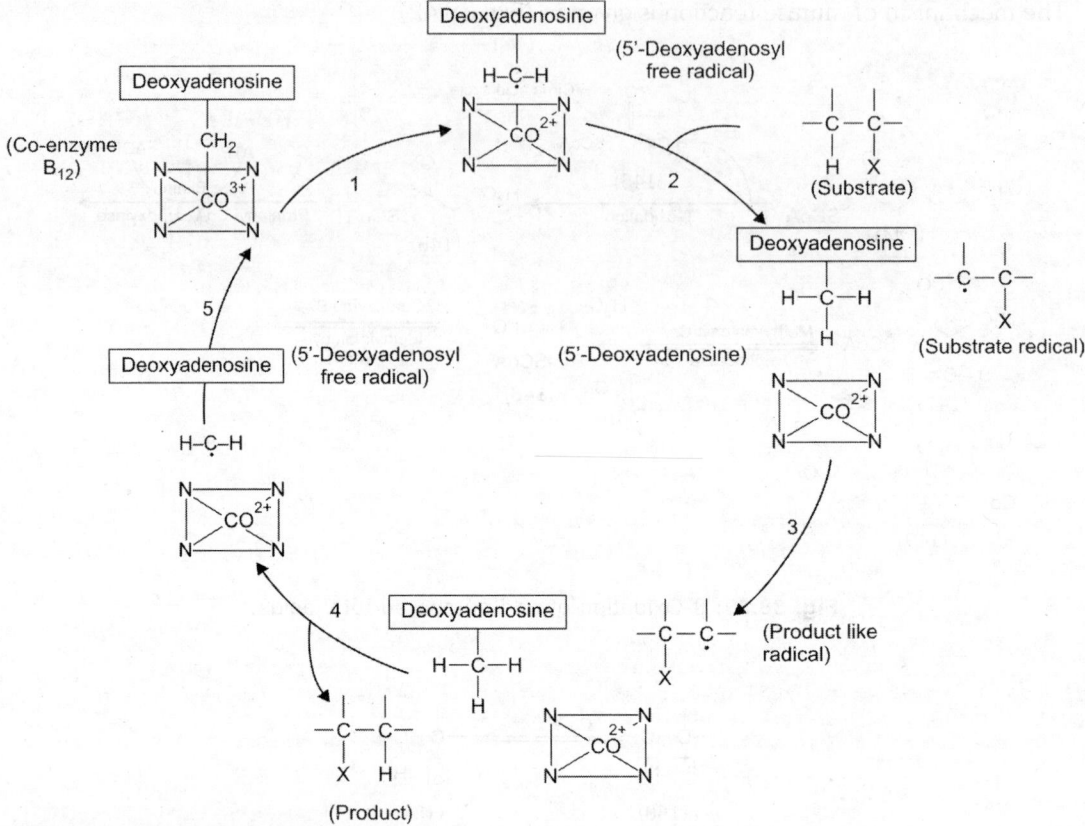

Steps involved in mutase reaction:
1. Formation of 5′-deoxyadenosyl radical by breaking of Co-C bond of coenzyme B_{12}.
2. Abstraction of hydrogen from substrate by 5′-deoxyadenosyl radical, formation of substrate free radical and 5′-deoxyadenosine.
3. Rearrangement of substrate free radical to product-like free radical.
4. Abstraction of hydrogen from 5′-deoxyadenosine by product-like free radical, formation of 5′-deoxyadenosyl radical and product.
5. Bond formation between carbon of 5′-deoxyadenosyl radical and cobalt resulting in regeneration of co-enzyme

Fig. 38.42: Mechanism of mutase reaction.

Ascorbic Acid (152)

3-Oxo-L-gulofuranolactone; Vitamin C; Antiscorbutic vitamin

Crystal, usually plates, mp 190-192°, $[\alpha]_D^{25}$ + 20.5° to + 21.5° (c = 1 in water).

Sources

Widely distributed in citrus fruits, paprikas, cabbages, and animals.

Deficiency Diseases

Deficiency of vitamin C results in scurvy which is charecterised by extreme weakness, spongy gums, and tendency to develop hemorrhages under the skin.

Structure

1. Molecular formula $C_6H_8O_6$.
2. Catalytic reduction of ascorbic acid gave a known compound L-idonic acid (153) indicating that the six carbon atoms present in ascorbic acid are arranged in a straight chain.

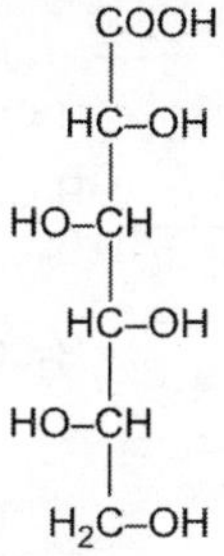

$$
\begin{array}{c}
\text{COOH} \\
|\\
\text{HC–OH} \\
|\\
\text{HO–CH} \\
|\\
\text{HC–OH} \\
|\\
\text{HO–CH} \\
|\\
\text{H}_2\text{C–OH}
\end{array}
$$

(153)

3. Aqueous iodine solution oxidizes acid to dehydroascorbic acid which on treatment with hydrogen sulphide gave back the ascorbic acid. Further, dehydroascorbic acid, which was found to be neutral behaved like a lactone of monobasic acid. Since conversion of ascorbic acid to dehydroascorbic acid and back takes place with mild oxidizing and reducing agents, it indicates that ascorbic acid like dehydroascorbic acid also must be a lactone. However, the properties of ascorbic acid could be due to enolic group. The presence of enolic function was confirmed by of violet colour formation with ferric chloride and phenyl hydrazone formation when treated with phenylhydrazine. These reactions can be explained by set of reactions shown in Fig. 38.43.

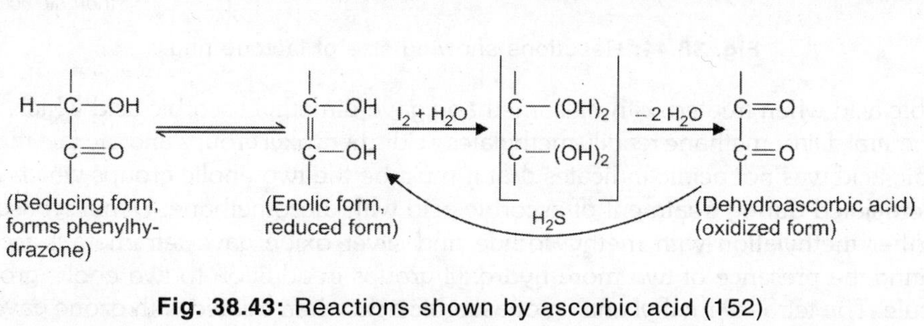

Fig. 38.43: Reactions shown by ascorbic acid (152)

4. When dehydroascorbic acid is treated with sodium hypoiodite, it gave oxalic acid (154) and L-threonic acid (155). The formation of these products indicate that dehydroascorbic is lactone of 2,3-diketo-L-gulonic acid (156) and accordingly, since ascorbic acid contains two enolic groups, it must be the lactone of structure (157).

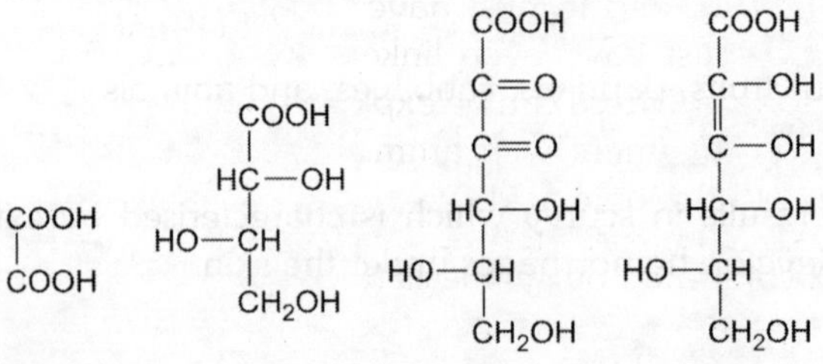

COOH
|
COOH
(154)

COOH
|
HC—OH
|
HO—CH
|
CH$_2$OH
(155)

COOH
|
C=O
|
C=O
|
HC—OH
|
HO—CH
|
CH$_2$OH
(156)

COOH
|
C—OH
||
C—OH
|
HC—OH
|
HO—CH
|
CH$_2$OH
(157)

5. The size of the lactone ring was ascertained by the following set of reactions (Fig. 38.44).

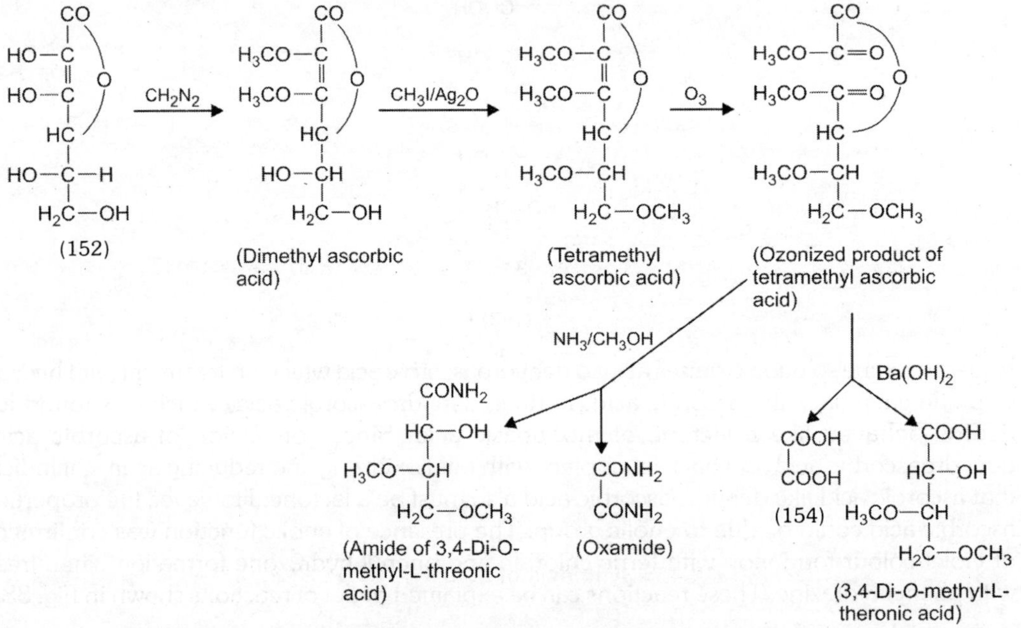

CO
|
HO—C
||
HO—C   O
|
HC
|
HO—C—H
|
H$_2$C—OH
(152)

→ CH$_2$N$_2$ →

CO
|
H$_3$CO—C
||
H$_3$CO—C   O
|
HC
|
HO—CH
|
H$_2$C—OH
(Dimethyl ascorbic acid)

→ CH$_3$I/Ag$_2$O →

CO
|
H$_3$CO—C
||
H$_3$CO—C   O
|
HC
|
H$_3$CO—CH
|
H$_2$C—OCH$_3$
(Tetramethyl ascorbic acid)

→ O$_3$ →

CO
|
H$_3$CO—C=O
|
H$_3$CO—C=O   O
|
HC
|
H$_3$CO—CH
|
H$_2$C—OCH$_3$
(Ozonized product of tetramethyl ascorbic acid)

NH$_3$/CH$_3$OH

CONH$_2$
|
HC—OH
|
H$_3$CO—CH
|
H$_2$C—OCH$_3$
(Amide of 3,4-Di-O-methyl-L-threonic acid)

CONH$_2$
|
CONH$_2$
(Oxamide)

Ba(OH)$_2$

COOH
|
COOH
(154)

COOH
|
HC—OH
|
H$_3$CO—CH
|
H$_2$C—OCH$_3$
(3,4-Di-O-methyl-L-theronic acid)

Fig. 38.44: Reactions showing size of lactone ring.

6. Ascorbic acid when treated with diazomethane gave dimethyl ascorbic acid which was found to be neutral. Diazomethane readily methylates acidic hydroxyl groups and the fact that dimethyl ascorbic acid was not acidic indicates that it must be the two enolic groups which must have got methylated during treatment of ascorbic acid with diazomethane. Dimethyl ascorbic acid on further methylation with methyl iodide and silver oxide gave tetramethyl ascorbic acid indicating the presence of two more hydroxyl groups in addition to two enolic groups in the molecule. The tetra -O-methyl analog of ascorbic acid when treated with ozone gave a neutral compound which had the same number of carbon atoms as its precursor. The ozonized product on hydrolysis with barium hydroxide gave oxalic acid (154) and dimethyl-L-threonic acid. The total number of carboxyl groups, accordingly, in the ozonized products are three. Further, since ozonization produces two carboxyl groups, so in the original molecule there must have been

present one carboxyl groups, and it must have been present as lactone. The free hydroxyl group in L-threonic acid must have been linked with this carboxyl group, accordingly the lactone must be a γ-lactone. All these can be explained if the structure of ascorbic acid is (152). The ozonized product on treatment with ammonia and methyl alcohol gave oxamide and amide of 2,4-di-O-methyl-I-threonic acid.

The structure is further confirmed by synthesis (Fig. 38.45).

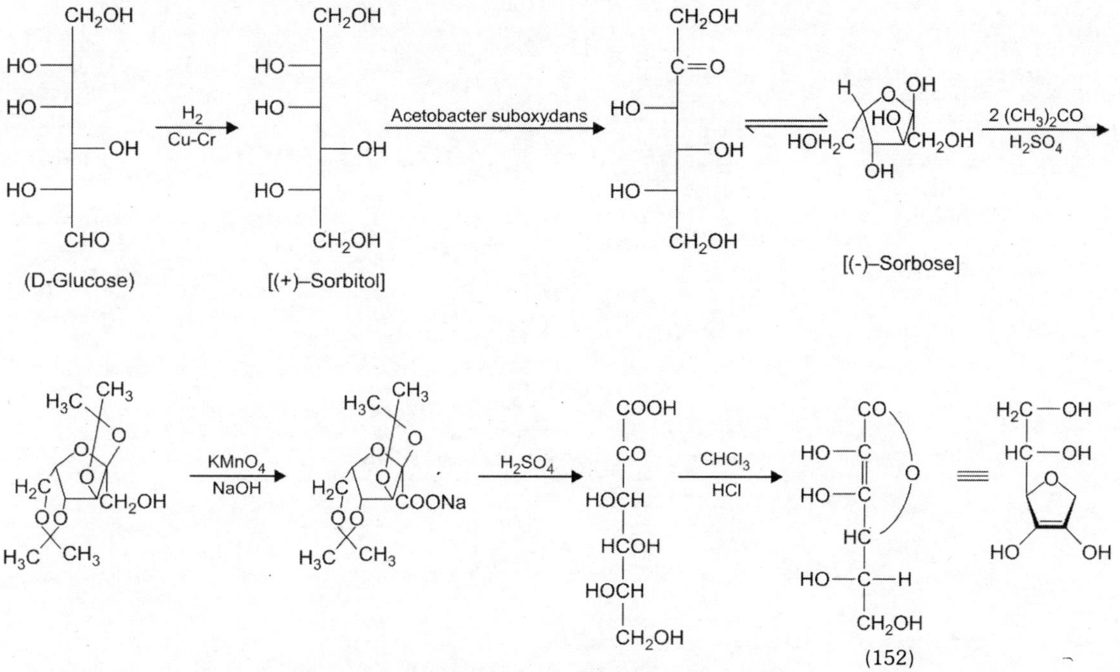

Fig. 38.45: Synthesis of ascorbic acid (152).

Biochemical Role

Co-enzyme complex of ascorbic acid (152) has not been yet isolated. However, ready conversion of ascorbic acid to dehydroascorbic acid and vice-versa plays an important role in oxidation-reduction of bio-system. Some of the reactions in which ascorbic acid is assumed to take part are given below.

1. Ascorbic acid + O_2 $\xrightarrow[\text{Hexaoxidase}]{\text{Cu}^{++}}$ Dehydroascorbic acid

2. Dehydroascorbic acid + Glutathione $\longrightarrow$ Ascorbic acid + oxidized glutathione

3. Oxidized glutathione + Glucose phosphate $\longrightarrow$ Glutathione + CO_2 + H_2O + Phosphate

present and acidic groups, and it must have been present as lactone. The free hydroxy
group (at the end) must have been linked with the carboxyl group; accounting the
lactone must be a lactone). All these can be explained if the structure of ascorbic acid is taken.
The ascorbic acid on treatment with ammonia and ethyl alcohol gave oxamide and
amide of 2,3,4-trihydroxy methylbutyl hreonic acid.

Hexauronic is further confirmed by synthesis (Fig. 36.15).

Fig. 36.15 Synthesis of ascorbic acid (1933)

Biochemical role

L-ascorbic acid (vitamin C and L-32) has not been yet pointed. However, ready conversion of
L-ascorbic acid and dehydroascorbic acid and vice versa play an important role in oxidation
reduction of biological system. Some of the reactions in which ascorbic acid is assumed to take part are
given below.

GLOSSARY

Acidosis
A metabolic condition in which the alkali reserves get reduced due to excess production of acidic metabolites which are incompletely oxidized or poorly eliminated.

Acne
Chronic inflammatory condition of pilosebaceous structures involving face, back, and chest occurring during adolescence.

Actin
Fiberous protein of the muscle.

Actinomycosis
Fungal disease caused by actinomycetes.

Active Site of Enzyme
The region on the surface of an enzyme where the substrate molecule binds and is catalytically transformed into products.

Acute
Sharp, severe, having a rapid onset with short duration. Opposite of chronic.

Addiction
The physical (physiological) dependence and psychological craving for a drug which is given continuously and then stopped suddenly.

Addison's Disease
Adrenocortical hypofunction charecterized by muscular weakness, low blood pressure, depression, anorexia, loss of weight, and hypoglycemia.

Adenoma
Benign tumor of glandular tissue.

Afferent
Carrying to e.g. afferent nerves which carry impulses to central nervous system.

Affinity
The charecteristics of a drug which enables it to bind to a receptor.

Agonist
A drug that binds to receptor and mimics the regulatory effects of endogenous signalling compound and possesses both affinity and intrinsic activity.

Agranulocytosis
Marked reduction or absence of granulocytes (mature granular leukocytes) due to bone marrow depression.Charecterized by high fever, ulcerative lesions of the mucous membrane of mouth, throat, and other areas.

Alkaloids
Nitrogenous organic compounds found in plants and animals.

Alkalosis
A condition when the capacity of body to buffer the hydroxyl ions is diminished.

Allosteric Site
The specific site other than the active site on the suface of an enzyme on which a modulator or effector binds.

Alopecia
Loss of hair.

Alzheimer Disease
Charecterized by marked atrophy of cerebral cortex and loss of cortical and subcortical neurons. This results in impairment of, short term memory, cognitive abilities such as ability to calculate, exercise visuo-spatial skills, and use of common objects and skills.

Amblyopia
Dimness of vision.

Amnesia
Partial or complete loss of memory.

Amphoteric
A substance that can act both as as an acid and a base.

Anabolism
Phase of intermediary metabolism in which small molecules are converted to more complex molecules.

Analogs
Compounds which show similar pharmacological activity but have different structures and origin. Such compounds can have similar electronic structures with different atoms.

Anaphylaxis
Hypersensitive state of body to foreign protein.

Anemia
Deficiency of haemoglobin due to deficiency of red blood corpuscles or dimunition of blood volume. It results because of loss of balance between the productive and destructive blood processes.

Angina
A condition marked by attacks of choking or suffocation.

Angina Pectoris
Severe pain in chest, arm, and neck due to insufficient blood supply to myocardium (myocardial ischemia).

Angioendothelioma
A tumor composed of endothelial cells and blood or lymph vessels.

Ankylosis
Stiffening of joints

Anomers
Diastereomers (diastereoisomers) of sugars, glycosides, or hemiacetals which differ in configuration at C_1 of aldoses or at C_2 of ketoses which are also known as anomeric centers.

Anorexia
Absence of appetite.

Antagonist
Molecules which inhibit or oppose the response of an agonist.

Anthralgia
Severe pain in joints which is not inflamed.

Antibiotic
Substance produced by plants or micro-organisms which is toxic to other plants or microorganisms.

Antibody
A protein (glycoprotein) synthesized by immune system of a vertebrate in response to antigen to which it binds.

Antigen
A molecule which elicits synthesis of a specific antibody in a vertebrate, also known as immunogen.

Antisense Molecules
Molecules which bind to specific regions of m-RNA and thus prevent them being used to code for protein synthesis.

Anxiety
A state of apprehension and fear accompanied by restlessness and uncertainities.

Aplastic
Structureless and incapable of forming new tissues.

Apnea
Transient suspension of breathing.

Apoptosis
Death and lysis of a cell brought out by itself by degrading its own macromolecules and brought out by signals from outside through programmed genes.

Arrhythmia
Absence of rhythm

Atrophy
Reduction in size of an organ or cell.

Autoimmune
Directed against body's own tissue.

Axetil
Ester with 1-acetyloxyethanol.

Bactericidal
Agents that kills bacteria.

Bacteriostatic
Agent that prevents the growth of bacteria

Baroreceptors
A sensory nerve ending that is stimulated by changes in blood pressure.

Benign
Not endangering health or life.

Benzathine
1,2-Bis(benzylamino)ethane.

Besylate
Benzenesulphonate. A compound with benzene sulphonic acid.

Bioisosteres
Isosteres that show agonistic or antagonistic activity.

Blood
The fluid tissue which circulates through heart, arteria, capillaries, and veins.

Blood Dyscrasia
Abnormality of blood cells due to toxic material in it.

Blood-Brain Barrier
Membrane between the circulating blood and brain composed of continuous layer of endothelial cells joined by tight junctions.

Bradycardia
Slowing of heart which is manifested in slow pulse rate.

Bronchitis
Inflammation of mucous membrane of bronchial tree

Calculus
A concrete mass composed chiefly of minerals and salts found in ducts, passages, hollow organs, and cysts.

Carcinoid
A benign tumor derived from enterochromaffin cells.

Carcinoma
Malignant growth of epidermal tissues e.g. skin, mucous memberane.

Cascade
A series of sequential interactions, as in physiological process, which once initiated continue to the final stage.

Catabolism
Phase of intermediary metabolism in which the complex molecules are broken down to small molecules and energy.

Cataract
Partial or complete opacity of lens of eye.

Chemical Antagonist
Compound which reacts with an agonist resulting in a pharmacologically inactive compound e.g. Ca^{++} and EDTA.

Chemoreceptor Trigger Zone
Area located in the 4th ventricle and associated with vomiting center.

Chiral
Molecule not superimposable on its mirror image.

Chiral Center
In a tetrahedral (or trigonal pyramidal) structure, the atom to which four (or three) different groups/atoms are attached.

Choriocarcinoma
A tumor containing cells of chorion (outermost of the fetal membrane).

Chronic
Of long duration, opposite to acute.

Cirrhosis
Chronic progressive inflammatory disease of liver.

Clonic
Series of involuntary movements of muscles charecterized by alternate contraction and relaxation e.g. clonic convulsions.

Cloning
Proliferation of a single cell to a large colony.

Clot
A semisolid coagulum of blood or Lymph.

Coagulum
A curd, a clot.

Colic
Paroxysmal abdominal pain due to smooth muscle spasm.

Colitis
Inflammation of colon.

Coma
Unconsciousness from which the patient cannot be aroused.

Complement
Complex protein formed in blood, plasma, or serum which in co-operation with antibody destroys the pathogenic organisms and other foreign substances. It has been fractionated into nine fractions.

Configuration
Three dimensional arrangement of atoms/groups around a chiral atom.

Conformation
Different arrangements of a molecule obtained by rotation around carbon carbon single bond.

Conformational Isomers
Stereoisomers that differ in conformations.

Congenital
Existing at birth.

Congenital Rubella
Disease since birth caused by rubella virus resulting in enlargement of lymph node.

Congestive Heart Failure
Chronic inability of heart to maintain adequate output of blood from one or both ventricles resulting in congestion and other distension of certain veins and organs with blood and in inadequate supply of blood to other body tissues.

Contraception
Prevention of conception

Convulsions
Involuntary paroxysm of muscular contraction. It can be either clonic or tonic or both.

Cretinism
Severe thyroid deficiency since birth charecterized by arrested physical and mental growth.

Crystalluria
Presence of crystals in urine which is normal. It can be serious if the crystals are of sulphonamides which may be formed in kidney tubules and cause blocking.

Cumulative Toxicity
Toxicity resulting from accumulation of drugs.

Cushing Disease
Charecterized by obesity, hyperglycemia, glycosuria, and hypertension. Caused by excessive secretion of corticoids by adrenal gland or by excessive administration of glucocorticoids.

Cushing Syndrome
Clinically similar to Cushing disease caused by overproduction of corticoids by adrenal gland due to hyperplasia or tumor of adrenal cortex.

Cycloplegia
Paralysis of ciliary muscles of eye resulting in paralysis of accommodation.

Cyst
A sac with memraneous wall enclosing fluid or semisolid matter.

Cytochrome
Colored proteins containing porphyrin-metal, usually iron, which readily undergoes oxidation-reduction in an organism.

Cytokines
Diverse group of soluble non-antibody proteins secreted by cell. They modulate the function of individual cells by interacting with specific plasma membrane receptors. Examples, interferons, interleukin.

Cypionic Acid
Cyclopentanepropanoic acid.

Cytotoxic
Toxic to cells.

Debility
Weakness.

Delirium
Mental excitement, confusion with hallucination.

Denaturation
Unfolding of protein or DNA by physical or chemical procedures.

Depolarization
When a cell is excited the sodium channels open and there is Inward flow of Na^+. The fast inward current of Na^+ increases the membrane potential from resting membrane of $-60\,mv$ to sodium equilibrium potential of $+40\,mv$ resulting in depolarization.

Depression
Emotional state of dejection associated with manic-depressive psychoses.

Dermatophyte
Fungal parasite which grows in or on the skin.

Diabetes Insipidus
Excessive urination caused by inadequate secretion of antidiuretic hormone, vasopressin.

Diabetes Mellitus
Excessive urination because of excess glucose in blood (hyperglycemia) and in urine (glucosuria) caused by disorder in carbohydrate metabolism which results because of inadequate production and utilization of insulin.

Diarrhoea
Frequent and loose evacuation of bowls.

Diastereoisomers
Stereoisomers which are not mirror images of each other. They differ in their physical and chemical properties.

Diastole
The rhythmic period of relaxation and dilation of heart chambers during which they are filled with blood. The diastolic blood pressure pertains to point of least pressure.

Dilation
Expansion of an organ.

Diolamine
Salt with diethanolamine.

Distention
A state of dilation.

Dizziness
Sensation of whirling (revolving rapidly) and having a feeling of tendency to fall.

Dysentry
Frequent evacuation of watery stools with blood and mucuous.

Dyspepsia
Disturbed digestion.

Edema
Excessive accumulation of fluid in tissue spaces.

Efferent
Carry away e.g Efferent nerves which carry impulses from central nervous system.

Eicosanoids
Collective term applied to substances derived from arachidonic acid such as prostaglandins, thromboxanes, leukotrienes, and lipoxins.

Embolism
Obstruction of blood vessels by a thrombi, fat globule, tumor cells, or an air bubble.

Enanthic Acid
n-Heptanoic acid.

Enanthate
Ester with n-heptanoic acid.

Enantiomers
Pair of molecules which are non-superposable mirror images of each other and possessing opposite type of optical activity but similar physical properties.

Endocarditis
Inflammation of endocardium.

Endocardium
Lining membrane of heart which covers valves.

Endocytosis
A process in which the cell membrane engulfs extracellular particles to form a coated vesicle in the interior of cell.

Endogenous
Developing or originating within the organism.

Endometrium
The mucous membrane of inner layer of uterine wall.

Endothelium
A layer of cells lining especially blood and lymph vessels and heart.

Endotoxins
Lipopolysaccharide protein complexes found in cell wall of gram negative bacteria.

Enterocolitis
Inflammation of mucous membrane of small and large intestines.

Enterohepatic
Pertaining to intestines and liver.

Enzyme
A catalytic molecule formed by a living cell which promotes a chemical reaction in the body by reducing the activation energy without affecting the equilibrium of the catalyzed reaction.

Eosinophile
White blood cells which have affinity for eosin dye.

Epigastric
Region lying directly over stomach and below lower ribbon.

Epimers
Diasteroisomers which differ in configuration at one of two or more chiral centers.

Epitope
An antigenic determinant on an antigenic molecule which can combine with antibody or T-cell receptors.

Essential Metabolite
Substances which cannot be synthesized by the cell and have to be provided from outside e.g vitamins.

Estolate
Salt with laurylsulphonic acid.

Euphoria
Feeling of well being.

Exocrine
Glands whose secretion reaches epithelial surface either directly or through a duct.

Exocytosis
Process of expelling cellular material from inside of the cell to the exterior of cell.

Exogenous
Developed or originating from outside of the cell.

Fibroma
Benign tumor of connective tissues.

Flatulance
The presence of excessive amount of gas in stomach and intestines.

Flavoproteins
Flavin dependent conjugated proteins, usually contain FAD or FMN as co-enzyme.

Gastroentritis
Inflammation of mucous membrane of stomach and intestines.

Genome
The genetic information as encoded in a cell or virus.

Geometrical Isomers
Molecules with differing arrangement of groups or atoms in which the free rotation around carbon- carbon bond is frozen (Ethylenic compounds and rings).

Glaucoma
Increased intraocular pressure of eye.

Gluconeogenesis
Formation of glucose from non-carbohydrate sources such as amino acids and fats.

Glycoprotein
Conjugated proteins containing covalently bond one or more sugar molecules.

Glycosuria
Excretion of glucose in urine.

Goitre
Enlargement of thyroid gland.

Granulation
Process of formation of granulation tissue (new capillaries and fibroblast) in or around inflammation.

Granulocyte
A mature granular leukocyte including neutrophilic, acidophilic, basophilic or morphonuclear leukocytes.

Granuloma
A nodule formed of inflammatory tissue in which granulation is significant.

Grave's Disease
Condition due to overactivity of thyroid gland.

Habituation
Psychological craving for a drug when it is given repeatedly and then stopped suddenly.

Hallucination
A false perception without objective reality. A common symptom in severe psychoses including schizophrenia.

Hapten
A small molecule which when combined with a large molecule acts as antigen and elicits an immune response.

Hard Drug
Drug which is resistant to biotransformation.

Hematoma
Swelling filled with blood which soon clots to form a solid mass.

Hemorrhage
Escape of blood from blood vessels

Hemostasis
Arrest of blood flow.

Hemostat
An agent/instrument which arrests hemorrhage.

Hepatitis
Inflammation of liver.

Hodgkin's Disease
Progressive disease of reticoendothelial system resulting in enlargement of lymphatic glands and spleen.

Homeostasis
The maintenance of dynamic study state by co-ordinated physiological processes involving brain, heart, nerves, etc., to compensate for changes in external environment.

Homozoin
A dark or red brown pigment found within plasmodia.

Hybridoma
A tumor of hybrid cells.

Hydrophobic
Non-polar.

Hydrophobic Interactions
The association of non-polar groups or molecules with each other in aqueous medium.

Hypercholesterolaemia
Increased levels of cholesterol in blood.

Hyperglycemia
Increased levels of glucose in blood e.g. in Diabetes mellitus.

Hyperplasia

Increase in size of tissue due to increase in number of cells.

Hypersensitive

Quantitative abnormality of an individual in resonse to a drug. The usual response in such cases being obtained with much lower dose.

Hypertrophy

Abnormal enlargement of an organ/tissue which is due to increase in size of its cellular content and not due to tumor.

Hypotensive

Denotes low blood pressure.

Hypocalcemia

Decreased calcium levels in blood.

Hypoglycemia

Decreased glucose levels in blood.

Idiopathic

Disease of unknown cause.

Idiosyncrasy

Qualitative abnormality of an individual to the response of a drug. Responses which are unexpected and different from the usual response to a drug e.g. morphine which is central nervous system depressant in human may act as excitant in some individuals.

Idiotype

The segment of immunoglobulin which determines its antigenic specificity.

Immunity, Active

Immunity which results from stimulation of host's tissue by an antigen.

Immunity, Passive

Immunity resulting because of transfer of pre-formed protective substances to the host e.g. injection of immune serum

Immunocyte

Leukocytes capable of producing antibodies or reacting in cell mediated immunity.

In Vitro

In glass – refers to process carried out in test tube.

In Vivo

In organism, in living cells.

Induced Fit

A change in conformation of an enzyme in response to binding of substrate that renders the enzyme catalytically active.

Inflammation

The reaction of tissue to infection, injury charecterized by swelling, redness, and heat.

Inotropy

The term used to describe the force of contraction of cardiac muscles.

Intercalation

Insertion between stacked aromatic or planar rings e.g. insertion of planar molecules between two successive bases in nucleic acids.

Interferon

A class of glycoproteins that modulate lymphocyte growth and activity. They possess antiviral effects and are used in hepatitis B andC.

Interleukin

Regulatory proteins that control lymphocyte development and activation. They also regulate immune and inflammatory responses. They are numbered as IL-1, IL-2 and so on.

Intermediary Metabolism

Constitutes the enzyme catalyzed reactions in cells involving extraction of chemical energy from nutrients and utilizing it for synthesizing cell components.

Intrinsic Activity

The ability to elicit a pharmacological response.

Ischaemia

Local dimunition of blood supply due to obstruction of inflow of arterial blood.

Isethionic Acid

2-Hydroxyethanesulphonic acid, $(HOCH_2CH_2SO_3H)$.

Isethionate

Compound with isethionic acid.

Isoelectric pH
The pH at which solute has no charge and does not move in an electric field.

Isoenzyme
Multiple forms of an enzyme that have same enzymatic activity but differ from each other in amino acid sequence.

Isoproxil
Ester with isopropyloxycarbonyloxy methanol.

Isosteres
Atoms, ions, and molecules in which the peripheral layer of electrons is identical.

Itching
An irritating sensation in skin.

Keratinisation
Conversion to a horny tissue.

Ketonemia
Presence of ketone bodies in blood.

Ketoneuria
Presence of ketone bodies in urine.

Ketosis
A condition in which there is high concentration of ketonic substances in body.

Leprosy
A chronic infectious disease caused by *Mycobacterium leprae.*

Lesion
Alteration of structure or functional capacity due to injury or disease.

Leukemia
Disease of blood forming organs in which there is uncontrolled proliferation of leukocytes.

Lumen
The space inside of a tube e.g blood vessel, duct.

Lyases
Enzymes that catalyze the removal of group from a molecule to form a double bond or addition of a group to a double bond.

Lymph
Yellowish basic liquid which is deived from tissue fluids.

Lymphoblast
A precursor of lymphocyte or monogranular white blood cell.

Lymphoblastoma
It is neoplastic diseases of lymph nodes and others not clearly neoplastic. It includes various forms of lymphocarcinoma and Hodgkin's disease.

Lymphocyte
White blood cells formed in lymphatic cell i.e lymph, spleen,thymus.

Lymphoma
A benign tumor of lymphatic tissue.

Lymphosarcoma
A malignant tumor of lymphatic tissues.

Lysis
Disintegration and dissolution of cell.

Lysosome
Cytoplasmic subcellular particle present in eukaryotic cells and contains hydrolytic enzymes.

Lysozyme
Enzyme which destroys the bacterial cell wall by hydrolyzing the 1,4-β-linkages between *N*-acetylmuramic acid and *N*-acetylglucosamine.

Malignant
Virulant and dangerous which results in fatal termination of life as malignant tumor.

Malnutrition
A state of being poorly nourished.

Mania
One phase of manic depressive psychosis.

Mast Cells
Connective tissue cells. Contain heparin and histamine.

Megablast
A large nucleated primitive red blood cell.

Meglumine
N-Methyl-D-Glucamine.

Meningitis
Inflammation of meninges.

Meso
Compounds with two or more asymmetric carbon atoms, whose mirror images are superimposable on original. They are optically inactive.

Mesylate
Methansulphonic acid salt.

Metabolite
Molecules which are involved in maintenance and formation of cell. All the biochemical processes lead to the formation of a metabolite.

Metaplasia
Conversion of one type of tissue to another. e.g. cartilage into bone.

Metastasis
The transfer of disease from one part of body to another, usually through blood.

Microfilaria
The embryonic and prelarvae form of filarial worms.

Migraine
Paroxysmal intense pain in head associated with vomiting and visual disturbances.

Morbid
Diseased.

Mucins
Various glycoprotein constituents of saliva and gastric juice which act as lubricants in body cavities and surfaces.

Mucopolysaccharides
General term for protein polysaccharide.

Mucus
A clear viscous secretion of mucous membrane.

Multidrug Resistance
The resistance to varied type of chemotherapeutic agents.

Mutagen
An agent that causes permanent inheritable change in DNA of an organism.

Myalgia
Muscular pain.

Myasthenia Gravis
An autoimmune disease charecterized by weakness in voluntary muscles.

Mycosis
Infection caused by fungi.

Mydriasis
Abnormal dilation of pupil of eye.

Myelin
White fatty substance forming sheath of some nerve fibres.

Myeloid
Pertaining to or derived from bone marrow

Myeloma
Malignant tumor of bone marrow also called myelosarcoma.

Myelomatosis
Multiple myeloma.

Myelopathy
Any disease of spinal cord or myeloid tissue.

Myeloplast
Leukocytes of bone marrow.

Myeloplegia
Paralysis of spinal origin.

Myelopoiesis
Process of formation and development of blood cells in bone marrow

Myeloseclorosis
Sclerosis of spinal cord.

Myelosis
Formation of myeloid tumors also called-myelocytosis.

Myoblastoma
Benign tumor of tongue, lip, or neck.

Myocarditis
Inflammation of myocardium.

Myocardium
Muscular tissue of heart.

Myopia
Near sightedness.

Myosin
One of the principal protein occurring in muscle.

Myxoedma
Decrease or absence of thyroid hormone resulting in constitutional disorder.

Nafate
An ester with formic acid.

Napsylate
Naphthalene -2-sulphonic acid salt.

Narcolepsy
Irresistible tendency to go to sleep.

Narcosis
State of unconsciousness, arrested activity or profound stupor.

Narcotic
Any substance which produces stupor.

Necrosis
The pathological death of a cell or group of cells in contact with living cell.

Neoplasm
Any new growth which is deviating from the normal in form or structure, usually denotes tumor – Neoplastic (adj.)

Nepherotoxic
Any substance which is toxic to kidney.

Nerve Block Anesthesia
Anesthetic injected into an area close to main nerve trunk supplying to the area where anesthesia is required.

Neuralgia
Severe paroxysmal pain along the path of nerve.

Neuritis
Lesion of a nerve or nerves.

Neuroblastoma
Malignant tumor of sympathetic system.

Neuroleptic
Also called antipsychotic or major tranquillizer. Neuroleptics affect behaviour and are used for psychotic disorders.

Neutrophils
The polymorphonuclear leukocyte of the blood which contains neutrophil granules in its cytoplasm and is stained readily by neutral dyes.

Nociceptive
Sensory neurons for pain sensation – pain receptors.

Nodule
A small aggregation of cells

Nootropics
Agents that improve nervous system functions.

Obstetrics
Care of women during pregnancy.

Obturation
Closing of an opening or passage, a form of intestinal obstruction involving obstruction of intestinal lumem by normal contents or by a foreign bodies.

Occlusion
Closing or shutting – up of an opening e.g coronary occlusion – occlusion of artery system that supplies blood to the heart.

Oncogene
A gene that induces uncontrolled cell proliferation.

Oncology
Science of neoplastic growth.

Oncosis
Any condition marked by development of tumor.

Ophthalmia
Inflammation of eye.

Opiates
Compounds which are structurally similar to morphine.

Opioids
All substances which possess pharmacological action similar to that of opium.

Opsonin
A substance that binds to antigen enhancing phagocytosis.

Optical Isomers
Molecules which rotate the plane of polarized light.

Orthostatic
Pertaining to or caused by standing e.g. orthostatic or postural hypotension.

Osteolysis
Resorption/degeneration of bone.

Osteomalacia
Osteoporosis resulting from lowered calcium absorption.

Osteomyelitis
Inflammation of bone marrow.

Osteoporosis
Loss of bone density.

Osteosarcoma
Sarcoma derived from the cells of bone and containing bone structures.

Otitis
Inflammation of ear.

Otosclerosis
Progressive impairment of hearing.

Paget's Disease
Charecterized by soft poorly mineralized bones which are prone to fracture.

Pagoplexia
Numbness due to cold.

Pallative
A drug relieving or soothing the symptoms of a disease but not curing it.

Pamoic Acid/ Embonic Acid
4,4'-Methylenebis(3-hydroxy-2-naphthoic acid).

Parallax
Apparent displacement of an object caused by looking at the object alternately first by one eye and then by other or by change of position of the observer.

Parkinsonism
A degenerative syndrome with four features which include bradykinesia (slowness and poverty of movement), muscular rigidity, resting tremors, and impairment of postural balance leading to gait and falling.

Paroxysm
Sudden and temporary attack which suddenly reappears.

Peritonitis
Inflammation of peritoneum.

Peritonium
A membrane which lines abdominal and pelvis cavities and the organs contained in them.

Phaeochromocytoma
Tumor of adrenal medulla.

Pharmacodynamics
The science of action of drugs.

Pharmacognosy
The science of crude drugs.

Pharmacokinetics
Involves the study of absorption, distribution, metabolism, and excretion (ADME) of a drug.

Pharmacology
The science of nature and properties of drugs.

Pharmacophore
Molecular charecteristics (electronic, steric) and functional groups of a drug that interact with target site to produce a pharmacological response.

Pharmacopeia
A collection of formulae, methods of preparation, quality control, and standards of drugs including dosage forms.

Physiological Antagonism
Balancing effects of hormones e.g. insulin and glucagon, which oppose the effects of each other by acting at different receptors.

Pivoxil
An ester with pivaloyloxymethanol.

Pneumonia
Inflammation of lungs.

Polycythemia
Increase in the number of red blood cells.

Postural
Pertaining to posture e.g postural hypotension.

Postural Hypotension
Hypotension caused because of posture or position e.g orthostatic hypotension.

Potentiation
When the pharmacological effect of combination of drugs is greater than the sum of their individual effects.

Pro-drug
Pharmacologically inert compound which upon biotransformation is converted to a pharmacologically active drug.

Prophylactic
An agent that acts as prophylaxis.

Prophylaxis
Prevention of disease.

Prostatic
Pertains to prostate gland.

Prosthetic group
A group of a compound that combines with a protein and is essential to its activity.

Prothrombin
A substance present in blood and essential for clotting.

Proxetil
An ester with isopropyloxycarbonyl-1-oxyethanol.

Pruritic
Itching due to irritation of the peripheral sensory nerves leading to scratching.

Pruritis
Itching due to irritation of peripheral nerve endings which is uncomfortable.

Pyrexia
Fever.

Racemic
An optically inactive mixture of equal parts of dextrorotatory and levorotatory forms of optical isomers.

Rash
Any skin eruption especially acute inflammatory dermatoses.

Rational Drug Design
A computer aided approach to drug design.

Receptor
A protein in the cell membrane of a nerve or organ to which a transmitter/drug binds to produce a pharmacological effect.

Receptor Antagonist
A receptor antagonist opposes the effects of an agonist either by competing with it for the active site (competitive) or by binding at the allosteric site (non-competitive), therby, changing the conformation of the receptor because of which agonist cannot bind to the receptor.

Repolarization
After depolarization, sodium channels close and potassium channels open. There is thus outward flow of K^+, this repolarizes the membrane towards potassium equilibrium potential of -100 mV.

Resting Membrane Potential
It is the potential difference between exterior and interior, exhibited by a cell. The interior is negative and the potential difference lies between -65 mV to -90 mV with an average of -70 mV.

Rh Factor
An agglutinogen first found in red blood cells of Rhesus monkey. Rh positive and Rh negative are the terms used to denote the presence or absence, respectively, of this factor.

Rheumatism
Disease of muscle joints, tendons, bones, or nerves resulting in discomfort.

Rickets
Skeletal deformity in children, due to deficiency of vitamin D.

Rubella
Viral disease charecterized by acute, contagious, eruptions, and spread by droplet infection. Also known as German measles.

Sarcoma
Malignant tumor of connective tissues composed of cells from non-epithelial tissues.

Schizophrenia
Psychic condition charecterized by lack of feelings, inappropriate mood, and unpredictable behaviour.

Sciatica
Neuralgic pain along the path of sciatic nerve.

Septicemia
Systemic disease produced by microorganisms and their poisonous products in blood.

Sinusitis
Inflammation of sinus.

Soft Drug
Drug which is biotransformed in vivo in a rapid and preditable manner into non-toxic moieties.

Spasm
A sudden muscular contraction.

Spondylitis
Inflammation of one or more of the vertebrae.

Sporozoa
Class of parasitic protozoa.

Sprain
Injury of soft tissue surrounding a joint and resulting in discoloration, swelling, and pain.

Stenosis
Contraction or narrowing of a duct or canal.

Stereoisomers
Isomers having similar constitution but differing in arrangement of atoms/ group of atoms in space e.g optical and geometrical isomers.

Stomatitis
Inflammation of soft tissues of mouth.

Strain
Excessive stretching, overuse of a part of body.

Stupor
A state of marked but not complete loss of consciousness

Substrate
A specific molecule/substance which is acted upon by an enzyme.

Summation
When the pharmacological effect of combination of drugs is equal to algebraic some of their individual effects

Syndrome
Group of symptoms which when considered together charecterize a disease.

Synergism
When the pharmacological effect of combination of drugs is greater than sum of their individual effects, synergistic (adj.).

Syphilis
Communicable veneral disease caused by spirochete, *Treponema pallidum.*

Systemic
Pertaining to or affecting the body.

Systole
The rhythmical contraction of heart and point of highest pressure in arterial vascular system.

Tachycardia
Excessive rapidity of heart's action.

Tebutate
Ester with *tert.* butyl acetic acid

Teoclate/Theocolate
Salt with 8-chlorotheophylline.

Teratogen
Any substance that causes abnormal fetal development.

Tetanus
A fatal infection caused by tetanus bacillus *Clostridium tetani* and charecterized by spasm of voluntary muscles, intense reflex activity, and convulsions.

Thecoma
Tumor of ovary, rarely malignant.

Thrombocytopenia
Decrease in number of platelets in circulating blood.

Thromboembolism
Obstruction of blood vessels with thrombus.

Thrombosis
Formation of thrombus.

Thrombus
A clot of blood formed within heart or blood vessel due to slowing of circulation or to alteration of blood or vessel walls.

Tocolytics
Uterine relaxants.

Tolerance
Reduction in response to a drug after repeated administration. As a result higher doses are required to produce the response similar to the response obtained after first administration of drug.

Tonic
Pertaining to tone e.g tonic convulsions-convulsions without relaxation.

Toxemia
Condition when the blood contains toxic substances, produced either by body or by the growth of microorganisms.

Toxin
A poisonous product of animal or plant origin which when given to an animal/man causes formation of antibodies.

Toxoid
A toxin whose toxic properties have been destroyed while retaining its ability to produce antibodies.

Transcription
Transfer of genetic information from DNA to RNA.

Transduction
Transfer of genetic material from one cell to another by a viral vector.

Translation
Synthesis of proteins from mRNA template.

Trismus
Tonic spasm of muscles of mastication.

Tromethamine
Compound with 2-amino-2-hydroxymethyl-1,3-propanediol.

Tubercle
Small aggregation of cells, a nodule.

Tussive
Pertaining to or caused by cough.

Typhoid Fever
Caused by acute infection due to *Salmonella typhosa.*

Uricacidemia
Presence of abnormal amount of uric acid in blood.

Uricosuric
Substances which increase the excretion of uric acid.

Urolith
Calculus in urine

Vasoconstriction
Narrowing of lumen of blood vessels.

Vasodilation
Widening of lumen of blood vessels.

Vector
A carrier of disease.

Veneral
Pertaining to or produced by sexual intercourse.

Venule
A small vein.

Vertigo
An unpleasant sensation of disturbed relation to surrounding objects in space or feeling that outer world is revolving.

Viscid
Semifluid, viscous, sticky, glutinous.

Vulnerary
Anything which is useful in healing of wounds.

Xeropthalmia
Dryness and ulceration of cornea leading to blindness due to deficiency of vitamin A.

Xinafoate
Salt with 1-hydroxy-2-naphthoic acid.

Yaws
Infectious non-veneral disease caused by *Treponema pertenue* found in hot moist tropics and charecterized by initial cutaneous lesions.

Zwitterion
Dipolar ion in which positive and negative charges are physically separated.

Zymogen
A proenzyme. An inactive precursor of an enzyme which shows enzymatic activity on activation by a catalysis e.g. pepsinogen.

SUBJECT INDEX

A

Acetylcholine
  receptors of 51
  stereochemistry and SAR in 53
  synthesis and release of 51
Acetylcholinestrase inhibitors 56
  reversible 57, 72
  irreversible 58, 76
  mechanism of 56
Acetylcholine receptors 51
  muscarinic receptors 52
  nicotinic receptors 52
Acetylcholine, stereochemistry and structure-activity
    relationship in 53
  alteration of alkylene chain 54
  alteration of quaternary ammonium head 54
  substitution of acetyl group with other acyl
    groups 54
  substitution or elimination of ester group 55
Adrenal cortex hormones 517
  biosynthesis of 518
  glucocorticoids 564
  mineralocorticoids 562
Adrenergic drugs 3
Adrenergic receptors 6
  disrribution in various organs and response to
    stimulation of 8
Adrenergic receptor agonists 12
  α_1-adrenergic receptor agonists 12, 27
  α_2-adrenergic receptor agonists 13, 30
  β_1- and β_2-adrenergic receptor agonists 14, 31
  β_2-adrenergic receptor agonists 14, 32
Adrenergic receptor antagonists 15
  α_1-adrenergic receptor antagonists 15, 37
  β-adrenergic receptor antagonists 169, 413, 424,
    442, 461

non-specific α_2-adrenergic receptor antagonists
  16, 39
non-selective β-adrenergic receptor antagonists
  18, 45
selective β_1-adrenergic receptor antagonists
  18, 41
mixed α- and β-adrenergic receptor antagonists
  19, 49
Adrenergic receptor blockers as
    antihypertensives 413, 424
  α_1-adrenergic receptor blockers as 413
  β-adrenergic receptor blockers as 413
  mixed α- and β-adrenergic blockers as 414,
Aldosterone antagonists as diuretics 390, 405
  mechanism of action 390
Aldosterone antagonists and inhibitors as diuretics 389
  aldosterone antagonists 390, 405
  aldosterone inhibitors 391
Alkylating agents as anticancer agents 886
  ethylenimines as 889, 907
  methanesulphonates as 889, 907
  miscellaneous agents as 890,908
  nitrogen mustards as 886, 903
  nitrogen mustard N-oxides as 888, 906
  nitrosoureas as 889, 907
Aminoglycoside antibiotics 725, 795
  antibacterial spectrum of 795
  mechanism of action of 795
  resistance to 795
p-Aminosalicylic acid and its derivatives as
    antitubercular drugs 812, 818
  antitubercular activity of 813
Amoeba, life cycle of 668
Amoebiasis, chemotherapy of 668
  natural drugs used in 669, 675
  synthetic drugs used in 670, 676

Amoebiasis, synthetic drugs used in 670
    aminoquinolines as 670, 676
    haloacetamides as 670, 676
    hydroxyquinolines as 670
    imidazole derivatives as 671, 676
    nitrothiazoles as 671
Analgesics 216, 335
    analgesics, antipyretics, and NSAIDs 335
    opioid 216
Analgesics, antipyretics, and nonsteroidal
    anti-inflammatory drugs (NSAIDs) 335, 338,
    anilines and aminophenols derivatives
        as 340, 351
    arylacetic and arylpropionic acids as 341, 355
    fenamates as 344, 365
    mechanism of action of 345
    oxicams as 344, 366
    pyrazolones and pyrazolidinediones as 340, 352
    salicylates as 338, 349
    structure-activity relationships in 345
Androgens 503
    antiandrogens 508, 534
    17α-hydroxylase/17, 20-lyase inhibitors 509, 537
    5α-reductase inhibitors and α1-adrenergic
        receptor antagonists 507, 530
    testosterone analogs and anabolic steroids 505, 521
Anesthetics, See *General and Local Anesthetics*
Angina 438
    drugs used for 438
    stable 438
    unstable 438
    variant 438
Anthelmintics drugs 684
    benzimidazoles as 684, 688
    miscellaneous compounds as 685, 690
    piperazines as 685, 689
Antianginal drugs 438
    β-adrenergic receptor blocking agents as 442, 461
    calcium channel blockers as 440, 455
    modulators of myocardial metabolism as 442, 462
    organic nitrites and nitrates as 438, 452
Antianginal, antiarrhythmic, and cardiotonic drugs 438
    antianginal drugs 438
    antiarrhythmic drugs 443
    cardiotonic drugs 445
Antiarrhythmic drugs 443
    class I drugs 443, 462
    class II drugs 444, 467
    class III drugs 444, 467
    class IV drugs 445, 470

Antibiotics 720
    aminoglycoside antibiotics 725, 795
    antibiotics with fused rings/tetracycline 725, 800
    chemical classification 720
    β-lactam antibiotics 720, 727
    macrolide antibiotics 724, 792
    miscellaneous antibiotics 726, 807
    peptide antibiotics 721, 789
    polyene antibiotics 723
Anticancer agents 885
    alkylating agents as 886
    antibiotics as 896
    antimetabolites as 892
    DNA cross linking agents as 892, 910
    hormones and antihormones as 900
    inhibitors of protein kinases as 901
    miscellaneous compounds as 903, 918
    plant products as 898
Anticholinergics, see *"Parasympatholytics"*
Anticoagulants, antiplatelet, and thrombolytic drugs 475
    anticoagulants 478
    antiplatelet drugs 482
    blood coagulation 475
    thrombolytic drugs 485
Anticoagulants 478
    charecteristics of an ideal anticoagulant 478
    injectable 479
    oral 481
Anticoagulants, injectable 479
    direct thrombin inhibitors 479, 486
    heparin based 479, 485
    selective factor Xa inhibitors 480, 487
Anticoagulants, oral 481
    coumarins as 481, 487
    indanediones as 482, 489
    mechanism of 482
Anticonvulsant drugs, see *Antiepileptic Drugs*
    Antidepressant drugs 258
    miscellaneous antidepressants 262, 283
    monoamine oxidase inhibitors 258, 271
    selective serotonin reuptake inhibitors 261, 280
    tricyclic antidepressants 259, 273
Antidiabetics, see *Hypoglycemic agents*
Antiemetic agents 615
    dopamine D_2-receptor antagonists as 617, 622
    histamine H_1-antagonists as 615, 619
    miscellaneous agents as 619, 624
    muscarinic antagonists as 616, 620
    neurokinin-1 receptor antagonists as 618
    5-HT_3 receptor antagonists as 616, 620

Antiepileptic drugs 199
    barbiturates as 200, 204
    benzodiazepines as 201, 211
    bromides as 200
    charecteristics of an ideal antiepileptic drug 199
    hydantoins as 200, 204
    imides as, 201, 209
    iminostilbenes as 202, 211
    miscellaneous agents as 202, 212
    2,4-oxazolidinediones as 200, 208
Antifungal agents 825
    amines as 830, 844
    antibiotics as 825
azoles as 827
    miscellaneous compounds as 830, 845
    phenols as 829, 843
Antifungal antibiotics 825
    griseofulvin as 825
    polyene antibiotics as 826
Antihistaminics and antiulcer agents 289
    antiulcer agents as 298
    biosynthesis, storage, and release of histamine 290
    histamine release inhibitors as 291, 301
    H_1-receptor antagonists as 291
    histamine release inhibitors with H_1-receptor antagonistic activity as 297, 327
    pharmacological effects of histamine 290
Antihypertensive drugs 408, 409
    angiotensin converting enzyme (ACE) inhibitors as 416, 426
    angiotensin II receptor antagonists as 418, 433
    calcium channel blockers as 415, 426
    diuretics as 410, 420
    sympatholytic agents as 410, 420
    vasodilators as 415, 424
Antimalarial drugs 645
    blood schizontocides 647
    gametocytocides 647
    natural 647
    sporontocides 647
    synthetic 652
    tissue schizontocides, primary 647
    tissue schizontocides, secondary 647
Antimalarial drugs, natural 647
    artimisnin and its synthetic analogs 651
    ch'ang shan 647
    cinchona alkaloids 648
Antimalarial drugs, synthetic 652
    acridines as 654, 661
    4-aminoquinolines as 654, 662

    8-aminoquinolines as 652, 660
    biguanides and 2,4-diamino-pyrimidines as 656, 664
    miscellaneous compounds as 659, 665
Antimetabolites as anticancer agents 892, 911
    folic acid analogs as 893, 911
    purine analogs as 895, 916
    pyrimidine analogs as 893, 912
Antiparkinsonian drugs 245
    anticholinergic drugs as 248, 254
    dopamine precursors as 247, 249
    dopamine receptor agonists as 247, 251
    dopamine release stimulants as 247, 251
    inhibitors of dopamine metabolism as 247, 250
    parkinsonism and dopamine 245
    peripheral dopa decarboxylase inhibitors as 247, 249
Antiplatelet drugs 475, 482
    cox-1 inhibitors as 482, 491
    glycoprotein IIb/IIIa receptor antagonists as 483, 493
    inhibitors of 2PY receptors as 484, 496
    phosphodiesterase inhibitors as 483, 491
Antiprotozoal drugs I:
    chemotherapy of malaria 645
Antiprotozoal drugs II 668
    chemotherapy of amoebiasis 668, 675
    chemotherapy of giardiasis 675, 682
    chemotherapy of leishmaniasis 675, 681
    chemotherapy of trichomoniasis 675
    chemotherapy of trypanosomiasis 672, 678
Antipsychotics, see *Neuroleptics*
Antitubercular drugs, synthetic 812, 818
    p-aminosalicylic acid and its derivatives 812, 818
    diamines as 815, 822
    hydrazides as 814, 821
    nicotinic acid and other heterocycles as, 813, 820
    thiosemicarbazones as 813, 819
Antiulcer agents 298
    Gastric acid secretion, mechanism of 298
    H_2-receptor antagonists as 300, 330
    proton pump inhibitors as 300, 332
Antiviral agents 847
    agents inhibiting virus attachment, penetration, and early viral replication as 850, 858
    DNA polymerase inhibitors as 851, 861
    HIV-protease inhibitors as 856, 876
    neuraminidase inhibitors as 850, 859
    nonnucleoside reverse transcriptase inhibitors (NNRTIs) as 855, 874

nucleoside reverse transcriptase inhibitors (NRTIs)
  as 853, 869
Anxiolytic agents 161, 166
  β-adrenoreceptor antagonists as 169
  barbiturates as 169
  benzodiazepines and GABAA receptor partial
    agonists as 166, 190
  miscellaneous agents as 170
  5-HT$_{1A}$ receptor partial agonists as 169, 196
Azoles as antifungal agents 827
  imidazoles as 827, 831
  triazoles as 827, 840

B

Barbiturates as sedatives and hypnotics 138, 144
  classification of 139
  mechanism of action of 141
  structure-activity relationship of 140
Benzodiazepines and GABAA receptor partial agonists
    as anxiolytics 166, 190
  mechanism of action of 167
  pharmacological activity of 167
  structure-activity relationship in 168
Blood coagulation 475
  factors involved in 476
  mechanism of 477
  vitamin K, mechanism of action of 477
Blood pressure and rennin-angiotensin system 408

C

Cardiac glycosides as cardiotonic drugs 445
  pharmacological action and mechanism of
    action of 450
  structure activity relationship in 450
Cardiotonic drugs 445, 470
  adenylyl cyclase stimulants as 451
  β-adrenergic receptor stimulants as 451, 471
  cardiac glycosides as 445
  drugs that increase calcium ion sensitivity to
    myocardium contractile proteins as 451
  phosphodiesterase inhibitors as 451, 470
Central nervous system stimulants 255
  analeptics 255, 263
  antidepressants 258, 271
  psychomimetics or hallucinogens 262
  psychomotor stimulants 256, 265
Cephalosporins 737
  degradation 741
  1st generation 738, 761
  2nd generation 739, 765

3rd generation 740, 774
4th generation 741, 782
mechanism of action of 742
spectrum of activity 742
Chemotherapy of acid fast infections 811
  leprosy 818
  tuberculosis 811
Cholinergic blockers 59
  ganglionic blocking agents as 66, 93
  neuromuscular blocking agents as 68
  parasympatholytic 59
Cholinergic drugs 50
Cholinergic receptors, distribution in various organs
    and response to stimulation of 53
Constipation, drugs used for 625
  luminally active agents as 625, 633
  non-specific stimulants and irritants as 627, 634
  prokinetic agents as 629
Coumarins as oral anticoagulants 481, 487
  structure activity relationship in 481
Cyclooxygenase-2 inhibitors as analgesics 345, 368

D

Diagnostic agents 923
  diagnostic dyes as 930
  miscellaneous agents as 933
  radiopaque substances as 923, 924
  agents used for examination of GI tract 924
Diagnostic dyes, used for
  hepatography 930
  kidney function 931
  miscellaneous functions 932
Diarrhea, drugs used for 629
  α$_2$-adrenergic receptor agonists as 631, 638
  adsorbents as 631
  antiinfective agents as 630, 635
  antimotility agents as 630, 636
  maintenance of fluid and electrolyte balance
    in 629
Dihydrofoliate reductase inhibitors (DHFRI) 700, 712
  synergism of DHFRI and sulphonamides 702
Disease modifying antirheumatoid drugs (DMARDs)
    346, 371
Diuretics 379
  acidifying salts as 381
  aldosterone antagonists and inhibitors as 389, 405
  high ceiling 391, 407
  organomercurials as 382
  phenoxyacetic acids as 383, 392

potassium sparing 391
purines and related heterocycles as 384
sulphonamides as 385
water and osmotic agents as 381
Drugs acting on adrenergic receptors, agonists 12
antagonists (blockers) 15
Drugs affecting norepinephrine biosynthesis 9
release 10, 22
storage 10, 22
Drugs affecting norepinephrine release 10
indirect acting sympathomimetics 11, 22
noradrenergic neurone blocking agents 10, 22
sympathomimetics with mixed action 12, 25
Drugs used for constipation, diarrhea, and inflammatory
bowl diseases 625
drugs used for constipation 625, 633
drugs used for diarrhea 629, 635
drugs used for inflammatory bowl diseases 631, 639

E

Endogenous catecholamines 20
Epinephrine, metabolism of 5
Estrogens 509
aromatase inhibitors 512, 550
estrogen antagonists 511, 546
mechanism of estrogen action 513
natural 538
non-steroidal estrogens 510, 544
synthetic analogs 540

F

Fungal diseases in man 825

G

General anesthetics 105
adjuvants to 114
charecteristics of an ideal 106
inhalation 106
intravenous 110
theories and mechanism of action of 114
General anesthetics, adjuvants to 114
basal anesthetics 114
control of pain 114
inhibition of salivation 114
prevention of nausea and vomiting 114
reduction of anxiety 114
skeletal muscle relaxant 114
General anesthetics, inhalation 106
ethers as 109
halogenated hydrocarbons as 107

hydrocarbons as 106
inorganic compounds as 106
General anesthetics, intravenous 110
ultrashort acting barbiturates as 110
miscellaneous compounds as 112
General anesthetics, theories and mechanism of
action of 114
biochemical theories 116
neurophysiological theory 115
physical theories 114
General anesthetics, physical theories 114
clathrate theory 115
colloid theory 114
lipid theory 115
molecular size theory 115
permeability theory 115
surface tension or adsorbent theory 115
Glycogen formation, mechanism of 591
Gout, drugs used in 347 373

H

H_1-Receptor antagonists 291
aminoalkyl ethers as 292, 304
ethylenediamines as 293, 308
piperazines as 294, 311
propylamines as 294, 315
second generation H_1-antagonists as 296, 322
tricyclic H_1-antagonists as 295, 318
Helmenthiasis 683
alimentary canal infections 683
other tissue infections 683
drugs used for, see Anthelmintics drugs
Histamine, biosynthesis, storage, and metabolism
of 290
conformations of 289
pharmacological effects of 290
Hormonal control of female reproductive system 516
Hormones and antihormones as anticancer
agents 900, 918
antiestrogens as 900, 918
gonadotropin releasing hormone
agonists and antiandrogens as 900, 918
Hydrazides as antitubercular drugs 814, 821
structure-activity relationship in 814
Hyperthyroidism and drugs used for 609, 610
Hypoglycemic agents 589
insulin and related analogs as 589
oral 593

Hypoglycemic agents, oral 593, 596
    biguanides as 595, 601
    α-glucosidase inhibitors as 596
    meglitinides as 594
    sulphonylureas as 593, 596
    thiazolidinediones as 595, 602
Hypothyroidism and drugs used for 609, 610

I

Inflammatory bowl diseases, drugs used for 631
    glucocorticoids as 632, 640
    immunosuppressive agents as 632, 641
    sulphasalazine and related compounds as
        631, 639
Insulin and related analogs as hypoglycemic agents 589
    amylin agonists as 592
    mechanism of action of insulin 590
    modified insulin 592

L

β-Lactam antibiotics 720, 727
    carbacephems 742, 783
    carbapenems 735, 758
    cephalosporins 737, 761
    monobactams 743, 785
    oxacephems 742, 783
    penicillins 727, 743
Leprosy, chemotherapy of 818
    antileprotic drugs 823
Leukotrienes, biosynthesis of 337
Local anesthetics 117
    administration of 124
    amide type 121, 131
    ester type 117, 125
    mechanism of action of 123
    miscellaneous compounds as 122,136
Local anesthetic administration of 124
    block anesthesia 124
    epidural anesthesia 124
    field block anesthesia 124
    infiltration anesthesia 124
    topical anesthesia 124
Local anesthetic, ester type 117, 125
    structure-activity relationship in 118
Luminally active agents for constipation 625
    bulk laxatives 625
    osmotic agents 626, 633
    stool softeners and emolients, 626, 633

M

Macrolide antibiotics 724, 792
    mechanism of action of 792
    resistance to 792
Malaria 645
    clinical cure of 647
    quartan 645
    radical cure of 647
    suppression of 647
    suppressive cure of 647
    tertian 645
Malarial parasite, life cycle of 645
Miscellaneous compounds as sedatives hypnotics 143, 158
    alcohols as 143
    aldehydes as 143, 159
    quinazolinones as 143, 158
Muscarinic agonists 55, 70
Muscle contraction, mechanism of 440

N

Neuroleptics and anxiolytics 161
    anxiolytic agents 166
    neuroleptics 161
Neuroleptics 161
    butyrophenones as 164, 182
    dibenzoazepines as 163, 178
    mechanism of action of 166
    miscellaneous compounds as 164, 185
    phenothiazines as 162, 170
    thioxanthenes as 163, 177
Neuromuscular blocking agents 68
    depolarizing 70, 101
    non-depolarizing 68, 94
Nicotinic agonists 56
Non-specific stimulants and irritants for constipation 627
    anthraquinones as 628
    diphenylmethane derivatives as 627, 634
    castor oil as 629
Norepinephrine 3
    biosynthesis, storage, and release of 4
    metabolism of 5

O

Opioid analgesics 216
    endogenous opioid peptides 224
    mechanism of action of 226
    narcotic antagonists as analgesics 224

opium and morphine analogs 216, 226
opioid receptors 225
synthetic opioids 219
Opioid analgesics, synthetic 219
6,7-benzomorphans as 220, 232
methadones and related analogs as 223, 241
morphinans as 219, 229
4-phenylpiperidines analogs as 220, 233
Opioid receptors 225
topography of 225
Opium and morphine analogs as opioid analgesics 216, 226
structure activity relationship in morphine 217
Oral contraceptives 515
long acting progestins only 516
once a week/once a month only 517

P

Parasympatholytics 59
semisynthetic analogs of solanaceous alkaloids 60, 77
solanaceous alkaloids 59, 77
synthetic 61
Parasympatholytics, synthetic 61
aminoalcohol esters as 62, 79
aminoalcohols as 64, 87
aminoamides as 64, 86
aminoethers as 65, 89
miscellaneous compounds as 65, 91
Parkinsonism and dopamine 245
biosynthesis of dopamine 245
metabolism of dopamine 246
Penicillins 727
allergy to 734
β-lactamase inhibitors 734, 756
mechanism of action of 732
natural 727
resistance to 734
semisynthetic 729
Penicillins, semisynthetic 729
with acid resistant properties 731, 755
with broad spectrum of activity 730, 748
with penicillinase resistant properties 730, 745
Peptide antibiotics 721, 789
actinomycins 721
bacitracins 721
linear gramicidins 721
polymixins 723

Phenoxyacetic acids as diuretics 383, 392
structure-activity relationship in 383
Progesterone and progestins 513
miscellaneous compounds as 513
progesterone and progesterone derivatives as 513, 551
progestin antagonists 515, 560
testosterone and 19-nortestosterone derivatives as 513, 555
Prostanoids, biosynthesis of 336
Pteridines as diuretics 384, 392
structure-activity relationships in 385
Purines and related heterocycles as diuretics 384, 392
pteridines as 384, 392
purines as 384, 392
pyrazines as 385, 393

Q

Quinolones as antibacterials 702, 712
antibacterial activity of 703
mechanism of action of 704
structure-activity relationships in 703

R

Radiopaques as diagnostic agents for 923, 924
angiography and urography 923, 924
bronchography, fistula, and sinuses 923, 930,
cholecystography 923, 928
gastrointestinal examination 924
myelography 923, 929
Renin-angiotensin system and blood pressure 409

S

Sedatives and hypnotics 138
barbiturates as 138, 144
benzodiazepines as 141, 150
miscellaneous compounds as 143, 158
non-benzenoid GABAA agonists as 142, 157
piperidinediones as 141, 149
Serotonin, metabolism of 258
Sex hormones 503
androgens 503
biosynthesis of 504
estrogens 509
progesterone and progestins 513
oral contraceptives 515
Smooth muscle relaxation due to organic nitrites and nitrates 439

Steroids and steroidal drugs 499
    adrenal cortex hormones 517
    bile acids 501
    cholesterol 500
    phytosterols and mycosterols 501
    sex hormones 503
Sulphonamides as antibacterials 695, 704
    antibacterial activity of 695
    mechanism of action of 697
    metabolism, protein binding, and distribution of 700
    nomenclature of 695
    resistance, development of 700
    structure-activity relationships in 696
Sulphonamides as diuretics 385
    carbonic anhydrase inhibitors as 385, 393
    thiazides and hydrothiazides as 388 , 402
Sulphonamides and quinolones 695
    dihydrofoliate reductase inhibitors 700
    quinolones 702, 712
    sulphonamides 695, 704
Suphonylureas as oral hypoglycemic agents 593
    first generation 593
    second generation 594
Sympatholytic agents as anti-hypertensives 410
    adrenergic receptor blocking agents as 413
    cenrally acting sympatholytic agents as 410, 420
    drugs affecting noradrenergic neurons as 412, 422
    ganglionic blocking agents as 412, 422

T

Tetracycline antibiotics 725, 800
    mechanism of action of, 802
    resistance to, 802
    spectrum of activity of, 802
    structure-activity relationship in, 801
Thiazides and hydrothiazides as diuretics, 388, 402
    structure-activity relationships in, 388, 389
Thyroid and antithyroid drugs, 607
    hyperthyroidism, 609
    hypothyroidism, 609
    thyroid hormones, 607

Thyroid hormones 607
    biosynthesis of 607
    mechanism of action of 608
Trypanosomiasis, chemotherapy of 672
    diamidines 672, 678
    miscellaneous compounds 673, 678
Tryptamine, metabolism of 259
Tuberculosis 811
    chemotherapy of 812
    synthetic antitubercular drugs 812, 818
    antibiotics for 815

U

Uric acid, biosynthesis and metabolism of 347

V

Viral infection, prevention of 849
    immunization 849
Virus, life history 847
    steps involved in replication of DNA virus 848
    steps involved in replication of RNA virus 848
Vitamins 937
    fat soluble 937
    water soluble 959
Vitamins, deficiency diseases due to and biochemical
    role of:
    ascorbic acid 993, 995
    biotin 979, 981
    cyanocobalamin 988, 990
    folic acid 983, 987
    niacin and niacinamide 970
    pantothenic acid 972, 973
    pyridoxamine, pyridoxal, and pyridoxine
      974, 978
    riboflavin 965, 968
    thiamine 959, 963
    vitamin A 938, 940
    vitamin D 941, 946
    vitamin E 948, 953
    vitamin K 954, 959

COMPOUND INDEX

A

Abarelix 901
Abacavir 854, 855
Abecarnil 168
Abiraterone 509
Acarbose 596
Acebutolol 18, 41, 43, 413
Acenocoumarol 481, 488
2-Acetamido-5-nitrothiazole 671
Acetaminophen, see Paracetamol
Acetanilide 340, 352
Acetazolamide 386, 393, 394, 395
Acetohexamide 593, 599
Acetophenazine 162, 176
2-Acetoxycyclopropyl-1-trimethyl ammonium iodide 53
Acetrizoate sodium 925
N-Acetyl p-aminosalicylic acid 813
Acetylcholine 3, 7, 50, 51, 52, 53, 54, 55, 59, 60, 66, 67, 68, 70, 245, 299, 300
Acetylcholine chloride 70
N-Acetylglucosamine 479, 486, 732
Acetyl isoniazid 821
Acetylhydrazide 821
6-Acetylmorphine 217
N-Acetylmuramic acid 732
Acetylsalicylic acid, see Aspirin
Acetyl sulphisoxazole 709
L-Acofriose 445
L-Acovenose, 445
Acoin 122
Acriquine 654
Acrivastine 296, 326
Acyclovir 851, 853, 863, 864
Adefovir 852, 853, 855, 867
Adefovir dipivoxil 868
Adenine 347

Adrenaline, see Epinephrine
Agar 625
Albendazole 684, 689
Albutoin 200, 207
Alclometasone 519, 571
Aldosterone 389, 390, 391, 392, 406, 408, 409, 415, 517, 518, 519
Alfentanil 222, 238
Alfuzosin 508, 533
Alitretinoin 903
Alizapride 617, 622
Allantoin 348
Allobarbital 139, 146
(±)-Allobiotin 981
Allocholanic acid 501
D-Allomethylose 445
Allopurinol 348, 373
Alloxanthine 348, 374
N-Allylnormorphine, see Nalorphine
Aloin 628
Aloxiprin 350
Alprazolam 167, 168, 195, 619, 624
Alteplase 485
Altretamine 890, 891, 909
Amantadine 247, 251, 850, 858
Ambenonium chloride 57, 58, 74
Amcinonide 520, 579
Amethocaine 119, 125, 126
Amethocaine hydrochloride 127
Amfenac 341, 356
Amikacin 725, 797
Amiloride 385, 391, 393
p-Aminobenzoic acid (PABA) 697, 699, 700
γ-Aminobutyric acid (GABA) 166
7-Aminocephalosporanic acid 737, 741
Aminoglutethimide 512
2-Amino-5-nitrothiazole 671

6-Aminopenicillanic acid 728, 729, 730, 731

p-Aminophenol 340

Aminophylline 257, 268, 384

Aminopterin 700

Aminopyrine 340, 341

p-Aminosalicylic acid (PAS) 812, 813, 814, 815, 818

5-Aminosalicylic acid 632, 639, 640

Amiodarone 444, 467

Amiphenazole 255. 256

Amitriptyline 260, 276

Amitryptyline N-oxide 277

Amlodipine 415, 441, 455, 456, 459

Ammonium chloride 381

Ammonium nitrate 381

Amobarbital 139, 146

Amodiaquine 655, 663

Amopyroquine 655

Amoxapine 163, 179, 180, 260, 275

Amoxicillin 730, 732, 751, 756, 763

Amphenone B 391

Amphetamine 11, 22, 23, 27, 265

Amphotericin B 723, 826

Ampicillin 730, 731, 732, 742, 748, 750, 751, 752, 755, 757, 764

Amprenavir 856, 880, 881

Amrinone 451, 470, 471

Amyl nitrite 438, 452

n-Amylpenicillin, see *Dihydro F penicillin Amylin* 592

Amylocaine 120

Analgin 340, 353

Anastrozole 512, 550, 551, 900, 918

Androsterone 503

Andrstenedione 504

Aneurin, see *Thiamine*

Angiotensin I 408, 409, 417

Angiotensin II 408, 409, 417, 418

Angiotensin III 408, 409

Anhydrodeacetylcephalosporoic acid 741

Anileridine 221, 235

Anisindione 482, 490

Antazoline 293, 308

Anthranilic acid 344

D-Antiarose 445

Antipyrine, see *Phenazone*

Antiscorbutic vitamin, see *Ascorbic acid*

Apraclonidine 13, 30, 31

Aprepitant 618

Argatroben 480, 486

Arachidonic acid 336, 337, 338

Arteether 651

Artemether 651

Artesunate 651

Artimisnin 651

Ascorbic acid 992

Aspirin 339, 340, 342, 343, 345, 349, 350, 351, 360, 482, 491

Aspirin aluminium salt 339

Aspirin calcium salt 339

Astemizole 296, 324, 329

Atazanavir 856

Atenolol 18, 41, 413, 442, 461

Atomoxetine 262

Atovaquine 660, 667

Atracurium besylate 68, 98

Atropine 50, 59, 60, 61, 77, 78, 248

Atropine methylbromide 60

Atropine methylnitrate 60

Atropine N-oxide 60

Atrial natriuretic peptide 409

Auranofin, 346

Aurothioglucose 346, 372

Azacitidine 893, 895

Azapropazone 341, 348

Azathioprine 632, 641

Azatidine 296, 321, 325

Azelastine 297, 329

Azithromycin 724

Azimilide 444, 470

Azosemide 387, 391, 398

Aztreonam 743,785, 787

B

Bacitracin 721, 789

Bacitracin A 721

Bacitracin B 721

Bacitracin C 721

Bacitracin D 721

Bacitracin E 721

Bacitracin F 721

Balsalazide 631, 640

Barbaloin, see *Aloin*

Barbital 139, 140, 144

Barbituric acid 138

Barium chloride 59

Barium sulphate 924
Becampicillin 750
Beclomethasone 519, 571
Bemidone 221, 236
Benazipril 416, 417, 426, 427, 428, 429, 430, 431
Benaziprilat 417, 427
Bendroflumethiazide 389, 404
Benorylate 339, 350
Benoxaprofen 343, 362
Benoxinate 120, 128
Benserazide 247, 250
Benznidazole 673, 674, 680
Benzocaine 118, 119, 124, 125
6,7-Benzomorphan 219, 220
Benzo [a] pyrene 885
Benzphetamine 11, 22, 256, 265
Benzthiazide 389, 402
Benztropine 248, 254
Benztropine mesylate 65, 89, 254
Benzyl alcohol 123
Benzylpenicillin, see Penicillin G
Bepridil 415, 441, 460
Betamethasone 519, 572
Betamethasone 21-acetate 573
Betamethasone 17α-benzoate 573
Betamethasone 17α, 21-dipropionate 573
Betamethasone 17α, 21-disodium-phosphate 573
Betamethasone 17α-valerate 573
Betaxolol 18 42, 413
Bethanechol chloride 55, 56, 71
Bethanidine 412, 413, 423
Biapenem 736, 758, 760, 761
Bicalutamide 508, 536, 901, 918
Bicuculline 255, 256
Biotin 978
(±)-Biotin 981
Biperiden 65, 89, 248, 254
Bisacodyl 627, 634
Bisoprolol 18, 42, 413
Bitolterol 14, 15, 35
Bivalirudin 480
Bleomycin 898
Bleomycin A₂ 898
Bleomycin B2 898
Bleomycinic acid 898
D-Boivinose 445
Bradykinin 335, 338, 409, 417

Bran 625
Bretazenil 168
Bretylium tosylate 10, 22, 444, 467
Brimonidine 13, 31
Bromides 138, 200
Bromindione 482, 490
Bromisovalium 144
Bromocriptine 248, 251
Bromodiphenhydramine 292, 305
Brompheniramine 295, 316
Buclizine 294, 313
Budesonide 520, 581
Bufotenine 262
Bumetanide 387, 391, 396, 397
Bupivacaine 121, 124, 133
Bupropion 262, 285
Burimamide 300
Buspirone 169, 196, 197
Busulfan 889, 907
Butabarbital 139, 147
Butacaine 119, 126
Butamin 119
Butanilicaine 121, 122
Butesine 118
Butethamine 120
Butoconazole 827, 834
Butorphanol 219
Butorphanol tartrate 231

C

Caffeine 256, 257, 267, 268, 384, 392
Calciferol, see Vitamin D₂
Calcitonin 607
Calcium chloride 381
Calcium nitrate 381
Calmodulin 440
Candesartan 418, 433, 434, 435, 436, 437
Canrenoate 390
Canrenone 390
Capecitabine 893, 894, 913
Captopril 417, 431
Carbachol 54, 55, 71
Carbamazepine 202, 203, 211, 214
Carbaryl 57, 58, 73
Carbenicillin 730, 752, 753, 757
Carbidopa 247, 249, 250
Carbimazole 609, 611

Carbinoxamine 292, 306
Carboplatin 892, 910
2-(6-Carboxyhexylamino)ethylguanide 423
Carbromal 144
Carbutamide 593, 596
Carebastine 296, 327
Carindacillin 730
Carmustine 889, 907
Carprofen 343
Carteolol 18, 45, 413
Carumonam 743, 787
Carvedilol 19, 20, 49, 414
Castor oil 627, 629
Cefaclor 739, 765, 784
Cefadroxil 738, 762
Cefamandole 739, 768. 770
Cefamandole nafate 768
Cefazolin 738, 765
Cefepime 741, 782
Cefixime 740, 778
Cefmetazole 739, 773
Cefonicid 739, 768
Cefoperazone 740, 780
Cefotaxime 740, 777
Cefotetan 739, 774
Cefoxitin 739, 770, 774
Cefpirome 741, 782
Cefpodoxime 739
Cefprozil 739, 767
Ceftazidime 740, 779
Ceftibuten 740, 774
Ceftizoxime 740, 775
Cefuroxime 739, 769
Celecoxib 345, 370
Cephalexin 738, 761, 767
Cephalosporin C 737
Cephalosporoic acid 741
Cephalothin 738, 764
Cephapirin 738, 764
Cephradine 738, 763
Cetrizine 296, 325
Chenodesoxycholic acid 502, 503
Chiniofon 670
Chloral hydrate 138, 140, 143, 159, 170
Chlorambucil 887, 904
Chloramphenicol 726, 730, 807, 808, 809, 810
Chloramphenicol palmitate 808, 810

Chloramphenicol sodium succinate 808, 810
Chlorcyclizine 294, 312
Chlordiazepoxide 141, 150, 166, 190
Chlorguanide 657, 658, 660, 664, 667, 701, 712
Chlormethiazole 160
Chlormidazole 827, 834
Chlorobutanol 143
Chlorodiphenhydramine 292, 305
8-Chlorofebrifugine 647
Chloroform 107
Chloroprocaine 120, 127
Chloroquine 655, 656, 658, 659, 662, 663, 664, 669, 670, 676, 712
4-Chlorotestosterone acetate 506
Chlorothiazide 388, 389, 402, 403, 404
Chlorotrianisene 510, 545
Chlorpheniramine 295, 315, 316, 317, 321
Chlorphenoxamine 65, 90, 308
Chlorphentermine 11, 24, 256, 266
Chlorpromazine 162, 164, 170, 174, 177, 335, 617, 622
Chlorpropamide 593, 598
Chlorprothixene 163, 177
Chlortetracycline 725, 800, 802, 803, 804
Chlortetracycline hydrochloride 803
Chlorthalidone 387, 399, 400, 401
Cholanic acid 501
Cholcalciferol, see *Vitamin D₃*
Cholesterol 500, 501, 503, 504, 517, 518
Cholic acid 502, 503
Choline 51, 54, 56
Choline theophyllinate 257, 268
Choline ethyl ether 55
6-Chromanol 946
Cidofovir 852, 853, 866
Ciglitazone 595, 602, 603, 604, 605, 606
Cilastatin 736, 758
Cilostazol 483, 491, 492
Cimetidine 300, 330
Cinchonidine 648
Cinchonine 648
Cinnarazine 615, 619
Cinoxacin 702, 719
Ciprofloxacin 630, 635, 702, 714, 718
Cisplatin 616, 892, 910
Citalopram 261, 282
Cladribine 895, 896, 917

Clarithromycin 724, 792, 793
Clavulanate potassium 734, 756
Clemastine 292, 293, 307
Clenbuterol 14
Clidinium bromide 62, 85
Clioquinol 670
Clobazam 167, 196, 201, 211
Clobetasol 519, 575
Clofarabine 895, 896
Clofazimine 818
Clometocillin 731, 756
Clomiphene 511, 546
Clomipramine 260, 276
Clonazepam 201, 211
Clonidine 13, 30, 410, 411, 420, 421, 631, 638
Clopidogrel 484, 496
Clorazepate potassium and dipotassium 167, 194, 201, 211
Clorindione 482, 489, 490
Clortermine 256, 266
Clothiapine 163, 180
Clotrimazole 827, 835
Cloxacillin 730, 732
Cloxacillin sodium 747
Clozapine 163, 166, 178, 182
Cocaine 117, 118, 120, 123, 125, 133, 256, 257, 412
Codeine 216, 217, 223, 227, 228, 234, 630, 631, 636
Co-enzyme R 898
Colcemid 898
Colchicine 348, 898
Colistin A 790
Colterol 15, 36
Corticosterone 391, 517, 518
Cortisol, see Hydrocortisone
Cortisol acetate, see Hydrocortisone acetate
Cortisol sodium succinate, see Hydrocortisone sodium succinate
Cortisone 517, 565
Cortisone acetate 566
Corynanthine 16
Coumarin 481, 482
Croconazole 827, 836
Cromolyn 291, 301, 303
Cyanocobalamine 988
Cyclazocine 220, 224, 233
Cyclizine 294, 311, 615, 619
Cyclobarbital 139, 147

Cyclobarbital calcium 148
Cycloguanil 657, 664, 701
Cyclomethycaine 120, 130
Cyclopentanoperhydrophenanthrene 499
1,2-Cyclopentenophenanthrene 499
Cyclopenthiazide 389, 404
Cyclopentolate hydrochloride 62, 80
Cyclophosphamide 887, 888, 906
Cyclopropane 106
Cyclorphan 224
Cycloserine 817
Cyclosporin A 632
Cyclosporin B 632
Cyclosporin C 632
Cyclosporin D 632
Cyclosporin G 632
Cymarin, 448
D-Cymarose 445
Cyproheptadine 296, 320, 330
Cyproterone 508
Cyproterone acetate 534
Cytarabine 893, 895, 914
Cytokines 335, 338, 519

D

Dacarbazine 890, 891, 909
Dactinomycin 721, 896, 897
Daltiparin 479
DDS, see Dapsone
Dapsone 812, 813, 818, 823, 824
Dasatinib 902
Daunorubicin 897
Deacetyl 7-aminocephalosporanic acid lactone 741
Deacetylcephalosporin 741,
Deacetylcephalosporin lactone 741
Deacetyldilitiazem 461
Decamethonium 56, 70
Decitabine 893, 895, 916
11-Dehydrocorticosterone 517
Dehydroemetine 669
Dehydroepiandrosterone 503, 504
11(4)-cis-3(3')-Dehydroretinal, see Vitamin A
all-trans-3(3')-Dehydroretinal, see Vitamin A
all-trans-3(3')-Dehydroretinol, see Vitamin A
Delavirdine 856, 874
Demecarium bromide 57, 58, 74
Demeclocycline 725, 800, 802, 804

N-Demethylphensuximide 209
N-Demethyltamoxifen 547
Demoxepam 166
2-Deoxy-2,3-dehydro-N-acetylamino-neuraminic acid (DANA) 850
L-Deprenyl, see Selegiline
Desipramine 260, 274
Desirudin 480
Desloratidine 296, 325
Desogestrel 514, 516, 558
Desonide 520, 580
Desoxycholic acid 502
Desoxycorticosterone 391, 517, 518
Desoxycorticosterone acetate 519, 562, 563
Desoxycorticosterone pivalate 519, 563
11-Desoxyhydrocortisone 391
Dexamethasone 391, 519, 619, 624
Dexamethasone acetate 573
Dexamphetamine 22, 256, 265
Dextromoramide 223, 242
Dextropropoxyphene 223, 243
Dextropropoxyphene napsylate, 244
Diacetylhydrazide 821
Diacetylmorphine 217, 227
Diacylglycerol (DAG) 7, 52, 291
2,4-Diamino-6,7-dimethylpteridine 384
Diaminodiphenylsulfone, see Dapsone
Diatrizoate meglumine 925
Diatrizoate sodium 924
Diazepam 166, 190, 201, 211
Diazoxide 415
Diazoxide sodium 425
3,5-Dibromosalicylaldehyde 829
Dibucaine 122, 134
Dichloroisoproterenol 18
3,4-Dichloro-α-methoxybenzyl-penicillin, see Clometocillin
Dichlorophen 685, 690
Dichlorphenamide 386, 395
Dichlorvos 687
Diclofenac 341, 345, 356
Diclofenac sodium 355
Dicloxacillin 730, 732
Dicloxacillin sodium 748
Dicoumarol 481
Dicyclomine hydrochloride 62, 81
Didanosine 854, 855, 871

Dideoxyadenosine 854, 855
Dienestrol 510, 545
Diel's hydrocarbon 499
5,5-Diethyl barbituric acid, see Barbital
Diethyl ether 109
Diethylcarbamazine citrate 685, 689
Diethylstilbestrol 510, 544, 545
Difenoxin 630, 631, 636, 637
Diflorasone 519, 575
Diflunisal 340, 351
D-Diginose 445
D-Digitalose 445
Digitoxigenin 447, 448
Digitoxin 447
D-Digitoxose 445
Digoxigenin 448,
Dihydroartimisnin 651
Dihydroavermectin B_{1a}, see Ivermectin,
Dihydroavermectin B_{1b}, see Ivermectin
1,4-Dihydro-3-carboxy-4-quinolone 702
Dihydrocodeine 218
Dihydrocodeine acid tartrate 228
Dihydrocodeinone 218
Dihydroergocalciferol, see Vitamin D4
Dihydrofolic acid 697, 702
Dihydrofoliate 697
Dihydro F-penicillin 727
Dihydromorphine 218
Dihydromorphinone 218
Dihydropteroate 697, 702
Dihydrostreptomycin 796, 815
4,5α-Dihydrotestosterone 504, 505, 507, 508
1,4-Dihydroxy-3-carboxy-4-quinolone 702
3,4-Dihydroxymandelic acid (DOMA) 5
Dihydroxy phenylacetaldehyde (DHPA) 246
Dihydroxyphenylacetic acid (DHPAA) 246
Dihydroxyphenylalanine, see Dopa
3,4-Dihydroxyphenylethyleneglycol, (DOPEG) 5
3,4-Dihydroxyphenylglycoaldehyde, (DOPGAL) 5, 6
N,N'-Diisopropyl ethylenediamine 815
Dilitiazem 415, 441, 445, 460, 470
Diloxanide 670
Diloxanide furoate 670, 676
Dimenhydrinate 305, 615, 619
Dimercaprol 382
Dimethadione 201
Dimethindene 295, 317

Dimethisoquin 123

Dimethisterone 514, 555

5,6-Dimethylbenzimidazolylcyanocoba-mide, see
Cyanocobalamin

Dimethylbiguanide, see Metformin

1,1-Dimethyl-4-phenylpiperazinium iodide 67

Dimethyltryptamine 262

Diminazine 672

Dionin 217, 227

1,3-Dioxolane 52

Diperodon 123, 136

Diphemanil methylsulphate 65, 91

Diphenadione 482, 491

Diphenhydramine 65, 292, 304, 307, 308, 309, 312,
318, 615, 619

Diphenhydramine theophyllinate, see Dimenhydrinate

Diphenoxylate 221, 630, 631, 636, 637, 638

Diphenylbutylpiperidine 164

Diphenylpyraline 292, 308

Dipipanone 223, 242

Dipivefrin 21

Diprophylline 257, 269

Dipyridamol 483, 492

Disopyramide 443, 463

Dobutamine 14, 32, 451, 471

Docetaxel 899

Docusate calcium 626

Docusate sodium 626, 633

Dofetilide 444, 468, 469

Dolasetron 616, 620

Domperidone 617, 623

Donepezil 57, 58, 75

Dopa 4, 9, 245, 411

Dopan 887

Dopamine 4, 10, 14, 21, 32, 161, 166, 245, 246, 247,
249, 250, 257, 258, 259, 261, 262, 265, 267,
285, 286, 413

Dothiepin 260, 278

Doxacurium chloride 68, 99

Doxapram 255, 256, 263

Doxazosin 16, 38, 413, 508, 532

Doxepin 260, 277, 278

Doxofylline 257, 270

Doxorubicin 896, 897

Doxycycline 660, 667, 725, 800, 801, 802, 805

Doxycycline hydrate 667, 804

Doxylamine 292, 293, 306

Dronabinol 619

Droperidol 164, 184, 617, 622

Drospirenone 515

Duloxetin 262, 284

Dutasteride 507, 532

Dyclonine 123, 136

Dynorphin 224

E

Ebastine 296, 326

Ecgonine 118

Econazole 827, 837

Echothiophate iodide 58, 76

Edrophonium chloride 57, 74

Efavirenz 856, 875

Eflornithine 673, 674, 681

Eicosanoids 335, 336, 346

Emedastine 297, 328, 329, 330

Emetine 669

Emtricitabine 854, 855, 872

Enalapril 416, 417, 427, 428

Enalaprilat 417, 427

Encainide 443, 465

Enclomiphene 511, 546

β-Endorphin 224

Englitazone 595, 606

Enkephalins, see Met-enkephalin and Leu-enkephalin

Enoxacin 702, 712

Enoxaparin 479

Entacapone 247

Ephedrine 12, 25, 27

(±)-Epiallobiotin 981

(±)-Epibiotin 981

Epicinchonidine 648

Epicinchonine 648

Epidihydroquinine 649

Epinastine 297

Epinephrine 3, 6, 16, 20, 50, 119, 126, 517

Epinephryl borate 21

Epiquindine 648

Epiquinine 648

Epirubicin 897

Eplerenone 390, 391, 392, 406

Eprosartan 418, 434

Eptifibatide 484

Equilin 510

Equilenin 510

Equilin sodium sulphate 510
Ergocalciferol, see *Vitamin D₂*
Ergocornine 17
Ergocristine 17
α-Ergocryptine 17, 252
Ergonovine 17
Ergosine 17
Ergosterol 501
Ergotamine 17
Erlotinib 902
Ertapenem 736,760
Erythrityl tetranitrate 438, 452
Erythromycin 296, 630, 635, 669, 675, 792, 793, 794
Erythromycin A 630, 724, 793
Erythromycin B 630, 793
Erythromycin C 630, 793
Erythromycin estolate 793
Erythromycin ethylsuccinate 793
Erythromycin stearate 793
Esmolol 18, 43, 413
Estazolam 142, 155
Estradiol 504, 509, 513, 538, 900
Estradiol 3-benzoate 509, 540
Estradiol cypionate 509, 542
Estradiol dipropionate 509, 540
Estradiol enanthate 509, 541
Estramustine 887, 905
Estramustine disodium phosphate 887
Estriol 509, 539
Estrone 504, 509, 539
Etamiphyllin 257, 269
Ethacrynic acid 383, 384, 391, 392, 396
Ethadione 200, 209
Ethambutol 815, 822
Ethchlorvynol 143
Ethinamate 144
Ethinyl estradiol 510, 516, 542, 543
17α-Ethinylestradiol 3-cyclopentyl ether,
    see *Quinestrol*
Ethionamide 814, 815, 820, 821
Ethisterone 514, 555
Ethoheptazine 222, 240
Ethopropazine 248, 254
Ethopropazine hydrochloride 65, 91, 254
Ethosuximide 201, 210
Ethotoin 200, 206
Ethoxzolamide 386, 394

Ethyl alcohol 138, 143
Ethyl p-aminobenzoate, see *Benzocaine*
Ethyl biscoumacetate 481
Ethyl chloride 108
Ethylene 107
Ethylestrenol 506, 527
β-(±)-5-Ethyl-2,9-dimethyl-2'-hydroxy-6,
    7-benzomorphan 220
Ethylnorepinephrine 36
17α-Ethyltestosterone 505
2-Ethyl thioisonicotinamide, see *Ethionamide*
Ethyl vanillate 829
Ethynodiol diacetate 514, 516, 557
Etidocaine 121, 132
Etodolac 341, 342
Etofylline 257, 269
Etofylline nicotinate 270
Etonogestrel 514, 559
Etoposide 899
Etoricoxib 345
α-Eucaine 118
β-Eucaine 118
Eucatropine hydrochloride 62, 84
Evans blue 933
Exemestane 512

F

Famciclovir 851, 853, 866
Famotidine 300, 330
Febrifugine 647
Felbamate 202, 203
Felodipine 415, 441, 456
Fenbufen 343, 364
Fenclofenac 341, 356
Fenfluramine 256, 265
Fenoprofen 342, 343
Fenoprofen calcium 361
Fentanyl 222, 237, 239
Fenticonazole 827, 838
Fermentation *L.casei* factor see *Folic acid*
Fexofenadine 296, 323
Finasteride 507, 531, 532
Flecainide 443, 465
Flomoxef 742
Floxuridine 893, 894, 913
Fluconazole 509, 537, 827, 840
Flucytosine 830, 845

Fludarabine 895, 896, 918

Fludrocortisone acetate 519, 564

Flufenamic acid 344, 366

Flumethasone 519, 577

Flunisolide 520, 582

Flunitrazepam 141, 151

Flunoxaprofen 343

Fluocinonide 520, 581

Fluorescein sodium 932

5-Fluorodeoxyuridine monophosphate 830, 846

Fluorometholone 519, 569

5-Fluorouracil, see *Fluorouracil.*

Fluorouracil 830, 893, 894, 912, 914

Fluoxetine 261, 280, 281, 282

Fluoxymestrone 505, 524

Fluphenazine 162, 176

Fluphenazine decanoate 176

Fluphenazine enanthate 176

Flurandrenolide 520, 583

Flurazepam 141, 152

Flurbiprofen 342, 345, 360

Fluspirilene 164,186

Flutamide 508, 536, 901, 918

Fluticasone propionate 520, 585

Flutrimazole 827, 835

Fluvoxamine 261, 280

Folic acid 697, 700, 893, 983

Fondaparinux 480, 487

Formestane 512

N^5-Formiminotetrahydrofoliate 987

N-Formyl isoleucine-gramicidine A 722

N-Formyl isoleucine-gramicidine B 722

N^5-Formyltetrahydrofoliate 697, 987

N^{10}-Formyltetrahydrofoliate 697, 987

N-Formyl valine-gramicidine A 722

N-Formyl valine-gramicidine B 722

Forskolin 451

Fosamprenavir 856

Foscarnet 853

Foscarnet sodium 852

Fosfomycin tromethamine 726

Fosinopril 417, 432

Fosinoprilat 417, 432

Fosphenytoin 200, 207

Fructose 626

D-Fucose 445

Fulvestrant 511, 512

Furazolidone, 675, 682

Furosemide, 386, 387, 391, 395, 396, 397, 398, 399

Fusidic acid, 725

G

Gabapentin 202, 203

Galactose 626

Gallamine triethiodide 68, 95

Ganciclovir 851, 853, 864

Gastrin 299, 300

Gatifloxacin 702, 716

Gefitinib 902

Gemcitabine 893, 895, 914, 915

Gentamicin 795, 798, 799

Gentamicin C_1 798

Gentamicin C_{1a} 798

Gentamicin C_2 798

Gentisic acid 340

Gepirone 169, 198

Gitoxigenin 447

Gitoxin, 447

Glibenclamide, see *Glyburide*

Glimepiride 593, 601

Glipizide 593, 600

Glucofrangulin A 628

Glucofrangulin B 628

Glucoscillaren A 450

D-Glucose 445, 629

Glucuronic acid 479, 486

Glutethimide 141, 150

Glyburide 593, 599

Glycerol 381, 626, 633

Glycine 255, 501

Glycopyrrolate 62, 82, 83

N-Glycyl p-aminosalicylic acid 813

Glyoxalic acid 347, 348

Goserelin 900

Gramicidins 721

Gramicidin A_2 721

Gramicidin, A_3 721

Gramicidin B_1 721

Gramicidin B_2 721

Gramicidin C 721

Granisetron 616, 621

Griseofulvin 725, 825

Guanabenz 13, 31, 410, 411, 421

Guanadrel 10, 22, 412, 413, 423

Guanethidine 10, 22, 412, 413, 420, 422, 423
Guanethidine N-oxide 423
Guanfacine 13, 31, 410, 411, 421
Guanine 347, 895

H

Halazepam 167, 191
Halcinonide 520, 585
Halobetasol propionate 520, 586
Halofantrine 659, 666
Haloperidol 164, 182, 617, 622
Haloprogin 829, 844
Halothane 108
Heparin 479, 485
n-Heptylpenicillin, see *Penicillin K*
Heroin, see *Diacetylmorphine*
Hetacillin 730, 754
Heterocodeine 217
Hexamethonium 67
n-Hexanol 143
Hexestrol 510, 544
Hexobarbital 139, 149
Hexylcaine 120, 130
Hirudin 480
Histamine 59, 289, 290, 291, 299, 302, 303, 304, 327, 335, 933
Histidine 290
HN2, see *Mechlorethamine*
HN2-oxide, see *Mechlorethamine oxide*
Homatropine 60, 78
Homatropine methobromide 60
Homovanillic acid (HVA) 246
Hydralazine 415
Hydralazine hydrochloride 424
Hydrochlorothiazide 389, 402, 403, 404, 405
Hydrocortisone 391, 517, 518, 564, 565, 566
Hydrocortisone acetate 565, 566
Hydrocortisone sodium succinate 565
Hydroflumethiazide 389, 403
Hydroxyamphetamine 11, 23
4-Hydroxy-1,2-benzothiazine carboxamide 344
p-Hydroxybenzylpenicillin, see *Penicillin X*
10-Hydroxycarbazepine 202
Hydroxychloroquine 346, 373, 655, 663
4-Hydroxycoumarin 481, 487
17α-Hydroxydesoxycorticosterone 517, 518
19-Hydroxydesoxycorticosterone 517

Hydroxydione sodim 112
2-Hydroxyiminostilbene 202
3-Hydroxy-N-methylmorphinan, see *Racemorphan*
Hydroxymethyldihydropterin 697
Hydroxymethyldihydropterinpyrophos-phate 697, 699
17α-Hydroxypregnenolone 504, 518
17α-Hydroxyprogesterone 504, 518
17α-Hydroxyprogesterone caproate 513, 552
Hydroxystreptomycin 796, 816
Hydroxyurea 903, 918
Hydroxyzine 294, 313, 326
Hyodesoxycholic acid 502
Hyoscine, see *scopolamine*
Hy oscyamine, 59

I

Ibuprofen 342, 343, 345, 359
Ibutilide 444, 469
Idarubicin 897
Idoxuridine 851, 852, 853, 861, 862
Iduronic acid 479, 486
Ifosfamide 887, 888, 906
Imatinib 902
Imidazenil 168
Imidazole acetic acid (IAA) 290
Imidazole acetic acid riboside (IAAR) 290
Imipenem 736, 758
Imipramine 260, 275, 276, 277, 278
Indane 1,3-dione 482
Indapamide, 387 400
Indigo carmine 931
Indinavir 856, 878
Indobufen 482, 483
Indomethacin 341, 342, 343, 345, 358
Indoramin 16, 39
Inositol triphosphate (IP3) 7, 52, 291, 299
Insulin 589, 590, 591, 592
Insulin Aspart 592
Insulin Detemir 592
Insulin Glargine 592
Insulin Glulisine 592
Insulin Lispro 592
Interferons 338, 850, 886
Interleukin 338, 346
Inulin 934
Iodipamide meglumine 926
Iodized oil 930

Iodophthalein sodium 929
Iodopyracet 928
Iodoquinol 670, 675
Iodoxamide 291
Iopanoic acid 928
Iophendylate 929
Iothalamate sodium 927
Ipratropium bromide 60, 78
Ipsapirone 169, 197
Irbesartan 418, 434
Isobucaine 120
Isocarboxazid 259, 272
Isoconazole 827, 838
Isoetharine 36
Isoflurophate 58, 76
Isomethadone 223, 224
Isoniazid 813, 814, 815, 817, 820, 821
Isonicotinic acid hydrazide, see *Isoniazid*
Isopentaquine 653
Isopropamide iodide 64, 86
5-Isopropyl-2-sulphanilamido-1,3,4-thiadiazole 593
Isoproterenol 6, 14, 18, 31
Isoquinine 649
Isosorbide 381
Isosorbide dinitrate 438, 454
Isphagula 625
Isradipine 415, 441, 457
Itraconazole 827
Ivermectin 685

K

Kallikrein 409
Kanamycin 795, 796
Kanamycin A 796, 797
Kanamycin B 796
Kanamycin C 796
Kaolin 631
Ketamine 112
Ketobemidone 221, 236
Ketoconazole 827, 833
Ketoprofen 342, 344, 360
Ketorolac 343, 364
Ketorolac tromethamine salt 364
Ketotifen 297, 329
Khellin 291
K-Strophanthiin-β 448
K-Strophanthoside 449

L

Labetalol 19, 49, 414
Lactoflavin, see *Riboflavin*
Lactulose 626
Lamifiban 484, 493, 495, 496
Lamivudine 854, 855, 872
Lamotrigine 202, 203, 213
Lanatoside A 448
Lanatoside C 448
Lanoconazole 827, 831, 832
Lansoprazole 301, 332
Lapatinib 902
Larocaine 119
Leflunomide 347, 373
Lefradafiban 484
Lepirudin, 480
Letrozole 512, 550, 900, 918
Leu-enkephalin 224
Leukotrienes 336, 338, 361
Leukotriene A_4, 337, 338
Leukotriene B_4, 337, 338, 348
Leukotriene C_4, 337, 338
Leukotriene D_4, 337, 338
Leukotriene E_4, 337, 338
Leukotriene F_4, 337, 338
Leuprolide 900
Levallorphan 219, 224, 230
Levamisole 347
Levetiracetam 202, 203
Levobunolol 18, 46
Levocabastine 297, 327, 329
Levodopa 247, 248, 249, 250, 251, 252, 253, 254
Levonorgestrel 514, 516, 560,
Levorphanol 219
Levorphanol tartrate 229
Liarozole 509, 537
Lidocaine, see *Lignocaine*
Lignocaine 121, 122, 124, 131, 443, 464
Linsodimine 440
Lisinopril 416, 427
Lithocholic acid 502
Liver *L.casei* factor, see *Folic acid*
Lobeline, 56, 67
Lodoxamide 291, 303
Lofepramine 260, 277
Lomefloxacin 702, 715
Lomustine 889, 908

Loperamide 221, 630, 631, 637
Lopinavir 856
Loprazolam 142, 155
Loracarbef 742, 783
Loratadine 296, 325
Lorazepam 167, 168, 194, 201, 211, 619, 624
Losartan 418, 435
Loxapine 163,179
Loxoprofen 342, 343
Lumiracoxib 345, 369
Lysergic acid 17
Lysergic acid diethylamide 262

M

Magnesium aluminium silicate (activated) 631
Magnesium citrate 626
Magnesium sulphate 626
Manesium hydroxide 626
Mannitol 381, 626
Maprotiline 262, 283
Mebendazole 684, 688
Mebeverine 62, 79
Mecamylamine 67, 412, 422
Mecamylamine hydrochloride 93, 422
Mechlorethamine 887, 889, 903, 904
Mechlorethamine oxide 888, 906
Meclizine 294, 312, 615, 619
Meclocycline 725, 800, 806
Meclofenamic acid 344, 365
Mecloqualone 143
Medrogestone 507, 530
Medroxyprogesterone acetate 513, 516, 553
Mefenamic acid 344, 365
Mefloquine 659
Mefloquine hydrochloride 665
Megestrol acetate 513, 554
Melarsoprol 673, 674, 681
Meloxicam 344, 367
Melphalan 887, 904,
Menadione, see *Vitamin K$_3$*
Menoquinone, see *Vitamin K$_2$*
Menoquinone 4, see *Vitamin K$_{2(20)}$*
Menoquinone 6, see *Vitamin K$_{2(30)}$*
Menoquinone 7, see *Vitamin K$_{2(35)}$*
Mepacrine, see *Quinacrine*
Mepenzolate bromide, 62, 84
Meperidine 164, 220, 221, 222, 223, 233, 234, 235, 236, 237, 241

Mephentermine 11, 12, 24
Mephenytoin 200, 206
Mephobarbital 139, 145, 200, 204
Mepivacaine 121, 133
Meprobamate 170
Meprylcaine 120
Merbaphen 382
Mercaptopurine 632, 641, 895, 916
6-Mercaptopurine, see *Mercaptopurine*
Meropenem 736, 759
Mersalyl 382
Mescaline 262
Mesoridazine 162, 172, 173
Mestranol 510, 516, 543
Metanephrine 5
Metaproterenol 14, 32
Metaraminol 12, 25, 26
Metazocine 220, 232
Met-enkephalin 224
Metformin 595, 602
Methacholine chloride 55, 70, 71
Methacycline 725, 800, 805
α-Methadol 224
β-Methadol 224
Methadone 223, 224, 241, 242, 243
Methamphetamine 11, 23, 256, 265
Methandrostenolone 524
Methantheline bromide 62, 81, 82
Methapyrilene 293, 294, 311
Methaqualone 143, 158
Metharbital 139, 140, 144, 200, 204
Methazolamide 386, 394
Methdilazine 295, 319
Methenolone acetate 506, 527
N^5,N^{10},-Methenyltetrahydrofoliate 697, 987
Methicillin 730, 783
Methicillin sodium 745
Methimazole 609, 610
Methixene 65
Methohexital sodium 110
Methoserpidine 424
Methotrexate 347, 373, 700, 701, 712, 893, 911
Methoxamine 13, 27
Methoxyflurane 109
3-Methoxy-4-hydroxymandelic acid, (MOMA) 5
3-Methoxy-4-hydroxyphenyl-acetaldehyde (MHPA) 246

3-Methoxy-4-hydroxyphenylethylene-glycol (MOPEG) 5

3-Methoxy-4-hydroxyphenylglyco-aldehyde (MOPGAL) 5

6-Methoxy-2-naphthylacetic acid 343

Methoxyphentermine 11, 24

6-Methoxyquinolyl-2-piperidylcarbinol 650

Methsuximide 201, 210

Methyclothiazide 389, 404

Methylcellulose 625, 631

β-Methyl choline ethyl ether, 55

N-Methylbarbital, see Metharbital

3-Methyldiazepam 168

Methyldopa 9, 14, 31, 410, 411

α-Methyldopa, see Methyldopa

Methyldopate 411

Methyldopate hydrochloride 31, 411, 420

Methylene blue 652

N5, N10-Methylenetetrahydrofoliate 697, 987

N-Methyl-L-glucosamine 816

N-Methylhistamine (NMH) 290

N-Methylimidazole acetic acid (NMIAA) 290

N-Methylisomorphinan 219

N-Methylmorphinan 219

α-Methylnorepinephrine 9, 14, 411

Methylparafynol 143

Methylparathion 58

Methylphenidate 256, 266

1-Methyl-4-phenyl-4-propionoxy-piperidine 222

N-Methyl-4-phenyl-1,2,3,6-tetrahydro-pyridine (MPTP) 245

6α-Methylprednisolone 519, 568, 619, 624

16β-Methylprednisone 519, 570

Methyl salicylate 339

17α-Methyltestosterone 505, 524

N5-Methyltetrahydrofoliate 987

α-Methyltyrosine, see *Metyrosine*

Methyl β-trimethylammonium-propionate 55

Methyprylon 141 149

Metiamide 300

Metiapine 163, 180

Metipranolol 18, 47

Metoclopramide 64, 87, 165, 188, 617, 623

Metocurine iodide 68, 94

Metolazone 387, 400

Metopon 218

Metoprolol 18, 44, 413, 442, 461

Metrifonate 687

Metronidazole 671, 672, 675, 676

Metronidazole benzoate 671, 677

Metyapone 391

Metyrosine 9, 410, 411

Mexiletine 443, 464

Mezlocillin 730, 753, 754

Mianserin 260, 278, 279

Miconazole 827, 836

Midazolam 142, 154, 201, 211

Mifepristone 515, 560, 562

Miglitol 596

Milnacipran 262

Milrinone 451, 471

Mineral oil 627

Minocycline 725, 800, 802, 805

Minoxidil 415, 425

Minoxidil N-O-sulphate, 425

Mirtazapine 260, 279

Misoprostol 629

Mitomycin C 897

Mitotane 903, 919

Mivacurium chloride 68, 100

Mizolastine 296

Moclobemide 259, 273

Moexipril 416, 417, 428

Moexiprilat 417, 428

Molindone 164, 188

Molsidomine 440, 454

Mometasone furoate 520, 587

Moricizine 443, 466

Morphinan 219

Morphine 216. 217, 218, 219, 220, 221, 222, 223, 224, 225, 226, 227, 228, 230, 231, 234, 238, 241, 290

Morphinone 218

Moxalactam 742, 784

Moxifloxacin 702

Moxonidine 411, 421, 422

Muscarine 50, 52, 55, 59, 71

Muscarone 52

Murein sacculus, 732

Mustard gas, 886

Mustine, see Mechlormethamine

Muzolimine, 391, 407

Myleran, see Busulfan

N

Nabilone 619
Nabumetone 343, 345
Nadolol 18, 47, 413
Naficillin 730, 732
Naficillin sodium 745
Naftifine 830, 844
Naldixic acid 702, 718
Nalorphine 219, 224, 228, 229
Naloxone 224, 228
Naltrexone 224, 229
Nandrolone 506, 525
Nandrolone decanoate 506, 526
Nandrolone phenylpropionate 506, 526
Naphazoline 13, 28
Naphthacaine 120
Naphthacene 800
Naproxen 342, 343, 345, 361
Narcotine 216, 217
Natamycn 826
Nateglinide 594
Nedocromil 291, 302
Nelfinavir 856, 879
Neomycin 797, 798
Neomycin A 797
Neomycin B 725, 797
Neomycin C 797
Neostigmine 57, 58, 73, 75
Neostigmine bromide 72
Neovitamin A, see *Vitamin A*
Neticonazole 827
Netilmicin 795, 798, 799
Netoglitazone 595, 605
Nevirapine 856, 874
Niacin see *Nicotinic acid*
Niacinamide see *Nicotinamide*
Nicardipine 415, 441, 457
Niclosamide 685, 690
Nicotinamide 813, 814, 969
Nicotine 50, 56, 67
Nicotinic acid 969
Nifedipine 415, 441, 458
Nifurtimox 673, 680
Nikethamide 255, 256, 264
Nilutamide 508, 537, 901, 918
Nimesulide 345, 368

Nimetazepam 141, 151
Nimodipine 415, 441, 459
Niquine 650
Niridazole 671
Nitrazepam 141, 150, 201, 211
Nitric oxide 51, 52, 415, 439, 440, 455
Nitroglycerin 438, 452, 453
Nitrosomethylurea 889
Nitrous oxide 106
Nizatidine 300, 331
Nociceptin 224
Nomifensine 262, 285
Noradrenaline, see *Norepinephrine*
Nordazepam 191
Norelgestromin 514
Norepinephrine 3, 4, 5, 6, 7, 8, 9, 10, 11, 12, 13, 16,
        17, 20, 36, 50, 66, 166, 257, 258, 259, 260,
        261, 262, 265, 267, 274, 283, 284, 285, 286,
        411, 412, 413
Norethandrolone 506, 526
Norethindrone 514, 515, 516, 556
Norethindrone acetate 3-cyclopentyl enol ether 517
Norethynodrel 514, 515, 516, 557
Norfloxacin 702, 714
Norgestimate 514
Normetanephrine 5
Nortriptyline 260, 274
Novembichin 887, 903
Novobiocin 726
Novocain 118
Nystatin A_1 723, 826

O

Ofloxacin 702, 718
Olanzapine 163, 182
Oleandomycin 724, 794
L-Oleandrose 445
Olmesartan 418
Olopatadine 297, 327, 328
Olsalazine 631, 639
Omeprazole 301, 332
Omoconazole 827, 832
Onapristone 515, 561
Ondansetron 616, 621
Opium 138, 216
Ornithine 674
Orphenadrine 65

Orphenadrine citrate 90
Oseltamivir 850, 860
Ouabagenin 449
Ouabain 449
Oxacillin 730, 732, 747
Oxacillin sodium 746
Oxaliplatin 892
Oxamniquine 687, 691
Oxandrolone 506 , 528
Oxaprozin 343, 363
Oxatomide 294, 314
Oxazepam 167, 168, 191, 193
Oxcarbazepine, 202, 212
Oxendolone, 508, 534
Oxethazaine, 122, 135
Oxiconazole, 827, 831
Oxilorphan, 219
Oxolinic acid, 702, 717
Oxymetazoline, 13, 28
Oxymetholone, 506, 528
Oxypertine, 164, 187
Oxyphenbutazone, 341, 354
Oxyphencyclimine hydrochloride, 62, 85
Oxyphenisatin acetate, 627, 635
Oxyphenonium bromide, 62, 79
Oxytetracycline, 725, 800, 801, 802, 806
Oxytetracycline hydrochloride, 803

P

Paclitaxel 899
Pamaquine 652, 653, 654
Pancuronium bromide 68, 95, 98
Pantoprazole 301, 333
Pantothenic acid 972
Papaverine 66, 89, 216, 217
Papaverine hydrochloride 92
Paracetamol 339, 340, 345, 350, 352
Paraldehyde 138, 140, 144, 159, 170
Paramethadione 200, 208
Paramethasone 519, 578
Parathion 58
Parecoxib 345, 371
Paromomycin 669, 675, 797
Paromomycin I 797
Paromomycin II 797
Paroxetine 261, 281
Pectin 631

Pemetrexed 893
Pemirolast 291, 304
Penaldic acid 728
Penbutolol 18, 413
Penciclovir 851, 853, 865, 866
Penfluridol 164, 186
Penicillamine 346, 372, 728
Penicillin I, see *Penicillin F*
Penicillin II, see *Penicillin G*
Penicillin III, see *Penicillin X*
Penicillin IV, see *Penicillin K*
Penicillin F 727
Penicillin G 126, 727, 729, 737
Penicillin G benzathine 744
Penicillin G procaine 744
Penicillin G sodium 743
Penicillin K 727
Penicillin N 730, 737
Penicillin V 727, 731, 732, 744
Penicillin X 727
Penilloaldehyde 728
Penicilloic acid 728, 734
Penillic acid 728
Pent-2-enylpenicillin see *Penicillin F*
Penilloic acid 728
Pentaerythritol chloral 143
Pentaerythritol tetranitrate 438, 453
Pentagastrin 299
Pentamidine 672, 675
Pentamidine isethionate 675, 678
Pentaquine 653
Pent-2-enylpenicillin see *Penicillin F*
Pentazocine 220, 224, 233
Pentobarbital 139, 148
Pentostatin 898
Pentoxifylline 257, 271
Pentylenetetrazole 255, 256, 264
Pergolide 248, 252
Perindopril 417, 431
Perindoprilat 417, 431
Peronin 217
Perphenazine 162, 175
Pethidine, see *Meperidine*
Phenacaine 122
Phenacetin 340, 351
Phenadoxone 223, 241
Phenazocine 220, 232s

Phenazone 340, 352
Phenbenzamine 293, 294, 309
Phencyclidine 262
Phenelzine 259, 271, 272
Pheneridine 234
Phenethicillin 731, 755
Phenformin 595, 601
Phenindamine 295, 318
Phenindione 482, 489, 490
Pheniprazine 259, 272
Pheniramine 295, 315
Phenobarbital 139, 140, 145, 169, 200, 203,
        204, 213
Phenolpthalein 627, 635
Phenolsulphonaphthalein 932
Phenoxybenzamine 17, 39
α-Phenoxyethylpenicillin, see *Phenethicillin*
Phenoxymethylpenicillin, see *Penicillin V*
α-Phenoxypropylpenicillin, see Propicillin
Phenprocoumon 481, 488
Phensuximide 201, 209
Phentermine 11, 23, 24, 25, 256, 265
Phentolamine 17, 40
Phenylbutazone 341, 343, 353, 355, 483
2-Phenyl-6,8-dichloro-4-quinolyl-2'-piperidylcarbinol
        650
Phenylephrine 13, 27
Phenylethanolamine 12, 26
Phenylethylbiguanide, see *Phenformin*
Phenylethylhydantoin 200, 204, 206
N-Phenylethylnormorphine 219
5-Phenylhydantoin 206
Phenylpropanolamine 12, 26
Phenyl salicylate 339
Phenytoin 200, 204, 205, 207, 214, 443, 464
Phethenylate 200
Phethenylate sodium 205
Pholedrine 11
Phosphatidylinositol-4,5-diphosphate (PIP2) 7, 52, 590
Phosphatidylinositol-4,5-triphosphate (PIP3) 590
Phthalylsulphathiazole 700
Phylloquinone, see *Vitamin K₁*
Physostigmine 57, 72
Picrotin 256, 263
Picrotoxin 256, 263
Picrotoxinin 255, 256, 263
Piketopofen 344
Pilocarpine 55, 56, 71

Piminodine 234
Pimobendan 451
Pimozide 164, 185
Pinazepam 167, 192
Pindolol 18, 48, 413
Pioglitazone 595, 604
Pipecurium bromide 68, 96
Piperacetazine 162, 171
Piperacillin 730, 753, 758
Piperazine citrate 685
Piperidolate hydrochloride 62
Piperocaine 120, 127
Pirarubicin 897
Pirbuterol 14, 35
Piretanide 387, 391, 396
Piritrexim 701
Piroxicam 344, 345, 366, 368
Plasmochin, see *Pamaquin*
Platelet activating factor 335, 338, 519
Podophyllotoxin 899
Polidine methylsulphate 62, 83
Polyethyleneglycol 626
Polymyxin 723, 790
Polymyxin, B₁ 723, 790
Polymyxin B₂ 723, 790
Polymyxin D₁ 723, 790
Polymyxin D₂ 723, 790
Polymyxin E₁ 723, 790
Polythiazide 389, 405
Potassium bromide 138
Practolol 18, 44
Pramilintide 592
Pramipexole 248, 253
Pramoxine 123, 137
Pranoprofen 343
Prazepam 167, 192
Praziquantel 686, 691
Prazosin 16, 37, 38, 413, 508, 532
Prednisolone 519, 567, 632, 640
Prednisolone acetate 567
Prednisolone disodium phosphate 567
Prednisolone sodium succinate 567
Prednisolone tebutate 567
Prednisone 391, 519, 568
Pregnenolone 504, 517, 518
Prilocaine 121, 131
Primaquine 653, 660
Primidone 202, 203, 212

Probenecid 348, 374, 750
Procainamide 443, 463
Procaine 118, 119, 122, 124, 125, 128, 132
Procaine hydrochloride, see *Novocain*
Procarbazine 890, 908, 909, 910
Prochlorperazine 162, 173, 617, 622
Procyclidine 248, 254
Procyclidine hydrochloride 64, 88, 254
α-Prodine 222, 237
β-Prodine 222
Progestrone 504, 509, 513, 515, 518, 551, 552
Proguanil, see *Chlorguanide*
Promazine 162, 170
Promethazine 295, 318, 319, 615, 616, 620
Pronethalol 18, 45
Prontosil 695
Propacetamol 340
Propafenone 443, 466
Propanidid 113
Propantheline bromide 62, 82
Proparacaine 120, 129
Propatyl nitrate 438, 453
Properidine 235
Propicillin 731, 755
Propipocaine 123
Propofol 113
Propoxycaine 120, 129, 130
Propranolol 18, 45, 413, 442, 444, 461, 467
Propyliodone 930
Propylthiouracil 609 , 611
Proscillaridin A 449
Prostacycline 338, 409
Prostaglandins 299, 336, 338, 345, 361, 362, 363, 364, 417, 519, 619
Prostaglandin D_2 (PGD2) 336, 338
Prostaglandin E_2 (PGE2) 336, 338, 409
Prostaglandin F_2 (PGF2) 336, 338
Prostaglandin G_2 (PGG2) 336
Prostaglandin H_2 (PGH2) 336
Prostaglandin I_2 (PGI2) 336, 338
Prostanoids 338
Prothionamide 814
Protriptyline 260, 273, 274, 275
Prourokinase 485
Proxyphylline 257, 270
Pseudoephedrine 12
Pteroylglutamic acid, see *Folic acid*
Purpurea glycoside A, 447

Purpurea glycoside B 447
Putrescine 674
Pyrantel pamoate 687, 692
Pyrathiazine 295, 320
Pyrazinamide 814, 820, 821
Pyrazinoic acid 821
3,5-Pyrazolidinedione 340
5-Pyrazolone 340
Pyrene 885
Pyridostigmine 57, 58, 75
Pyridostigmine bromide 72
Pyridoxal 974, 977
Pyridoxamine 974, 977
Pyridoxine 974, 977
Pyridylmethylsulfinylbenzimidazole 301
Pyrilamine 293, 294, 310
Pyrimethamine 658, 664, 701, 702, 712
Pyrogallol triacetate 829, 843
Pyrrobutamine 295, 316
Pyrrocaine 121, 132

Q

Quazepam 141, 153
Quetiapine 163, 181
Quinacrine 654, 661
Quinapril 416, 417, 429
Quinaprilat 417, 429
Quinestrol 517, 543
Quinethazone 387, 401
Quinidine 443, 462, 648, 649
Quinine 648, 649, 650, 651, 654, 656, 658, 712
Quinotoxines, 650

R

Rabeprazole 301, 333
Racemorphan 219
Radioiodine 609
Raloxifene 511, 549
Ramipril 416, 417, 429
Ramiprilat 417, 430
Ranitidine 300, 331
Ranolazine 442, 462
Reboxetine 262, 283
Remifentanil 222, 240
Remoxipride 165, 166, 189
Repaglinide 594
Reserpine 10, 22, 165, 188, 245, 412, 413, 424
Reteplase 485

Retinal, see *Vitamin A*
11(4)-*cis*-Retinal, see *Vitamin A*
all-*trans*-Retinoic acid, see *Vitamin A*
Retinol, see *Vitamin A₁*
all-trans-Retinol, see *Vitamin A₁*
L-Rhamnose 445
Ribavirin 852, 853, 868
Riboflavin 964
Ricinoleic acid 629
Rifabutin 816
Rifampin 816, 818
Rifamycin B 816
Rifamycin S 816
Rifamycin SV 816
Rifamycin X 816
Rilmenidine 411, 422
Rimantadine 850, 858
Ritonavir 856, 877
Rivastigmine 57, 73
Rivoglitazone 595, 605
Rofecoxib 345, 369
Rolitetracycline 725, 800, 802, 806
Ropinirole 248, 253
Ropivacaine 134
Rosiglitazone 595, 604
Roxifiban 484, 494
Rubane 648

S

Salbutamol 14, 33, 314
Salicylamide 339, 349
Salicylanilide 829, 843
Salicylic acid 338, 339, 340, 344, 349
Salmeterol 14, 34
Salol, see *Phenyl salicylate*
Salsalate 339, 350
Sancycline 800
Saperconazole 827, 841
Saquinavir 856, 876
Saralasin 418
L-Sarcolysine, see *Melphalan*
D-Sarmentose 445
Satraplatin 892
Scillaren A 449
Scillarenin 449, 450
Scopine 60
Scopolamine 59, 60, 77, 616, 620
Scopolamine methobromide 60

Scopolamine N-oxide 60
Secobarbital 139, 140, 148
Selegiline 247, 259
Sennosides 628
Sennoside A 628
Sennoside B 628
Serotonin 10, 59, 166, 169, 257, 258, 259, 261, 262, 265, 273, 280, 286, 413, 615
Sertaconazole 827, 839
Sertraline 261, 281
Setastine 292, 305
Sialic acid 850
SIN-1A 440
Sisomicin 798, 799
Sodium antimony gluconate, see *Sodium stibogluconate*
Sodium aurothiomalate 346, 371
Sodium gentisate 340
Sodium iodomethamate 927
Sodium nitroprusside 415, 426
Sodium phosphate 626
Sodium salicylate 339, 349
Sodium stibogluconate 675, 681
Solapsone 823
Sontoquine 655
Sorafenib 902
Sorbitol 381, 626
Sotalol 444, 469
Sparfloxacin 702, 716
Spectinomycin 795, 799
Spermine 674
Spermidine 674
Spiperone 164, 183
Spirapril 416, 417, 430
Spiraprilat 417, 431
Spironolactone 390, 391, 392, 405, 407
Stanozolol 506, 529
Stavudine 854, 855, 870, 871
Sterculia gum 625
Stigmasterol 501
trans-Stilbene 510
Streptidine 816
Streptokinase 485
Streptose 816
Streptomycin 725, 795, 796, 813, 814, 815, 816
Streptozocin 896
Strophanthidin 448, 449
K-Strophanthin β 448

K-Strophanthoside 449
Strychnine 255, 263
Substance P 519, 618
Succinylcholine chloride, see *Suxameth-onium chloride*
Succinylsulphathiazole 705
Sufentanil 222, 239
Sulbactam 734, 756
Sulconazole 827, 837
Sulfazecin 743
Sulindac 341, 342, 345, 357
Sulmazole 451
Sunitinib 902
Sulphacetamide sodium 710
Sulphachlorpyridazine 710
Sulphadiazine 697, 702, 705, 706, 707, 712
Sulphadimidine 706
Sulphadoxine 658, 665, 666, 702, 711
Sulphamerazine 697, 706, 707
Sulphamethazine 697
Sulphamethizole 707
Sulphamethoxazole 697, 702, 707, 712
Sulphanilamide 385, 695, 704, 706, 712, 812
Sulphapyridine 632, 708
Sulphasalazine 631, 632, 639, 640
Sulphathiadiazole 813
Sulphathiazole 704
Sulphinpyrazone 341, 348, 374, 482, 483, 491
Sulphisoxazole 697, 708, 709, 710
Sulphisoxazole diolamine 709
Sulphobromophthalein sodium 930
Sulpiride 165, 166, 188
Sunitinib 902
Sultopride 165
Suprofen 343, 363
Suramin sodium 673, 678
Suxamethonium chloride 56, 70, 101
Synthalin 672

T

T_3, see *Triiodothyronine*
T_4, see *Thyroxine*
Tacrine 57, 58, 75
Tachykinins 225
L-Talomethylose 445
Tamoxifen 511, 547, 548, 900, 918
Tamsulosin 16, 508, 533
Taurine 501
Tazobactam 734, 757

Tegafur 893, 894, 912
Teicoplanin 790
Teicoplanin A_2-1 790
Teicoplanin A_2-2 790
Teicoplanin A_2-3 790
Teicoplanin A_2-4 790
Teicoplanin A_2-5 790
Telmisartan 418, 436
TEM, see *Triethylenemelamine*
Temazepam 141, 153
Temozolomide 890, 891, 910
Tenecteplase 485
Teniposide 899
Tenitramine 438, 453
Tenofovir 854, 855, 873
Tenofovir disoproxil 855, 873
Tenoxicam 344, 367
TEPA, see *Triethylenephosphoramide*
Terazosin 16, 38, 413, 508, 532
Terbinafine 830, 845
Terbutaline 14, 33
Terconazole 827, 842
Teriflunomide 373
Terfenadine 296, 322, 324, 327
TESPA, see *Thiotepa*
Testolactone 507, 512, 529, 550
Testosterone 503, 504, 505, 507, 508, 509, 521, 523, 524, 525, 900
Testosterone cypionate 505, 523
Testosterone enanthate 505, 523
Testosterone phenylpropionate 523
Testosterone propionate 505, 522
Tetracaine hydrochloride, see *Amethocaine hydrochloride*
Tetracycline 725, 800, 802
Tetraethylammonium 67
Tetraethylpyrophosphate 58
Tetrahydrofolic acid 697, 702, 893, 987
Tetrahydrozoline 13, 29
Thebaine 216, 217
Theobromine 256, 257, 268, 384, 392
Theophylline 256, 257, 267, 384, 392
D-Thevetose 445
Thiabendazole 684, 688
Thiacetazone 813, 819
Thiamine 959
Thiamylal 139, 140, 149
Thiamylal sodium 111, 149

Thienamycin 735, 736
Thiethylperazine 162, 174, 617, 622
Thioguanine 895, 917
Thioisonicotinamide 813
Thiopental 139, 149, 169
Thiopental sodium 111, 149
Thioridazine 162, 172
Thiotepa 889, 907
Thiothixene 163, 177
Thonzylamine 293, 310
Thromboxanes 336
Thromboxane A$_2$, 336
Thyroxine 607, 608, 609, 610
Tiagabine 202, 203, 214, 215
Ticarcillin 730, 752, 753, 756
Ticlopidine 484, 496
Tigemonam 743, 787, 788
Timolol 18, 48, 413, 442, 461
Tinidazole 671, 672, 675, 677
Tinzaparin 479
Tioconazole 827, 839
Tipranavir 856
Tirofiban 484, 495
Tobramycin 798
Tocainide 443, 464
Tocol 946
Tocopherol, see *Vitamin E*
α-Tocopherol, see *Vitamin E*
β-Tocopherol, see *Viamin E*
γ-Tocopherol, see *Vitamin E*
δ-Tocopherol, see *Vitamin E*
Tocotrienol, see *Vitamin E*
α-Tocotrienol, see *Vitamin E*
β-Tocotrienol, see Vitamin E
γ-Tocotrienol, see *Vitamin E*
δ-Tocotrienol, see *Vitamin E*
Tolazamide 593, 598
Tolazoline 17, 40
Tolbutamide 593, 597, 598
Tolcap one 247, 250
Tolfenamic acid 344, 366
Tolmetin 341, 342, 358
Tolnaftate 829, 844
Toremifene 511, 548, 900, 918
Torsemide 387, 391, 397
Trandolapril 416, 417
Trandolaprilat 417

Tranylcypromine 259, 273
Trazodone 262, 286
Tretinoin 903
Triamcinolone acetonide 520, 584
Triamcinolone acetonide 21-acetate 584
Triamcinolone acetonide 21-disodium phosphate 584
Triamcinnolone acetonide 21-hemi-succinate 584
Triamterene 385, 391, 392, 393
Triazolam 142, 156
Trichlormethiazide 389, 403
Trichloroethanol 143, 159
Trichloroethylene 108
Triclofos 143
Triclofos sodium 159
Tridihexethyl chloride 64, 87
Triethylenemelamine 889
Triethylenephosphoramide 889
Triethylenethiophosphoramide, see *Thiotepa*
Trifluoperazine 162, 174, 617, 622,
Trifluperidol 164, 183
Triflupromazine 162, 171
Trifluridine 851, 853, 861
Triflusal 482
Trihexyphenidyl 248, 254
Trihexyphenidyl hydrochloride 65, 88, 254
2, 3, 5-Trihydroxybenzoic acid 340
Triiodothyronine 607, 608, 609
Trimegestone 515
Trimeprazine 295, 319
Trimethadione 200, 201, 208
Trimethaphan camsylate 67, 93, 412, 422
Trimethobenzamide 617, 623
Trimethoprim 700, 701, 702, 708, 712
Trimetrexate 701
Trimipramine 260, 275
Tripamide 387, 391, 398
Tripelennamine 293, 309, 310, 311
Triprolidine 295, 317, 326
Troglitazone 595, 603
Troleandomycin 794
Tropacocaine 118
Tropic acid 60
Tropicamide 64, 86
Tropine 60
Tropine mandelate, see *Homatropine*
Tropisetron 616, 622
Trovafloxacin 702

ryptamine 258
ubocurarine chloride 68, 94, 95, 96, 99
ramine 12, 27
rocidine A 722
rocidine B 722
yrocidine C 722
Tyrocidine D 722
L-Tyrosine, 4 245, 411

U

Ubiquinones 653, 660
Urea 138, 347, 348, 381
Urethane 138
Urokinase 485
Uric acid 347, 348

V

Valacyclovir 851, 853, 863
Valdecoxib 345, 370, 371
Valproic acid 202, 203, 213
Valrubicin 897
Valsartan 418, 437
Vancomycin 791
Vecuronium bromide, 68, 97
Venlafaxine 262, 284
Verapamil 415, 441, 445, 461, 470
Vidarabine 851, 853, 862, 895, 896, 917
Vinblastine 898, 899
Vincristine 898
Vinorelbine 898
Vinyl ether 110
Vitamin A 937
Vitamin A aldehyde, see *Vitamin A*
13(2)-*cis*-Vitamin A, see *Vitamin A*
Vitamin A₁ 903 937, 938
Vitamin B₁ see *Thiamine*
Vitamin B₂ see *Riboflavin*
Vitamin B₃ see *Nicotinic zcid and Nicotinamide*
Vitamin B₅, see *Pantothenic acid*
Vitamin B₆, see *Pyridoxine, Pyridoxal, and Pyridoxamine*
Vitamin B₇, see *Biotin*
Vitamin B₉, see *Folic acid*
Vitamin B₁₂, see *Cyanocobalamine*
Vitamin C, see *Ascorbic acid*
Vitamin D 940
Vitamin D₁ 940

Vitamin D₂ 941
Vitamin D₃ 941, 944
Vitamin D₄ 941, 945
Vitamin E 946
Vitamin G, see *Riboflavin*
Vitamin H, see *Biotin*
Vitamin K 476, 953,
Vitamin K₁ 476, 953, 954,
Vitamin K₂ 476, 953
Vitamin K₂(₂₀) 954
Vitamin K₂(₃₀) 954, 957
Vitamin K₂(₃₅) 476, 954
Vitamin K₃ 476, 954
Vitamin K- 2,3-epoxide 477, 478
Vitamin KH₂ 477, 478
Vitamin K-quinone 477, 478
Vitamin M, see *Folic acid*
Vofopitant 618
Voglibose 596
Voriconazole 827, 840, 842

W

Warfarin 481
Warfarin sodium 487

X

Xanthine 347, 348, 374
Xanthopterin 384
Xipamide 387, 399
Xylometazoline 13, 29

Y

allo-Yohimbine 16

Z

Zalcitabine 854, 855, 869, 872
Zaleplon 142, 157
Zanamivir 850, 859
Ziconotide 415
Zidovudine 854, 855, 869, 870, 871,
Zinc undecenylate 830, 846
Zolpidem 142, 157
Zomepirac 341, 342, 359
Zonisamide 202, 203, 214
Zopiclone 142
Zuclomiphene 511, 546